C0-ARE-332

Third Edition

OPHTHALMIC PATHOLOGY

An Atlas and Textbook

Volume 2

WILLIAM H. SPENCER, M.D.
Department of Ophthalmology
Pacific Medical Center
San Francisco, California

Published under the Sponsorship of
The American Academy of Ophthalmology
and the Armed Forces Institute of Pathology

1985 W. B. SAUNDERS COMPANY
Philadelphia London Toronto
Mexico City Rio de Janeiro Sydney Tokyo

W. B. Saunders Company West Washington Square
Philadelphia, PA 19105

1 St. Anne's Road
Eastbourne, East Sussex BN21 3UN, England

1 Goldthorne Avenue
Toronto, Ontario M8Z 5T9, Canada

Apartado 26370—Cedro 512
Mexico 4, D.F., Mexico

Rua Coronel Cabrita, 8
Sao Cristovao Caixa Postal 21176
Rio de Janeiro, Brazil

9 Waltham Street
Artarmon, N.S.W. 2064, Australia

Ichibancho, Central Bldg., 22-1 Ichibancho
Chiyoda-Ku, Tokyo 102, Japan

Library of Congress Cataloging in Publication Data

Spencer, William H.
Ophthalmic pathology.

1. Eye—Diseases and defects. 2. Eye—Diseases and defects—Atlases. I. Title. [DNLM: 1. Ophthalmology—Atlases. WW 17 061]
RE66.S7 1985 617.7′1 82—42620
ISBN 0-7216-8510-2 (set)
0-7216-8505-6 Vol. I
0-7216-8507-2 Vol. II
0-7216-8508-0 Vol. III

Volume 1	ISBN	0–7216–8505–6
Volume 2	ISBN	0–7216–8507–2
Volume 3	ISBN	0–7216–8508–0
Complete Set	ISBN	0–7216–8510–2

Ophthalmic Pathology

Last digit is the print number: 9 8 7 6 5 4 3 2 1

We wish to dedicate this book to the memory of four outstanding ophthalmic pathologists: Michael J. Hogan, Georgiana D. Theobald, Algernon B. Reese, and Frederick H. Verhoeff, who have shown us the way.

FOREWORD

As Col. Frank M. Townsend observed in his Foreword to the second edition of *Ophthalmic Pathology*, the work was made possible by the remarkably close liaison that had developed between the American Academy of Ophthalmology and Otolaryngology and the Armed Forces Institute of Pathology (AFIP) dating back to 1921. That Foreword was written after a beautiful 40 year marriage between organized American ophthalmology and the AFIP. I am pleased to report that this eminently successful union continues to be extremely rewarding to all concerned today, 63 years after the contract was established.

The then-novel idea to establish at an Army installation a highly specialized pathology laboratory to support the civilian sector provided a precedent-setting model that would subsequently be copied by most of the other specialty groups. Soon after the Ophthalmic Pathology Laboratory was established at the Army Medical Museum, the registry concept was introduced for long-term clinicopathologic and follow-up study of well-documented pathologic conditions. Thus, almost from the beginning, these specialized laboratories sponsored by various national societies were named Registries. At the present time there are 27 Registries and a total of 31 Sponsoring Societies at the AFIP.

In 1976, Congress officially noted that the AFIP offers unique pathologic support to national and international medicine, that its contributions are of vital importance in support of the civilian health care system as well as of the Armed Forces, and that it was important for all concerned that the Institute continue its activities in serving both the civilian and military sectors in education, consultation, and research in the medical, dental, and veterinary sciences. Accordingly, the 94th Congress passed Public Law 94-361, which not only provided a Congressional Charter for the AFIP but also provided for the establishment of a nonprofit corporation to be known as the American Registry of Pathology (ARP), authorized to do many things to assist the AFIP in accomplishing its missions. Specifically mentioned were the entering into contracts with public and private organizations for the preparation of books, and the formation of agreements with professional societies for the maintenance of the Registries of Pathology.

Soon after the passage of PL 94-361, the American Academy of Ophthalmology and Otolaryngology again exhibited its outstanding leadership in helping to speedily implement the law. Drs. Bradley R. Straatsma and Paul Henkind initially were the responsible representatives for ophthalmology; Dr. W. Richard Green is the current representative for the American Academy of Ophthalmology, serving also as Treasurer of the ARP. As this is being written, word has been received that two other medical societies have indicated their desire to become cosponsors of the Registry of Ophthalmic Pathology: the American Association of Ophthalmic Pathologists and the Verhoeff Society (of ophthalmic pathologists).

During the 22 years since publication of the second edition, several smaller but more up-to-date books on ophthalmic pathology have appeared. Those who planned the third edition felt the need for a much more comprehensive treatise than was available anywhere. They considered the facts that transmission electron microscopy, introduced into ophthalmic pathology only shortly before the preparation of the second edition, has now been exploited and that much new information has also been obtained by scanning electron microscopy, ultrasonography, computed tomography, vitreous cytology, and, most recently, immunohistochemical and quantitative morphometric studies. To incorporate into the text a good bit of this new information—and to illustrate it—has required much more space. Also, the authors wished to heed the advice of critics of the second edition who complained about the absence of documentation for many statements made in the text and who felt that most chapters had too few references.

Ophthalmic Pathology has grown immense and will now require three volumes for the new information and accompanying illustrations, additional references, and changes made to satisfy the critics. The authors, who have labored for years in the preparation of these books, will receive no royalties for their time, effort, and expertise. I admire and commend them for their dedication. This third edition of three volumes should be enthusiastically welcomed by pathologists and ophthalmologists alike and also should prove very helpful for Residents and Fellows in training.

Robert R. McMeekin, M.D.
Colonel, MC, USA
The Director, Armed Forces Institute of Pathology

PREFACE

In 1938 the American Academy of Ophthalmology and Otolaryngology, as part of its educational activity, sponsored preparation and publication of the first edition of the *Atlas of Ophthalmic Pathology* and a companion *Atlas of Otolaryngic Pathology*. The *Atlas of Ophthalmic Pathology* was jointly written by Captain Elbert DeCoursey, pathologist at the Registry of Ophthalmic Pathology, and Lieutenant Colonel James E. Ash, curator of the Army Medical Museum. It represented an expansion of the syllabus prepared to accompany the museum's loan set of slides on ophthalmic pathology and contained contributions from Roy M. Reeve, Lawrence P. Ambrogi, and Helenor C. Wilder. The first edition was an immediate success, and the same authors subsequently prepared a second and third edition, published respectively in 1939 and 1942. Following World War II, the Education Committee of the Academy asked Dr. Jonas S. Friedenwald to oversee preparation of a combined atlas and textbook not only incorporating photographs of individual cases but also providing discussions of normal ocular physiology and of mechanisms influencing pathologic alterations in ocular tissues. The first edition of *Ophthalmic Pathology—An Atlas and Textbook* ("the green atlas") was published in 1952 by W. B. Saunders Company and was cosponsored by the Academy and by the Armed Forces Institute of Pathology. Dr. Friedenwald's coauthors included Helenor C. Wilder, A. Edward Maumenee, Theodore E. Sanders, John E. L. Keyes, Michael J. Hogan, and W. C. and Ella U. Owens. Several authoritative ophthalmic pathologists, including Frederick H. Verhoeff, James E. Ash, Georgiana D. Theobald, Algernon B. Reese, John S. McGavic, Brittain F. Payne, and Benjamin Rones, acted as consultants. The new format was enthusiastically received, and it has served as the basis for all later editions.

In 1956, Michael J. Hogan, Chairman of the Academy's Committee on Ophthalmic Pathology, and Lorenz E. Zimmerman, Chief of the Ophthalmic Pathology Branch and Registrar of the Registry of Ophthalmic Pathology at the Armed Forces Institute of Pathology, again enlisted the aid of influential ophthalmic pathologists in this country in preparation of the second edition of *Ophthalmic Pathology—An Atlas and Textbook* ("the blue atlas"). This extensive work, first published in 1962, re-used from the first edition many illustrations that had been initially selected and prepared by Helenor C. Wilder. The text was completely revised, and it incorporated advances in virtually every aspect of the field of ophthalmic pathology. Emphasis was placed not only on ocular pathologic alterations but also on their clinical manifestations. This was found by practicing ophthalmologists and pathologists to be very valuable, and the book has enjoyed great popularity.

More than two decades have elapsed since publication of the second edition. During this interval many important observations have been made and much has been learned about the pathogenesis, course, and treatment of a wide array of ocular illnesses. New work continues to be produced in quantity, and in some areas entirely new concepts have emerged. Accordingly, the American Academy of Ophthalmology has provided its steadfast and enthusiastic support for the development and publication of a new edition of this book.

The Board of Directors and the staff of the Academy have shown admirable patience with authors who have experienced difficulties in meeting production schedules, and we are grateful for their forbearance during the long gestation of this book. Grant funds from the Academy were used to provide technical assistance in preparing the text and photographs. In keeping with the tradition initiated by contributors to previous editions of the atlas, the authors have received no monetary compensation for their efforts, and royalties will be received by the Academy.

The third edition, now expanded to three volumes, is organized in the same anatomic format as the second edition, beginning with a discussion of general principles of pathology and pathologic alterations affecting all tissues and followed by chapters concerned with individual ocular and adnexal structures. In the preface to the second edition, Drs. Hogan and Zimmerman noted that the anatomic method of discussing and describing pathologic changes in the eye necessitates a certain amount of repetition and often requires the reader to refer to several chapters to obtain a complete picture of a specific ocular disease. We have tried to minimize this shortcoming in the third edition by duplicating certain illustrations and also by permitting significant amounts of redundancy and overlap in the content of the text from one chapter to another, to enable the reader to visualize the essence of each disease process without the necessity of too much cross-referencing.

We would not have been able to complete this effort without the invaluable aid provided by Dr. Lorenz Zimmerman and his staff at the Armed Forces Institute of Pathology. A large proportion of the photographs in the book were obtained from the files of the Registry of Ophthalmic Pathology at the Armed Forces Institute of Pathology, and we thank Mrs. Alice Masten for her help in locating them. We especially wish to thank the staff and faculty members of each of our departments for their cooperation and encouragement during the preparation and completion of this book. Clinical photographs and correlative photomicrographs of histologic sections have been freely provided by a great number of our colleagues. We are grateful for their generosity and have made every effort to acknowledge their contribution in the legends describing each figure. Mrs. Carolyn Strecker, editor, worked long and hard to check all bibliographic references and to make the manuscript clear and readable. Mr. Carroll Cann and Ms. Wynette Kommer of the Saunders Company provided amiable and sound editorial advice and guidance.

All the chapters have been reviewed by friends and colleagues with special areas of knowledge, and we are indebted to them for their valuable suggestions. We hasten to note that surviving imperfections are the responsibility of the authors. The text and galleys of Chapters 1 through 7 and 11 have been laboriously and patiently read and reviewed by David G. Cogan, Bethesda, Maryland; William F. Hoyt, San Francisco; J. Brooks Crawford, San Francisco; John C. Cavender, Atlanta; Robert N. Shaffer, San Francisco; Jin Kinoshita, Bethesda, Maryland; and G. Richard O'Connor, San Francisco. Mr. J. Michael Coppinger at Pacific Medical Center, Department of Ophthalmology, kindly prepared photographs for many of these chapters and we thank him for his careful contributions which have added greatly to the value of these portions of the book. Dr. Heinrich Konig of Bern, Switzerland, graciously assisted in translating foreign articles and in preparation of their bibliographic references. Hedy Krasnobrod at the Pacific Medical Center, Benjamin Goldfeller and Winifred Slauson at the University of California Medical Center in San Francisco, and Virginia Cruse at the Department of Pathology of the San Francisco General Hospital provided valuable assistance in preparation of light microscopic sections, electron micrographs, and drawings. We are indebted to Ms. Mary Dessau, who spent many hours typing and re-typing these chapters, and to Ms. Elizabeth Ahlers and Ms. Judith Peck, who typed the initial drafts of Chapters 3 and 4.

At the end of Chapters 8 and 9, Dr. W. Richard Green has acknowledged the assistance and encouragement he received from his colleagues in the preparation and review of these chapters.

Drs. T. P. Dryja (Boston), B. L. Gallie (Toronto), and A. L. Murphree (Los Angeles) reviewed the manuscript dealing with retinoblastoma and retinocytoma and were especially helpful in providing critical evaluations of the section on the genetics of retinoblastoma.

We thank Ms. Donna Murphy of Houston, Texas, for her photographic expertise and for preparation of several of the electron micrographs that appear in Chapter 10. Ms. Janice Bryant, Ms. Joyce Samuel, and Ms. Sharan Francis are thanked for their secretarial assistance in preparation of this chapter.

Dr. Takeo Iwamoto provided electron micrographs used in Chapter 12. Without his fine technical work, the task of producing this chapter would have been much more difficult.

William H. Spencer, *Editor*

Ramon L. Font
W. Richard Green
Edward L. Howes, Jr.
Frederick A. Jakobiec
Lorenz E. Zimmerman

AUTHORS

WILLIAM H. SPENCER, MD, Editor
Director, Ophthalmic Pathology Laboratory, Pacific Medical Center, San Francisco, California

RAMON L. FONT, MD
Director, Ophthalmic Pathology Laboratory, Cullen Eye Institute
Professor of Pathology and Ophthalmology, Baylor College of Medicine
Consultant in Pathology, The Methodist Hospital, Baylor College of Medicine, and M.D. Anderson Hospital and Tumor Institute, Texas Medical Center, Houston, Texas

W. RICHARD GREEN, MD
Professor of Ophthalmology and Associate Professor of Pathology, Johns Hopkins University School of Medicine
Ophthalmologist and Pathologist, Eye Pathology Laboratory, Johns Hopkins Hospital, Baltimore, Maryland

EDWARD L. HOWES, Jr., MD
Professor of Pathology and Ophthalmology, University of California, San Francisco, School of Medicine
Co-Director, Eye Pathology, University of California, San Francisco, Medical Center
Assistant Chief of Pathology, San Francisco General Hospital, San Francisco, California

FREDERICK A. JAKOBIEC, MD
Professor of Clinical Ophthalmology and Clinical Pathology, Columbia University College of Physicians and Surgeons
Chairman, Department of Ophthalmology, and Director of Laboratories, Manhattan Eye, Ear and Throat Hospital, New York, New York

LORENZ E. ZIMMERMAN, MD
Professor of Pathology and Ophthalmology, Georgetown University School of Medicine
Emeritus Chairman, Department of Ophthalmic Pathology, The Armed Forces Institute of Pathology
Consultant Ophthalmic Pathologist, Washington Hospital Center, Washington, DC

Volume I

Volume II

Volume III

CONTENTS
Volume II

Selected Aspects of the Pathology of the Retinal Pigment Epithelium (RPE) 1227
Neuroepithelial Tumors of Ciliary Body 1246
Retinoblastoma and Retinocytoma, by Lorenz E. Zimmerman 1292

OPHTHALMIC PATHOLOGY
An Atlas and Textbook

Volume 2

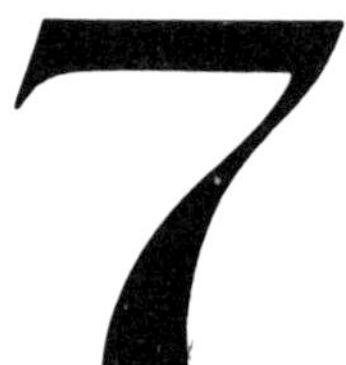

CHAPTER 7 VITREOUS

William H. Spencer

The vitreous body is a transparent, gelatinous structure, situated behind the lens and surrounded by the inner surface of the retina, ciliary body, and optic nerve head. Nearly all the normal adult vitreous volume (approximately 4 ml) and weight (approximately 4 gm) is due to its water content, which allows passage of metabolites to and from adjacent structures and plays a role in changes in viscosity associated with advancing age or pathologic conditions. The vitreous transmits light to the retina (its index of refraction is similar to that of the aqueous) and, because of its bulk, it assists in supporting surrounding structures and in maintaining intraocular pressure and the configuration of the eye.

ANATOMY AND HISTOLOGY

Gross Anatomy

Posterior to the ora serrata, the vitreous is spherical and is in contact with the inner limiting membrane of the retina, except over the surface of the optic disc (Fig. 7–1). Anterior to the ora serrata, the lateral aspect of the vitreous is in contact with the ciliary epithelium and with the zonule (Fig. 7–2). The anterior surface of the vitreous is indented, forming the patellar fossa in which the lens rests. The lens is attached to the anterior vitreous surface along a circular zone approximately 1 to 2 mm in width and 8 to 9 mm in diameter (hyaloideocapsular ligament, ligamentum pectinatum) (Fig. 7–3). This circular attachment is firm in youth and tenuous to absent in older individuals. Berger's space lies at the center of the anterior vitreous within the hyaloideocapsular ligament. In most adults, this is a potential rather than a true space.

The outer portion of the vitreous, particularly where it is close to the ciliary body and retina, is relatively dense (Fig. 7–4). This zone, which is about 100 microns thick, is referred to as the vitreous cortex to distinguish it from the central vitreous, which is more fluid and less fibrillar. The surface of the vitreous cortex constitutes the hyaloid. The hyaloid anterior to the ora serrata is often referred to clinically as the anterior vitreous face or anterior border layer. Posterior to the ora serrata, the surface of the vitreous is referred to as the posterior hyaloid or posterior border layer. When this separates from the retina (Fig. 7–5), it is visible clinically and is referred to as the posterior vitreous face.

The attachment of the vitreous to contiguous structures varies in firmness. It is strongest at the vitreous base and at the periphery of the optic disc. The vitreous base straddles the ora serrata as a circular band, varying in width from 2 to 6 mm. This attachment remains firm throughout life, and displacement or traction of the vitreous base produces a pull on the inner aspect of the retina immediately behind the ora serrata and along the posterior portion of the pars plana of the ciliary body. The peripapillary attachment of the vitreous is not as firm or broad as that at the vitreous base; with advancing age, it becomes more tenuous. The vitreous is loosely attached to the macular region over a zone 3 to 4 mm in diameter. This attachment is more substantial in fetal eyes and in the eyes of young adults than in older eyes (Hogan, 1963). Foos (1972a) studied

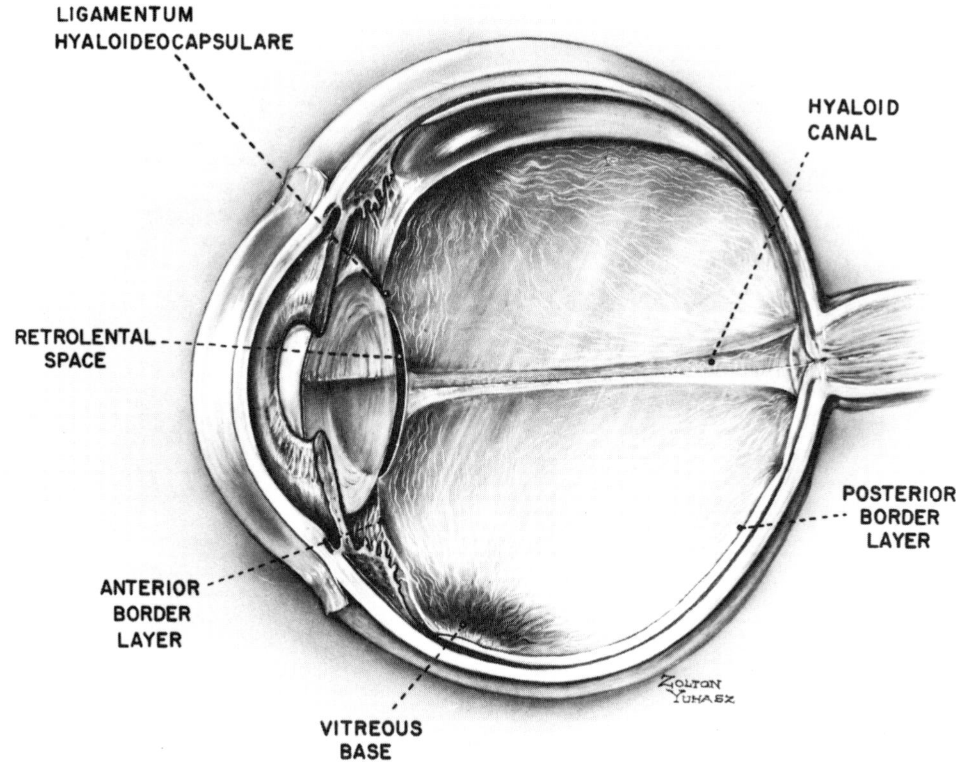

Figure 7–1. Relationship of vitreous to surrounding structures. The anterior border layer (anterior hyaloid) is in contact with the posterior surface of the lens at the ligamentum hyaloideocapsulare. The potential retrolental space of Berger is diagrammatically exaggerated. Vitreous adheres to the ciliary body and peripheral retina at the broad vitreous base. The posterior border layer (posterior hyaloid) is in contact with the inner retinal surface. The narrow peripapillary attachment of the vitreous to the retina lies at the posterior margin of the hyaloid canal (Cloquet's canal).

the ultrastructural features of anterior (basal), equatorial, and posterior vitreous fibrils at their junction with the retinal internal limiting lamina and found focal condensations where vitreous fibrils traverse the lamina to attach to the cell membrane of the underlying Müller cells (''attachment plaques''). The plaques were present in the basal and equatorial zones but not posteriorly.

The canal of Cloquet represents the residual structure of the primary vitreous (see pages 556 and 557). It extends from the optic nerve head to a point slightly nasal and inferior to the posterior pole of the lens. It is 1 to 2 mm wide, spreading anteriorly to 4 to 5 mm at Berger's space. Posteriorly, it broadens as it approaches the disc in the area of Martegiani. It appears to have a serpentine shape at slit lamp examination, dipping down centrally and rising posteriorly. When the patient is sitting, it lies mostly below the horizontal meridian.

Microscopic Anatomy and Physical Properties

The vitreous gel is composed of a liquid phase (the vitreous humor) and a solid phase (residual protein). The solid components of the vitreous constitute only 1 per cent of its weight. They include collagen fibrils, peripheral cells (hyalocytes), and minute amounts of protein. The liquid phase is primarily water (99 per cent), but it also contains inorganic salts, sugar, ascorbic acid, soluble proteins, and hyaluronic acid.

Descriptions of the collagen component differ with the varying methods used to study vitreous structure (e.g. gross observation, slit lamp microscopy, standard light microscopy, phase contrast microscopy, dark field microscopy, x-ray diffraction, and electron microscopy). Light microscopy of fixed and stained vitreous shows a series of netlike, fibrous membranes extending centrally from the vitreous base and also parallel to the retina; however, these membranes appear to be processing artifact. By electron microscopy, fresh vitreous is a structureless gel (Hogan, Alvarado, Weddell, 1971), and no fibers are found in fresh vitreous until 15 to 20 minutes after removal or when the vitreous is stored at 2.0°C for 2 to 8 hours (Rossi, 1953). Other ultrastructural studies (Schwarz, 1961; Fine, Tousimis, 1961; Hogan, 1963; Brini, Porte, Stoeckel, 1968) have confirmed the absence of fibers and the presence of collagen fibrils varying from 10 to 25 nm in di-

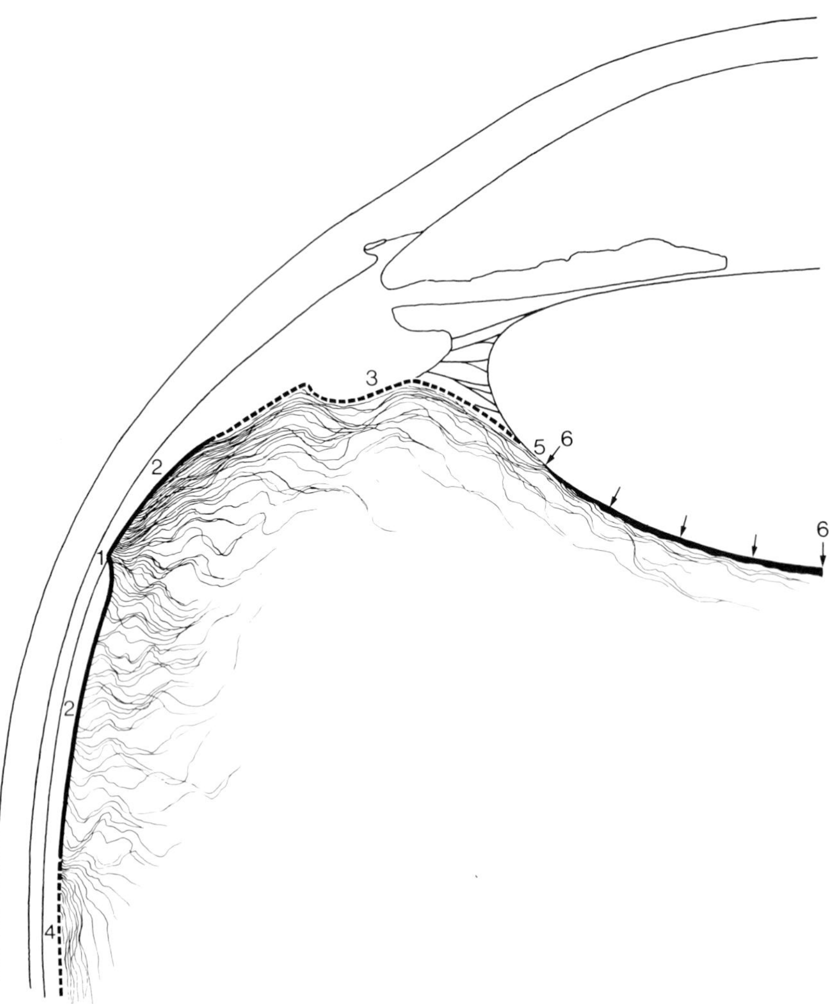

Figure 7–2. Vitreous relations in the anterior eye. The ora serrata (1) is the termination of the retina. The vitreous base (2) extends forward about 2 mm over the ciliary body and posteriorly about 4 mm over the peripheral retina. The collagen in this region is oriented at a right angle to the surface of the retina and ciliary body, but anteriorly over the pars plana it is more parallel to the inner surface of the ciliary body. The posterior hyaloid (4) is continuous with the retina, and the anterior hyaloid (3) with the zonule and lens. The hyaloideocapsular ligament is at 5 and the space of Berger is at 6.

(From Hogan MJ, Alvarado JA, Weddell JE: Histology of The Human Eye. Philadelphia, W. B. Saunders Company, 1971.)

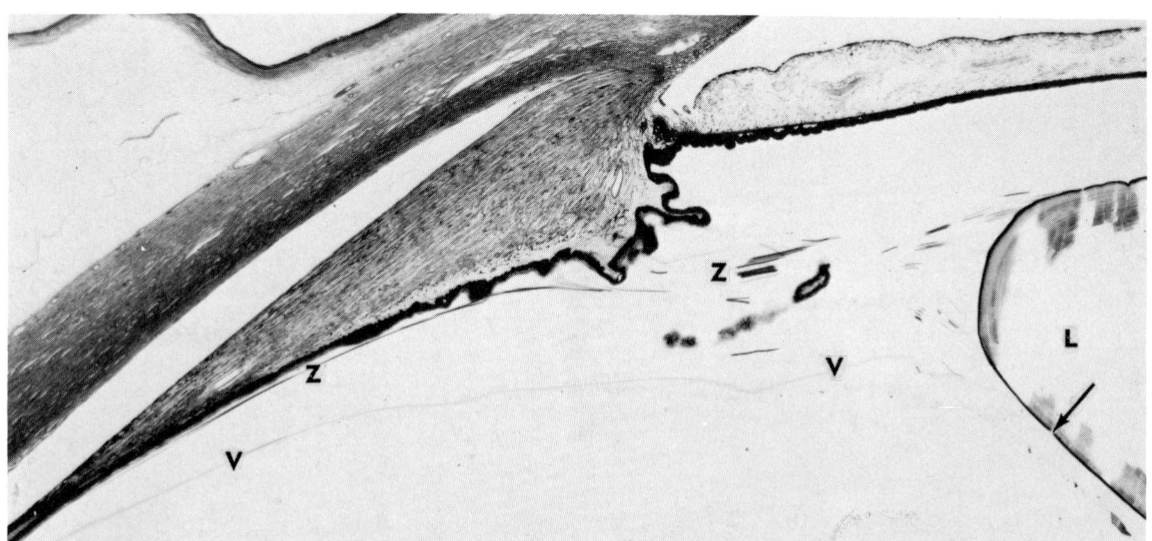

Figure 7–3. Vitreous relations in the anterior aspect of a normal human eye. *L,* lens; *V,* anterior hyaloid. *Z,* zonular fibers; Arrow, attachment of vitreous to posterior lens capsule (hyaloideocapsular ligament). ×28. AFIP Acc. 630832.

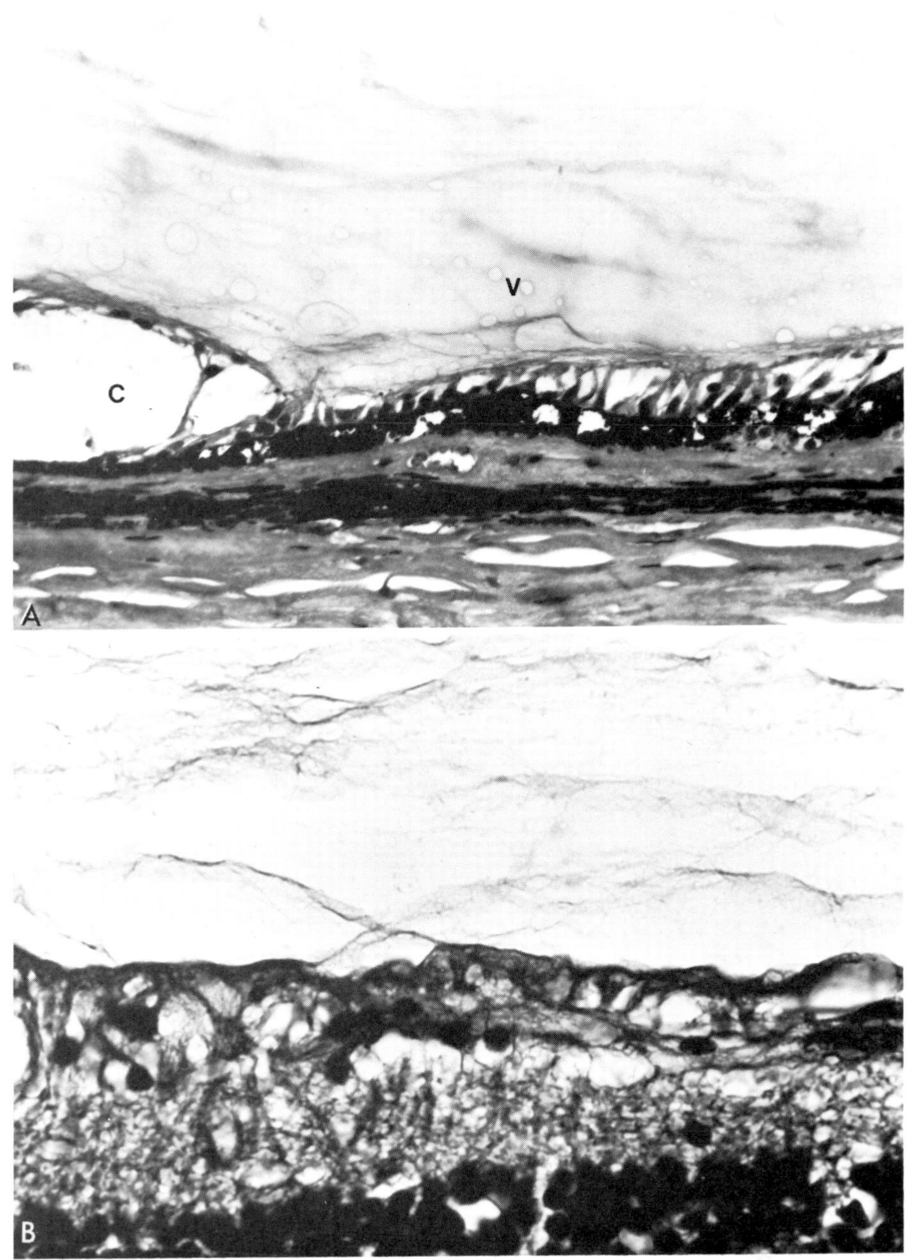

Figure 7–4. Normal vitreous attachment to ciliary body and retina. *A,* Relatively dense vitreous cortex *(V)* adheres to the ciliary epithelium and inner surface of the retina at the ora serrata. *C,* Pars plana cyst. H and E, ×25. *B,* Junction of vitreous and retina anterior to the equator. H and E, ×25.

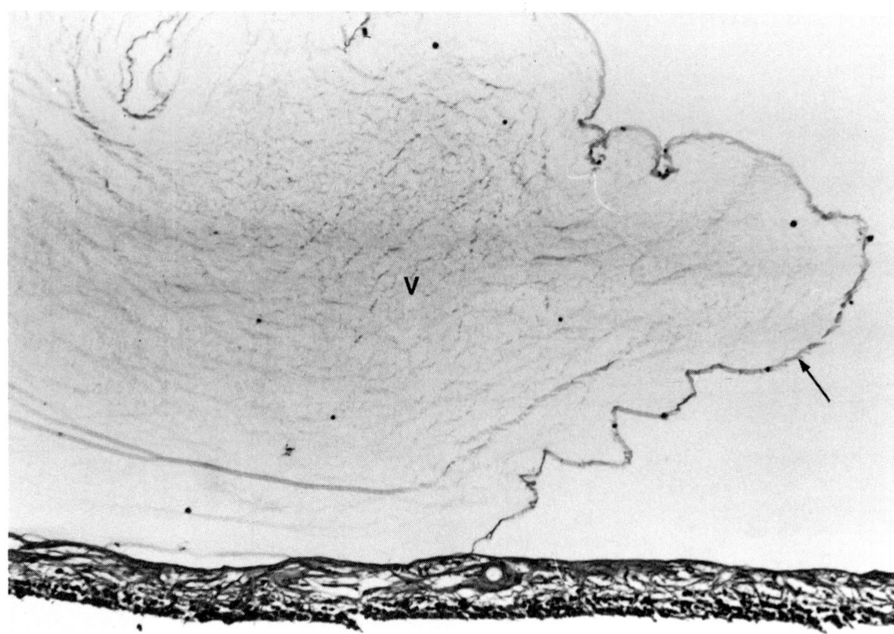

Figure 7–5. Posterior vitreous detachment. The posterior portion of the vitreous *(V)* has separated from the postequatorial retina (right side of photograph). The posterior hyaloid (arrow) is artifactitiously convoluted. H and E, ×25.

ameter, with a periodicity of about 22 nm (Fig. 7–6).

The fibrils are somewhat condensed in the vitreous cortex, where they are randomly arranged and contact the inner limiting membrane of the retina. They are particularly numerous at the vitreous base, where the fibrils lie at right angles to the basement membrane of the ciliary epithelium, and in the zone of peripapillary attachment of the vitreous to the Müller cells of the retina. The cen-

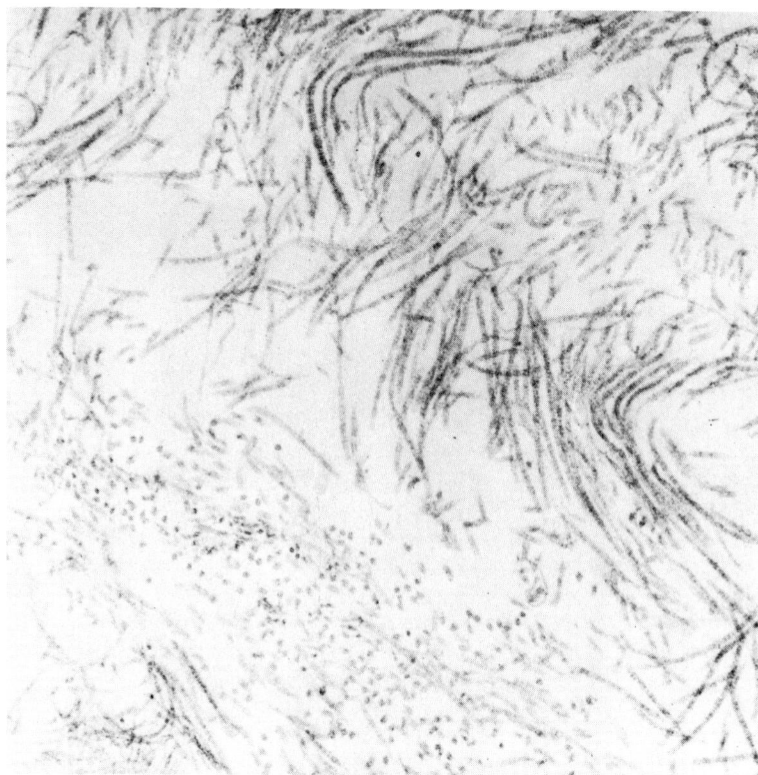

Figure 7–6. Collagen fibrils in normal vitreous cortex. Randomly arranged fibrils in longitudinal and cross-section. The fibrils vary only slightly in diameter and show periodic banding. TEM, ×52,500.

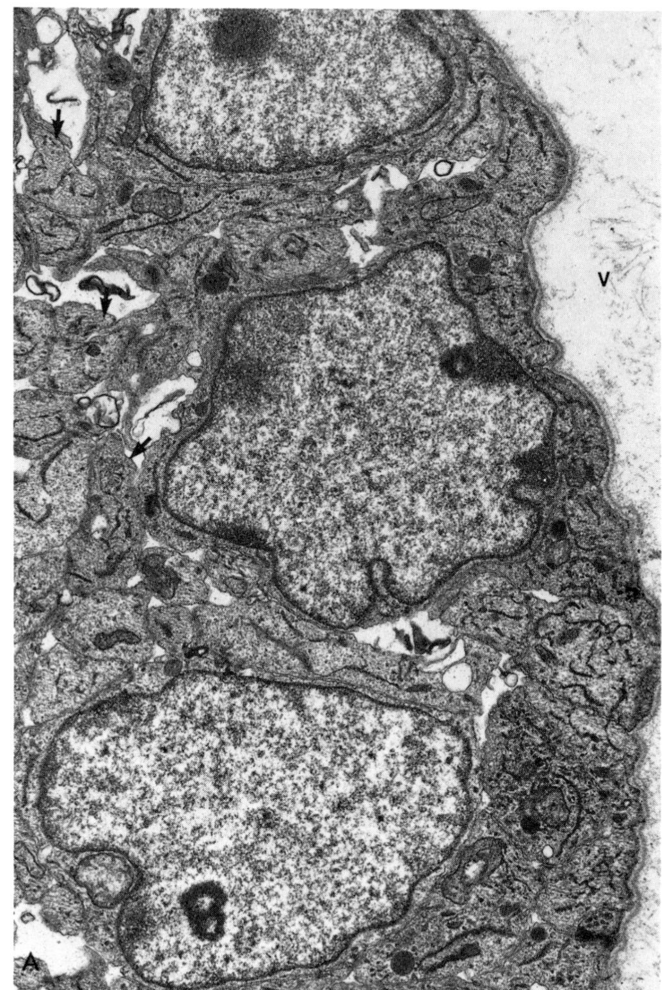

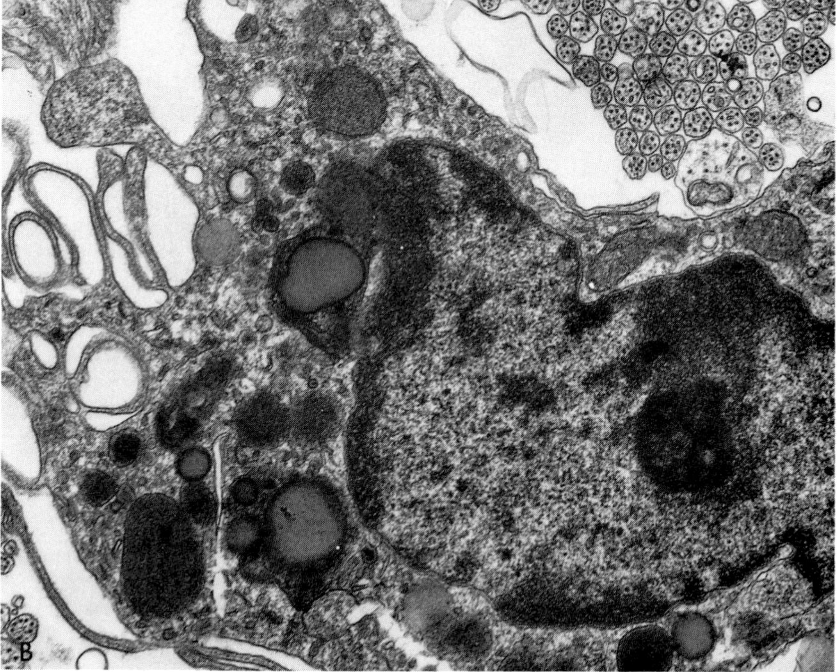

Figure 7–7. Hyalocytes in the fetal eye. *A,* Sixteen week fetal eye (110 mm human embryo). Three hyalocytes with lobulated nuclei lie in contact with glial cells (arrows) at the margin of the canal of Cloquet. Vitreous collagen fibrils *(V)* lie close to the hyalocytes. TEM, ×23,030. *B,* Twenty week fetal eye (150 mm human embryo). Hyalo cyte in the nerve fiber layer of the peripapillary retina. Lobulated nucleus is surrounded by abundant cytoplasm containing small vacuoles (thought to contain mucopolysaccharide). Larger, membrane-bound vacuoles contain electron-dense material of undetermined type. TEM, ×28,200. (Courtesy of I. Wood.)

tral vitreous contains many fewer collagen fibrils than does the cortex.

At and just beneath the anterior and posterior hyaloid surface, there are condensations of collagen fibrils arranged parallel to the surface. By light microscopy, these appear to form a membrane; however, no true membrane exists (Fine, Tousimis, 1961). It is likely that reformation of the vitreous face, which is observed clinically in aphakic eyes in which the vitreous face has "broken" during or shortly after surgery, is in part due to reaggregation and realignment of the collagen fibrils in accordance with physical factors governing the formation of surface tension membranes at an interface between substances of differing viscosity (i.e., similar to a membrane forming on the surface of pudding). Reformation of the face also may be modified by contraction of the surface collagen and possibly by proliferation of hyalocytes or, in the case of the posterior face, by cellular elements derived from the nerve fiber layer and the internal limiting membrane of the retina.

Cells (hyalocytes), variously described by light microscopy as being spindle-shaped, rounded, or even star-shaped, are a normal component of the vitreous. Ultrastructurally, they are oval or spindle-shaped and 10 to 15 microns in size. Their nuclei are lobulated, and the cytoplasm is characterized by the presence of many secretory granules and a well-developed Golgi complex (Bloom, Balazs, 1965). Hyalocytes are more numerous in the embryonic and fetal vitreous than in the adult vitreous (Fig. 7–7) (Hogan, Alvarado, Weddell, 1971, p 632) and are found in greater numbers close to the retina and at the vitreous base. The precise nature and function of the hyalocytes is not known. They may be associated with the secretion of hyaluronic acid, since the concentration of this material is greater in the cortical vitreous where most of the hyalocytes are found. Balazs (1961) observed negative staining for glia; the presence of cytoplasmic inclusions, denoting phagocytic activity, led him to suggest that the cells may be connective tissue macrophages. However, in a study of monkey vitreous, Hogan found cells believed to be hyalocytes which, because of their paucity of lysosomes, did not resemble macrophages. Cells that do have the characteristics of macrophages and fibroblasts can be found in the vitreous of adults in the region of the ora serrata and near the optic nerve head. It is not known whether these are normal components of vitreous or whether they are derived from contiguous structures reacting to a pathologic stimulus.

Hyaluronic acid is a mucopolysaccharide polymer that is weakly bound to the vitreous collagen (Balazs, 1961). The hyaluronic acid is formed into coiled chains, which in the hydrated state incorporate water as in a sponge (1 gm of hyaluronic acid encloses approximately 65 ml of water). Hyaluronic acid appears blue when stained with colloidal iron or alcian blue. If a section is pretreated with the enzyme hyaluronidase, the blue-staining material disappears, thus allowing one to differentiate hyaluronic acid from other forms of mucopolysaccharide.

The water content of the vitreous is believed to have a high turnover rate (half the water in the vitreous of animals is replaced every 10 to 15 minutes [Kinsey, Grant, Cogan, 1942]) and to carry substances between the vitreous and aqueous by diffusion (Maurice, 1957; Suran, McEwen, 1961). When hyperosmotic agents are given orally (e.g., glycerin) or intravenously (e.g., urea or mannitol), the volume of the vitreous is transiently decreased. The vitreous is normally fully hydrated and, therefore, does not swell in response to conditions causing hypotonicity of the blood (Tolentino, Schepens, Freeman, 1976, p. 26).

The residual protein of the vitreous, in combination with the hyaluronic acid, is believed to be responsible for its gel state and for its viscosity and elasticity. The transparency of vitreous results from high water content, absence of color, localization of most of the residual protein in areas away from the pupillary axis, and lack of significant diffraction produced by the few collagen fibrils located in the central vitreous.

EMBRYOLOGY

The embryologic development of the vitreous is generally stated to have three phases: formation of the primary, secondary, and tertiary vitreous. It also may be viewed as a biphasic process, since the tertiary vitreous develops into the suspensory ligament of the lens, which is anatomically separate from the adult vitreous.

The primary vitreous begins to form during the third to fourth week (4 to 7 mm stage) and ends its growth by the ninth week (40 mm stage). Its precise source is uncertain. Its earliest components are tenuous protoplasmic processes that lie between the lens plate (derived from surface ectoderm) and the innermost retina (derived from neural ectoderm). By the sixth week (13 mm), the posterior aspects of these processes are identifiable as vitreous fibers. They are continuous with the footplates of the Müller cells of the retina.

During the third to fourth week, vasoformative cells (derived from mesoderm) become visible behind the lens as part of the capsula perilenticularis fibrosa (Fig. 7–8). The vascular components of the primary vitreous (hyaloid artery, vasa hyaloidea propria, and the posterior portion

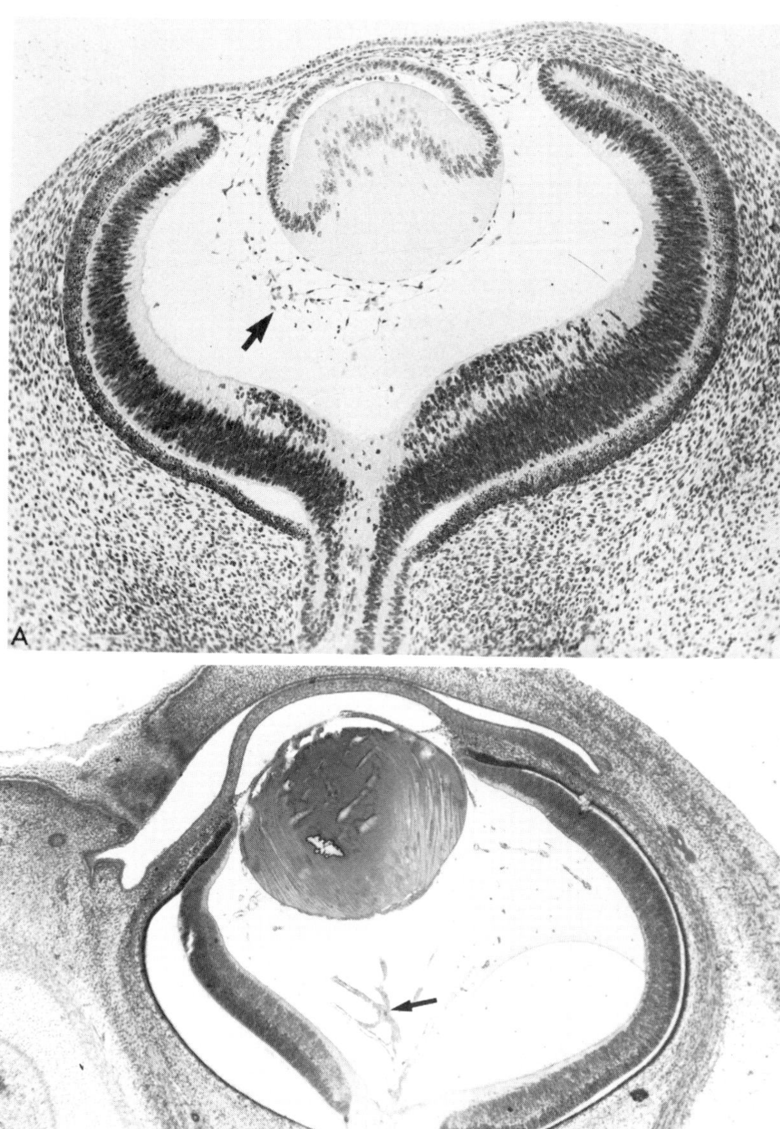

Figure 7–8. Vascular elements of embryonic vitreous. *A,* Five week fetal eye (12 mm human embryo). Vasoformative cells (arrow) are visible behind the lens. H and E, ×115. AFIP Neg. 60-4414. *B,* Nine week fetal eye (40 mm human embryo). Vessels of the primary vitreous (arrow) extend from the optic nerve head toward the lens. H and E, ×30.

of the tunica vasculosa lentis) continue to develop throughout early embryonic life, but then undergo regression. Regression is particularly marked during the seventh and eighth months (240 to 290 mm stage), and by birth all vessels in the vitreous normally have disappeared.

The secondary vitreous is destined to become the main portion of the postnatal and adult vitreous. It begins to form during the ninth week (40 mm stage), and it apparently continues to develop as the eye enlarges throughout early childhood. It is derived from the inner retina (neural ectoderm), although mesodermally derived cells from the primary vitreous also may play a minor role in its formation. The developing secondary vitreous has a firm consistency and is transparent. As it encroaches upon the vascular primary vitreous, which becomes displaced centrally, a delimiting condensation layer forms along the junction between the primary and secondary vitreous. This layer will become the wall of Cloquet's canal (see Fig. 7–1). At the anterior aspect of the secondary vitreous, the marginal bundle of Druault forms (commencing during the tenth week, 48 mm stage). This bundle of condensed fibers runs parallel to the wall of the optic cup along the lens equator and extends to the mesoderm of the iris.

Shortly after the 12th week (65 to 70 mm stage), fibers derived from the inner aspect of the growing optic cup margin (future internal limiting membrane of the nonpigmented ciliary epithelium) pass at a right angle through the marginal bundle. These fibers form the tertiary vitreous, which will become the suspensory ligament of the lens (zonular lamella of the lens capsule). The marginal bundle atrophies, and surface condensations form along the anterior aspect of the secondary vitreous, separating it from the future suspensory ligament. The paracentral aspect of the anterior condensations of the secondary and primary vitreous remains in contact with the posterior lens capsule over a narrow circular zone known as Egger's line in embryonic life and as the hyaloideocapsular ligament thereafter. It surrounds the central space of Berger at the anterior, widened end of Cloquet's canal. At the posterior aspect of Cloquet's canal, there is a peripapillary condensation of primary and secondary vitreous adherent to the disc margins, which delimits the area of Martegiani, wherein remnants of the hyaloid vessels may occasionally be observed in the adult eye.

NORMAL GROWTH AND AGING

The volume of the eye increases 3.25 times from birth to adult life, and after the first year the greatest change is in the posterior segment. It must be assumed that the fluid portions of the vitreous, as well as the soluble and insoluble components, increase after birth, although little is known of the mechanism or qualitative changes of this growth. Until young adulthood, the vitreous is intimately united with the retina. With increasing age the attachment weakens, and separation from the retina (posterior vitreous detachment) may occur (Fig. 7–9). The space between the detached vitreous and the retina is filled with nonviscous fluid resembling aqueous. Often the attachment of the vitreous to the optic nerve head persists until quite late in the process (Fig. 7–10). It may then separate and can be seen with the ophthalmoscope or slit lamp as a circular or oval opacity on the posterior surface of the detached vitreous.

Foos (1972b) found evidence of posterior vitreous detachment in 16 per cent of 786 postmortem eyes from patients 45 to 65 years old and in 41 per cent of eyes from patients over age 65. Only eight eyes from patients under 55 years of age had posterior vitreous detachment, and seven of these had predisposing conditions such as surgical aphakia. A subsequent quantitative study of a larger number of postmortem eyes has confirmed the age-related incidence of posterior vitreous detachment, with the highest percentage (63 per cent) occurring in the eighth decade (Foos, Wheeler, 1982). These findings are consistent with those of Pischel (1952), Favre and Goldmann (1956), Wadsworth (1956), and Linder (1966). Posterior vitreous detachment is preceded by liquefaction (synchysis) of the central portion of the vitreous. Foos and Wheeler (1982) found an increase in synchysis with age and also noted a statistical correlation between the rate of posterior vitreous detachment and the degree of synchysis. This was especially notable in the seventh decade. It has been suggested that synchetic vitreous is "unstable" and is thus likely to undergo age-related posterior vitreous detachment. Presumably the latter can be precipitated by a tear in the posterior vitreous cortex (often

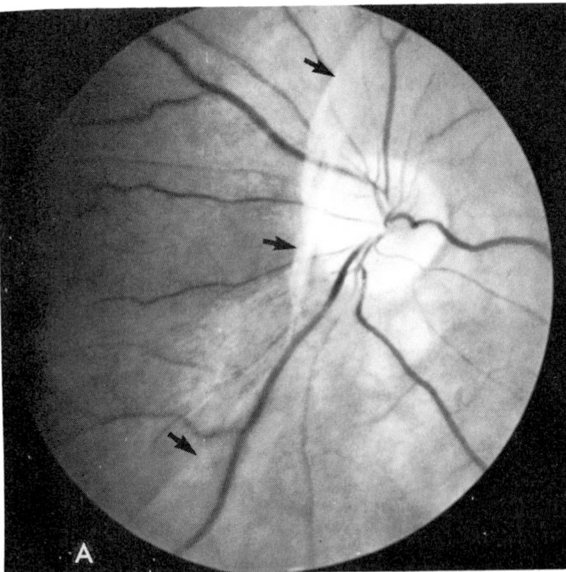

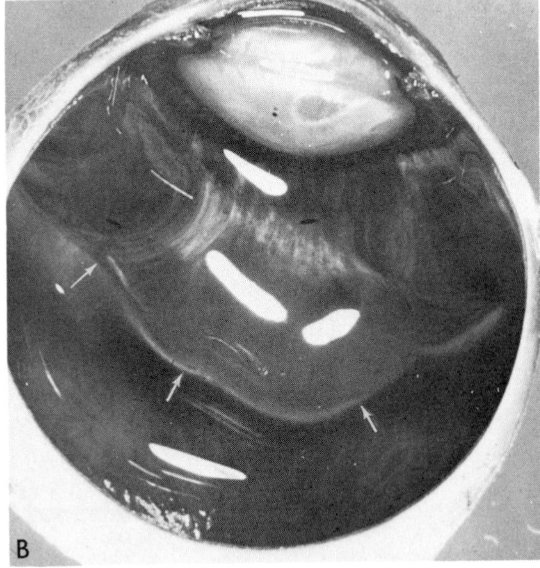

Figure 7–9. Posterior Detachment and Condensation of Vitreous. *A,* Clinical appearance: Vitreous is separated from temporal aspect of retina. Arrows indicate posterior surface of condensed vitreous. (Courtesy of Dr. W. Fung.) *B,* Gross appearance in enucleated eye. Arrows indicate posterior surface of condensed vitreous.

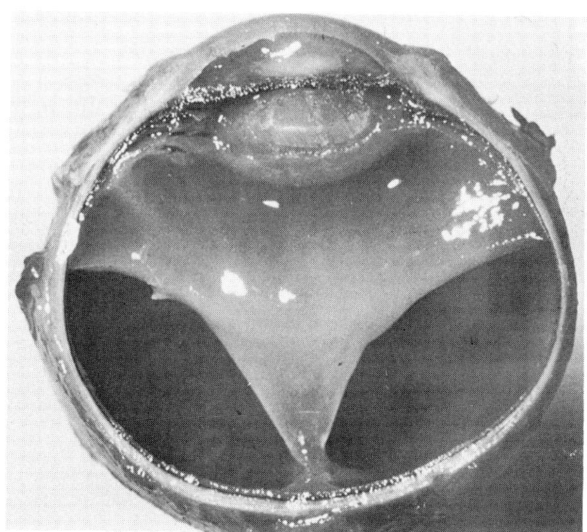

Figure 7–10. Partial posterior detachment and condensation of vitreous. The vitreous remains adherent about the optic disc.

overlying the macula) and can be followed by dissection of synchetic fluid from the central portion of the vitreous through the break in the posterior hyaloid (Linder, 1966; Foos, Wheeler, 1982). Posterior vitreous detachment also may occur in the absence of a break in the vitreous cortex. The latter appears to occur more frequently in patients with diabetes mellitus (Foos, Kreiger, Forsythe, Zakka, 1980).

When the vitreous first detaches, the patient is aware of "lightning flashes" resulting from the vitreous contacting the retina during change in body position or rapid eye movements. These symptoms also may result from focal traction on the retina at the posterior margin of the detachment of the vitreous. As further separation of the vitreous occurs, these symptoms may resolve. Occasionally, a thin layer of the cortical vitreous remains attached to the inner aspect of the retina. This may contract and cause the internal limiting membrane of the retina to wrinkle (cellophane retinopathy) (Fig. 7–11). Focal condensations of protein and collagen in the main portion of the detached vitreous frequently lie in the visual axis. These "floaters" are visible to the patient and are frequently described as "flying flies" (muscae volitantes).

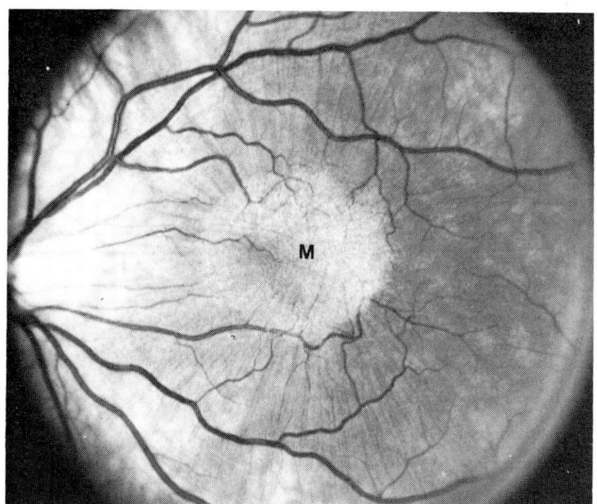

Figure 7–11. Surface wrinkling caused by cortical vitreous membrane. Ophthalmoscopic appearance of a thin membrane *(M)* adherent to the inner surface of the retina. The bulk of the posterior vitreous has detached and is not seen in the photograph.

Posterior detachment and liquefaction of the vitreous are common in myopic patients and undoubtedly contribute to the greater incidence of retinal detachment occurring in these individuals than in emmetropes and hypermetropes.

DEVELOPMENTAL ANOMALIES

Virtually all developmental anomalies of the vitreous are due to persistence in the adult eye of all or part of the vascular components of the primary vitreous or to hyperplastic changes in its connective tissue and vascular components. Dysembryogenesis of the secondary vitreous has not been recognized or described, and most hereditary processes affecting the secondary vitreous are classified as degenerations. Anomalies of the zonule, derived from the tertiary vitreous, are described in Chapter 5.

Persistent Vessels and Associated Changes

Persistence of Hyaloid Vessels and Vascular Loops. All or part of the embryonic vascular system may fail to regress and remain in the adult eye, although the remnants rarely result in significant visual symptoms. The vessels, particularly those located posteriorly, often contain blood. Occasionally, the entire hyaloid artery will persist and remain attached to the posterior aspect of the lens (Fig. 7–12), but more often this attachment is interrupted and the posterior portion of the vessel moves freely with rotations of the eye

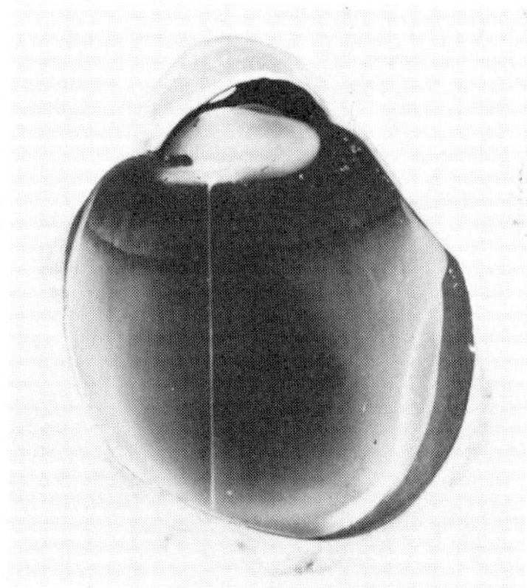

Figure 7–12. Persistence of hyaloid artery. AFIP Acc. 721733.

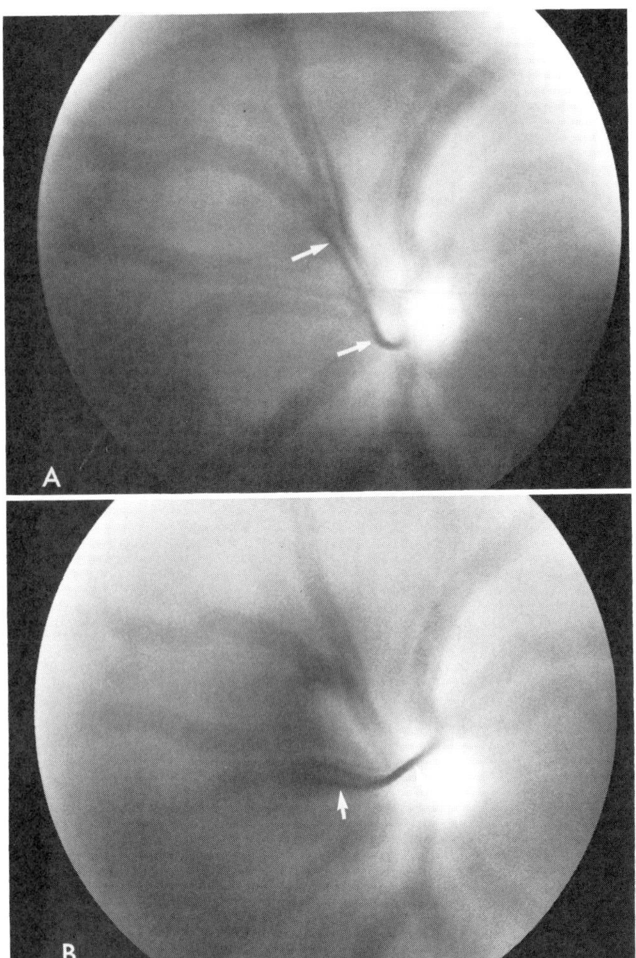

Figure 7–13. Persistence of hyaloid artery. Ophthalmoscopic appearance of hyaloid artery attached to optic nerve head but not to the lens. The focus is on the anterior portion of the persistent vessel, which moves freely with rotations of the eye. In *A*, the hyaloid artery (arrows) is displaced superiorly. In *B*, it is displaced nasally.

(Fig. 7–13). Vascular loops overlying the optic disc appear to be continuous with the central retinal artery. They are most likely derived from the hyaloid artery. Remnants of the tunica vasculosa lentis or of the anterior aspect of the hyaloid artery can adhere to the posterior surface of the lens and lie within Berger's space and the anterior aspect of Cloquet's canal.

Mittendorf's Dot and Bergmeister's Papilla. During embroynic development, the principal attachment of the hyaloid vessel to the posterior aspect of the lens lies slightly inferior and nasal to the posterior pole of the lens. A focal opacity on the surface of the lens capsule at this site is frequently seen in adult eyes and is known as Mittendorf's dot or as spurious posterior polar cataract. (See Chapter 5, Lens, page 439, for further discussion.)

Bergmeister's papilla has the clinical appearance of a veil overlying the optic disc and adjacent retina. It is composed of occluded remnants of the posterior portion of the hyaloid artery surrounded by glia (see Figs. 11–13, 11–14).

Vitreous Cysts. Congenital cysts have been reported in the anterior as well as the posterior vitreous (Bullock, 1974; Feman, Straatsma, 1974). They usually occur in otherwise normal eyes, and their origin is unknown. Some contain hyaloid remnants, leading to speculation that the cysts are dilations of remnants of the hyaloid artery. In five of nine patients with posterior vitreous cyst reported by François (1950), vessels were associated with the cysts. Cysts of the anterior vitreous lie just behind the lens or near the ciliary body (Hilsdorf, 1965). They do not seem to be related to vessels, although threadlike connections to the lens are occasionally seen. It is possible that anterior cysts are derived from the ciliary epithelium.

Vitreous cysts can be fixed (François, 1950) or free-floating (Donaldson, Hagler, 1967), bilateral (Bullock, 1974), or unilateral (Feman, Straatsma, 1974); they vary in size from 1 to 12 mm. Several have been found to be speckled with pigment, while others are reported as having a clear, glistening surface. As noted, most occur in otherwise normal eyes, but some have been found in eyes with retinitis pigmentosa. The latter may represent examples of acquired rather than congenital cysts.

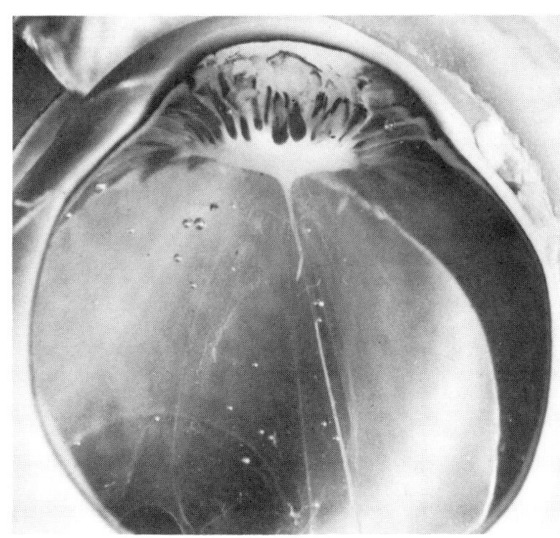

Figure 7–14. Persistent hyperplastic primary vitreous and persistent hyaloid artery. Gross photograph. An opaque plaque adheres to the posterior aspect of the lens and extends laterally to attach to elongated, centrally displaced ciliary processes. Hyaloid vessel inserts into posterior aspect of the plaque.

Persistent Hyperplastic Primary Vitreous (PHPV)

Reese (1949, 1955) described the spectrum of clinical and pathologic features of this unilateral (occasionally bilateral) congenital malformation of the anterior portion of the primary vitreous. Subsequently, others observed rare posterior forms of PHPV (Manschot, 1958; Pruett, Schepens, 1970; Nissim, Ivry, Oliver, 1972).

In the typical anterior form, a plaque of fibrovascular connective tissue occupies the retrolental portion of the vitreous and extends laterally to attach to elongated, centrally displaced ciliary processes (Fig. 7–14). At the posterior aspect of the plaque, the hyaloid artery and surrounding connective tissue occasionally can be traced posteriorly to the optic disc (Fig. 7–15). Blood may be supplied by the hyaloid artery or from arterioles of the ciliary processes. The anterior aspect of the plaque usually adheres to the lens capsule (Fig. 7–15 and 7–16), and it may extend through a capsular interruption into the lens cortex (see (Figs. 7–15 and 7–16), and it may extend through and become opaque later, suggesting that capsular wrinkling and interruption associated with cortical degeneration are secondary phenomena. The retina usually is not involved, but occasionally secondary traction occurs near the ora serrata. Rarely, the retina will exhibit dysplastic changes not directly related to PHPV (Balaglou, 1965). In mild forms of PHPV the retrolental plaque may be small and the lens clear, permitting clinical observation of the hyaloid artery extending back to the disc (see Fig. 5–15). These eyes may show only minimal clinical evidence of ciliary process elongation, and the eyes are usually of normal size. In more advanced forms of PHPV, the eyes are often smaller than normal, with anterior displacement of the lens-iris diaphragm and shallowing of the anterior chamber. Secondary glaucoma may occur, and this in turn may result in enlargement of the eye owing to stretching of the sclera and cornea. Because PHPV produces leukokoria, clinically it may be mistaken for retinoblastoma. This diagnostic error has occurred less frequently in recent years.

Adipose tissue, cartilage, and smooth muscle have been observed in the retrolental mass, in the lens, and in the vitreous (Reese, 1949, 1955; Manschot, 1958; Reese, Payne, 1964; Font, Yanoff, Zimmerman, 1969) (Fig. 7–17). Ten of 47 eyes with PHPV studied at the Armed Forces Institute of Pathology contained mature adipose tissue in these structures, and one contained cartilage (Font, Yanoff, Zimmerman, 1969). These eyes also exhibited related ocular malformations, such as microphthalmia, cataract, persistent hyaloid vessels, retinal detachment, and abnormal differentiation of the anterior chamber angle. Font and coworkers suggest that the adipose tissue and cartilage result from metaplasia of mesenchymal elements. Cartilage has been found in the eye of an otherwise healthy child (Yanoff, Font, 1969). It also may occur in association with trisomy 13 (Cogan, Kuwabara, 1964) and with medulloepitheliomas of the ciliary body (Anderson, 1962).

Several forms of posterior persistent hyperplastic primary vitreous have been described. These vary in extent, and in some cases may show opaque connective tissue membranes, believed to be derived from Bergmeister's papilla and the hyaloid vessels, overlying the optic nerve head. More severe cases may develop tentlike retinal folds that can lie in any meridian and usually contain vessels believed to be derived from the hyaloid artery. In some cases of posterior PHPV there is coexistent anterior PHPV, suggesting that the two conditions are related (Fig. 7–18). In the posterior form, leukokoria is infrequent; however, the retinal folds may result in poor vision, strabismus, and occasionally nystagmus. Vitreoretinal adhesions may lead to retinal breaks and detachment (Manschot, 1958).

DEGENERATIONS

Syneresis and Vitreous Detachment

Although syneresis and vitreous detachment are considered to be normal consequences of growth and aging, they also occur as a result of numerous pathologic processes that cause depolymerization of hyaluronic acid and breakdown of the collagen-like network. In addition, adhesions may form between the vitreous and retina as a result of pathologic processes, such as chorioretinitis. Liquefaction and detachment of the vitreous adjacent to such adhesions may cause traction on

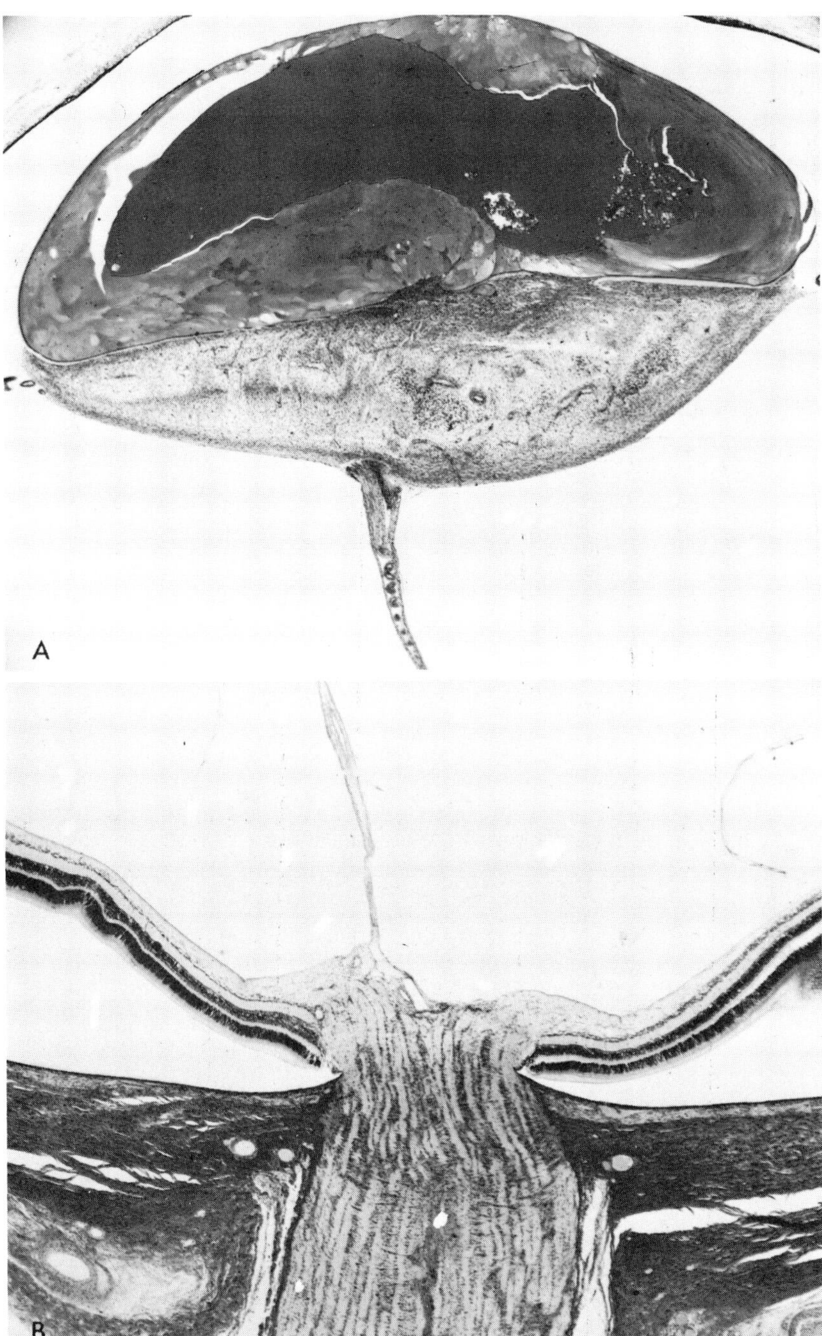

Figure 7–15. Persistent hyperplastic primary vitreous and persistent hyaloid artery. *A,* Insertion of hyaloid vessel into retrolental fibrovascular mass (hyperplastic primary vitreous). Posterior aspect of lens capsule is interrupted with formation of advanced cataract. H and E, ×50. AFIP Acc. 79594. *B,* Same patient. Origin of hyaloid vessel from optic disc. H and E, ×50. AFIP 79594.

Figure 7–17. Persistent hyperplastic primary vitreous with adipose tissue. *A,* Persistence of hyaloid vessel (arrow) is evident. Retina is artifactitiously detached. Extensive anterior synechiae are present. Lens has been replaced by adipose tissue. Note elongated ciliary processes drawn inward and reaching lens equator, H and E, ×4.5. AFIP Neg. 67-5562. *B,* Higher magnification. Lens has been almost entirely replaced by adipose tissue. Portions of wrinkled lens capsule (arrow) are still visible. Stretched ciliary processes are evident on left. H and E, ×28. AFIP Neg. 67-4974. *C,* Another patient. Vitreous is occupied by adipose tissue and capillaries. Retina is totally detached. H and E, ×6. AFIP Neg. 67-5281. (All figures from Font RL, Yanoff M, Zimmerman LE: Intraocular adipose tissue and persistent hyperplastic primary vitreous. Arch Ophthalmol *82*:43–50, 1969.)

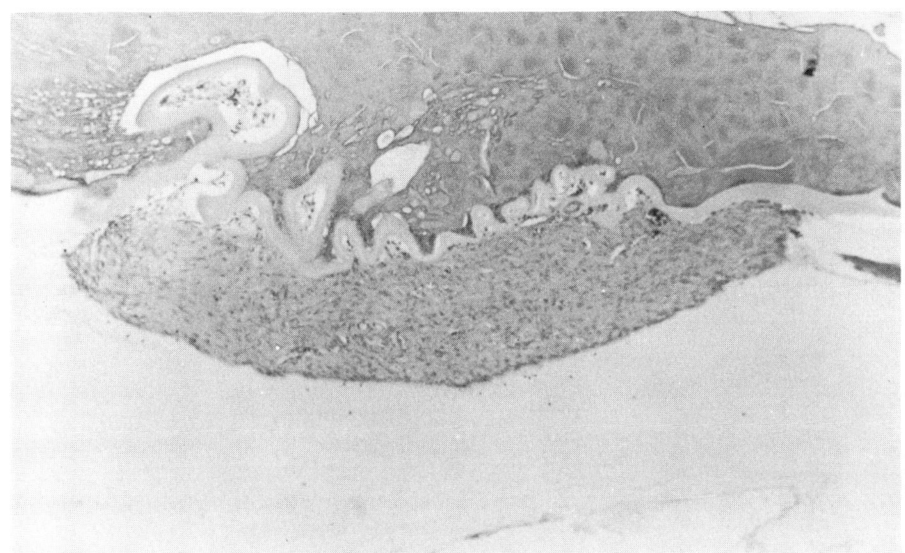

Figure 7–16. Persistent hyperplastic primary vitreous with posterior subcapsular cataract. The posterior aspect of the intact lens capsule is thrown into folds by an adherent retrolental fibrovascular mass (hyperplastic primary vitreous). The subcapsular cortex is degenerated. H and E, ×17.

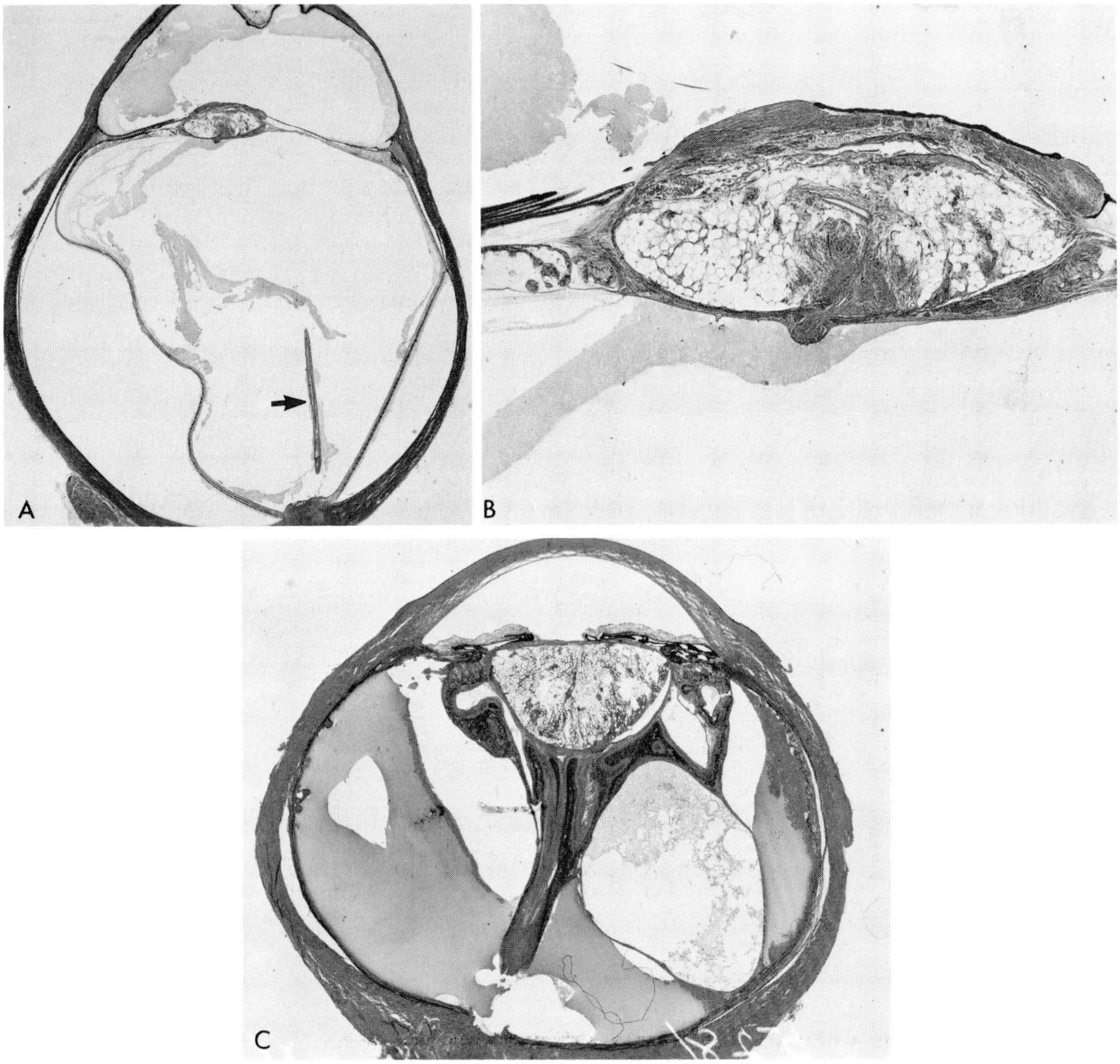

Figure 7–17 *See legend on opposite page*

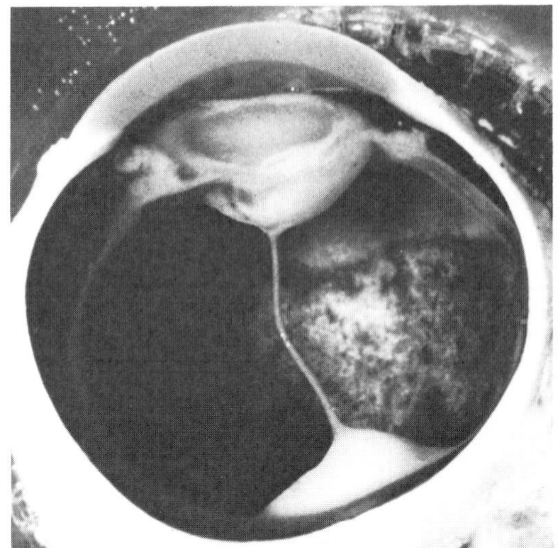

Figure 7–18. Coexistent anterior and posterior hyperplastic primary vitreous. Gross photograph of microphthalmic eye showing retrolental plaque and centrally displaced ciliary processes, persistent hyaloid vessel, and posterior plaque. (Courtesy of Dr. H. Ben-Moshe.)

the retina and lead to a number of pathologic changes in the retina, such as pits, tears, hemorrhages, folds, cystoid degeneration, and preretinal membrane formation. These are discussed in detail in Chapter 8.

Asteroid Hyalosis
(Asteroid Hyalitis)

Asteroid hyalosis is an innocuous degenerative process occurring in vitreous that appears otherwise normal. The condition is characterized clinically by the presence of large numbers of minute spherical or disc-shaped opacities suspended throughout the vitreous. There is little or no evidence of liquefaction of the vitreous immediately surrounding these particles, and they do not appear to aggregate as a result of gravity. When viewed with the slit lamp or the ophthalmoscope, they have a glistening, polychromatic appearance (Fig. 7–19). When the opacities are concentrated in the central vitreous, they may interfere with observation of fundus detail. It is surprising that they are usually asymptomatic, although some patients complain of an intermittent "film" obscuring their vision. This seems to occur in eyes in which the opacities are centralized in the visual axis, or following intracapsular cataract extraction with anterior displacement of the vitreous into the pupil.

Asteroid hyalosis is unilateral in over 75 per cent of the patients and is usually found in the eyes of patients over 60 years of age. It occurs in all races and with equal frequency in both sexes (Luxenberg, Sime, 1969). In earlier editions of this text, the condition was stated to be rare; however, all ophthalmologists encounter asteroid hyalosis in their practices, and it is likely a relatively common condition. The etiology is unknown. At present there is no good evidence that asteroid hyalosis is related to any systemic disease process, although it has been speculated that it occurs more frequently in patients with hypercholesterolemia and with diabetes mellitus (Smith, 1958). Other studies (Hatfield, Gastineau, Rucker, 1962; Luxenberg, Sime, 1969), however, have disclosed no differences in incidence of asteroid hyalosis in patients with and without diabetes.

The histologic features of asteroid hyalosis were described in 1921 by Verhoeff, who suggested that the opacities consist chiefly of calcium soap. They are roughly spherical, are 0.01

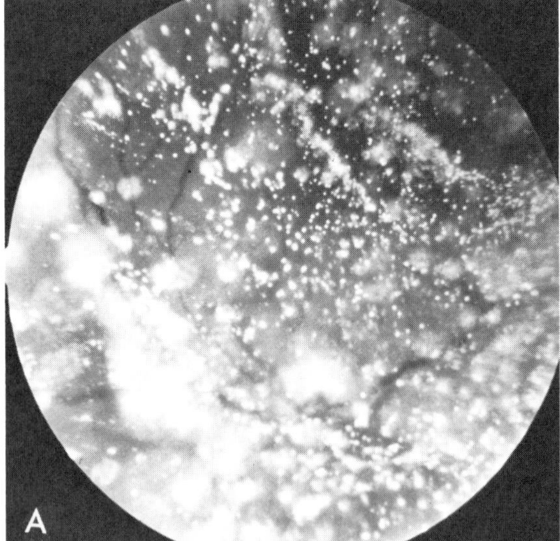

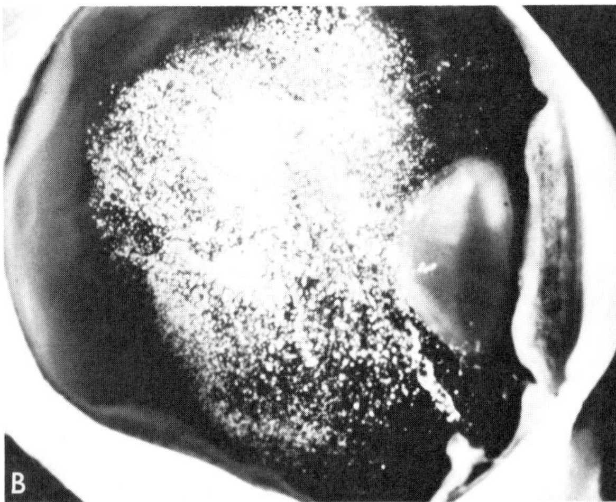

Figure 7–19. Asteroid hyalosis. *A,* Clinical appearance. Details of the retina are obscured by glistening spherical vitreous opacities. *B,* Gross appearance. The opacities are limited to the vitreous, and in this case they are predominantly axial in distribution. Vitreous has separated from retina posteriorly.

to 0.1 mm in diameter, and appear weakly basophilic with hematoxylin-eosin stains. They are stained by lipid stains (oil red O, Sudan black B, Scharlach R, Nile blue sulfate); however, they resist the usual fat solvents. They stain intensely with stains for acid mucopolysaccharide (alcian blue, colloidal iron), and this stain reaction is not affected by hyaluronidase (Fig. 7–20). Rodman, Johnson, and Zimmerman (1961) showed that these bodies stain metachromatically. This finding, plus the presence of sudanophilia and the results of additional studies ruling out the presence of protein components, nucleic acids, and sulfated mucopolysaccharides, lends support to Verhoeff's suggestion that the bodies consist of a calcium-containing lipid. Histochemical analysis (March, Shoch, O'Grady, 1974) and x-ray absorption studies have confirmed the presence of calcium and of phosphorus (Topilow, Kenyon, Takahashi, et al, 1983; Miller, Miller, Rabinowitz, et al, 1983) (Fig. 7–21). Under polarized light, the asteroid bodies appear to be composed of fine, birefringent spicules embedded in a matrix of nonbirefringent material that is intimately associated with vitreous fibrils. This finding suggests that the asteroid bodies may arise from vitreous fibril degeneration (Rodman, Johnson, Zimmerman, 1961). The relationship between the asteroid bodies and the surrounding vitreous fibrils is readily seen in scanning electron micrographs (Fig. 7–21). The asteroid bodies have been observed to have a lamellar arrangement with a periodicity of 4.6 nm. The configuration is considered to be characteristic of liquid crystalline

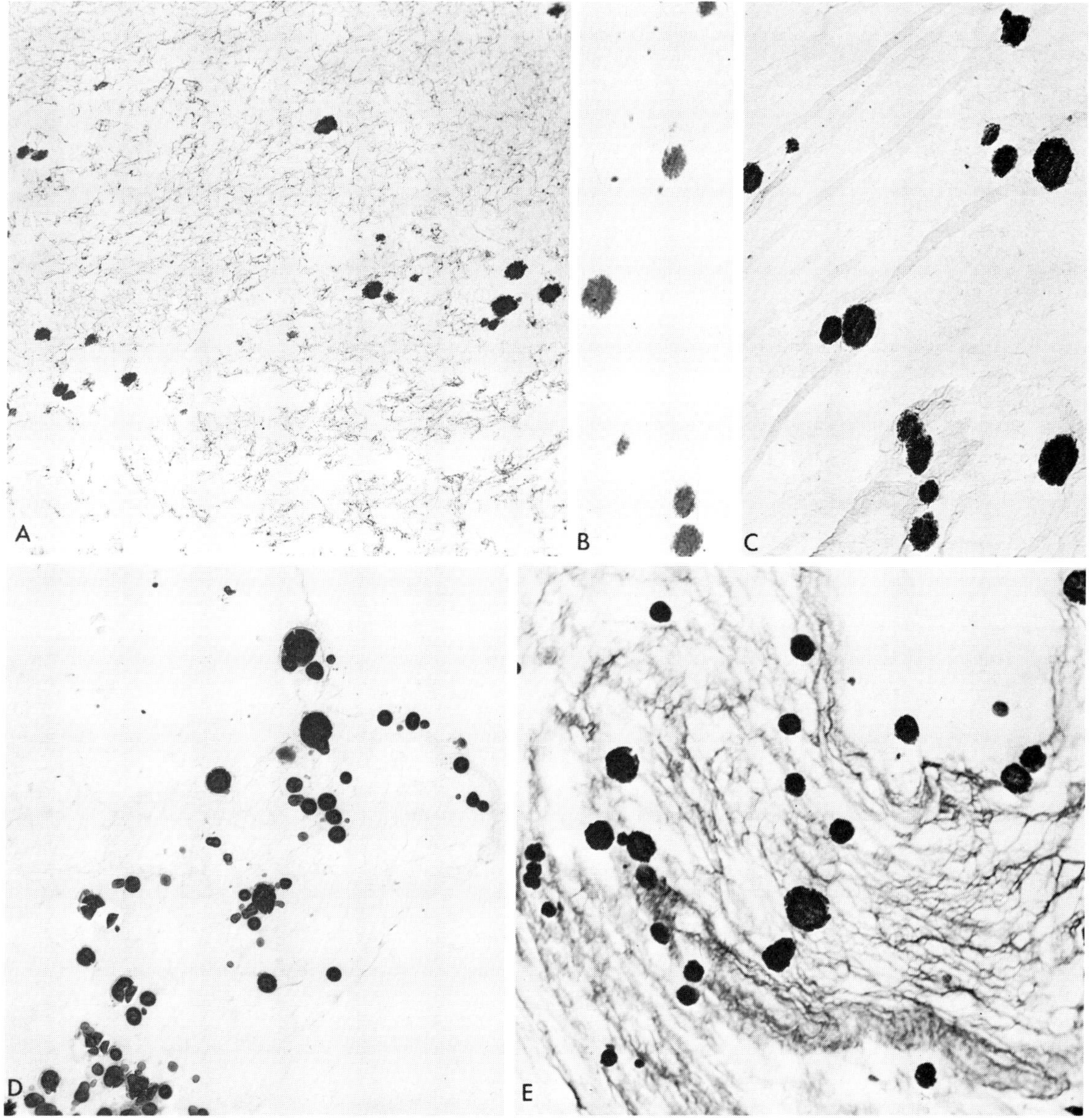

Figure 7–20. Asteroid hyalosis. *A,* H and E, ×80. AFIP Acc. 906582. *B,* Oil red O, ×160. AFIP Acc. 330261. *C,* Sudan black B, ×160. AFIP Acc. 523342. *D,* Alizarin red after microincineration, ×105. AFIP 715044. *E,* Colloidal iron, ×95. AFIP Acc. 523342.

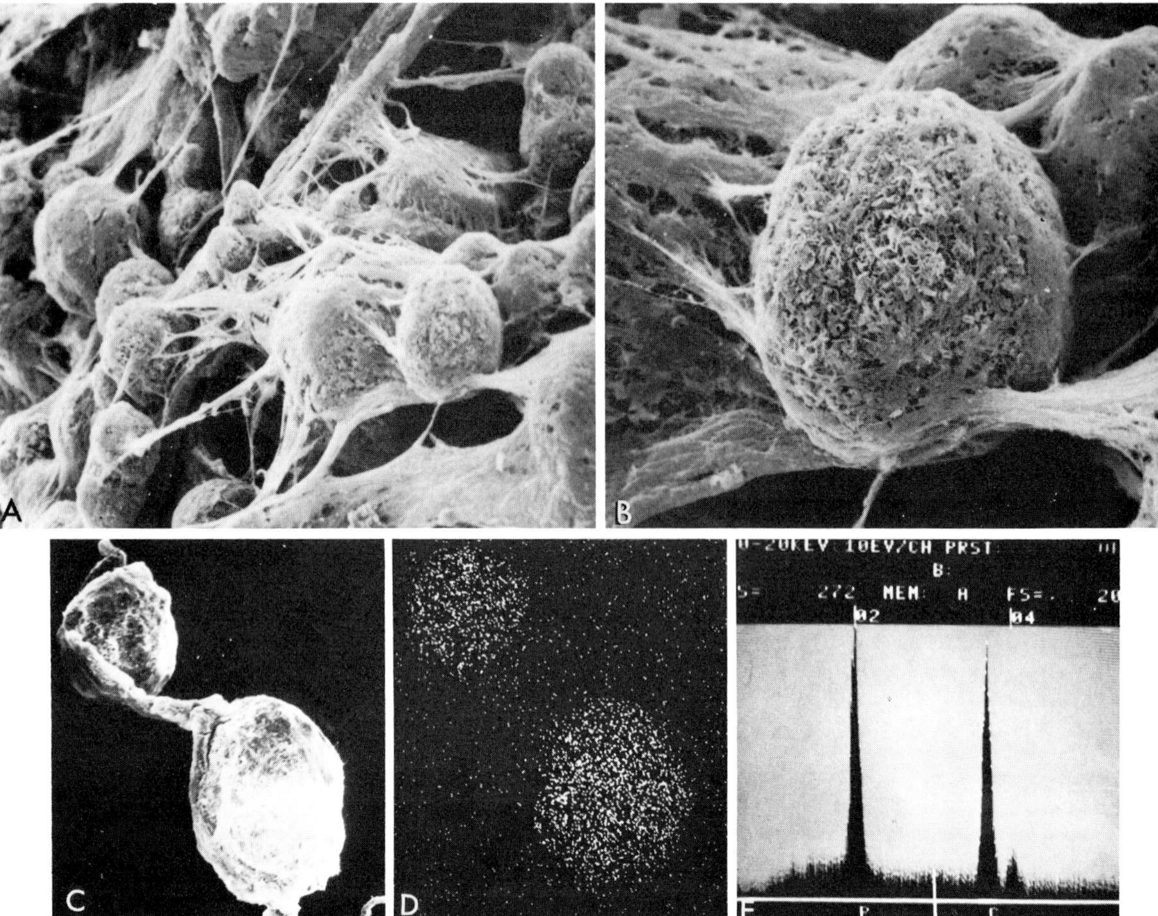

Figure 7–21. Asteroid hyalosis. *A,* Scanning electron microscopic appearance of asteroid bodies enmeshed within vitreous. ×500. *B,* Higher magnification showing pitted surface of asteroid body and adhesion to vitreous collagen strands. ×1450. *C,* Scanning electron micrograph of two asteroid bodies connected by a vitreous strand. ×500. *D,* Same asteroid bodies viewed by energy dispersive x-ray mapping denotes calcium concentrated within asteroid opacities. ×500. *E,* X-ray spectrograph of asteroid bodies demonstrates sharp peaks for phosphorus and calcium. (From Topilow HW, Kenyon KR, Takahashi M, et al: Asteroid hyalosis: Biomicroscopy, ultrastructure, and composition. Arch Ophthalmol, in press. Courtesy of Dr. K. R. Kenyon.)

phases of lipids in water, and it has been proposed that asteroid bodies are phospholipid liquid crystals in an intermediate state between true crystals and a true liquid (Miller, Miller, Rabinowitz, et al, 1983).

In recent years, the term *asteroid hyalosis* has supplanted the older term *asteroid hyalitis* because the bodies do not ordinarily stimulate an inflammatory cellular response; however, occasionally a foreign body type of giant cell reaction does occur (Rodman, Johnson, Zimmerman, 1961) (Fig. 7–22). Transmission electron microscopy has shown intracytoplasmic complex lipid inclusions within these cells (Topilow, Kenyon, Takahashi, et al, in press).

Cholesterosis Bulbi
(Synchysis Scintillans)

Incomplete resolution of extensive vitreous hemorrhage occasionally results in syneresis and the accumulation of highly refractile cholesterol crystals (Andrews, Lynn, Scobey, Elliott, 1973) (Fig. 7–23). In contrast to the particles in asteroid hyalosis, the cholesterol crystals are freely moveable and settle to the bottom of the vitreous chamber when the eye is at rest. They vary in size and number and appear somewhat larger than the glittering particles seen in asteroid hyalosis. This condition frequently appears in eyes with poor vision as a result of pathologic processes leading to hemorrhage (e.g., trauma). In aphakic eyes or in those with dislocated lenses, cholesterol and surrounding hemorrhagic debris may become displaced into the anterior chamber (Wand, Gorn, 1974; Gruber, 1955) (Fig. 7–23).

In routine paraffin-embedded sections of vitreous, the locations of the cholesterol crystals appear as slitlike spaces devoid of content because the cholesterol esters dissolve in processing (Fig. 7–23). In frozen sections, the cholesterol esters are retained, and the birefringent nature of the

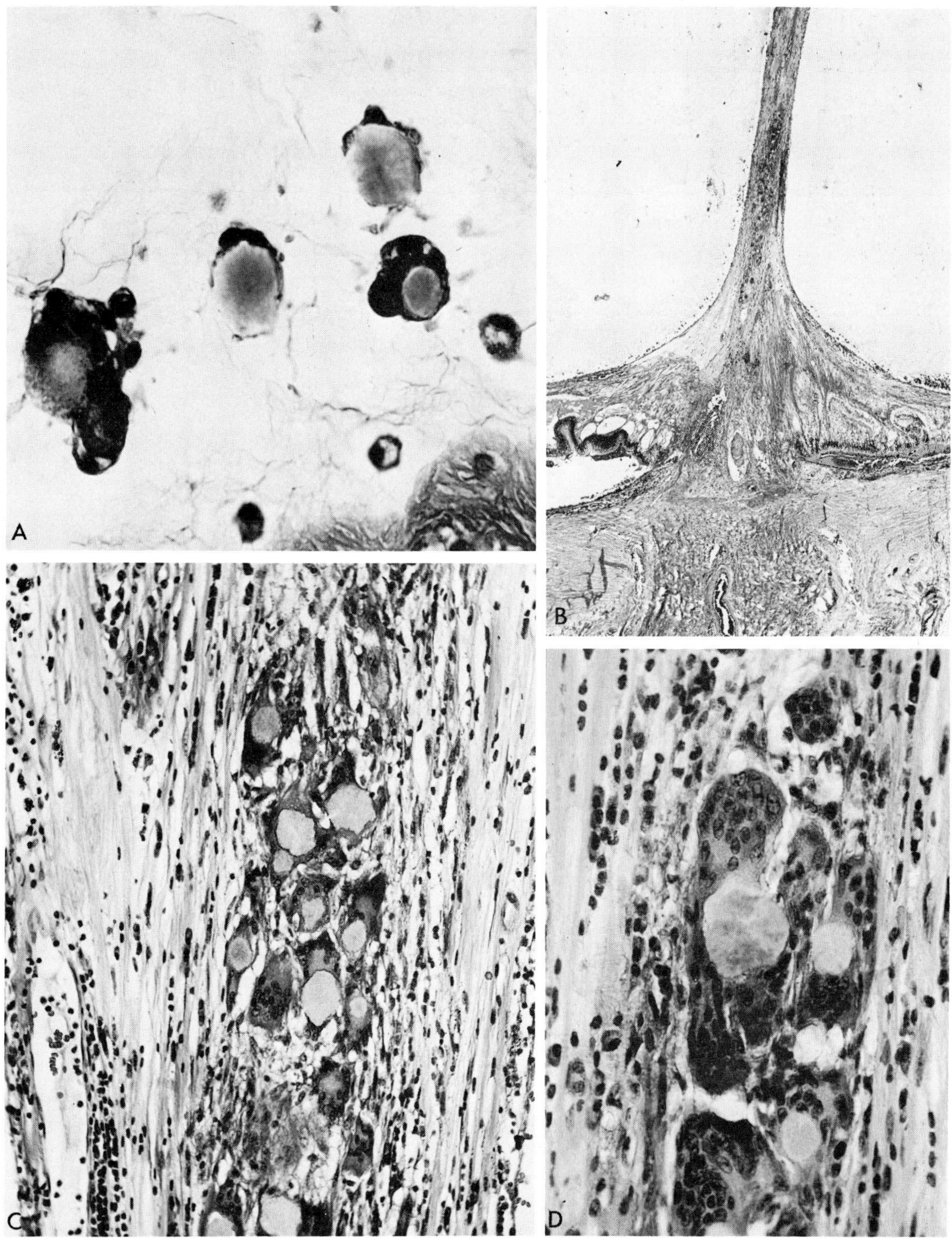

Figure 7–22. Asteroid hyalosis with giant cell reaction. *A,* The vitreous opacities are surrounded by foreign body giant cells. H and E, ×530. AFIP Acc. 269271. *B,* Projecting from the optic disc is a mass of shrunken vitreous containing asteroid bodies. H and E, ×14. AFIP Acc. 955663. *C and D,* The asteroid bodies have provoked a foreign body giant cell reaction. H and E, ×180 and 305, respectively.

crystals can be observed with polarized light (Fig. 7–23). The vitreous surrounding the crystals degenerates and liquefies, with displacement of collagen to remote portions of the vitreous. The latter may stain somewhat more strongly than usual with eosin because of the presence of protein derived either from the hemorrhage or from leakage of protein into the vitreous from the retina. The crystals may elicit a low-grade inflammatory response characterized primarily by foreign body giant cells (Fig. 7–23). Breakdown products of persistent or recurrent hemorrhage

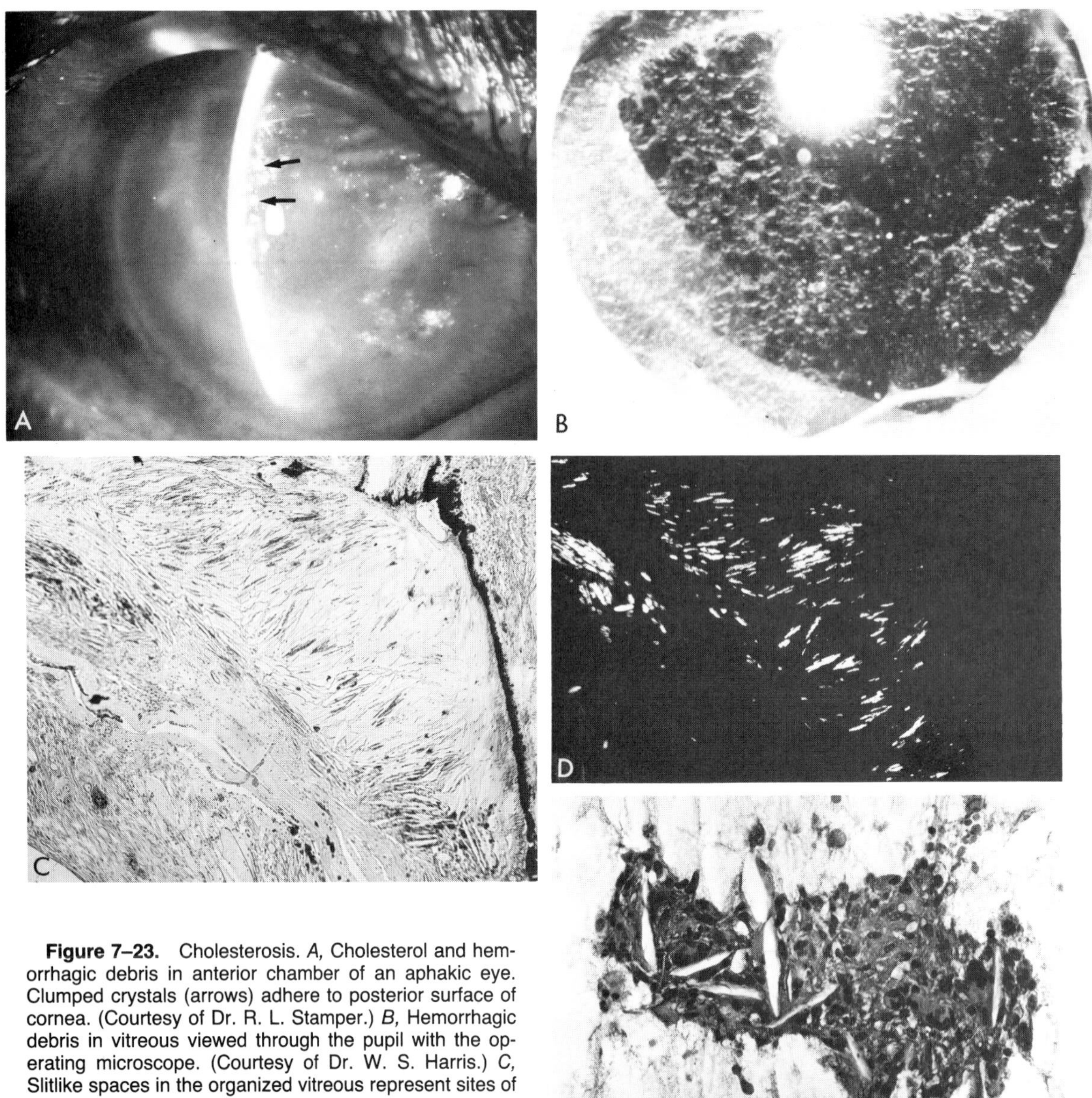

Figure 7–23. Cholesterosis. *A,* Cholesterol and hemorrhagic debris in anterior chamber of an aphakic eye. Clumped crystals (arrows) adhere to posterior surface of cornea. (Courtesy of Dr. R. L. Stamper.) *B,* Hemorrhagic debris in vitreous viewed through the pupil with the operating microscope. (Courtesy of Dr. W. S. Harris.) *C,* Slitlike spaces in the organized vitreous represent sites of cholesterol ester crystal deposition. H and E, ×50. AFIP Acc. 929200. *D,* The cholesterol ester crystals are birefringent when viewed with polarized light. Frozen section, ×50. AFIP Acc. 929200. *E,* Inflammatory response elicited by cholesterol ester crystals in the vitreous. Histiocytes and giant cells partially surround slitlike spaces. H and E, ×250.

also may undergo organization and contraction in conjunction with proliferation of fibrovascular tissue arising from the retina. Further breakdown of the hemoglobin may result in hemosiderosis (see Chapter 8, Retina, page 795).

Focal Protein and Collagen Condensations
(Floaters)

When liquefaction of the vitreous occurs because of insidious processes such as aging or myopia, focal condensation or coagulation of the remaining vitreous produces opacities visible to the examiner and also (entoptically) to the patient. Similar opacification may be produced by detachment of the vitreous, particularly by the condensation ring surrounding the optic nerve head.

Plasma proteins may enter the vitreous as a result of inflammation of retinal, optic nerve head, or ciliary body vessels. This process can cause either localized or diffuse turbidity and opacification of the vitreous, and it is often accompanied by vitreous condensation and shrinkage (see section on vitreous inflammation, page 574).

Hereditary Vitreoretinal Degenerations
(Hyaloideoretinopathies)

Because of the intimate relationship between the vitreous and retina, it is often impossible to determine which structure is responsible for pathologic processes occurring at their junction. Those that are transmitted genetically are known as the hyaloideoretinopathies and are considered in this section. Additional discussion may be found in Chapter 8 on the retina.

Lattice Degeneration, Radial Perivascular Lattice Degeneration, and Snail Track Degeneration. The term *lattice degeneration of the retina* was introduced by Schepens in 1952. The hereditary nature of this disorder is not clearly understood. Several pedigrees of families with lattice degeneration have been published (Everett, 1968; Lewkonia, Davies, Salmon, 1973); however, these studies do not pertain to lattice degeneration alone but rather to the condition as it occurs in association with retinal detachment and other intraocular diseases. Byer (1965) found an incidence of 7.1 per cent in a clinical study of 1300 consecutive patients, and Straatsma and Allen (1962) found lattice degeneration in 6 per cent of autopsy eyes. In an extensive clinical and pathologic study of a large number of eyes, Straatsma and coworkers found lattice degeneration to be least common in the first decade, most common in the second decade, and distributed rather evenly throughout subsequent decades. This study found bilateral involvement in 48.1 per cent of eyes with a striking symmetry in the location and appearance of lesions in bilateral cases. There appears to be no sex predilection. Lattice degeneration seems to occur more frequently in myopic eyes (Straatsma, Zeegan,

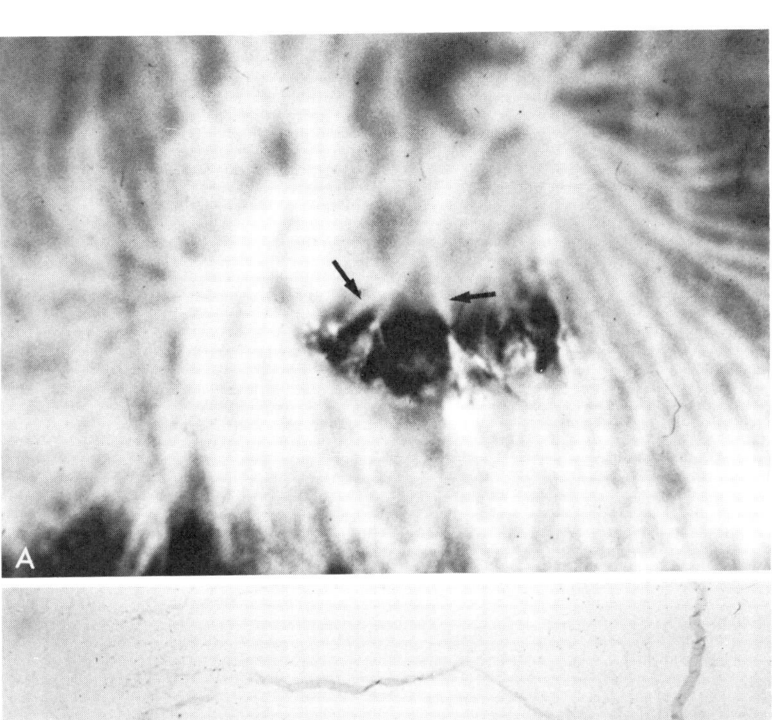

Figure 7–24. Lattice degeneration. *A,* Gross appearance of typical lesions lying parallel to the ora serrata. The retina is focally thinned and the subjacent retinal pigment epithelium appears irregular and mottled. Lattice-like white lines (arrows) represent fibrosed or occluded retinal vessels.

B, Microscopic appearance. The retina is focally thinned, with partial loss of cellular elements. Note thick-walled vessel (arrow) and retinal pigment epithelial irregularity *(R)*. The retinal separation *(S)* is artifactitious. The vitreous immediately overlying the lesion is liquefied *(LV)* and separated from the retina. It appears condensed and firmly adherent to the retina at the margins of the lesion. PAS, ×40.

Foos, et al, 1974); however, Byer's study suggests that refractive error is not a contributing factor.

The average number of lesions per eye is 2 to 2.4. They are usually oval and average slightly over 2 mm in length and 0.5 mm in width. Most are situated in the pre-equatorial region and are circumferential (parallel to the ora serrata) in orientation (Fig. 7–24). In Byer's study, the lower temporal quadrant was most commonly involved, and most lesions were distributed within 1 clock hour of the vertical meridian, both superiorly and inferiorly. The lesions are nonprogressive or very slowly progressive throughout life, and only a small number lead to retinal detachment, usually associated with posterior vitreous detachment. Detachment occasionally follows the gradual development of an atrophic retinal hole within a zone of lattice degeneration.

Histologically, there is a discrete area of retinal thinning associated with liquefaction and separation of the overlying vitreous (Fig. 7–24). The vitreous appears condensed at the border of the liquefied area, with exaggerated vitreoretinal attachments along the margins of the degenerated area. Most lattice lesions are associated with abnormalities of the retinal pigment epithelium. All studies have remarked on a decreased number of retinal capillaries associated with fibrotic degeneration of larger vessels in the region. This is readily seen in trypsin-digested flat retinal preparations (Streeten, Bert, 1972). The lumina of larger vessels often show obliterative fibrosis, and the adjacent retina thins as a consequence of cell loss and fibrosis. This is frequently associated with disruption of the inner limiting membrane.

Within the area of retinal thinning, the fibrosed or occluded retinal vessels are visible clinically as a series of white lines. Punched-out holes or focal hemorrhages may occur where thinning is severe. Straatsma and coworkers postulate that ischemia initiates the process, followed by focal vitreous liquefaction and detachment and condensation of vitreous at the margins of the lesion. At the same time, the ischemic portion of retina undergoes thinning and scarring; this, in turn, stimulates retinal pigment epithelial changes characterized by depigmentation and clumping of pigment.

Retinal circulatory disturbance may be the primary cause of the process (Straatsma, Zeegan, Foos, et al, 1974). In one study (Sato, Tsunakawa, Inaba, Yangisawa, 1971), fluorescein angiography of vessels surrounding areas of lattice degeneration showed extravasation of dye in 61 per cent, delayed filling in 54 per cent, arteriovenous shunts in 33 per cent, capillary dilation in 33 per cent, and formation of microaneurysms in 16 per cent of cases.

Radial perivascular lattice degeneration of the retina is identical histopathologically to typical lattice degeneration (Parelhoff, Wood, Green, et al, 1980). It is associated with cataracts, myopia, glaucoma, and retinal detachment and seems to be inherited as a dominant trait (Hagler, Crosswell, 1968).

Snail track degeneration of the retina is a crinkled or frostlike change of the inner retinal surface reminiscent of the tracks made by a snail (Gonin, 1904). The condition may be related to lattice degeneration, although the typical lesions of lattice degeneration are not usually seen. Aaberg and Stevens (1972) studied four families with this condition. It affected both sexes and appeared to be inherited either as a recessive trait or as a dominant trait with limited penetrance. The median age was 18 years. Of 21 eyes studied, 19 were myopic and 10 developed retinal detachment. Unlike lattice degeneration, the white line appearance of vessels was not seen, and generally there was no pigmentation within or surrounding the lesions. No histopathologic studies of this entity are available.

Snowflake Degeneration. Hirose, Lee, and Schepens (1974) described 15 members of three successive generations of one family with a peculiar type of vitreoretinal degenerative process that appears to have an autosomal dominant inheritance pattern. All patients over 32 years of age had cataract. Impaired vision also was attributed to myopia and to retinal detachment (five eyes). Retinal breaks and holes were noted only in eyes with detachment.

Bilateral fundus changes occurred in four stages. In stage 1, which was characteristic of patients less than 15 years of age, minute, yellow-white spots were seen in areas that were "white with pressure" (an asymptomatic grayish translucency of the peripheral fundus, possibly related to vitreous traction, visible with the indirect ophthalmoscope in the portion of the retina indented by scleral depression). In stage 2, the "white with pressure" areas showed minute, snowflake–like yellow-white spots, some of them brilliant as if crystalline, located in the superficial layers of the retina and extending as far anteriorly as the ora serrata. Stage 3 was characterized by sheathing of peripheral retinal vessels and irregular pigmentation around the equator near the posterior margin of snowflake degeneration. Stage 4, which occurred in patients over age 58, was characterized by increased pigmentation as well as disappearance of retinal vessels. The snowflakes were less apparent, and there were areas of chorioretinal atrophy. Most of the patients in this series showed vitreous abnormalities; the younger individuals had fine, swirling vitreous strands and liquefaction of the gel.

Robertson, Link, and Rostvold (1982) studied

ten asymptomatic patients (age range, 9 to 70 years) in four families with dominantly inherited white or yellow-white granular deposits (100 to 200 microns in size) of the equatorial retina. These were believed to be consistent with the deposits seen in the published figures of Stage 2 snowflake degeneration in the family reported by Hirose, Lee, and Schepens in 1974. Robertson and coworkers did not observe progression of the deposits nor did they note patchy pigmentation of the peripheral retina, vessel sheathing, retinal breaks, vitreous liquefaction, or vitreous strand formation. Some of the eyes described in this report had no evidence of coexisting lattice degeneration ("pure snowflake degeneration"), while others showed areas of potentially troublesome lattice degeneration. No histopathologic studies of this condition have been reported.

Wagner's Disease. In 1938, Wagner described a large family that had changes in the vitreous and the subjacent retina. All patients were mildly to moderately myopic (4 diopters or less). The vitreous space was optically empty except for a few strands or threads. Preretinal avascular membranes were noted in the equatorial region, even in first-decade patients. The membranes appeared whitish-gray and occasionally were perforated. The peripheral retina showed progressive perivascular pigment accumulations of pigment epithelial origin that were less well delineated than those of retinitis pigmentosa. Patchy areas of peripheral retinal vessel sheathing and posterior choroidal atrophy were found. The macula appeared normal, and most young patients had normal corrected visual acuity. In the 22 to 40 year age group, the visual acuity was reduced, owing to lens changes characterized by dotlike opacities in the anterior and posterior lens cortex. After age 40 years, the cataracts were sufficiently dense to require surgery. Dislocated lenses were reported in two patients. Other studies of the same family (Bohringer, Dieterle, Landolt, 1960; Ricci, 1961; Maumenee, Stoll, Mets, 1982) have confirmed Wagner's observations and also have detected a moderate reduction of the electroretinogram with abnormal night vision. Dark adaptation rates and final thresholds have shown a slowly progressive decline, initially involving rods and later cones. The electroretinogram at this late stage shows greatly reduced responses. Maumenee, Stoll, and Mets (1982) noted that advanced cases of Wagner's disease are difficult to differentiate from those seen in typical retinitis pigmentosa; however, the vitreous changes are more severe. None of the members of Wagner's original family (now followed for five generations) developed retinal detachment, and no systemic anomalies were reported (Maumenee, Stoll, Mets, 1982). Bohringer, Dieterle, and Landolt (1960) concluded that the degeneration results from a developmental defect of the secondary vitreous. The disease is transmitted as an autosomal dominant trait with 100 per cent penetrance.

Since the original reports, additional families believed to have Wagner's disease have been studied. Alexander and Shea (1965) reported a 50 per cent rate of retinal detachment, but it is likely that these researchers and others (Frandsen, 1968; Hirose, Lee, Schepens, 1973) were studying families with variants of Stickler's syndrome (described later).

Histopathologic studies have been performed on only a few eyes (Bohringer, Dieterle, Landolt, 1960; Manschot, 1971; Maumenee, Stoll, Mets, 1982). Most of the vitreous is liquefied, with only a thin membrane covering the inner aspect of the retina from the equator to the posterior pole. The subjacent retina exhibits thinning, with photoreceptor degeneration and cystoid changes peripheral to the equator. Clusters of pigment occur in a perivascular distribution, and there is atrophy of the choriocapillaris, especially in areas of chorioretinal adhesions.

Hereditary Arthro-Ophthalmopathy (Stickler's Syndrome). In 1965, Stickler, Belau, Farrell, and associates described a five-generation family with ocular, orofacial, and general skeletal (epiphyseal dysplastic) abnormalities inherited in an autosomal dominant fashion, with variable expressivity and almost complete penetrance. The ocular manifestations consist of high myopia (8 to 18 diopters) and, in over 50 per cent of affected individuals, retinal detachment believed to be related to vitreoretinal degeneration. Other ocular findings include cataract, glaucoma, amblyopia, and strabismus. Additional families with varying degrees of ocular and skeletal abnormalities have since been designated as having different forms of the Stickler syndrome. Herrmann, France, Spranger, and coworkers (1975) reviewed 64 affected patients from 6 families and found myopia (usually greater than 10 diopters) in 46 (72 per cent).

The most common orofacial abnormalities of Stickler's syndrome are those of the Pierre Robin syndrome (mandibular hypoplasia, glossoptosis, and U-shaped palatoschisis) (Schreiner, McAlister, Marshall, Shearer, 1973; Turner, 1974; Blair, Albert, Liberfarb, Hirose, 1979; Van Balen, Falger, 1970). Approximately 50 per cent of children with the Pierre Robin anomaly in fact have Stickler syndrome (Herrmann, France, Spranger, et al, 1975). Knobloch (1975) described five families with vitreoretinopathy and mild to moderately severe spondyloepiphyseal dysplasia characterized by hyperextendable joints (knees, wrists, fingers), hypotonia and relative muscular hypoplasia. Maumenee (1979) has been able to identify six distinct single gene-inherited dysplastic disorders of bone associated with vitreoretinal degeneration: all appear to have an autosomal dominant inheritance pattern.

The subgroup originally described by Stickler and coworkers has a marfanoid habitus, whereas other subgroups have short stature and identifying radiographic characteristics, such as epiphyseal flattening, broad metaphyses, and spondyloepiphyseal dysplasia. The severity of the ocular manifestations also seems to vary with the subgroup and in families within each subgroup. Maumenee (1979) has observed that Type II collagen is present in both secondary vitreous and in cartilage. She has suggested that separate mutations involving Type II collagen chains (which are long and have multiple sites at which mutations can occur) may account for each of the subgroups within the arthro-ophthalmopathies. Her studies and those of her coworkers (Maumenee, Stoll, Mets, 1982) have greatly aided in differentiating the arthro-ophthalmopathies (which are frequently associated with retinal detachment) from Wagner's disease (which is not associated with skeletal disease nor retinal detachment).

The histologic findings in the eyes of patients with hereditary ophthalmopathy have not yet been reported.

Vitreoretinal Dystrophy of Goldmann-Favre (Favre's Microfibrillar Vitreoretinal Degeneration). Goldmann (1957) studied a brother and sister with peripheral retinoschisis, chorioretinal atrophy, and extensive vitreous abnormalities. The macula had a microcystoid appearance associated with a delicate membrane that appeared to be detached from the retina. The condition was progressive, with decreasing visual acuity and expanding retinoschisis. Both patients later developed cataracts.

François and coworkers reviewed this syndrome in 1974. The vitreous shows syneresis, fibrillar degeneration, punctate deposits, and whitish strands. The fundus exhibits pigmentary changes similar to those seen in retinitis pigmentosa, except that the characteristic bone spicule type of pigmentation is not always present. The vessels appear attenuated and the discs, waxy and pale. The peripheral retina and macula have a coarse microcystic pattern, and sometimes there are large holes in the inner leaf of the retina in the temporal periphery. Visual acuity is usually decreased at an earlier age than in typical retinitis pigmentosa, although retinal function studies are very similar in the two conditions. Fluorescein angiography (Fishman, Jampol, Goldberg, 1976) shows pronounced leakage of dye from several vessels, while others in the retinal periphery appear opaque. The areas of schisis occur where vessel opacity, leakage, and nonperfusion are found. Cystoid macular edema appears to be a major cause of decreased central acuity.

Peyman, Fishman, Sanders, and Vichek (1977) obtained a 4 mm biopsy specimen of the superior temporal peripheral sclera, choroid, and retina from one eye of a 27 year old woman with longstanding night blindness, slowly progressive decreased central visual acuity, high hypermetropia, early posterior subcapsular cataracts, areas of vitreous liquefaction and condensation, atypical pigmentary retinopathy, midperipheral sclerotic vessels, pre-equatorial retinoschisis, and a nondetectable electroretinogram. Despite a negative family history of night blindness, the patient was diagnosed as having Goldmann-Favre disease. Histopathologically, there was attenuation of the outer nuclear layer of the retina and absence of photoreceptor outer segments adjacent to normal-appearing pigment epithelium and choriocapillaris, suggesting a "primary degeneration of the sensory retina." The inner retina contained vessels with a thickened basement membrane, stated to correlate with the clinical appearance of vascular "sclerosis." Electron microscopy showed a preretinal glial and fibrous membrane without evidence of retinoschisis, although the area biopsied appeared to be schitic clinically.

Hereditary Vitreoretinal Degeneration and Night Blindness. Feiler-Ofry, Adam, Regenbogen, et al (1969) studied two affected generations of a nonmyopic consanguineous family with early-onset night blindness, vitreous degeneration (syneresis and posterior detachment), retinal holes without detachment, lattice degeneration, and electroretinographic abnormalities. The mode of inheritance could not be established. No histopathologic studies have been reported.

Familial Exudative Vitreoretinopathy. Criswick and Schepens (1969) described six members of two families with bilateral, slowly progressive abnormalities of the retina and vitreous that simulated retrolental fibroplasia, although there was no history of prematurity or oxygen administration during the neonatal period. Gow and Oliver (1971) identified an autosomal dominant inheritance pattern with almost complete penetrance of the abnormal gene. They divided the disease into three stages: stage 1 is characterized by peripheral retinal degeneration, posterior vitreous detachment, and snowflake vitreous opacities. Stage 2 shows peripheral retinal neovascularization, elevation of a fibrovascular mass in the temporal periphery, dragging of the disk and macula, and localized retinal detachment. In stage 3, there is total retinal detachment. In some eyes these changes are followed by anterior segment disease, including iris atrophy, cataract, angle closure, band keratopathy, and eventual blindness. Fluorescein angiography (Canny, Oliver, 1976) shows closure of peripheral retinal vessels temporally, which resembles the findings seen in retrolental fibroplasia.

Additional studies (Slusher, Hutton, 1979; Nijhuis, Deutman, Aan de Kerk, 1979; Ober, Bird, Hamilton, 1980; Schulman, Jampol, Schwartz, 1980; Gasman, Russburger, Shields, et al, 1981; Brockhurst, Albert, Zakov, 1981; Miyakubo, Inohara, Hashimoto, 1982; Van Nouhuys, 1982; Bergen, Glassman, 1983) have confirmed these observations and have identified mild, nonprogressive forms of the disease. Seven of the twelve patients studied by Ober, Bird, and Hamilton had no ocular symptoms and were only mildly affected by the disease. All seven had nonperfusion of pre-equatorial retinal vessels. These investigators concluded that there is great variability in the phenotypic expression of the abnormal gene, so that many patients may have mild disease that is detectable only by fluorescein angiography. In their study, progression of fundus changes was rare after age 20 years.

The pathogenesis of familial exudative vitreoretinopathy is unknown; however, the sharply demarcated zone of peripheral retinal blood vessel closure and the pattern of arteriovenous anastomoses suggest that the disease is of retinal rather than vitreous origin. The similarity of these findings to those seen in retrolental fibroplasia also suggests that affected individuals have a hematologic abnormality (perhaps associated with decreased oxygen-carrying capacity of their red blood cells); however, to date no such abnormality has been found. Histopathologic studies of eyes enucleated because of suspected retinoblastoma or secondary angle-closure glaucoma have shown a total retinal detachment and a folded vitreous membrane in close proximity to the inner surface of the retina that is composed of an amorphous acellular component and a fibroglial cellular component (Brockhurst, Albert, Zakov, 1981; Van Nouhuys, 1982; Gass, 1983; Egbert, 1983). Brockhurst and coworkers emphasize that the membrane forms posterior to the ora serrata, and, on the basis of clinical observations, they suggest that preretinal membrane formation precedes the development of retinal vessel abnormalities.

X-Linked Juvenile Retinoschisis. This vitreoretinal degenerative process also has been called congenital vascular veils (Mann, MacRae, 1938; Balian, Falls 1960), inherited retinal detachment (Juler, 1947; Levy, 1952), congenital hereditary retinoschisis (Tolentino, Schepens, Freeman, 1976), and juvenile sex-linked retinoschisis (Forsuis, Vainio-Mattilla, Eriksson, 1962; Harris, 1969). The disease occurs almost exclusively in young boys. Only one girl has been reported, and she was the daughter of an affected man and his second cousin (Sabates, 1966). The condition is usually bilateral, although visual acuity may be affected differently in each eye. The process may be present at or shortly after birth, but the diagnosis is rarely made before school age when visual problems are first noticed. Associated conditions, such as strabismus or nystagmus, occasionally trigger earlier examination and diagnosis.

The process is characterized by bilaterally symmetric splitting of the retina, often involving the macula and the inferior temporal quadrant of the peripheral retina. In approximately half the affected eyes, macular retinoschisis is the only finding. Peripheral retinoschisis may extend posteriorly into the macula. The visual loss is primarily related to the extent of foveal involvement. Ophthalmoscopically, the fovea has a microcystoid appearance, which has been likened to "beaten copper." The cystoid change may slowly progress to form a larger cyst or a macular hole. In the periphery, the split inner retina may resemble a veil waving in the vitreous as the eye moves. Vessels within this portion of the retina appear sheathed by connective tissue. The vitreous cortex adjacent to areas of retinoschisis appears condensed, while other areas liquefy and cavitate. Strands of condensed vitreous, sometimes mistaken for the inner layer of split retina, adhere to the split retina, and their movement may cause secondary tears, holes, and hemorrhage.

Histopathologically, the intraretinal splitting occurs in the nerve fiber layer rather than in the outer plexiform layer, as occurs in senile retinoschisis. Acid mucopolysaccharide, which is present in senile retinoschisis, is not found in X-linked juvenile retinoschisis (Yanoff, Rahn, Zimmerman, 1968; Manschot, 1972). Retinoschisis is nonprogressive in areas of the fundus with posterior vitreous detachment, but it is progressive if the vitreous is not detached, suggesting that retinal traction may be a pathogenetic factor (Tolentino, Schepens, Freeman, 1976, pages 255–286).

Systemic Primary Amyloidosis. Bilateral vitreous opacification can occur as an early manifestation of the dominantly inherited form of familial amyloidosis (Kaufman, 1958; Kaufman, Thomas, 1959; Wong, McFarlin, 1967; Crawford, 1967; Paton, Duke, 1966). Other clinical manifestations of this condition include upper and lower extremity polyneuropathy and central nervous system abnormalities. Amyloidosis involving the vitreous has rarely been observed in nonfamilial cases (Brownstein, Elliott, Helwig, 1970; Schwartz, Green, Michels, et al, 1982). The extracellular vitreous opacities initially appear to lie adjacent to retinal vessels posteriorly and then they develop anteriorly (Wong, McFarlin, 1967). At first they appear granular with wispy fringes, but as they enlarge and aggregate the vitreous takes on a "glass wool" appearance. When the posterior vitreous detaches, the opacities may be displaced into the visual axis, causing reduction in visual acuity accompanied by photophobia. Removal of the opacified vitreous is the accepted method of treating this condition. Recurrent opacities may later develop in residual vitreous (Irvine, Char, 1976). Histologic examination of removed vitreous has shown material with a fibrillar appearance and staining reaction characteristic of amyloid (Kaufman, 1958; Paton, Duke, 1966; Kasner, Miller, Taylor et al, 1968). Electron microscopic studies are confirmatory (Hitchings, Tripathi, 1976). Immunocytochemical studies have shown the major amyloid constituent to be protein resembling prealbumin (Doft, Rubinow, Cohen, 1984).

Retinitis Pigmentosa

Although the site of primary pathology in retinitis pigmentosa is the junction between the percipient elements and the retinal pigment epithelium, the peripheral portions of the vitreous frequently contain, "cells," which cause no symptoms. They have a gray or gray-brown ophthalmoscopic appearance, thus sometimes are termed "tobacco flecks" (Tolentino, Schepens, Freeman, 1976). Their origin and composition are not fully understood. Possibly they are acellular. Possibly they represent retinal pigment epithelial granules that have migrated through the degenerating retina into the vitreous. They vary somewhat in size and configuration. The larger particles may be aggregated pigment granules or possibly macrophages that have engulfed pigment. The vitreous may have areas of syneresis and detachment, although this may not be specifically related to retinitis pigmentosa.

INFLAMMATION

General Pathologic Considerations

Inflammations of the vitreous are largely passive and are usually characterized by liquefaction, opacification, and shrinkage. Inflammatory cells, pigment granules, or pigment-bearing cells may enter following primary inflammation of contiguous structures or as a result of an intravitreous inflammatory stimulus, such as a foreign body. When the retina or ciliary body becomes inflamed, the blood-vitreous barrier, normally effective in regulating and limiting the entrance of serum proteins into the vitreous, breaks down. The resulting increase in the amount of vitreous protein alters the colloidal structure of the vitreous, resulting in condensation in some areas and liquefaction in others. In the liquefied areas there is an increase in the ability of substances to move through the vitreous.

When infectious organisms are introduced into the vitreous, they appear to grow in relatively unimpeded fashion. The avascularity and relative acellularity of the vitreous may account for its susceptibility to infection. The viscosity of the vitreous undoubtedly modifies the rapidity of the inflammatory response. The anterior hyaloid transiently may restrict extension of inflammation from vitreous into the aqueous. Abscess formation is common, and even organisms of low pathogenicity, such as nonhemolytic staphylococci, can grow rapidly.

Acute inflammatory exudates quickly become necrotic in the vitreous, and, when studied histopathologically, the polymorphonuclear leuko-

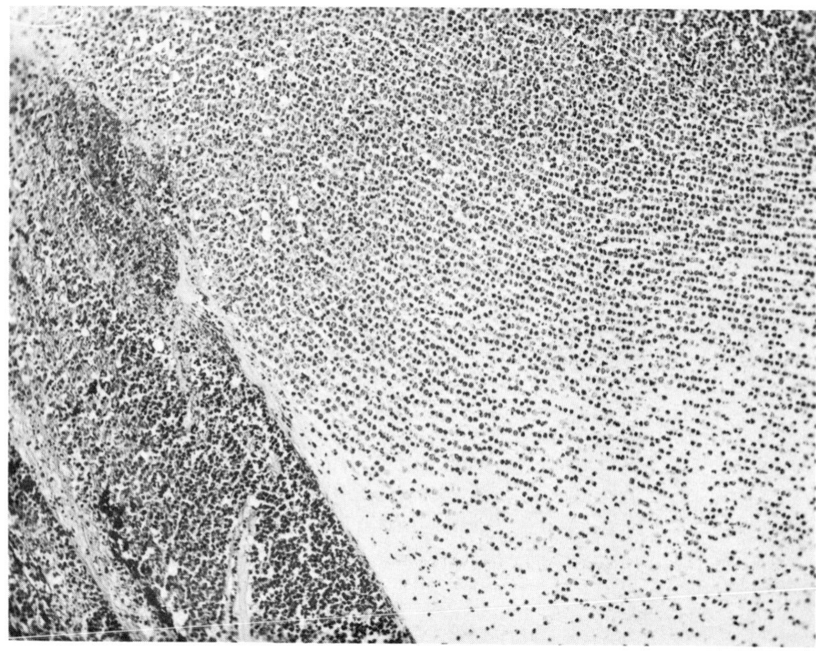

Figure 7–25. Purulent exudate in vitreous. The polymorphonuclear leukocytes appear in single file arrangement because their migratory activity is curbed by the vitreous collagen fibrils. H and E, ×115. AFIP Acc. 76528.

cytes are often degenerative. Inflammatory cells tend to aggregate along the course of the collagenous fibrils (Fig. 7–25), particularly adjacent to the retina and ciliary body where the vitreous is relatively dense. Abscesses may remain discrete, occasionally laying down an encapsulating wall of connective tissue, or they may become diffuse and invade the entire vitreous. In the early stages of an acute inflammatory process, most cells appear to be polymorphonuclear leukocytes. Large mononuclear phagocytes, lymphocytes, and plasma cells may appear later.

Following the acute phase of inflammation, varying degrees of capillary proliferation and connective tissue infiltration extend into the vitreous from adjacent structures. The volume of the vitreous is reduced by connective tissue contraction and loss of fluid. Traction of this tissue upon the retina and choroid often produces a detachment of these structures. A membrane derived from the ciliary body (cyclitic membrane) may form in the anterior portion of the vitreous and along its anterior surface. Contraction of this membrane frequently results in detachment of the ciliary body and anterior choroid. This is accompanied by hypotony, presumably due to secondary reduction in aqueous production, and eventually leads to phthisis. (For further discussion, see Vitreal Membranes, page 581.)

Causes

Vitreous inflammations may be grouped into those that are due to ocular causes and those that are part of a systemic disease. Each of these groups may further be subcategorized into infec-

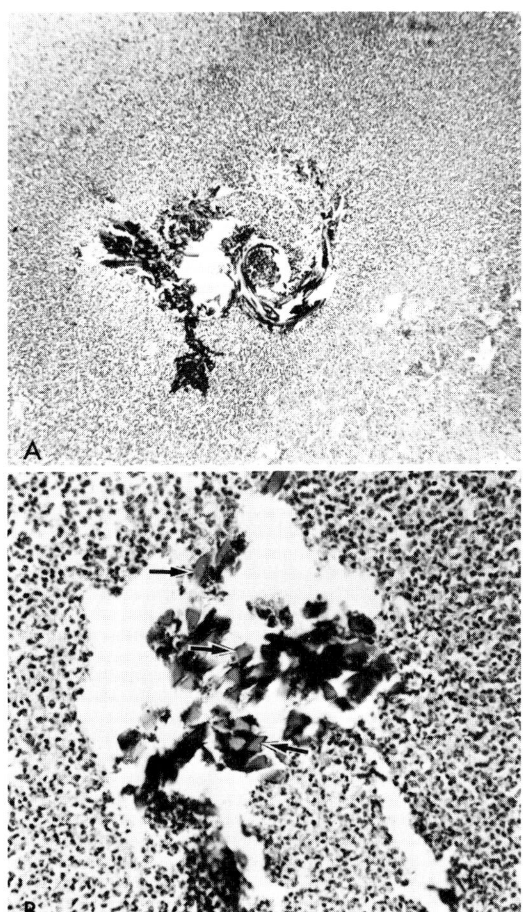

Figure 7–26. Exogenous bacterial infection of vitreous. *A,* An infected suture has eroded into the vitreous following surgery for repair of retinal detachment. Acute inflammatory cells surround the strands of suture material. H and E, ×175. *B,* Higher magnification showing suture (arrows) and surrounding inflammatory cells. H and E, ×250.

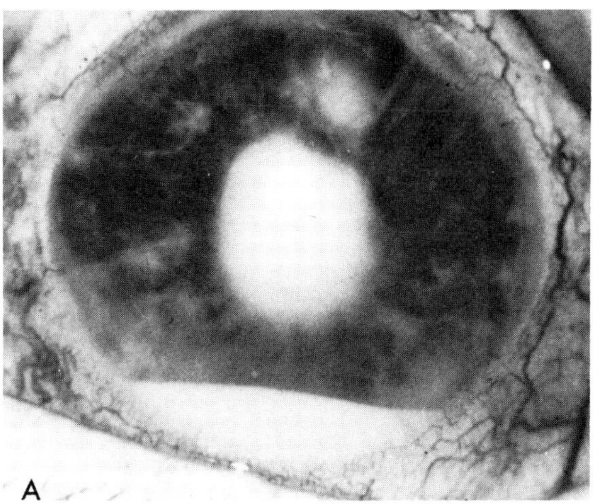

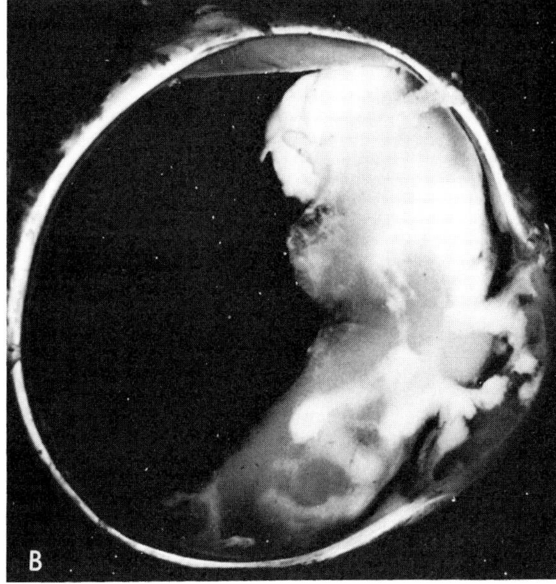

Figure 7–27. Mycotic infection following cataract extraction. *A,* Slit lamp appearance. Opaque milky white vitreous is visible through the pupil and the iridectomy. Hypopyon partially fills inferior portion of anterior chamber. Episclera is injected. *B,* Gross photograph of same eye after enucleation. Vitreous is detached posteriorly and is anteriorly displaced. Whitish opacities represent separate and confluent microabscesses, some of which have been artifactitiously displaced into the anterior chamber.

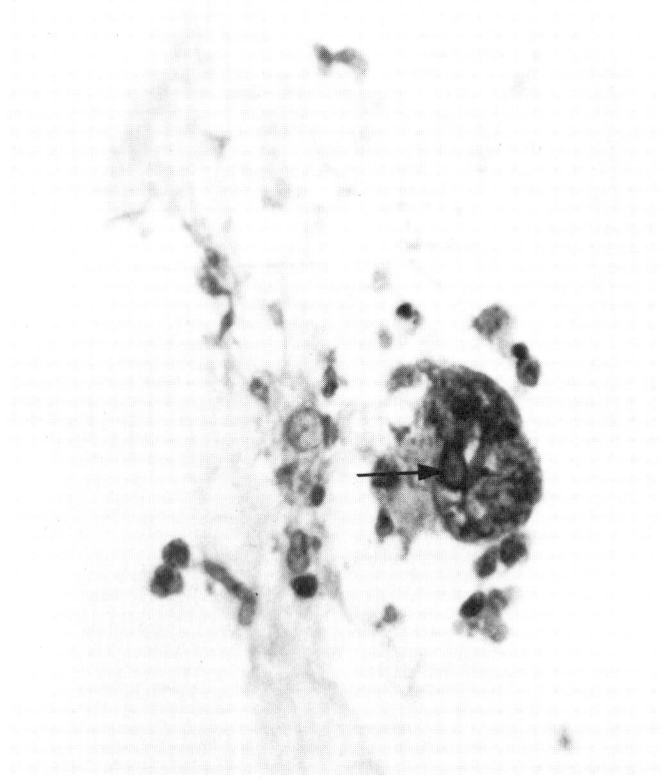

Figure 7–28. Endogenous mycotic infection of vitreous. Cortical vitreous. Organisms morphologically consistent with a species of *Candida* (arrow) have been partially surrounded by histiocytes. Specimen was obtained at autopsy from an immunosuppressed patient with systemic candidiasis. PAS, ×150.

tious and noninfectious causes, and into those that are exogenous and endogenous. Examples of infectious vitreous inflammations include those caused by bacteria, fungi, or parasites. Noninfectious inflammations may result from nongranulomatous or granulomatous inflammation of the uveal tract, necrosis of neoplasms, or inflammation produced by foreign particles lodged in the vitreous.

Infectious

Bacterial. Bacteria may be carried to the eye endogenously as part of a systemic septicemia or be introduced exogenously by surgical or nonsurgical trauma (Fig. 7–26). Bacterial infections of the vitreous usually develop and progress rapidly, although their course is modified by the pathogenicity of the individual organism and by the local vitreous structural factors already mentioned.

Mycotic. Mycotic infections of the vitreous progress more slowly and tend to remain localized much longer than do bacterial infections (Fine, Zimmerman, 1959). Saprophytic fungi like *Aspergillus, Cephalosporium, Fusarium,* and *Candida* are most often encountered. Exogenous mycotic infection may result from an accidental penetrating injury (especially in an agricultural setting) or as a consequence of surgery. The latter tends to follow anterior segment procedures, and the inflammation is usually localized to the anterior portions of the eye (Fig. 7–27). Clinical signs and symptoms may not arise for a period of weeks to months, depending upon the size and location of the mycotic inoculation. Organisms lying in the midvitreous may proliferate and form a microabscess that does not elicit an appreciable inflammatory response until it becomes large enough to approach vascularized structures within the eye, such as the iris or ciliary body. At this point, the clinical signs and symptoms of endophthalmitis (pain, redness, photophobia) become exacerbated. Multiple inoculations of mycotic organisms may cause many microabscesses that become confluent as they enlarge. This often is associated with gradual extension of a fibrinopurulent membrane on the vitreous face. Often a single microabscess will develop satellite lesions.

Endogenous mycotic infections of the vitreous usually follow localized retinitis. This form of infection is most likely to occur in immunosuppressed or debilitated individuals or in drug addicts who inject contaminated material into their blood. Most often, saprophytic fungi are causative, particularly the various species of *Candida* (Edwards, Foos, Montgomerie, Gutz, 1974; Michelson, Stark, Reeser, Green, 1971) (Fig. 7–28). The process starts as a localized perivascular retinitis that then extends into the vitreous, producing a fluffy white opacity. Occasionally there are multiple foci. The ophthalmoscopic appear-

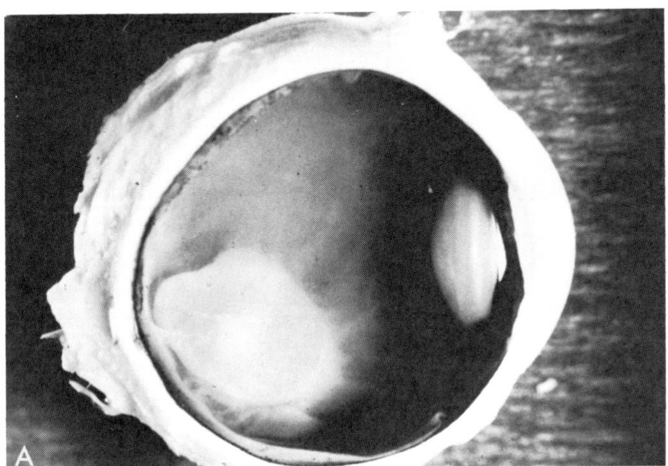

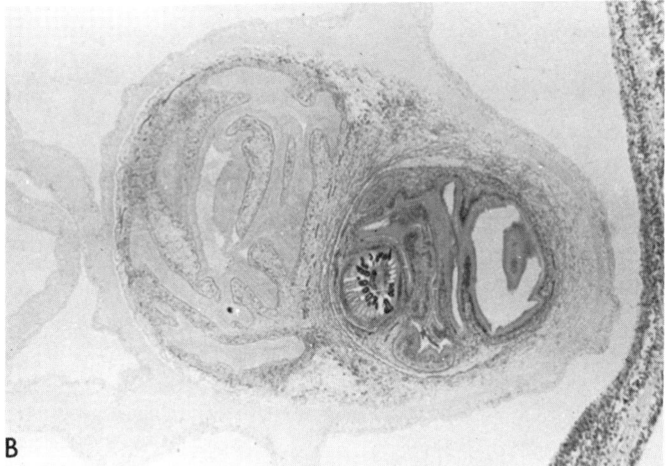

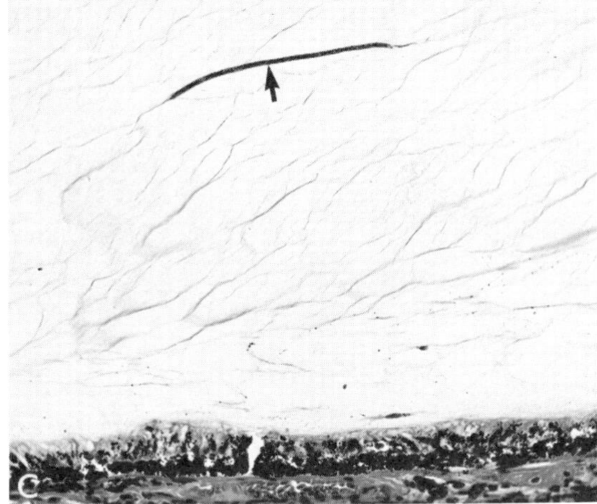

Figure 7–29. Parasitic infection of the vitreous. *A,* Gross appearance of *Cysticercus* in posterior vitreous. (Courtesy of Dr. F. C. Contreras.) *B,* Microscopic section of *Cysticercus* in posterior vitreous adjacent to retina. H and E, ×13. *C,* Onchocerciasis. Microfilaria (arrow) in anterior vitreous. Pars plana ciliaris is seen below. H and E, ×195. AFIP Neg. 66-7544. (From Paul EV, Zimmerman LE: Some observations on the ocular pathology of onchocerciasis. Hum Pathol *1*:581–594, 1970.)

ance, combined with documentation of mycotic septicemia or mycotic infection in other organs, is usually sufficient to establish a clinical diagnosis. Definitive diagnosis may be accomplished through needle aspiration of the vitreous or other forms of vitrectomy (Snip, Michels, 1976).

Parasitic. Parasitic infections of the vitreous occur more frequently in the Orient, Africa, and portions of Central and South America than they do in the United States. Several types of parasites have been found, including cysticerci, onchocerci, and the larvae of insects and nematodes (Dixon, Winkler, Nelson, 1969; Hunt, 1970; Manschot, 1968; Paul, Zimmerman, 1970; Tudor, Blair, 1971; Anderson, Font, 1976) (Fig. 7–29).

Nematode infections in the eye were first documented histopathologically by Wilder (1950). Most of these are apparently caused by second-stage larvae of *Toxocara canis* (Nichols, 1956; Beaver, 1956). The organisms incite little inflammation when they are alive; however, as they disintegrate, they cause an intense, acute inflammatory reaction often associated with localized eosinophilia (Fig. 7–30). The associated connective tissue response may produce a whitish mass behind the lens, which must be differentiated from other causes of leukokoria. The parasite enters the vitreous from contiguous structures and also has been reported in the posterior and anterior retina (Ashton, 1960; Hogan, Kimura, Spencer, 1965; Byers, Kimura, 1974; Wilkinson, Welch, 1971).

The natural hosts of the worms are dogs *(T. canis)* and cats *(T. cati)*, and in humans the infection is acquired by the ingestion of eggs from contaminated pets, clothes, soil, and so on. After the ova are ingested, they hatch in the stomach and intestine, and the larvae migrate through the walls of these organs and are disseminated via the blood, lymphatics, and tissue spaces. The larvae do not complete their life cycle within the human host, but they may survive for many months

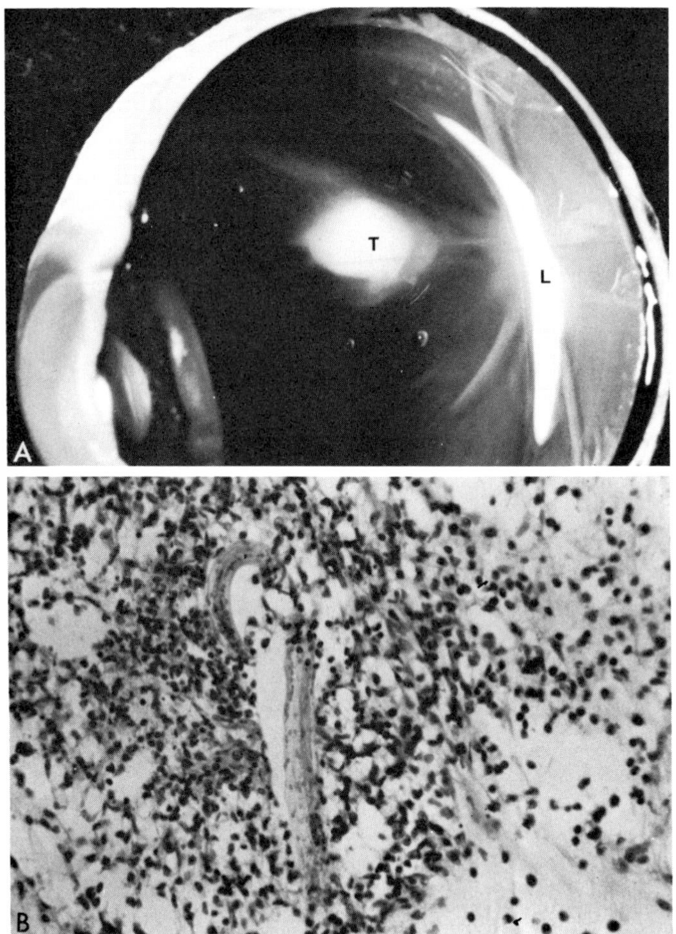

Figure 7–30. Nematode infection of the vitreous. *A,* Gross appearance of focal vitreous abscess caused by *Toxocara canis (T). L,* Light reflex. *B,* Microscopic section through abscess. Larva, morphologically compatible with *Toxocara canis,* is curled upon itself and is surrounded by polymorphonuclear leukocytes and eosinophils.

in human viscera. In humans, *T. canis* infestation occurs almost exclusively in children and young adults. There is often a history of dirt eating or close contact with puppies.

Although fever, general debility, and pulmonary and hepatic involvement are frequently present in disseminated worm infections, the ocular cases have been peculiar in that there has been no history of such generalized symptoms. Patients with ocular lesions typically have no eosinophilia. Since the larvae rarely develop to an adult stage in humans, examination of the stool for ova is fruitless. A variety of relatively nonspecific diagnostic tests has been suggested (e.g., use of isohemagglutinins, skin tests, using antigens from adult worms, fluorescent antibody test) (Duguid, 1961; Huntley, Lyerly, Patterson, 1969; Woodruff, 1970). The enzyme-linked immunosorbent assay (ELISA) is sensitive and useful in the diagnosis of visceral larva migrans (Cypess, Karrol, Zidian, et al, 1977; Pollard, Jarrett, Hagler, et al, 1979). Luxenberg (1979) used ELISA to evaluate systemic as well as intraocular responses to experimental infection with *T. canis*. Positive serum responses were obtained, but intraocular fluids gave a negative response.

Glickman and coworkers (1979) found the ELISA titer to be lower in the aqueous (1:16) than in the serum (1:2048) in a patient with systemic visceral larva migrans and suspected iris lesion. Since most organisms are located in the vitreous or retina, vitreous aspiration may provide more spe-

Figure 7–31. Noninfectious vitreous changes associated with "pars planitis." *A,* Slit lamp appearance of retrolental vitreous opacities in the eye of a 9 year old girl. *B,C, and D,* Vitrectomy specimen containing "snowballs" composed of epithelioid cells (small arrows) and multinucleated giant cells (large arrows). Millipore filter, modified Papanicolaou stain. *B* and *C,* ×500; *D,* ×1000. *E,* Ultrastructural appearance of a large macrophage with numerous inclusions of varying size and type. Some appear to be lipofuscin granules. Cellular debris and degenerating lysosomes are present around the cell. ×10,800. (From Green WR, Kincaid MC, Michels RG, et al: Pars planitis. Trans Ophthalmol Soc UK *101*:361–367, 1981. Courtesy of Dr. W. R. Green.)

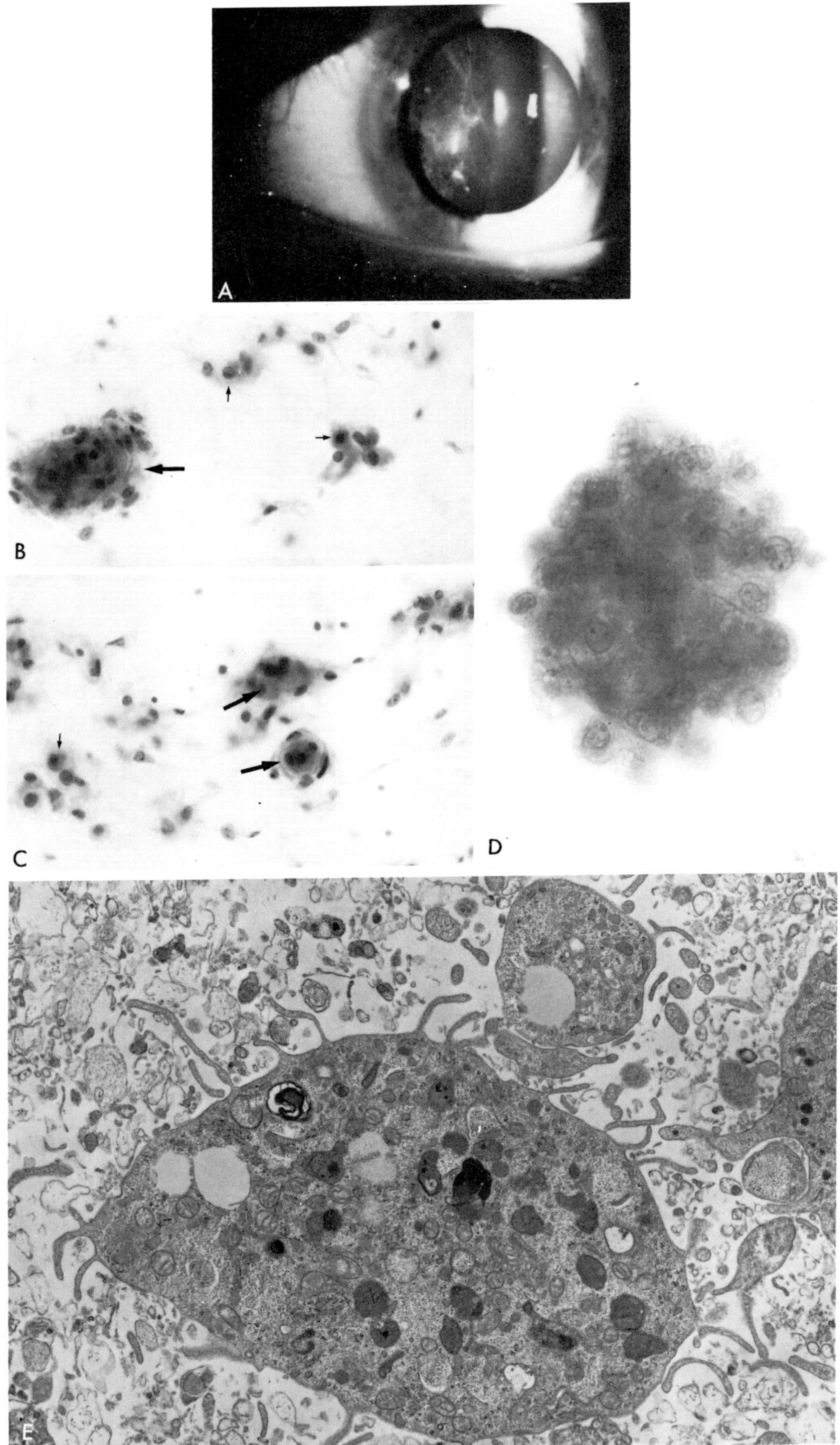

Figure 7–31 *See legend on opposite page*

cific information than does aqueous or serum sampling. Biglan, Glickman, and Lobes (1979) reported higher ELISA titers in the vitreous than in the serum of five patients with clinical diagnoses of nematode endophthalmitis. Berrocal (1980) surveyed serum ELISA titers in 312 healthy Puerto Rican children and 303 healthy adults. He found a 0 titer in infants younger than 6 months, increasing to 1 per cent by 12 months, to 6 per cent between 1 and 2 years, to 8.3 per cent up to 9 years, and to 10 per cent in patients from 10 to 80 years of age. The high prevalence of positive blood tests may reflect environmental and sociologic factors in Puerto Rico. The study suggests

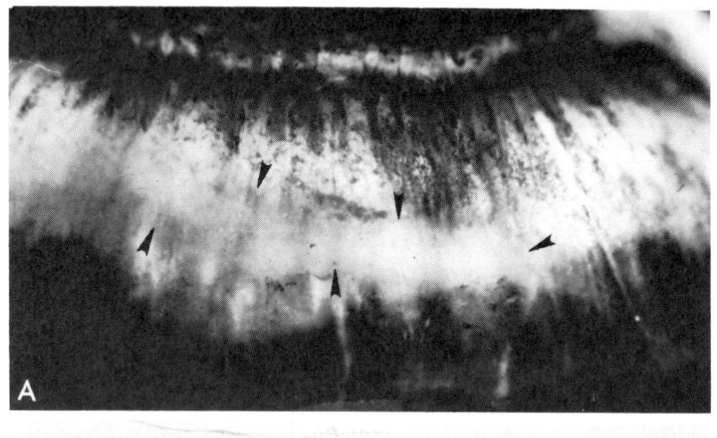

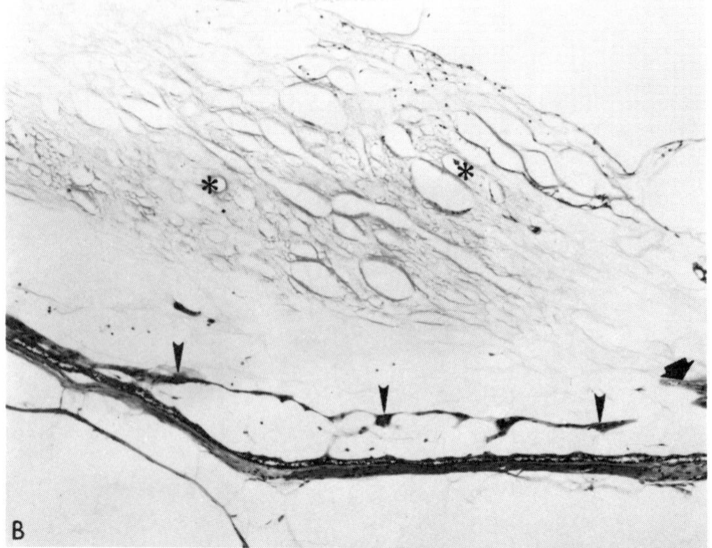

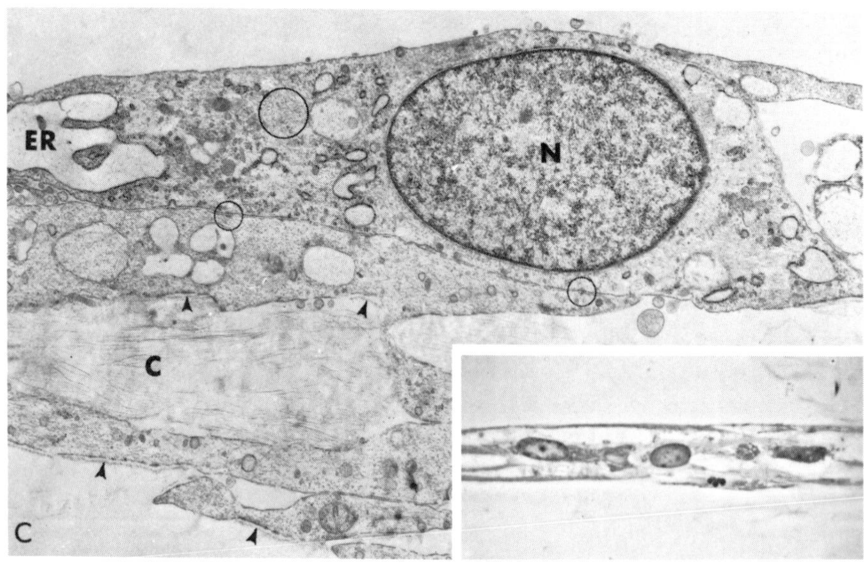

Figure 7–32. Noninfectious vitreous changes associated with "pars planitis." *A,* Gross appearance of "snowbank" of the vitreous base (arrowheads), which overlies the pars plana and ora serrata inferiorly. ×10. *B,* Snowbank composed of vitreous condensate, blood vessels (asterisks), scattered lymphocytes, spindle-shaped cells, and proliferated nonpigmented ciliary epithelium (arrowheads). Peripheral retina, arrow. H and E, ×100.

C, Inset: Light micrograph of intravitreal "snowbank" opacity includes elongated, fibrocytic-appearing cells within a fibrous matrix. Phase contrast, paraphenylenediamine, ×1200. Electron micrograph shows these cells to include fine microfilaments (large circle), dilated cisternae of rough-surfaced endoplasmic reticulum *(ER),* prominent nucleus *(N),* and desmosomal connections (small circles). Basement membrane (arrowheads) appears incomplete, and the cells appear to have secreted fibrillar collagen *(C).* ×24,500. (From Pederson JE, Kenyon KR, Green WR, Maumenee AE: Pathology of pars planitis. Am J Ophthalmol *86*:762–774, 1978. Courtesy of Dr. W. R. Green.)

that a negative serum ELISA is evidence against infection with *T. canis*.

Histopathologic identification of the larva or its remnants often requires examination of multiple sections. The organism induces a focal, necrotizing, granulomatous inflammation characterized by an accumulation of eosinophils, epithelioid cells, multinucleated giant cells, plasma cells, and lymphocytes surrounding the larva or its remnants. Rarely, a relatively intact larva surrounded by only minimal reaction is found. More often, the organism has been entirely destroyed and the diagnosis must be presumptive, based on the characteristic tissue reaction.

Noninfectious

Noninfectious inflammations of the vitreous result from inflammation of the retina, ciliary body, and iris. The most common form of nongranulomatous inflammation accompanies inflammation of the peripheral choroid, ciliary body, and iris. This condition has been termed peripheral uveitis (Brockhurst, Schepens, Okamura, 1961), pars planitis (Welch, Maumenee, Wahlen, 1960), cyclitis with peripheral chorioretinitis (Hogan, Kimura, 1961), and chronic cyclitis (Kimura, Hogan, 1963). The disease occurs primarily in children and young adults. It is often bilateral and is characterized by minimal anterior chamber reaction and nongranulomatous inflammation in the anterior and inferior vitreous, where the accumulation of cells and debris often resembles a "snowbank" that is composed of condensed vitreous containing mononuclear cells ("snowballs") intermixed with fibroglial tissue, vessels, nonpigmented ciliary epithelium, and occasional fibrocyte-like cells (Kenyon, Pederson, Green, Maumenee, 1975; Pederson, Kenyon, Green, Maumenee, 1978; Green, Kincaid, Michels, et al, 1981) (Figs. 7–31, 7–32). Ultrastructural study has shown condensed vitreous collagen and large-diameter (about 24 nm) collagen fibrils produced by cells resembling fibrous astrocytes (Pederson, Kenyon, Green, Maumenee, 1978). (For further discussion, see Vitreal membranes, page 581, and, in Chapter 8, Retinal and Periretinal Proliferations, page 710.) The posterior retina frequently shows a phlebitis associated with peripapillary and macular edema.

Noninfectious granulomatous inflammation of the vitreous occurs in patients with systemic sarcoidosis who develop retinitis. The clinical manifestations are described in Chapter 8. Occasionally, the inflammatory material collects in the inferior aspect of the vitreous, and this can resemble the "snowbank" seen in nongranulomatous peripheral uveitis. Histologically, the aggregates in sarcoidosis are composed of histiocytes often interspersed with connective tissue derived from the adjacent retina and ciliary body.

TRAUMA

Blunt Injury

The vitreous may transmit the effects of blunt injury to surrounding structures. The extent of the injury depends on mechanical factors relating to the direction and severity of the trauma, the firmness of the vitreoretinal interface, and the status of the eye prior to injury. For example, a myopic eye with a pre-existing lattice degeneration of the retina or abnormal vitreoretinal attachments is more likely to develop a retinal tear and detachment following blunt trauma than is an emmetropic eye without pre-existing retinal degeneration. Uveal and retinal pigment granules or hemorrhage may be seen in the vitreous following blunt trauma, especially if there is a retinal tear (Hamilton, Taylor, 1972). Dialysis of the retina may be produced by traumatic displacement of the base of the vitreous where the vitreoretinal adhesion is quite firm.

Penetrating Injury

The vitreous tends to prolapse through, or become incarcerated in, the entry and exit sites of wounds that either penetrate or perforate the eyeball posterior to the limbus. Frequently, the track of the missile can be seen in appropriately sectioned, enucleated eyes. Secondary fibrovascular ingrowth may occur along the course of the injury, and this contributes to subsequent vitreous traction and its related complications. (See Chapter 8.) Retained foreign bodies elicit varying degrees of inflammatory and connective tissue infiltration, depending upon their composition, proximity to the retina, and sterility. Following surgical procedures, such as intracapsular cataract extraction, the vitreous may become adherent to or prolapse through the wound margins (Fig. 7–33). Subsequently, iridovitreal adhesions also may occur at the pupillary margin. The adhesions are believed to contribute to the development of mild or subclinical uveitis and retinitis with retinal edema. The latter is particularly evident in the macula, which undergoes cystoid changes (Irvine-Gass syndrome) (see Chapter 8). Anteriorly displaced vitreous may obstruct aqueous flow through the pupil and produce secondary glaucoma. The vitreous also may contact the posterior surface of the cornea, causing the endothelium to degenerate or to undergo fibrous metaplasia with formation of a retrocorneal membrane.

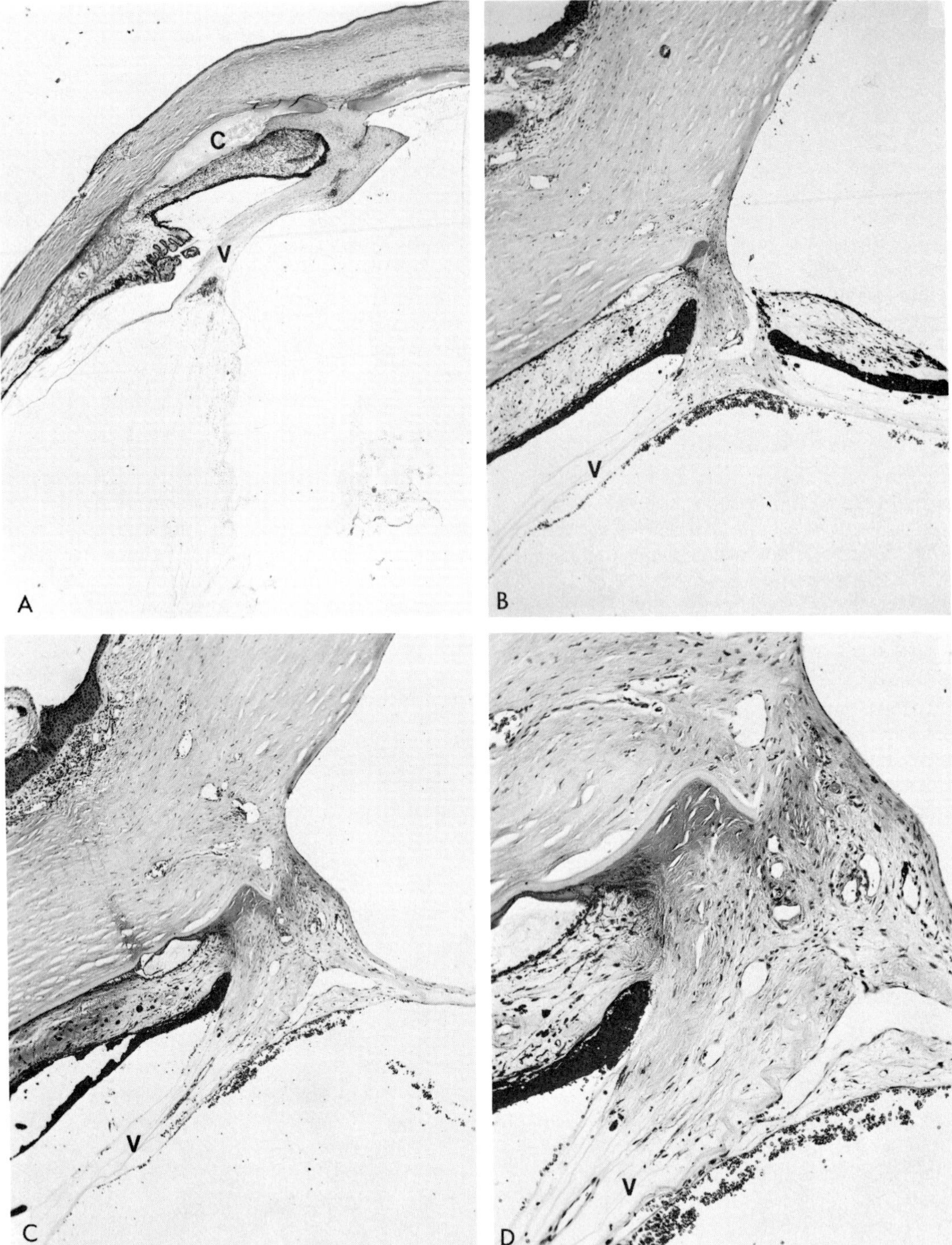

Figure 7–33. Postoperative vitreous adhesions. *A,* A band of dense connective tissue binds the anteriorly displaced vitreous *(V)* to the cornea and iris. The very shallow anterior chamber *(C)* contains serous exudate. H and E, ×12. AFIP Acc. 924896.

B, C, and *D,* Dense fibrovascular connective tissue extends from the vitreous *(V)* through a surgical coloboma of the iris to the inner aspect of a vascularized surgical scar. H and E, ×50, 50, and 115, respectively. AFIP Acc. 822983.

HEMORRHAGE

Causes

Vitreous hemorrhage may be the result of a large variety of local and systemic disease processes. Bleeding can extend posteriorly from the anterior segment of the globe or may arise from vessels of the optic nerve head, retina, or choroid. Small hemorrhages may not obscure fundus detail, and the initiating site may be visible. With larger hemorrhages, the origin cannot be seen un-

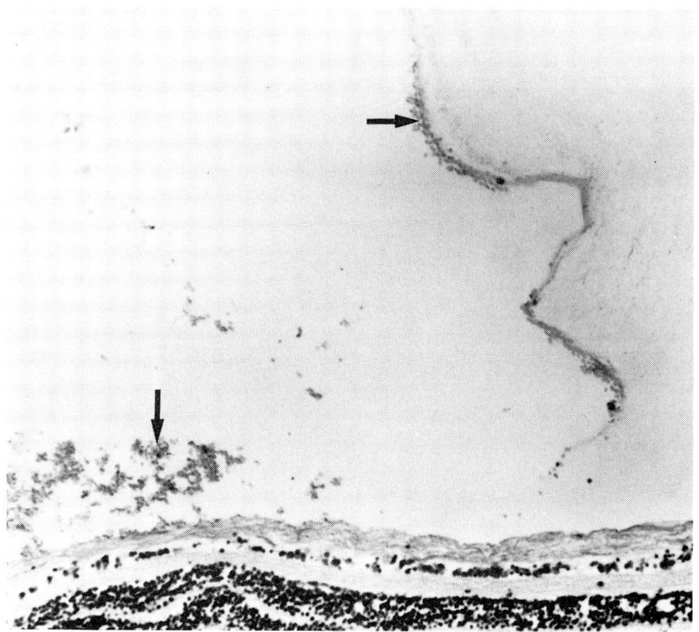

7–34. Retrovitreal hemorrhage and vitreous detachment. Red blood cells (arrows) are dispersed within the space between the retina and the posterior face of the detached vitreous. Several red blood cells adhere to the posterior vitreous face. H and E, ×25.

til the hemorrhage has settled, resolved, or been removed by vitrectomy. Only the more common causes of vitreous hemorrhage are discussed here.

Vitreous detachment, either spontaneous or following blunt trauma, may produce a retinal tear of varying severity. The resulting hemorrhage may be large and can cause visual loss when the macula is involved (Cibis, Watzke, Chua, 1975). Hemorrhage caused by spontaneous vitreous detachment is usually small. In most cases the blood does not extend into the vitreous but is dispersed between the retina and the posterior face of the detached vitreous (Fig. 7–34).

Anterior segment bleeding (following, for example, cataract surgery or iris and ciliary body contusion) may extend posteriorly into the vitreous, particularly in aphakic eyes. The vitreous hemorrhage may be slower to resolve than the one in the anterior chamber.

The proliferative phase of advanced diabetic retinopathy is one of the most common causes of vitreous hemorrhage. This and other forms of proliferative retinopathy, such as retinopathy of prematurity, and the sickle hemoglobinopathies are discussed in Chapter 8. Vitreous hemorrhage also may arise as a result of systemic hypertension, central or branch retinal vein occlusion, retinal vasculitis, and Eales' disease. A sudden increase in venous pressure resulting from a precipitous increase in intracranial pressure also may lead to intraretinal and vitreous hemorrhage (Terson, 1926; Vanderlinden, Chisholm, 1974; Khan, Frenkel, 1975). Necrotic choroidal melanomas, retinoblastomas, and some forms of metastatic intraocular tumor also may cause vitreous hemorrhages that can obscure the underlying process.

Sequelae

Very small vitreous hemorrhages can resolve without apparent sequelae. As noted in the discussion of cholesterosis bulbi (page 566), most large vitreous hemorrhages are associated with liquefaction of some portions of the vitreous and condensation, detachment, and organization of other portions. Dissolution of the blood may result in the development of cholesterosis, hemosiderosis, or hemolytic and ghost cell glaucoma (Fenton, Zimmerman, 1963; Fenton, Hunter, 1965; Campbell, Simmons, Grant, 1976). Persistent or recurrent hemorrhage can act as a stimulus for inflammation and lead to further organization of the vitreous clot, followed by proliferation of fibrovascular tissue into the vitreous and traction upon the retina.

VITREAL MEMBRANES

Membranes may form on and within the anterior or posterior portions of the vitreous following a variety of stimuli, such as surgical or accidental trauma, inflammation, hemorrhage, retinal vein occlusion, diabetic retinopathy, or longstanding retinal detachment. During the course of their development, many membranes undergo contraction, resulting in pupillary displacement, ciliary body detachment, or retinal detachment. It has been shown that the primary contractile component of these membranes is cellular rather than extracellular (Sugita, Tano, Machemer, et al, 1980; Grierson, Forrester, 1980; Grierson, Rahi, 1981). The vitreous may stimulate cellular proliferation when it touches structures that it does not normally contact (such as the posterior

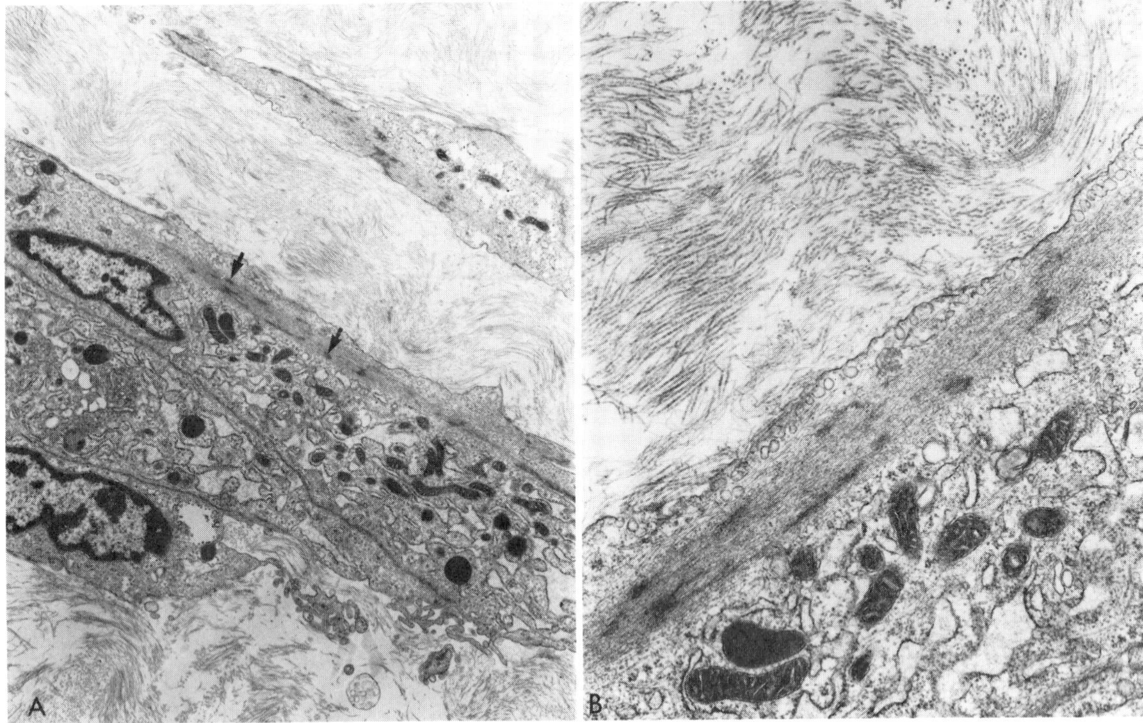

Figure 7–35. Myofibroblasts in vitreous membranes. *A,* Ultrastructural appearance of cellular preretinal membrane removed by vitrectomy. Spindle-shaped cells resembling fibroblasts contain bundles of myofilaments with dense bodies (arrows) lying parallel to the long axis of the cell. ×27,500. *B,* At higher magnification, the cells are seen to be surrounded by and intimately connected with collagen fibrils. ×29,500.

surface of the cornea or the iris), and it may also serve as a scaffold upon which the cellular membranes proliferate and contract. The cells originate from the injured or inflamed surrounding structures, and the membranes that form may be composed of one or several types of cells. Thus a poorly apposed surgical limbal wound with incarcerated vitreous may give rise to an anterior noncontractile membrane composed only of epithelial cells (epithelial downgrowth) or to a more complex contractile membrane containing limbal stromal fibroblasts, vessels, and proliferating corneal endothelial cells.

Following intracapsular cataract extraction, vitreous that has prolapsed through the pupil may adhere to the pupillary margin and the limbal wound, with eventual formation of a contractile membrane along the vitreous surface derived from connective tissue cells of the cornea and the iris stroma (updrawn pupil). Contractile membranes may arise from the inner aspect of the ciliary body and peripheral retina and proliferate along the anterior hyaloid surface (cyclitic membrane). They are often complex and may contain epithelial cells derived from the ciliary body, vessels, inflammatory cells, fibroblasts, and glial cells.

Posterior membranes (epiretinal or epipapillary membranes) arise from the retina or optic nerve head. These membranes vary in extent and complexity, ranging from a single layer of connective tissue cells lying along a small portion of the inner retinal surface (epiretinal membrane) to larger, multilayered structures containing combinations of fibroblasts, astrocytes, retinal pigment epithelial cells, macrophages, and vessels. These large membranes subsequently may contract and detach the retina (fixed retinal folds, massive vitreal retraction). (For further discussion see Chapter 8, Retinal and Periretinal Proliferations, page 710.)

Electron microscopic and immunofluorescent studies of membranes excised during vitrectomy procedures (Engel, Green, Michels, et al, 1981) and of experimentally induced membranes (Grierson, Rahi, 1981) have shown that they contain contractile cells known as myofibroblasts (Gabbiani, Ryan, Majno, 1971; Majno, Gabbiani, Hirschel, et al, 1971; Majno, 1979) (Fig. 7–35). These cells are converted fibroblasts containing bundles of compacted and contractile intracytoplasmic myofilaments (Gabbiani, Ryan, Majno, 1971; Majno, Gabbiani, Hirschel, et al, 1971; Majno, 1979). The myofilaments contain dense bodies resembling those seen in smooth muscle cells. However, in the latter, the myofilaments are dispersed throughout the cytoplasm, while in myofibroblasts they usually run parallel to the axis of the cell (Bhawan, 1981). Immunofluorescent staining has shown the presence of actomyosin within these cells (Hirschel, Gabbiani, Ryan, Majno, 1971), and in pharmacologic studies the myofibroblasts behave like smooth muscle cells

(Majno, Gabbiani, Hirschel, et al, 1971). During wound healing in the skin, myofibroblasts tend to diminish in number as the wound matures and contraction ceases (Rudolph, Guber, Suzuki, Woodward, 1977). It is likely that similar changes occur in myofibroblasts in mature vitreous membranes.

Experimental studies of the activity and morphology of fibroblasts in the vitreous have shown that they undergo sequential structural changes, with maximum organization and compaction of the microfilaments 3 to 6 weeks after the cells are introduced (Grierson, Rahi, 1981). The vitreous cells appear to be linked by gap junctions and form compact sheets. Studies of myofibroblasts in granulation tissue have shown that they are able to synthesize type III collagen (Gabbiani, LeLous, Bailey, et al, 1976). In membranes excised via vitrectomy, the myofibroblasts appear to secrete extracellular collagen fibrils (approximately 20 nm in diameter) that mingle with normal vitreous fibrils (approximately 10 nm in diameter) (Engel, Green, Michels, et al, 1981). The large-diameter vitreous collagen has not been typed.

NEOPLASMS AND THE VITREOUS

The clinical appearance and the effects of tumor cells upon the vitreous closely parallel those produced by inflammation. Large collections of neoplastic cells can produce liquefaction, increased protein content, clouding, detachment, and condensation of the vitreous. Small neoplastic infiltrates often cause local opacities resembling those seen with granulomatous inflammation, with little or no disturbance of the clarity or consistency of the surrounding vitreous. Many neoplasms are associated with intraocular inflammation and hemorrhage, so that the cellular infiltrate is mixed.

Tumor cells are commonly dispersed into the vitreous in eyes containing retinoblastoma, par-

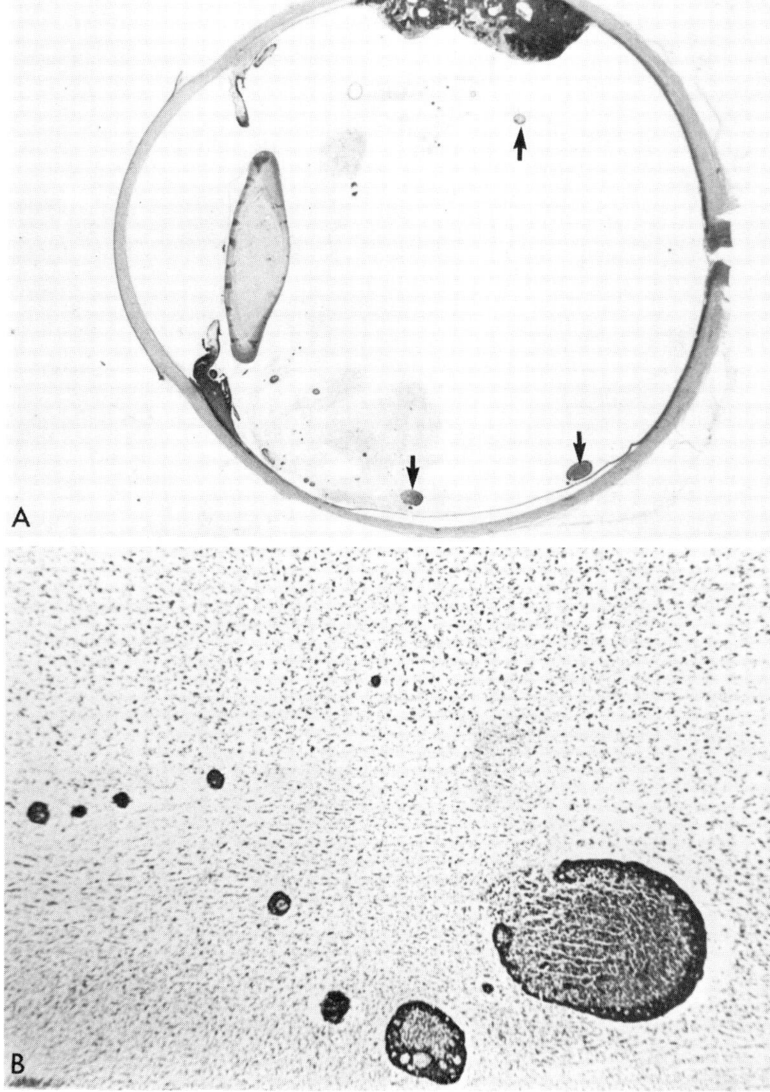

Figure 7–36. Tumor cells in the vitreous—retinoblastoma. *A,* Endophytic retinoblastoma located at the superior equator has dispersed "seeds" of tumor cells into the vitreous (arrows). Iris and ciliary body are invaded by tumor. H and E, ×1.5. *B,* At higher magnification, the tumor "seeds" are seen to vary in size, with relatively viable cells at their periphery; the center appears necrotic. Adjacent vitreous contains eosinophilic-staining proteinaceous material. H and E, ×10.

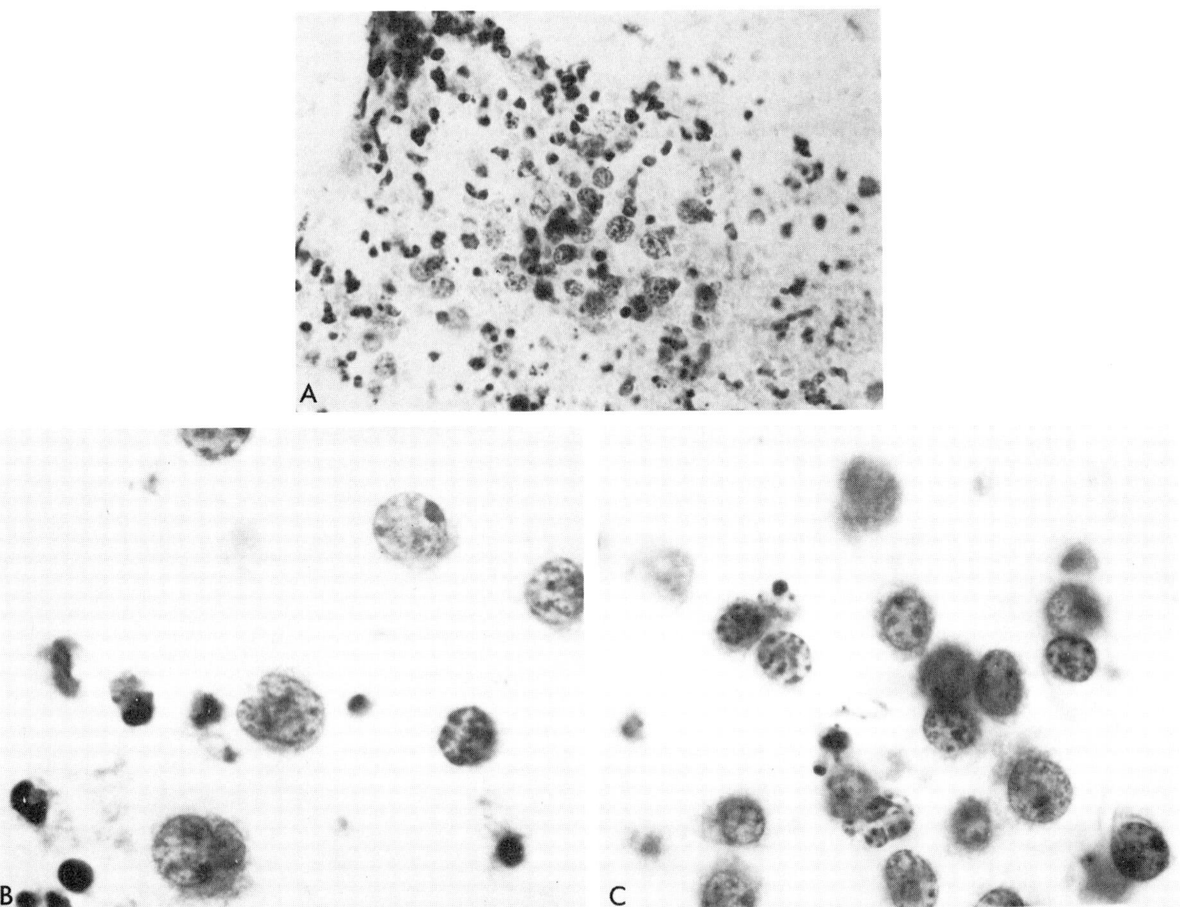

Figure 7–37. Tumor cells in the vitreous—diffuse histiocytic lymphoma (reticulum cell sarcoma). *A,* A large collection of tumor cells and cellular debris obtained by vitrectomy. Membrane filter, modified Papanicolaou stain, ×375. *B* and *C,* Cytoplasm of tumor cells is relatively scanty. Nuclei are round, oval, or bean-shaped, with prominent nucleoli. Membrane filter, modified Papanicolaou stain, ×1500. (Courtesy of Dr. W. R. Green.)

ticularly the endophytic type (Fig. 7–36). Viable "seeds" may be transported through the vitreous to other portions of the retina where they adhere to the internal limiting membrane and result in secondary tumors. Clumps of tumor cells are occasionally carried into the anterior chamber. Rarely, fragments of tumor cells may be dispersed into the vitreous from the inner surface of medulloepitheliomas of the ciliary body. These do not appear to result in secondary neoplasms.

Reticulum cell sarcoma (histiocytic lymphoma) involving the eye and brain may cause unilateral or bilateral cellular deposition in the posterior vitreous (Vogel, Font, Zimmerman, Levine, 1968; Neault, Van Scoy, Okazaki, et al, 1973; Barr, Green, Payne, et al, 1975). Tumor cells are seen often in the vitreous of eyes containing similar cells within and beneath the retina; however, vitreous cellular infiltrate may be the only ocular manifestation of this process (Barr, Green, Payne, et al, 1975). When there are associated neurologic signs, histologic diagnosis may be achieved by vitreous aspiration, vitrectomy, or both (Fig. 7–37) (Michels, Knox, Erozan, Green, 1975; Engel, Green, Michels, et al, 1981).

Most cases occur in the fifth and sixth decades and present as a unilateral posterior or anterior "uveitis" that is refractory to therapy and eventually becomes bilateral. Ocular disease may antedate neurologic symptoms for periods ranging from 3 months to 8 years (Vogel, Font, Zimmerman, Levine, 1968). Patchy cellular infiltrates of varying size occur in the choroid, optic nerve head, and retina and beneath the retinal pigment epithelium. The vitreal cells apparently arise from the retina and optic nerve head and initially are most numerous in the cortical vitreous, where they form fluffy, nondiscrete opacities. In severe cases the cells extend into the central vitreous, where they interfere with vision.

The tumor cells are often pleomorphic (Fig. 7–37). The round-to-oval nuclei frequently have an irregular contour, with small, finger-like protrusions and irregular multiple nucleoli. The scanty cytoplasm is delicate, and in vitreous aspirates it is often poorly preserved.

The cells may initially appear to be inflammatory rather than neoplastic. Kennerdell, Johnson and Wisotzkey (1975) reported a fatal case with reticulum cell sarcoma of the brain in which inflammatory cells were found throughout the vitreous and no intraocular sarcoma was present. They speculated that an inflammatory cell infiltrate may precede the infiltration of the eye by malignant histiocytic cells. This report demonstrates the difficulty in classifying the vitreous cells solely upon their morphologic characteristics. Diagnostic reliability can be augmented by immunologic studies of the vitreous cell surface markers and their in vitro functional activity. Complete characterization usually requires a larger number of cells than can be obtained via vitrectomy. However, microtechniques have now been developed that allow partial immunologic characterization with a limited number of cells (Kaplan, Meredith, Aaberg, Keller, 1980), and it is likely that technical improvements will soon permit more complete designations of cellular origin from vitreous samples containing relatively few cells.

Necrotic uveal melanomas, particularly those associated with intraocular hemorrhage and glaucoma, may disperse viable and nonviable tumor cells into the vitreous. Similar dispersion may occur with necrotic metastatic neoplasms. For further discussion, see Chapters 6 and 9.

References

Aaberg TM, Stevens TR: Snail-track degeneration of the retina. Am J Ophthalmol *73*:370–376, 1972.

Alexander RL, Shea M: Wagner's disease. Arch Ophthalmol *74*:310–318, 1965.

Anderson J, Font RL: Ocular onchocerciasis, *in* Binford CH, Connor DH (eds): Pathology of Tropical and Extraordinary Diseases. An Atlas. Vol 2. Armed Forces Institute of Pathology, Washington, DC, 1976, pp 373–381.

Anderson JR; Medulloepithelioma of the retina. Int Ophthalmol Clin *2*:483–506, 1962.

Andrews JS, Lynn C, Scobey JW, Elliott JH: Cholesterosis bulbi: Case report with modern chemical identification of the ubiquitous crystals. Br J Ophthalmol *57*:838–844, 1973.

Ashton N: Larval granulomatosis of the retina due to toxocaria. Br J Ophthalmol *44*:129–148, 1960.

Balaglou PJ: Persistent hyperplastic primary vitreous: An unusual case associated with a dysplastic retina. Surv Ophthalmol *10*:360–364, 1965.

Balazs EA: Molecular morphology of the vitreous body; *in* Smelser GK (ed): Structure of the Eye. New York, Academic Press, 1961, pp 291–310.

Balian JV, Falls HF: Congenital vascular veils in the vitreous. Arch Ophthalmol *63*:92–101, 1960.

Barr CC, Green WR, Payne JW, et al: Intraocular reticulum cell sarcoma. Clinical pathologic study of 4 cases and review of the literature. Surv Ophthalmol *19*:224–239, 1975.

Beaver PC: Larva migrans. Exp Parasitol *5*:587–621, 1956.

Berrocal J: Prevalence of *Toxocara canis* in babies and in adults as determined by the ELISA test. Trans Am Ophthalmol Soc *78*:376–413, 1980.

Bergen RL, Glassman R: Familial exudative vitreoretinopathy. Ann Ophthalmol *15*:275–276, 1983.

Bhawan J: The myofibroblast. Am J Dermatopathol *3*:73–78, 1981.

Biglan W, Glickman LT, Lobes LA: Serum and vitreous *Toxocara* antibody in nematode endophthalmitis. Am J Ophthalmol *88*:898–901, 1979.

Blair NP, Albert DM, Liberfarb RM, Hirose T: Hereditary progressive arthro-ophthalmopathy of Stickler. Am J Ophthalmol *88*:876–888, 1979.

Bloom G, Balazs E: An electron microscopic study of hyalocytes. Exp Eye Res *4*:249–255, 1965.

Bohringer HR, Dieterle P, Landolt E: Zur Klinik und Pathologie der Degeneratio hyaloideoretinalis hereditaria (Wagner). Ophthalmologica *139*:330–338, 1960.

Brini A, Porte A, Stoeckel NE: Morphology and structure of the vitreous, *in* Biology and Surgery of the Vitreous Body. Paris, Masson et Cie, 1968.

Brockhurst RJ, Albert DM, Zakov ZN: Pathologic findings in familial exudative vitreoretinopathy. Arch Ophthalmol *99*:214342146, 1981.

Brockhurst RJ, Schepens CL, Okamura ID; Uveitis. III. Peripheral uveitis: Pathogenesis, etiology, and treatment. Am J Ophthalmol *51*:19–26, 1961.

Brownstein MH, Elliott R, Helwig EG: Ophthalmologic aspects of amyloidosis. Am J Ophthalmol *69*:423–430, 1970.

Bullock JD: Developmental vitreous cysts. Arch Ophthalmol *91*:83–84, 1974.

Byer NE: Clinical study of lattice degeneration of the retina. Trans Am Acad Ophthalmol Otolaryngol *69*:1064–1081, 1965.

Byers B, Kimura SJ: Uveitis after death of a larva in the vitreous cavity. Am J Ophthalmol *77*:63–66, 1974.

Campbell DG, Simmons RJ, Grant WM: Ghost cells as a cause of glaucoma. Am J Ophthalmol *81*:441–450, 1976.

Canny CLB, Oliver GL: Fluorescein angiographic findings in familial exudative vitreoretinopathy. Arch Ophthalmol *94*:1114–1120, 1976.

Cibis GW, Watzke RC, Chua J: Retinal hemorrhages and posterior vitreous detachment. Am J Ophthalmol *80*:1043–1046, 1975.

Cogan DG, Kuwabara T: Ocular pathology of the 13–15 trisomy syndrome. Arch Ophthalmol *72*:246–253, 1964.

Crawford JB: Cotton wool exudates in systemic amyloidosis. Arch Ophthalmol *78*:214–216, 1967.

Criswick VG, Schepens CL: Familial exudative vitreoretinopathy. Am J Ophthalmol *68*:578–594, 1969.

Cypess RH, Karrol MH, Zidian JL, et al: Larva specific antibodies in patients with visceral larva migrans. J Infect Dis *135*:633–640, 1977.

Dixon JM, Winkler CH, Nelson JH: Ophthalmomyiasis interna caused by cuterebra larva. Trans Am Ophthalmol Soc *67*:110–115, 1969.

Doft BH, Rubinow A, Cohen AS: Immunocytochemical demonstration of prealbumin in the vitreous in heredofamilial amyloidosis. Am J Ophthalmol *97*:296–300, 1984.

Donaldson D, Hagler WS: Free-floating cysts. Arch Ophthalmol *78*:400–401, 1967.

Duguid IM: Chronic endophthalmitis due to toxocara. Br J Ophthalmol *45*:705–717, 1961.

Edwards JE Jr, Foos RY, Montgomerie JA, Gutz LB: Ocular manifestations of Candida septicemia: Review of 76 cases of hematogenous Candida endophthalmitis. Medicine *53*:47–75, 1974.

Egbert PR: Familial exudative vitreoretinopathy; case presented at the Verhoeff Society meeting, Washington, DC, April, 1983.

Engel HA, Green WR, Michels RG, et al: Diagnostic vitrectomy. Retina *1*:121–149, 1981.

Everett WG: Study of a family with lattice degeneration and retinal detachment. Am J Ophthalmol *65*:229–232, 1968.

Favre M: À propos de deux cas de dégénérescence hyaloideo-retinienne. Ophthalmologica *135*:604–609, 1958.

Favre M, Goldmann H: Zur Genese der hinteren Glaskörperabhebung. Ophthalmologica *132*:87–97, 1956.

Feiler-Ofry V, Adam A, Regenbogen L, et al: Hereditary vitreoretinal degeneration and night blindness. Am J Ophthalmol *67*:553–558, 1969.

Feman SS, Straatsma BR: Cyst of the posterior vitreous. Arch Ophthalmol *91*:328–329, 1974.

Fenton RH, Hunter WS: Hemolytic glaucoma. Surv Ophthalmol *10*:355–364, 1965.

Fenton RH, Zimmerman LE: Hemolytic glaucoma: An unusual cause of acute open-angle glaucoma. Arch Ophthalmol *70*:236–239, 1963.

Fine BS, Tousimis AJ: The structure of the vitreous body and the suspensory ligaments of the lens. Arch Ophthalmol *65*:95–110, 1961.

Fine BS, Zimmerman LE: Exogenous intraocular fungus infections. Am J Ophthalmol *48*:151–165, 1959.

Fishman GA, Cunha-Vaz JG, Travassos AC: Vitreous fluorophotometry in patients with fundus flavimaculatus. Arch Ophthalmol *100*:1086–1088, 1982.

Fishman GA, Jampol LM, Goldberg MF: Diagnostic features of the Favre-Goldmann syndrome. Br J Ophthalmol *60*:345–353, 1976.

Font RL, Yanoff M, Zimmerman LE: Intraocular adipose tissue and persistent hyperplastic primary vitreous. Arch Ophthalmol *82*:43–50, 1969.

Foos RY: Vitreoretinal juncture: Topographical variations. Invest Ophthalmol *10*:801–808, 1972a.

Foos RY: Posterior vitreous detachment. Trans Am Acad Ophthalmol Otolaryngol *76*:480–497, 1972b.

Foos RY, Kreiger AE, Forsythe AB, Zakka KA: Posterior vitreous detachment in diabetic subjects. Ophthalmology *87*:122–128, 1980.

Foos RY, Wheeler NC: Vitreoretinal juncture synchysis senilis and posterior vitreous detachment. Ophthalmology *89*:1502–1512, 1982.

Forsuis H, Vainio-Mattilla B, Eriksson A: X-linked hereditary retinoschisis. Br J Ophthalmol *46*:678–681, 1962.

François J: Pre-papillary cyst developed from remnant of the hyaloid artery. Br J Ophthalmol *34*:365–368, 1950.

François J: Degenerescence hyaloideotapetoretinienne de Goldmann-Favre. Ophthalmologica *168*:81–96, 1974.

Frandsen E: Hereditary hyaloideoretinal degeneration (Wagner) in a Dutch family. Acta Ophthalmol *44*:223–232, 1966.

Gabbiani G, LeLous M, Bailey AJ, et al: Collagen and myofibroblasts of granulation tissue. A chemical, ultrastructural and immunologic study. Virchows Arch Cell Pathol *21*:133–145, 1976.

Gabbiani G, Ryan GB, Majno G: Presence of modified fibroblasts in granulation tissue and their possible role in wound contraction. Experientia *27*:549–550, 1971.

Gasman W, Russburger, JJ, Shields JA, et al: Familial exudative vitreoretinopathy. Trans Am Ophthalmol Soc *79*: 211–226, 1981.

Gass JDM: Familial exudative vitreoretinopathy; case presented at the Verhoeff Society meeting, Washington, DC, April 1983.

Glickman L, Cypess R, Hiles D, Gessner T: *Toxocara*-specific antibody in the serum and aqueous humor of a patient with presumed ocular and visceral toxocariasis. Am J Trop Med Hyg *28*:29–35, 1979.

Goldmann H: Biomicroscopie du corps vitré et du fond de l'oeil. Bull Mem Soc Fr Ophtalmol *70*:265–272, 1957.

Gonin J: La pathologenie du decollement spontane de la retine. Ann Ocul *32*:30–55, 1904.

Gow J, Oliver GL: Familial exudative vitreoretinopathy. Arch Ophthalmol *86*:150–155, 1971.

Green WR, Kincaid MC, Michels RG, et al: Pars planitis. Trans Ophthalmol Soc UK *101*:361–367, 1981.

Grierson I, Forrester JV: Vitreous hemorrhage and vitreal membranes. Trans Ophthalmol Soc UK *100*:40–50, 1980.

Grierson I, Rahi AHS: Structural basis of contraction in vitreal fibrous membranes. Br J Ophthalmol *65*:737–749, 1981.

Gruber E: Crystals in the anterior chamber. Am J Ophthalmol *40*:817–827, 1955.

Hagler WS, Crosswell HH Jr: Radial perivascular chorioretinal degeneration and retinal detachment. Trans Am Acad Ophthalmol Otolaryngol *72*:203–216, 1968.

Hamidi-Toosi S, Maumenee IH: Vitreoretinal degeneration in spondyloepiphyseal dysplasia congenita. Arch Ophthalmol *100*:1104–1107, 1982.

Hamilton AM, Taylor W: Significance of pigment granules in the vitreous. Br J Ophthalmol *56*:700–702, 1972.

Harris GS: Juvenile sex-linked retinoschisis. Mod Probl Ophthalmol *8*:363–370, 1969.

Hatfield AE, Gastineau CF, Rucker CW: Asteroid bodies in the vitreous: Relationship to diabetes and hypercholesterolemia. Mayo Clin Proc *37*:513–514, 1962.

Hermann J, France TO, Spranger JW, et al: The Stickler syndrome (hereditary arthro-ophthalmopathy). Birth Defects *11*:76–103, 1975.

Hilsdorf C: Über einen Fall einer einseitgen Glaskörpercyste. Ophthalmologica *149*:12–20, 1965.

Hirose T, Lee KY, Schepens CL: Wagner's hereditary vitreoretinal degeneration and retinal detachment. Arch Ophthalmol *89*:176–185, 1973.

Hirose T, Lee KY, Schepens CL: Snowflake degeneration in hereditary vitreoretinal degeneration. Am J Ophthalmol *77*:143–153, 1974.

Hirschel BJ, Gabbiani G, Ryan GB, Majno G: Fibroblasts of granulation tissue: Immunofluorescent staining with anti-smooth muscle serum. Proc Soc Exp Biol Med *138*:466–469, 1971.

Hitchings RA, Tripathi RC: Vitreous opacities in primary amyloid disease. A clinical, histochemical and ultrastructural report. Br J Ophthalmol *60*:41–54, 1976.

Hogan MJ: The vitreous: Its structure in relation to the ciliary body and retina. Invest Ophthalmol *2*:418–445, 1963.

Hogan MJ, Alvarado JA, Weddell JE: Histology of the Human Eye. Philadelphia, W. B. Saunders Company, 1971.

Hogan MJ, Kimura SJ: Cyclitis and peripheral chorioretinitis. Arch Ophthalmol *56*:667–677, 1961.

Hogan MJ, Kimura SJ, Spencer WH: Visceral larva migrans and peripheral retinitis. JAMA *194*:1345–1347, 1965.

Hunt EW Jr: Unusual case of ophthalmomyiasis interna posterior. Am J Ophthalmol *70*:978–980, 1970.

Hunter WS, Zimmerman LE: Unilateral retinal dysplasia. Arch Ophthalmol *74*:23–30, 1965.

Huntley CC, Lyerly AD, Patterson MV: Isohemagglutinins in parasitic infections. JAMA *208*:1145–1148, 1969.

Irvine AR, Char DH: Recurrent amyloid involvement in the vitreous body after vitrectomy. Am J Ophthalmol *82*:705–708, 1976.

Juler F: An unusual form of retinal detachment (? cystic). Trans Ophthalmol Soc UK *67*:83–96, 1947.

Kaplan HJ, Meredith TA, Aaberg TM, Keller RH: Reclassification of intraocular reticulum cell sarcoma (histiocytic lymphoma). Immunologic characterization of vitreous cells. Arch Ophthalmol *78*:707–710, 1980.

Kasner D, Miller GR, Taylor WH, et al: Surgical treatment of amyloidosis of the vitreous. Trans Am Acad Ophthalmol Otolaryngol *72*:410–418, 1968.

Kaufman HE: Primary familial amyloidosis. Arch Ophthalmol *60*:1036–1043, 1958.

Kaufman HE, Thomas LB: Vitreous opacities diagnostic of familial primary amyloidosis. N Engl J Med *261*:1267–1271, 1959.

Kennerdell JS, Johnson BL, Wisotzkey HM: Vitreous cellular reaction: Association with reticulum cell sarcoma of brain. Arch Ophthalmol *93*:1341–1345, 1975.

Kenyon KR, Pederson JE, Green WR, Maumenee AE: Fibroglial proliferation in pars planitis. Trans Ophthalmol Soc UK *95*:391–396, 1975.

Khan SG, Frenkel M: Intravitreal hemorrhage associated with rapid increase in intracranial pressure. Am J Ophthalmol *80*:37–43, 1975.

Kimura SJ, Hogan MJ: Chronic cyclitis. Trans Am Ophthalmol Soc *61*:397–417, 1963.

Kinsey VE, Grant M, Cogan DG: Water movement and eye. Arch Ophthalmol *27*:242–252, 1942.

Knobloch WH: Inherited hyaloideoretinopathy and skeletal dysplasia. Trans Am Ophthalmol Soc *73*:417–451, 1975.

Levy J: Inherited retinal detachment. Br J Ophthalmol *36*:626–636, 1952.

Lewkonia I, Davies MD, Salmon JD: Lattice degeneration in a family with retinal detachment and cataract. Br J Ophthalmol *57*:566–571, 1973.

Linder B: Acute posterior vitreous detachment and its retinal complications. A clinical biomicroscopic study. Acta Ophthalmol (Koh) Suppl *87*:1–108, 1966.

Luxenberg MN: An experimental approach to the study of intraocular *Toxocara canis*. Trans Am Ophthalmol Soc *78*:542–602, 1979.

Luxenberg MN, Sime D: Relationship of asteroid hyalosis to diabetes mellitus and plasma lipid levels. Am J Ophthalmol *67*:406–413, 1969.

Majno G: The story of the myofibroblasts. Am J Surg Pathol *3*:535–542, 1979.

Majno G, Gabbiani G, Hirschel BJ, et al: Contraction of granulation tissue in vitro: Similarity to smooth muscle. Science *173*:548–550, 1971.

Mann I, MacRae A: Congenital vascular veils in the vitreous. Br J Ophthalmol *22*:1–10, 1938.

Manschot WA: Persistent hyperplastic primary vitreous. Arch Ophthalmol *59*:188–203, 1958.

Manschot WA: Intraocular cysticercus. Arch Ophthalmol *80*:772–774, 1968.

Manschot WA: Pathology of hereditary conditions related to retinal detachment. Ophthalmologica *162*:223–234, 1971.

Manschot WA: Pathology of hereditary juvenile retinoschisis. Arch Ophthalmol *88*:131–138, 1972.

March W, Shoch D, O'Grady R: Composition of asteroid bodies. Invest Ophthalmol *13*:701–705, 1974.

Maumenee IH: Vitreoretinal degeneration as a sign of generalized connective tissue diseases. Am J Ophthalmol *88*:432–449, 1979.

Maumenee IH, Stoll HU, Mets MB: The Wagner syndrome versus hereditary arthroophthalmopathy. Trans Am Ophthalmol Soc *81*:349–365, 1982.

Maurice DM; The exchange of sodium between the vitreous body and the blood and aqueous humor. J Physiol *137*:110–125, 1957.

Michels RG, Knox DL, Erozan YS, Green WR: Intraocular reticulum cell sarcoma. Diagnosis by pars plana vitrectomy. Arch Ophthalmol *93*:1331–1335, 1975.

Michelson PE, Stark WJ, Reeser F, Green WR: Endogenous Candida endophthalmitis. Report of 13 cases and 16 from the literature. Int Ophthalmol Clin *11*:125–147, 1971.

Miller H, Miller B, Rabinowitz H, et al: Asteroid bodies—an ultrastructural study. Invest Ophthalmol Vis Sci *24*:133–136, 1983.

Miyakubo H, Inohara N, Hashimoto K: Retinal involvement in familial exudative vitreoretinopathy. Ophthalmologica *185*:125–135, 1982.

Neault RW, Van Scoy RE, Okazaki H, et al: Uveitis associated with isolated reticulum cell sarcoma of the brain. Am J Ophthalmol *73*:431–436, 1973.

Nichols RL: The etiology of visceral larva migrans: Diagnostic morphology of infective second-stage toxocara larvae. J Parasitol *42*:349–362, 1956.

Nijhuis FA, Deutman AF, Aan de Kerk AL: Fluorescein angiography in mild stages of dominant exudative vitreoretinopathy. Mod Probl Ophthalmol *20*:107–114, 1979.

Nissim J, Ivry M, Oliver M: Persistent hyperplastic primary vitreous at the optic nerve head. Am J Ophthalmol *73*:580–583, 1972.

Ober RR, Bird AC, Hamilton AM, et al: Autosomal dominant exudative vitreoretinopathy. Br J Ophthalmol *64*:112–120, 1980.

Parelhoff ES, Wood WJ, Green WR, et al: Radial perivascular lattice degeneration of the retina. Ann Ophthalmol *12*:25–32, 1980.

Paton D, Duke JR: Primary familial amyloidosis: Ocular manifestations with histopathologic observations. Am J Ophthalmol *61*:736–747, 1966.

Paul EB, Zimmerman LE: Some observations on the ocular pathology of onchocerciasis. Hum Pathol *1*:581–594, 1970.

Pederson JE, Kenyon KR, Green WR, Maumenee AE: Pathology of pars planitis. Am J Ophthalmol *86*:762–774, 1978.

Peyman GA, Fishman GA, Sanders DR, Vichek J: Histopathology of Goldmann-Favre syndrome obtained by full thickness eye-wall biopsy. Ann Ophthalmol *9*:479–484, 1977.

Pischel DK: detachment of vitreous as seen with slit lamp examination. Trans Am Ophthalmol Soc *50*:329–346, 1952.

Pollard ZF, Jarrett WH, Hagler WS, et al: ELISA for diagnosis of ocular toxocariasis. Ophthalmology *86*:743–749, 1979.

Pruett R, Schepens CL: Posterior hyperplastic primary vitreous. Am J Ophthalmol *69*:535–543, 1970.

Reese AB: Persistence and hyperplasia of primary vitreous: Retrolental fibroplasia—two entities. Arch Ophthalmol *41*:527–549, 1949.

Reese AB: Persistent hyperplastic primary vitreous. Am J Ophthalmol *40*:317–331, 1955.

Reese AB, Payne F: Persistence and hyperplasia of the primary vitreous. Am J Ophthalmol *29*:1–19, 1964.

Ricci MA: Clinique et transmission hereditaire des degenerescences vitreo-retiniennes. Bull Soc Ophthalmol Fr *9*:618–662, 1961.

Robertson DM, Link RP, Rostvold JA: Snowflake degeneration of the retina. Ophthalmology *89*:1513–1517, 1982.

Rodman HI, Johnson FB, Zimmerman LE: New histopathological and histochemical observations concerning asteroid hyalitis. Arch Ophthalmol *66*:552–563, 1961.

Rossi A: Structure of the vitreous body. Br J Ophthalmol *37*:343–348, 1953.

Rudolph R, Guber J, Suzuki M, Woodward M: The life cycle of the myofibroblast. Surg Gynecol Obstet *145*:389–394, 1977.

Sabates FN: Juvenile retinoschisis. Am J Ophthalmol *62*:683–688, 1966.

Sato K, Tsunakawa N, Inaba K, Yanagisawa Y: Fluorescein angiography on retinal detachment and lattice degenerations. I. Equatorial degeneration with idiopathic retinal detachment. Acta Soc Ophthalmol Jap *75*:635–642, 1971.

Schepens CL: Subclinical retinal detachments. Arch Ophthalmol *47*:593–606, 1952.

Schreiner RL, McAlister WH, Marshall RE, Shearer WT: Stickler syndrome in a pedigree of Pierre Robin syndrome. Am J Dis Child *126*:86–90, 1973.

Schulman J, Jampol LM, Schwartz H: Peripheral proliferative retinopathy. Am J Ophthalmol *90*:509–514, 1980.

Schwartz MF, Green WR, Michels RG, et al: An unusual case of ocular involvement in primary systemic non-familial amyloidosis. Ophthalmology *89*:394–401, 1982.

Schwarz W: Electron microscopic observations in the human vitreous body, *in* Smeltzer GK (ed): The Structure of the Eye. New York, Academic Press, 1961, pp 283–291.

Slusher MM, Hutton WE: Familial exudative vitreoretinopathy. Am J Ophthalmol *87*:152–156, 1979.

Smith JL: Asteroid hyalitis: Incidence of diabetes and hypercholesterolemia. JAMA *168*:891–893, 1958.

Snip RC, Michels RG: Pars plana vitrectomy in the management of endogenous *Candida* endophthalmitis. Am J Ophthalmol *82*:699–704, 1976.

Stickler GB, Belau PG, Farrell FJ, et al: Hereditary progressive arthro-ophthalmopathy. Mayo Clin Proc *40*:443–455, 1965.

Straatsma BR, Allen RA: Lattice degeneration of the retina. Trans Am Acad Ophthalmol Otolaryngol *66*:600–613, 1962.

Straatsma BR, Zeegan PD, Foos RY, et al: Lattice degeneration of the retina (XXX Edward Jackson Memorial Lecture). Am J Ophthalmol *77*:619–649, 1974.

Streeten BW, Bert M: The retinal surface in lattice degeneration of the retina. Am J Ophthalmol *74*:1201–1209, 1972.

Sugita G, Tano Y, Machemer R, et al: Intravitreal autotransplantation of fibroblasts. Am J Ophthalmol *89*:121–130, 1980.

Suran AA, McEwen WK: Diffusion studies with ox vitreous body. Am J Ophthalmol *51*:814–819, 1961.

Terson A: Le syndrome de l'hématome du corps vitré et de l'hémorragie intracranienne spontanée. Ann Ocul *163*:666, 1926.

Tolentino FI, Schepens CL, Freeman HM: Vitreoretinal Disorders. Philadelphia, W. B. Saunders Company, 1976.

Topilow HW, Kenyon KR, Takahashi M, et al: Asteroid hyalosis: Biomicroscopy, ultrastructure and composition. Arch Ophthalmol, in press.

Tudor RC, Blair E: *Gnathostoma spinigerum*: An unusual cause of ocular nematodiasis in the Western hemisphere. Am J Ophthalmol *72*:185–190, 1971.

Turner G: The Stickler syndrome in a family with the Pierre Robin syndrome and severe myopia. Aust Paediatr J *10*:103–108, 1974.

Van Balen ATM, Falger ELF: Hereditary hyaloideoretinal degeneration and palatoschisis. Arch Ophthalmol *83*:152–162, 1970.

Vanderlinden RG, Chisholm LD: Vitreous hemorrhages and sudden increased intracranial pressure. J Neurosurg *41*:167–176, 1974.

Verhoeff FH: Microscopic findings in a case of asteroid hyalitis. Am J Ophthalmol *4*:155–160, 1921.

Vogel MH, Font RL, Zimmerman LE, Levine RA: Reticulum cell sarcoma of the retina and uvea. Am J Ophthalmol *66*:205–215, 1968.

Wadsworth JAC: The vitreous: Gross and microscopic observations seen in age and disease with special emphasis on the role of vitreous in detachment of the retina. Trans Am Ophthalmol Soc *54*:709–728, 1956.

Wagner H: Ein bisher unbekanntes Erbleiden des Auges (Degeneratio hyaloideo-retinalis hereditaria), beobachtet im Kanton Zurich. Klin Monatsbl Augenheilkd *100*:840–857, 1938.

Wand M, Gorn RA: Cholesterolosis of the anterior chamber. Am J Ophthalmol *78*:143–144, 1974.

Welch RB, Maumenee AE, Wahlen HE: Peripheral posterior segment inflammation, vitreous opacities and edema of the posterior pole: Pars planitis. Arch Ophthalmol *64*:540–549, 1960.

Wilder HC: Nematode endophthalmitis. Trans Am Acad Ophthalmol Otolaryngol *55*:99–109, 1950.

Wilkinson CP, Welch RB: Intraocular *Toxocara*. Am J Ophthalmol *71*:921–930, 1971.

Wong VG, McFarlin DE: Primary familial amyloidosis. Arch Ophthalmol *78*:208–213, 1967.

Woodruff AW: Toxocariasis. Br Med J *3*:663–669, 1970.

Yanoff M, Font RL: Intraocular cartilage in a microphthalmic eye of an otherwise healthy girl. Arch Ophthalmol *181*:238–240, 1969.

Yanoff M, Rahn EH, Zimmerman LE: Histopathology of juvenile retinoschisis. Arch Ophthalmol *79*:49–53, 1968.

CHAPTER

8

RETINA

W. Richard Green

ANATOMY AND HISTOLOGY

The retina is composed of the tissues arising from the optic vesicle and consists of a pigment layer derived from the outer wall of the optic cup and a complex sensory layer derived from the inner wall.

Retinal Pigment Epithelium (RPE)

The retinal pigment epithelium (RPE) (Zinn, Benjamin-Henkind, 1979) is a single layer of hexagonal-shaped cells with a quite regular arrangement (Fig. 8–1). This epithelium extends from the margin of the optic disk to the ora serrata. From that point forward in the eye, the RPE is continuous with the pigment epithelium of the ciliary body. Internally, the epithelial layer is adjacent to the photoreceptors, and, externally, it is attached to Bruch's membrane. At the margin of the disk, the epithelial layer gradually becomes thinner, and it ends slightly before the termination of Bruch's membrane. In the posterior part of the eye, the RPE cells are fairly uniform in size and shape and measure approximately 16 microns in diameter. In the midperiphery and equatorial area, the cells are thinner and larger in diameter. In the far periphery, the RPE cells are quite variable in size, and some are enlarged. RPE cells have a rounded nucleus that is situated close to the base in the posterior part of the eye; in the peripheral portion, many cells contain two or more nuclei. Each cell has an apical surface that faces the rods and cones and a basal surface adjacent to Bruch's membrane (Fig. 8–2).

The lateral surfaces of each of the cells are closely applied to each other and are joined by junctional complexes. The basal surface of each cell has a convoluted cell membrane with infoldings. Along the entire basal surface of the RPE cells is a basal lamina, which is separated from

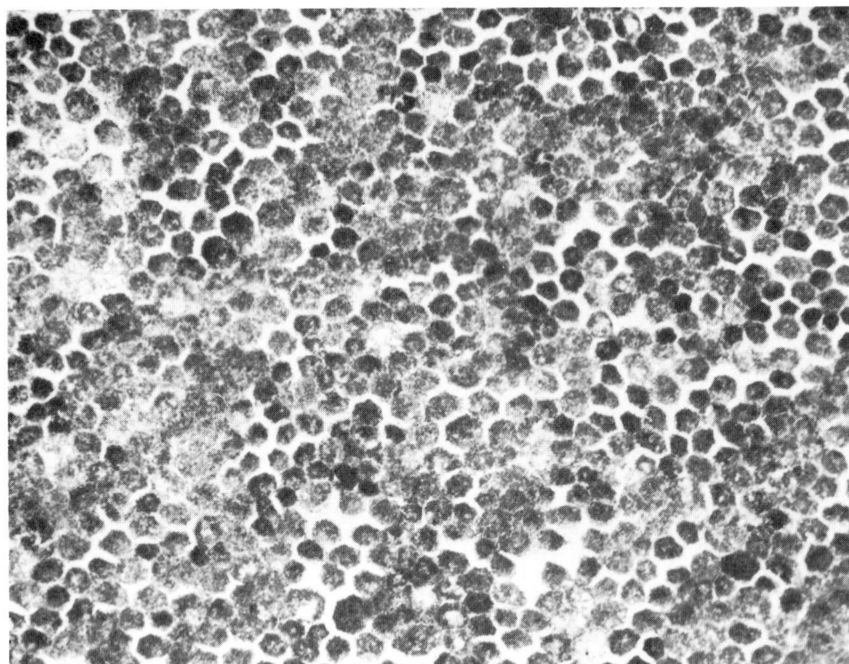

Figure 8–1. Flat preparation of **retinal pigment epithelium (RPE)**. Unstained, ×225. EP 29544.

the convoluted infoldings by a narrow space. The basal lamina is closely applied to the collagenous tissue in Bruch's membrane. The apical surface of each cell possesses complex foldings, or villi, directed toward the photoreceptors. These frondlike villi extend internally to surround the external portion of the outer segments of the photoreceptor system. The outer segments of the rods extend to the surface of the cell, where they are surrounded by the RPE villi; this is in contrast to the cones, which terminate at a greater distance from the cell surface so that the villi that extend in to surround their outer segments are much longer and more complex than those of the rods. The lateral surfaces between the RPE cells are characterized by occluding junctions (or zonulae occludentes) near the apical surfaces, but the intercellular space is narrow and open in the external third of the intercellular region.

The cytoplasm of the RPE cells contains oval or rounded pigment granules that mostly are located near the apical side. The granules often extend into the apical villi around the photoreceptor outer segments. The cytoplasm contains numerous organelles, including an abundant content of smooth endoplasmic reticulum. With increasing age, a number of other pigment granules composed of lipofuscin are found in the cytoplasm (Feeney-Burns, 1980). Also present in the cytoplasm of the RPE cells are structures known as phagosomes, which are produced by phagocytosis of groups of discs from the rod and cone outer segments by the apical villi. These phagosomes are gradually digested by enzymes derived from the organelles in the cytoplasm of the RPE cells, and their products are often cast off into Bruch's membrane or are retained in the cytoplasm to become lipofuscin granules. In the fovea of the macular region, the epithelial cells are taller, narrower, and darker.

Sensory Retina

The sensory retina is a delicate, transparent layer. It is firmly attached only at two points: posteriorly at the optic disc and anteriorly at the ora serrata, where it terminates. Elsewhere the attachment to the underlying retinal pigment epithelium is rather weak, and is maintained by the intraocular pressure and by the contacts between the photoreceptor outer segments and the RPE villi, a mucopolysaccharide cementing substance surrounding the photoreceptors and probably active transport processes. The internal surface of the retina is adjacent to the vitreous at the internal limiting membrane of the retina. In young persons, the two structures are rather firmly bound to each other by collagenous filaments; with increasing age and syneresis of the vitreous, the connections between the two become tenuous.

Anatomically, the retina gradually terminates at the optic disk by reduction of the nuclear and synaptic layers and the Müller cells and disappearance of the photoreceptors. The nerve fiber layer, however, increases in thickness at the edge of the disc and is the only retinal structure that continues into the disc and eventually becomes the optic nerve.

It is not easy to picture the complex microscopic anatomy of the retina because of the delicacy and perishability of the tissue. Postmortem

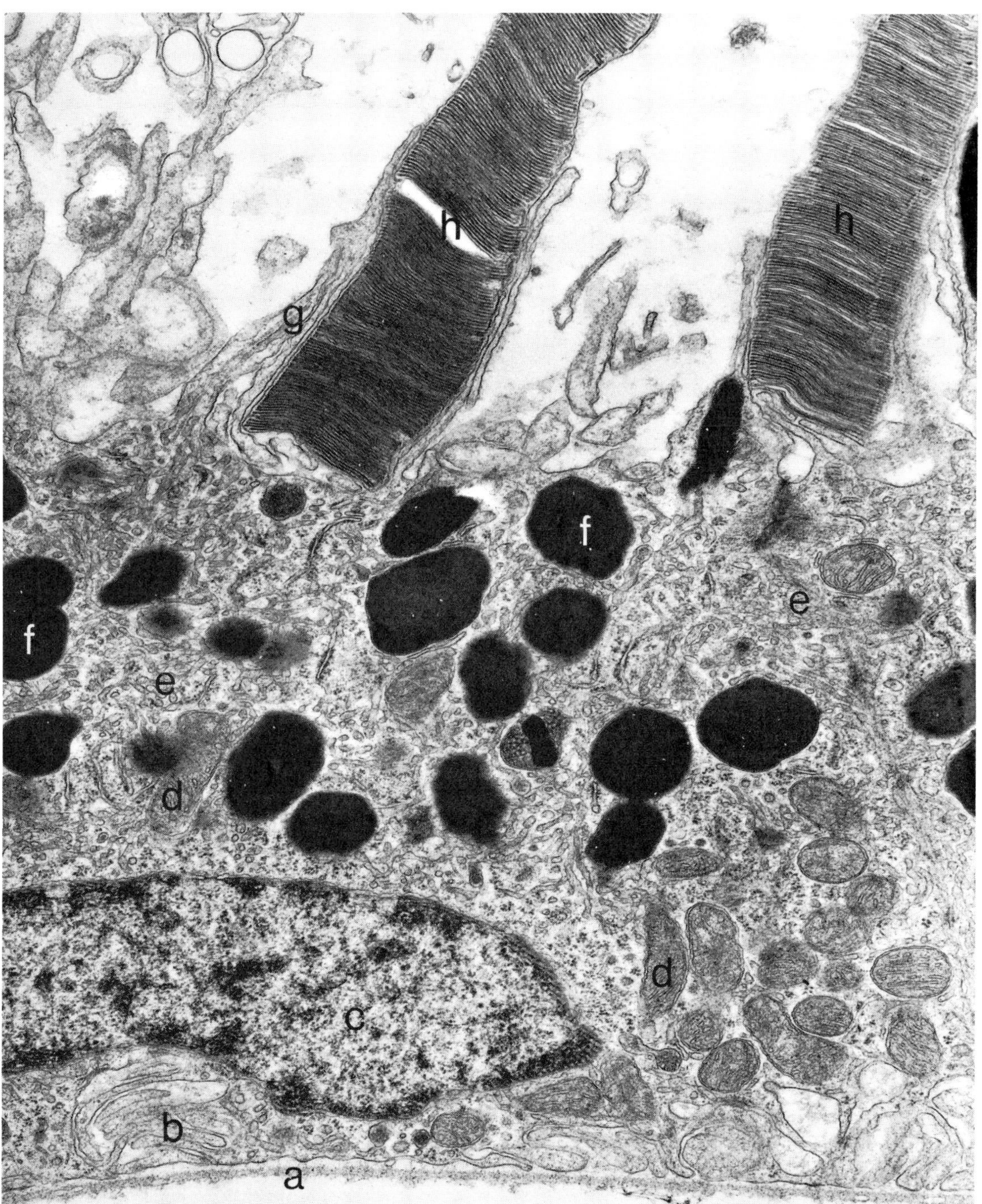

Figure 8–2. Electron micrograph of the **retinal pigment epithelium (RPE)** to show its relation to the rod outer segments. The RPE basement membrane is at *(a);* the basal infoldings of its cell membrane are at *(b);* the nucleus is at *(c);* and the external cytoplasm contains numerous mitochondria *(d)*. Characteristically, there is a large amount of reticulum *(e)*. The pigment granules *(f)* are located mainly in the apical portion of the cell. Microvilli *(g)* along the apical surfaces of these cells extend internally to surround the outer segments of the photoreceptors *(h)*. ×18,000. (Courtesy of Hogan MJ, Alvarado JA, Weddell JE: Histology of the Human Eye. Philadelphia, W.B. Saunders Company, 1971, p 409.)

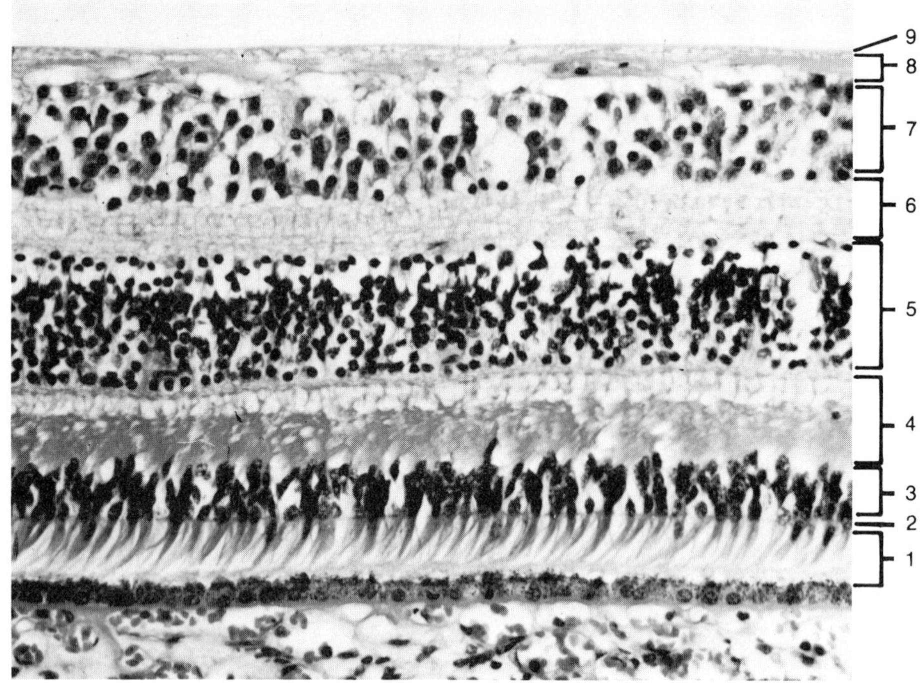

Figure 8–3. The nine layers of the sensory retina. (1) Layer of the outer and inner segments of the photoreceptors of the rods and cones; (2) the external limiting membrane; (3) outer nuclear layer; (4) outer plexiform layer; (5) inner nuclear layer; (6) inner plexiform layer; (7) ganglion cell layer; (8) nerve fiber layer; and (9) internal limiting membrane. H and E, ×170. EP 36477.

changes and artefacts are common in many retinal specimens, and for this reason ordinary histologic techniques and staining methods do not adequately reveal its structural details. Special stains, employing silver and gold, customarily have been used to demonstrate the glia and neurons. Additionally, a combination of thin serial sectioning of plastic-embedded tissue and the study by both light and electron microscopy have revealed much about the structure of the retina and the interconnections of the various layers.

The sensory retina is considered to be made up of nine layers (Fig. 8–3). From outside inward, these are (1) the layer of photoreceptors of the rods and cones, (2) the external limiting membrane, (3) the outer nuclear layer, (4) the outer plexiform layer, (5) the inner nuclear layer, which contains nuclei of horizontal cells, bipolar cells, amacrine cells, and Müller cells; (6) the inner plexiform layer, (7) the ganglion cell layer, (8) the nerve fiber layer, and (9) the internal limiting membrane.

The retinal layers are connected to each other by a complex of axons and dendrites, which forms synaptic connections in the inner and outer plexiform layers and to the ganglion cells. The neurons are supported by a system of supporting fibers composed of the Müller cells and astrocytes in the inner portion of the retina.

The layer of **rods and cones** has a layered arrangement of their constituent elements. Each rod and cone is composed of an outer and inner segment. The outer segments contain the disks, and the inner segments contain the mitochondria and other enzyme-producing organelles. The inner segments of the cones are large and are filled with mitochrondria, whereas the rods are longer and more cylindrical and contain fewer mitochondria. The outer segment of the rod is long and extends to the apical side of the RPE, whereas that of the cone is shorter and terminates earlier. Different areas of the retina contain different proportions of rods and cones. At the fovea, only cones are found, and these are long and slender, resembling rods. The cones become relatively scarcer toward the retinal periphery.

A mucoid extracellular interstitial substance surrounds the rod and cone outer and inner segments and also the villi of the RPE. This mucopolysaccharide is complex and is composed of a variety of mucoprotein substances. The mucopolysaccharide does not stain with ordinary dyes but can be detected by special stains, such as the Alcian blue and colloidal iron techniques. The mucopolysaccharide is mostly resistant to digestion by hyaluronidase.

The **external limiting membrane** (Fig. 8–4) is not a true membrane. It is formed by junctional complexes uniting the Müller cells to the photoreceptor cell inner segments (Fig. 8–5). A junc-

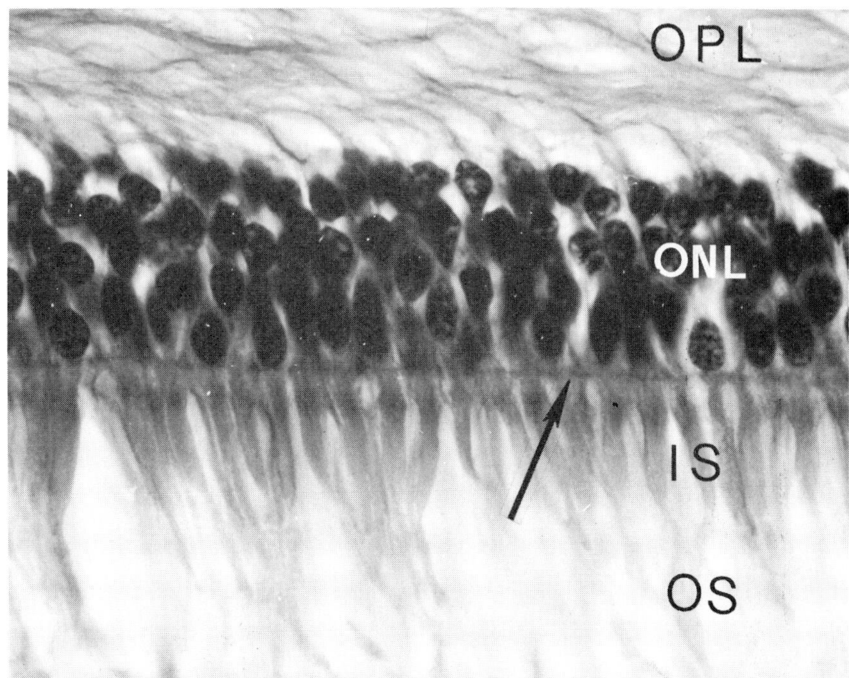

Figure 8–4. Outer nuclear layer *(ONL),* external limiting membrane (arrow), outer plexiform layer *(OPL),* inner segments *(IS),* and outer segments *(OS)* of photoreceptor cells. H and E, ×900. EP 46511.

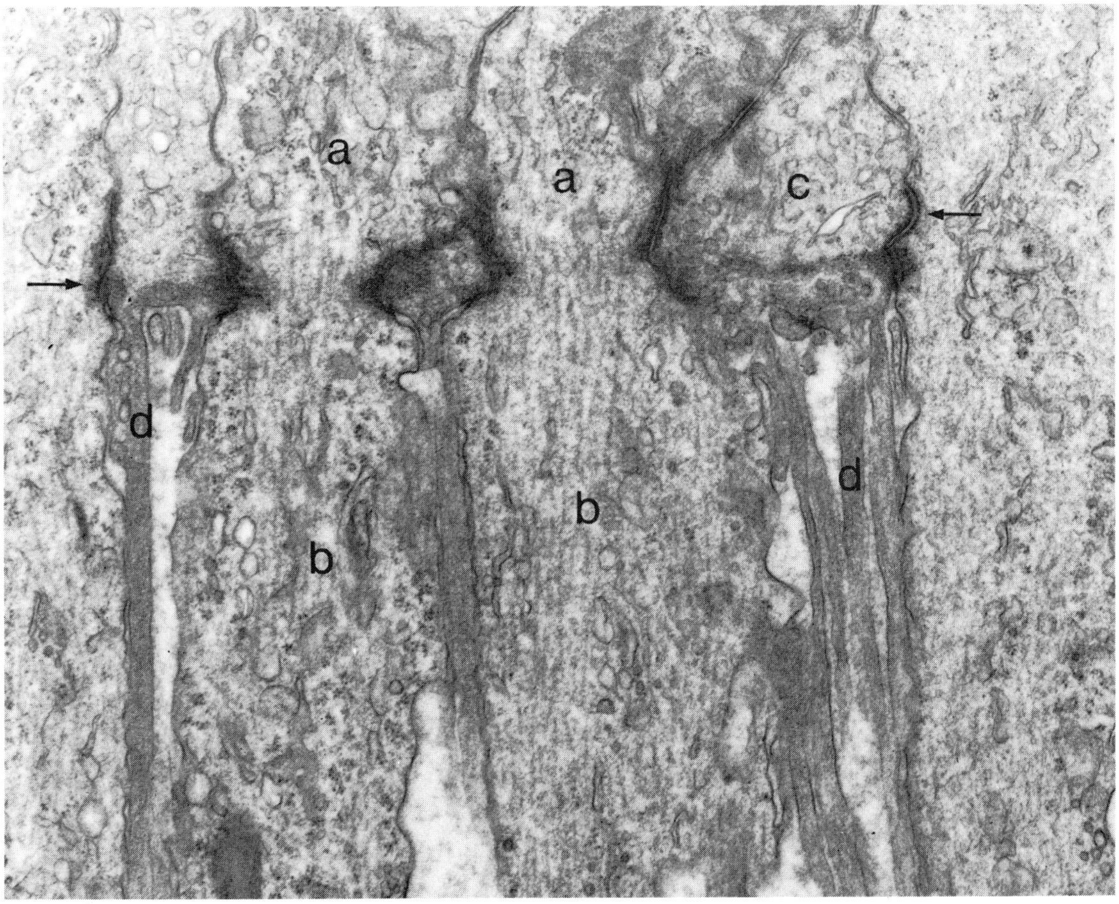

Figure 8–5. The external limiting membrane (arrows) in meridional section. The external receptor fibers *(a)* of the rods and cones are continuous with the inner segments of the photoreceptors *(b)*. These fibers are separated from each other by Müller cell processes *(c)* that are continuous with the Müller cell fiber baskets *(d)* and continue beyond the external limiting membrane. ×18,000. (Courtesy of Hogan MJ, Alvarado JA, Weddell JE: Histology of the Human Eye. Philadelphia, W.B. Saunders Company, 1971, p 482.)

tional complex like this is known as a zonula adherens. Occasionally, the connections are between Müller cells themselves or between neurons. The inner segments of the rods and cones extend past these junctional complexes to the external nuclear layer of the retina.

The Müller cells extend fine fibrils externally between the inner segments of the rod and cone photoreceptors for a short distance. These fibrils are believed to play a part in the formation of the complex mucopolysaccharides that lie in this region.

The **outer nuclear layer** is composed of eight or nine layers of cells with densely staining nuclei—the cell bodies of the photoreceptor cells. Two kinds of cells can be identified on the basis of nuclear morphology. The smaller, more densely staining nuclei belong to the rods; the larger, more weakly stained nuclei, which tend to lie just within the external limiting membrane, belong to the cones. Occasionally, cone nuclei are found to be displaced into the rod and cone layer as a normal variation (Fig. 8–6; see also Figs. 8–92,*B*, 8–106, 8–428,*C*, and 8–474,*A*). Gartner and Henkind

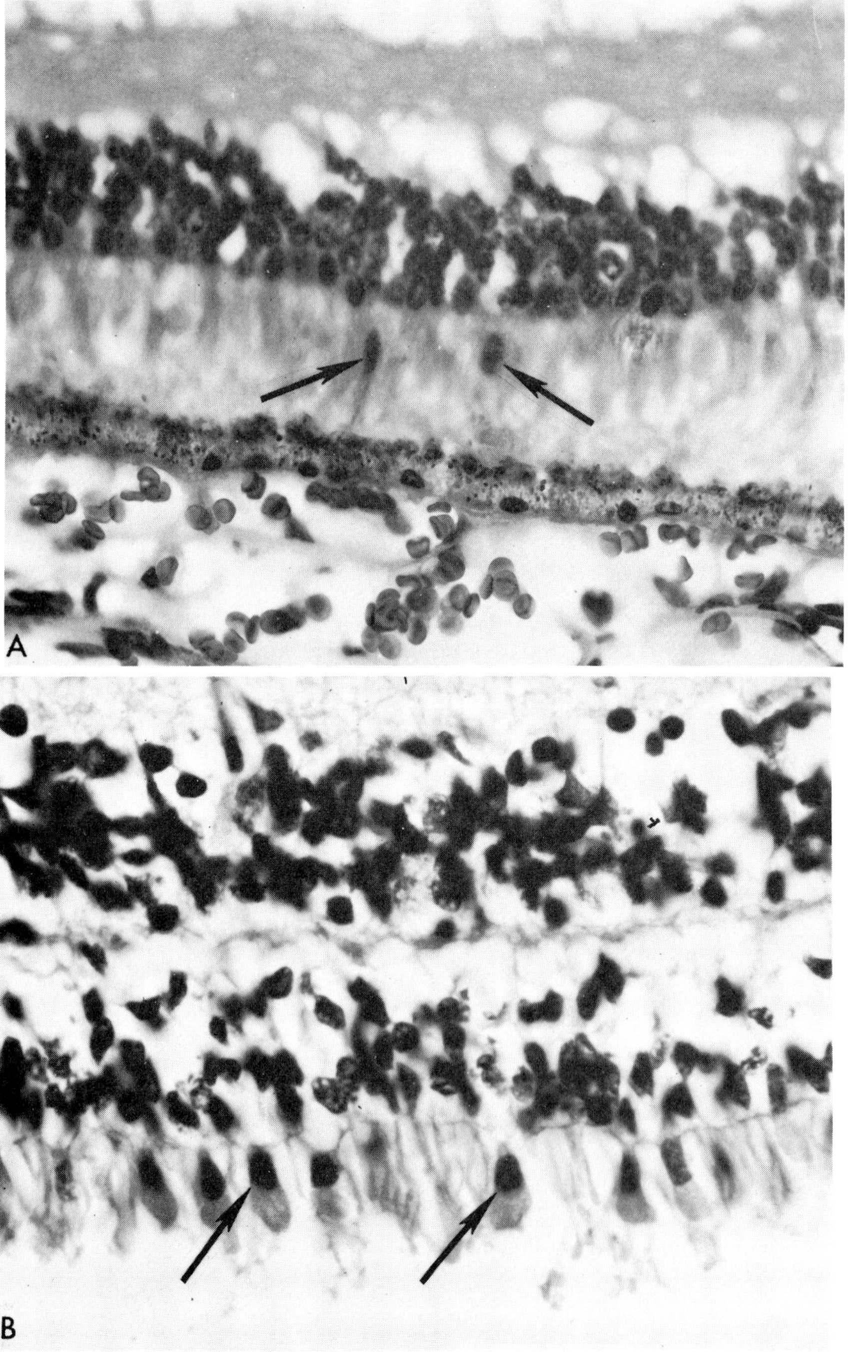

Figure 8–6. Peripapillary *(A)* and macular area *(B)* showing migration of cone nuclei (arrows) in the inner segment area. *A,* H and E, ×575; EP 5174. *B,* H and E, ×750; EP 51159.

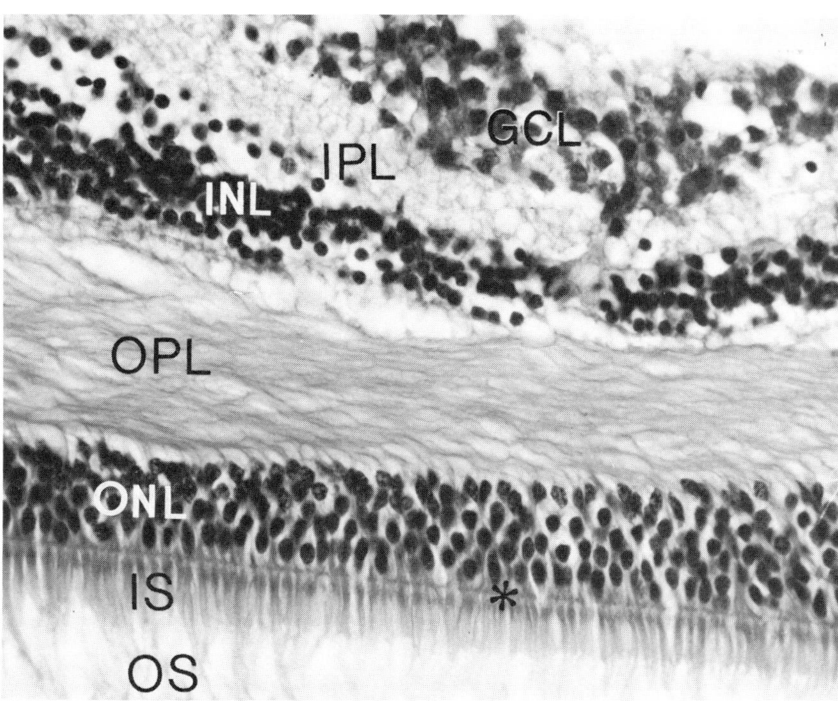

Figure 8–7. Parafoveal area showing tangential orientation of the fibers in the outer plexiform layer *(OPL)* (Henle's fiber layer), ganglion cell layer *(GCL),* inner plexiform layer *(IPL),* inner nuclear layer *(INL),* outer nuclear layer *(ONL),* external limiting membrane (asterisk), inner segments *(IS),* and outer segments *(OS)* of photoreceptor cells. H and E, ×500. EP 46511.

(1981a) have attributed such displacement of nuclei to an aging change. Dendrites extend from both types of outer nuclear cells into the outer plexiform layer, where they synapse with the rod and cone bipolar cells and also with horizontal cells and other bipolar cells. The rod dendrites terminate in a spherule, and the cone dendrites terminate in a peduncle. The Müller cells fill out all the space between the processes of the rods and cones and also between the bipolar and horizontal cells.

The **outer plexiform layer** (Fig. 8–7) consists of axons, from the rod and cone cells, forming synaptic junctions with dendrites from the bipolar cells and horizontal cells. The fibers in this layer are loosely arranged and form a delicate network when viewed with the light microscope. In the macular region, the axons and dendrites of the outer plexiform layer are greatly elongated and radiate outward from the foveal region, to form the fiber layer of Henle (Fig. 8–7).

The **inner nuclear layer** is a closely packed mass of cells resembling the outer nuclear layer, but it is generally thinner. The complicated structure of this layer has been revealed by special staining methods and by electron microscopy. Three types of neurons are present in this layer. The *bipolar cells* have dendrites that are in contact with the axons of the rod and cone cells in the outer plexiform layer. Their axons extend into the inner plexiform layer, forming synapses with the dendrites of the ganglion cells and with the amacrine cells. The *horizontal cells* lie at the external surface of this layer and have long and complex arborizing processes in the outer plexiform layer that synapse with the spherules and peduncles of the rod and cone axons and also with adjacent bipolar cells. Occasional processes extend from the horizontal cells into the inner plexiform layer. The *amacrine cells* are pear-shaped and lie at the inner aspect of the inner nuclear layer. They have processes that extend into the internal plexiform layer, where they synapse widely with the dendrites of the ganglion cells and with the bipolar axons. The nuclei and cell bodies of the Müller cells are also found in the inner nuclear layer. The Müller cells send fibers internally to form the internal limiting membrane and externally to form the zonulae adherens that compose the external limiting membrane.

The **inner plexiform layer** consists of a fine reticulum of axons and dendrites; several sublayers may be recognized. This layer is formed by the synapses of the bipolar cells, the amacrine cells, and the ganglion cells.

The **ganglion cell layer** consists of a row of ganglion cells separated from each other by the processes of Müller cells and neuroglia. The ganglion cells are multipolar, with large nuclei and prominent Nissl granules. Their numerous dendrites arise in the inner plexiform layer, and their long axons extend along the nerve fiber layer of the retina, eventually constituting the optic nerve at the disc. In the macular region of the retina, the ganglion cells are much more numerous, forming a layer two to eight cells deep, but elsewhere mostly they form a single cell layer.

The **nerve fiber layer** is composed almost entirely of the axons of the ganglion cells, which extend via the optic nerve to the brain. This layer

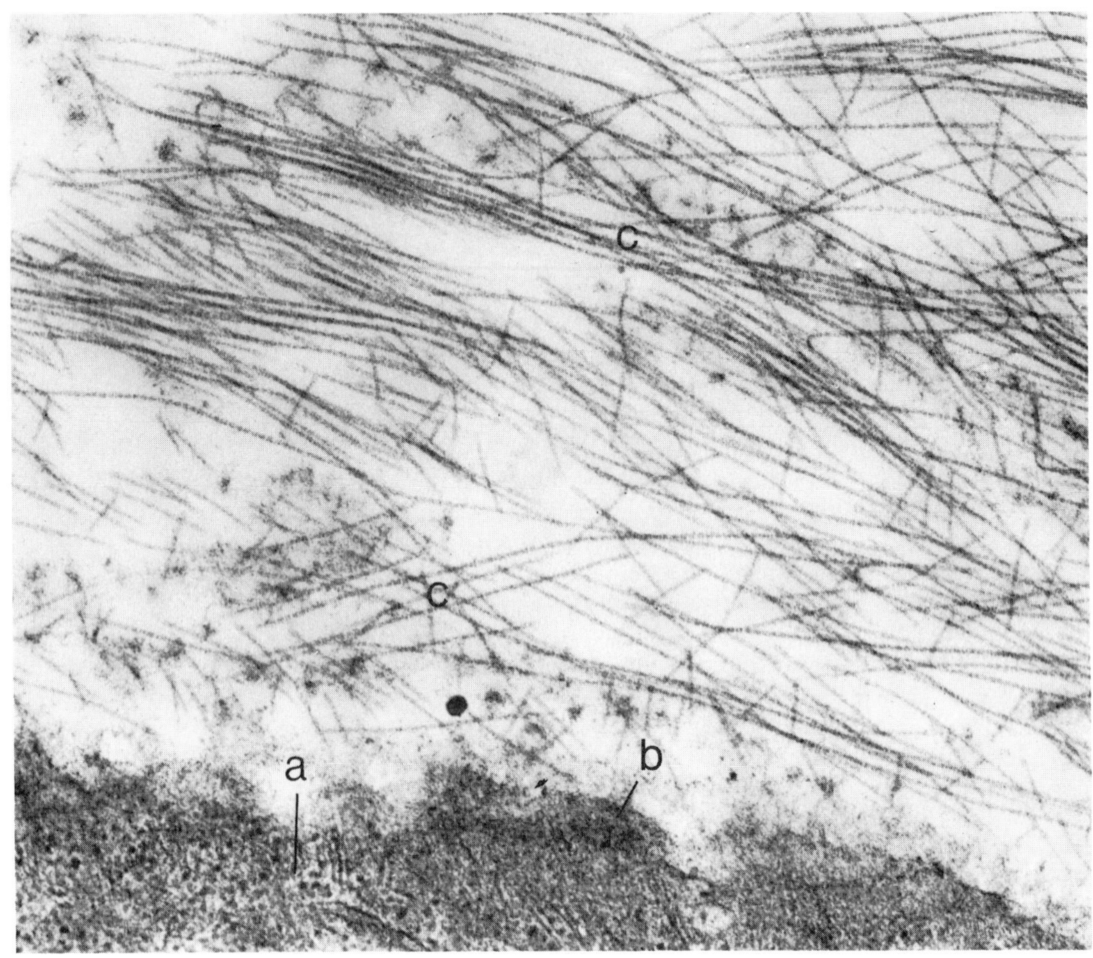

Figure 8–8. The vitreous base in the region of the peripheral retina. The Müller cells *(a)* have a basement membrane *(b)* that forms the inner limiting membrane of the retina. The collagen fibrils *(c)* of the vitreous base form a meshwork internal to the retina. These fibrils join the internal limiting membrane. ×50,000. (Courtesy of Hogan MJ, Alvarado JA, Weddell JE: Histology of the Human Eye. Philadelphia, W.B. Saunders Company, 1971, p 442.)

also contains some neuroglia, mainly astrocytes, of varying sizes and shapes. Because the nerve axons radiate toward the optic disk, it follows that this layer is thickest near the disk because of the accumulation of the fibers from the retina as they converge on the disk.

The **internal limiting membrane (ILM)** in the normal eye of a young person is a very delicate, basement membrane structure applied to the footplate-like extensions of the Müller fibers. The ILM is actually the basal lamina of the Müller cells, but occasionally the basal lamina is formed by astrocytic processes. The ILM becomes attenuated or is absent in the foveola, over major retinal vessels, and at the optic nerve head. The fine collagenous fibrils from the cortical vitreous are attached to and blend with this basal lamina (Fig. 8–8). Occasionally, broad, flat cells containing rod-shaped and reniform nuclei are present along the inner surface of the inner limiting membrane, but these are probably identical with the vitreous cells (hyalocytes), which may be macrophages or fibrocyte-like cells in the cortical vitreous, as described by Szirmai and Balazs (1958).

Special staining methods and electron microscopy reveal several types of glia in the retina:

(1) Müller's fibers form a protoplasmic skeleton or framework throughout the thickness of the retina to support and surround the nerve cells and their axons and dendrites (Fig. 8–9). The inner ends of the **Müller cells** form a mosaic pattern known as the internal limiting membrane. The outer processes form the outer limiting membrane, through which the rod and cone inner segments extend. Kuwabara and Cogan (1959) and Cogan and Kuwabara (1959b) have found Müller's fibers to reduce tetrazolium, indicating the presence of dehydrogenase and suggesting a further function of these scaffolding cells. The cytoplasm also contains a considerable amount of glycogen.

(2) Large numbers of cells have processes in the nerve fiber layer, ganglion cell layer, and inner plexiform layer. The branching processes of these cells run in a plane at right angles to the

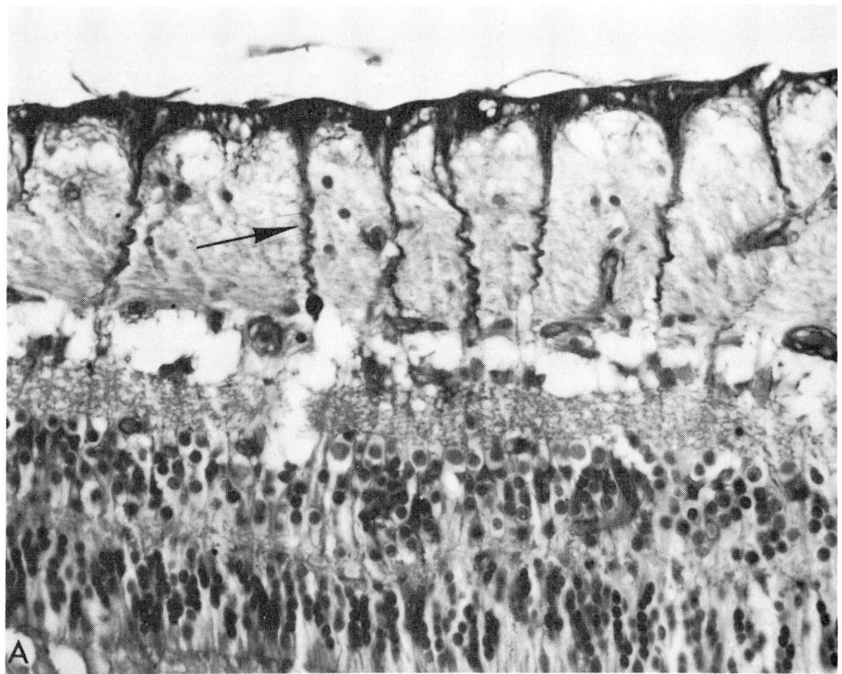

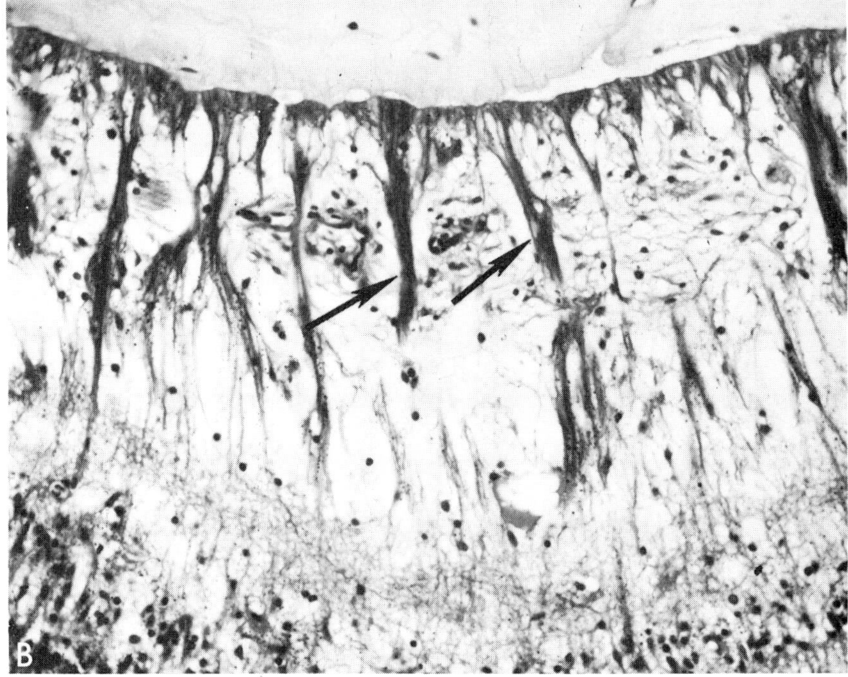

Figure 8–9. Müller cells (arrows) with broad footplates as they approach and become continuous with the internal limiting membrane. *A,* Peripapillary area from a patient with diabetes. PAS, ×330. EP 20652. *B,* Edema of posterior retina in eye with peripheral vascular changes of Coats' disease. PAS, ×210. EP 51883.

Müller fibers and have no close connection with them. With the electron microscope, these cells have all the characteristics of astrocytes.

(3) Occasional astrocytes are present in the ganglion cell and inner plexiform layers. They are star-shaped, with round nuclei and a number of slender processes. They also are arranged horizontally and surround the vessels with a dense network of fibers. They form an archlike, honeycomb structure that surrounds and supports the nerve axons derived from the ganglion cells. They frequently have strong attachments to the surfaces of the blood vessels.

The structure of the **macular region** affords maximal visual acuity, and thus several modifications in retinal architecture have taken place. The area centralis encompasses a zone measuring 5.85 mm that is located in the posterior pole. This zone is subdivided into the foveola, fovea, parafoveal, and perifoveal areas on the basis of morphologic features (Hogan, Alvarado, Weddell, 1971, pages 491–498; Warwick, 1976). There are

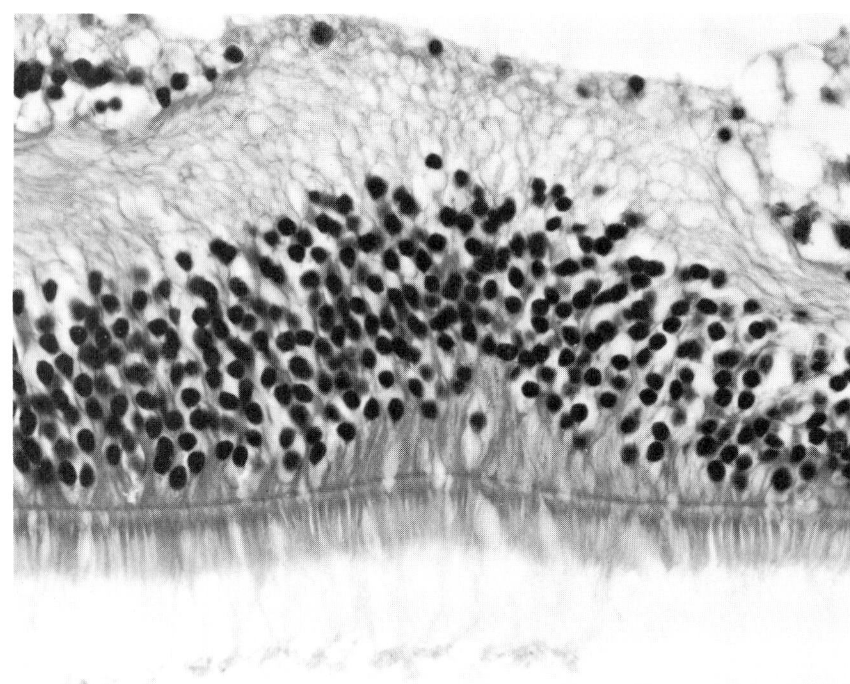

Figure 8–10. Accumulation of specialized cones in the center of the fovea causes a bow-shaped configuration—the umbo. H and E, ×110. EP 46511.

no retinal vessels in the fovea to hinder photic reception or to cast shadows. There are no rods in the fovea, but the cones have become so modified that they resemble rods in form. The external segments of the cones are long and approach the apical side of the retinal pigment epithelial cells. The accumulation of a large number of these specialized cones in the foveola causes a forward, bow-shaped configuration—the umbo (Fig. 8–10). At the edge of the fovea and extending away from it, there is thickening of the ganglion cell layer and the inner nuclear layer, but both layers disappear within the fovea (Fig. 8–11). In the foveola area, only photoreceptor cells are present; the design is such as to afford the highest functional capacity. Each cone is united with but a single bipolar cell and possibly with a single ganglion cell, thus yielding maximal transmission of the stimulus.

The retina terminates at the ora serrata. Here, the many layers resolve themselves into a single layer of cells that is continued into the ciliary body as the nonpigmented epithelium. As the **retinal periphery** is approached, the external segments of the rods and cones disappear and the inner segments persist as deformed and swollen bulbous structures. There is a relative increase in the number of cones in the far periphery, as compared with the equatorial area. The nuclear layers blend into one, and the ganglion cells and fiber layer end, while the neuroglia and Müller cells increase.

The **vascular system of the retina** is composed of arterial and venous channels with intervening arterioles, capillaries, and venules. A capillary-free zone is present around the arteries (Fig. 8–12). Four main branches of the arteries and veins supply the upper nasal and upper temporal and also the lower nasal and lower temporal areas of the retina. Arterioles branch from the main arteriolar channels near the optic disc and elsewhere in the retina and quickly form a capillary net that is densely distributed throughout the retina, except for the peripheral millimeter near the ora serrata. The venules form a similar pattern and join the capillaries in the spaces between the main branches and also between the arterioles and larger venules. In the peripapillary region are several distinct layers of capillaries: one in the nerve fiber layer (the radial peripapillary capillary network) (Fig. 8–13) and the others distributed in the ganglion cell and internal plexiform layers, but elsewhere in the retina the capillaries are diffusely distributed and do not seem to form definite layers.

Shimizu and Ujiie (1978) have shown by scanning electron microscopy of plastic casts that the retinal capillaries are arranged in well-defined, layered patterns in the lateral and posterior aspects of the retina (Fig. 8–14). In the normal eye, the capillaries have a one-to-one ratio of pericytes and endothelial cells (Fig. 8–15).

The arterial and venous blood vessel system of the retina extends into the retina as far as the inner portion of the inner nuclear layer. Because of this, the inner portion of the retina derives its nutrition from the retinal arterial system; the outer layers, including the outer portion of the inner nuclear layer, derive their nutrition from the choriocapillaris of the choroid.

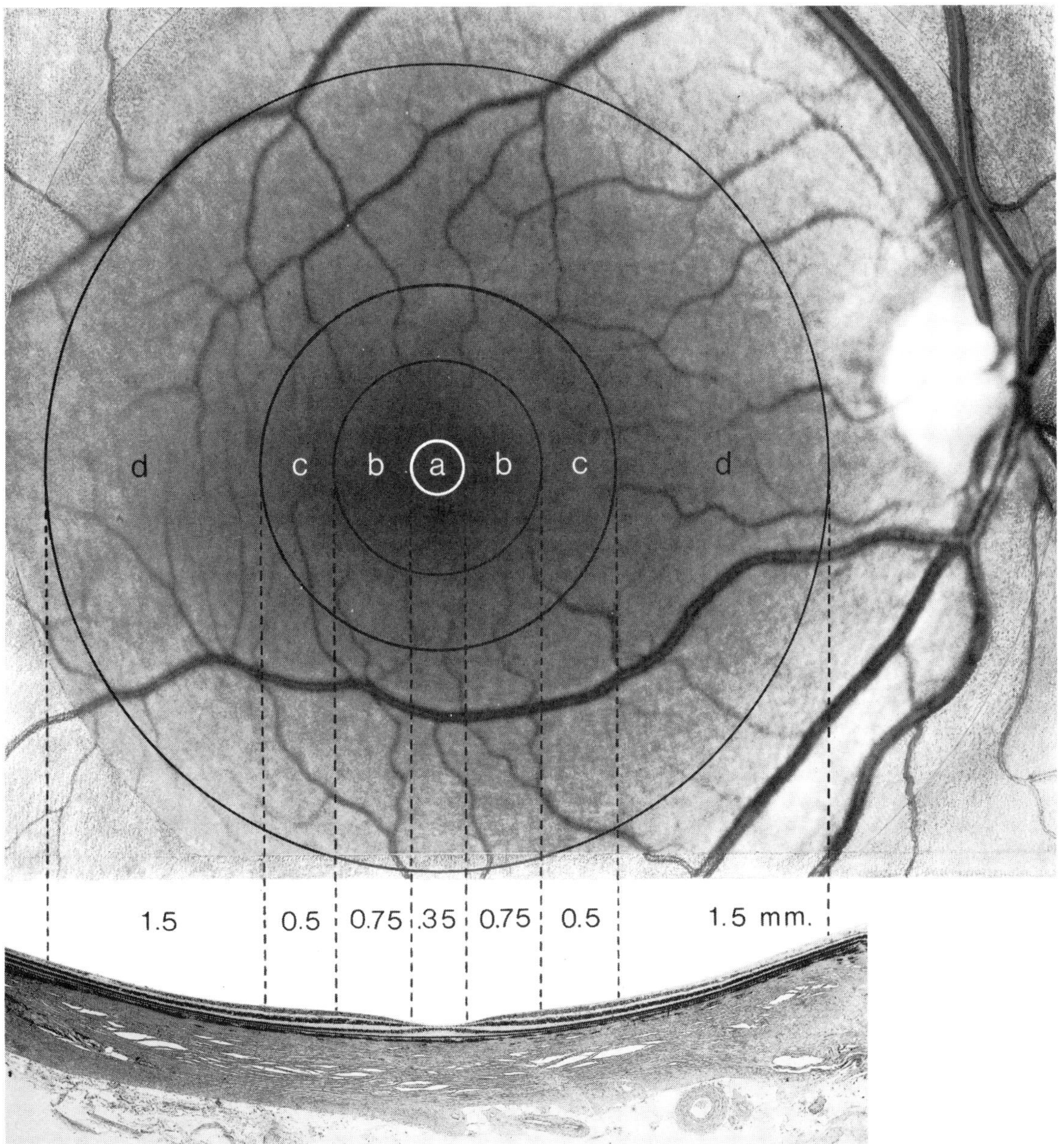

Figure 8–11. This fundus photograph is matched with a meridional light micrograph of the macular region. The fundus photograph shows the foveola *(a)*, fovea *(b)*, parafoveal area *(c)*, and perifoveal region *(d)*. (Courtesy of Hogan MJ, Alvarado JA, Weddell JE: Histology of he Human Eye. Philadelphia, W.B. Saunders Company, 1971, p 491.)

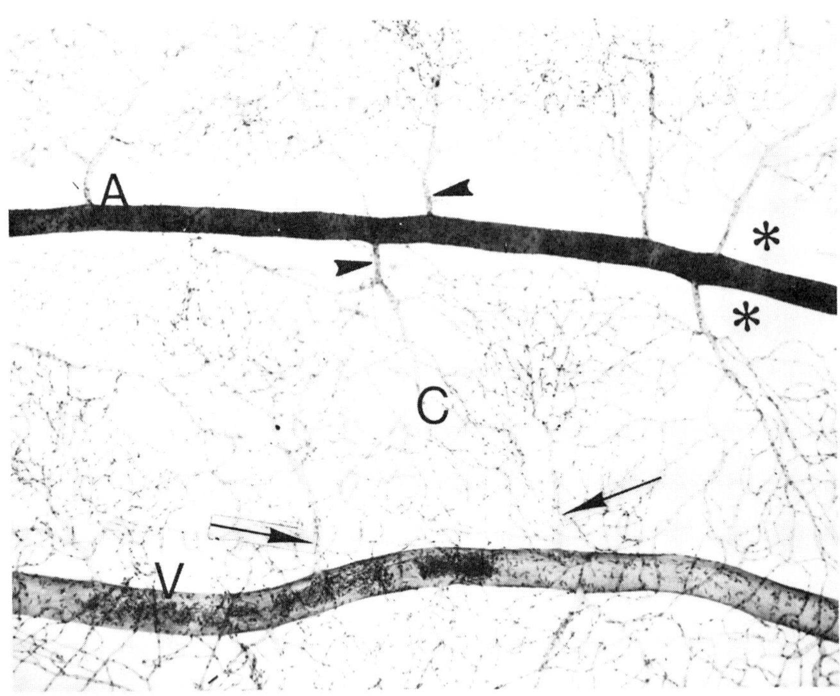

Figure 8–12. Trypsin digestion retinal preparation showing artery *(A),* periarterial capillary-free zone (asterisks), precapillary arterioles (arrowheads), capillaries *(C),* post-capillary venules (arrows), and vein *(V).* H and E; PAS, ×65. EP 44923.

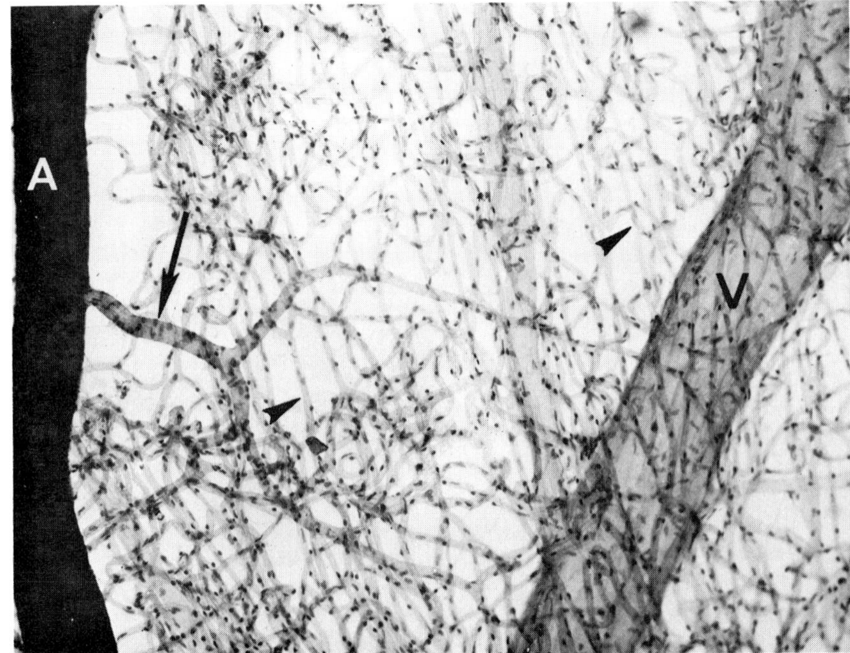

Figure 8–13. Trypsin digestion retinal preparation showing peripapillary area, radial peripapillary capillaries (arrowheads), artery *(A),* vein *(V),* and precapillary arteriole (arrow). H and E; PAS, ×110. EP 44923.

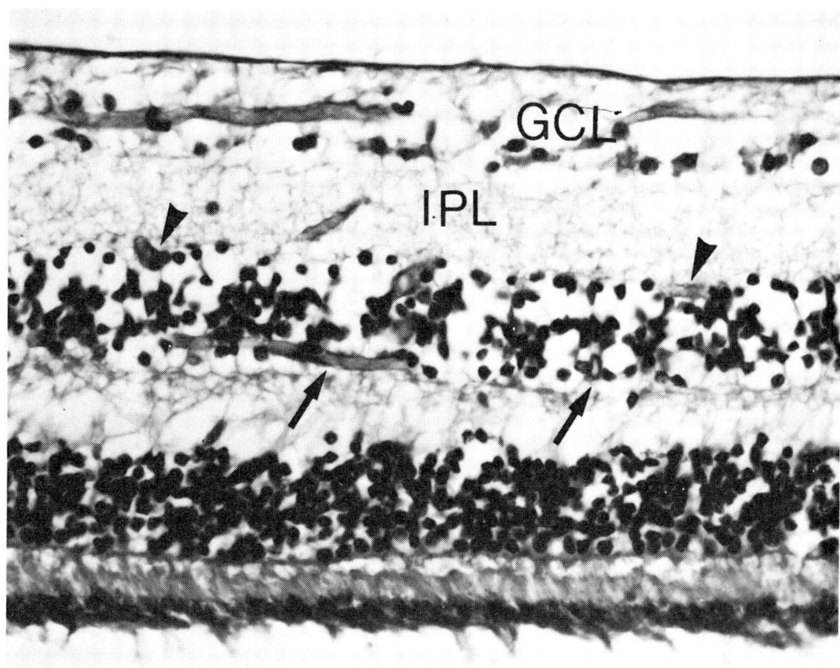

Figure 8–14. Peripapillary retina showing four strata of capillaries: one each in the nerve fiber layer, ganglion cell layer *(GCL)* complex, inner plexiform layer *(IPL)*, and inner (arrowheads) and outer (arrows) portions of the inner nuclear layer. PAS, ×300. EP 45244.

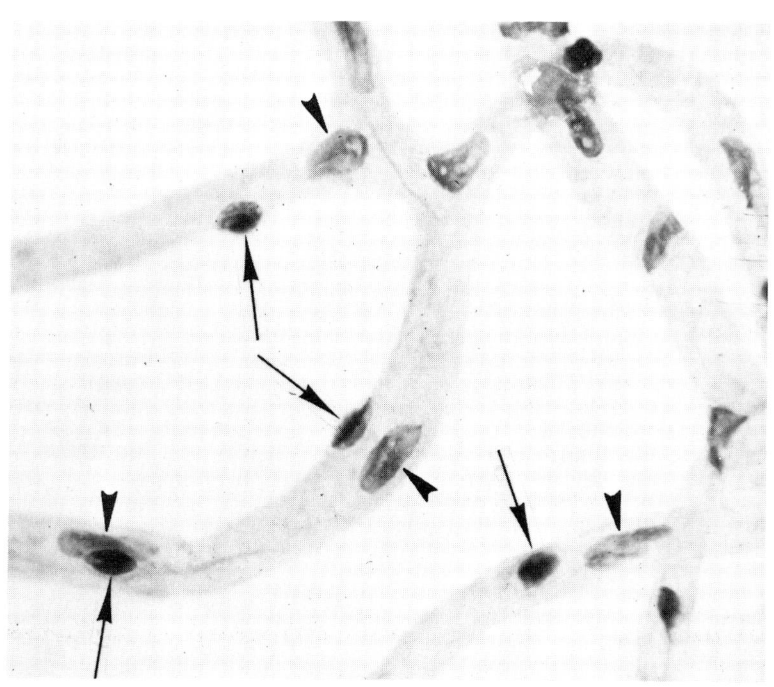

Figure 8–15. Trypsin digestion retinal preparation showing retinal capillaries with a 1:1 ratio of pericytes (arrows) to endothelial cells (arrowheads). H and E; PAS, ×900. EP 44923.

The center of the macular area is free of blood vessels (Fig. 8–16). This capillary-free zone measures 300 to 500 microns and is an important landmark to consider in laser photocoagulation.

GROWTH AND AGING

The human retina is almost fully differentiated at birth. This is quite different from the development of the subprimate retina, in which rod and cone formation takes place after birth. The human macula and fovea, however, complete their differentiation during the first few months after birth. At birth, the fovea contains most of the retinal layers but is incompletely differentiated. At the periphery, the ora serrata is less well developed than in the adult retina, and in the eyes of premature and newborn infants there is a characteristic fold of redundant retina (Lange's fold) on histopathologic examination. This fold appears to be an artefact (Gartner, Henkind, 1981b), caused by either delayed fixation or mild shrinkage of the sclera, and is not observed in the eye of a living infant (Kalina, 1971).

The Retinal Pigment Epithelium

Some differentiation of the the retinal pigment epithelial cells occurs after birth, especially in the macular region. An increase in cell density of the

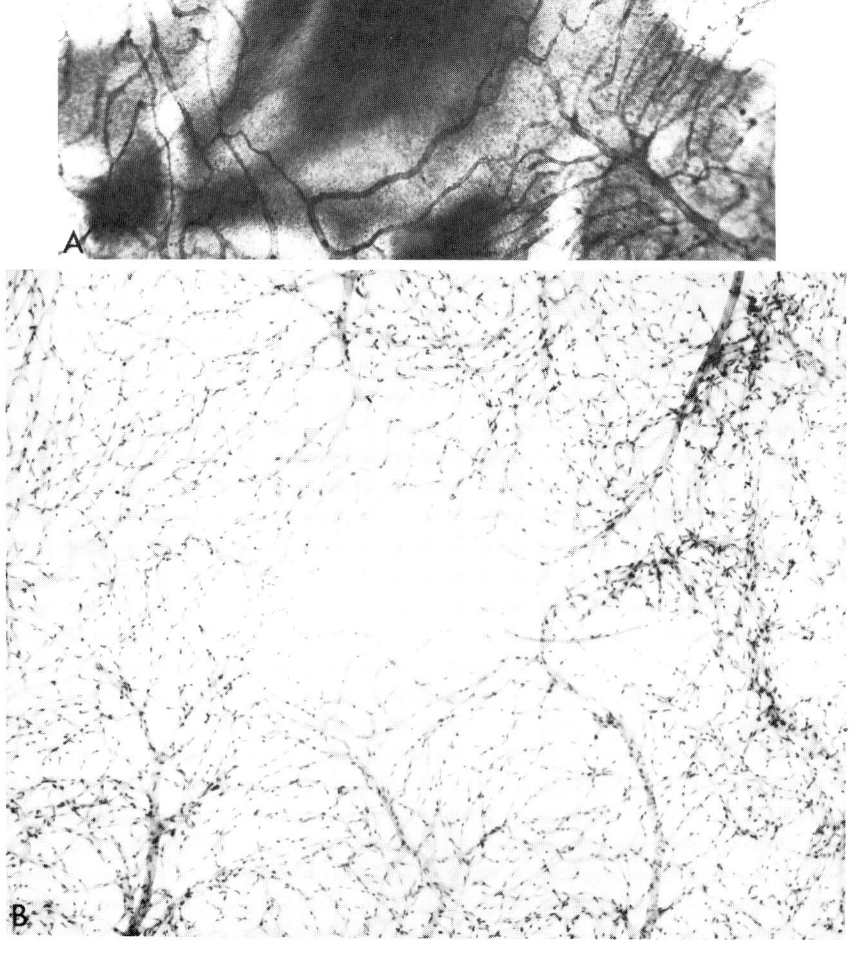

Figure 8–16. Foveal capillary-free zone. *A,* Flat retinal preparation. AFIP 219548. (From Friedenwald JS: New approach to some problems of retinal vascular disease [Jackson Memorial Lecture]. Am J Ophthalmol *32*:487–498, 1949.) *B* and *C,* Trypsin digest preparation, ×60; ×200. EP 44923. *D,* India ink preparation of monkey eye, unstained, ×40. EP 47482.

Illustration continued on opposite page

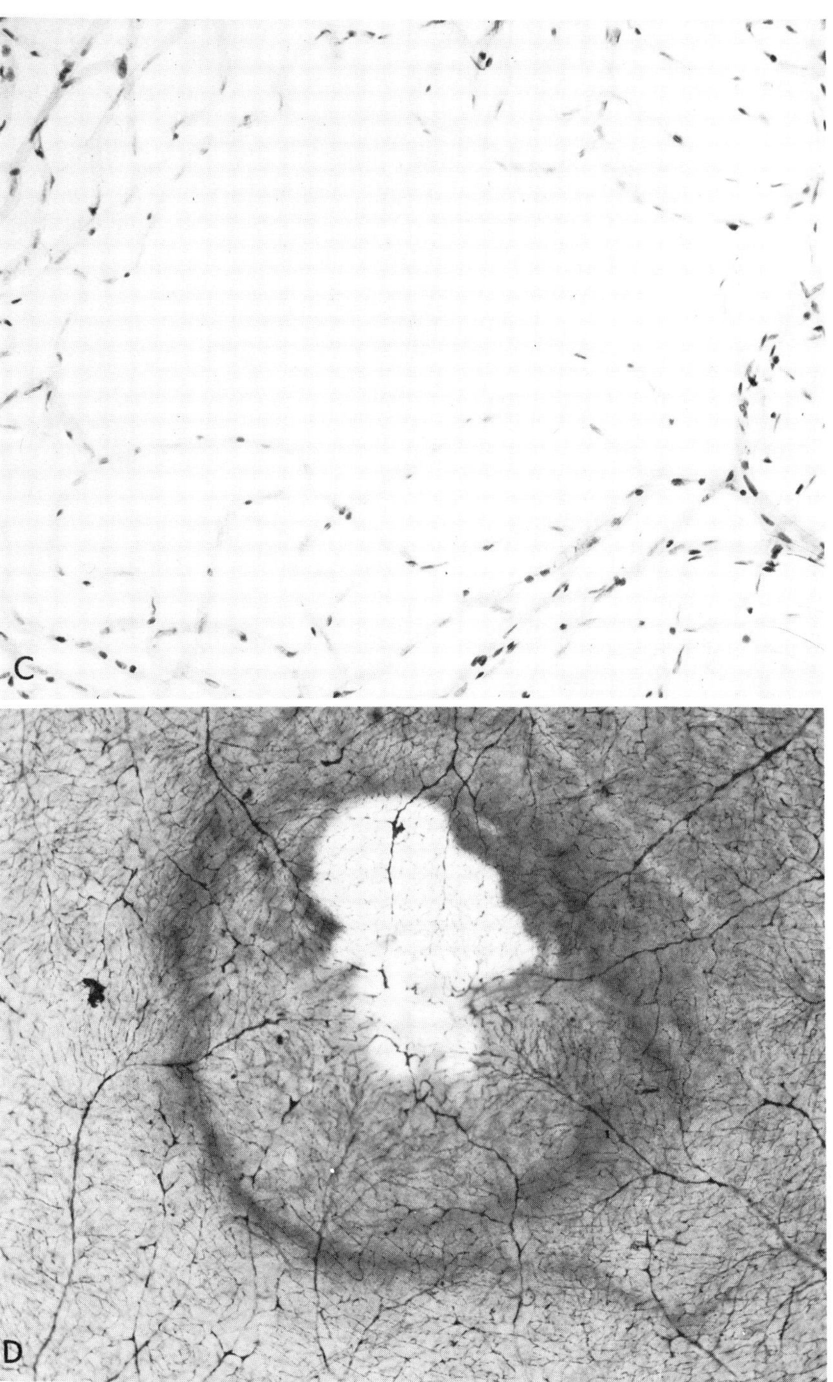

Figure 8–16 *Continued*

retinal pigment cells occurs between birth and 2 years of age, when the adult range is achieved (Streeten, 1969). In fetal and postnatal eyes, the entire retinal pigment epithelium (RPE) increases slowly in size. This nonuniform enlargement of cells occurs at the ora serrata region, from infancy to adolescent life, in a zone that gradually enlarges from 1 to 4 mm wide. By age 3 to 6 years, growth is largely confined to the region anterior to the equator (Streeten, 1969). Between the second and third years of life, the total number of RPE cells increases only slightly, even though the surface area of the retina increases by 37 per cent. Friedman and T'so (1968) found only a 20 per cent increase in the number of equatorial cells, but the area covered by the cells in the periphery was found to be doubled as a result of thinning and stretching. At the same time, however, the cells in the macular region showed a decrease in the area covered in the eyes they studied.

Aging. With aging, a significant degree of pleomorphism occurs in the RPE. This involves the size and shape of the cells and their nuclei and pigment granules (Friedman, Tso, 1968). The pigment cells in healthy eyes appear normal-sized with aging, but their nuclei become smaller and more basophilic. The RPE in the macular area increases in height and becomes narrower in adult life. The opposite has been found to occur in the peripheral cells. The amount of pigment also seems to be less in the cytoplasm of the cells of the young, compared with older eyes centrally, but the reverse seems to be true in the periphery. In the periphery, however, the cells seem to become broader, lower, more vacuolated, and markedly pleomorphic.

The cytoplasm of the pigment cells, especially in the posterior retina, gradually accumulates lipid and granular particles with increasing age. This lipid material is known as lipofuscin, and it accumulates secondary to metabolic activities in the cells. This pigment in its various forms migrates from the cells and is deposited in the adjacent Bruch's membrane, frequently contributing to masses of sub-RPE material that are called drusen. Thinning, depigmentation, or atrophy of the pigment cells over the drusen is a consistent finding. Pigmentary changes in the peripheral RPE cells are a universal finding in older age, some being related to depigmentation or atrophy and others to hypertrophy, hyperplasia, and migration. The changes may be so marked that the condition is called senile peripheral pigmentary degeneration.

Several forms of linear degeneration of the peripheral pigment epithelium have been encountered in older eyes. Most of these are related to changes in the pigment epithelium secondary to changes occurring in Bruch's membrane in older age groups (Morris, Henkind, 1979), especially neovascularization of Bruch's membrane (Daicker, 1973; Bec, Secheyron, Arne, Aubry, 1979). Peripheral intra-Bruch's membrane vascularization has been observed in young children and may represent a congenital variation (Spitznas, 1977).

Drusen

Drusen (colloid bodies) (also see page 936) are excrescences formed on the inner aspect of Bruch's membrane as a result of activity of the RPE cells. Most often drusen represent degenerative changes that occur in the cells, but in younger persons they may represent a product of abnormal metabolism within the pigment cell. Clinically, the typical druse is a small, yellowish-white lesion that lights up early during fluorescein angiography and stains late with no leakage. The extent to which drusen are seen ophthalmoscopically, without fluorescein, depends on their size, the degree of effacement or loss of the overlying RPE, and the degree of surrounding RPE hypertrophy.

Histologically, drusen have a fairly characteristic structure, being composed of granular ground substance, degenerating lipid and protein particles, crystalline deposits of calcium and amino acids, residual bodies, and also partially digested photoreceptor outer segment discs. These drusen lie adjacent to the basal lamina of the pigment epithelial cell, lifting it up and causing some secondary atrophy of the cells. Other drusen appear to be crystalline in nature, are uniform in appearance, and are composed of lipid and protein. Clinically, some small RPE detachments are mistaken for drusen.

Bruch's Membrane

Localized and diffuse thickening of the inner aspect of Bruch's membrane is also a commonly observed aging change, which has been clinically and histopathologically interpreted as a form of drusen. Ultrastructural studies have shown the main constituent of the thickened material to be aggregates of widely spaced collagen and abnormal basement membrane (Green, Key, 1977; Green, 1980a). This material has been referred to as "basal laminar deposit" by Sarks (1973). As early as 1855, H. Mueller also noted generalized thickening of the cuticular (inner) portion of Bruch's membrane in eyes of older individuals, and he believed that drusen originate from this substance.

Sensory Retina

In the sensory retina, the Müller cells and the limiting membranes become somewhat thickened with increasing age, and atrophic changes can be seen in the peripheral retina, with diminution of the neuronal elements and secondary glial proliferation. This leads to extensive disorganization of the retina in the ora serrata region, and pigment cells from the RPE may wander into the sensory retina in this region. The retinal neurons show very few changes as a result of increasing age; however, there is a substantial accumulation of lipids in the nerve cells, especially in the ganglion cells, in which the pigment lipofuscin increases considerably. Similar changes are seen in the bipolar layer of cells.

Gartner and Henkind (1981a) have observed drop-out of nuclei in the outer nuclear layer with age.

Hyalin bodies (corpora amylacea) (Fig. 8–17) are observed in the peripapillary retinal nerve fiber layer, the optic nerve head, and the optic nerve as an aging process and may be increased in various pathologic conditions. The origin of corpora amylacea has been attributed to nerve fibers (Wolter, Liss, 1959), ganglion cells (Wolter,

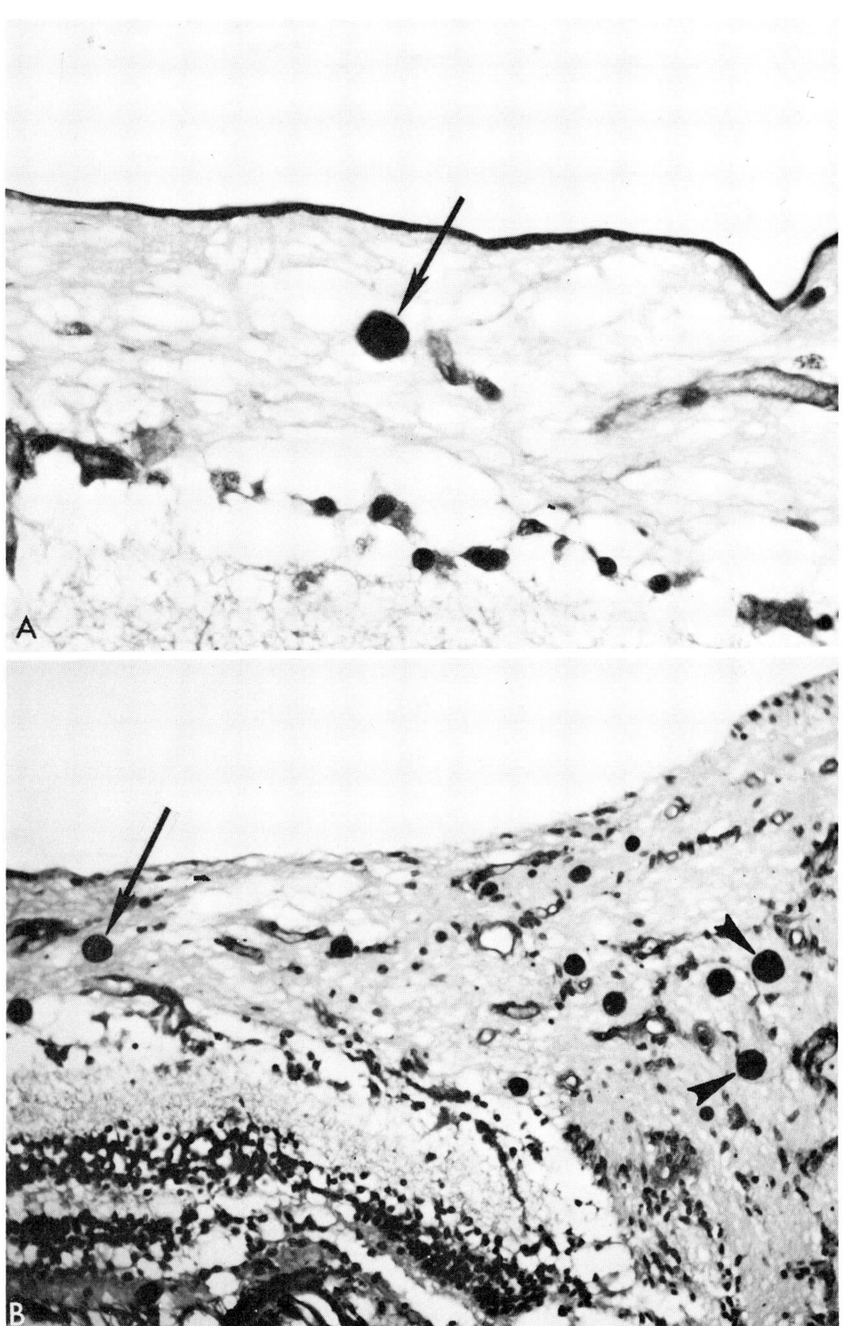

Figure 8–17. *A,* **Corpora amylacea** (arrow) in the nerve fiber layer of peripapillary retina and *B,* in the optic nerve head (arrowheads). *A,* PAS, ×500; *B,* PAS, ×205. EP 51578.

1959a), and fibrous astrocytes (Ramsey, 1965). Woodford and Tso (1980) (Fig. 8–18) and Avendano, Rodrigues, Hackett, and Gaskins (1980) have presented convincing electron microscopic studies that show that corpora amylacea are intracellular organelles (neurotubules, mitochondria, and dense bodies) found in axonal swellings. (See Chapter 11 on the optic nerve.)

The Retinal Vessels

The peripheral retinal circulation develops during the last trimester of gestation. Occasionally in the full-term and always in the premature neonate the retina is incompletely vascularized. The temporal periphery is farther from the optic disk; therefore, incomplete vascularization is more often observed on the temporal side. During the last several months of fetal life, the vessels have extended almost to the ora serrata nasally and to the retinal equator on the temporal side. The early retinal vasculature is characterized by its "chicken-wire" pattern, but in the last month of fetal life this pattern becomes less uniform and there are larger meshes, especially in the posterior retina. Pericytes, or mural cells, are not evident up to this time, and they do not seem to be

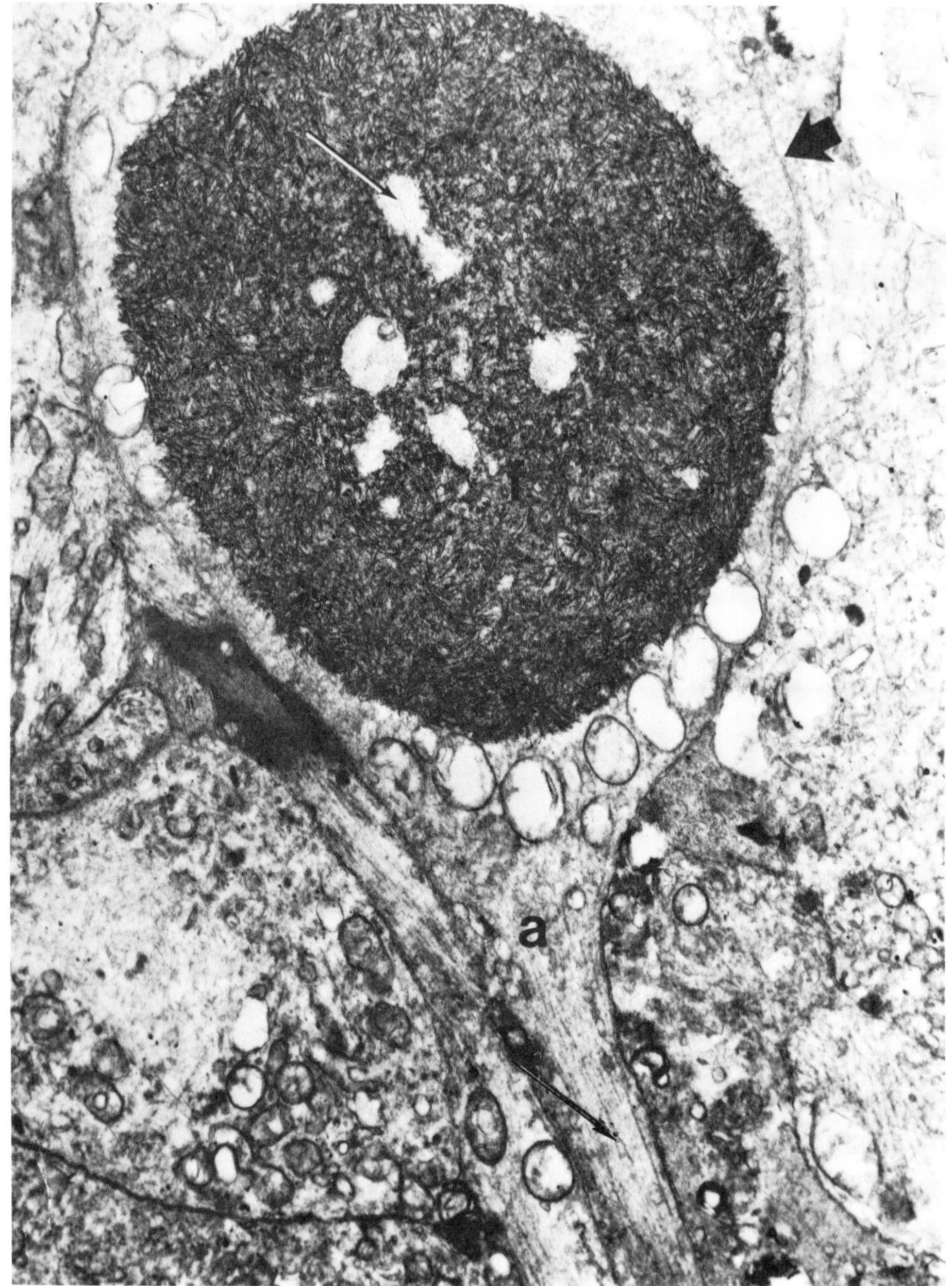

Figure 8–18. A swollen segment of an axon (thick arrow) contains a corpus amylaceum and merges into a narrow axonal segment *(a)*. Normal neurotubules (thin black arrow) are present in the normal axonal segment. Central areas of loose ground substance within the filamentous tangle *(f)* also contain similar tubules (black and white arrow). ×17,600. (Courtesy of Woodford B, T'so MOM: An illustrated study of the corpora amylacea of the optic nerve head and retina. Am J Ophthalmol *90*:492–502, 1980.)

present until about 2 months after birth. The retinal vasculature achieves the adult pattern by about the fifth month after birth, and at this time the chicken-wire mesh pattern is gone but some peripheral vessels still lack mural cells. After the fifth postnatal month, the capillaries differ from those of the adult retina only by their greater cellularity and more intense staining properties.

The retinal vessels show rather characteristic aging changes, apart from the arterial sclerosis which is commonly seen in senile eyes. The principal changes affect the capillaries. Cogan (1963) and Kuwabara and Cogan (1965) found widespread loss of cellularity to be a constant occurrence in the peripheral capillaries of elderly people. The loss of cellularity occurs initially by loss of endothelial cells and later by loss of pericytes. Eventually the affected areas may become totally acellular. Associated with this, the internal limiting membrane becomes attached to the peripheral vascular arcades. These investigators noted that if the pericytes disappeared prior to the endothelial cells, vascular shunts, loops, and microaneurysms tended to form. Similar changes may be seen in the posterior eye but never as severe as peripherally. Kornzweig, Eliasoph, and Feldstein (1964, 1966), in the study of flat preparations of the eyes of elderly patients, found that nearly 60 per cent of the specimens showed a diminution in the number of capillaries around the fovea, with a reduced number of capillary cells and poorer staining of the vessel walls.

A number of more specific types of retinal degenerations generally also can be classified as aging changes. These include pavingstone degeneration (cobblestone or peripheral chorioretinal atrophy), typical and reticular peripheral cystoid degeneration, typical and reticular degenerative retinoschisis, retinal pits, and lattice degeneration. These degenerative lesions and others are discussed in detail in the section on retinal degenerations (page 814).

CONGENITAL VARIATIONS AND ABNORMALITIES

Congenital abnormalities restricted to the retina are not as common as in the uveal tract. Most abnormalities are related to changes in the adjacent choroid.

Lange's Fold

This folding has been described in the previous section (page 602). Eyes obtained post mortem from fetuses and infants frequently show an inward folding of the retina at the ora serrata. This originally was believed to be related to the development of the retina but has been shown to be an artefactitious change (Kalina, 1971).

Meridional Folds and Complexes

These lesions are not congenital abnormalities, strictly speaking, but normal variations in the structure of the peripheral retina. They are discussed in detail elsewhere (pages 893 and 900).

Albinism

Albinism is a general term that refers to a congenital pigmentary dilution of the skin, or skin and eyes, or just the eyes (Witkop, 1971). True albinism has been subdivided into two major types: (1) oculocutaneous albinism, when the skin and eyes are affected, and (2) ocular albinism, when only the eye is affected. This is somewhat helpful to the clinician, but it is important to know that this clinical classification is not accurate histopathologically. All forms of so-called ocular albinism are probably oculocutaneous—it is just that the cutaneous pigmentary dilution is mild.

The pathophysiologic cause of oculocutaneous albinism is a reduction in the amount of primary melanin deposited in each of the pigment organelles (melanosomes). The pathophysiologic cause of ocular albinism is a reduction of the numbers of melanosomes, although each melanosome may be fully pigmented (melanized).

Many different types of albinism have been described; a simple concept helps formulate a clinical approach. Regardless of the type of albinism, the ocular involvement conforms to one of two clinical patterns: (1) congenitally subnormal visual acuity and nystagmus, or (2) normal or only minimally reduced visual acuity and no nystagmus. The latter clinical pattern has been called albinoidism because the visual consequences are much milder than in a typical albinism. Both patterns share clinical features, such as photophobia, iris transillumination, and hypopigmented eye grounds. They differ because the effects on foveal differentiation are drastically different. In albinoidism (pattern 2) the fovea is normal or nearly so, whereas in true albinism (pattern 1) the

Table 8–1. TYPES OF ALBINISM WITH OCULAR INVOLVEMENT

Types
Oculocutaneous Albinism
Tyrosinase-positive (AR)
Tyrosinase-negative (AR)
Yellow-mutant (AR)
Albinism with hemorrhagic diathesis (Hermansky-Pudlak syndrome) (AR)
?Albinism–oligophrenia–microphthalmia (Cross-McKusick syndrome) (AR)
Ocular Albinism*
Nettleship-Falls X-linked
Autosomal recessive (Witkop)
Chediak-Higashi syndrome (AR)
Autosomal dominant with deafness and lentigines (Lewis)
Albinoidism†
Autosomal dominant oculocutaneous (Donaldson-Fitzpatrick)
Punctate oculocutaneous (Bergsma-Kaiser-Kupfer) (AD)
Apert's syndrome (AD)
Waardenburg-like syndrome (Bard) (AD)

*Classification as "ocular" is based on clinical signs. Actually, all these disorders are "oculocutaneous."

†These patients lack nystagmus and the significant visual impairment typical of true albinism.

AR, autosomal recessive; AD, autosomal dominant.

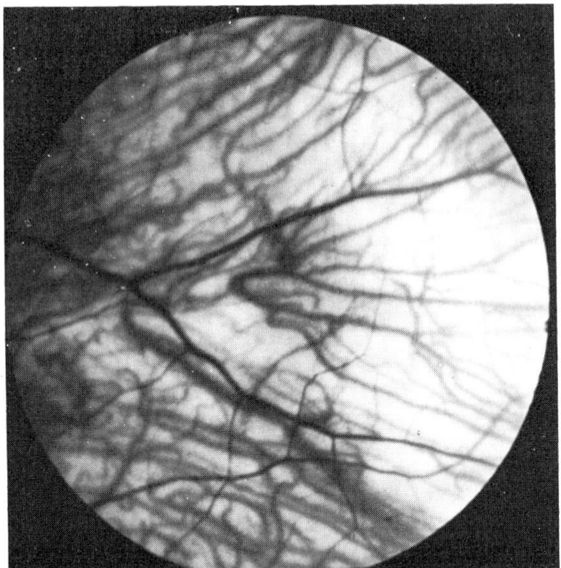

Figure 8–19. Albinotic fundus of a male with sex-linked recessive **ocular albinism**.

fovea is hypoplastic. The ophthalmoscopic appearance of foveal hypoplasia, therefore, is the sine qua non of true albinism. In addition, although clinically inapparent, the passage of temporal hemiretinal nerve fibers through the chiasm is atavistic; that is, many of these temporal hemiretinal nerve fibers decussate rather than project to the ipsilateral geniculate body. This seems to obviate the possibility of binocular vision and perhaps explains the high incidence of strabismus in true albinism.

Diagnosis of the exact type of albinism is important for accurate genetic counseling and detection of two life-threatening types of albinism.

Table 8–1 summarizes the inheritance pattern of the types of albinism. The general rule to remember is: True albinism is inherited as an autosomal recessive trait, whereas albinoidism is inherited as an autosomal dominant trait with incomplete penetrance. The exception to this rule is that one form of albinism is inherited as an X-linked trait, which is diagnosed by (1) carrier findings in the mother or a daughter, (2) an affected male with a pedigree compatible with X-linked inheritance, and (3) macromelanosomes found upon biopsy of clinically normal skin.

The tyrosinase test has been used to successfully divide oculocutaneous albinism into two major types, tyrosinase-positive and tyrosinase-negative, on the basis of the presence or absence of tyrosinase enzyme activity. This enzymatic reaction is an important step in the biosynthesis of melanin. The clinician should be aware that the value of this test is limited. Tyrosinase-negative albinos lack any pigment in the skin, hair, or eyes, so it is relatively easy to make a clinical differentiation between older children and adults with tyrosinase-negative versus tyrosinase-positive albinism. Furthermore, with the exception of tyrosinase-negative oculocutaneous albinism, all other types of albinism or albinoidism are tyrosinase-positive, as are all normally pigmented individuals. So the tyrosinase test does not help greatly to identify the exact subtype of albinism. More sophisticated biochemical tests and ultrastructural studies are needed to make laboratory

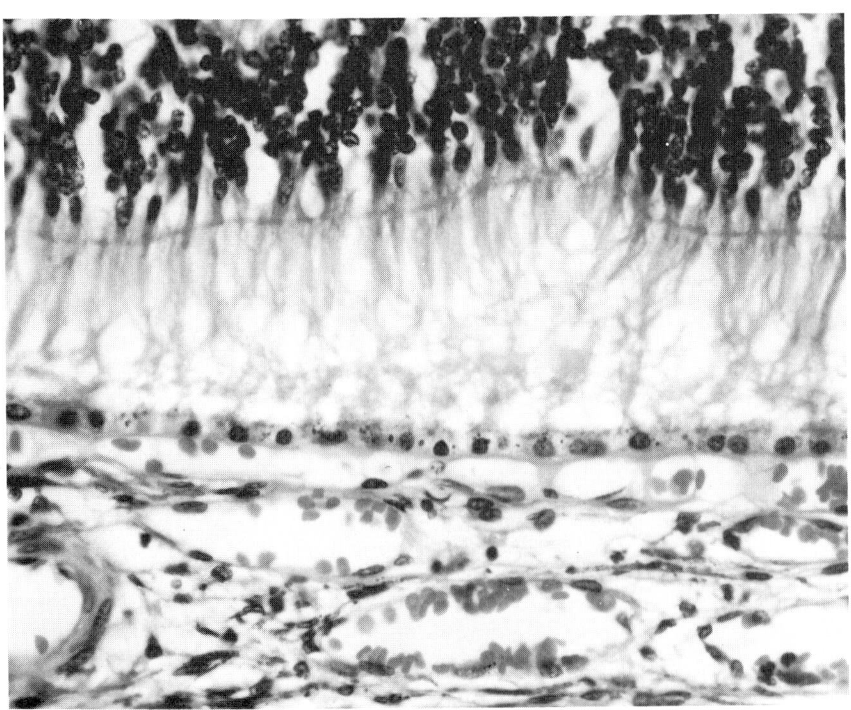

Figure 8–20. Parafoveal area of male with sex-linked **ocular albinism,** showing an intact retinal pigment epithelium with sparse pigment granules and hypopigmented choroid. H and E, ×430. EP 33307.

confirmation of a clinical diagnosis of the exact type of albinism (see Table 8–1).

The detection of the two potentially lethal forms of albinism depends largely on historical information: (1) The Chediak-Higashi syndrome is characterized by an easy susceptibility to infections in a young child. (2) The Hermansky-Pudlak syndrome is characterized by an easy susceptibility to bruising and bleeding. When either of these two types of albinism is suspected, hematologic consultation is imperative.

Ocular Albinism

Ocular albinism is most often transmitted as an X-linked recessive trait—the Nettleship-Falls type. Autosomal recessive and dominant transmission also have been observed.

Affected males have photophobia, reduced visual acuity, translucent irides (although iris color may be quite dark), ocular deviations, normal color vision, apparent macular hypoplasia with absent foveal reflex, and clearly visible choroidal vasculature, especially in areas outside the area centralis (Fig. 8–19). The RPE is only sparsely pigmented (Fig. 8–20). Carrier females are typically asymptomatic but often have partial iris translucency, mottling of RPE in the macula, and pigmentary mosaicism in the periphery.

O'Donnell, Hambrick, Green, et al (1976) have observed the presence of macromelanosomes in the iris (Fig. 8–21,*A*), in ciliary (Fig. 8–21,*B*) and

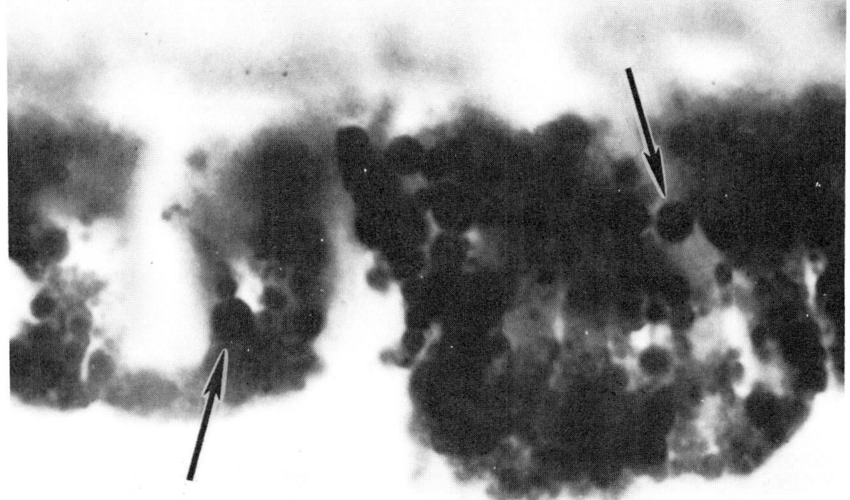

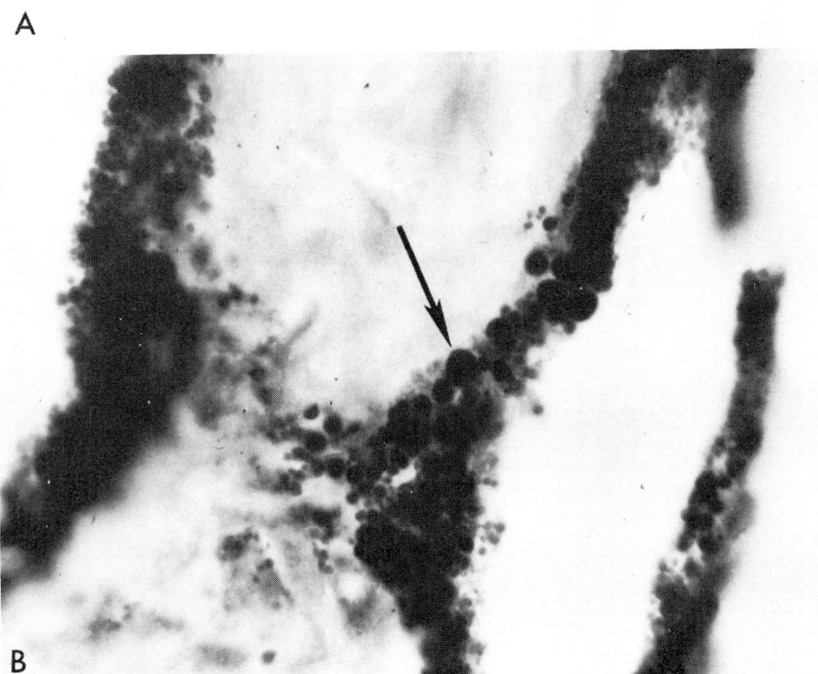

Figure 8–21. *A,* Iris and *B,* ciliary pigment epithelium showing giant pigment granules (arrows) from a patient with sex-linked **ocular albinism**. Both, H and E, ×700. EP 33307. (From O'Donnell FE Jr, Hambrick GW Jr, Green WR, et al: X-linked ocular albinism: An oculocutaneous macromelanosomal disorder. Arch Ophthalmol *94*:1883–1892, 1976.)

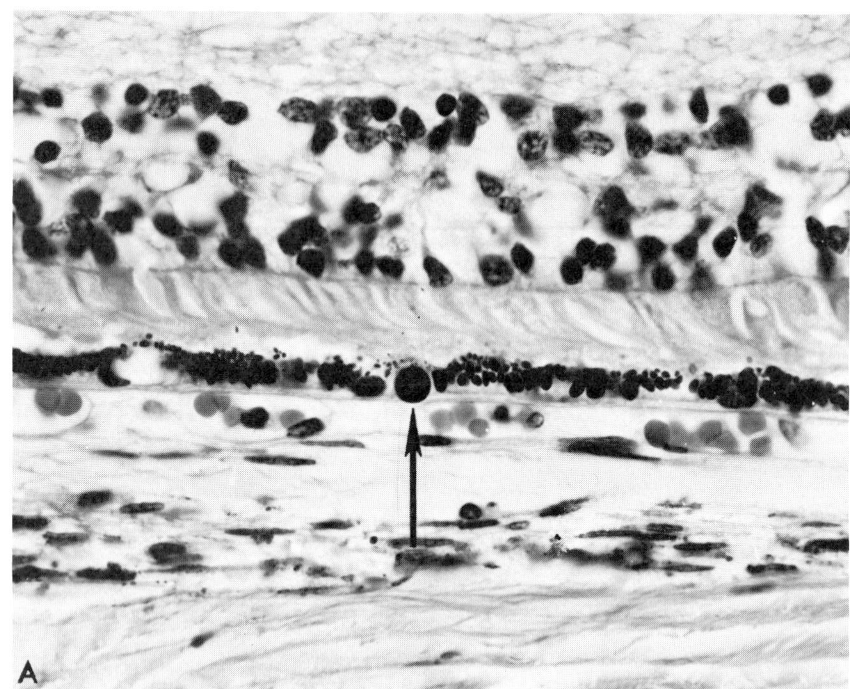

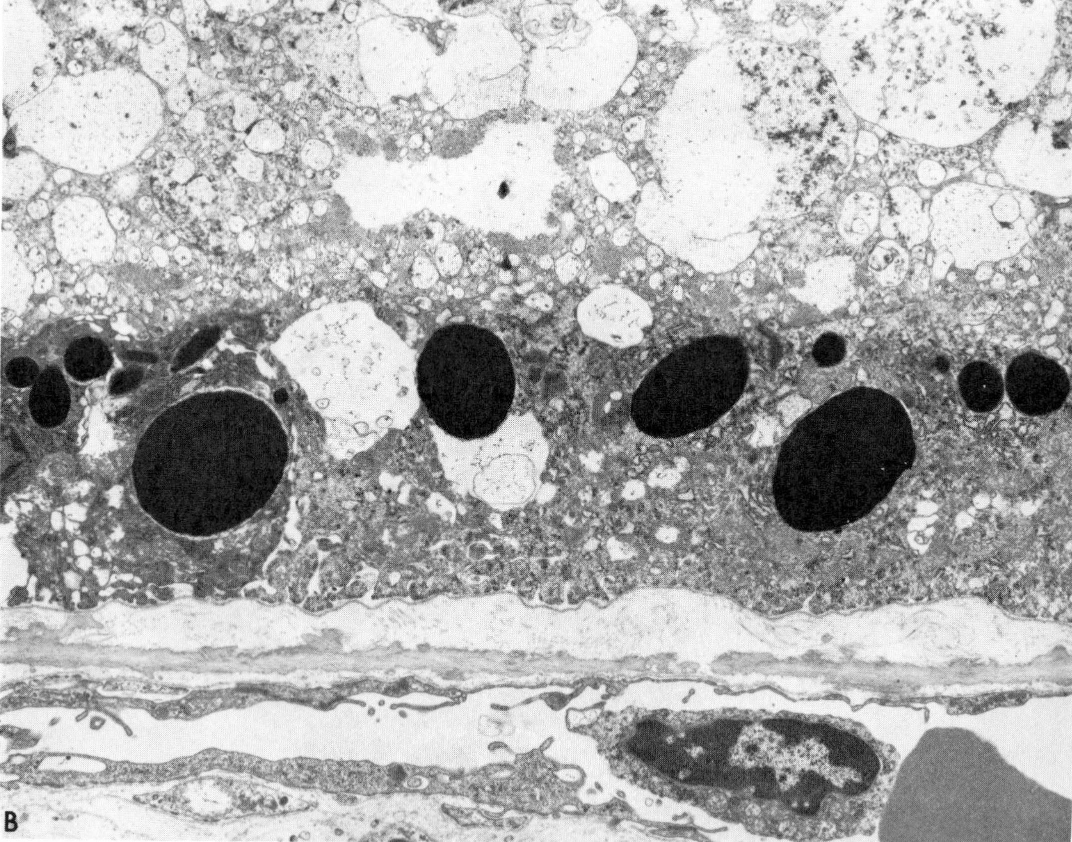

Figure 8–22. *A,* Light and *B,* electron microscopic appearance of giant pigment granules (arrow) in RPE of patient with sex-linked **ocular albinism**. *A,* H and E, ×750; *B,* ×7000. EP 33307. (From O'Donnell FE Jr, Hambrick GW Jr, Green WR, et al: X-linked ocular albinism: An oculocutaneous macromelanosomal disorder. Arch Ophthalmol *94*:1883–1892, 1976.)

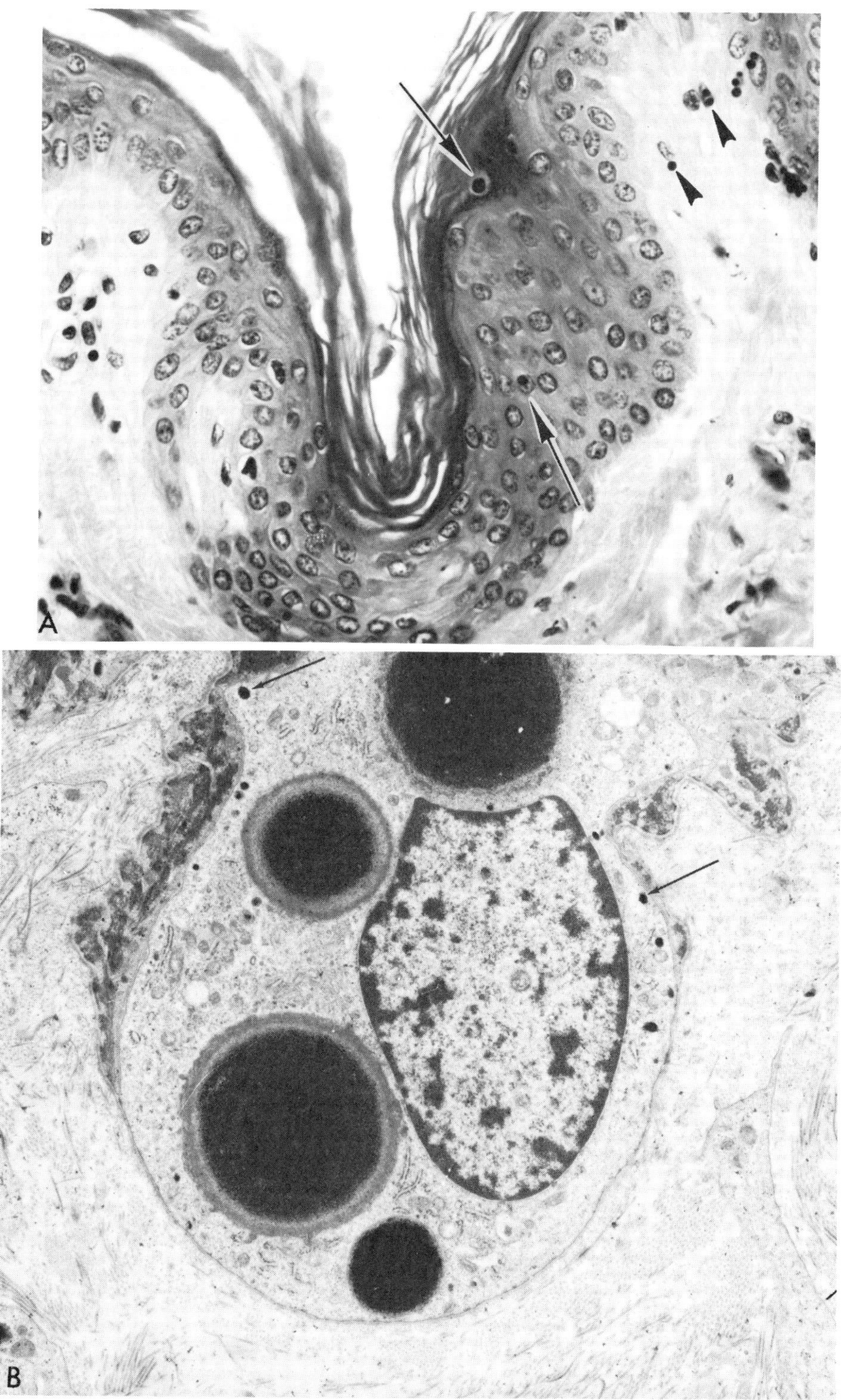

Figure 8–23. *A,* Skin biopsy from patient with sex-linked **ocular albinism,** showing giant pigment granules in dermal melanocytes (arrowheads) and keratinocytes (arrows). H and E, ×430. *B,* Electron micrograph of dermal melanocytes from patient with sex-linked ocular albinism. Four macromelanosomes and some normal-sized melanosomes (arrows) are shown. ×8000. EP 33307. (From O'Donnell FE Jr, Hambrick GW Jr, Green WR, et al: X-linked ocular albinism: An oculocutaneous macromelanosomal disorder. Arch Ophthalmol *94*:1883–1892, 1976.)

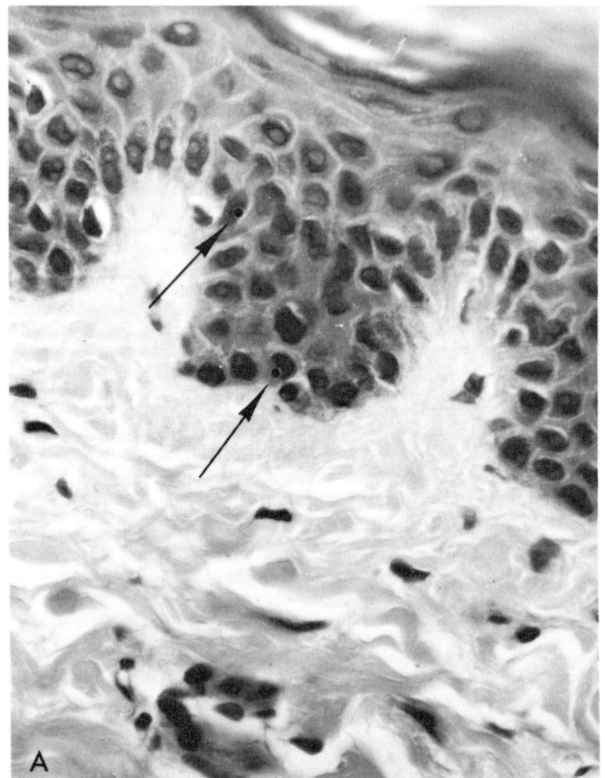

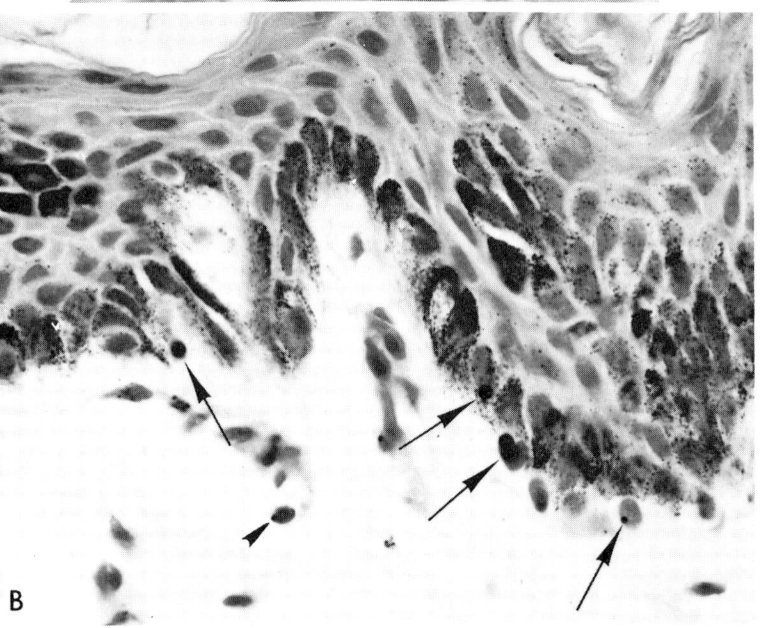

Figure 8–24. Skin biopsy from female carrier of sex-linked **ocular albinism,** showing giant pigment granules in epithelial cells (arrows) and dermal melanocyte (arrowhead). *A,* H and E, ×650; B, Fontana, ×750. EP 40063. (From O'Donnell FE Jr, Hambrick GW Jr, Green WR, et al: X-linked ocular albinism: An oculocutaneous macromelanosomal disorder. Arch Ophthalmol *94*:1883–1892, 1976.)

retinal pigment epithelia (Fig. 8–22), and in keratinocytes and dermal melanocytes (Fig. 8–23). These abnormal pigment granules are also evident in the skin of carrier females (Fig. 8–24), as well as affected males. Therefore this allows one to document the female carrier state. Histopathologic studies of eyes from a patient with the Nettleship-Falls type of ocular albinism have disclosed the lack of foveal differentiation (O'Donnell, Hambrick, Green, et al, 1976), which explains the absence of a foveal reflex and is probably a factor in the reduced visual acuity of these patients.

In blacks, X-linked ocular albinism can be an unexpected cause of congenital nystagmus. In the first two black kindreds reported with ocular albinism (O'Donnell, Green, Fleischman, Hambrick, 1978), eight of ten affected males lacked appreciable iris transillumination, and they had nonalbinotic, moderately pigmented fundi. All these patients had a subnormal visual acuity (range: 20/25 to 20/200), congenital nystagmus, and foveal hypoplasia on ophthalmoscopic examination. Regardless of the degree of fundus pigmentation, none of the patients had the normal relative hyperpigmentation of the RPE at the fovea, suggesting that hyperpigmentation of the RPE may normally induce foveolar differentiation. As in white ocular albinos, skin biopsy of affected black males and carrier females with X-linked ocular albinism revealed macromelanosomes.

In a study of the retinal pigment epithelium of a 21 week old fetus with X-linked ocular albinism, Wong, O'Donnell, and Green (1983) found giant pigment granules (macromelanosomes) with a vesiculoglobular substance in the equator and posterior regions. Anteriorly, compound granules and melanosomes of unusual appearance were present and were interpreted as possible precursors of macromelanosomes. Lack of pigmentation from autophagocytosis could not be totally excluded.

Forsius and Eriksson (1964) described an X-linked type of ocular albinism that differed from the more common type in that the males had protanomalous color blindness and female carriers had a slight disturbance in color vision and lacked the characteristic mosaic pattern of fundus pigment. Skin biopsy specimens of six patients with this syndrome did not show any macromelanosomes (O'Donnell, Schaltz, Reid, Green, 1979).

Bergsma and Kaiser-Kupfer (1974) have described a mother and two children with a different form of ocular albinism (albinoidism). These patients have diffuse, fine, punctate depigmentation of the iris and RPE, slightly reduced visual acuity, elevation of central cone thresholds, light-colored skin and hair, and positive tyrosinase hair bulb tests.

The precise pathophysiology of visual impairment in albinism is unknown. Suggested factors are light scatter, light-induced retinal damage, macular hypoplasia, and abnormal retinogeniculostriate projections. (For discussion, see O'Donnell and Green, 1979).

Oculocutaneous Albinism

This form of albinism may be complete or incomplete, depending on whether tyrosinase activity is partially or completely lacking.

In the complete, or perfect, type, the tyrosinase test is negative. Some of the patients also may have a hemorrhagic diathesis; this condition is referred to as the albinism–hemorrhagic diathesis type, or the Hermansky-Pudlak syndrome. These types are most often inherited as an autosomal trait and are characterized by a total absence of pigment.

Oculocutaneous albinism with a positive tyrosinase test is an attenuated form and is characterized by lightly pigmented skin and blond or straw-colored hair. The iris, skin, and hair may darken with age. The fundus is lightly pigmented. Vision is usually reduced and the macula hypoplastic. Recent histopathologic studies (Naumann, Lerche, Schroeder, 1976; Fulton, Albert, Craft, 1978) have confirmed macular hypoplasia in oculocutaneous albinism.

Histopathologic study discloses the iris, ciliary, and retinal pigment epithelia to be normal but with few melanin pigment granules.

Four types of incomplete tyrosinase-positive oculocutaneous albinism are recognized:

1. Tyrosinase-positive oculocutaneous albinism
2. Chediak-Higashi syndrome (see page 1154)
3. Cross syndrome: hypopigmentation, microphthalmos, oligophrenia syndrome
4. Yellow mutant: the tyrosinase test is variable in this type

Colobomas

Colobomas of the retina are usually associated with an accompanying coloboma of the choroid (see page 1415). Colobomas occur as the result of dysembryogenesis of the fetal fissure and include localized defects ranging from involvement of only the RPE to microphthalmos with cyst.

They can be divided into two types: typical and atypical. The *typical* coloboma involves the region of the fetal fissure and is usually located inferonasally. It is bilateral in about 60 per cent of patients and may extend from the optic disk into the anterior portion of the eye or be localized. Histologically, the RPE is absent in the area of the coloboma. The sensory retina may be absent or may be present as hypoplasic strands; it may show dysplasia in the area of the cleft. These lesions are discussed more fully in the section on the choroid. *Atypical* colobomas occur in positions other than the inferonasal fundus and resemble typical colobomas, but are usually incomplete. Many cases of so-called macular colobomas probably are not real colobomas but are secondary to a pre-existing ocular inflammation, such as toxoplasmosis or cytomegalic inclusion disease.

Retinal Cysts

In the retina, discrete cysts have been described in various positions, including the macula. The cysts are usually sharply circumscribed and of varying size; some are quite large, but usually they are about 2 to 3 disk-diameters in dimension. Most often they are nonprogressive. Histologically, the cysts are intraretinal and oc-

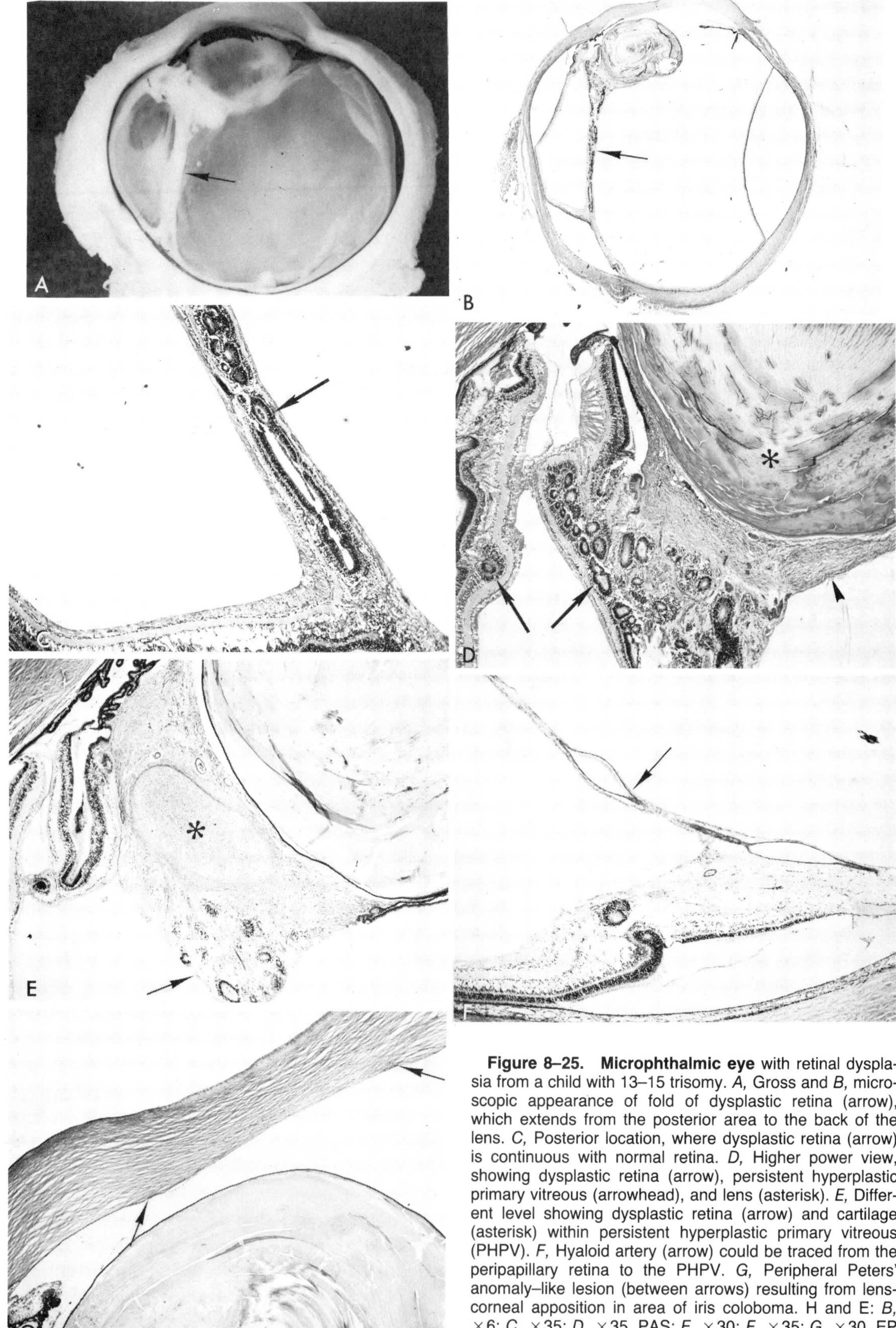

Figure 8–25. Microphthalmic eye with retinal dysplasia from a child with 13–15 trisomy. *A,* Gross and *B,* microscopic appearance of fold of dysplastic retina (arrow), which extends from the posterior area to the back of the lens. *C,* Posterior location, where dysplastic retina (arrow) is continuous with normal retina. *D,* Higher power view, showing dysplastic retina (arrow), persistent hyperplastic primary vitreous (arrowhead), and lens (asterisk). *E,* Different level showing dysplastic retina (arrow) and cartilage (asterisk) within persistent hyperplastic primary vitreous (PHPV). *F,* Hyaloid artery (arrow) could be traced from the peripapillary retina to the PHPV. *G,* Peripheral Peters' anomaly–like lesion (between arrows) resulting from lens-corneal apposition in area of iris coloboma. H and E: *B,* ×6; *C,* ×35; *D,* ×35. PAS: *E,* ×30; *F,* ×35; *G,* ×30. EP 42258.

cupy the area between the inner limiting membrane and the outer nuclear layer. The intervening elements are degenerated, and the margins of the cyst are formed by surrounding neurons and Müller cells. The congenital nature of retinal cysts is questioned, since most occur in the inferotemporal area and develop from reticular degenerative retinoschisis. Those in the macular area usually develop from coalescence of cystoid macular edema.

Retinal Dysplasia

Retinal dysplasia is an inherited condition in which developing retina, without the normal influences of RPE, proliferates in an abnormal fashion, leading to tubular, acinar, rosette-like configurations (Fig. 8–25). It is a conspicuous feature of the Patau syndrome (trisomy 13–15, trisomy D). The retinal rosettes may have one or two layers of differentiated cells or may be composed of undifferentiated cells (Lahav, Albert, Wyand, 1973). Experimental studies have shown that intrauterine trauma (Silverstein, 1974) and intrauterine viral infection (Silverstein, Parshall, Osburn, Prendergast, 1971) can also produce dysplastic retina. One of the important features of retinal dysplasia is that it is a cause of leukocoria and in the past has been confused clinically with retinoblastoma, even though there are microphthalmia and a constellation of other findings with dysplasia.

The term *retinal dysplasia* originally was used in a general sense to describe abnormalities in development of the retina. Reese and Blodi (1950), however, used the term to designate a syndrome consisting of congenital anomalies involving the brain, heart, extremities, mouth, and eye. They gave this syndrome that name because the dysplastic retina was the principal feature common to all cases. In all eight patients, the ocular abnormality was bilateral and occurred in newborn full-term infants, thus distinguishing it from retrolental fibroplasia. The eyes were usually microphthalmic, and on clinical examination a white mass consisting of persistent primary vitreous and dysplastic retina could be seen behind the lens.

Hunter and Zimmerman (1965) reviewed a number of additional cases, including some of those reported by Reese and Straatsma in 1958. Hunter and Zimmerman preferred to use the term *retinal dysplasia* as designating a retinal lesion and not a clinical syndrome. These investigators found that dysplastic retina often was observed in unilaterally malformed eyes (Figs. 8–26 and 8–27) in which there were none of the features of the syndrome described by Reese and Blodi (1950). In 16 of 73 cases surveyed, they found unilateral ocular lesions with dysplastic changes in the retina. In only 2 of the 16 cases were there congenital anomalies in addition to those in the eye. They concluded that dysplasia of the retina is a nonspecific finding common to many examples of ocular maldevelopment, with or without systemic abnormalities.

Later, Miller, Robbins, Fishman, et al (1963); Sergovich, Madronich, Barr, et al (1963); and Cogan and Kuwabara (1964) described chromosomal abnormality in the 13–15 or D group–paired chromosomes (trisomy 13–15). In these patients, the dysplastic changes in the retina were bilateral and persistent primary vitreous and a fetal configuration of the anterior chamber angle were seen. Cogan and Kuwabara (1964) commented on the frequency with which microphthalmic eyes from persons with trisomy 13–15 contain cartilage within the retrolental fibrous tissue mass, which often extends to the sclera through a coloboma of the ciliary body. Other reports (Yanoff, Frayer, Scheie, 1963; Hunter and Zimmerman, 1965) indicate that patients with trisomy 13–15 do not always show retinal dysplasia but that there may be other abnormalities in the eye. It seems evident that, whatever the causative insult, the appearance of dysplastic retina is a nonspecific result of disturbed retinal growth and differentiation. The dysplasia may be severe or mild and unilateral or bilateral, depending on the type of insult occurring in the differentiating retina.

The affected eyes in retinal dysplasia associated with trisomy 13–15 are smaller than normal, although the degree of microphthalmos may vary. Cataractous changes may be present, but the lens often is sufficiently clear to visualize a white, vascularized, retrolental tissue. Elongated ciliary processes may be seen to insert into the periphery of a retrolental mass composed of fibrous tissue, retinal elements, and sometimes persistent hyperplastic primary vitreous (PHPV). In some cases, the membrane covers only a part of the lens, permitting visualization of the dysplastic retinal folds. Secondary glaucoma may develop from malformation of the anterior chamber angle.

The common feature of the ocular abnormality is the developmental defect involving the inner layer of the optic cup. It seems to result from a proliferation and folding of the outer layers of the stroma. Microscopically, a series of straight branching tubes is present, composed of abortive elements of the rod and cone layer, external limiting membrane, and outer nuclear layer. Serial sections reveal a communication between the lumen of these tubes and the subretinal space. The late stages show an obliteration of the tubes, with formation of rosettes similar to those seen in retinoblastoma. Neoplastic rosettes, however, are usually small, spherical clusters, while elliptical rosettes and tubes are characteristic of dysplasia. Dysgenesis of the entire retina, including the gan-

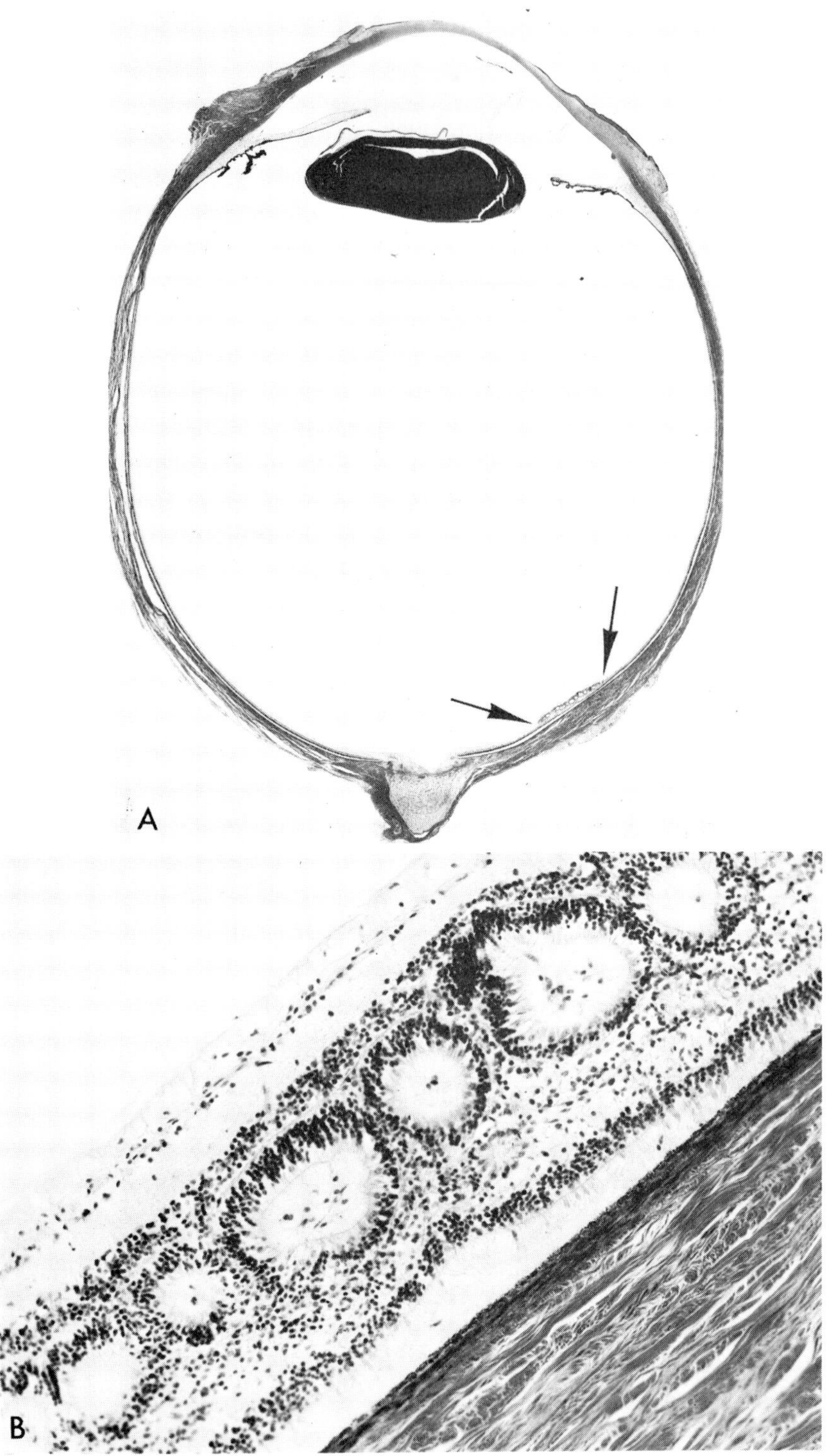

Figure 8–26. Localized **retinal dysplasia** (between arrows) associated with congenital abnormalities of the anterior segment and an orbital encephalocele. *A,* H and E, ×6. AFIP Neg. 64-1163. *B,* H and E, ×180. AFIP Neg. 64-1166. (From Hunter WS, Zimmerman LE: Unilateral retinal dysplasia. Arch Ophthalmol *74*:23–30, 1965.)

glion cells, may account for the reduced vision, even in the nondetached areas. Gliosis of the retina may be extensive. Persistence of the primary vitreous and failure in the formation of the secondary vitreous may accompany retinal dysplasia.

Other abnormalities, such as microphthalmos, a fetal type of filtration angle with congenital glaucoma, peripheral Peters' anomaly of the cornea, and coloboma of the uveal tract and optic nerve, may accompany retinal dysplasia. The central nervous, respiratory, gastrointestinal, cardiovascular, and genitourinary systems may be severely affected. The condition is sometimes familial, suggesting that the retinal dysplasia is due to an environmental disturbance or a genetic defect. In trisomy 13–15, the genetic defect is ev-

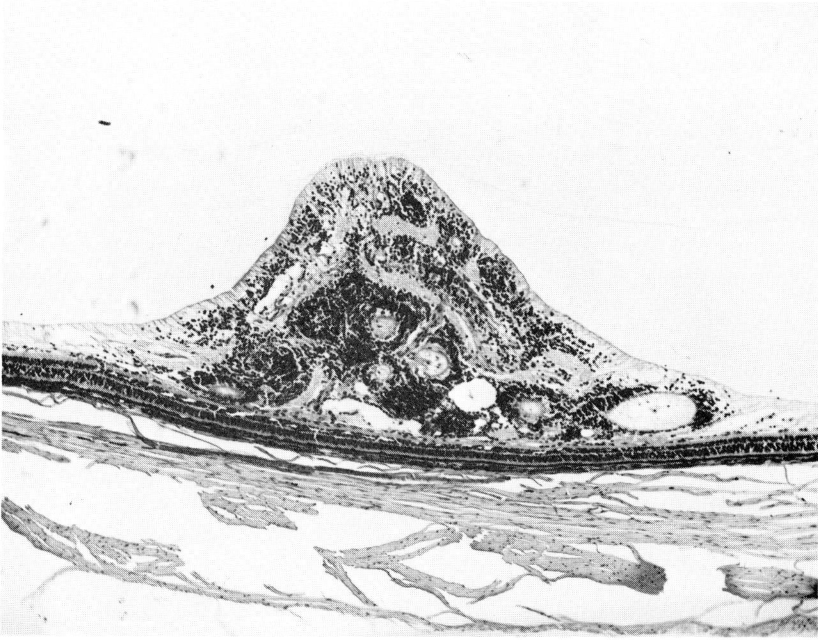

Figure 8–27. Localized **retinal dysplasia** unassociated with any other ocular or systemic abnormality. H and E, ×70. AFIP Neg. 64-1176. (From Hunter WS, Zimmerman LE: Unilateral retinal dysplasia. Arch Ophthalmol *74*:23–30, 1965.)

ident. In otherwise healthy individuals, minor changes may be found in the retina that greatly resemble retinal dysplasia. These isolated changes, however, are rarely sufficient for a diagnosis of retinal dysplasia.

Retinal dysplasia, along with many other ocular anomalies, may occur from the dysembryogenic effects of D-lysergic diethylamide (LSD) on the developing fetus when ingested by the mother (Chan, Fishman, Egbert, 1978).

Myelinated Nerve Fibers

When myelinated nerve fibers are of marked degree, they may present a startling ophthalmoscopic picture. The feathery edge and the conformity to the configuration of the nerve fiber layer are diagnostic. These myelinated fibers usually show continuity with the optic disk but may be located away from the disk (Fig. 8–28). Normally, myelinization of the optic nerve starts at the lateral geniculate body at about the fifth month of gestation, extends centrifugally, and reaches the optic chiasm from the sixth to seventh month and the optic nerve head at 8 months. In some instances, this myelinizing process extends abnormally into the retina.

The number of fibers that are myelinated varies from minimal to a very extensive amount that may seriously affect vision. In more extensive cases there is loss of transparency of the affected portions of retina, producing a scotoma. Ophthalmoscopically, the lesions do not progress (even after prolonged observation), and, therefore, it seems certain that this is a congenital defect. Microscopically, the axons in the retina show typical myelinization in the affected zones. Myelin production and metabolic turnover are a function of the glial oligodendrocytes.

In a study of 3968 consecutive autopsy cases, Straatsma, Foos, Heckenlively, and Taylor (1981) found myelinated retinal nerve fibers in 39 cases (0.98 per cent).

Baarsma (1980) has observed the unique occurrence of acquired myelinated nerve fibers in a 23 year old man.

Schachat and Miller (1981) observed the disappearance of myelinated nerve fibers following anterior ischemic optic neuropathy.

Astrocytic (Glial) Hamartomas

Glial tumors of the retina and optic nerve head are considered to be congenital and are therefore classified as hamartomas. Rarely, new tumors have been observed to develop in clinically normal retinas (Harley and Grover, 1970). Glial tumors are most frequently seen in association with tuberous sclerosis, rarely with Von Recklinghausen's disease (neurofibromatosis) (Bloch, 1948; Martyn and Knox, 1972), and, rarely, unassociated with either disease (McLean, 1937; Ganley and Streeten, 1971; Reeser, Aaberg, Van Horn, 1978).

Ophthalmoscopically, the early lesions are rather flat and appear translucent (Fig. 8–29). The lesion may enlarge, becoming dome-shaped. Older lesions have a tendency to undergo calcification, which gives the lesion a focal chalky-white appearance that may be confused clinically with re-

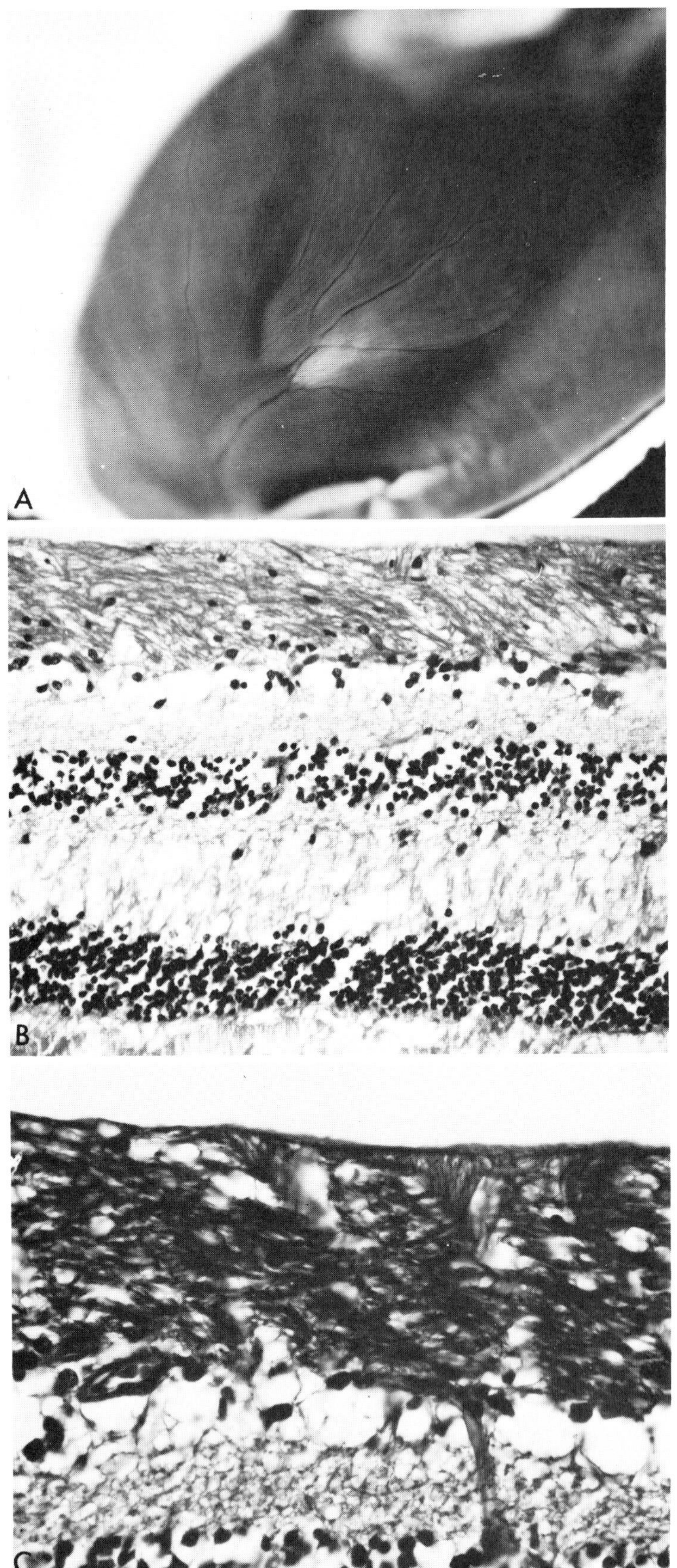

Figure 8–28. *A,* Gross appearance of myelinated nerve fibers in midperiphery of retina. *B,* Histologic section through area shows a thickened nerve fiber layer. H and E, ×300. *C,* Special staining for myelin is positive in the thickened nerve fiber layer. Verhoeff von Gieson, ×510. EP 31488.

tinoblastoma (Cleasby, Fung, Shekter, 1967). Astrocytes at the optic nerve head may become quite large and calcified, with a tapioca- or mulberry-like appearance (Fig. 8–30).

These slow-growing glial tumors do not metastasize or extend out of the eye; however, larger optic nerve head tumors may lead to loss of vision (Wolter and Mertus, 1969) from vitreous hemorrhage and retinal detachment (Atkinson, Sanders, Wong, 1973).

Histologically, most of the tumors are composed of elongated fibrous astrocytes, containing small oval nuclei, and interlacing cytoplasmic processes (Reeser, Aaberg, Van Horn, 1978; Ramsay, Kinyoun, Hill, et al, 1979; Font, Ferry, 1972) (Figs. 8–31 and 8–32). Foci of calcification may be observed. Larger lesions, especially those at the optic nerve head, may have large, moderately pleomorphic, gomistocytic (large, round) astrocytes (Fig. 8–33).

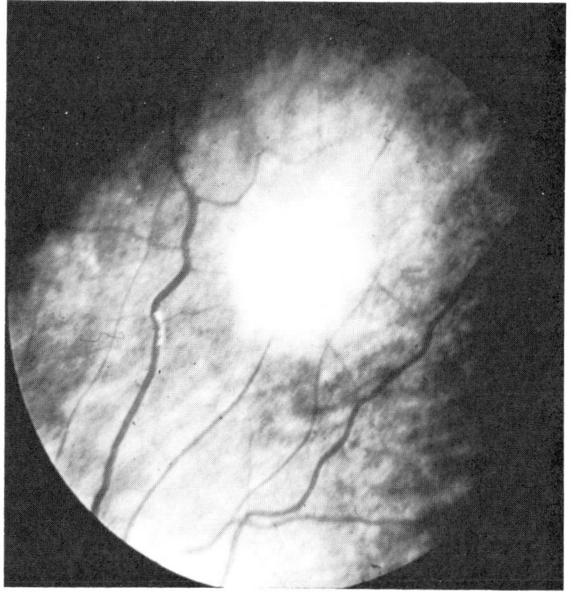

Figure 8–29. Glial (astrocytic) hamartoma of retina in child with tuberous sclerosis. (Courtesy of Dr. Robinson D. Harley.)

Vascular Abnormalities

Various congenital defects of the retinal vessels, both on the arterial and venous sides, have been described as developmental abnormalities. These include abnormal, dilated, tortuous vessels unassociated with any other disease. Arteriovenous anastomoses have been described within the retina, involving vessels in one or several quadrants. These anastomoses may be quiescent and unassociated with retinal disease, or there may be some leakage of fluid from the vessels with secondary loss of retinal function.

Proliferative Retinopathy in Anencephalic Babies. Cogan (1963); Andersen, Bro-Rasmussen, and Tygstrup (1967); and Addison, Font, and Manschot (1972) published definitive papers on retinal changes that occur in anencephalic babies. Some of the changes in these eyes relate to the degree of prematurity of the babies; others, to the anencephalic state. Features of the anencephaly are well documented and include hypoplasia of the ganglion cell layer, nerve fiber layer, and optic nerve head. The ganglion cells are much fewer than normal, with pyknosis of the nuclei of the persisting cells. The nerve fiber layer shows extensive loss of nerve axons and only occasional glial cells. The optic disk shows an absence of most of the prelaminar tissue, and the sensory retina on either side encroaches on the disk's edges. The optic nerve is much smaller than normal, and it shows loss of axons and marked secondary gliosis.

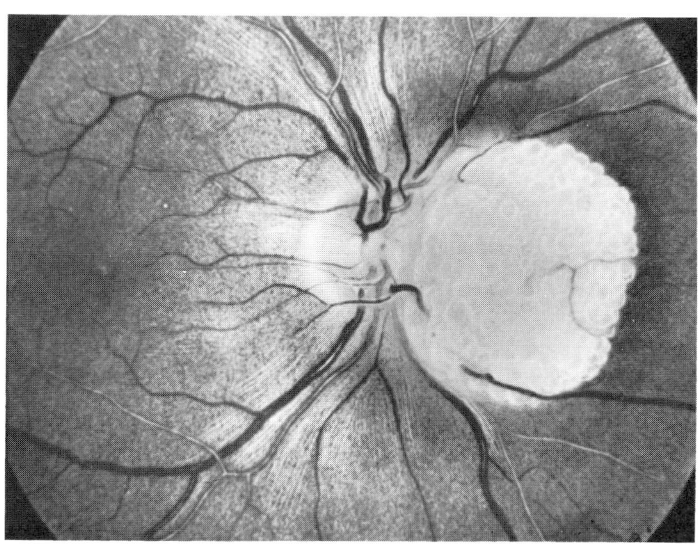

Figure 8–30. Partially calcified **astrocytic hamartoma** of optic nerve head associated with tuberous sclerosis.

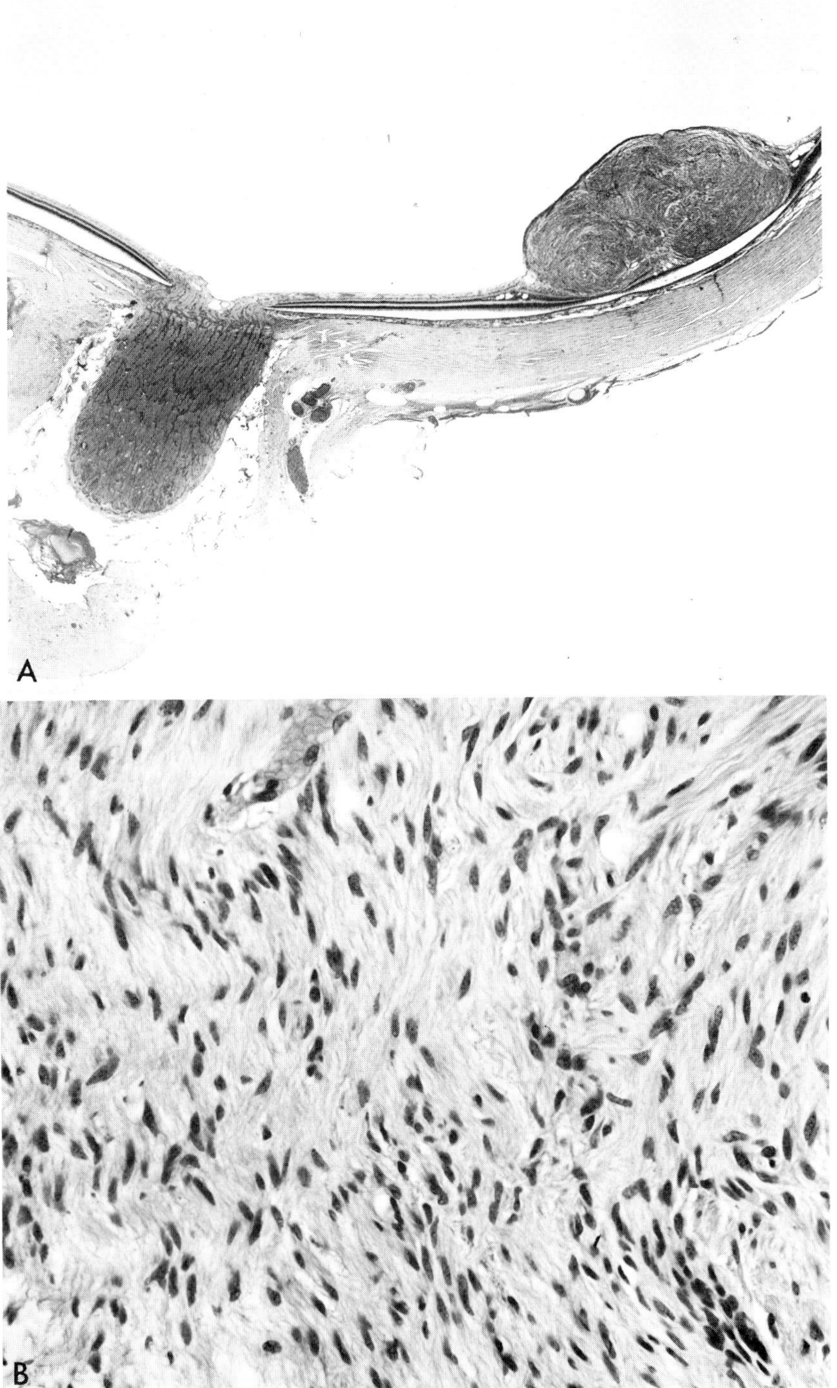

Figure 8–31. Glial hamartoma composed of spindle-shaped cells with abundant fibrillar cellular processes. H and E: *A,* ×8; *B,* ×290. EP 3711. (From Nicholson DH, Green WR: Tumors of the eye, lids, and orbit in children, *in* Harley RD (ed): Pediatric Ophthalmology. Philadelphia, W.B. Saunders Company, 1975, p 923.)

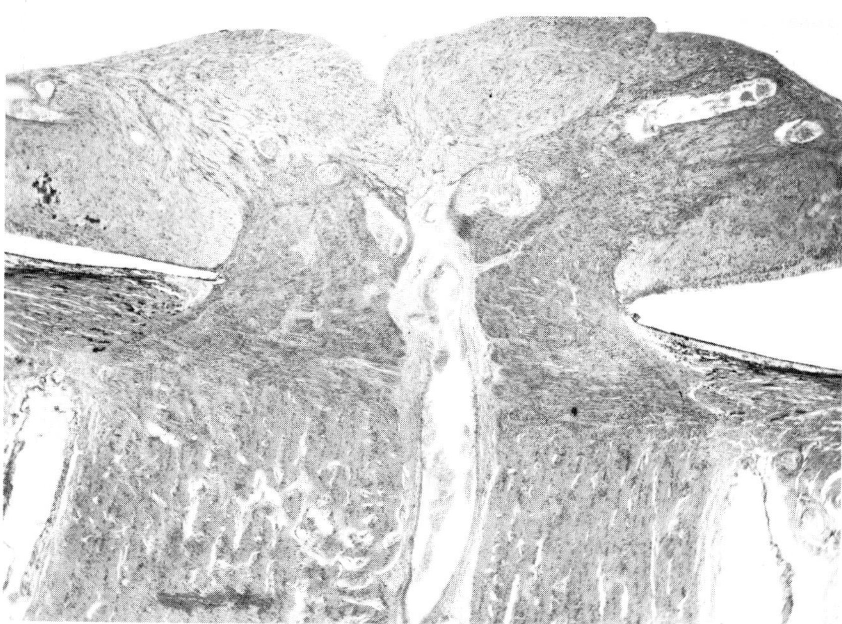

Figure 8–32. Glial hamartoma of optic nerve head associated with von Recklinghausen's disease. H and E, ×30. (Courtesy of Dr. M.J. Hogan; case presented at the Ophthalmic Pathology Club, Washington, DC, April, 1955.)

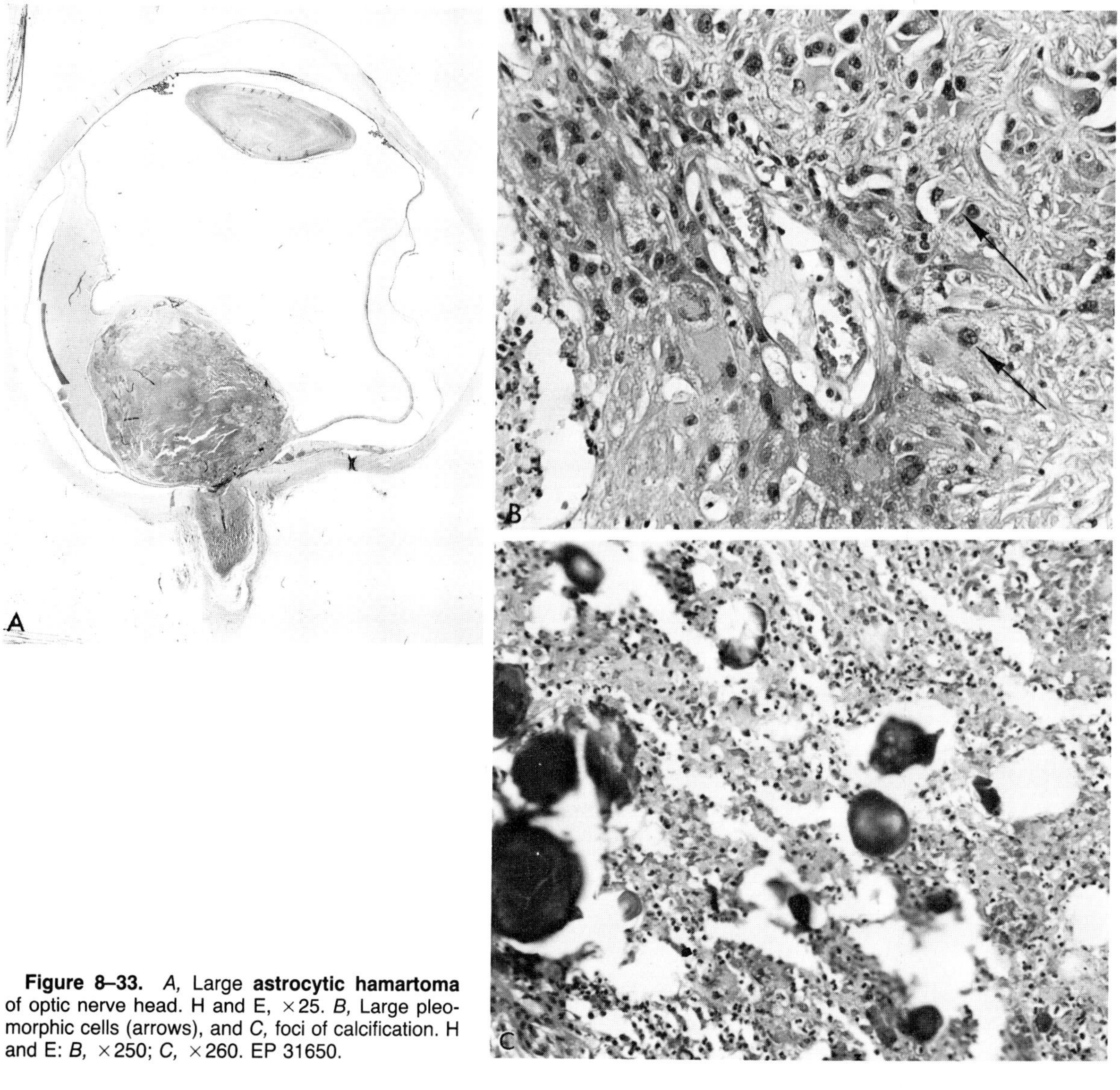

Figure 8–33. *A,* Large **astrocytic hamartoma** of optic nerve head. H and E, ×25. *B,* Large pleomorphic cells (arrows), and *C,* foci of calcification. H and E: *B,* ×250; *C,* ×260. EP 31650.

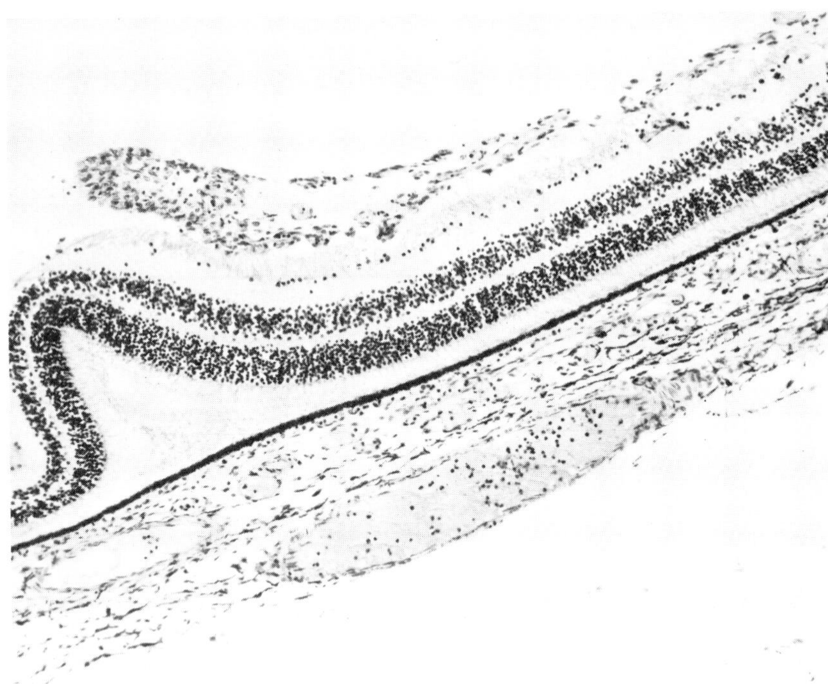

Figure 8–34. Retinal neovascularization extending into vitreous in an anencephalic neonate. H and E, ×120.

The outstanding retinal finding in this condition is the broad range of defects in the retinal blood vessels. All the reported eyes showed incomplete vascularization of the peripheral retina. In some eyes there was a proliferation of spindle-shaped cells, the vanguard of retinal vascularization of the nerve fiber layer; in others, frank intraretinal neovascularization was seen. In some eyes the proliferation of new vessels can be seen to pass through the internal limiting membrane, producing varying degrees of intravitreal neovascularization. Bleeding can occur from these intravitreal vessels and may lead to retinal detachment. The occurrence of retinal vascular proliferation, however, is not a constant feature of anencephaly. Only one definite case in 41 eyes was reported by Andersen and coworkers (1967). However, among 73 eyes from anencephalic babies studied by Addison and coworkers (1972), nine eyes from six infants showed varying degrees of vascular proliferative changes in the retina and vitreous that strikingly resembled those seen in the retinopathy of prematurity (Fig. 8–34). It is believed that in those eyes that develop retinal neovascularization, the process is secondary to hypoxia related to an abnormal blood supply to the retina.

Retinal Arteriovenous Communication (Retinal Arteriovenous Aneurysm) (Racemose Hemangioma of Retina). This lesion may be present on the optic disk and in the retina and may present a distinctive ophthalmoscopic appearance. The vessels on the disc and surrounding retina are hugely dilated and tortuous. It is believed that there is a direct connection between the arteries and veins, without an intervening capillary bed (Henkind, Wise, 1974). Blood passes directly from the artery to the vein, and this is best demonstrated by fluorescein angiography. Some workers prefer the term *racemose hemangioma* because the arteriovenous feature of the lesion is not always apparent. The lesion does not progress. There is no leakage of fluorescein and usually no tendency to bleeding or exudation. Visual impairment depends on the location of the lesion.

Some of these arteriovenous communications are related to similar vascular communications within the optic nerve and intracranially. One group of cases that was initially described by Wyburn-Mason (1943) had arteriovenous aneurysms of the midbrain and retina and also facial hemangioma and mental changes. This association of retinal and midbrain vascular hamartomata is now referred to as the Wyburn-Mason syndrome (Font, Ferry, 1972). However, some cases of these congenital retinal arteriovenous aneurysms have been described in which there was no associated central nervous system disease (Rundles and Falls, 1951).

Cameron and Greer (1968) described the histologic findings in a patient with arteriovenous aneurysm of the right retina (Fig. 8–35), optic nerve, optic tract, and midbrain. The lesion had resulted from a malformation of the right middle cerebral vessels, which occupied most of the third ventricle and extended into the upper end of the aqueduct. Large abnormal supernumerary retinal vessels were found running from the disk toward the equator. It was not possible to distinguish arteries and veins, because all the vessels had fibromuscular medial coats of variable thickness and wide, almost acellular, fibrohyaline adventitial coats. Some of the abnormal vessels occupied the whole thickness of the retina and were adherent to Bruch's membrane. In all sections examined, the retina showed marked loss of nerve axons and a reduced number of ganglion cells.

An additional case studied histopathologically was interpreted as showing a venous angioma of the retina, optic nerve, chiasm, and brain (Krug and Samuels, 1932).

Similar arteriovenous malformations have been observed in monkeys (Fig. 8–36) (Bellhorn, Friedman, Henkind, 1972; Horiuchi, Gass, David, 1976).

Cavernous Hemangioma of Retina. This uncommon congenital malformation is characterized by isolated clusters of vascular globules in which plasma and erythrocyte sedimentation may be present. Fluorescein angiography shows a nor-

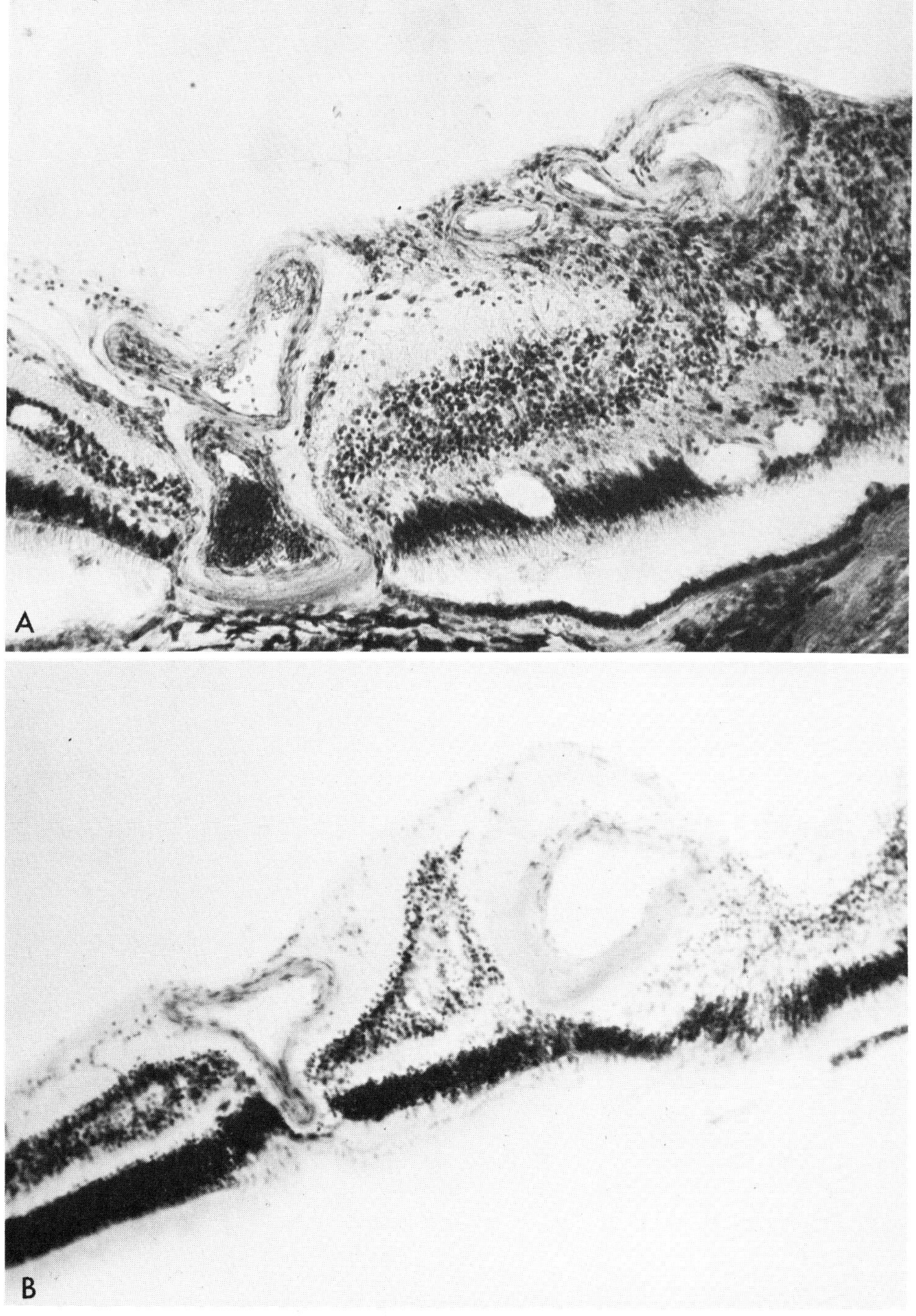

Figure 8–35. Arteriovenous malformation of retina *(A* and *B)* **and optic nerve.** *(C).*

Illustration continued on following page

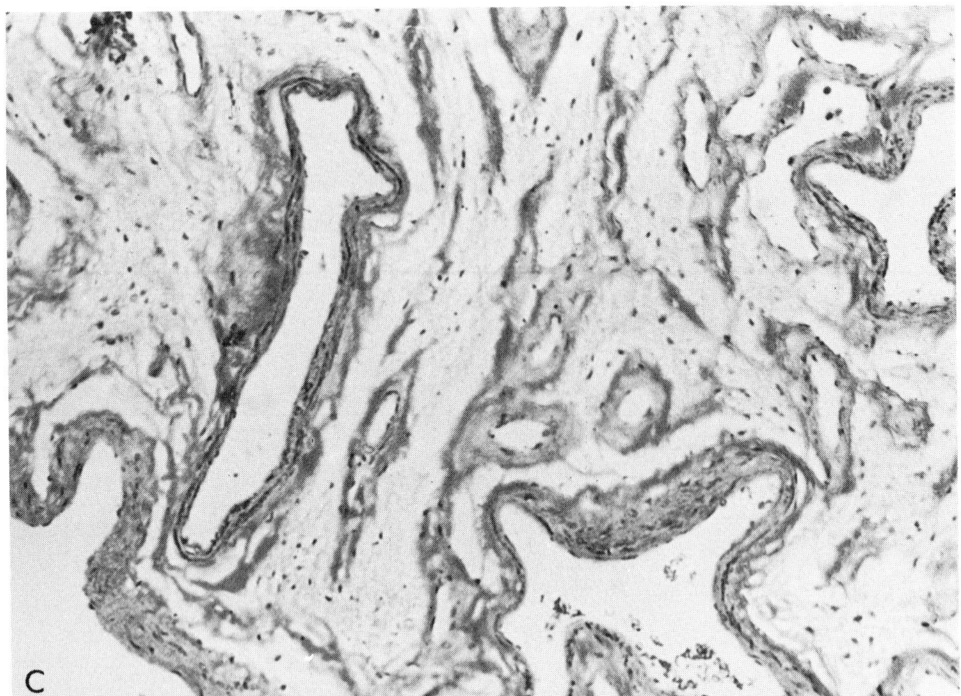

Figure 8–35 *Continued A,* Masson trichrome, ×100; *B,* Masson trichrome, ×80; *C,* phosphotungstic acid–hematoxylin, ×100. (From Cameron ME, Greer CH: Congenital arteriovenous aneurysm of the retina: A post-mortem report. Br J Ophthalmol *52*:768–772, 1968.)

mal arterial supply, slowed transmission of dye, and slowed venous drainage. There are no arteriovenous shunting and no disturbance in vascular permeability (Lewis, Cohen, Wise, 1975). The lesions are nonprogressive and are rarely a source of bleeding. The study of one four-generation pedigree of patients with this lesion disclosed the association of seizures or cranial nerve palsies and cutaneous hemangiomas with retinal cavernous hemangiomas (Goldberg, Pheasant, Shield, 1979). These investigators noted a probable autosomal dominant inheritance pattern with incomplete penetrance. Colvard, Robertson, and Trautmann (1978) reported two patients with cavernous hemangioma, one of whom had features suggestive of a hemangioma of the brain stem.

Histopathologically, the retina is greatly thickened by large vascular channels with normal walls (Fig. 8–37,*A*). The inner retinal layers are discontinuous in the area of the vascular lesions. Vitreous condensations may occur over the lesion; with posterior vitreous detachment, traction on the retina in the area of the hemangioma may occur and can lead to retinal and vitreous hemorrhage (Fig. 8–37,*B*). Davies and Thumin (1956) reported the histopathologic features of a case of cavernous hemangioma of the optic disk and retina.

Miliary Retinal Aneurysms. Miliary retinal aneurysms were first described by Leber in 1912. The aneurysms usually affect only a small area of the fundus in one or another sector. The involved area is usually peripheral in location and elevated and contains numerous small, reddish to red-white globules or globular vascular dilatations in the more superficial layers of the retina. The condition is usually present in only one eye. Ophthalmoscopically, it is usually easily detected by the presence of a discrete area in the fundus outlined by numerous hard-appearing, whitish exudates resembling those seen in circinate retinopathy in the macula.

As more patients have been studied with the use of fluorescein angiography, it has become evident that this condition shows a spectrum of changes and has telangiectatic vessels and areas of nonperfusion present. Leber's disease (retinal microaneurysms) is thought by many to be the forerunner of Coats' disease. Others (Paufique, Ravault, Bonnet, Istre, 1964) consider Leber's miliary angiomatosis to be distinct and believe that it does not lead to the picture of Coats' disease. Although considered here under Congenital Lesions, it is not certain that miliary retinal aneurysms are congenital.

Coats' Disease. Coats' disease is of unknown cause. It consists of an exudative detachment of the retina, associated with vascular abnormalities, including telangiectatic vessels, microaneurysms, areas of nonperfusion, and saccular "light bulb" venous dilatations. It is usually unilateral but rarely may occur bilaterally (Green, 1967).

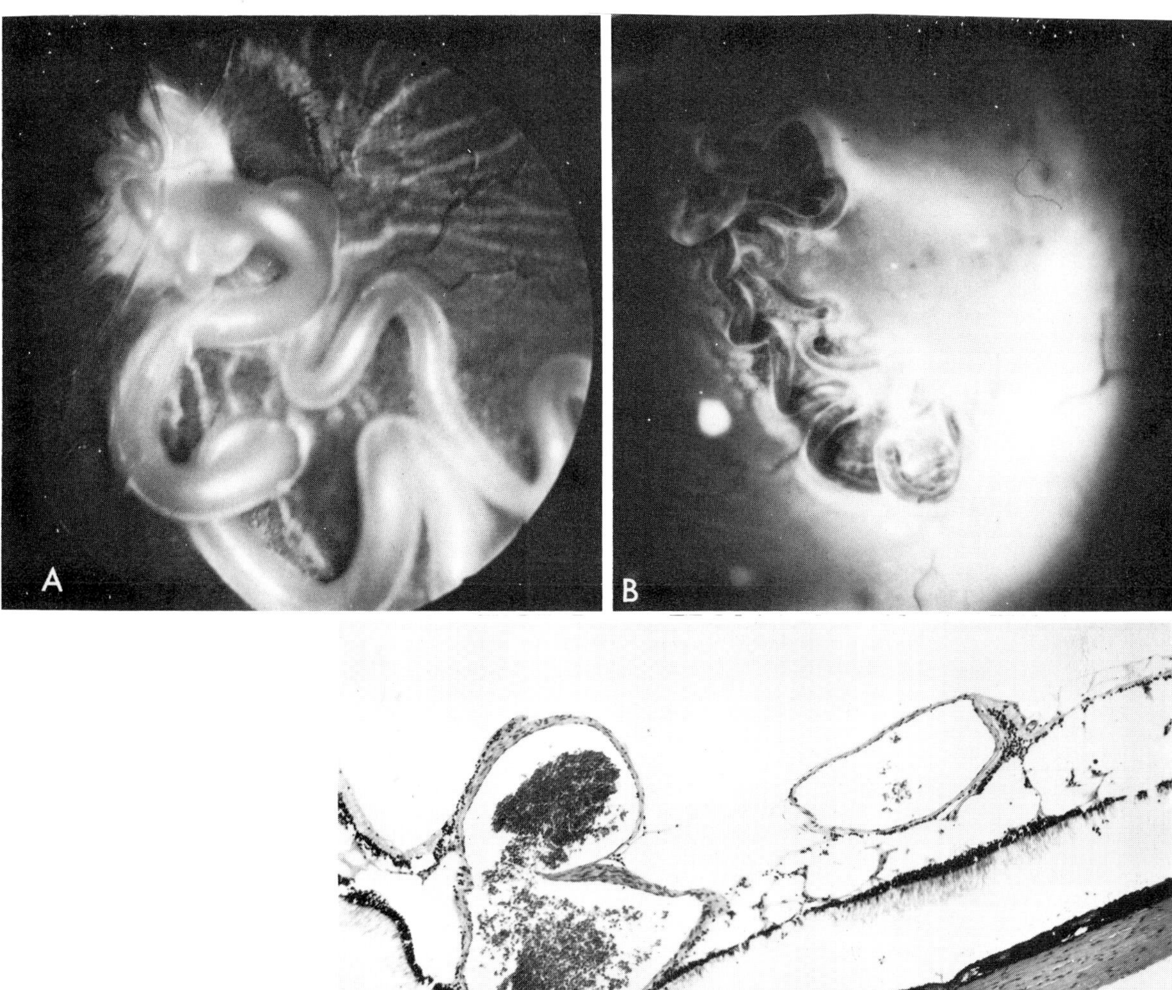

Figure 8–36. *A,* Ophthalmoscopic, *B,* gross, and *C,* microscopic appearance of **retinal arteriovenous malformation** in a monkey. (From Bellhorn RW, Friedman AH, Henkind P: Racemose (cirsoid) hemangioma in Rhesus monkey retina. Am J Ophthalmol *74*:517–525, 1972.)

Coats, in 1908 and 1912, described a type of retinopathy in which there was a collection of intraretinal and external retinal exudates leading to retinal detachment. He recognized that some cases were related to abnormalities of the retinal vessels, but that in other cases the clinical examination showed no abnormality of the retinal vessels. Reese, in 1956, described this entity and indicated that it was almost always related to abnormal vessels that were telangiectatic. Henkind and Morgan (1966) found vascular and neovascular anomalies near the periphery in four adult cases. It now seems that Coats' disease is related to congenital vascular abnormalities and that (sooner or later) changes occur in the walls of the vessels that lead to leakage of plasma and cellular elements, with secondary degeneration of the vessel and neuronal tissue, causing an accumulation of massive exudate in and under the retina, thus separating it from the RPE.

With the light microscope, areas of abnormal vessel telangiectasia are seen (Fig. 8–38), with alterations in the walls of the vessels, leakage of plasma, accumulation of exudates, and edema and degeneration of the retinal tissues (Fig. 8–39). There is accumulation of much fluid under the retina and large numbers of macrophages containing lipid pigment and other substances. These macrophages presumably come from the retinal vessles and migrate through the tissues into the subretinal region. Some of them, however, may come from the choroidal side; also,

Text continued on page 630

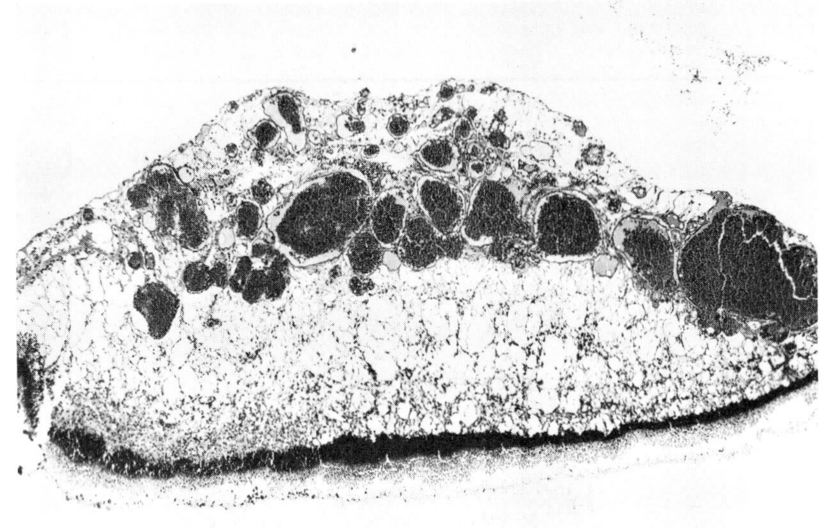

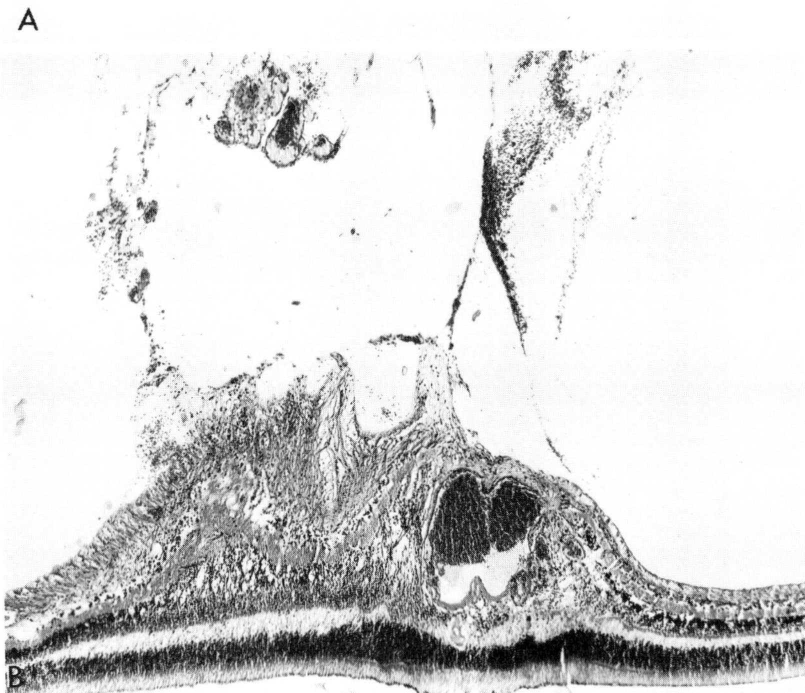

Figure 8–37. Cavernous hemangioma of retina. *A,* Retina is greatly thickened by edema and large, normal-appearing vessels in the inner layers. H and E, ×4. *B,* Different area, showing strands of vitreous with entrapped blood exerting traction on retina containing cavernous hemangioma. H and E, ×40. AFIP Acc. 960712; Neg. 60-6819.

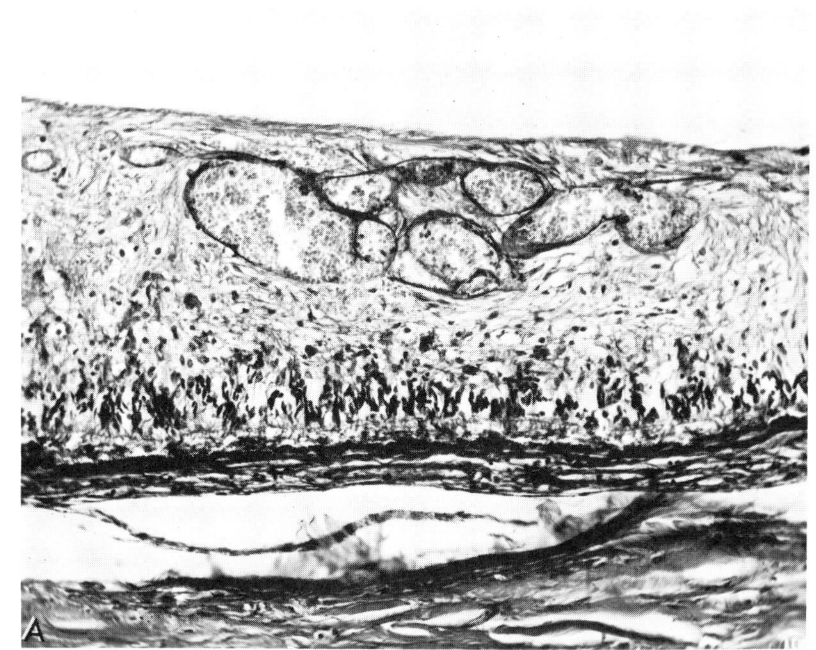

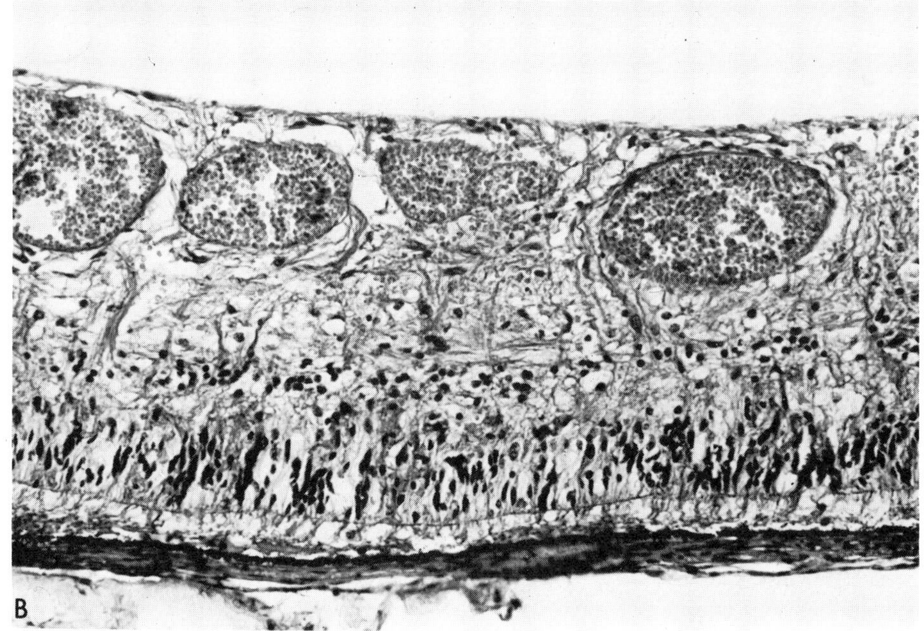

Figure 8–38. Retinal telangiectatic vessels in Coats' disease. *A,* PAS, ×145; *B,* H and E, ×250. (From Green WR: Bilateral Coats' disease. Arch Ophthalmol *77*:378–385, 1967.)

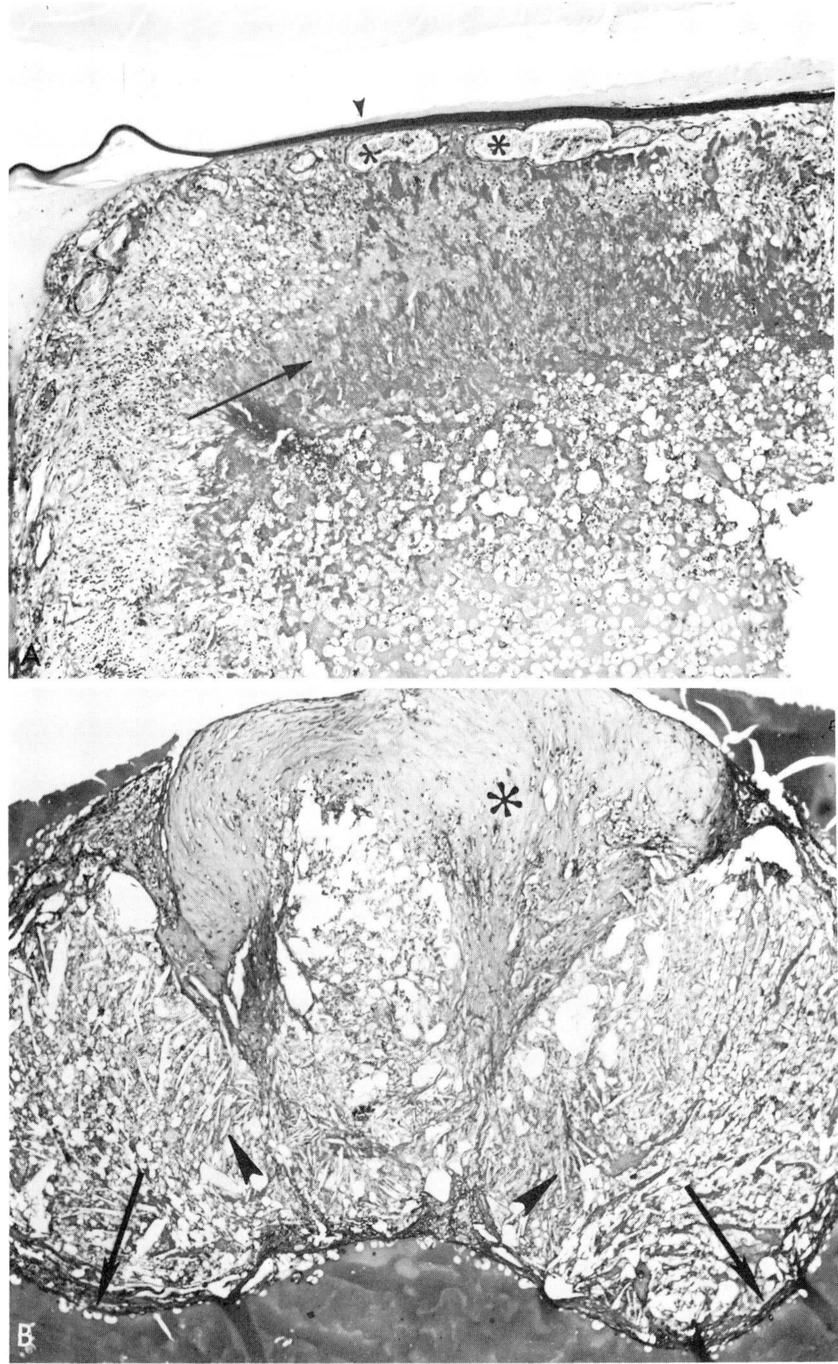

Figure 8–39. Coats' disease. *A,* Retina with telangiectatic vessels (asterisks) and marked degeneration is greatly distended by a dense, proteinaceous material, is detached, and rests against the posterior surface of the lens (arrowhead marks the posterior lens capsule). PAS, ×45. *B,* Nodule with fibrous tissue (asterisk), a fibrocellular capsule (arrows), and a lipid-rich exudate containing some cholesterol slits (arrowheads). PAS, ×55. EP 48472. (From Nicholson DH, Green WR: Pediatric Ocular Tumors. New York, Masson, 1981, p 11.)

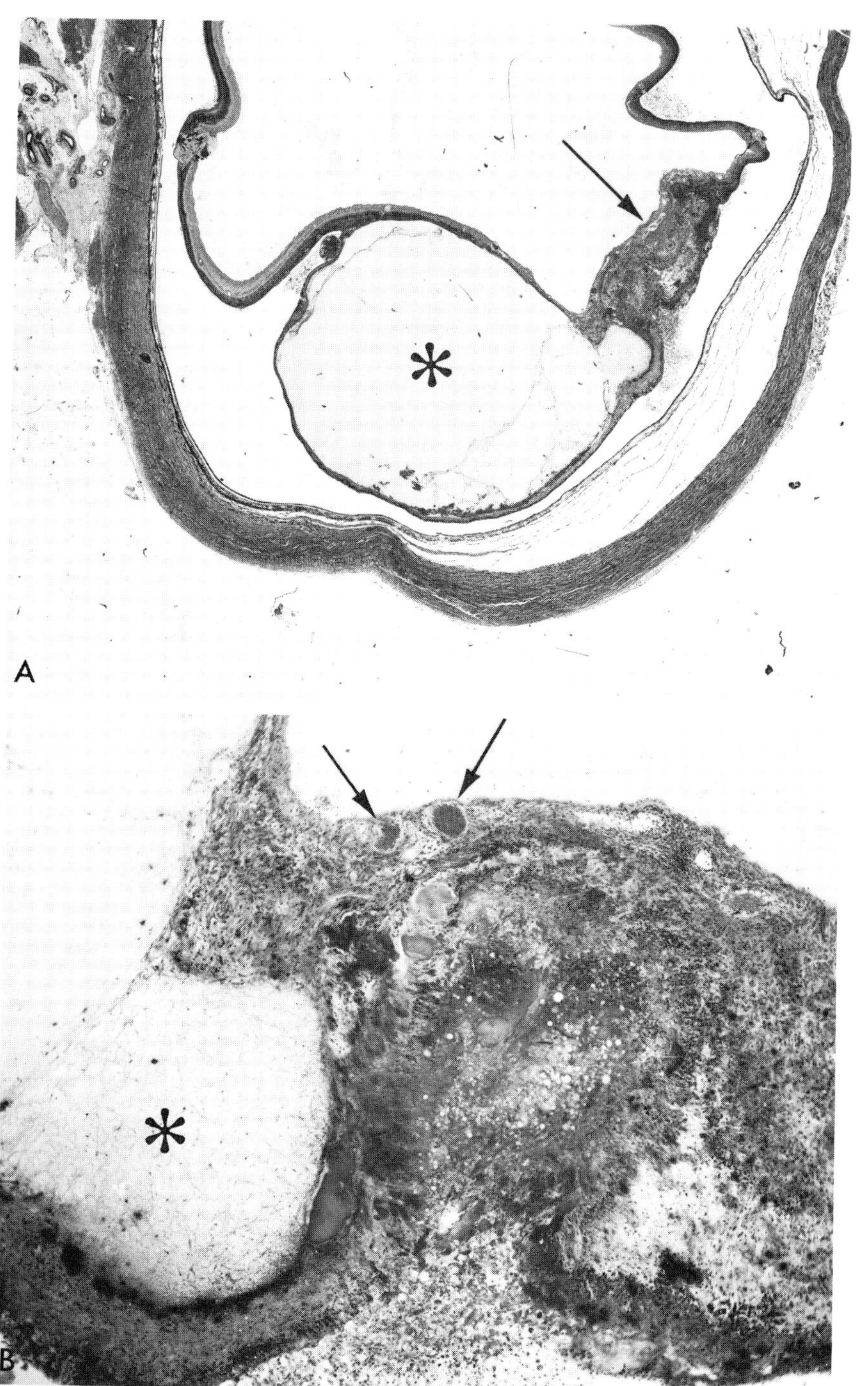

Figure 8–40. Coats' disease with secondary retinoschisis. *A,* Retina (arrow) containing telangiectatic vessels is thickened by exudate and is adjacent to a large area of retinoschisis containing proteinaceous material (asterisk). H and E, ×7.5. *B,* Higher power view of thickened retina with telangiectatic vessels (arrows) and margin of the area of retinoschisis (asterisk). H and E, ×35. (From Klien B; case presented at the Ophthalmic Pathology Club, Washington, DC, April, 1949.)

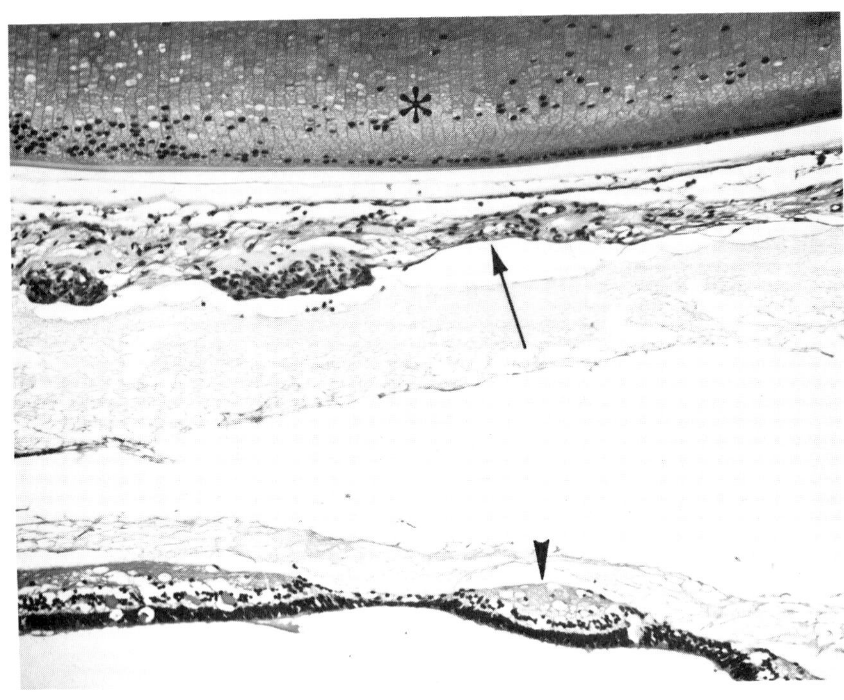

Figure 8–41. Coats' disease with retinoschisis. A proteinaceous material is present between inner (arrow) and outer (arrowhead) layers of secondary retinoschisis in a retina that is detached and rests against the posterior surface of the lens (asterisk). H and E, ×100. EP 46866.

some of them may be secondary to detachment and proliferation of the RPE cells.

Tripathi and Ashton (1971), by electron microscopic study, confirmed the widely held view that an abnormal permeability of the retinal vessels is basic to the pathogenesis of Coats' disease. According to them, there is a breakdown in the blood-retina barrier at the endothelial level, causing leakage of plasma into the wall and disorganization of the walls of the vessels, followed by aneurysmal dilatations and telangiectasis. Plasma then leaks into the adjacent tissues and produces the classic intraretinal and subretinal exudates.

In some instances the marked exudation may lead to splitting of the retina into two layers and formation of a large area of retinoschisis (Figs. 8–40 and 8–41). Under certain conditions, hemorrhages occur; and if fluid is absorbed from the lipid-filled exudate, the classic fatty deposits occur in and under the retina. Fibrin precipitates also are present in the vessel walls, around the vessels, and in the retinal tissue. In some cases, a fibrous tissue nodule is present under the macular area, even with the vascular changes located in the periphery (Figs. 8–39, 8–42, and 8–43). This nodule is composed of hyperplastic RPE and fibrovascular tissue, which results from organization of the lipid-rich subretinal exudate. In some instances vessels from the choroid can be traced into the disciform submacular retinal nodule.

Trypsin digestion studies (Egbert, Chan, Winter, 1977) of patients with Coats' disease disclosed large aneurysms and thick periodic acid–Schiff-positive deposits in vessel walls. The aneurysms ranged from 50 to 350 microns and frequently formed large, sausage-like or beaded outpouchings (Fig. 8–44). Some areas are interpreted as showing some capillaries that become dilated and telangiectatic, while others become acellular strands (Fig. 8–45).

Treatment of Coats' disease can result in resolution of the process in some eyes. Of 7 eyes of patients under the age of 4 years with severe disease treated with cryotherapy or photocoagulation, one eye was stabilized with no light perception and 6 improved (Ridley, Shields, Brown, Tasman, 1982). These investigators reported treatment results of 29 eyes of persons aged 4 to 45 years. Of these 29, 8 deteriorated, 15 were stabilized, and 6 improved.

Retinal Telangiectasis in Adults. This vascular condition has features similar to those seen in Coats' disease. Although familial cases have been observed, it is not at present considered to be congenital.

Coats'-Like Response in Retinitis Pigmentosa. A Coats'-like response has been described in 15 patients with retinitis pigmentosa. Fogle, Welch, and Green (1978) found in the study of one case that the retinal vasculature was sclerotic, acellular, and occluded (Fig. 8–46,*A*) and that the exudative material apparently was coming from multiple areas of choroidal neovascularization in the equatorial area. The new vessels were traced from the choroid, through a break in Bruch's membrane, through the retina, and into the vitreous as a rete mirable–like configuration (Fig. 8–46,*B–D*).

Parafoveal Telangiectasia. The familial occurrence of telangiectasis in the parafoveal area apparent by fluorescein angiography has been described by Hutton, Snyder, Fuller, and Vaiser (1978). Similar, but hereditary, cases have been reported by Gass (1968b) and Schatz (1975).

Clinicopathologic studies of one patient (Green, Quigley, de la Cruz, Cohen, 1980) have demonstrated thickening of the wall of the capillaries, with multilamination of the basement membrane, narrowing of the capillary lumen, extensive degeneration of pericytes, lipid deposits in the capillary wall, focal endothelial cell degeneration, and no telangiectasis (Figs. 8–47 through 8–49). These changes were greatest in the area of involvement, as determined by fluorescein angiography. Similar but milder changes were observed throughout the retina. The changes were interpreted as being caused by endothelial cell degeneration and regeneration, with successive basement membrane production and secondary degeneration of pericytes.

Capillary Hemangioma. The retinal lesions of angiomatosis retinae (von Hippel tumors) are benign vascular tumors. The cellular constituents (by light microscopy and histochemical and ultrastructural studies) are similar to those of cerebel-

Text continued on page 637

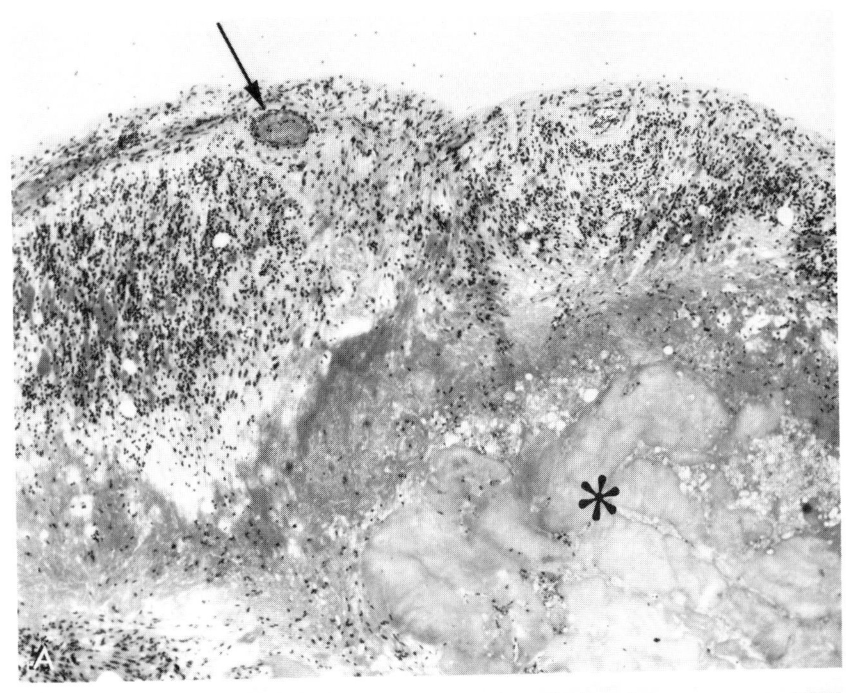

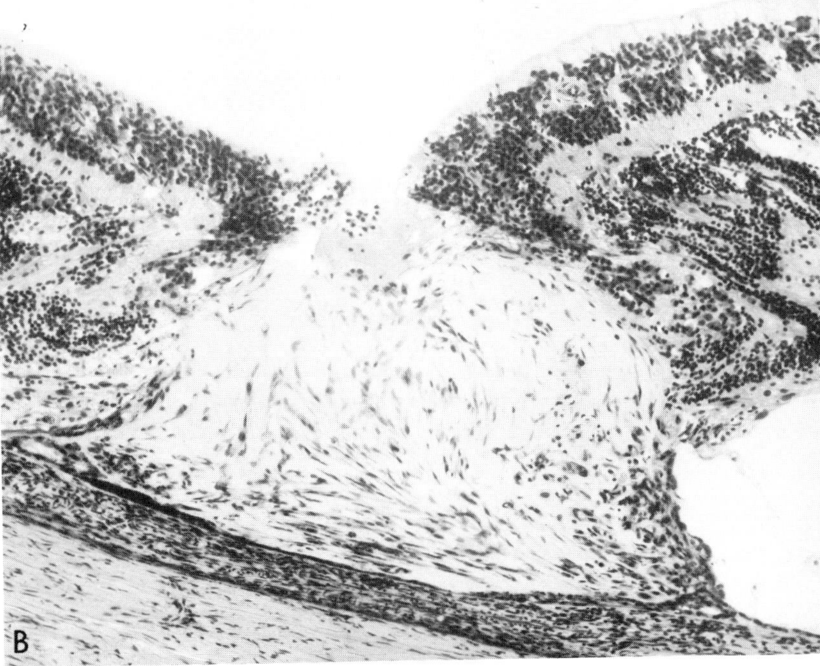

Figure 8–42. Coats' disease with fibrous scar under macula. *A,* Peripheral retina is greatly thickened by a dense proteinaceous material (asterisk) and contains telangiectatic vessels (arrow). H and E, ×65. *B,* A fibrous nodule composed of laminated, hyperplastic RPE is present under the foveal area. H and E, ×100. EP 43898. (From Green WR: Pathology of the Retina, *in* Frayer WC (ed): Lancaster Course in Ophthalmic Histopathology. Unit 9. Philadelphia, F.A. Davis, 1981.)

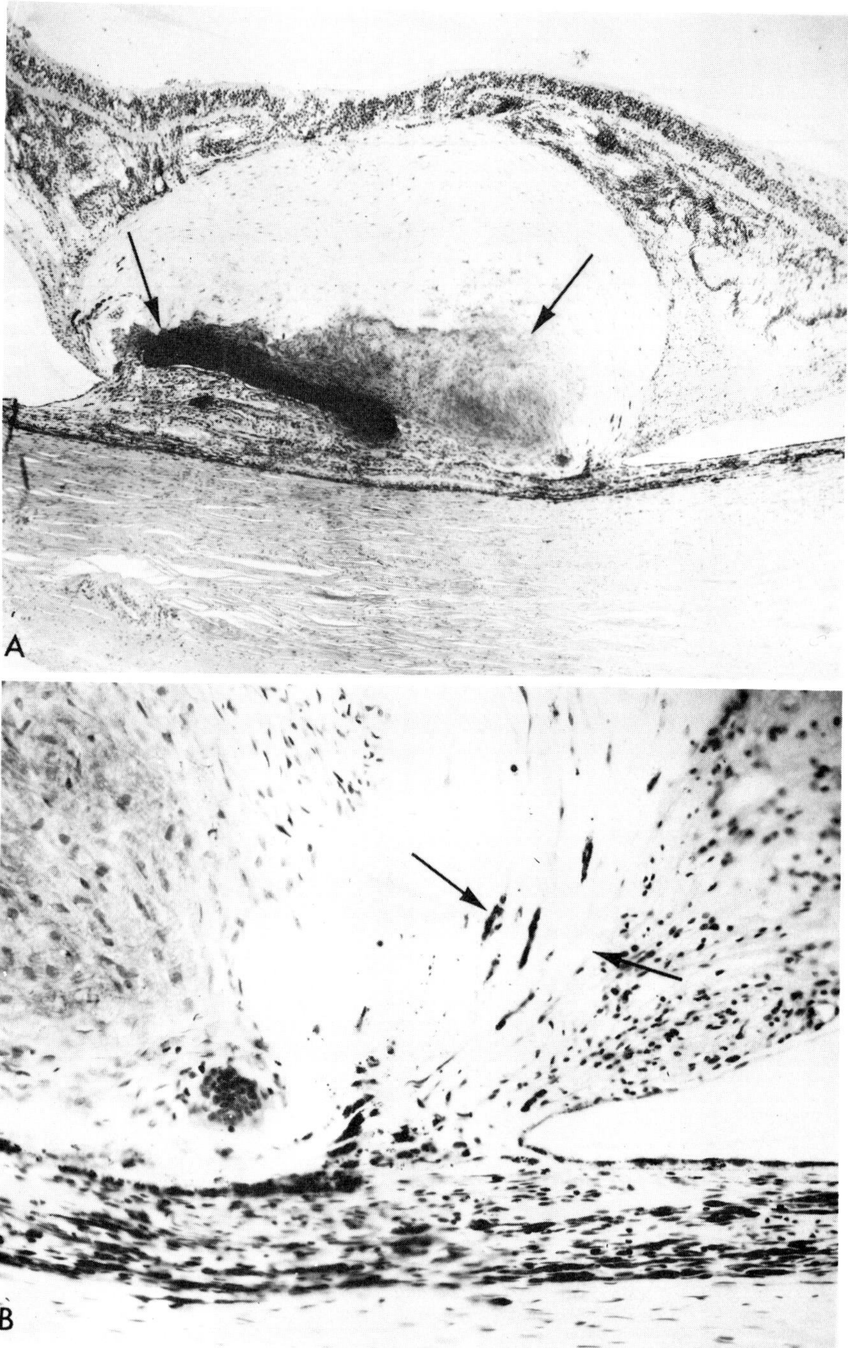

Figure 8–43. *A,* Disciform scar in macular area associated with **Coats' disease**. The laminated appearance is suggestive of old RPE hyperplasia. An area of calcification (arrows) is present. H and E, ×40. *B,* Higher power view of margin of the nodule shows the layered appearance of hyperplastic, pigment-containing cells (arrows). H and E, ×205. (From McGavic J; case presented at the Ophthalmic Pathology Club, Washington, DC, April, 1948.)

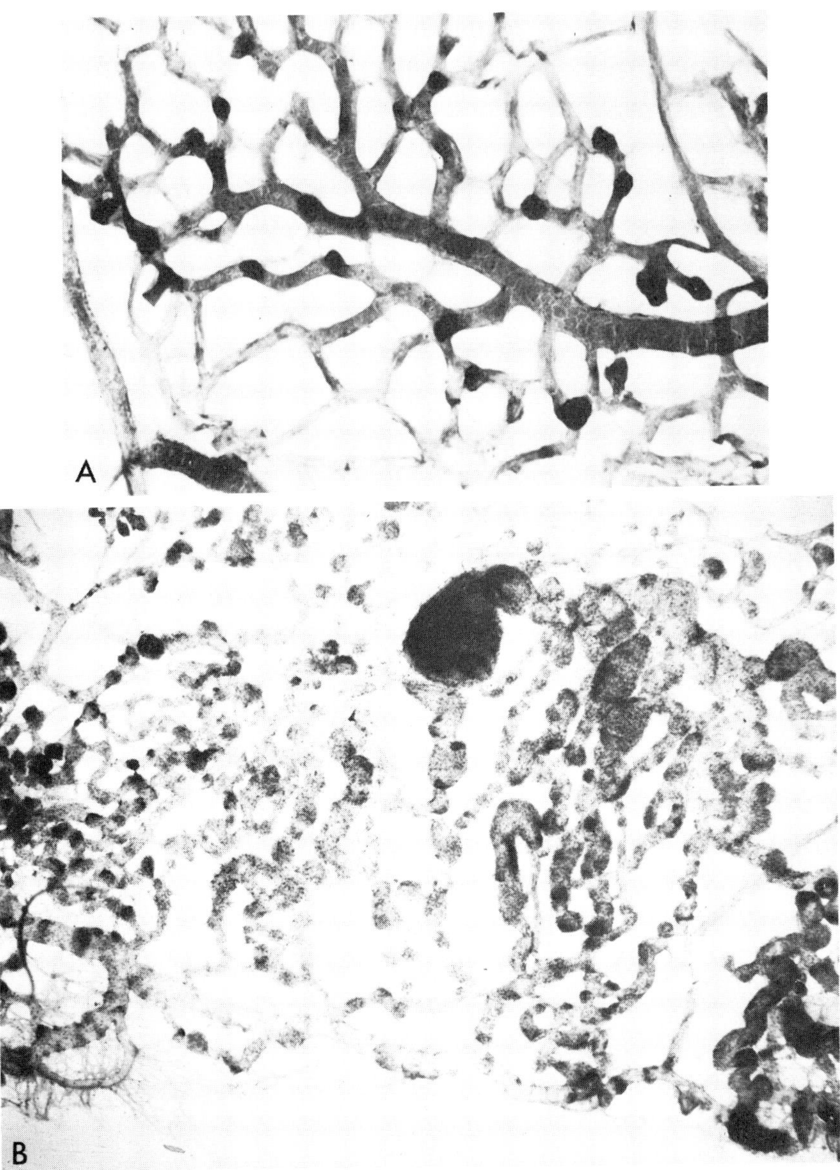

Figure 8–44. Trypsin digestion preparation of retina in **Coats' disease**. *A,* Dilated capillaries with numerous small microaneurysms. PAS, ×122. *B,* Large aneurysms and sausage-like beading of vessels. PAS, ×44. (From Egbert PR, Chan CC, Winter FC: Flat preparations of the retinal vessels in Coats' disease. J Pediatr Ophthalmol *14*:336–339, 1977.)

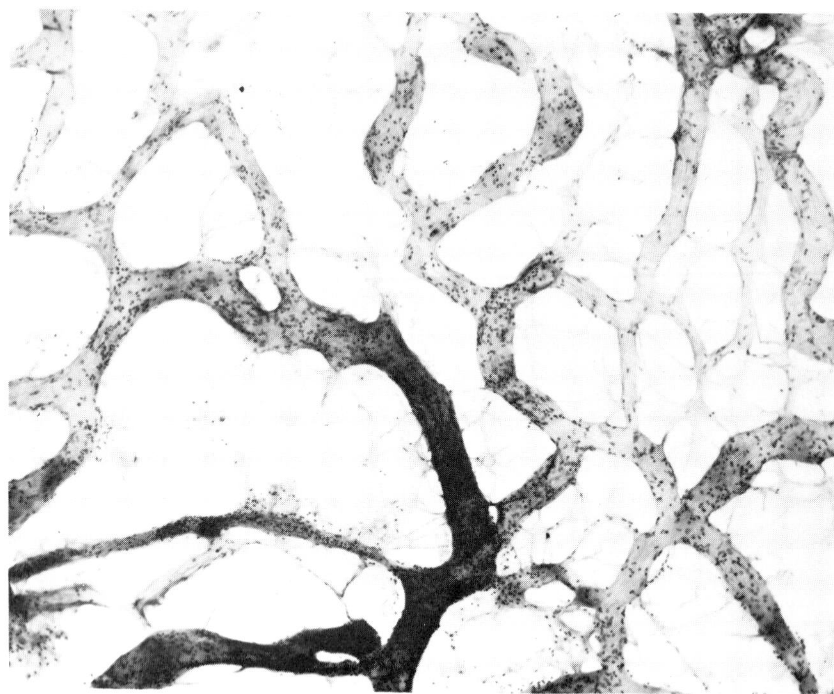

Figure 8–45. Trypsin digestion preparation of retina in **Coats' disease**. The capillary background is largely acellular. Some capillaries have become dilated and telangiectatic. H and E; PAS, ×60. EP 48472.

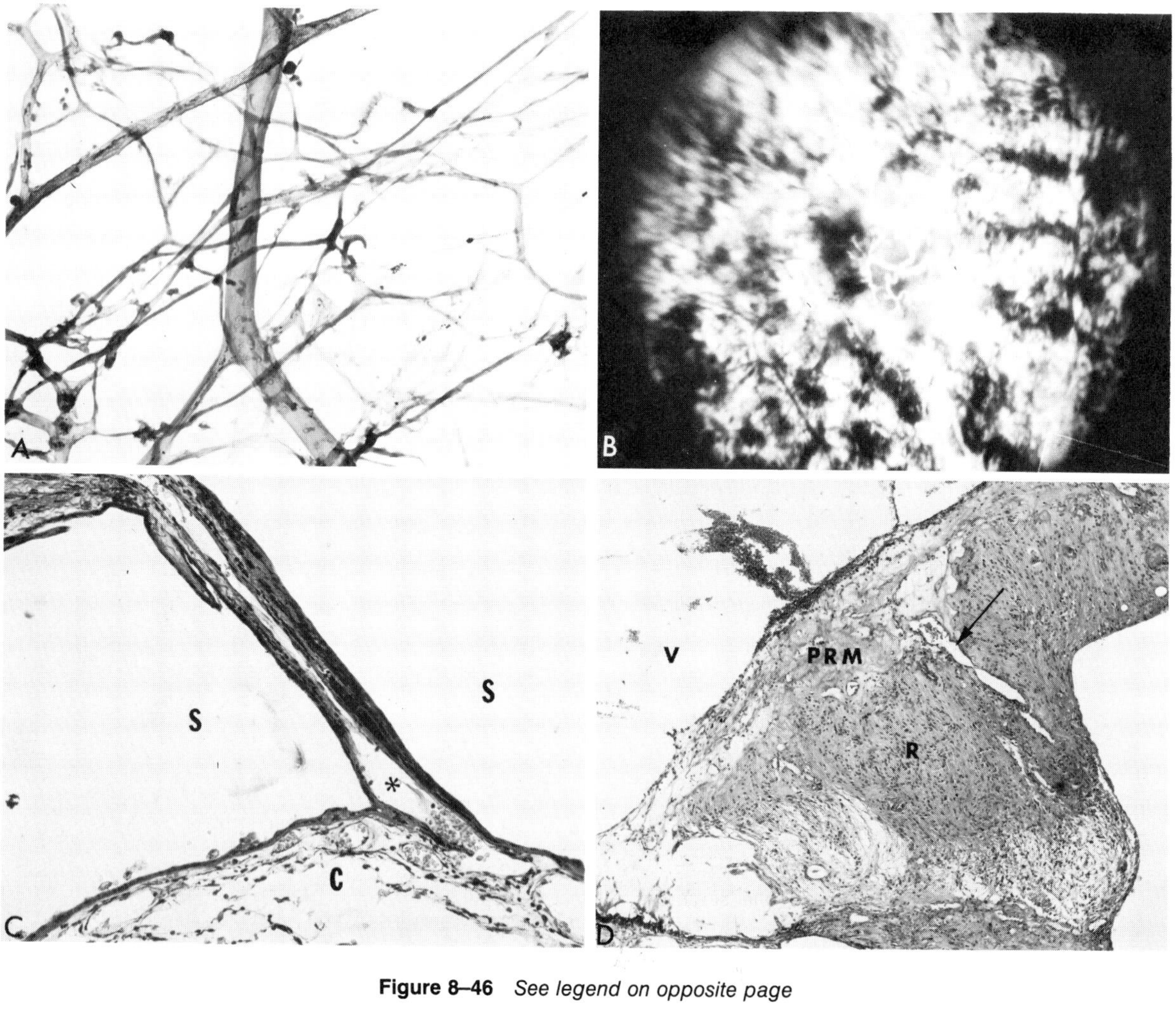

Figure 8–46 *See legend on opposite page*

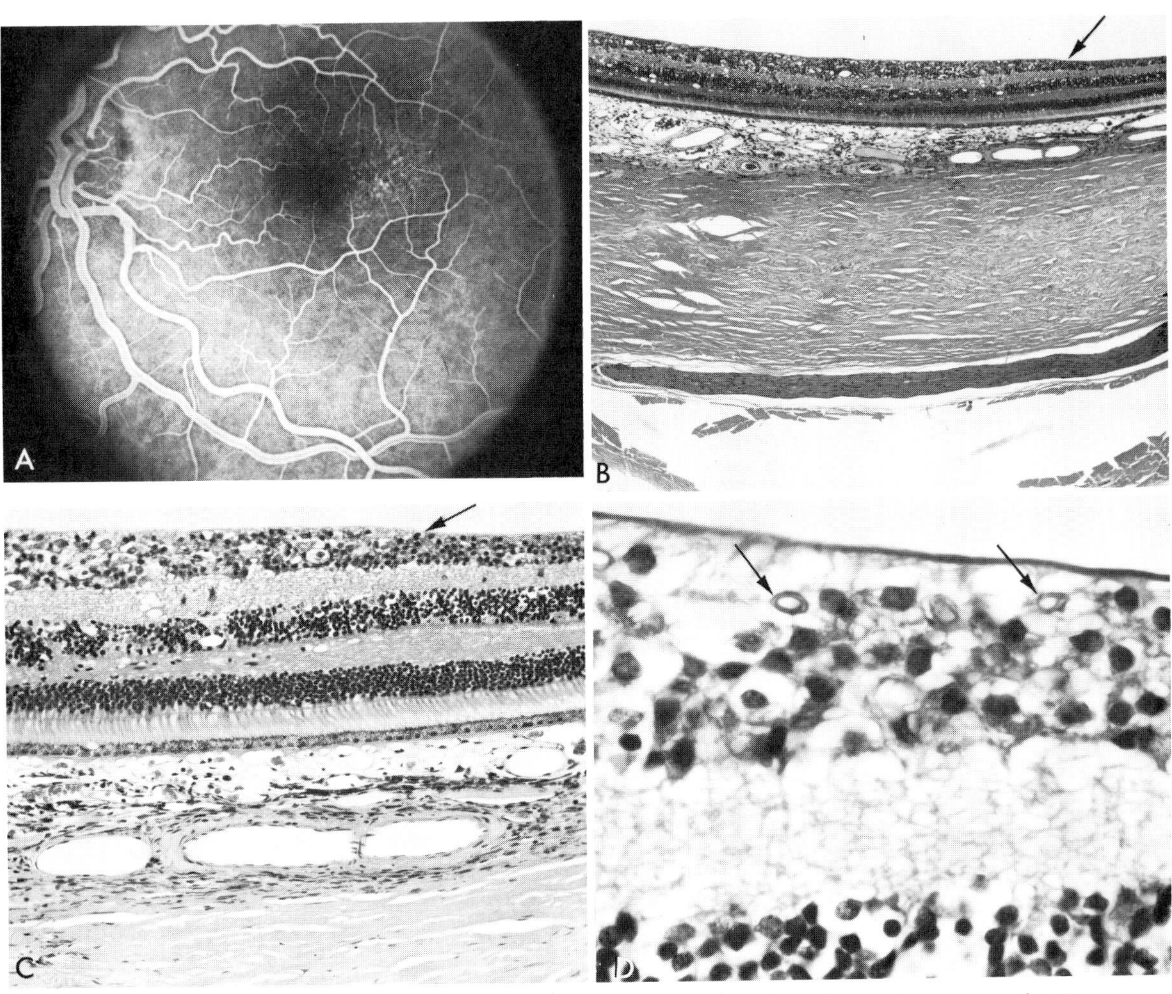

Figure 8–47. Parafoveal telangiectasis. *A,* Fluorescein staining of capillary walls in temporal parafoveal area at 20 seconds. *B,* Temporal margin (arrow) of abnormal area observed by fluorescein angiography. The retina is thicker, from edema and mild microcystic changes. H and E, ×50. *C,* Higher power magnification showing temporal margin (arrow) of temporal parafoveal area of involvement. The retina is thickened by edema, mainly involving retinal layers internal to the outer nuclear layer. A few microcystic cavities are present. The RPE is normal. H and E, ×180. *D,* Capillaries (arrows) with thickened walls, multiple layers of basement membrane, and no pericytes in the temporal parafoveal area. PAS, ×900. EP 46601. (From Green WR, Quigley HT, de la Cruz Z, Cohen B: Parafoveal retinal telangiectasis: Light and electron microscopy studies. Trans Ophthalmol Soc UK *100*:162–170, 1980.)

Figure 8–46. Retinitis pigmentosa with Coats'-like response secondary to choroidal neovascularization. *A,* Trypsin digest preparation revealing severe sclerosis, hypocellularity, and partial loss of retinal capillaries. PAS, ×155. *B,* Fluorescein angiograph of vascular lesion. No retinal feeder vessels are apparent because retina is nonperfused. *C,* Close detail of vessel (asterisk) from choroid *(C)* and subretinal space *(S)*. Van de Grift, ×175. *D,* Serial sectioning of temporal periphery of left eye, proving continuity between choroidal vessel and thin-walled vessels of preretinal membrane *(PRM)* via the gliotic retina *(R)*. Arrow denotes entry of vessel from retina into preretinal membrane; *V* indicates vitreous cavity. Van de Grift, ×60. EP 42254. (From Fogle JA, Welch RB, Green WR: Retinitis pigmentosa and exudative vasculopathy. Arch Ophthalmol *96*:696–702, 1978.)

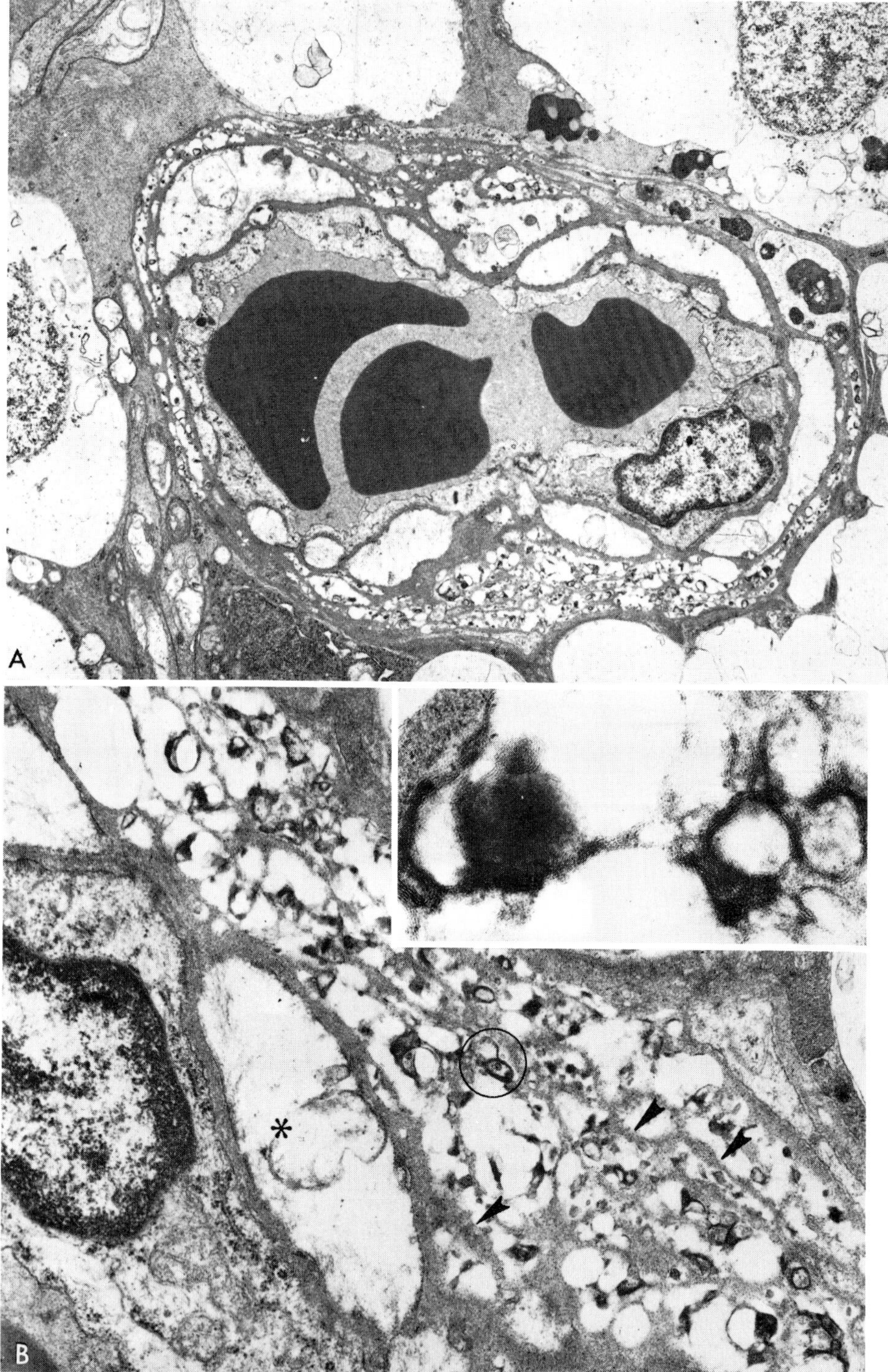

Figure 8–48. *A,* **Retinal capillary** in temporal parafoveal area with endothelium that is intact but with early degenerative appearance. Multiple layers of basement membrane are separated by cellular debris and multimembranous lamellar material. No pericyte is observed. ×8000. *B,* Higher power view of wall of capillary, showing layers of basement membrane (arrowheads), cellular debris (asterisk), and laminated lipid material (circle). ×36,000. *Inset,* Higher power view (×107,900) illustrates the membranous lamellar material. EP 96601. (From Green WR, Quigley HT, de la Cruz Z, Cohen B: Parafoveal retinal telangiectasis: Light and electron microscopic studies. Trans Ophthalmol Soc UK *100*:162–170, 1980.)

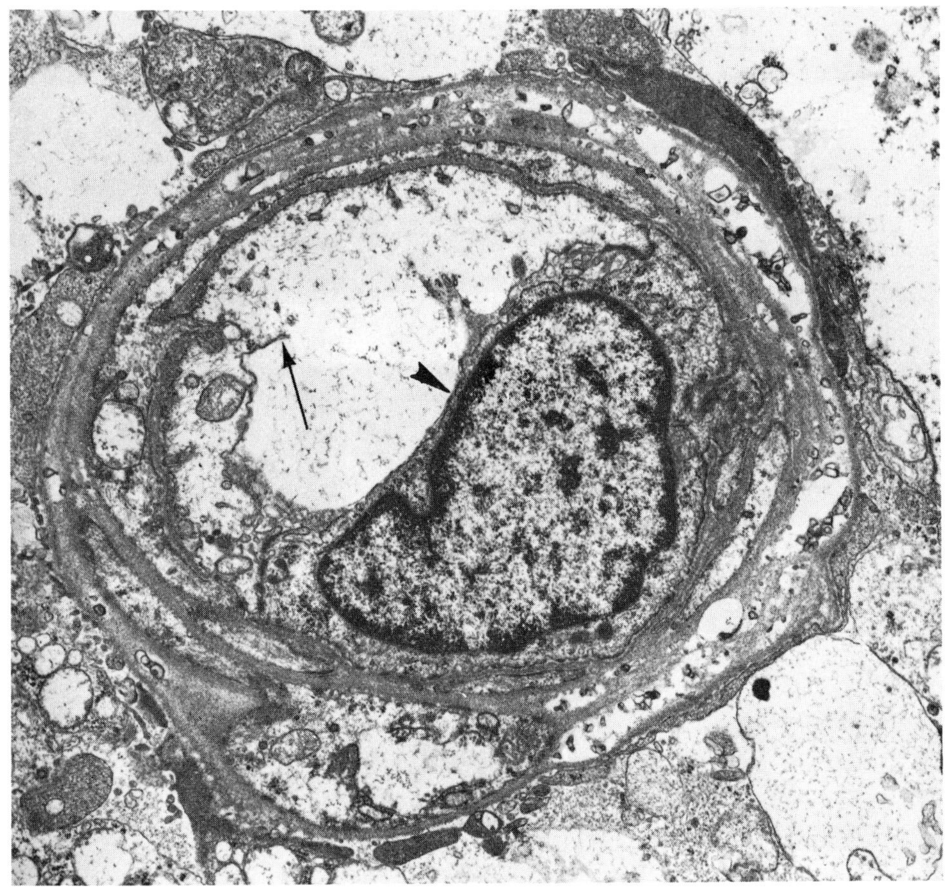

Figure 8–49. Capillary in temporal parafoveal area, showing disrupted and degenerating endothelial cell on one side (arrow) and an intact endothelial cell on the other side (arrowhead). Cellular debris and membranous material are deposited between the multiple layers of basement membrane. No intact pericytes remain. ×12,400. EP 46601. (From Green WR, Quigley HT, de la Cruz Z, Cohen B: Parafoveal retinal telangiectasis: Light and electron microscopic studies. Trans Ophthalmol Soc UK *100*:162–170, 1980.)

lar hemangioblastoma. The retinal tumor is associated with the cerebellar tumor in about 25 per cent of the patients (Font, Ferry, 1972), and this is known as von Hippel-Landau disease. These tumors traditionally have been considered to be congenital and therefore hamartomatous in nature. Welch (1970), however, has observed the apparent de novo origin of a retinal angioma.

The early lesions are small, red-to-gray, and not associated with abnormal afferent and efferent vessels (Fig. 8–50,*A*). These very small lesions may not stain with fluorescein. As the lesion enlarges, it may appear as a small capillary cluster or as a small pink nodule that stains with fluorescein. Next, the feeler vessels become dilated, and the tumor develops the classic "pink balloon" configuration (Fig. 8–50,*B*). The tumor may be partially masked ophthalmoscopically if the lesion is predominately exophytic in relation to the peripapillary retina. The fluorescein angiographic pattern, however, is typical. Yimoyines, Topilow, Abedin, and McMeel (1982) have reported the clinical features of a patient with bilateral peripapillary exophytic retinal hemangiomas. The temporal periphery is the most common site, but these tumors also have been described in the juxtapapillary retina (Manschot, 1968d), at the optic disk (Figs. 8–51 and 8–52), and near the macula (Horowitz 1971; Welch, 1970). Bilateral tumors occur in 30 to 50 per cent of the cases, and multiple tumors in one eye occur in about one third of patients.

Vision may be affected by various mechanisms—lipid deposition in the macula, vitreous hemorrhage, exudative retinal detachment, or, rarely, rhegmatogenous retinal detachment.

In histopathologic study of cross-sections of the tumor, a fusiform thickening is found, which generally replaces the normal architecture of the entire thickness of the retina (Fig. 8–53). The tumor is composed of small, capillary-like or slightly larger blood vessels, lined by endothelium and a delicate reticulum (Fig. 8–54). Larger lesions have numerous vaculated cells in the stromal interstitium between the blood vessels (Goldberg, Duke, 1968).

The nature of these cells was obscure until electron microscopic studies (Nicholson, Green,

Text continued on page 642

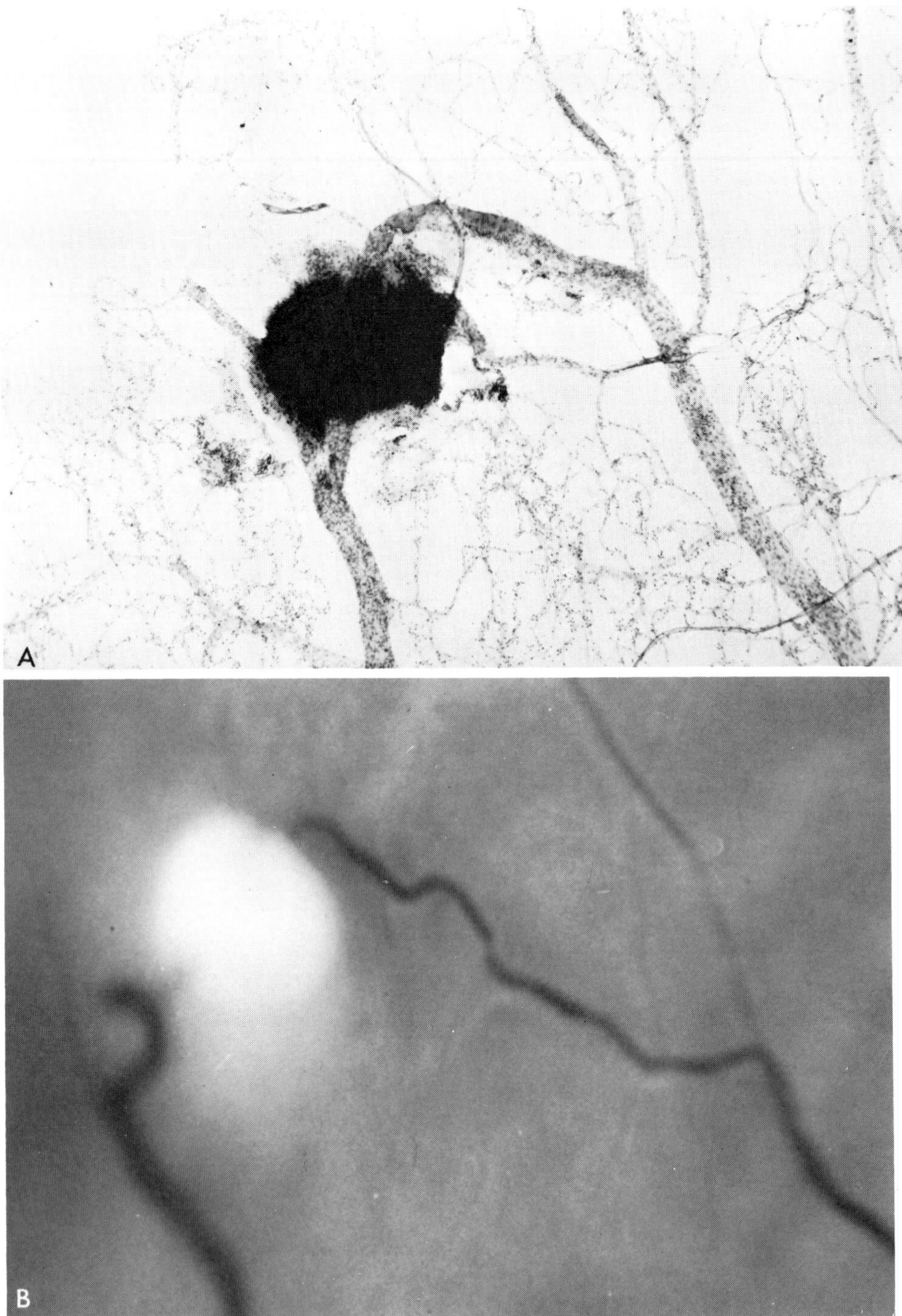

Figure 8–50. Lindau–von Hippel disease. *A,* Small retinal hemangioma without dilated or tortuous artery and vein. Trypsin digest preparation (H and E; PAS) ×45. *B,* Gross appearance of slightly larger retinal hemangioma with dilated and slightly tortuous afferent and efferent blood vessels. EP 33611. (From Nicholson DH, Green WR, Kenyon KR: Light and electron microscopic study of early lesions in angiomatosis retinae. Am J Ophthalmol *82*:193–204, 1976.)

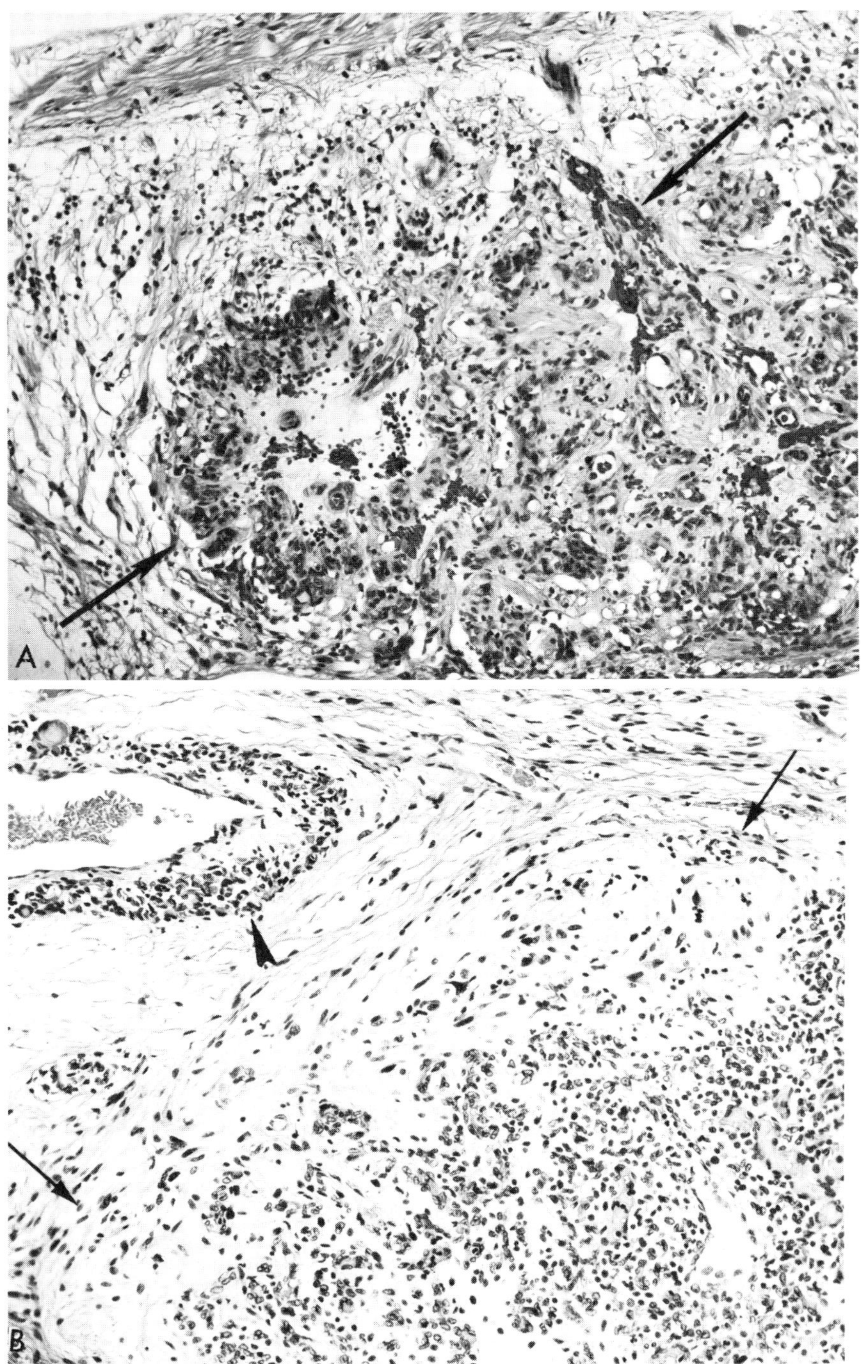

Figure 8–51. Small hemangioma of optic nerve head and peripapillary retina (between arrows). Angiomatous tissue surrounds a branch of central retinal vein (arrowhead). H and E: *A,* ×90; B, ×200. EP 47681.

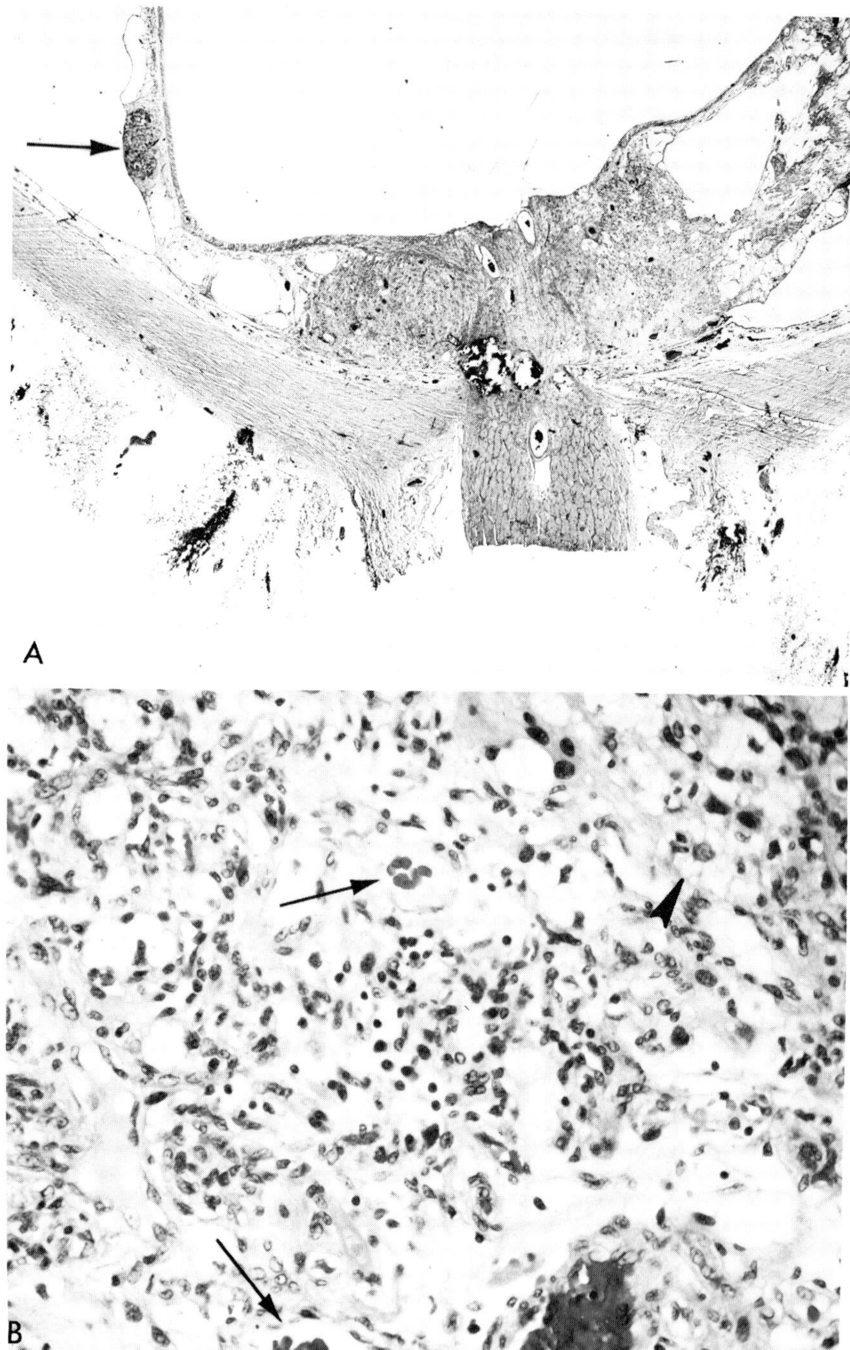

Figure 8–52. *A,* **Large hemangioma of optic nerve head and peripapillary retina,** plus small hemangioma (arrow) in the midperiphery. There is marked secondary cystic degeneration and detachment of retina. H and E, ×10. *B,* Higher power view of angioma. The vascular component (arrows) is observed by cellular proliferation, some cells of which are large with vacuolated cytoplasm (arrowhead). H and E, ×300. EP 47910.

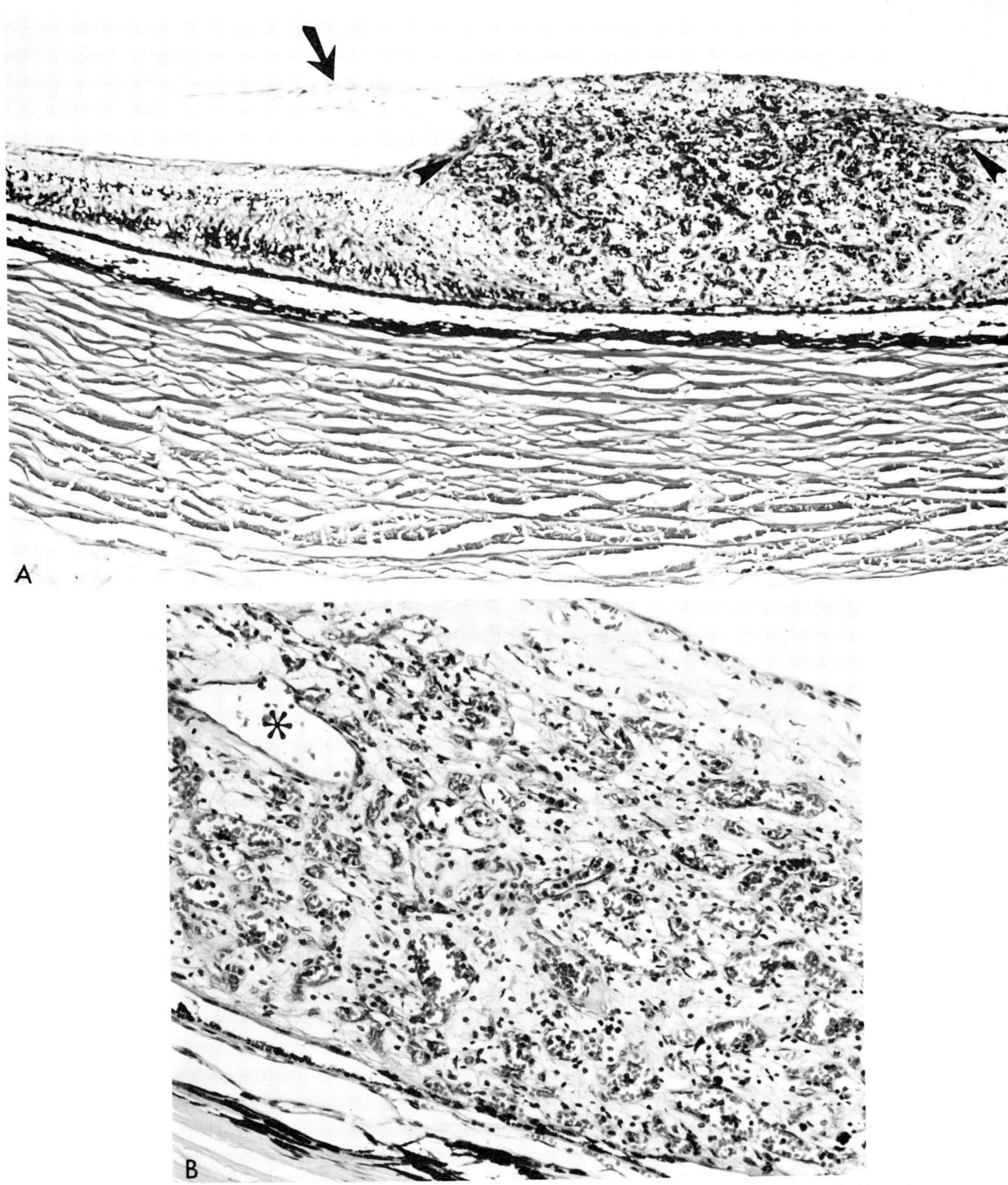

Figure 8–53. *A,* **Retinal hemangioma** involving full thickness of retina. The tumor extends through a defect in the internal limiting membrane (ILM) (between arrowheads), and a neovascular tuft (arrow) extends from the anterior and posterior edges of the inner tumor surface onto the posterior surface of detached vitreous. H and E, ×70. *B,* Higher power view of retinal hemangioma. Large vessel (asterisk) is at anterior aspect of the tumor. Numerous capillary vessels are present. H and E, ×180. EP 33611. (From Nicholson DH, Green WR, Kenyon KR: Light and electron microscopic study of early lesions in angiomatosis retinae. Am J Ophthalmol *82*:193–204, 1976.)

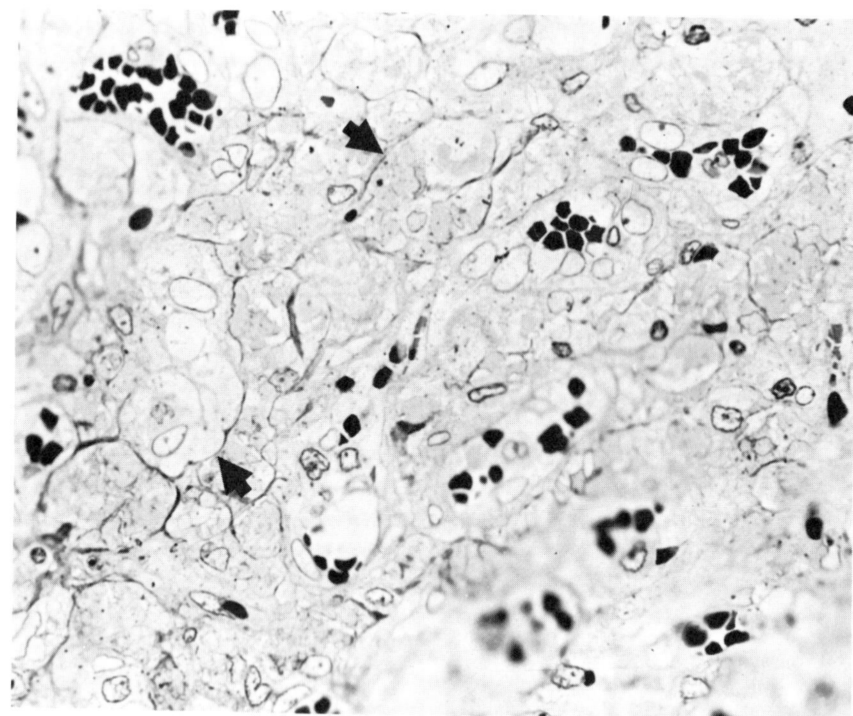

Figure 8–54. Retinal hemangioma showing clusters of cells surrounded by a fine reticulum (arrows). Reticulin stain, × 550. EP 33611.

Kenyon, 1976; Jakobiec, Font, Johnson, 1976) showed the ultrastructural features of fibrous astrocytes that have become lipidized (Figs. 8–55 and 8–56). Larger tumors may have a marked indentation and cystic degeneration within the tumor and surrounding retina. Marked exudation may lead to a nonrhegmatogenous and exudative retinal detachment. Exudate accumulation in and under the retina in the macular area may be striking, and it appears to cause a submacular disciform scar in some instances.

Some retinal hemangiomas may extend through

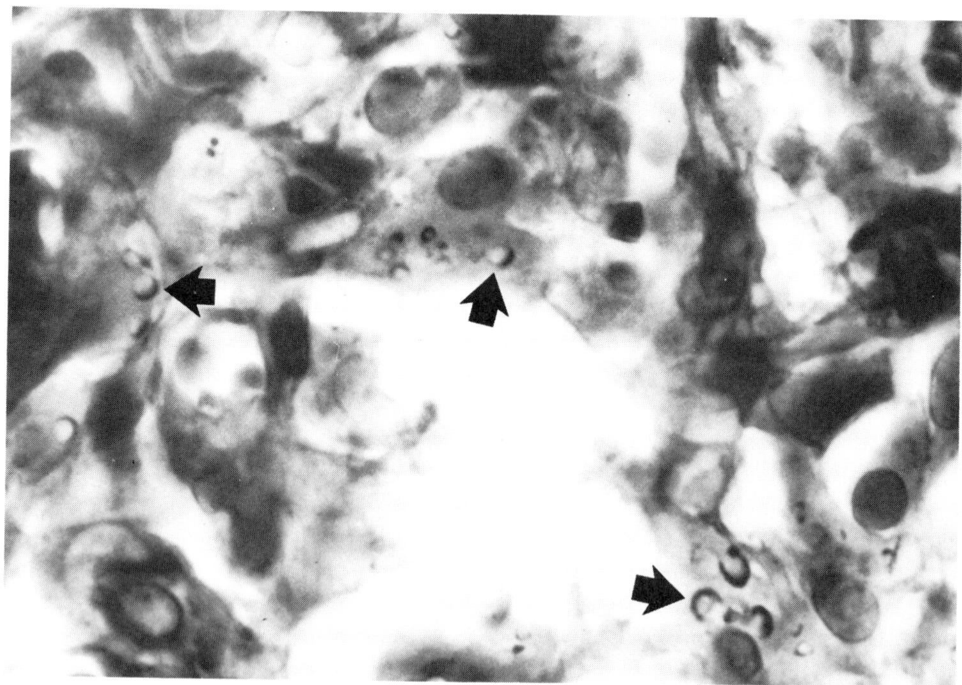

Figure 8–55. Lipid droplets (arrows) in cytoplasm of interstitial cells of **retinal angioma**. Frozen section, Sudan black-B, ×1050. EP 33611. (From Nicholson DH, Green WR, Kenyon KR: Light and electron microscopic study of early lesions in angiomatosis retinae. Am J Ophthalmol *82*:193–204, 1976.)

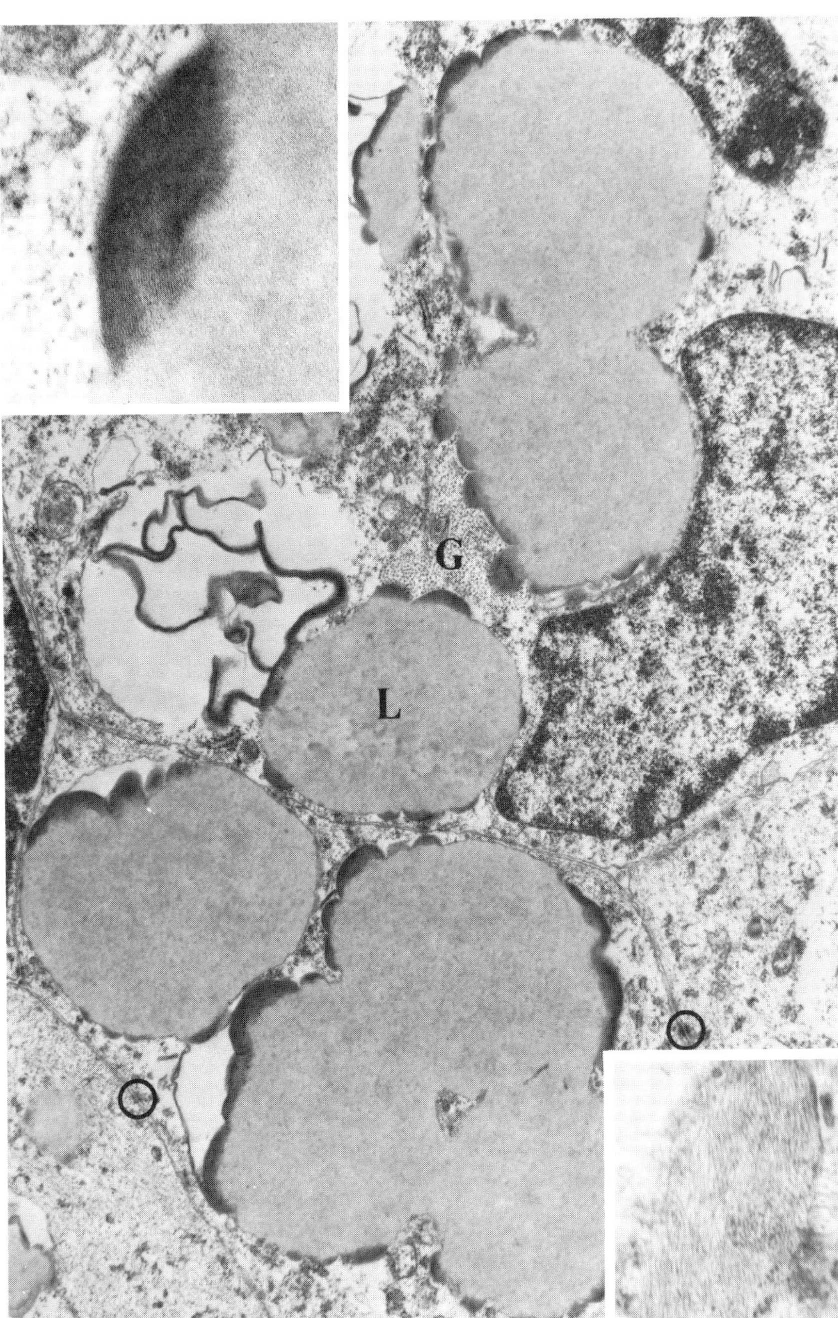

Figure 8–56. Retinal hemangioma. Electron micrograph of clustered interstitial cells shows large vacuolar intracytoplasmic lipid inclusions *(L)* that are of homogeneous, medium electron density. Glycogen granules *(G)* and occasional desmosomes (circled) are also seen. ×17,000. Upper inset: At high magnification, the highly electron-dense material at the periphery of vacuoles had 6 to 7 nm periodicity, typical of complex lipids. In the adjacent cytoplasm, multiple fine filaments (lower inset) of approximately 8 nm diameter are evident. ×90,000. EP 33611. (From Nicholson DH, Green WR, Kenyon KR: Light and electron microscopic study of early lesions in angiomatosis retinae. Am J Ophthalmol *82*:193–204, 1976.)

a discontinuity in the internal limiting membrane, with strands of condensed vitreous attached. The overlying vitreous changes can be a source of traction, which may be a factor in rare hemorrhage from the tumor and also in rhegmatogenous retinal detachment.

Electron microscopic studies have confirmed that the vessels of this tumor have endothelial cells, pericytes, and, rarely, multilaminar pericytes with smooth muscle differentiation (Jakobiec, Font, Johnson, 1976). In one ultrastructural study, the endothelium of the tumor's blood vessels was found to have fenestrations, which possibly explains the basis of the extravasated exudate that is characteristic of the larger tumors (Jakobiec, Font, Johnson, 1976). The investigation also found that extracts of lipid from the tumor consisted mostly of cholesterol stearate. They suggested that leaky fenestrated endothelium of the tumor capillaries allows for passive imbibition of plasma lipid by the fibrous astrocytes, leading to their gradual transformation into the lipidized stromal cells.

Retinal Vascular Abnormality Associated with Angioma Serpiginosum. Gautier-Smith, Sanders, and Sanderson (1971) have observed "an-

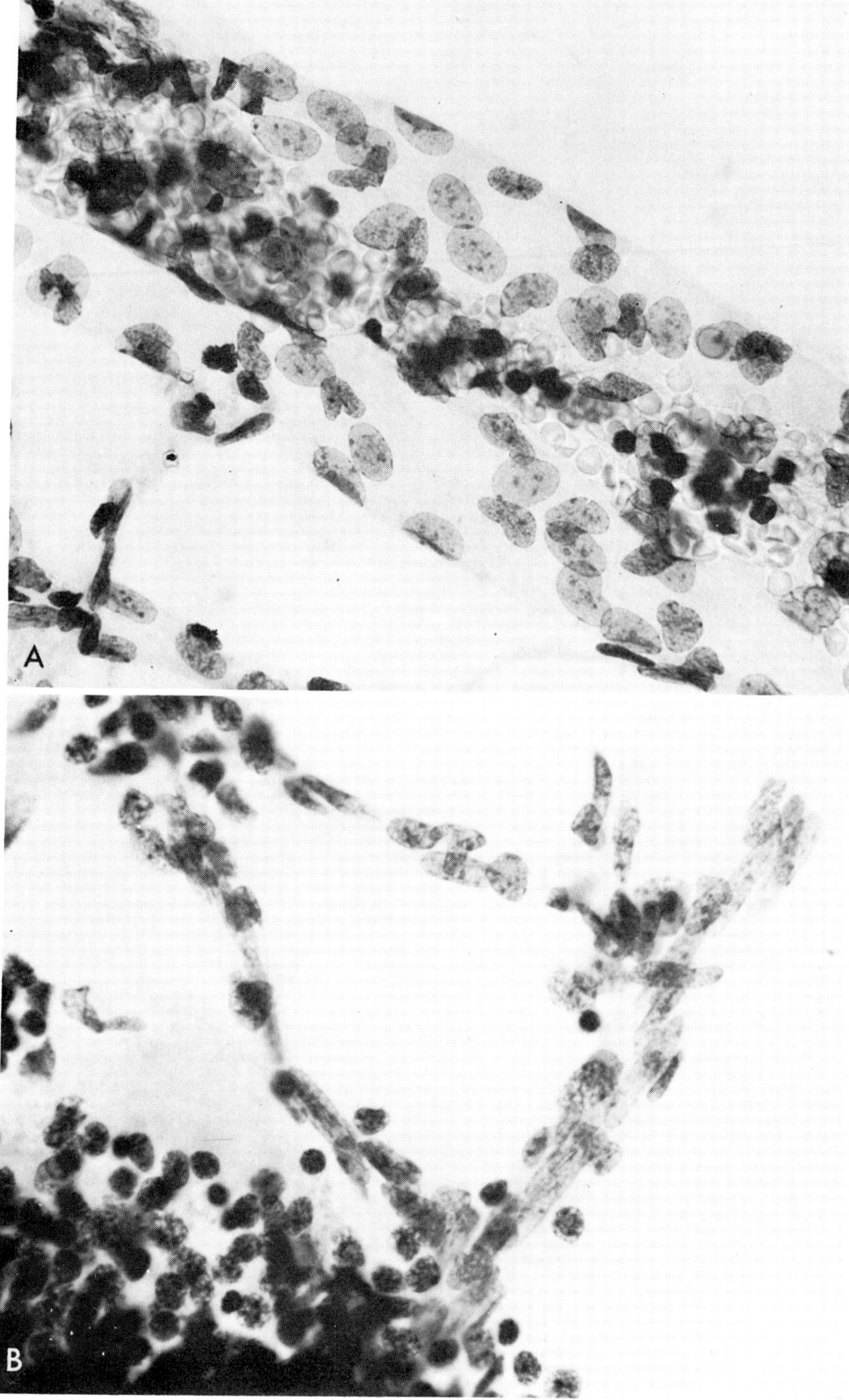

Figure 8–57. Abnormal retinal vasculature associated with diffuse **congenital hemangiomatosis**. *A,* Larger retinal blood vessel, with very thin wall containing only endothelium and no pericytes. Trypsin digestion; H and E, PAS, ×600. *B,* Retinal capillaries, with prominent endothelium and no pericytes. H and E, PAS, ×875. EP 30306. (From Naidoff MA, Kenyon KR, Green WR: Iris hemangioma and abnormal retinal vasculature in a case of diffuse congenital hemangiomatosis. Am J Ophthalmol *72*:633–644, 1971.)

giomatous involvement'' of the retina, particularly the venous system, in association with extensive cutaneous and central nervous system angioma.

Abnormal Retinal Vasculature Associated with Diffuse Congenital Hemangiomatosis. Naidoff, Kenyon, and Green (1971) have reported the clinical and histopathologic features of a neonate with congenital generalized cutaneous and visceral hemangiomas, cavernous hemangioma of the iris, and almost total absence of intramural pericytes in the retinal (Fig. 8–57) and hemangiomatous lesions.

Congenital Hypertrophy of the Retinal Pigment Epithelium

This abnormality is considered elsewhere (p. 1227).

Congenital Retinal Fold
(Falciform Retinal Fold)

This congenital abnormality consists of an inferotemporal fold of retina that extends from the optic disk to the back of the lens. A prominent blood vessel occupies the apex of the fold. Whether this is a true congenital anomaly is disputed. Manschot (1958) suggested that these folds may be considered as a form of posteriorly located persistent hyperplastic primary vitreous (PHPV). The fact that posteriorly located PHPV can occur is supported by observation of a similar process in mice (Badtke, Damke, 1966). Similar retinal folds may be seen as a result of traction in PHPV, retrolental fibroplasia, the familial exudative vitreoretinopathy of Criswick and Schepens (1969), and peripherally located nematode inflammatory lesions.

Macular Folds

These are discussed elsewhere (p. 924).

Macular Hypoplasia/Aplasia

This topic is discussed elsewhere (p. 924).

Congenital Night Blindness

Stationary congenital night blindness has been classified into two groups—one with a normal fundus appearance and one with abnormal findings on ophthalmoscopic examination. Oguchi's disease, fundus albipunctatus, and the flecked retina of Kandori are three conditions in which there are night blindness and abnormal fundus findings.

Carr (1974) has suggested that the basic abnormality in these conditions is in neural transmission at certain levels of the outer retina. He concluded this on the basis of electrophysiologic and psychophysical tests and a study of the visual pigments in vivo. That investigation found that patients with congenital stationary night blindness with normal fundi and those with Oguchi's disease had normal amounts and kinetics of visual pigments. In fundus albipunctatus, visual pigment kinetics and electrophysiologic tests of retinal function were greatly retarded, indicating a retardation in the formation of the visual pigments.

Oguchi's Disease. Patients with this condition have difficulty with night vision, and psychophysical testing reveals retardation of dark adaptation. The fundus findings in Oguchi's disease are characterized by a peculiar grayish-white discoloration of the retina, with a change from dark-to-light adaptation (Mizuo's phenomenon).

Few histologic studies have been done in patients with Oguchi's disease. The light and electron microscopic study by Kuwabara, Ishihara, and Akiya (1963) showed an abnormal layer between the RPE and photoreceptors (Fig. 8–58), and the outer segments of photoreceptors had abnormal microvacuolar or tubular internal structures instead of the normal lamellae. The pigment granules in the RPE were crowded toward the apex of the cells, while the basal portions were rich in lipid, probably lipofuscin granules.

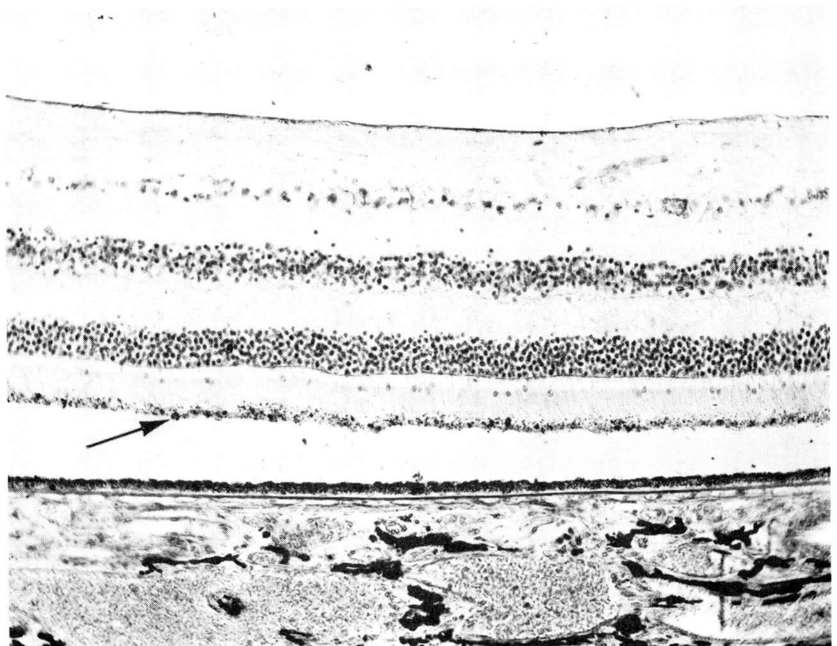

Figure 8–58. Oguchi's disease. The retina is normal except for the accumulation of pigment (arrow) between the photoreceptors and the retinal pigment epithelium and migration of photoreceptor cell nuclei into the inner segment area. AFIP Neg. 65-13094. H and E, ×130.

Other studies (Yamanaka, 1969) have demonstrated changes interpreted as similar to those in primary pigmentary degeneration of the retina.

Fundus Albipunctatus. This stationary disorder reveals a myriad of deep-seated yellowish-white spots, more pronounced in the posterior pole; they have a less atrophic appearance than is seen in retinitis punctata albescens. Patients with this disorder have night blindness and normal visual acuity. The retinal vessels are normal. The electro-olfactogram is abnormal and the electroretinogram is normal. Histopathologic studies have not been conducted in patients with this condition.

Flecked Retina of Kandori. This is a rare form of congenital, nonprogressive night blindness in which there are ophthalmoscopic abnormalities, including sharply defined, dirty yellow, deep, irregular flecks in the equatorial or midperipheral areas. No macular lesions are observed (Kandori, 1959; Kandori, Tamai, Kurimoto, Fukunaga, 1972). Although this condition is classified as a congenital night blindness, there is only a slight retardation in reaching normal dark-adapted levels.

Congenital Night Blindness with Normal Fundi. Three modes of inheritance have been recognized (Carr, 1974): autosomal recessive, autosomal dominant, and sex-linked recessive.

Vaghefi, Green, Kelley, et al (1978) reported the presence of a normal pattern and proportion of rods and cones (Fig. 8–59) in a patient with congenital stationary night blindness and a normal fundus. This indicates that the abnormality was not due to an absence of rods and supports the view of Carr (1974) that the abnormality is probably in the neural transmission within the retina.

Other congenital retinal diseases include congenital hypertrophy of the RPE (bear tracks, grouped pigmentation), macular folds, and macular aplasia or hypoplasia. These are discussed in detail elsewhere.

Juvenile Retinoschisis

(Sex-Linked Retinoschisis, Congenital Retinoschisis)

This condition has also been referred to as vitreous veils, congenital vascular veils in the vitreous, congenital cystic retinal detachment, and inherited retinal detachment. It is considered to be one of the hereditary hyaloideoretinopathies. This group of conditions is considered on page 870 and in Chapter 7, Vitreous.

In juvenile retinoschisis, the splitting of the retina is usually most marked in the inferotemporal area (Forsius, Eriksson, Vainio-Mattila, 1963; Sarin, Green, Dailey, 1964; Bengtsson, Linder, 1967; Burns, Lovrien, Cibis, 1971). The thin inner layer contains blood vessels, and it often develops oval areas of dehiscence. Only blood vessels may bridge some areas of the inner layer, and the vessels also may extend from one layer to the other. Such vessels may be the source of bleeding into the vitreous or schisis cavity or both. The macular lesions are thought clinically to be a combination of cystic cavities and retino-

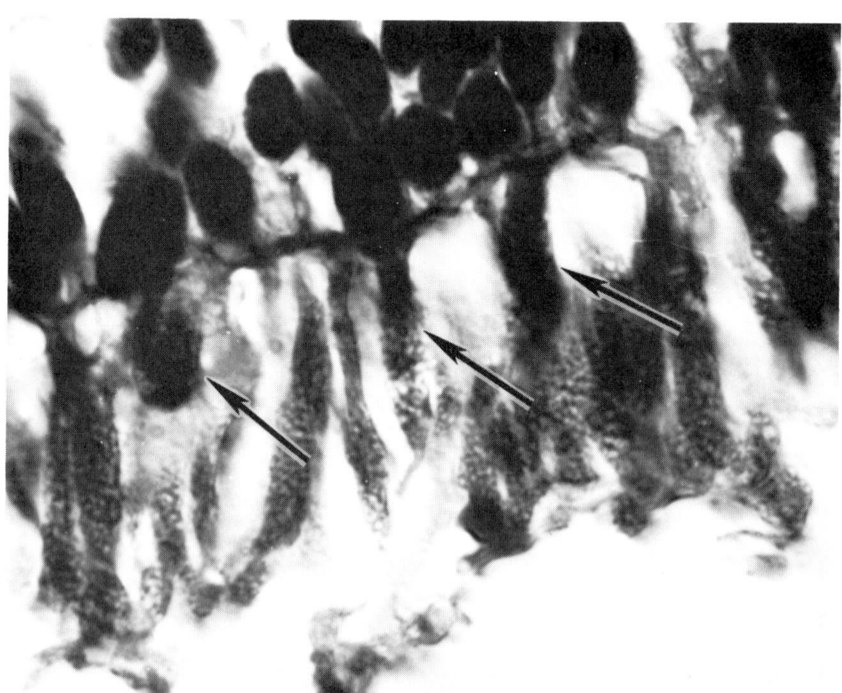

Figure 8–59. Congenital night blindness. Perifoveal area of retina showing rod and cone (arrows) inner segments. Van de Grift, ×1650. EP 40584. (From Vaghefi HA, Green WR, Kelley JS, et al: Correlation of clinicopathologic findings in a patient. Congenital night blindness, branch retinal vein occlusion, cilioretinal artery, drusen of optic nerve head, and intraretinal pigmented lesion. Arch Ophthalmol *96*:2097–2104, 1978.)

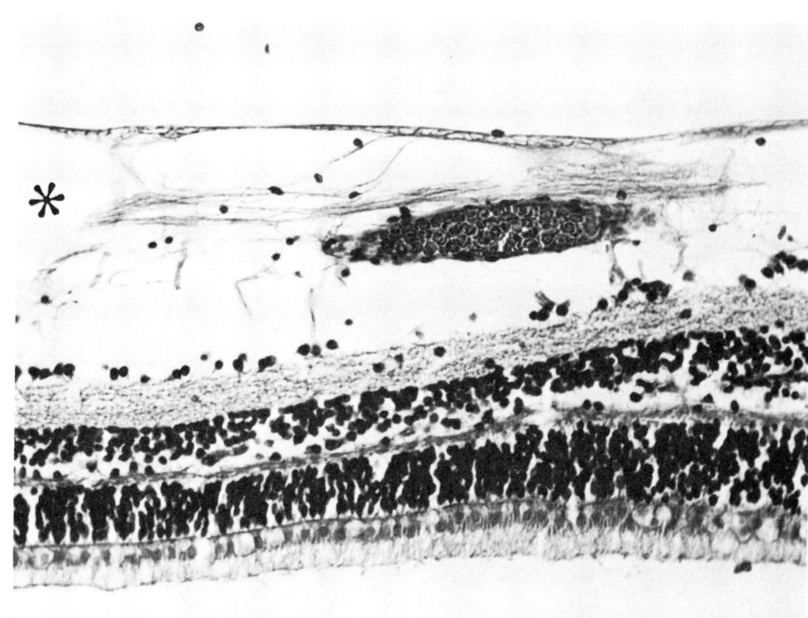

Figure 8–60. Juvenile retinoschisis. Splitting occurs in the nerve fiber layer (asterisk). H and E, ×445. AFIP Neg. 65-5582.

schisis. Pigmentary changes in the macula also may be observed. The macular changes have not been documented histopathologically.

The splitting of the retina in the periphery occurs in the nerve fiber layer (Fig. 8–60) (Yanoff, Rahn, Zimmerman, 1968; Zimmerman, Nauman, 1968; Manschot, 1972). Extensive splitting may occur, so that retinal tissue may be at or near the posterior surface of the lens.

DEVELOPMENTAL ABNORMALITIES

Retrolental Fibroplasia (RLF)
(Retinopathy of Prematurity)

The most important retinal disease that may be classified as an intoxication is retrolental fibroplasia (RLF), the oxygen-induced retinopathy of premature infants. The incompletely vascularized peripheral retina of premature infants and newborn animals is most sensitive to variations in oxygen concentration of the circulating blood (Ashton, 1953). According to Campbell (1951), a lowered oxygen tension causes a reduction of the capillary-free zone around the arteries. Experimentally, oxygen in high concentrations has been shown to obliterate immature terminal arterioles by vasoconstriction. The effect spreads to involve the whole capillary bed, and finally the entire vasculature (arterioles, capillaries, and veins) closes down. This phenomenon is peculiar to the incompletely vascularized retina.

Once the developing retinal vessels have reached the periphery and attained maturity, they no longer are susceptible to oxygen-induced vaso-obliteration. Were it not for the diffusion of oxygen from the choriocapillaris, the retinal reaction would be self-limiting; Ashton, Graymore, and Pedler (1957) have shown that this is why the reaction is not observed when the immature retina is detached from the choroid.

In the kitten, the immediate vasoconstriction induced by excessive oxygen is transient, and after about 10 minutes the retinal vessels dilate again. Despite continuous hyperoxygenation, they remain dilated for about 6 hours. Then a delayed vaso-obliteration occurs, which at first is reversible after normalization of oxygen tension. Gradually the process becomes irreversible. At this stage, the vessel walls have become adherent to each other or show degeneration. By this time, regardless of whether oxygen tension is made normal or not, vasoproliferative changes occur from the vessels that are immediately adjacent to the obliterated areas.

Retrolental fibroplasia thus has three clinicopathologic phases: vaso-obliterative, active (proliferative), and cicatricial. Only the vaso-obliterative phase is related directly to the oxygen concentration. In the earliest proliferative stage, the pathologic change consists of tiny endothelial nodules in the inner portion of the retina (Fig. 8–61). These nodules have the appearance of glomeruloid capillary tufts. After this, there is proliferation of capillaries within the retina, directed away from the tufts. The newly formed capillaries break through the internal limiting membrane and then line the surface of the retina, or, if the process is more aggressive, they may extend into the vitreous (Kushner, Essner, Cohen, Flynn, 1977) (Figs. 8–62 and 8–63). In later stages, the proliferating vitreal capillaries can lead to vitreous hemorrhage, fibrous organization, and traction and retinal detachment (Fig. 8–64).

In cases in which oxygen therapy is diminished or discontinued early, the RLF process may stop at the point where the changes have taken place. Spontaneous recovery from mild proliferative RLF may occur in as many as 90 per cent of patients (Kinsey, Arnold, Kalina, 1977).

In the most severe cases, the completely detached retina and organized vitreous may form an opaque, retrolental mass that produces a white pupil when examined clinically and a cat's eye type of reflex when the pupil is illuminated in the dark. For this reason, and because both conditions are often bilateral, retrolental fibroplasia and retinoblastoma may be difficult to differentiate clinically. In most advanced cases, the eye eventually becomes phthisical. Transient secondary glaucoma may be observed, but buphthalmos is unusual.

Histopathologic diagnosis is difficult in these advanced cases because secondary changes tend to obscure the basic vasoproliferative and obliterative processes. If the examination of the peripheral fundus reveals an absence of capillaries, this provides important circumstantial evidence of prematurity and therefore of susceptibility to oxygen toxicity.

In the less severe cases, only a part of the retina may be involved. Reese and Stepanik (1954) showed the retina to be affected on the temporal side in 90 per cent of such patients. This is believed to reflect the longer period required for vascularization of the retina to occur on the temporal side, compared with the nasal retina.

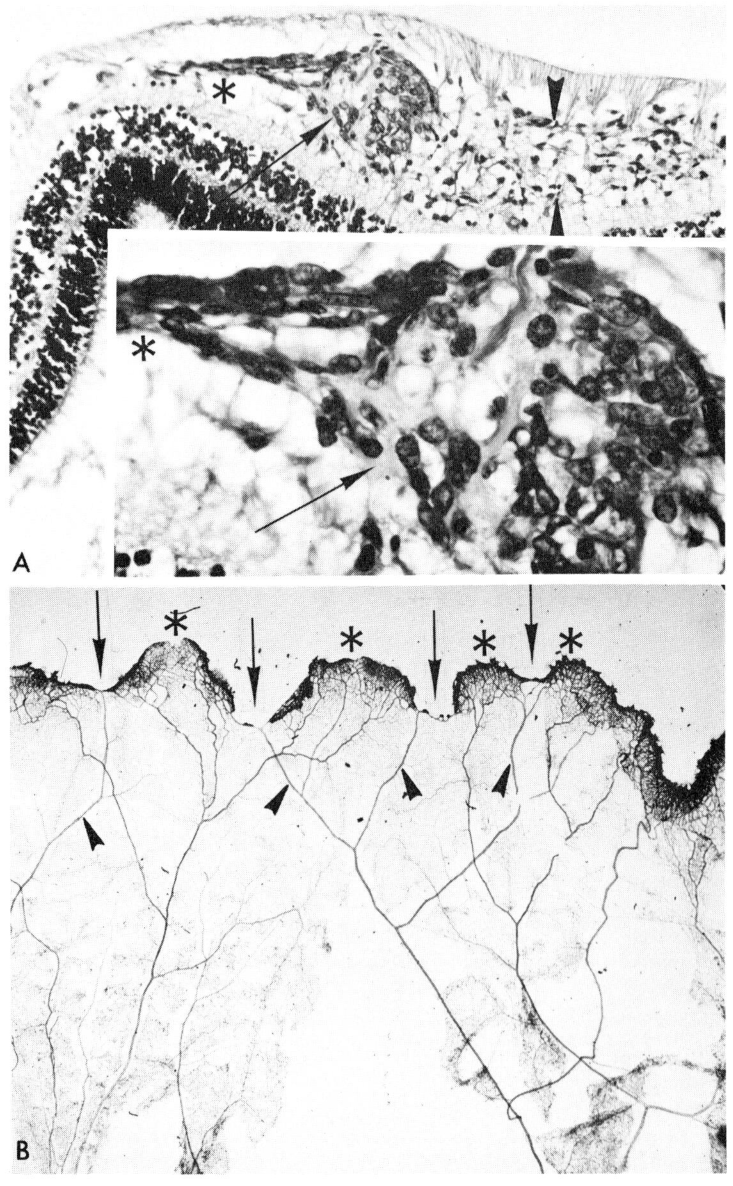

Figure 8–61. *A,* Equatorial area temporally with retinal vessel (asterisk) extending into a large zone of endothelial cell proliferation (arrow and inset). A wedge-shaped area of spindle-shaped mesenchymal cells (arrowheads) is present anterior to the nodule of endothelial cell proliferation. H and E, ×185; inset, ×300. *B,* Peripheral temporal retina showing hypercellular and hypervascular venous areas (asterisks) alternating with more posterior arterial zones of hypocellular and hypovascular retina (arrows). A retinal arteriole (arrowheads) enters each of the hypocellular and hypovascular areas. Trypsin digest preparation, ×7.

Illustration continued on opposite page

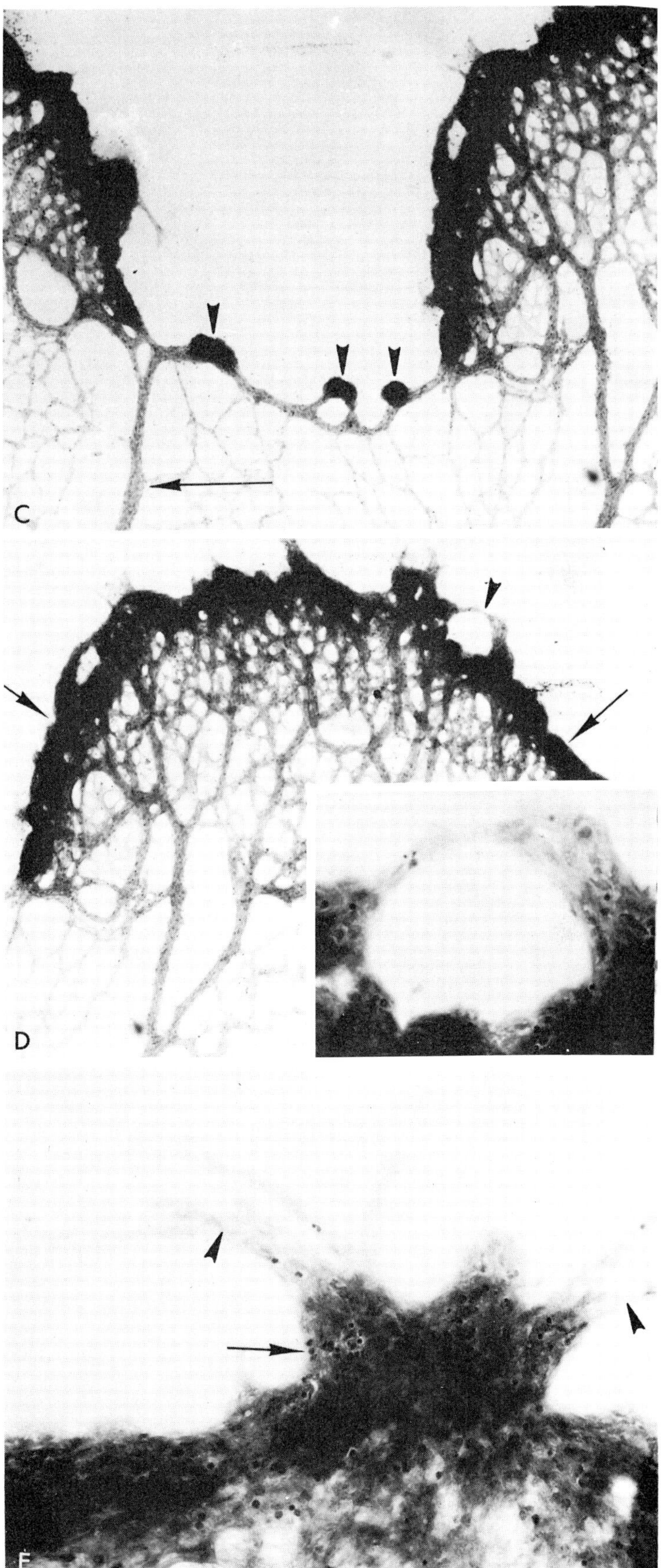

Figure 8–61 *Continued C,* Higher power view of one of the hypocellular and hypovascular areas present in *B*. There are only three small endothelial cell nodules (arrowheads). A retinal arteriole (arrow) enters the area posteriorly. Trypsin digest preparation, ×60.

D, Peripheral hypervascular and hypercellular venous area with progressively increasing vascular anastomoses and arcades merging with dense zone of endothelial cell proliferation (arrows). Nonvascularized strands of mesenchymal cells extend anteriorly from the endothelial zone, and some of these join to form an arcade (arrowhead and inset). Trypsin digest preparation, ×60; inset, ×250. *E,* Nodular anterior extension of proliferative endothelial zone (arrow), with strands of mesenchymal cells streaming from its anterior extent (arrowheads). Trypsin digest preparation, ×250. EP 45313. (From Naiman J, Green WR, Patz A: Retrolental fibroplasia in hypoxic newborn. Am J Ophthalmol *88*:55–58, 1979.)

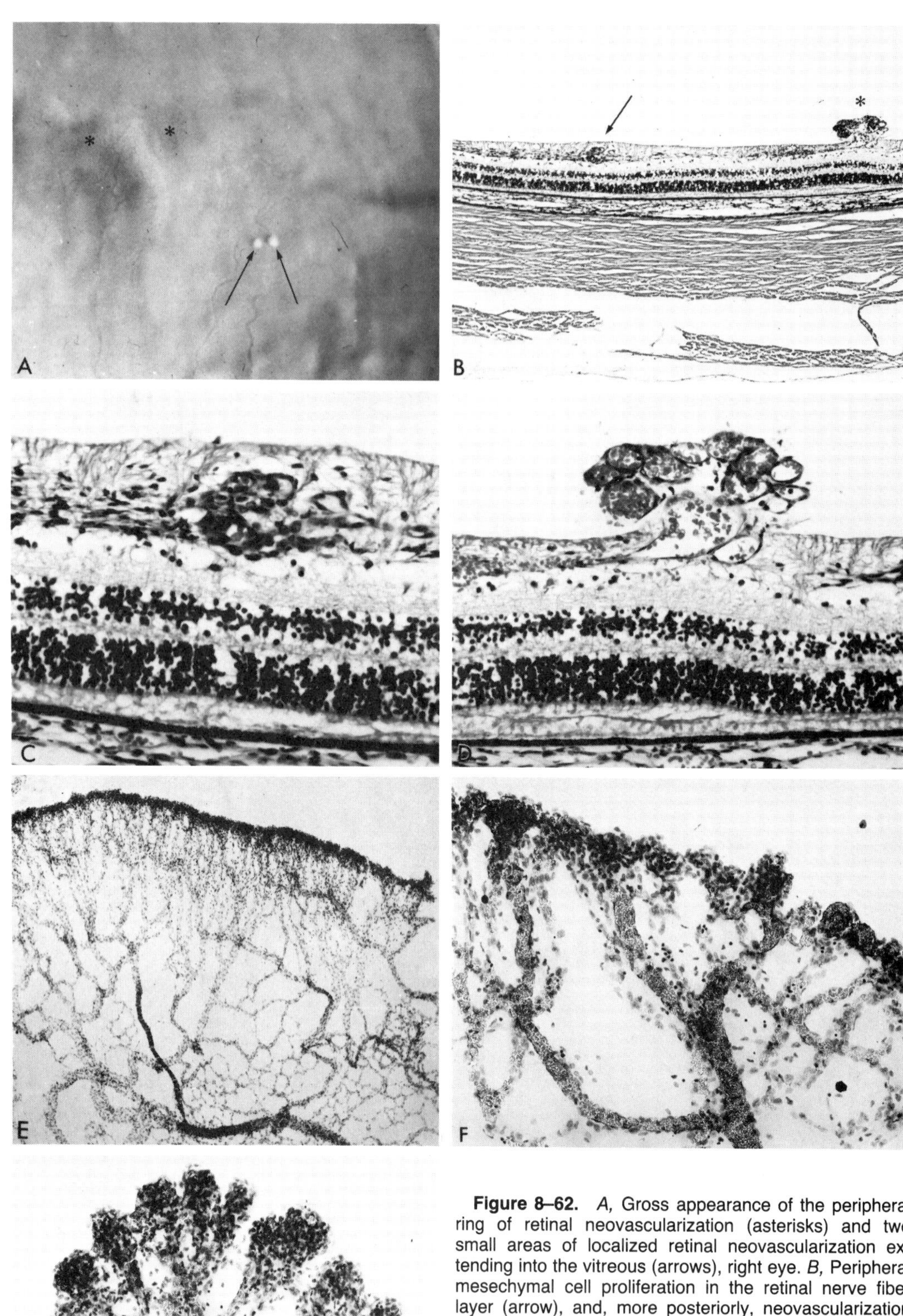

Figure 8–62. *A,* Gross appearance of the peripheral ring of retinal neovascularization (asterisks) and two small areas of localized retinal neovascularization extending into the vitreous (arrows), right eye. *B,* Peripheral mesechymal cell proliferation in the retinal nerve fiber layer (arrow), and, more posteriorly, neovascularization budding through the internal limiting membrane (ILM) (asterisk), temporal equatorial region of right eye. H and E, ×60. *C,* Mesenchymal cell proliferation in the retinal nerve fiber layer. H and E, ×330.

D, Area of neovascularization extending through the ILM into the vitreous. H and E, ×320. *E,* Increasing arborization of retinal vessels in periphery, forming a band of active neovascularization. Trypsin digest; PAS, H and E, ×60. *F,* Neovascular network demonstrating glomerular-like tufts of mesenchymal and endothelial cells, with abundant red blood cells within thin-walled capillaries. Trypsin digest; PAS, H and E, ×100. *G,* Intraretinal neovascularization arranged in a sea fan–like configuration. Trypsin digest; PAS, ×110. EP 34417.

(From Chui HC, Green WR: Acute retrolental fibroplasia: A clinicopathologic correlation. Md Med J *26*:71–74, 1977.)

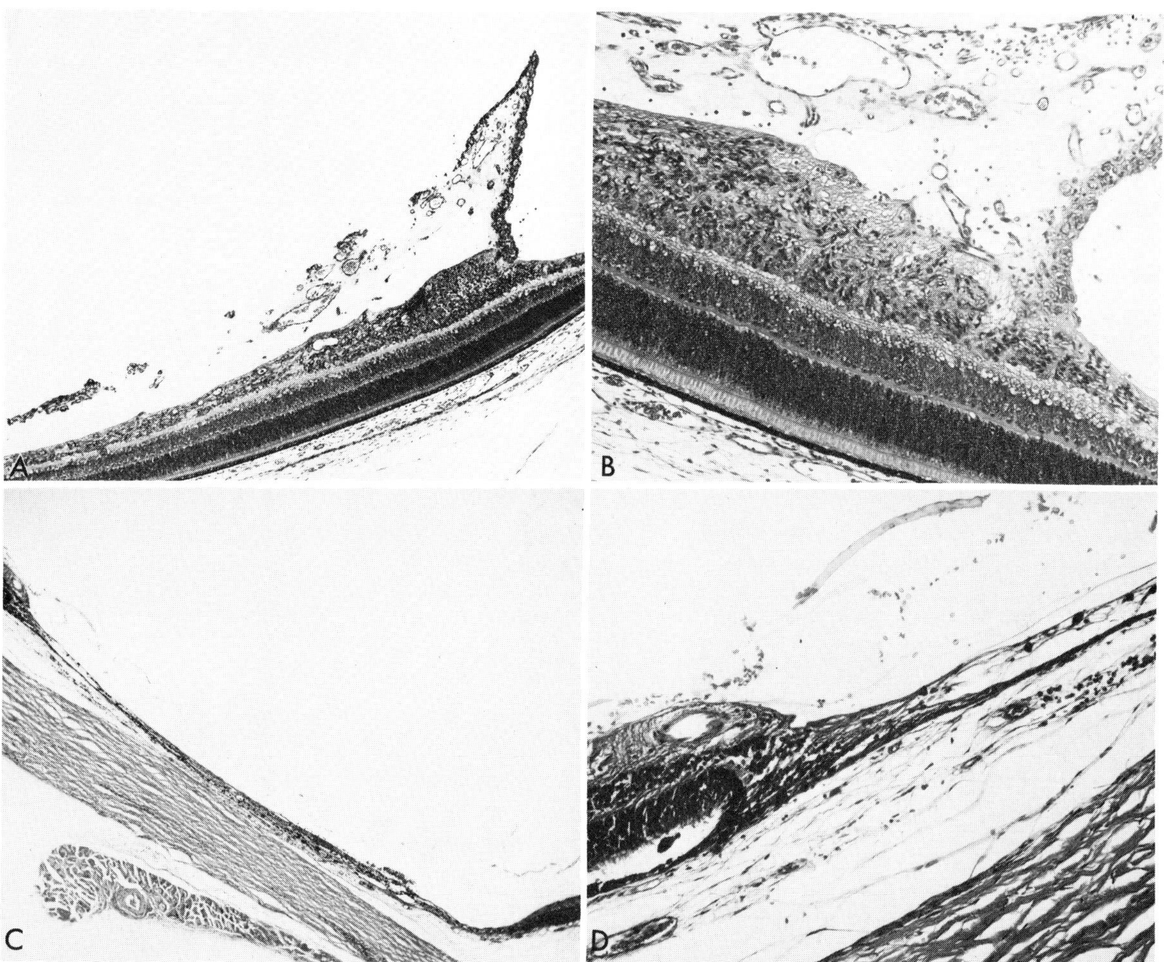

Figure 8–63. Retrolental fibroplasia, with area of extensive neovascularization extending into vitreous (*A* and *B*) and area of chorioretinal scar with eradication of neovascular tissue by cryotherapy (*C* and *D*). *A*, PAS, ×55; *B*, H and E, ×140; *C* and *D*, H and E, ×35. EP 41280.

Faris, Tolentino, Freeman, et al (1971) studied 71 patients with RLF, most of whom were between ages 6 and 15 years. The characteristic changes were usually located in the temporal fundus periphery. Most often there was proliferation of retinal pigment epithelium (RPE), chorioretinal scarring, translucent vitreous membrane overlying the temporal periphery of the fundus, retinal folds, dragged disk, and macular lesions. The vitreous often contained dense, organized bands and membranes, especially near the temporal base. Vitreal retinal traction was considered to be a major cause of the fundus changes.

Although oxygen is now considered to be the primary factor stimulating neovascularization in the premature retina, some cases have been observed at birth without exogenous oxygen administration (Karlsberg, Green, Patz, 1973; Brockhurst, Chishti, 1975; Stefani, Ehalt, 1974) and other cases have been noted with apparently acceptable and closely monitored Po_2 levels (Naiman, Green, Patz, 1979). Schulman, Jampol, and Schwartz (1980) have suggested that RLF occurring in healthy full-term infants, without supplemental oxygen, could possibly represent sporadic cases of familial exudative vitreoretinopathy. Also, experimental studies have shown significantly less intravitreal neovascularization when there was treatment with vitamin E (Phelps, Rosenbaum, 1979). Flower (1980) has shown experimentally that the vasoconstriction caused by oxygen apparently is a protective mechanism. When the vasoconstriction is blocked, the intensity of the neovascularization is greater, thus suggesting a direct toxicity of the oxygen on the developing retinal vessels. Kalina (1980) recently has reviewed the therapy of RLF.

Heterotopia of Macula and/or Optic Disc

This is an acquired condition that occurs from traction on the retina by preretinal tissue outside the macular area. Some conditions that produce

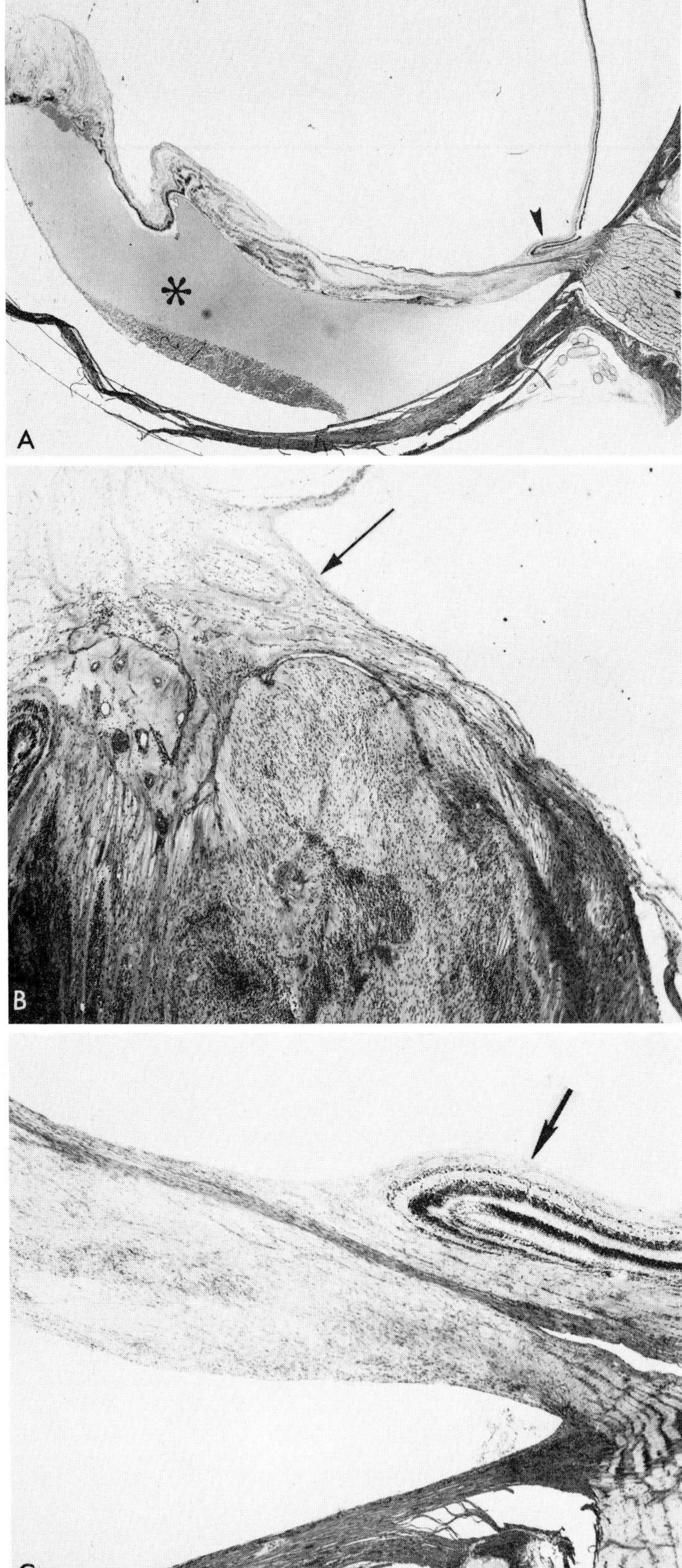

Figure 8–64. Retrolental fibroplasia with traction retinal detachment and dragging of optic disc and macula. *A,* Neovascular tissue (arrow) in temporal periphery. A proteinaceous material (asterisk) with some blood occupies the subretinal space. The nasal retina has been drawn over the optic nerve head (arrowhead). H and E, ×5.5. *B,* Higher power view of fibrovascular tissue in vitreous (arrow). The retina has been drawn into folds. H and E, ×35. *C,* Higher power view showing dragging of the disc. The nasal peripapillary retina (arrow) has been pulled over the optic nerve head. H and E, × 35. EP 44003. (From Nicholson DH, Green WR: Pediatric Ocular Tumors. New York, Masson, 1981, pp 14–15.)

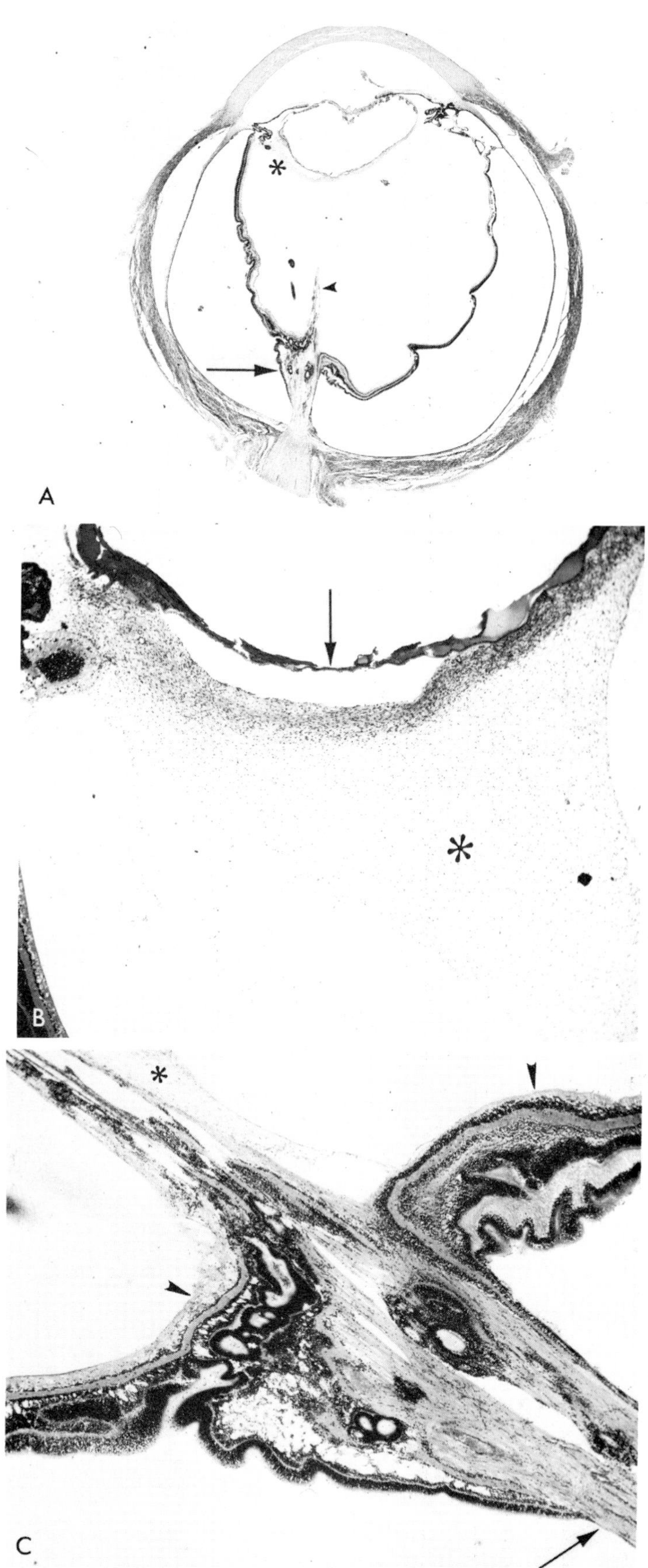

Figure 8–65. Persistent hyperplastic primary vitreous (PHPV) with marked dragging of the disc. *A,* PHPV (asterisk), hyaloid vessel (arrowhead), and traction on optic nerve head and peripapillary retina (arrow). H and E, ×7. *B,* Higher power view of PHPV (asterisk) posterior to lens (arrow indicates lens capsule). H and E, ×55. *C,* Higher power view showing the optic nerve head (arrow) and peripapillary retina (arrowheads) in a pulled-forward position by PHPV (asterisk). H and E, ×35. EP 44000. (From Nicholson DH, Green WR: Pediatric Ocular Tumors. New York, Masson, 1981, pp 4–5.)

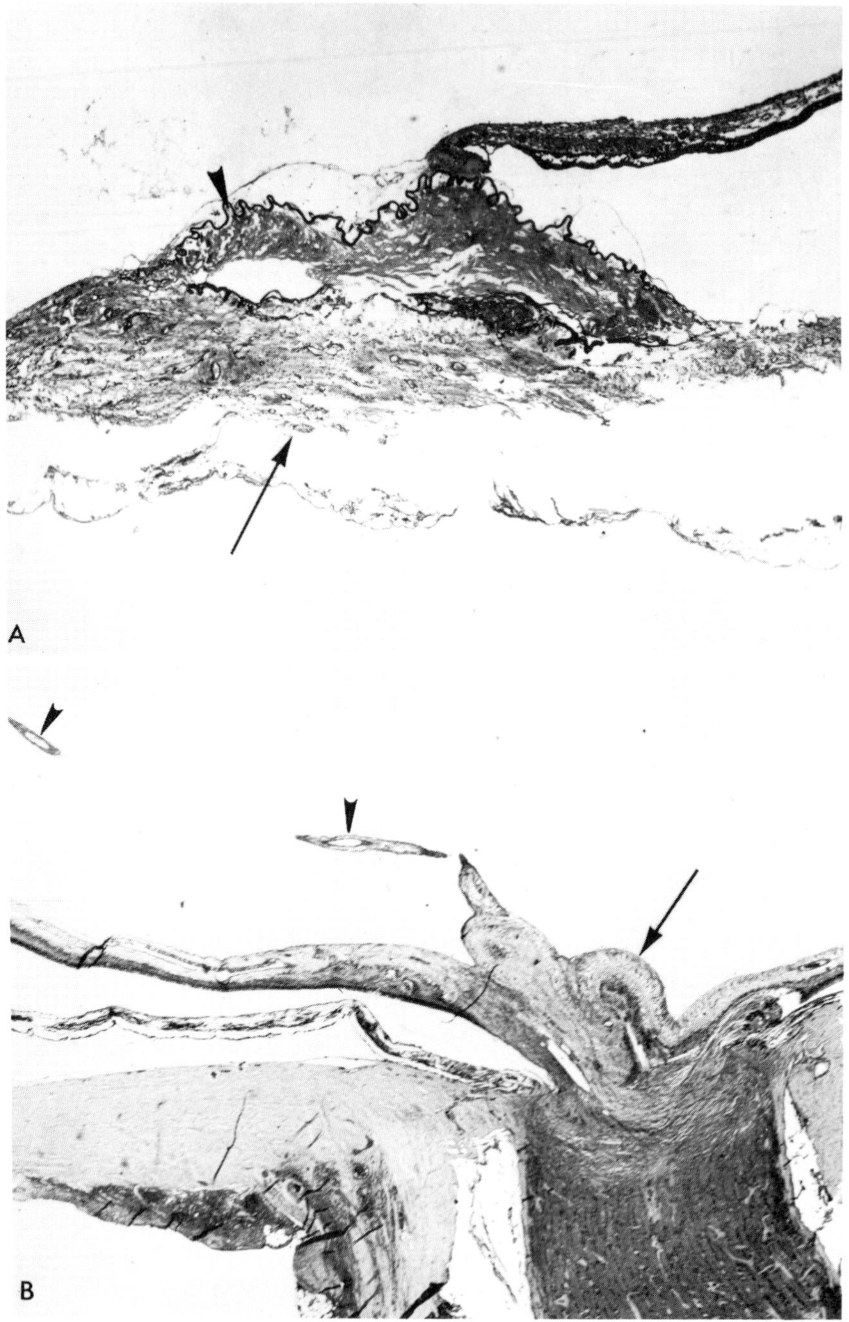

Figure 8–66. *A,* Persistent hyperplastic primary vitreous (PHPV) (arrow) with one leaf of the iris adherent to the lens remnants (arrowhead). PAS, ×40. *B,* Hyaloid artery (arrowheads). The optic nerve head and peripapillary retina (arrow) have been pulled toward one side. H and E, ×17. EP 6691.

this are retrolental fibroplasia (Fig. 8–64), peripheral nematode inflammatory lesions, persistent hyperplastic primary vitreous (PHPV) (Figs. 8–65 and 8–66), proliferative diabetic retinopathy, and familial exudative vitreoretinopathy of Creswick and Schepens.

RETINAL ISCHEMIA; VASCULAR AND CIRCULATORY CONDITIONS AND DISEASES

Etiology

Retinal ischemia is observed in a variety of conditions, including arterial sclerosis, systemic vascular hypertension, hypertensive retinopathy (carotid occlusive disease, pulseless disease), venous congestion, collagen vascular diseases, embolism, and vasculitis.

Histopathology of Retinal Ischemia

The retina has a high oxidative capacity and an unusually high glycolytic activity and is therefore extremely susceptible to hypoxia. Permanent retinal damage was formerly thought to occur as early as 15 minutes after arterial blood supply is totally interrupted. Hayreh, Kolder, and Weingeist (1980) have observed the retina of monkeys to survive even after 90 minutes of mechanical occlusion of the central retinal artery before it enters the optic nerve.

The retina derives its blood supply from two distinct sources. The intrinsic retinal vessels supply the inner two thirds, while the avascular outer layers depend on the choriocapillaris for their sustenance. Pathologic changes produced in the retina by vascular lesions, therefore, will vary with the capillary system affected. They will also differ according to the size of the vessel affected, the nature and rate of development of the primary disease process, and the part of the vascular tree (arterial or venous) involved.

The initial effect is anoxic damage to the retinal capillary endothelium, which leads to intercellular and intracellular edema. The retinal cells destroyed by anoxia undergo autolysis, releasing macromolecules that increase the tissue osmotic pressure and the edema, which increases the capillary closure.

Various constituents of the retina react to ischemia, as follows:

Neurons. The **nuclei** and **axons** of the neurons may survive if the ischemia is mild and transient. With more severe and protracted ischemia, the neurons degenerate, are phagocytosed, and disappear.

With central retinal artery occlusion, for example, the inner retinal neurons—the ganglion cells and the cells of the inner part of the inner nuclear layer—show nuclear pyknosis at 2 hours. With time, these neurons disappear, as well as glia, microglia, and vascular pericytes and endothelium. This leads to the picture of inner retinal ischemic atrophy, with loss of the nerve fiber, ganglion cells, inner plexiform layers, and the inner portion of the inner nuclear layer (Fig. 8–67). With total ischemia, there is also generally no attempt at repair with gliosis or neovascularization. Minor glial cell proliferation may be observed with localized inner ischemic atrophy of the retina.

Cotton-Wool Spots (Microinfarctions of Nerve Fiber Layer, Cytoid Bodies). Cotton-wool spots are microinfarcts from arteriolar occlusion. Clinically, they are called cotton-wool spots; however, they were initially observed with the microscope as a characteristic lesion of the retina and given the name cytoid bodies (Ashton, Harry, 1963; Ashton, 1969, 1970; Dollery, 1969; Ferry, 1972). Clinically, cotton-wool spots are gray and semiopaque, with feathery edges; they lie either internal to or around the blood vessels, or they may be deep to these vessels in the nerve fiber layer. They are usually small in size but some very large ones have been seen. Cotton-wool spots disappear in 4 to 12 weeks (longer in diabetes, according to Kohner, Dollery, and Bulpitt, 1969) and leave a localized area of inner ischemic atrophy, with loss of the nerve fiber, ganglion cell, inner plexiform, and inner portion of the inner nuclear layers. In some instances, minor glial cell proliferation may produce a slight scar.

Histologically and with flat preparations of the retina, these microinfarcts are found in the nerve fiber layer of the retina and are usually less than 300 microns in size. They occur both at the optic disk and in that portion of the retina where numerous vessels supply the nerve fiber layer. In flat preparations, the lumina of the capillaries in the cotton-wool spot are devoid of blood, and their walls show marked loss of both endothelial cells and pericytes (Ashton, 1970; Ashton, Harry, 1963).

Angiographic studies of the retina after the cotton-wool patch has cleared show the circulation to be renewed in the area of the former patch, possibly as a result of reopening of the capillaries but more likely from ingrowth of new vessels (Ashton, Harry, 1963).

By light microscopy, the lesion of a cotton-wool patch involves chiefly the innermost layers of the retina. The ganglion cell and nerve fiber layers are greatly thickened by a disciform, sharply circumscribed lesion. Within the lesion are cytoid bodies, which are globular structures 10 to 20 microns in diameter, each somewhat resembling a cell because of the nucleoid central

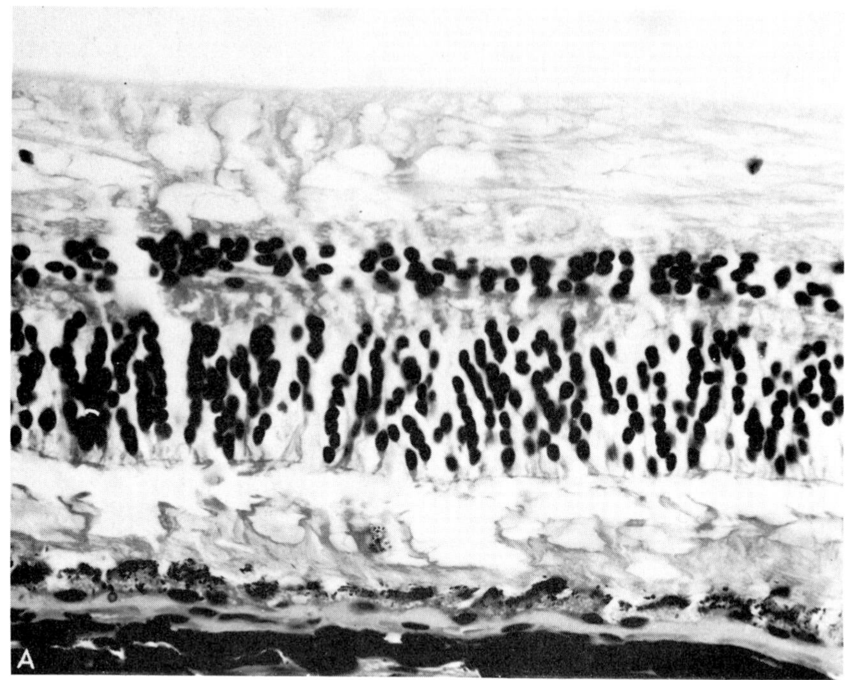

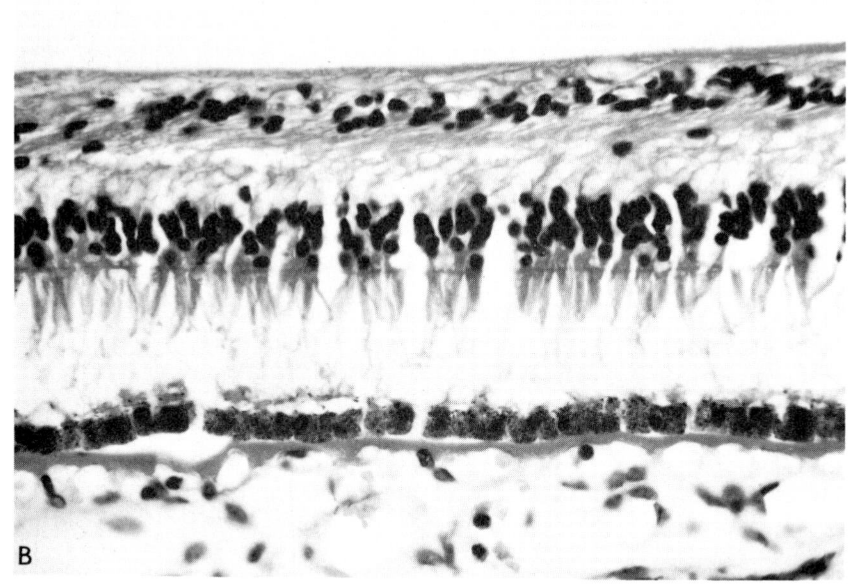

Figure 8–67. Inner ischemic atrophy of the retina, with loss of all the inner layers, down to and including the inner portion of the inner nuclear area in the macular area *(A)* and midperiphery *(B)*. *A,* H and E, ×575. EP 51825. *B,* PAS, ×500. EP 30762.

structure (Fig. 8–68; see also Figs. 8–427,*E* and *F*). Localized inner ischemic atrophy of the retina is thought to be the sequela of a cotton-wool patch (Fig. 8–69).

Wolter (1959b, 1968), using the silver carbonate method of del Rio Hortoga, showed that cytoid bodies are axonal enlargements and that some nerve fibers were interrupted as they passed through the cotton-wool spot. The proximal ends of the interrupted nerves, on the ganglion cell side, were swollen and formed bulbous endings. Wolter likened these end bulb swellings to those described initially by Cajal (later known as Cajal's end bulbs) in his work on degeneration and regeneration of the nervous system.

Ashton and Harry (1963) showed that both the arterioles leading to the cotton-wool spots and adjacent capillaries contained fat within their lumina. This is evidence of a causal relation between the cotton-wool spot and the partially occluded arteriole.

With the electron microscope, the "nucleus" (or pseudonucleus) of the cytoid body has been shown to be formed by proliferation and degen-

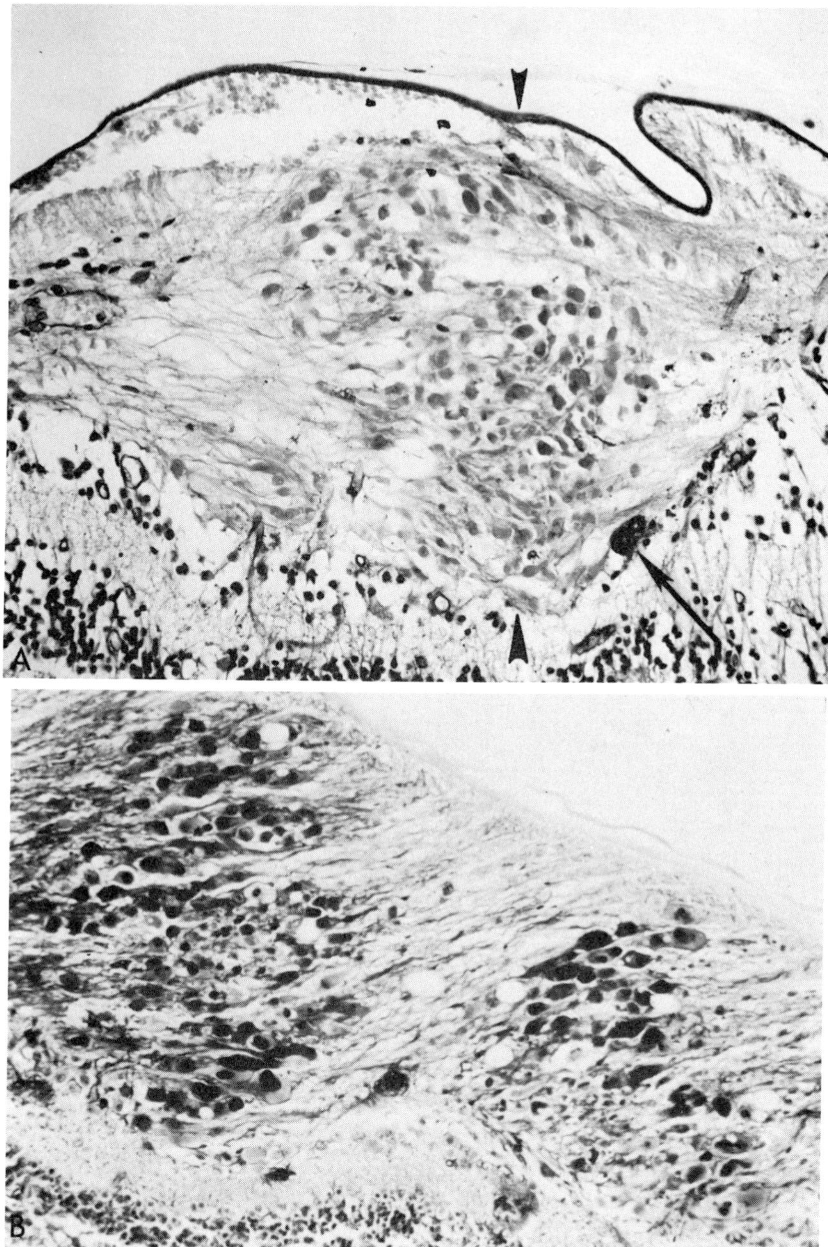

Figure 8–68. Microinfarctions of nerve fiber layer. *A,* Microinfarction showing thickening with edema and cytoid bodies (between arrowheads) and an occluded arteriole (arrow). PAS, ×265. EP 47147. *B,* Two microinfarctions in nerve fiber layer in malignant hypertension. PAS, ×150. EP 4036.

eration of axoplasmic organelles, such as mitochondria, neurofilaments, and endoplasmic reticulum (Shakib, Ashton, 1966; Inomata, Ikui, Kimura, 1967). This pseudonucleus, therefore, consists of aggregates of newly formed and degenerating organelles. The nucleus-like structure is embedded in axoplasm that has flowed from the region of the ganglion cell into the swollen nerve ending.

In experimental studies, McLeod, Marshall, Kohner, and Bird (1977) induced localized retinal ischemic necrosis by argon laser photocoagulation. Two days after coagulation there was necrosis in the inner retina in the territory of occluded arterioles. Swollen axon terminals packed with cytoplasmic organelles were found in the retinal nerve fiber layer in the margin of the infarcted area. These swellings corresponded to the zones of opacification (cotton-wool spots). Utilizing tritiated leucine, these investigators showed that the swellings were the result of interruption of orthograde and retrograde axoplasmic flow. They suggested that cotton-wool spots should be redefined as accumulations of cytoplasmic debris in the retinal nerve fiber layer caused by obstruction of orthograde and retrograde axoplasmic flow in ganglion cell axons.

Since cotton-wool patches occur under various conditions but occlusion of the afferent vessel cannot be demonstrated in all instances, it seems

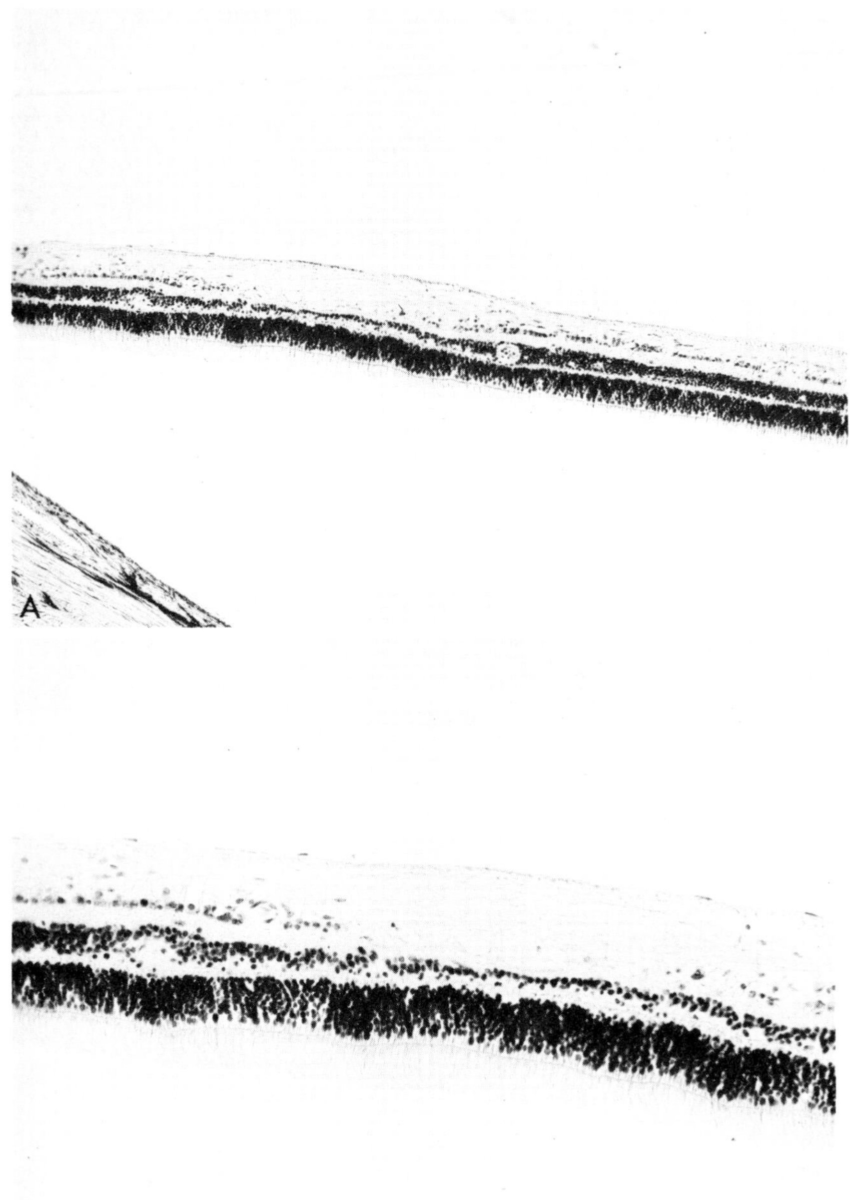

Figure 8–69. Localized area of inner ischemic atrophy that presumably followed a microinfarction with cytoid bodies. *A,* H and E, ×75; *B,* ×160. AFIP Acc. 625745. (From Green WR: Pathology of the Retina, *in* Frayer WC (ed): Lancaster Course in Ophthalmic Histopathology. Unit 9. Philadelphia, F.A. Davis, 1981.)

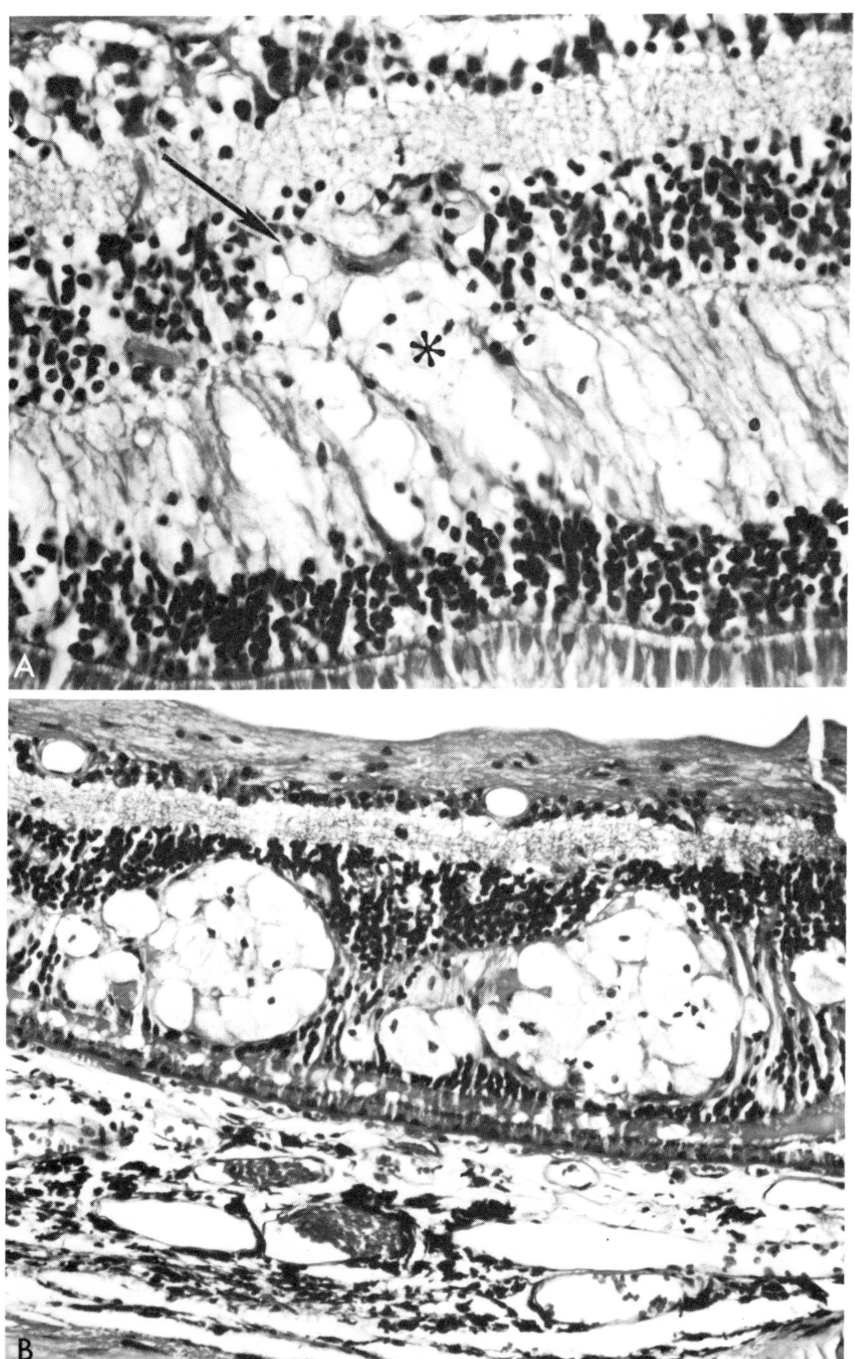

Figure 8–70. *A,* Lipid-laden histiocytes in outer plexiform (arrow) and inner nuclear (asterisk) layers in a diabetic patient. H and E, ×350. EP 30632. *B,* Two aggregates of histiocytes in outer plexiform layer, with crowding of inner and outer nuclear layers, in an eye with an arterial macroaneurysm. H and E, ×225. EP 42728.

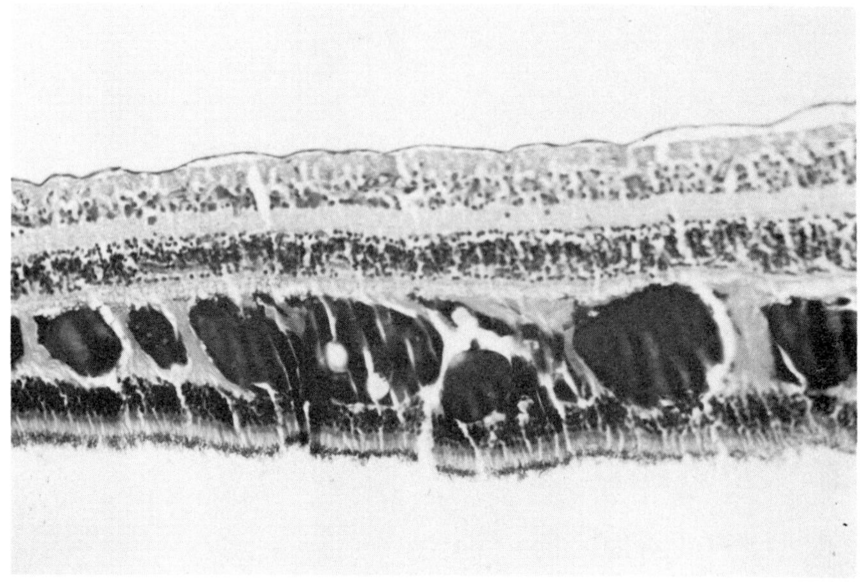

Figure 8–71. Exudate residues in outer plexiform layer in macular area in a diabetic patient. PAS, ×140. EP 29890. (From Green WR: Pathology of the Retina, *in* Frayer WC (ed): Lancaster Course in Ophthalmic Histopathology. Unit 9. Philadelphia, F.A. Davis, 1981.)

likely that, in addition to arteriolar occlusion, any condition causing ischemia of the retina in a localized area can lead to infarction and formation of a cotton-wool patch. Cotton-wool patches are a common feature of systemic hypertension, diabetic retinopathy, and some collagen vascular diseases, with or without hypertension.

The experimental use of microsphere embolization has demonstrated the sequence of the clinical (Dollery, Henkind, Paterson, et al, 1966) and morphologic changes in retinal microinfarctions (Dollery, 1969).

Glia. In totally ischemic lesions, **astrocytes** degenerate and disappear. In less severe situations, astrocytes may undergo proliferation (gliosis) and produce a fibroglial scar.

Microglia are not truly glial cells, but rather are tissue macrophages derived from the perivascular mesodermal tissue or blood monocytes. These cells correspond to the reticuloendothelial cells in the liver, spleen, and lymph nodes. Microglia are relatively resistant to hypoxia, but, with total anoxia, they degenerate, like the astrocytes. Their function is phagocytosis and removal of extravascular blood, exudates, and cellular debris. Such materials are usually rich in lipid, which mainly comes from the serum via the damaged and leaky vascular endothelium. Most of the exudate (protein and cellular debris) is usually cleared away by the microglia without much difficulty. The lipid material, however, is taken up by the microglia. The lipid material and the microglia with phagocytosed lipid are not cleared from the retina as readily as are other exudate constituents.

The swollen microglia with phagocytosed lipid are known as lipid histiocytes (lipoidal histiocytes, foamy macrophages, bladder cells, gitter cells, and others). Such histiocytes have a tendency to accumulate in the outer plexiform layer (Fig. 8–70). The deep, "hard-waxy" exudates observed ophthalmoscopically are various combinations of lipid-rich exudate residues (Fig. 8–71) and aggregates of these cells. Accumulation of these constituents in the outer plexiform layer (Henle's layer) of the posterior pole region is responsible for the ophthalmoscopic appearance of the macular wing or star.

Blood Vessels. ***Edema.*** Retinal edema is one of the earliest signs of disturbance of the retinal vascular system. Clinically, the edema may escape early ophthalmoscopic recognition, but, as the retina becomes more edematous, retinal opacification and haziness develop, obscuring the vessels. Edema that is primarily extracellular (Henkind, Bellhorn, Schall, 1980) may be localized or diffuse, depending on the vascular area affected. Eventually, the edema may lead to degeneration of the neurons, and glial tissue and cell debris accumulate in spaces occupied by the edema. The edema fluid tends to accumulate in the plexiform layers as localized collections of fluid that produce cystoid spaces (Fig. 8–72; also see Fig. 8–102). Edema fluid also collects in the inner nuclear and ganglion cell layers to produce similar but much smaller spaces.

In Henle's fiber layer, where the axons and dendrites lie almost parallel to the retina, there is a strong tendency for pocketing of the edema fluid. With time, the lipid and proteinaceous fluid that has collected in the cystoid spaces becomes inspissated to produce soft or hard exudates. Clinically, these appear as whitish to yellow-white, sharply circumscribed opacities in various layers of the retina. The greater the lipid content, the yellower the exudate.

In the macular region, the exudates become

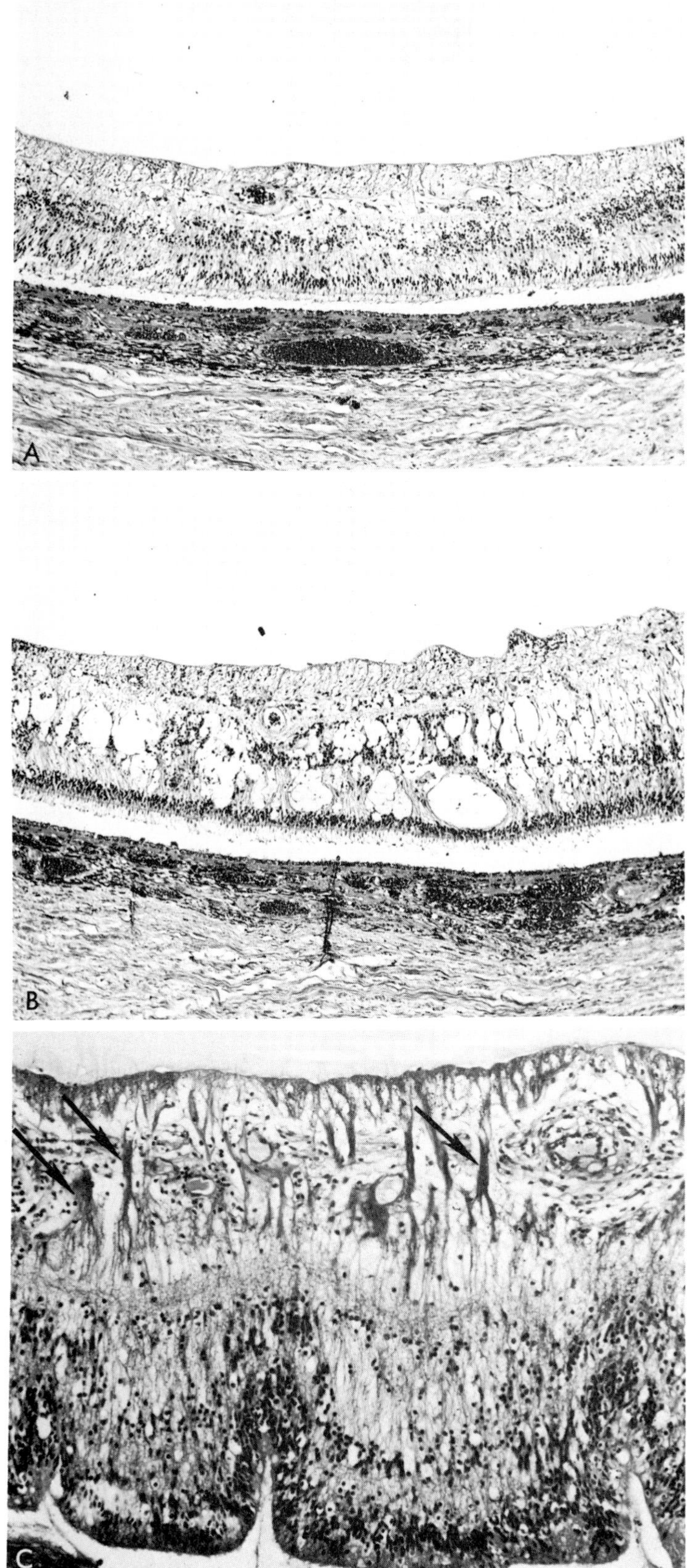

Figure 8–72. Diffuse retinal edema associated with central retinal vein occlusion *(A* and *B)* and Coats' disease *(C)*. Müller cells (arrows) are prominent in *C. A,* H and E, ×60; AFIP Neg. 70-1184. *B,* H and E, ×60; AFIP Neg. 70-1183. *C,* PAS, ×150; EP 51883.

aligned along Henle's layer in a radial fashion to produce a star figure at the macula. Histologically, these exudates and the star figure are eosinophilic, are sharply circumscribed, and may be surrounded by small amounts of fluid. The Müller cells and axons at the margins of the exudates are crowded together to form a boundary. The exudates and the star figure are long and linear in the outer plexiform layer. As more and more fluid is absorbed from the coagulated protein and lipid in the exudates, they become "harder," and "waxier," and more sharply circumscribed.

Appropriate staining will show that these exudates contain lipid. Commonly, macrophages containing phagocytized exudate, and perhaps the degenerating axons, accumulate around and within these exudates.

Hemorrhages. Hemorrhages are a common accompaniment of ischemic, hypertensive, and other vascular disorders in the retina, and their clinical appearance depends in part upon the retinal level at which they occur. Some of them are produced by extravasation through the severely damaged vascular wall; others are smaller and produced by diapedesis. Hemorrhages are usually observed clinically as either linear or rounded, but there are numerous variations.

Hemorrhages in the nerve fiber layer of the retina are linear, since the blood is aligned parallel to the axons (Fig. 8–73). Rounded (dot-and-blot) hemorrhages lie in the nuclear and plexiform layers, where they displace the neurons and glial cells, and are limited at the periphery by undamaged neurons and Müller cells (Fig. 8–74). Some retinal hemorrhages have a white center

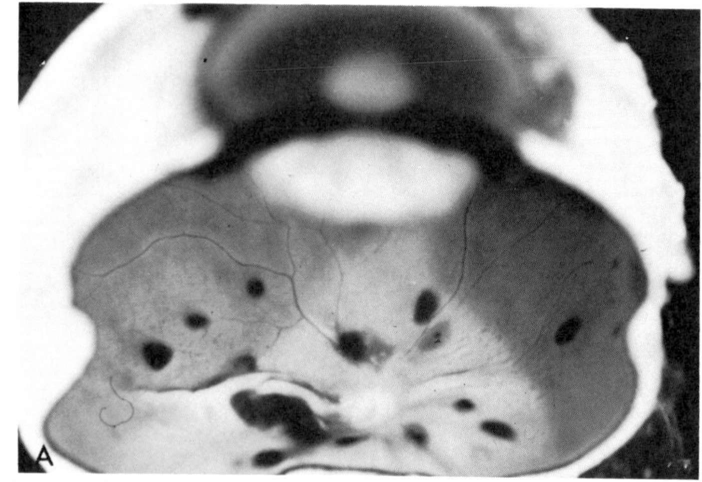

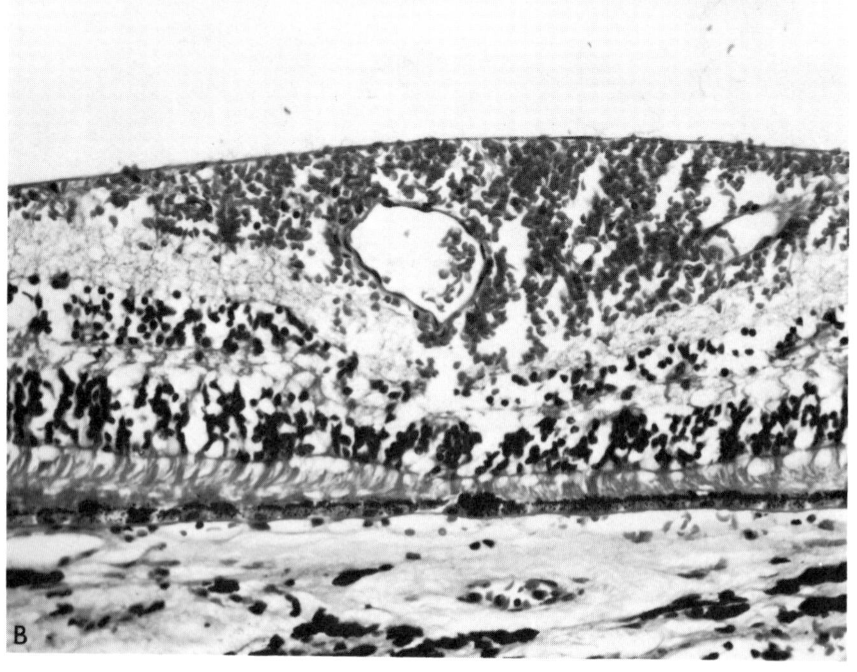

Figure 8–73. *A,* Gross and *B,* microscopic appearance of splinter-shaped **retinal hemorrhages** around optic nerve head. *B,* H and E, ×250. EP 30956. (From Green WR: Pathology of the Retina, *in* Frayer WC (ed): Lancaster Course in Ophthalmic Histopathology. Unit 9. Philadelphia, F.A. Davis, 1981.)

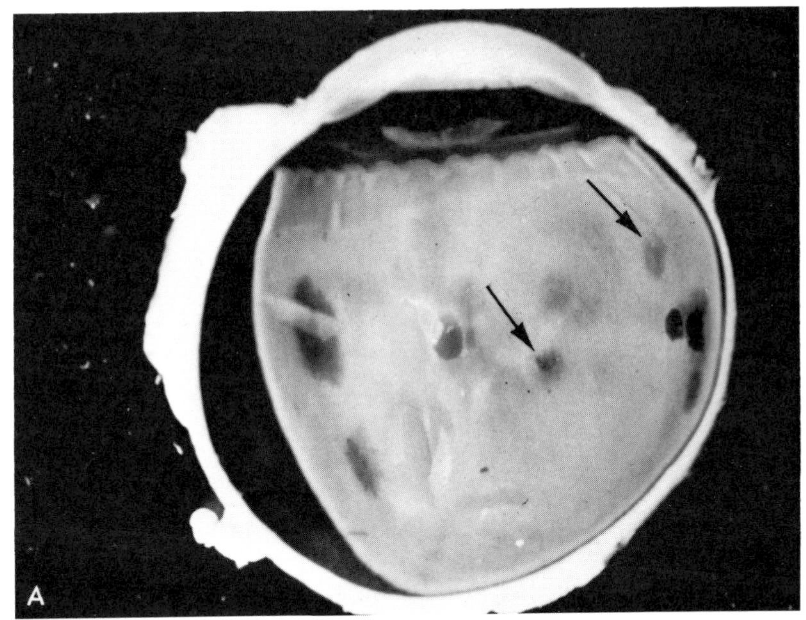

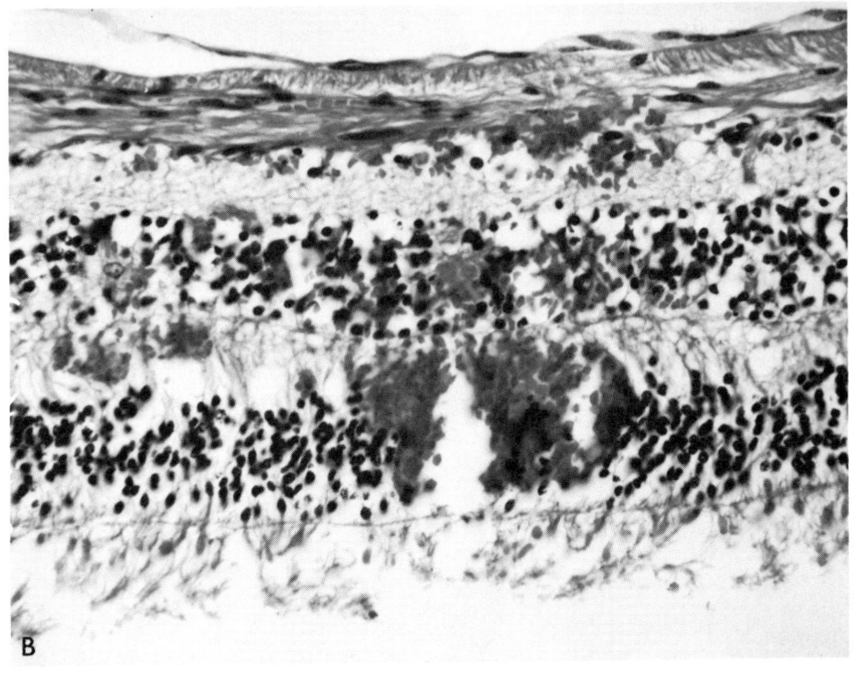

Figure 8–74. *A,* Gross and *B,* microscopic appearance of dot-and-blot type of **retinal hemorrhages** (arrows). *A,* EP 31151. *B,* H and E, ×110. EP 43889.

(so-called Roth spots) (Fig. 8–75), caused by the accumulation of platelets and fibrin (Fig. 8–76) (Duane, Osher, Green 1980).

In a clinical study of patients with thrombocytopenia and/or anemia or hemophilia, Rubenstein, Yanoff, and Albert (1968) found retinal hemorrhages in the following percentages: anemia alone, 10 per cent; thrombocytopenia alone, 0 per cent; Cooley's anemia, 10 per cent, hemophilia, 10 per cent; anemia and thrombocytopenia, 44 per cent. When severe anemia was associated with severe thrombocytopenia, 70 per cent of the patients had ocular hemorrhage.

Retinal hemorrhages may occur in persons subjected to high altitude. Acute mountain sickness is related to the speed and height of ascent and becomes manifest 6 to 96 hours after ascent. Lubin, Rennie, Hackett, and Albert (1982) have reviewed the association of retinal hemorrhages and high altitude and reported the clinicopathologic features of one case.

Retinal hemorrhages have been observed in patients with overdose of methaqualone (Trese, 1981).

Hemorrhages may be massive, in which case they may extend under the retina (Fig. 8–77) into the vitreous (Fig. 8–78) and may infiltrate the retina diffusely and extend to detach the inner lim-

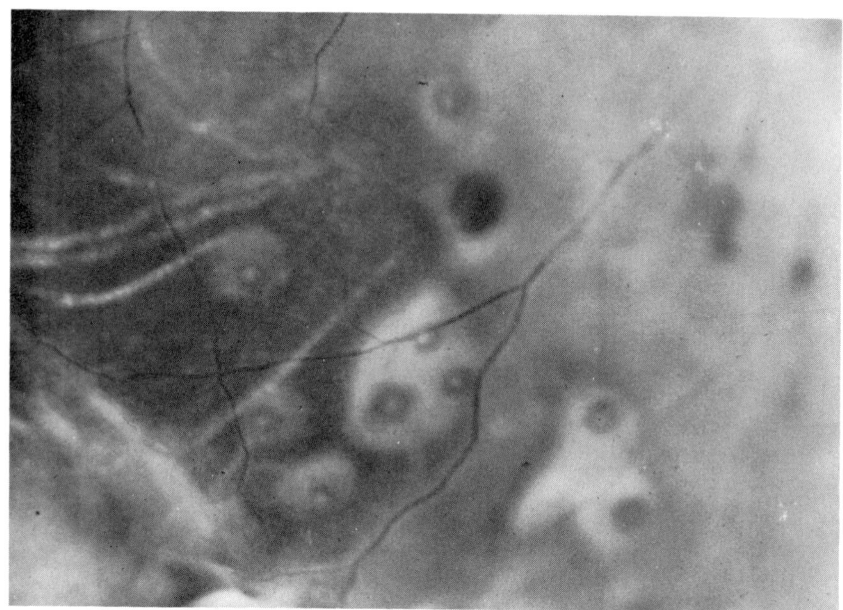

Figure 8–75. White-centered retinal hemorrhages. EP 30956.

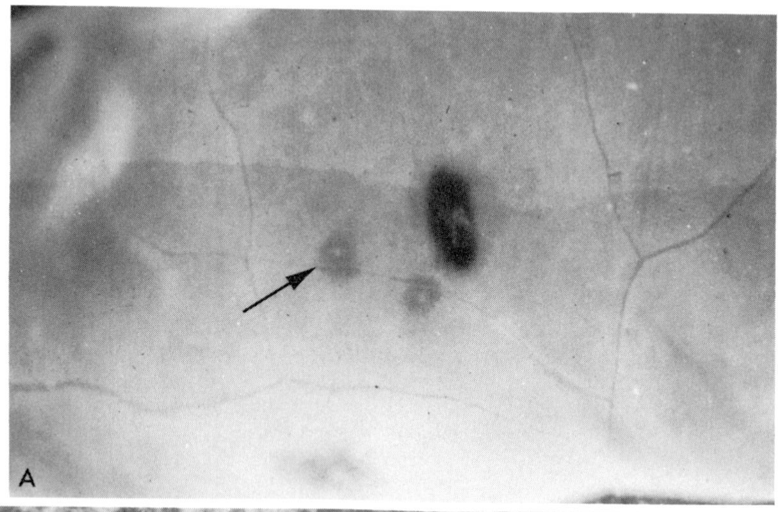

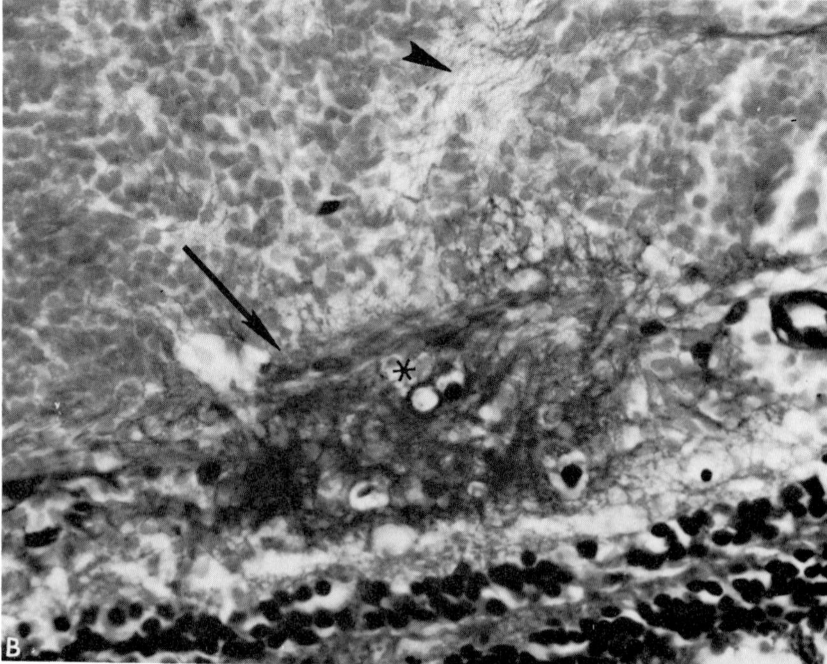

Figure 8–76. *A,* Gross appearance of several small, white-centered retinal hemorrhages (arrow) in a 51 year old anemic woman who died of metastatic pulmonary carcinoma. *B,* Section through center of retinal hemorrhage noted in *A.* Fibrin (arrowhead) and fibrin platelet aggregates (arrow) are present around a capillary with a disrupted wall (asterisk). PAS; original magnification, ×450. EP 7609. (From Duane TD, Osher RH, Green WR: White-centered hemorrhages: Their significance. Ophthalmology *87*:66–69, 1980.)

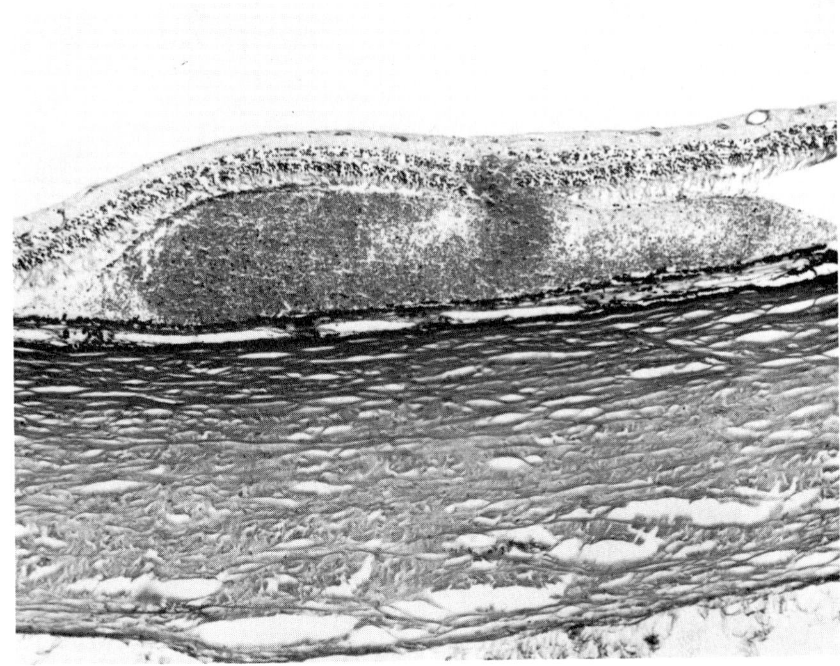

Figure 8–77. Retinal hemorrhage that extends into the subretinal space in a patient with sickle cell hemoglobinopathy. H and E, × 60. EP 32867. (From Romayananda N, Goldberg MF, Green WR: Histopathology of sickle cell retinopathy. Trans Am Acad Ophthalmol Otolaryngol 77:652–676, 1973.)

iting membrane (Fig. 8–79). This type of hemorrhage may be mistaken for preretinal (subhyaloid) hemorrhage. Observation of Gunn's dots is helpful in determining whether the hemorrhage is under the internal limiting membrane (ILM).

Retinal hemorrhages generally clear, but the period of time varies from several days to many months. Eventually, gradual lysis of the red cells occurs, with also a migration of macrophages into the hemorrhagic region in an attempt to remove the debris. Eventually all the blood is absorbed into undamaged vessels. The macrophages migrate to the blood vessels, where they accumulate in the perivascular region, and eventually their products or the cells enter the blood stream and are carried away.

Minor hemorrhages usually fade away and leave no detectable ophthalmoscopic signs. As

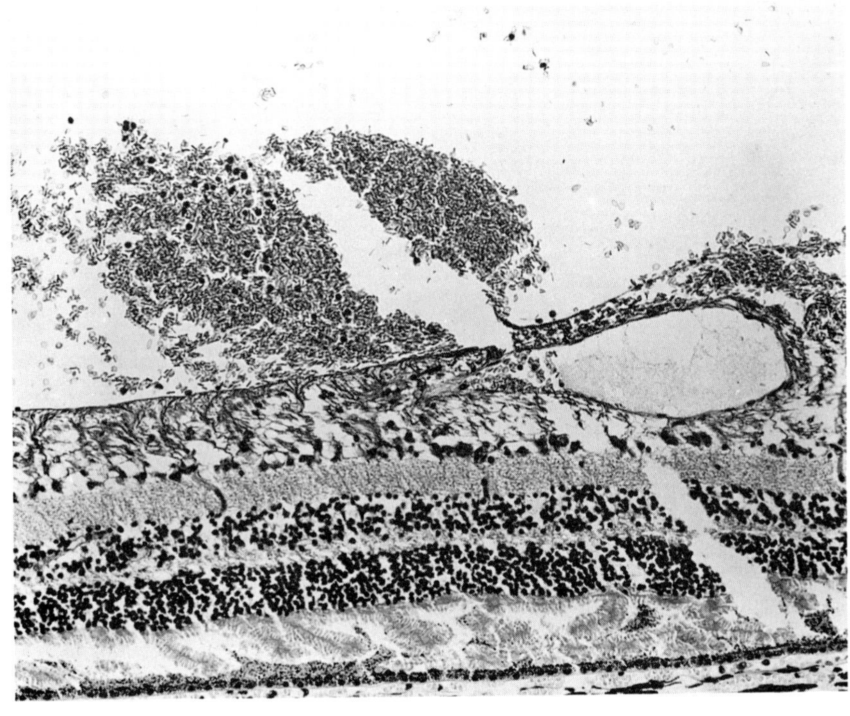

Figure 8–78. Retinal hemorrhage, with extension into vitreous cavity in a patient with sickle cell–hemoglobin C disease. H and E, ×110. EP 40439. (From Romayananda N, Goldberg MF, Green WR: Histopathology of sickle cell retinopathy. Trans Am Acad Ophthalmol Otolaryngol 77:652–676, 1973.)

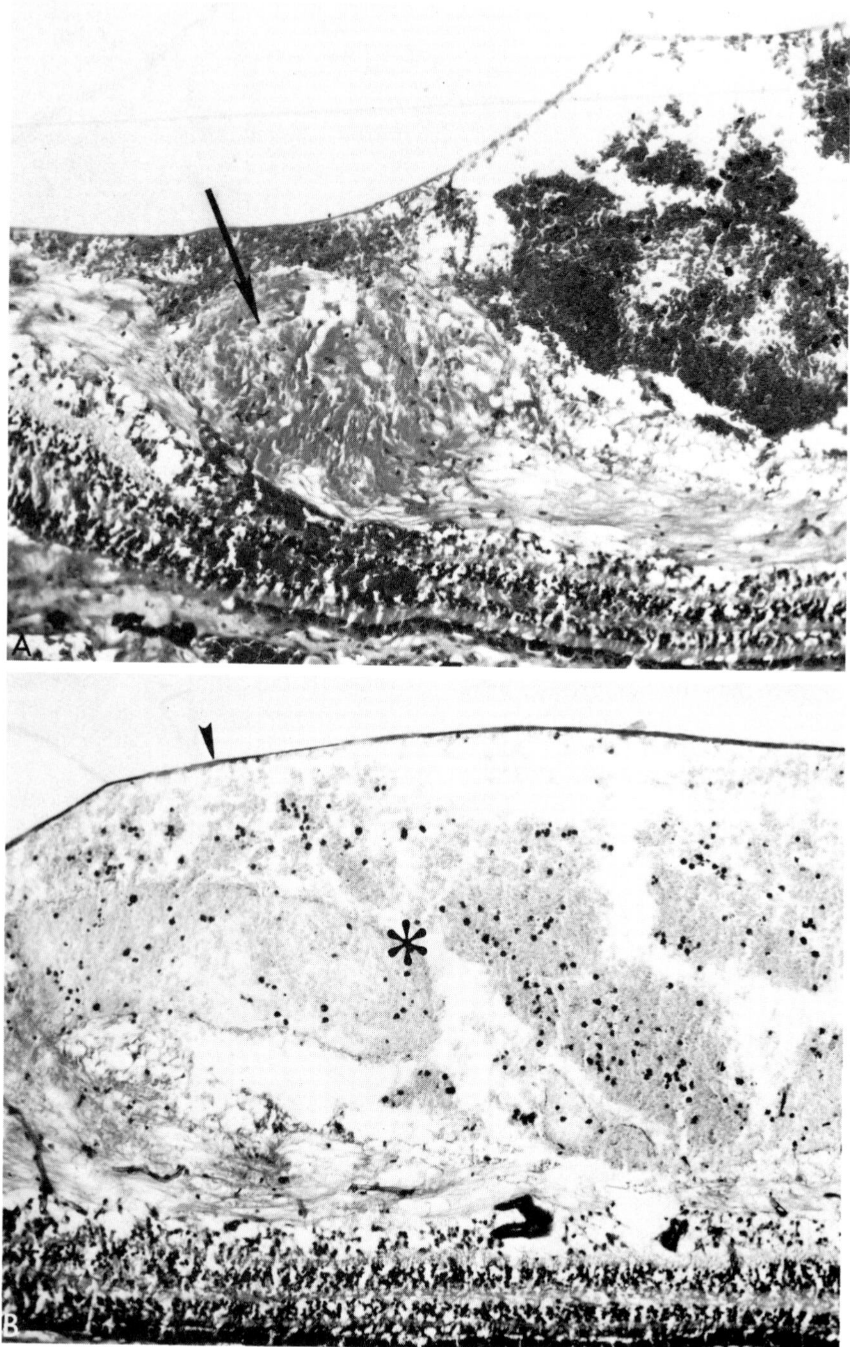

Figure 8–79. *A,* Retinal hemorrhage in the vicinity of a microinfarction of a nerve fiber layer with cytoid bodies (arrow) and hemorrhage extension and separation of the internal limiting membrane (ILM). H and E, ×125. *B,* Retinal hemorrhage (asterisk) located under the ILM (arrowhead). This is an older hemorrhage with partial breakdown of the erythrocytes and hemosiderin deposition. PAS, ×110. EP 30956.

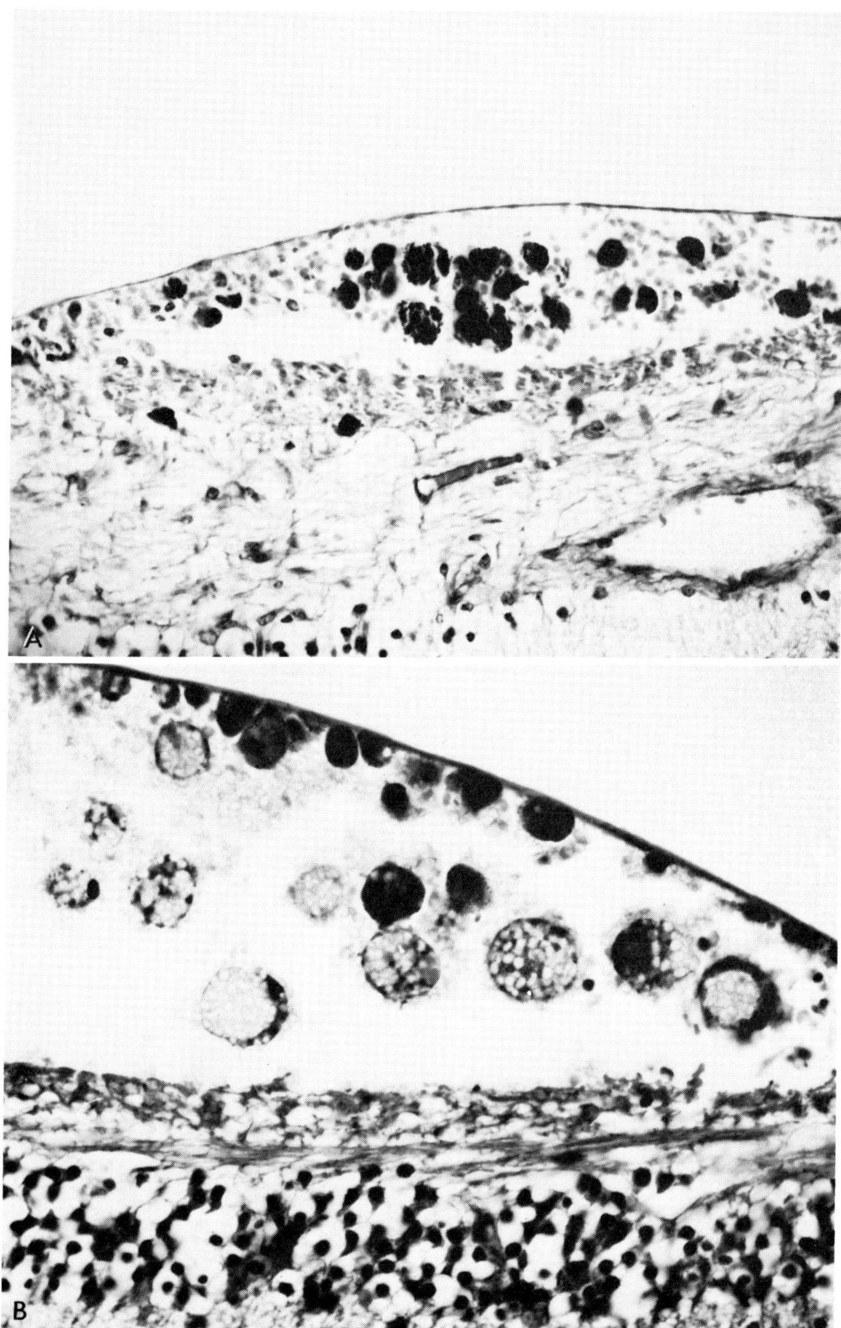

Figure 8–80. Acquired schisis cavity from resolving sub-internal limiting membrane (ILM) hemorrhage, with breakdown of erythrocytes and macrophages and phagocytosed erythrocytic debris and hemosiderin. *A,* PAS, ×300; EP 47060. *B,* PAS, ×360; EP 40655.

the blood undergoes hemolysis, iron is released and is taken up by retinal cells or macrophages. In more marked cases this may give a rusty color to the area, known as hemosiderosis (Fig. 8–80). Minor glial proliferation may be associated with some hemorrhages. As sub-ILM and subhyaloid hemorrhages clear, color changes occur; when sufficient hemosiderin is present, the lesion may appear iridescent, as has been observed in sickle cell retinopathy (Fig. 8–81) (Romayananda, Goldberg, Green, 1973).

Capillary Microaneurysms. Capillary microaneurysms are generally 50 to 100 microns in size, and only the larger one or the ones with associated bleeding are visible ophthalmoscopically without fluorescein angiography. Capillary microaneurysms are occasionally found in the periphery of the retina of elderly persons, when studied by the trypsin digestion technique.

Microaneurysms occur in increased numbers in disease states in which retinal hypoxia is thought to occur.

In diabetes mellitus, capillary microaneurysms are seen mainly in the posterior pole region (Fig. 8–82). In central retinal vein occlusion, microaneurysms are found throughout the retina. In Coats' disease, microaneurysms are present in localized areas. In a number of conditions, such as hypertension, arteriosclerosis, hyperviscosity states, hypotensive retinopathy (venous stasis retinopathy), and chronic leukemia, microaneurysms occur in increased numbers in the anterior portion of the retina.

Capillary microaneurysms often have an increased number of endothelial cells. Whether this increase is due to proliferation or to migration from adjacent capillaries is not known. The wall of the microaneurysm is thin at first and leaks fluorescein. The wall then thickens by the deposition of a hyaline, periodic acid–Schiff-positive

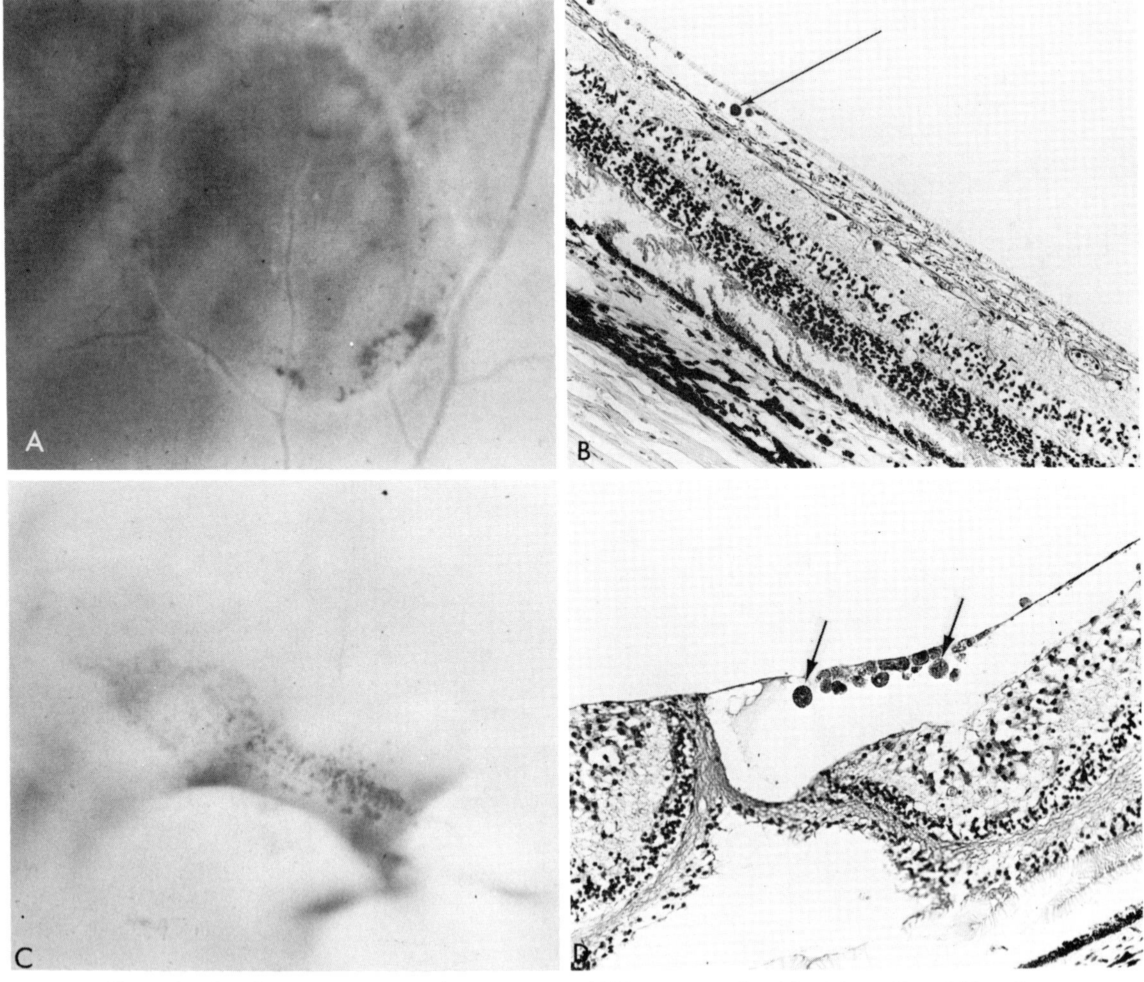

Figure 8–81. Gross and microscopic appearance of iridescent spot in midperiphery *(A* and *B)* and macular area *(C* and *D)* in **sickle cell–hemoglobin C retinopathy**. Both show resolving sub–internal limiting membrane (ILM) hemorrhages with hemosiderin-laden macrophages (arrows) in an acquired schisis cavity. Prussian blue; B, ×50; D, ×60. (From Romayananda N, Goldberg MF, Green WR: Histopathology of sickle cell retinopathy. Trans Am Acad Ophthalmol Otolaryngol *77*:652–676, 1973.)

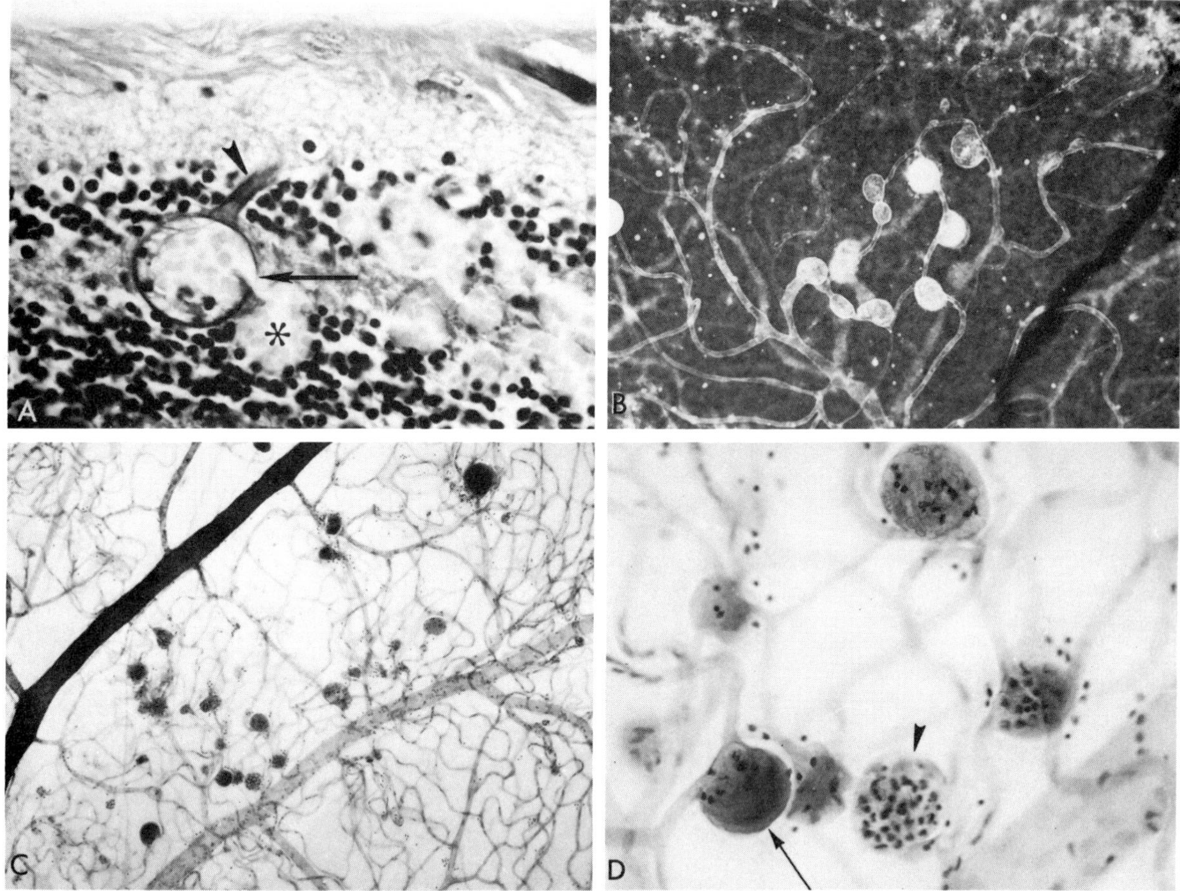

Figure 8–82. Capillary macroaneurysms in diabetes. *A,* Light microscopic appearance. Capillary (arrowhead) is continuous with microaneurysm that is disrupted (arrow) and produced mild hemorrhage (asterisk). PAS, ×575. EP 30498. *B,* Flat preparation of retina. AFIP Acc. 219548. (From Friedenwald JS: A new approach to some problems of retinal vascular disease. The Jackson Memorial Lecture. Am J Ophthalmol *32*:487–498, 1949.) *C* and *D,* Trypsin digest preparation of retina showing microaneurysms between artery and vein at margin of a zone of capillary acellularity. *D,* Higher power view shows one microaneurysm with a dense periodic acid–Schiff-positive material (arrow) and another with neutrophils present (arrowhead). PAS; hematoxylin. *C,* ×50; *D,* ×350. EP 39108.

material. The microaneurysms eventually may become occluded by this hyaline material or by thrombosis.

Retinal Neovascularization. The development of new vessels originating from and contiguous with the pre-existing retinal vascular bed constitutes retinal neovascularization (Henkind, Wise, 1974). The stimulus for this process appears to be related to poor retinal nutrition resulting in retinal hypoxia or the accumulation of metabolic products or both. Retinal neovascularization is a feature of diabetic retinopathy, retrolental fibroplasia, some hemoglobinopathies, sarcoidosis, branch retinal vein occlusion, Eales' disease, and others.

Figure 8–83 illustrates a localized area of nonvascularization from a retinal vein, with extension into the vitreous, in an eye from a patient with diabetes.

Retinal Collaterals. These are vessels that develop within the framework of the existing vascular network (Henkind, Wise, 1974). Collaterals develop adjacent to areas of nonperfusion. At first these involve capillaries but collaterals may evolve to *arterioarteriolar (A-A),* after branch artery occlusion; *venovenular (V-V),* after vein occlusion; and *arteriovenous (A-V),* after capillary bed obstruction.

Retinal Vascular Shunts. These are arteriovenous (A-V) communications without an intervening capillary bed (Henkind, Wise, 1974). These shunts may be congenital or acquired. Acquired A-V shunts may occur in retinal angiomatosis, Coats' disease, and others.

Patterns of Ischemic Disease of the Retina

In the foregoing, we have considered the general categories of conditions in which retinal ischemia is observed. We also have reviewed

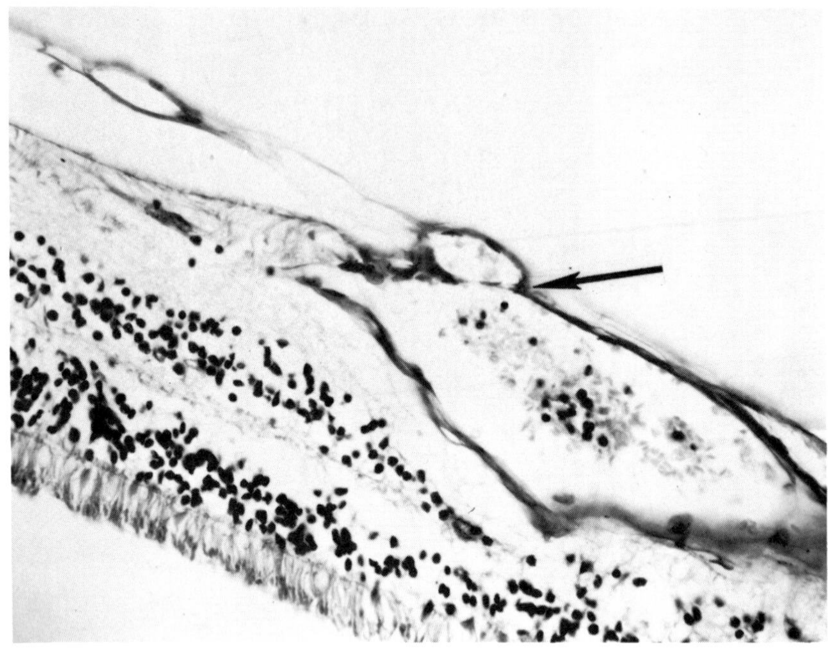

Figure 8–83. Neovascularization (NVE) with direct extension from a retinal vein (arrow) into the vitreous cavity in a diabetic patient. PAS, ×300. EP 30498. (From Green WR: Pathology of the Retina, *in* Frayer WC (ed): Lancaster Course in Ophthalmic Histopathology. Unit 9. Philadelphia, F.A. Davis, 1981.)

briefly the various cellular constituents of the retina and how they react to ischemia.

Discussed next are various patterns of ischemia that are encountered and some of the specific disease entities involved.

Focal Arteriolar Occlusion

Focal arteriolar occlusion of the retina is observed in diabetes mellitus, collagen vascular diseases, embolism, vasculitis, sickle cell retinopathy, arteriosclerosis, hypertension, and others.

In most of these instances, the focal arteriolar occlusion is evident clinically by the occurrence of microinfarctions (cotton-wool exudate) (see page 655). In some instances, especially in sickle cell retinopathy, the tertiary and quaternary branches of the central retinal artery are occluded, and cotton-wool exudates are not usually evident. Larger areas of infarction show slight thickening of the retina as it gains a milky-gray color. After a few days, the retina repairs to normal transparency (Wise, Dollery, Henkind, 1971).

Embolism is an important cause of focal, as well as more extensive, arteriolar occlusion. Some of the various types of emboli and selected references to histopathologic studies are —atrial myxoma (Anderson, Lubow, 1973; Jam-

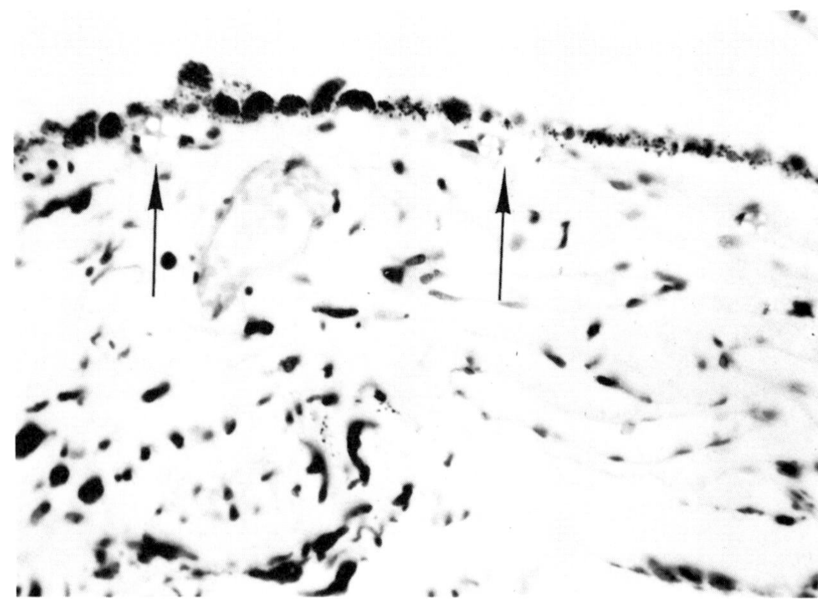

Figure 8–84. Talc emboli in choriocapillaris (arrows). H and E, polarized light, ×500. EP 28117.

pol, Wong, Albert, 1973; Manschot, 1959; Cogan, Wray, 1975)
—calcific emboli (Penner, Font, 1969; Baghdassarian, Crawford, Rathbun, 1970; Patrinely, Green, Randolph, 1982)
—cholesterol emboli (McBrien, Bradley, Ashton, 1963; Ball, 1966; Wolter and Ryan, 1972; Wolter, 1972; McKibbin, Bulkley, Green, et al, 1976)
—platelet fibrin embolus (Zimmerman, 1965)
—fat emboli (Cogan, Kuwabara, Moser, 1964)
—metastatic tumor embolus (Tarkkanen, Merenmies, Mäkinen, 1973).
—metastatic chondrosarcoma tumor emboli (Burde, Smith, Black, 1982)

Clinical studies of additional types of emboli include
—amniotic fluid (Fischbein, 1969)
—talc (Fig. 8–84) (Brucker, 1979; Friberg, Gragoudas, Regan, 1979; Michelson, Whitcher, Wilson, O'Connor, 1979; Kresca, Goldberg, Jampol, 1979; Schatz, Drake, 1979; Tse, Ober, 1980)
—corticosteroids (Whiteman, Rosen, Pinkerton, 1980; Evans, Zahorchak, Kennerdell, 1980)
—cloth particles from artificial cardiac valves (Pluth, Danielson, 1974; Rush, Kearns, Danielson, 1980)

In a clinical study of 70 patients with retinal embolism, Arruga and Sanders (1982) considered 40 to have cholesterol emboli, 8 platelet-fibrin emboli, 6 calcific emboli, and 1 possible myxomatous embolus. Retinal periarteriolar sheathing was observed in 41 cases. The carotid artery or other major arteries was felt to be the source of 67.5 per cent of the cholesterol emboli, and the heart was felt to be the source of 67 per cent of the calcific emboli.

Thromboembolism is considered to be the basis of retinal and choroidal occlusions observed in the hypereosinophilic syndrome (Chaine, Davies, Kohner, et al, 1982).

Branch Retinal Artery Occlusion

Most branch retinal artery occlusions are caused by embolism, which frequently occurs at a bifurcation of a retinal arteriole. Obstruction of the arteriole usually results. With cholesterol crystals, however, a blood flow around the embolus may persist. Branch retinal artery occlusion also may occur in late, severe arteriosclerosis, diabetes mellitus, arteritis, dysproteinemias, collagen vascular diseases, and malignant hypertension. Cholesterol emboli may appear in the retina and choroid from ulcerated atheromatous disease of the carotid arteries and an aortotomy for bypass at the time of cardiac valvular surgery (Fig. 8–85) (David, Klintworth, Friedberg, Dillon, 1963; McKibbin, Bulkley, Green, et al, 1976).

Penner and Font (1969) reported the clinicopathologic features of a retinal calcareous embolus in a 45 year old woman with inactive calcific aortic valvulopathy of rheumatic origin. Clinicopathologic studies of ocular calcific emboli in a 41 year old man with rheumatic heart disease also have been reported (Baghdassarian, Crawford, Rathbun, 1970). Similar features are illustrated in Figure 8–86. Ulcerated atheromatous plaques of the carotid are a source of calcific and cholesterol emboli (Pfaffenbach, Hollenhorst, 1972; Ball, 1966).

With branch retinal artery occlusion, central retinal artery occlusion, and localized inner retinal infarction, there is loss of the inner retinal layers, including the nerve fiber, ganglion cell, and inner plexiform layers and the inner aspect of the inner nuclear layer (Fig. 8–87).

Platelet emboli have a whitish-gray appearance and may appear in "showers." They usually pass through the retinal circulation without causing obstruction (Fig. 8–88).

Septic emboli, as in subacute bacterial endocarditis (SBE), may produce branch retinal artery occlusion. Figure 8–89 illustrates a branch retinal artery occlusion in a right eye and a single Roth spot in the left eye, which were the initial manifestations of SBE in a 54 year old man. A Roth spot (Roth, 1872) is defined as a white-centered hemorrhage from a septic embolus. Histopathologic examination of a Roth spot of a different patient with SBE (Fig. 8–90) shows localized thickening of the retina, with an infiltration of polymorphonuclear leukocytes and some surrounding hemorrhage.

Atrial myxomas also may be a source of emboli to the eye. Figure 8–91 illustrates myxoma emboli to the choroid and outer retinal ischemic atrophy in a 26 year old woman with a 3 year history of an "arteritis" picture. Retinal vascular occlusion was observed prior to death.

Choroidal arteriolar occlusion by thrombus (Fig. 8–92) and by calcific and myxomatous emboli can affect the retina. This leads to a round, oval, or sometimes sectorial area of RPE atrophy. These lesions have been referred to as Elschnig's spots (Elschnig, 1904; Klien, 1968; Morse, 1968).

The gross and microscopic appearance of a choroidal infarct (Elschnig's spot) is illustrated in Figure 8–93. There is outer ischemic retinal atrophy, with loss of the RPE, photoreceptor cell layer, outer plexiform layer, and outer portion of the inner nuclear layer.

A similar process may be diffuse, without discrete, punched-out lesions; this has been observed clinically in giant cell arteritis (Wang, Henkind, 1979). Granato, Abben, and May (1981) and Novak, Green, and Miller (1982) have observed temporal arteritis in a father and daughter (Fig. 8–94). Examination of the surgically enucleated eye of the father disclosed giant cell ar-

Text continued on page 684

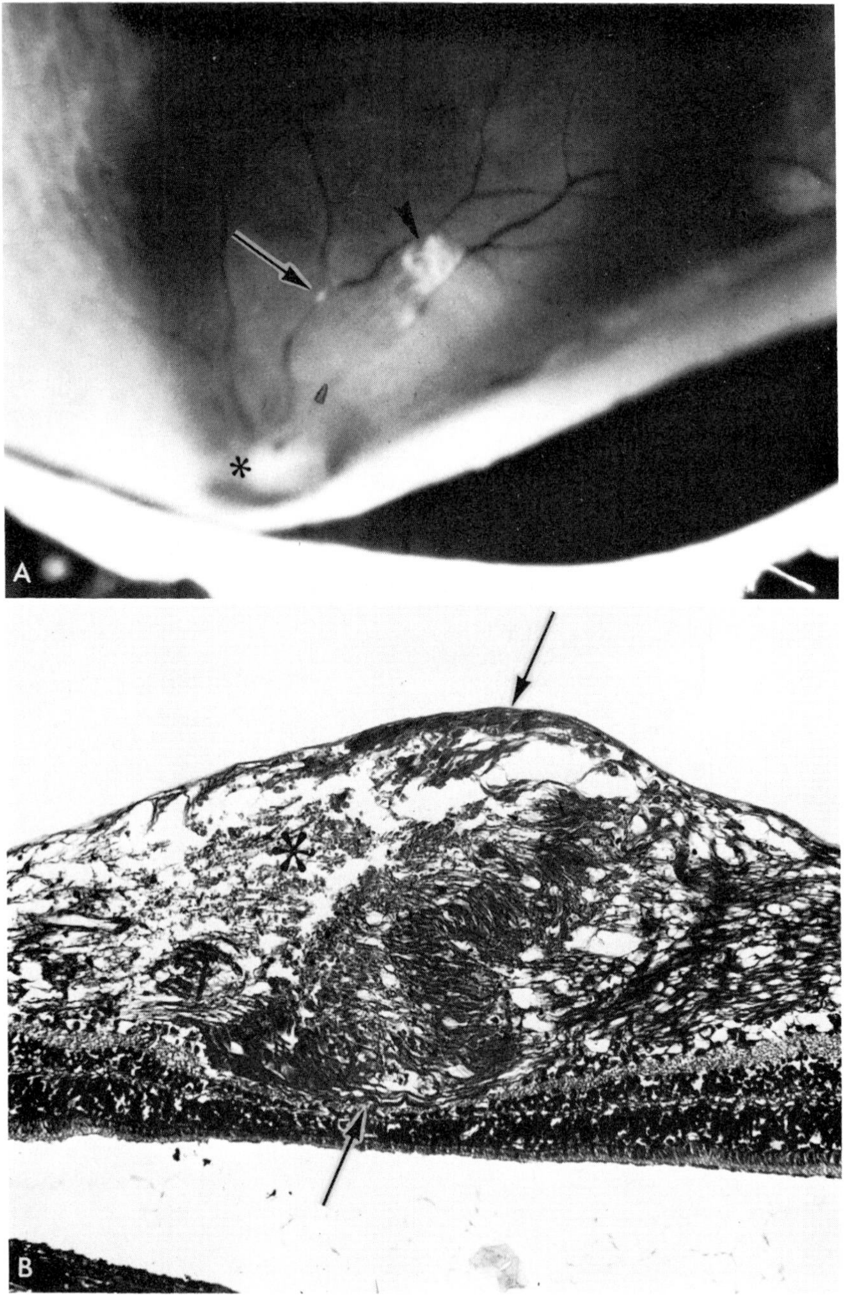

Figure 8–85. Cholesterol emboli in eye. *A,* Gross appearance of embolus at point of bifurcation of artery (arrow) and microinfarction (arrowhead); the optic nerve head is at the asterisk. *B,* Area of microinfarction showing marked thickening of nerve fiber layer with cytoid bodies (between arrows) and mild hemorrhage (asterisk). Verhoeff–van Gieson, ×150.

Illustration continued on opposite page

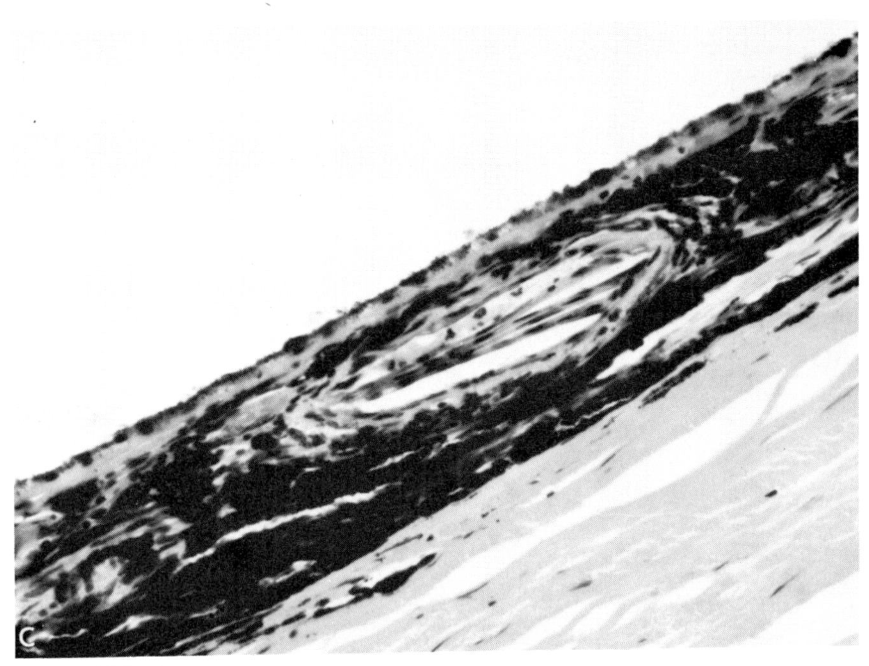

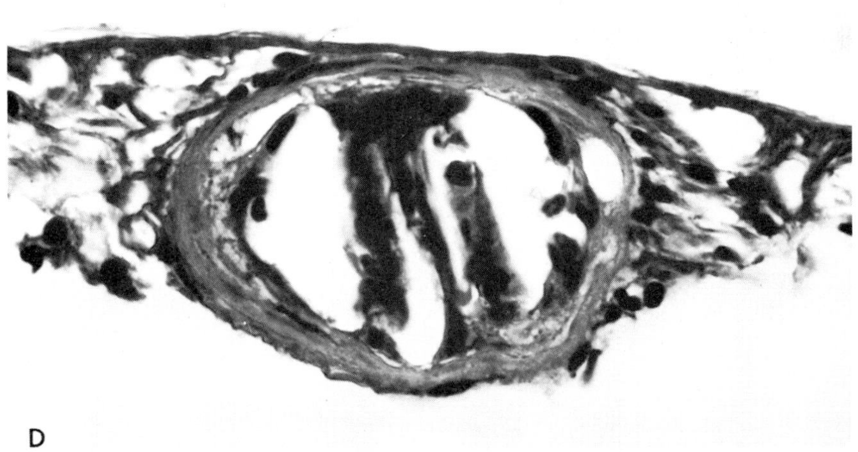

Figure 8–85 *Continued C,* Cholesterol embolus in choroidal vessels. The cholesterol slit is surrounded by foreign body giant cell. H and E, ×325. *D,* Cholesterol embolus in retinal artery. H and E, ×500. EP 39960. (From McKibbin DW, Gott VL, Hutchins GM: Fatal cerebral atheromatous embolization after cardiopulmonary bypass. J Thorac Cardiovasc Surg *71*:741–745, 1976.)

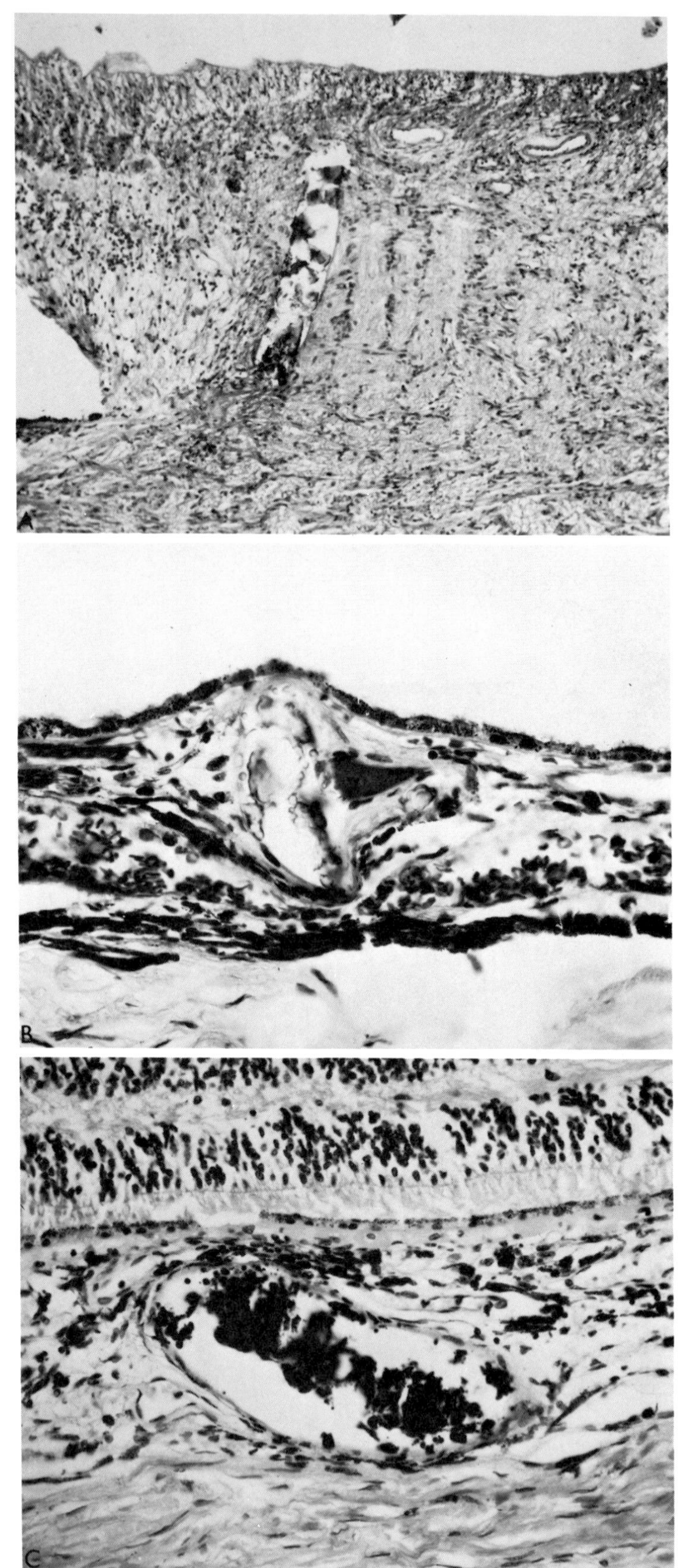

Figure 8–86. Calcific emboli in branch of central retinal artery *(A)* and choroidal artery *(B* and *C)*. *A,* H and E, ×110; EP 28337. *B,* H and E, ×550; EP 28337. *C,* PAS, ×800; EP 30176.

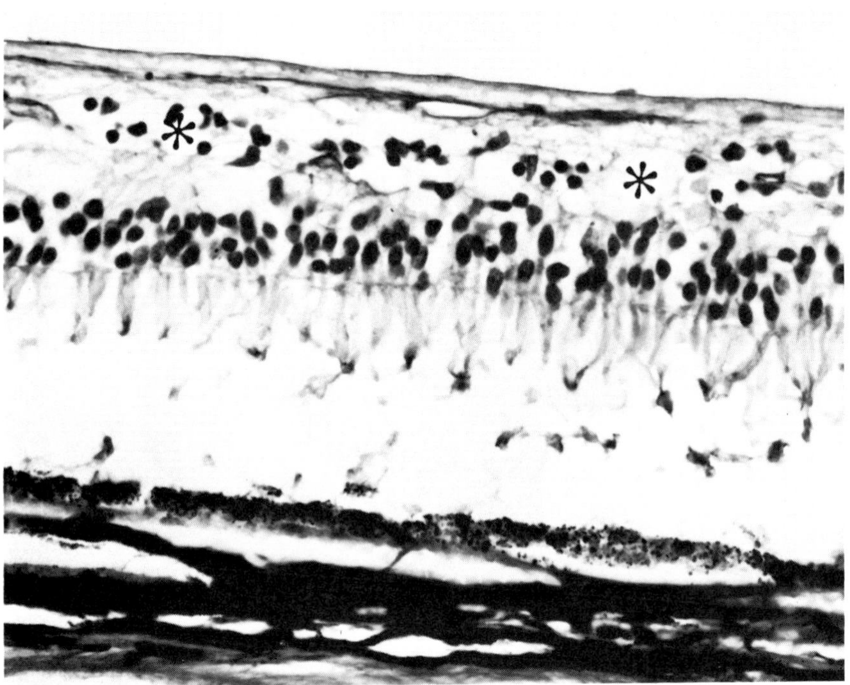

Figure 8–87. Inner ischemic atrophy associated with cholesterol embolus. There is loss of all inner retinal layers, down to and including the inner aspect of the inner nuclear layer; remaining portion of outer aspect of the inner nuclear layer is shown by asterisks. PAS, ×450. EP 40584.

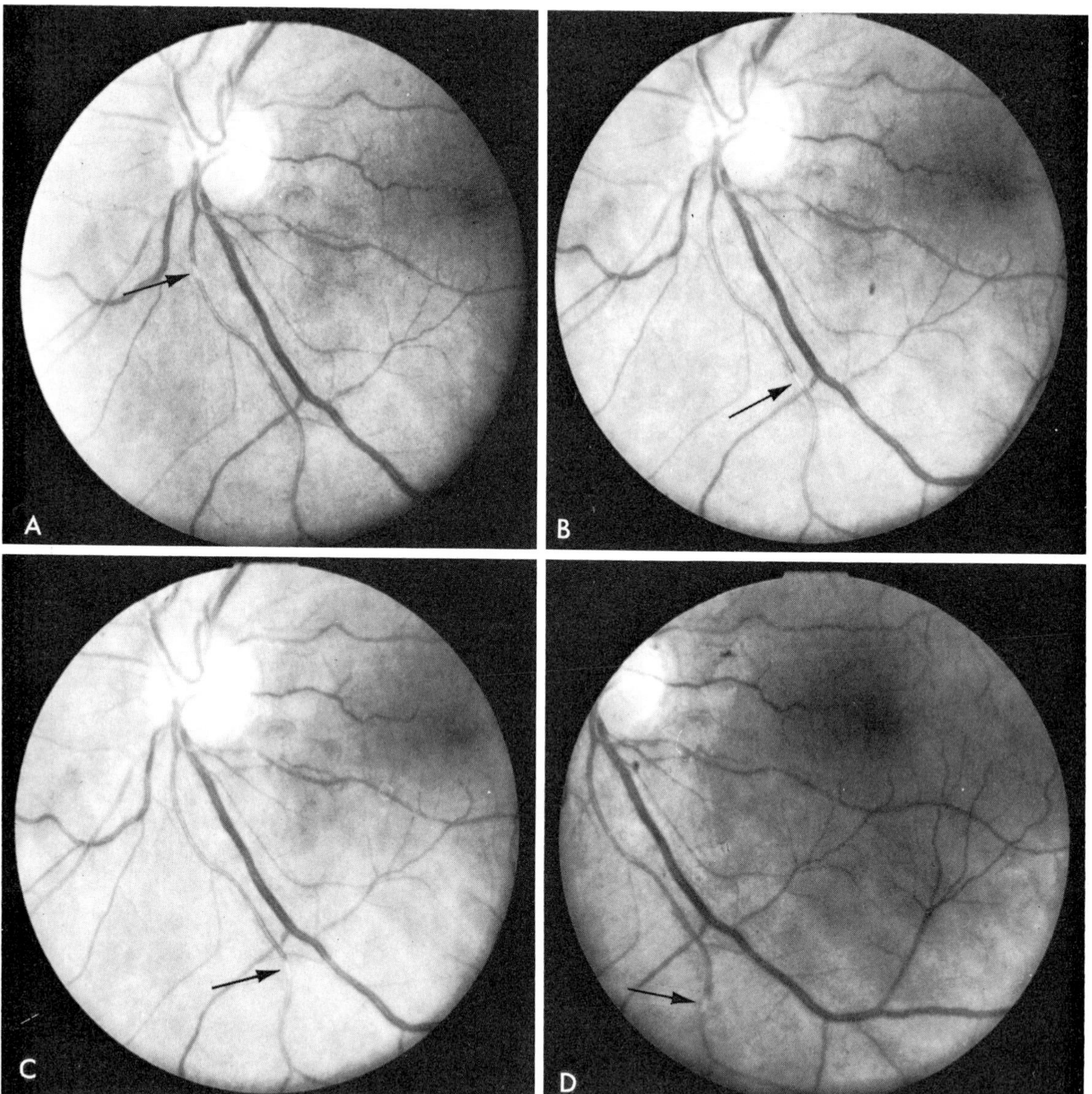

Figure 8–88. *A–D,* Sequence of photographs showing different **platelet emboli** (arrows) in the same retinal vessel. (Courtesy of Dr. Alvin North.)

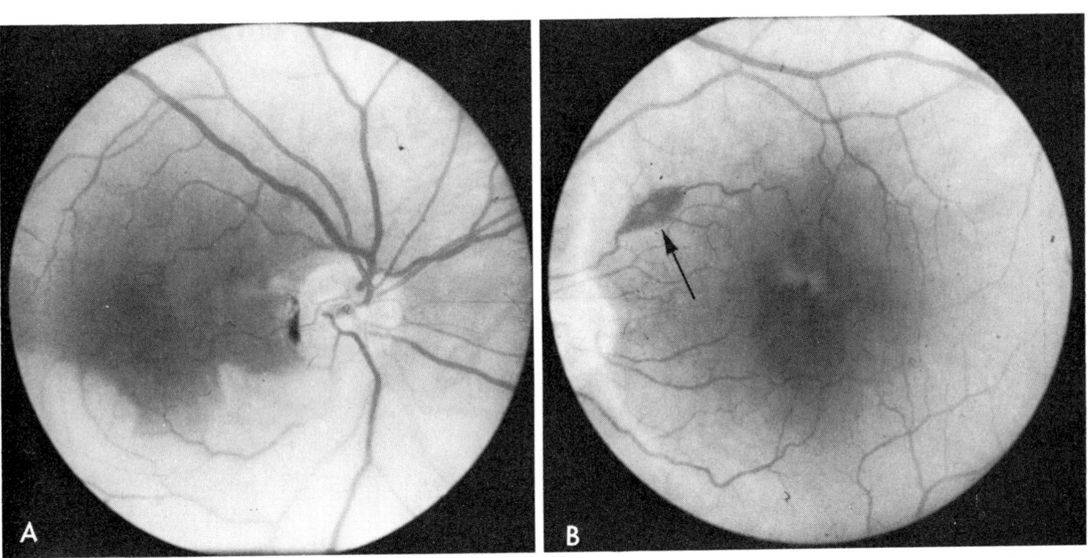

Figure 8–89. Septic emboli in a patient with subacute bacterial endocarditis, showing *A,* branch retinal artery occlusion in the right eye and *B,* Roth spot (arrow) in the left eye. (Courtesy of Dr. P. Robb McDonald.)

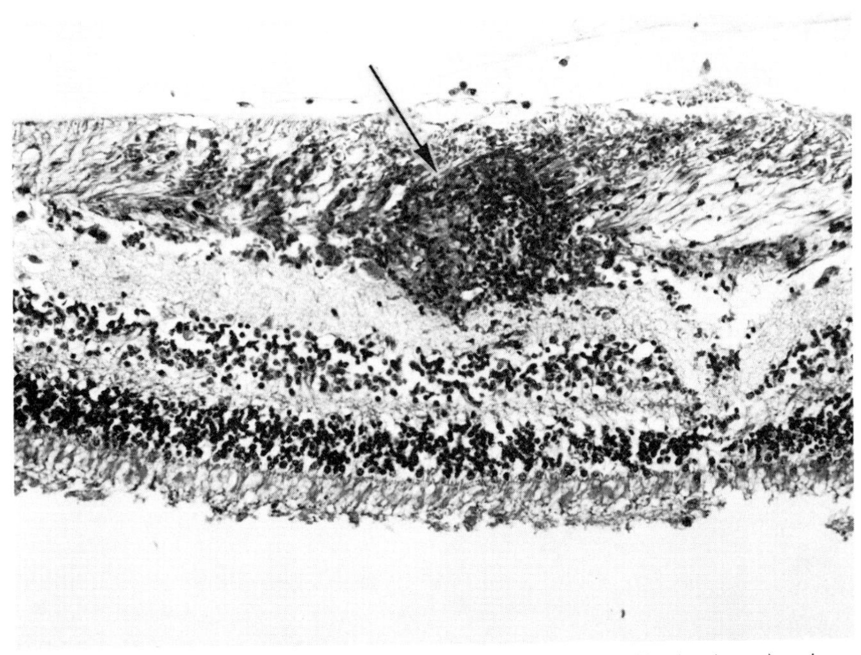

Figure 8–90. Roth spot, with central area of acute inflammatory cell infiltration (arrow) and surrounding hemorrhage. H and E, ×210. EP 3305.

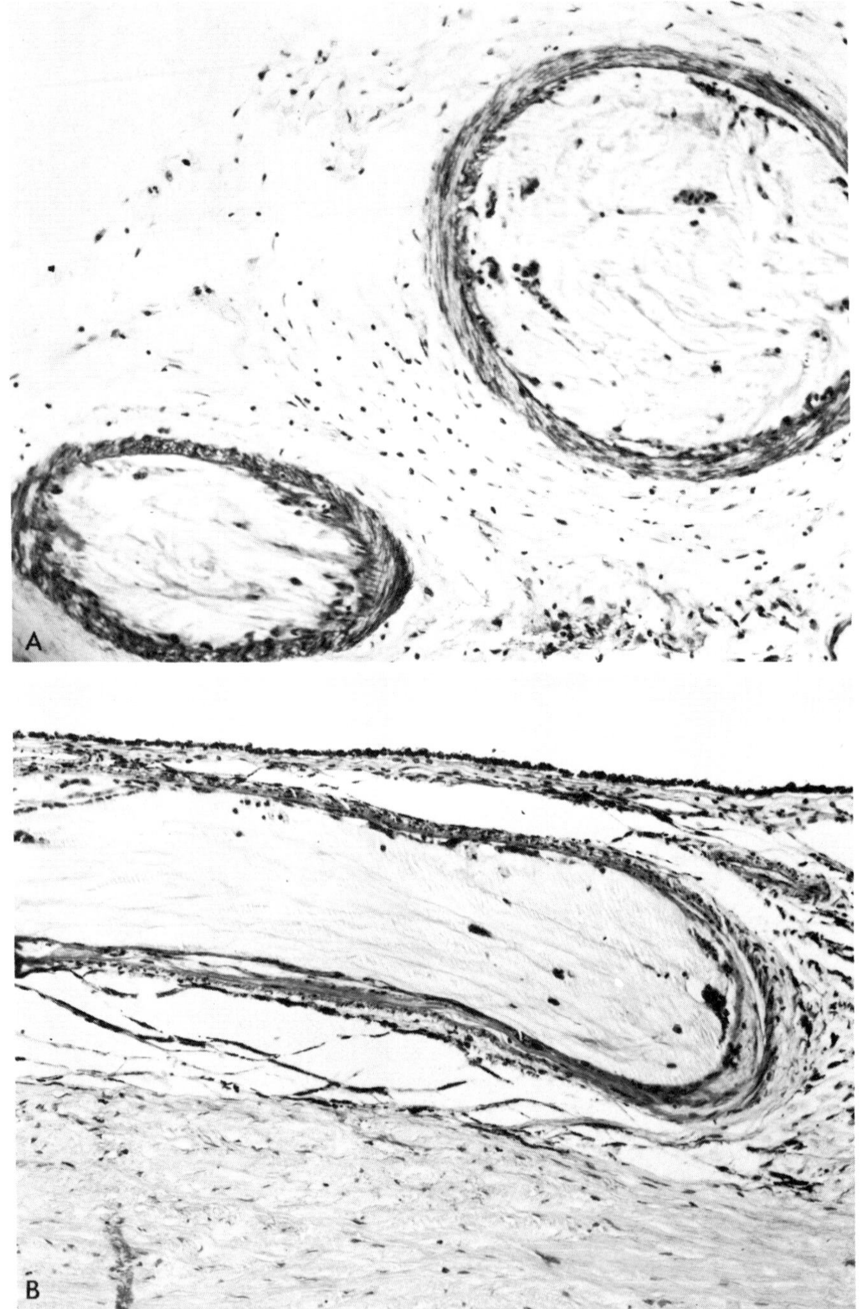

Figure 8–91. Atrial myxoma emboli in eye. *A,* Short ciliary arteries. PAS, ×190. *B,* Choroidal artery. PAS, ×135.

Illustration continued on opposite page

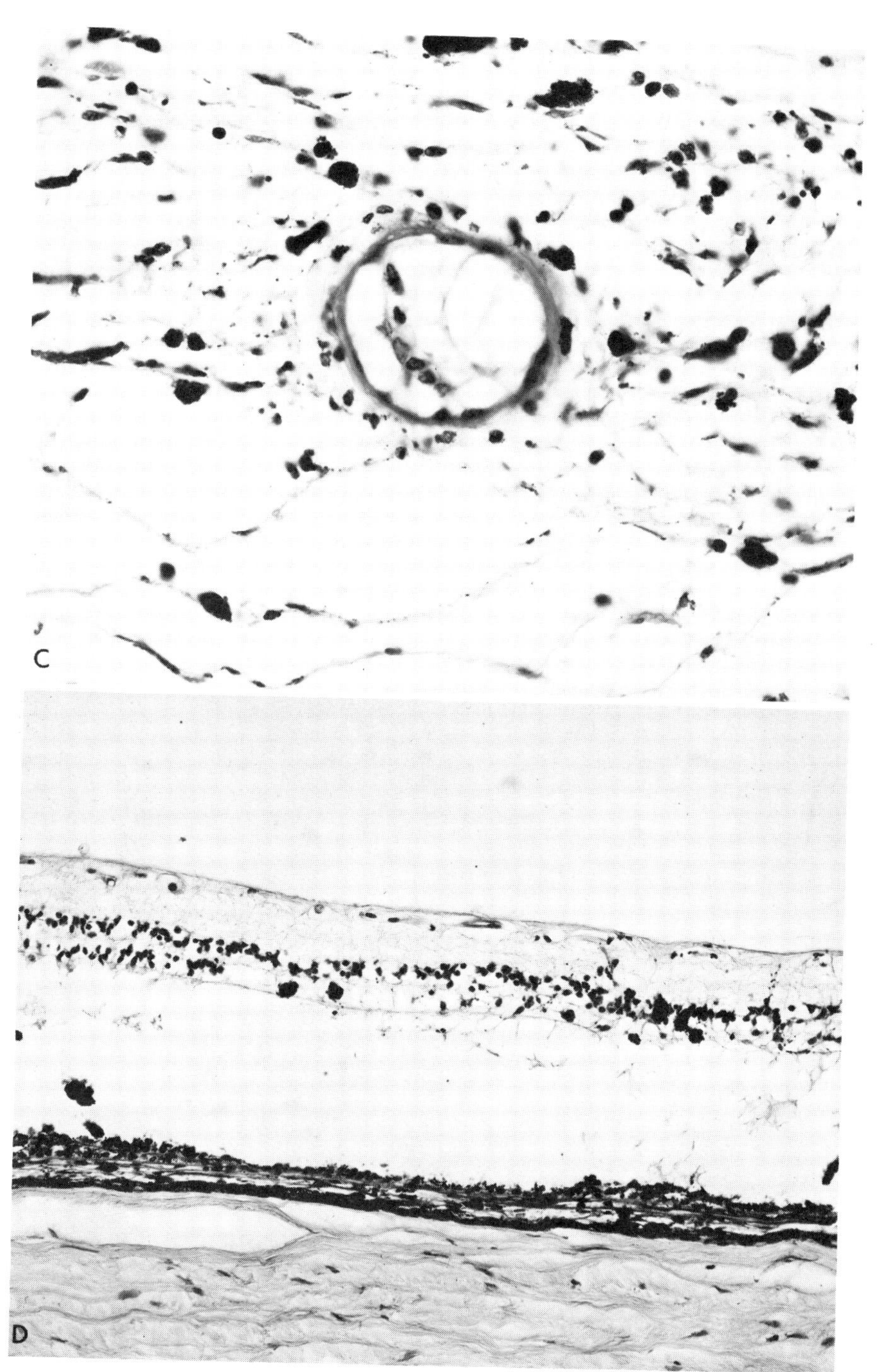

Figure 8–91 *Continued C,* Choroidal artery. PAS, ×550. *D,* Outer ischemic atrophy of retina with loss of photoreceptors, outer nuclear layer, outer plexiform layer, and outer aspect of inner nuclear layer. The retinal pigment epithelium (RPE) is relatively intact and shows some hypertrophy, hyperplasia, and migration into the retina. PAS, ×210. (Courtesy of Dr. Taylor Smith; case presented at the Eastern Ophthalmic Pathology Society, New York, May, 1969.)

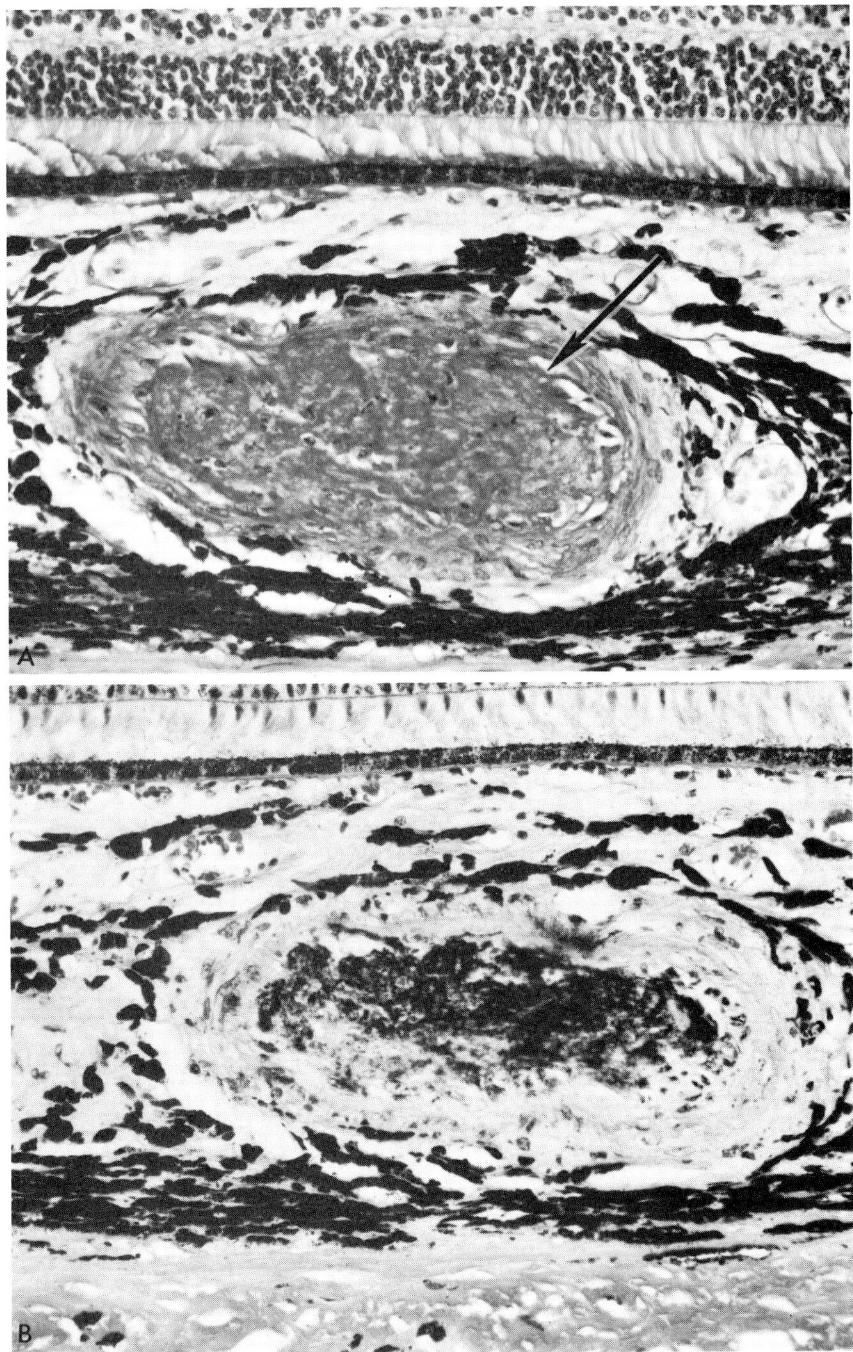

Figure 8–92. *A,* **Thrombus** (arrow) in choroidal artery. H and E, ×250. *B,* Special staining shows the fibrinous component of the thrombus. Phosphotungstic acid–hematoxylin, ×250. EP 51443.

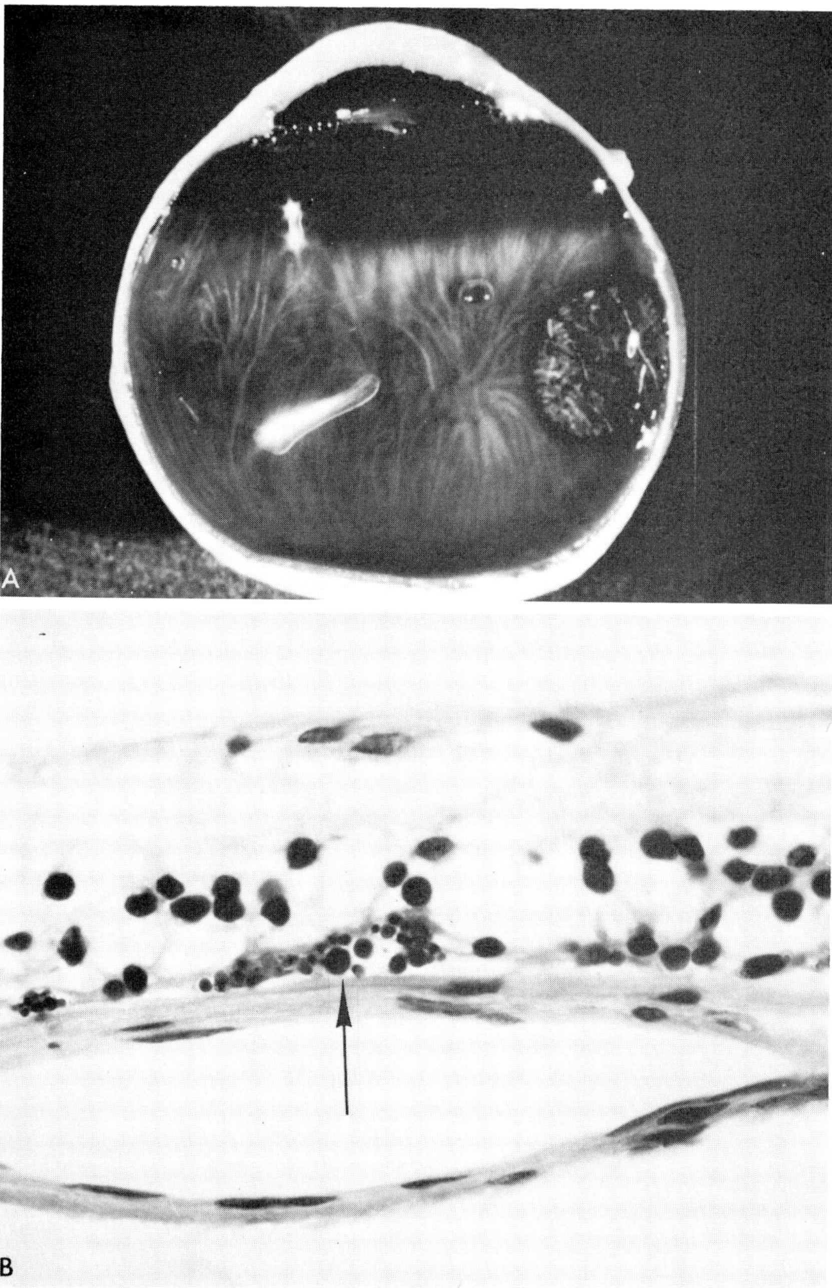

Figure 8–93. *A,* Gross appearance of a **choroidal infarct.** *B,* The lesion is characterized by loss of the choriocapillaris, retinal pigment epithelium (RPE), and outer retinal layers, including the photoreceptor cell and outer plexiform layers and the outer portion of the inner nuclear layers. An occasional area of preserved hypertrophic RPE with giant pigment granules (arrow) is present. H and E, partially bleached, ×900. EP 44344.

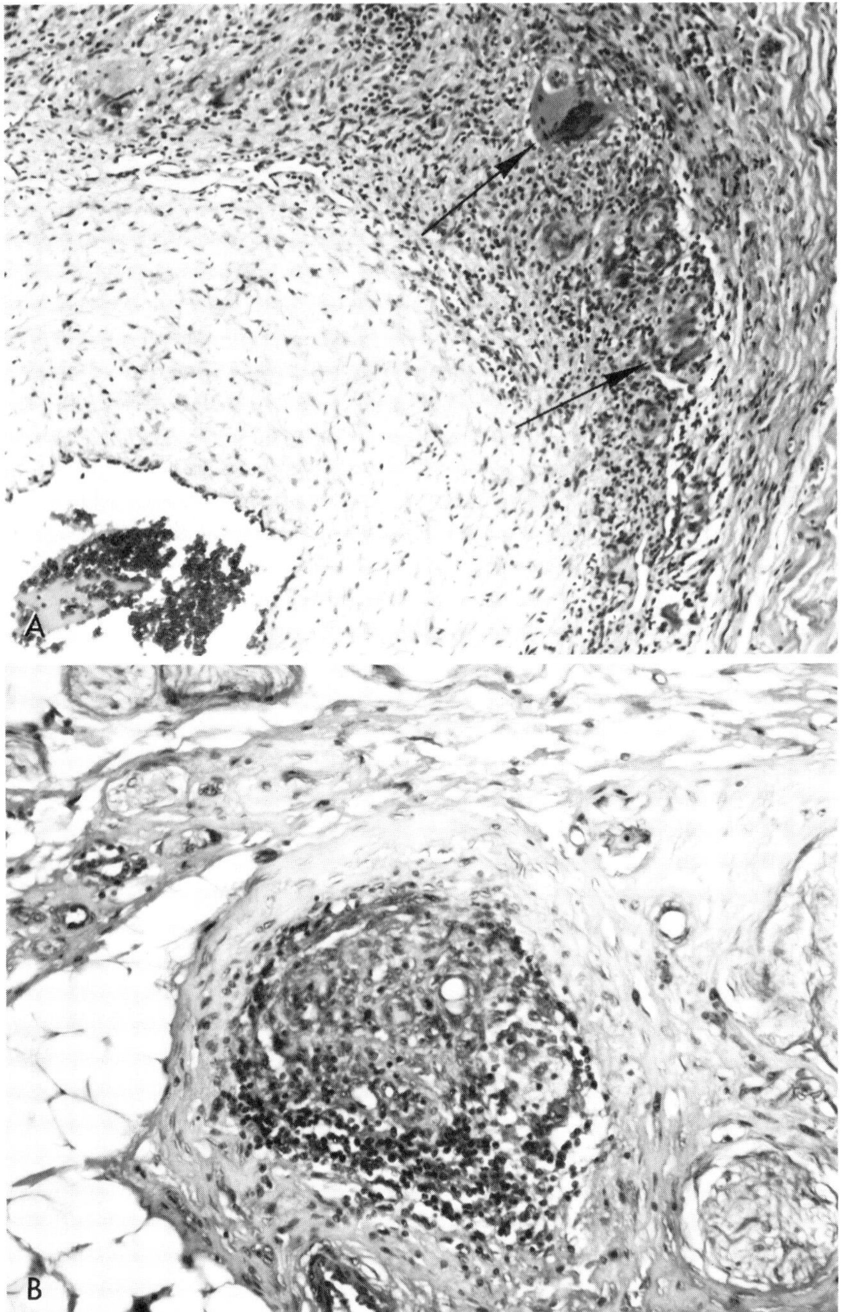

Figure 8–94. Familial temporal arteritis in a father and daughter. *A,* Temporal artery biopsy specimen of daughter, showing arteritis with giant cells (arrows) in vicinity of the fragmented elastic membrane. H and E, ×135. EP 45572. *B,* Short ciliary artery of father, showing a nonspecific occlusive vasculitis of one short ciliary artery. H and E, ×240.

Illustration continued on opposite page

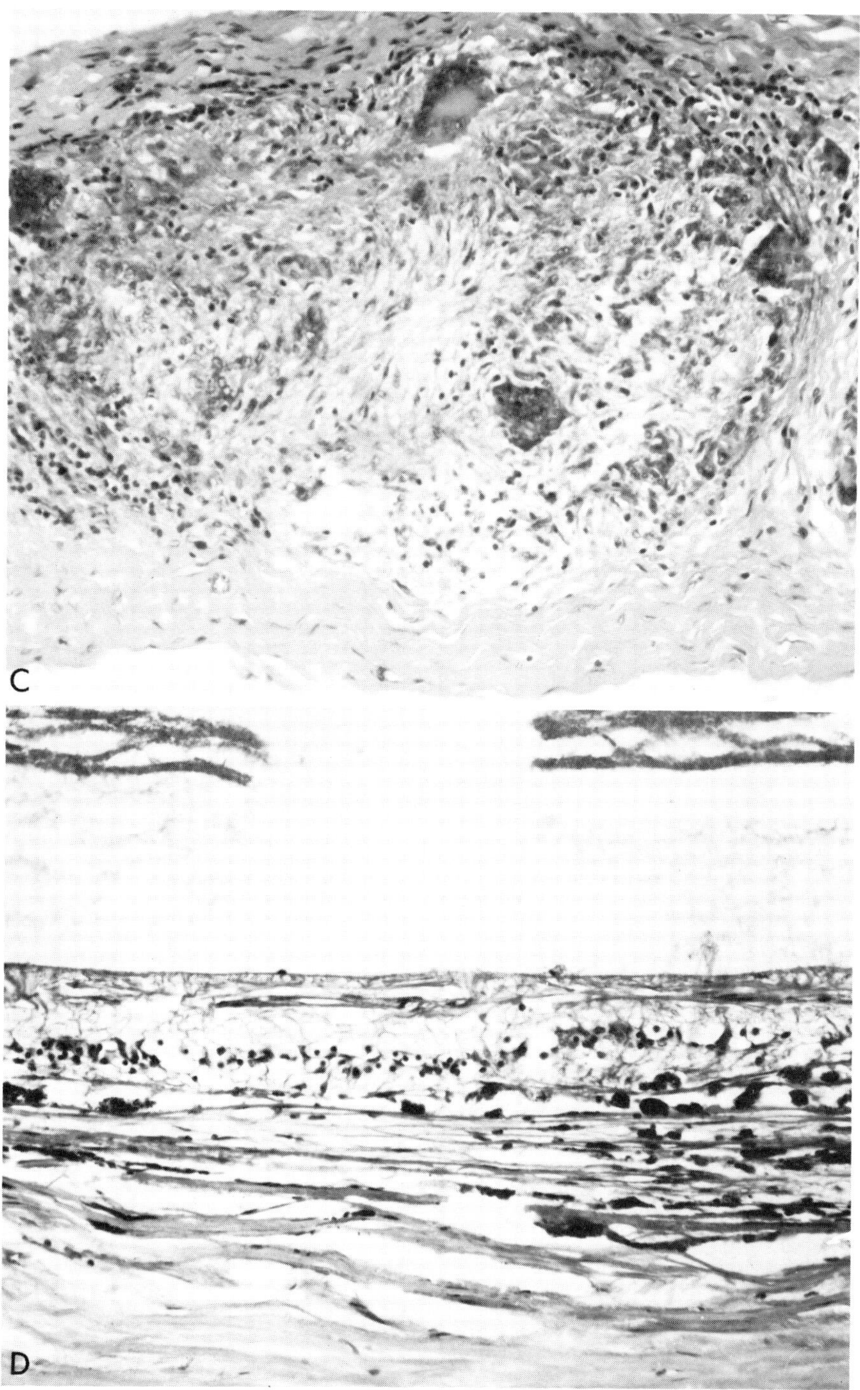

Figure 8–94 *Continued C,* Typical giant cell arteritis, with occlusion of a short ciliary artery of father. H and E, ×240. *D,* Eye of father, showing outer ischemic atrophy of retina with loss of retinal pigment epithelium (RPE) and all outer retinal layers, including the outer portion of the inner nuclear layer. H and E, × 240. EP 11479.

teritis involving the short ciliary arteries and associated outer ischemic atrophy of the retina.

Outer retinal ischemic atrophy also may be observed with nonspecific vasculitis (Fig. 8–95) or the vasculitis that occurs in several of the collagen vascular disorders. Figure 8–96 illustrates partial outer ischemic retinal atrophy that was observed in a patient with Wegener's granulomatosis, who was seen with peripheral corneal furrows, ciliochoroidal effusion, and episcleritis.

Uhthoff's Symptom. The reduction of vision with exercise or hyperthermia occurs in multiple sclerosis and is referred to as Uhthoff's symptom. Raymond, Sacks, Choromokos, and Khodadad (1980) have observed transient visual blurring in two patients—one with carotid artery occlusion and the other with temporal arteritis. In both cases, choroidal filling defects were observed with fluorescein angiography. This symptom was elicited by exercise in the first patient and from a hot bath in the second patient.

Hypereosinophilic Syndrome. Chaine, Davies, Kohner, et al (1982) observed vascular occlusive changes in the choroid of 8 (66 per cent) and in

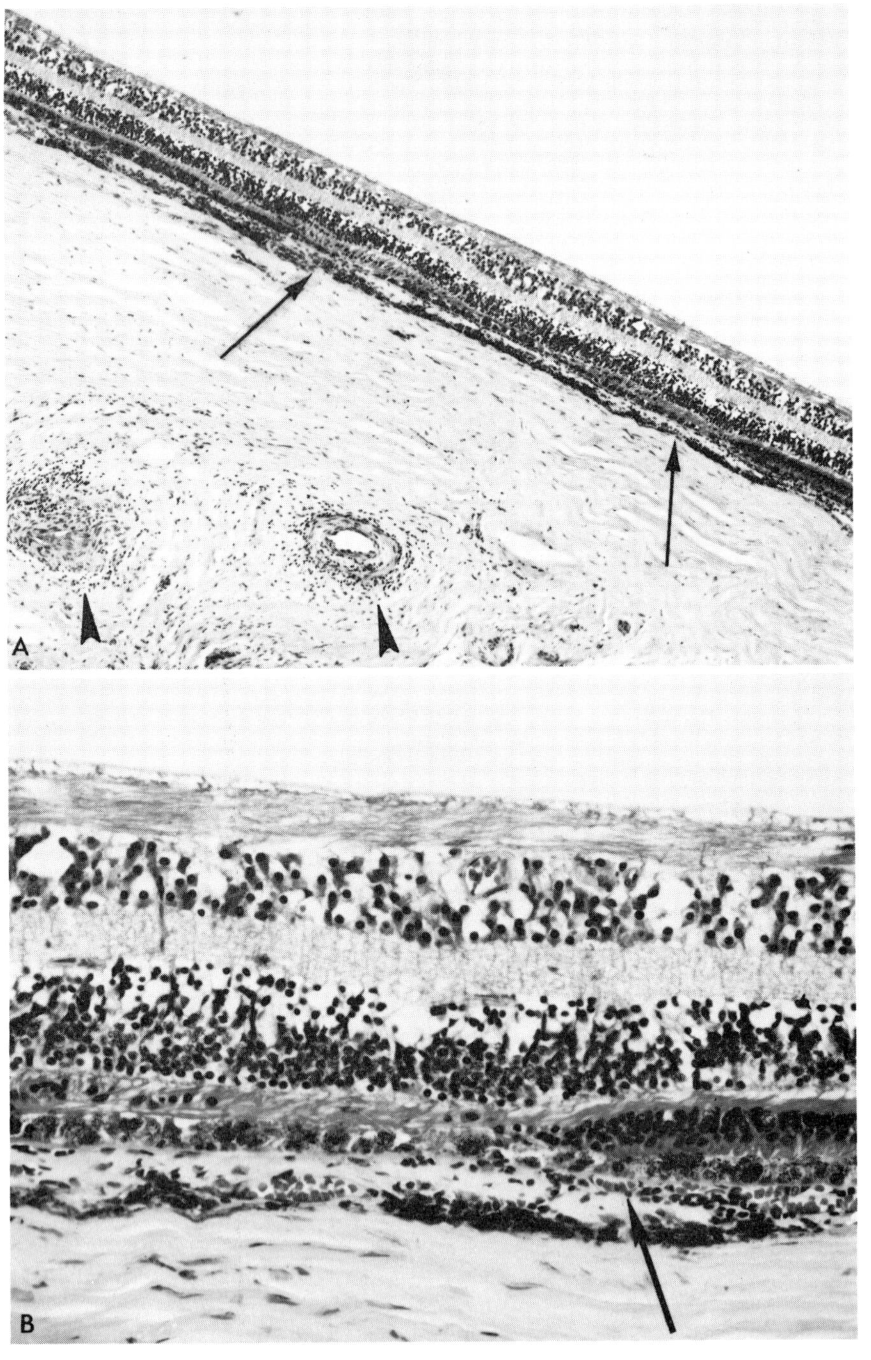

Figure 8–95. Incomplete outer ischemic atrophy of the macular retina associated with a vasculitis (without giant cells) involving the temporal short ciliary artery (arrowheads). *A,* Lymphocytes in wall and surrounding area of temporal short ciliary artery. The adjacent macular retina shows partial outer ischemic atrophy (between arrows). H and E, ×65. *B,* Higher power view of temporal margin (arrow) of lesion. H and E, ×250. AFIP Acc. 1295165. (From Zimmerman LE; case presented at the Verhoeff Society, Washington, DC, April, 1970.)

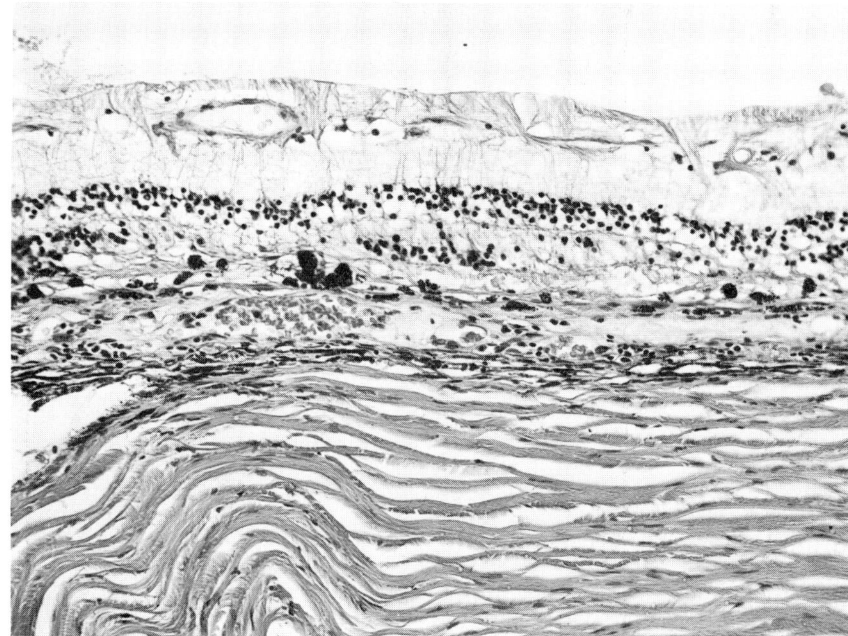

Figure 8–96. Partial outer ischemic atrophy of the retina in a patient with Wegener's granulomatosis. The retinal pigment epithelium (RPE) and photoreceptor cell layer are partially absent. H and E, ×210. EP 41141.

the retina in 7 (58 per cent) of 12 patients with this condition. These changes were attributed to thromboembolism and included delayed choroidal infarcts in 2 patients, branch retinal artery occlusion in 3 patients, and areas of retinal nonperfusion in 6 patients—one of which involved the parafoveal area.

Central Retinal Artery Occlusion

Most occlusions of the central retinal artery (CRA) are caused by atheromatous disease or emboli. Some investigators stress the association of central retinal artery occlusion with carotid atheromatous disease (Kollaritis, Lubow, Hissong, 1972). Histopathologic studies of calcific (Wolter, Ryan, 1972; Wolter, 1972) and platelet fibrin (Zimmerman, 1965) thrombi to the CRA have been reported. Ulcerative atheromatous plaques of the carotid artery with mural thrombus are also a source of emboli (Gunning, Pickering, Robb-Smith, Russell, 1964).

Central retinal atheromatous disease sometimes occurs in patients with hypertension and advanced systemic arteriosclerosis. The CRA occlusion usually occurs at the level of, or at the posterior aspect of, the lamina cribrosa (Fig. 8–97) but also may occur anterior to the lamina cribrosa (Fig. 8–98). With buildup of subendothelial atheromatous material, the CRA lumen is narrowed and may become occluded. Abrupt occlusion can occur as the result of bleeding into the atheromatous plaque. Histopathologic studies of such a case have been reported by Dahrling (1965).

With CRA occlusion, the retina first becomes diffusely edematous, with a cherry red spot. The latter is due to the visualization of choroidal vasculature through the thin foveolar area. In an eye with a cilioretinal artery and CRA occlusion, variable preservation of the retina is noted. The inner retinal layers show pyknosis of the nuclei. With time, all the retinal layers supplied by the CRA degenerate and disappear, leaving inner ischemic atrophy. The nerve fiber, ganglion cell, and inner plexiform layers, and also the inner two thirds of the inner nuclear layer (Foos, 1976) are totally lost. This pattern of atrophy is illustrated in Figure 8–99; it was caused by a thrombus of a branch of the CRA. Variable portions of the retina may be spared when a cilioretinal artery (Fig. 8–100) is present.

In a study of 27 patients under the age of 30 years with retinal arterial obstruction, Brown, Magargal, Shields, and associates (1981) found the most common associated systemic factors of etiologic significance to be migraine and coagulation abnormalities. Less frequently associated conditions included trauma, sickle cell hemoglobinopathies, cardiac disorders, use of oral contraceptives, pregnancy, systemic lupus erythematosus, and intravenous drug abuse.

Hypotensive Retinopathy

The entire eye has a reduced blood supply in this condition, which can occur in carotid occlusive disease and pulseless disease and is discussed in detail elsewhere (page 1046).

Iris neovascularization (see Fig. 8–104) does not usually occur after arterial occlusive disease of the retina, but has been observed after both

Text continued on page 691

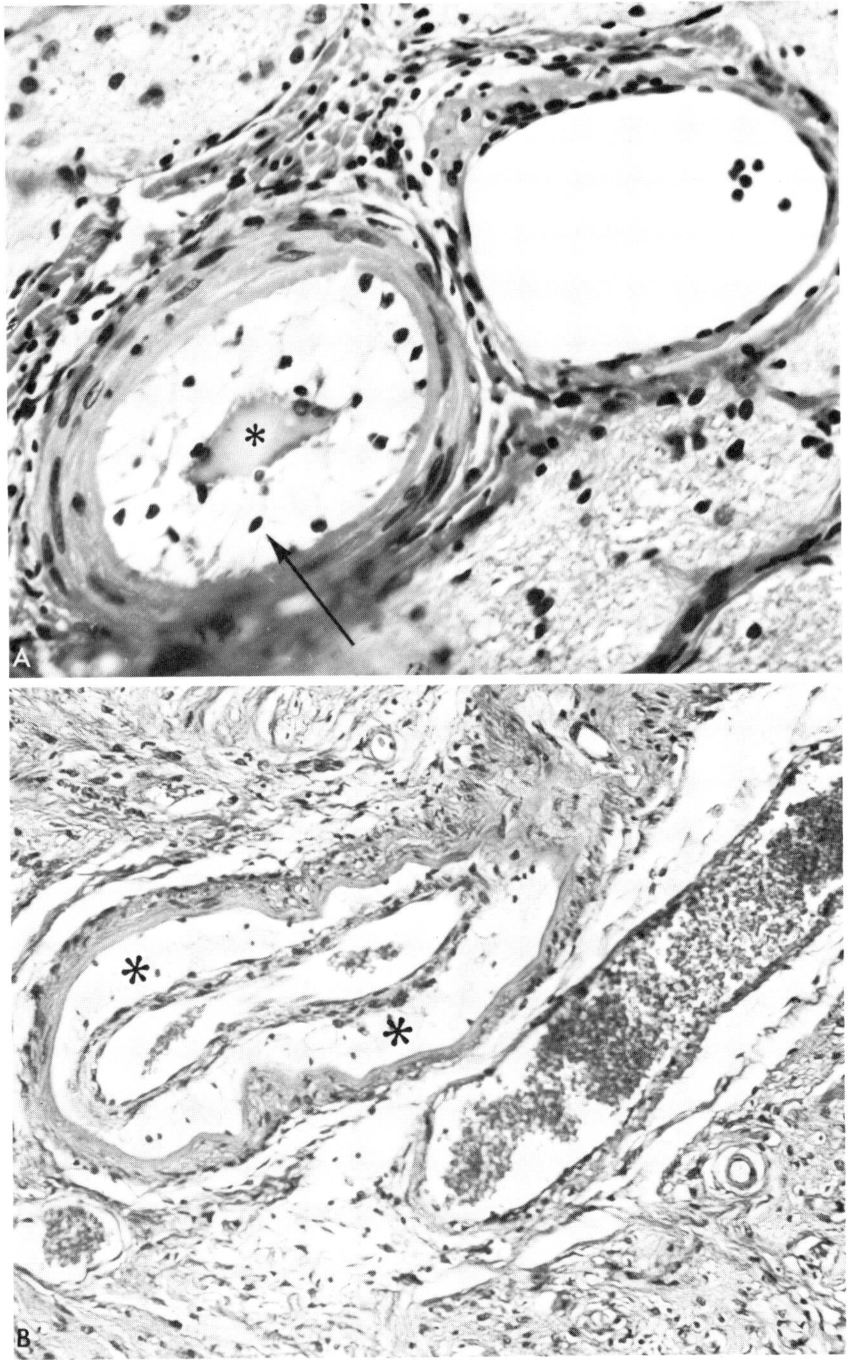

Figure 8–97. Atherosclerosis of the central retinal artery. A, Cross-section of optic nerve showing extreme narrowing of the lumen of the central retinal artery (CRA) (asterisk) by accumulation of subendothelial lipid-laden histiocytes (arrow). Hematoxylin and eosin, ×320. EP 51825. *B,* Longitudinal section, showing atheromatous plaque (asterisks) in the CRA at the level of the lamina cribrosa. Van de Grift, ×150. EP 43457.

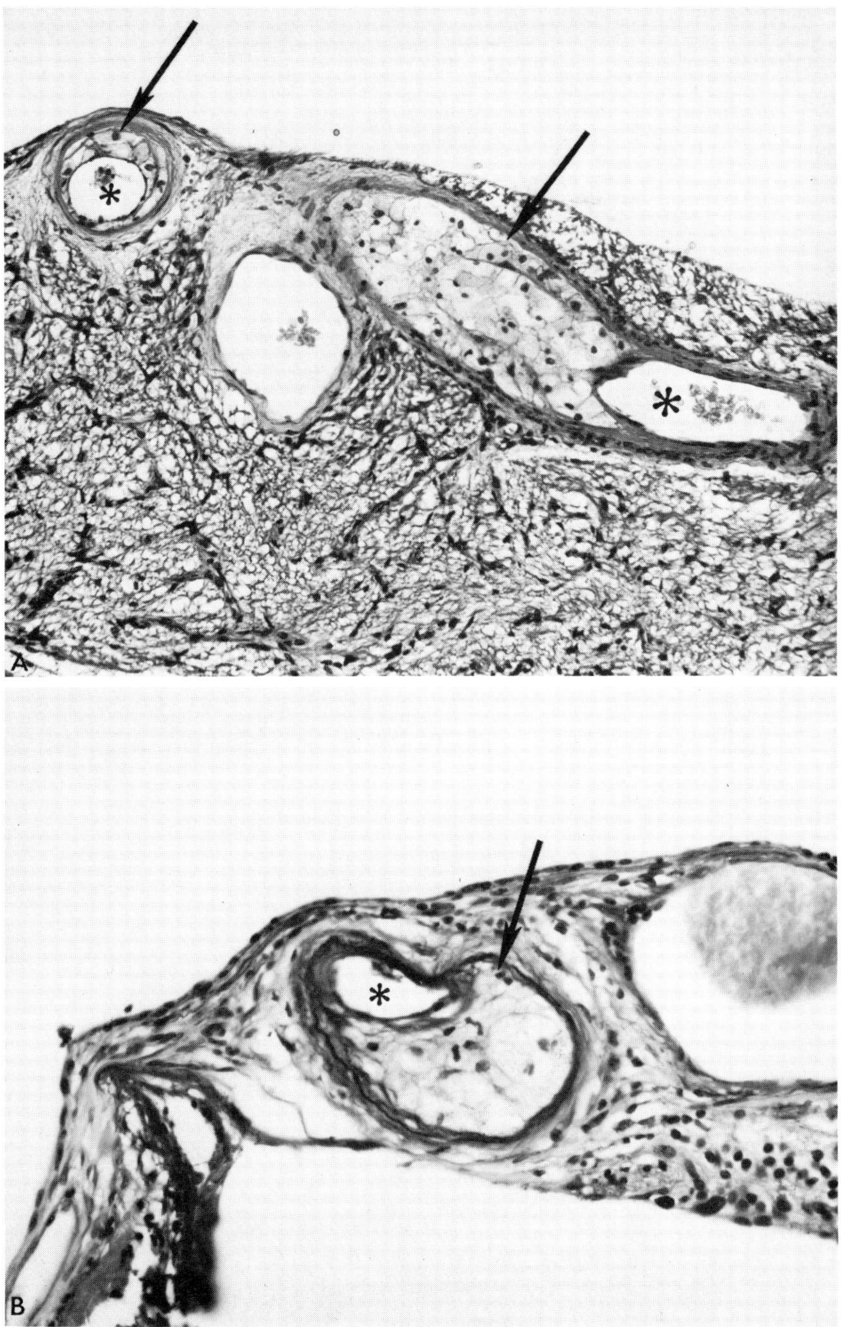

Figure 8–98. Atheromatous process involving a branch of the central retinal artery (CRA) within the optic nerve head. The lumen (asterisks) is narrowed by the accumulation of subendothelial lipid-laden histiocytes (arrows). A, H and E, ×185. *B*, ×310. EP 41451. Courtesy of Dr. M. Spiritus.

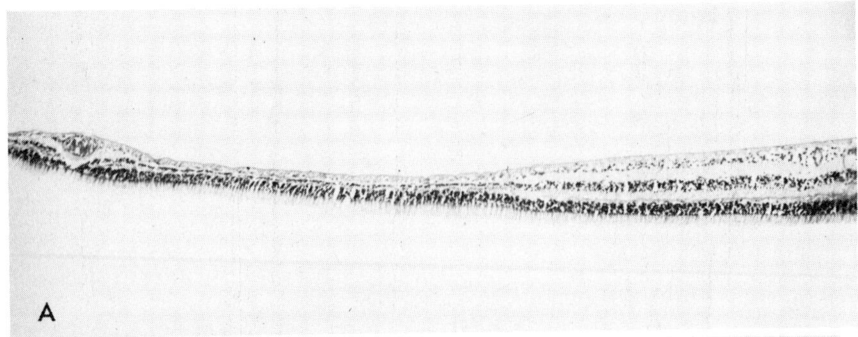

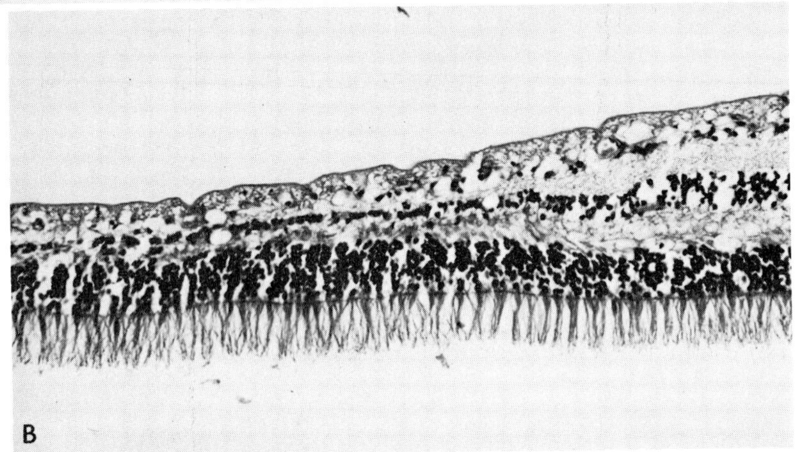

Figure 8–99. Inner ischemic retinal atrophy from branch retinal artery occlusion. There is loss of all inner retinal layers, including the inner aspect of the inner nuclear layer. A, H and E, ×40. B, ×210. EP 32655.

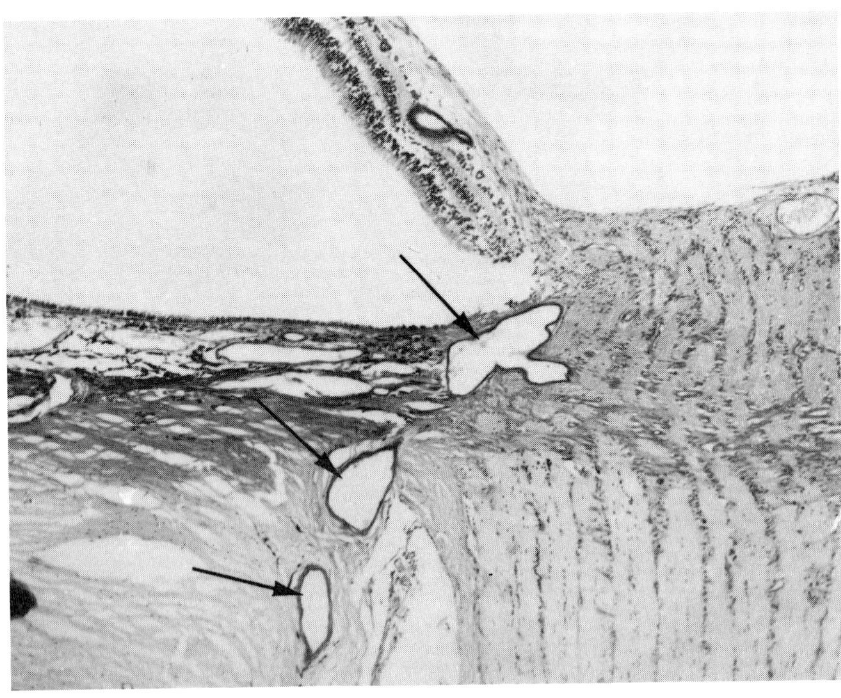

Figure 8–100. Cilioretinal artery (arrows). PAS, ×50. EP 40103.

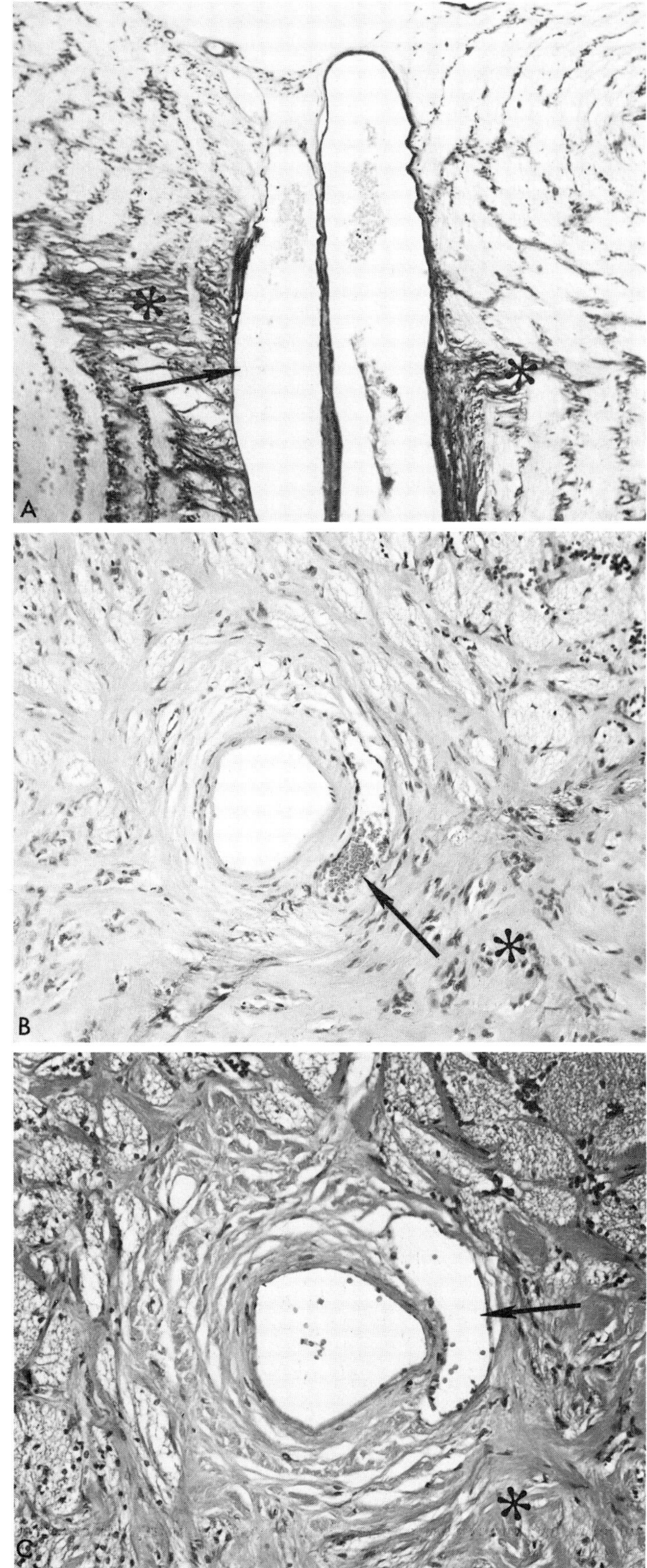

Figure 8–101. *A,* Longitudinal and *B* and *C,* cross-sections of the **central retinal artery and vein** (arrow) as they traverse the lamina cribrosa (asterisks). At this point the vessels have a common wall and are confined by the dense connective tissue of the lamina cribrosa. The cross-sections demonstrate how the vein is molded by the sturdier structure of the artery. *A,* PAS, ×100; EP 51165. *B,* H and E, ×200; EP 48231. *C,* H and E, ×185; EP 51165. (From Green WR, Chan CC, Hutchins GM, Terry JM: Central retinal vein occlusion. A prospective histopathologic study of 29 eyes in 28 cases. Retina *1*:27–55, 1981, and Trans Am Ophthalmol Soc *79*:371–422, 1981.)

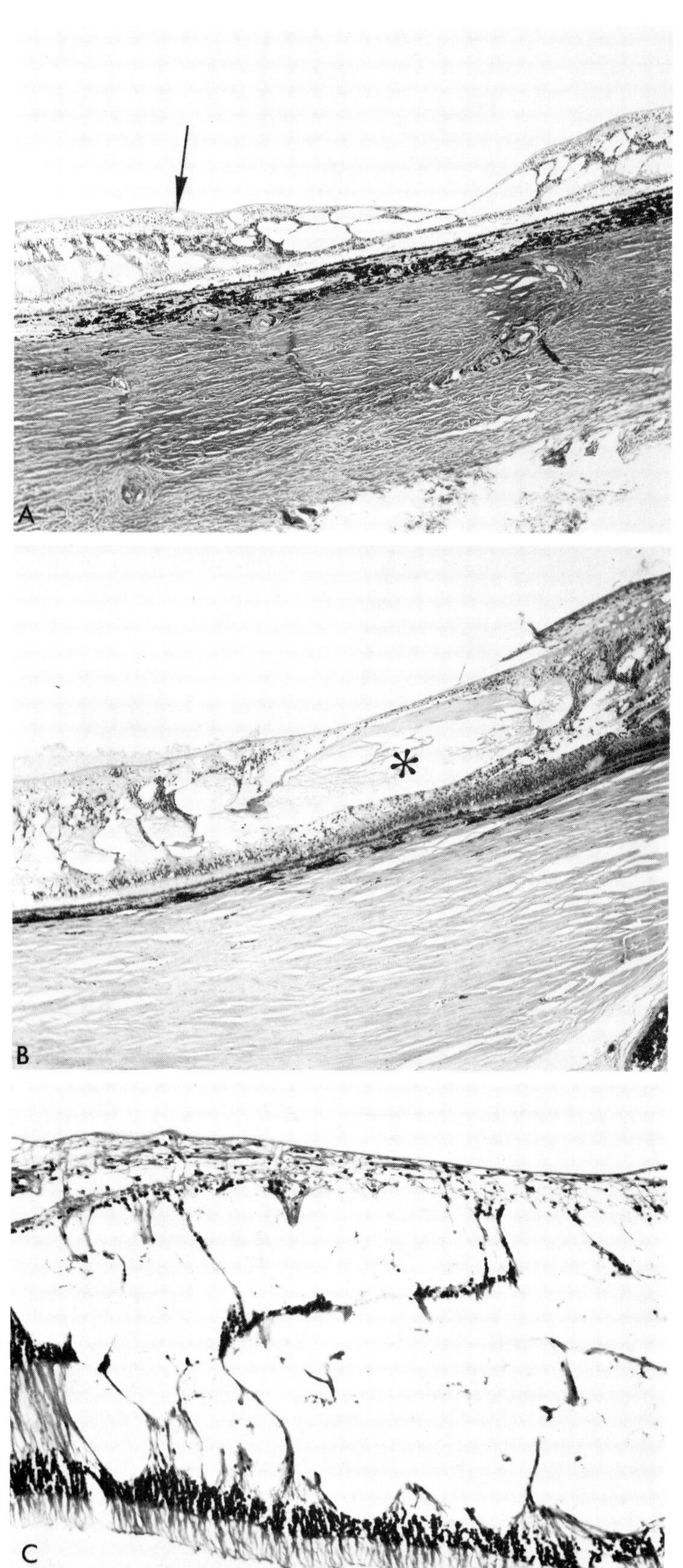

Figure 8–102. Macular changes with central retinal vein occlusion. *A,* Cystoid macular edema. The cystic spaces are present in the outer plexiform and inner nuclear layers. A few spaces (arrow) involve the ganglion cell layer. H and E, ×40. EP 39595. *B,* Cystic edema of macula. Coalescence of cysts form a large cyst or small schisis cavity in the foveal area (asterisk). A light-staining proteinaceous material is present in the cystic spaces. H and E, ×50. EP 42384. *C,* Retinoschisis in the macular area. H and E, ×125. EP 39853. (From Green WR, Chan CC, Hutchins GM, Terry JM: Central retinal vein occlusion. A prospective histopathologic study of 29 eyes in 28 cases. Retina *1*:27–55, 1981, and Trans Am Ophthalmol Soc *79*:371–422, 1981.)

CRA occlusion (Perraut, Zimmerman, 1959) and branch artery occlusion (Bresnick, Gay, 1967). The various conditions with which rubeosis irides has been associated have been reviewed by Gartner and Henkind (1978). Rubeosis is frequently followed by endothelialization and descemetization across peripheral anterior synechiae and on the anterior iris surface.

Retinal Venous Occlusions

Retinal venous occlusions can be grouped into the central variety and the tributary form. About 85 per cent of retinal venous occlusions are of the tributary type, and the superior temporal vein is affected more often, in about 70 per cent of cases. Central and tributary venous occlusions occur mainly in patients with arteriosclerosis, hypertension, and diabetes mellitus, who are over age 50 years. These occlusions occur more often in men.

The clinical onset of central and tributary vein occlusions is often less dramatic than that of arterial occlusions. There is usually a period of incipient closure, with venous dilatation and occasional obscurations of vision, but eventually the occlusion becomes complete, at which time clinical examination shows dilated, tortuous retinal veins and extensive retinal hemorrhages. In the early stage, the hemorrhages are small and located in the nerve fiber. They tend to be perivenous, but, as the process continues, they become more extensive and larger, involving most of the layers of the retina. This process is associated with clinical evidence of edema and cotton-wool patches; on fluorescein angiography massive leakage of fluid into the retina and the diffuse presence of microaneurysms are noted.

The cause of central and branch venous occlusions is generally considered to be related to arterial disease. Some cases, however, may be due to primary disease of the vein, such as phlebitis. Pre-existing glaucoma (Dryden, 1965) and compression from orbital tumors may predispose to central retinal vein (CRV) occlusion.

At the lamina cribrosa, normally there is a narrowing of the lumina of the central artery and vein. Both vessels are confined by the connective tissue of the lamina cribrosa (Fig. 8–101). In this area, a portion of this wall is common. If arteriosclerosis occurs in the artery, it can produce secondary changes in the vein—with narrowing of the blood column and disturbance and slowing of the venous blood flow. The induced turbulence of venous flow may then lead to endothelial damage and secondary thrombosis and occlusion.

The course after venous occlusion is one of restoration of partial circulation by recanalization and by formation of venous collaterals through the capillary system. Commonly, one sees new vessels around the optic disk that have developed as a result of the occlusion.

Secondary macular changes are likely to occur after CRV or tributary vein occlusions. Edema fluid that collects in Henle's layer and in the inner portion of the retina is very slow to absorb. Extensive cystic degeneration (Fig. 8–102) and, rarely, retinoschisis (Fig. 8–102,*C*) may develop

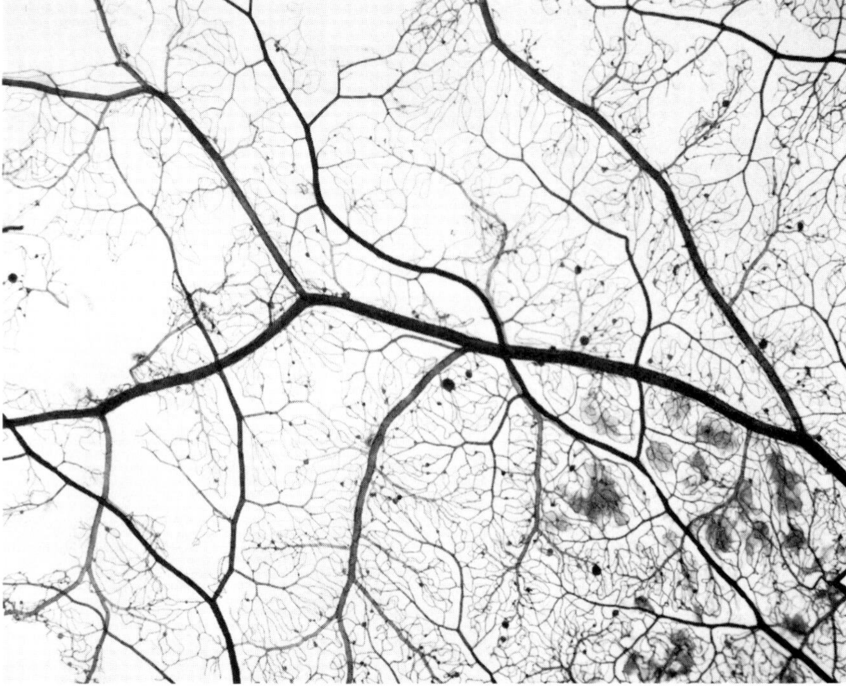

Figure 8–103. Capillary microaneurysms scattered throughout the retina in an eye with central retinal vein occlusion (CRVO). PAS, ×10. EP 49053. (From Green WR, Chan CC, Hutchins GM, Terry JM: Central retinal vein occlusion. A prospective histopathologic study of 29 eyes in 28 cases. Retina *1*:27–55, 1981, and Trans Am Ophthalmol Soc *79*:371–422, 1981.)

in the macular area. Capillary microaneurysms may develop and are present throughout the retina (Fig. 8–103).

Histologically, in recent central and branch vein occlusions, there are marked edema and superficial and deep hemorrhages. Superficial hemorrhages follow the plane of the nerve fibers and form linear streaks and flame-shaped configurations. Deeper hemorrhages are often delimited by Müller's fibers and tend to be rounded. Larger hemorrhages involve the full thickness of the retina and erupt through the internal limiting membrane to form preretinal hemorrhages or dissect posteriorly, separating the sensory retina from the pigment epithelium. Focal necroses may develop in scattered areas and lead to invasion of the tissues by microglia (macrophages). Sometimes edema fluid collects in large, irregular cystic areas, and it may escape subretinally to produce a localized flat detachment of the retina. Eventually the hemorrhages and exudates are absorbed, although this may take a long time. Hemosiderin staining of the retina and hemosiderin-laden macrophages usually persist. These, to-

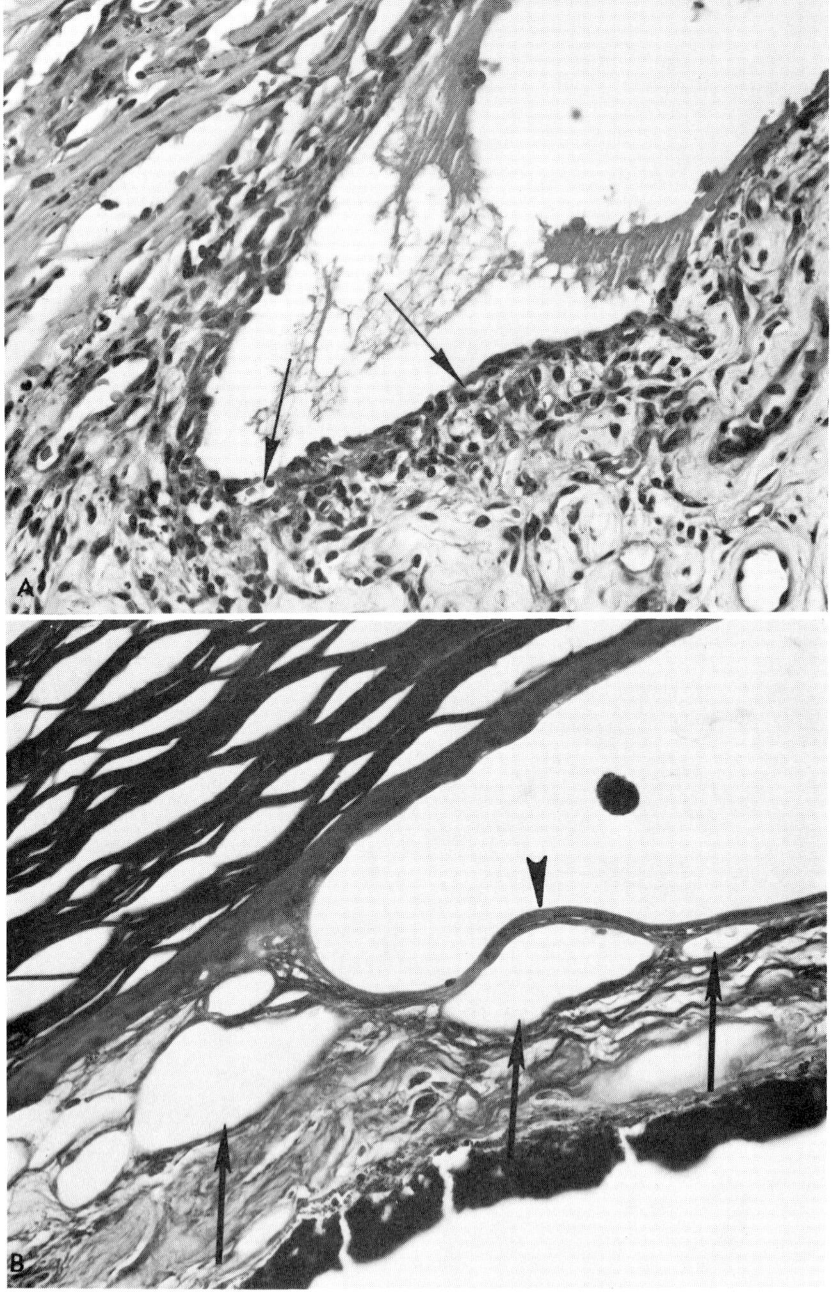

Figure 8–104. Iris neovascularization following central retinal vein occlusion (CRVO). *A,* Open angle with early neovascularization (arrows). H and E, ×300. EP 38375. *B,* Rubeosis iridis (arrows), with peripheral anterior synechia and endothelialization and descemetization (arrowhead) of the false angle. Van de Grift, ×350. EP 41223. (From Green WR, Chan CC, Hutchins GM, Terry JM: Central retinal vein occlusion. A prospective histopathologic study of 29 eyes in 28 cases. Retina *1*:27–55, 1981, and Trans Am Ophthalmol Soc *79*:371–422, 1981.)

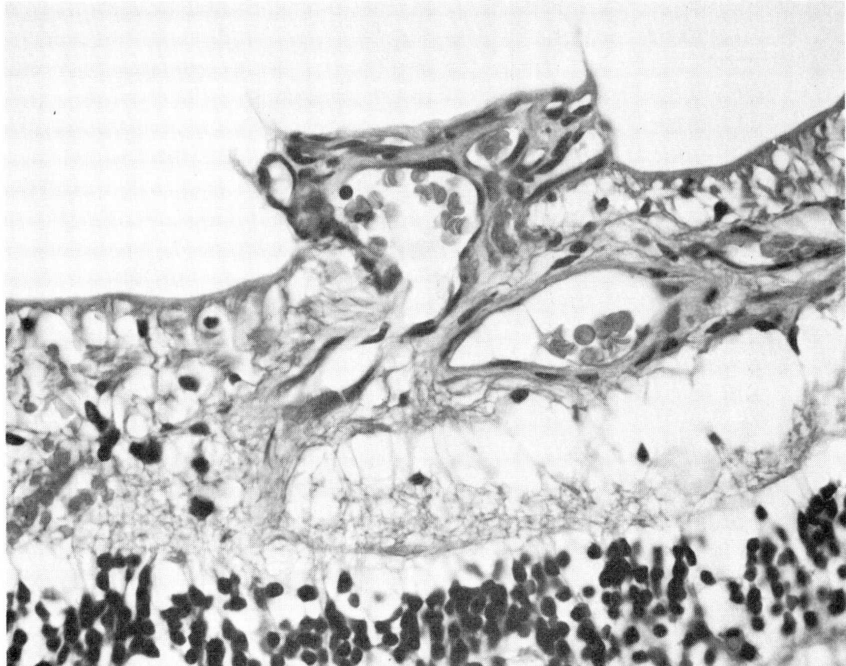

Figure 8–105. Retinal neovascularization after central retinal vein occlusion (CRVO). H and E, ×430. EP 49053. (From Green WR, Chan CC, Hutchins GM, Terry JM: Central retinal vein occlusion. A prospective histopathologic study of 29 eyes in 28 cases. Retina *1*:27–55, 1981, and Trans Am Ophthalmol Soc *79*:371–422, 1981.)

gether with some disorganization of retinal architecture and the marked gliosis, help differentiate the final histopathologic picture from that seen after central retinal artery occlusion. Occlusions that involve only a branch of the retinal vein generally heal, with some functional recovery of the affected area.

In cases of CRV occlusion, the damage is not only more extensive but also more destructive. About 20 per cent of patients with CRV occlusion develop rubeosis iridis and neovascular glaucoma ("90 day glaucoma") about 3 months after the initial venous occlusion. The angle may be open early, but peripheral anterior synechiae with descemetization ensue in most cases (Fig. 8–104). Those eyes that develop neovascularization of the iris are likely to show areas of retinal nonperfusion by angiography (Laatikainen, Kohner, 1976). While iris neovascularization occurs in about 20 per cent of eyes with CRVO, disk and

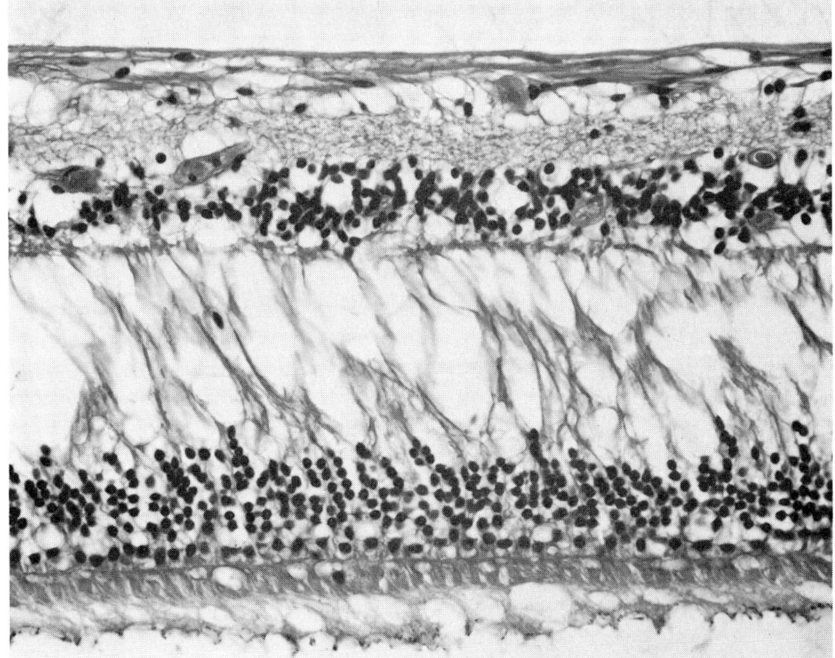

Figure 8–106. Retina from eye with central retinal vein occlusion (CRVO), showing glaucomatous atrophy but the absence of inner ischemic atrophy. H and E, ×300. EP 38375. (From Green WR, Chan CC, Hutchins GM, Terry JM: Central retinal vein occlusion. A prospective histopathologic study of 29 eyes in 28 cases. Retina *1*:27–55, 1981, and Trans Am Ophthalmol Soc *79*:371–422, 1981.)

retinal neovascularization (Fig. 8–105) are much less frequent (Chan, Little, 1979; Green, Chan, Hutchins, Terry, 1981).

Occlusive arterial disease is not a consistent feature of CRVO. Most eyes studied histopathologically do not show inner ischemic atrophy. Those with glaucoma show loss of the nerve fiber and ganglion cell layers, but there is preservation of the inner plexiform and inner nuclear layers (Fig. 8–106).

Green and coworkers (1981) studied 29 eyes from 28 patients with central retinal vein occlusion (CRVO). Twenty eyes were surgical specimens—all enucleated because of neovascular glaucoma. Nine eyes were obtained post mortem. One autopsy case had CRVO in both eyes. A fresh or recanalized thrombus was observed in each eye. That study considered the chronologic aspects of the cases, and it noted the different morphologic features at different intervals after the occlusion. Their results explained the variability of the changes observed in previous reports. The different features were judged by Green and coworkers to be stages in the natural evolution of a thrombus—that is, thrombus with fibrin and platelets and adherence to the wall of the vein (Figs. 8–107 through 8–109); fibrovascular organization with recanalization (Figs. 8–110 through 8–112) and endothelial cell proliferation (Fig. 8–113); inflammation in the area of throm-

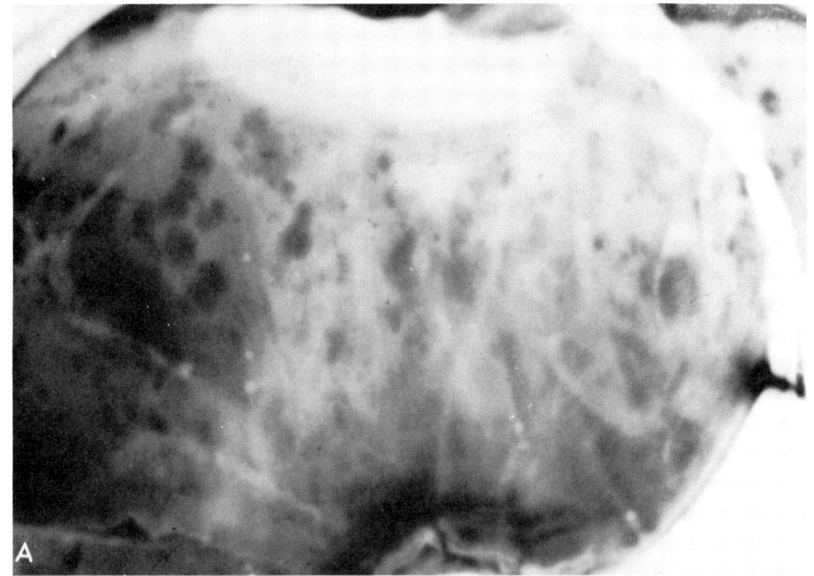

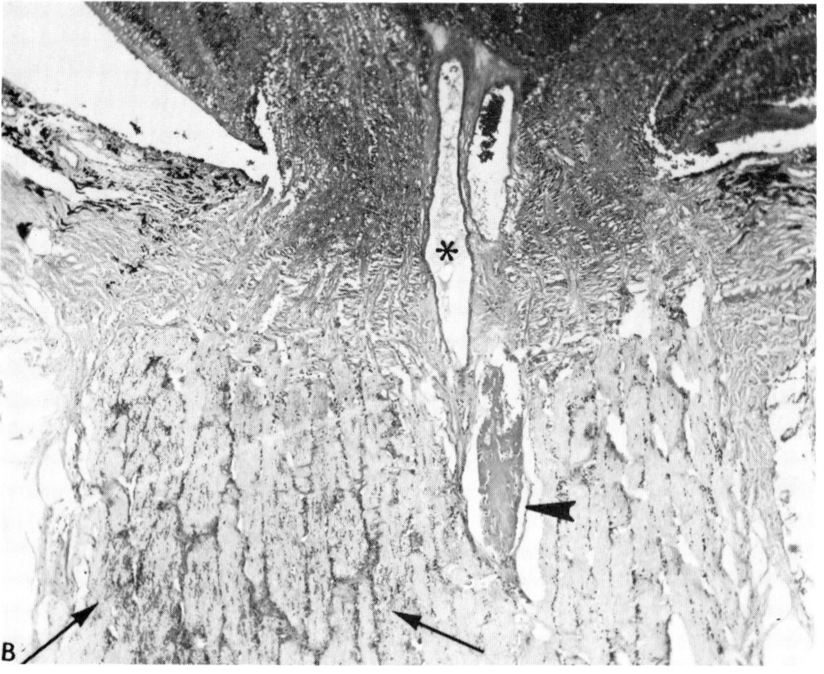

Figure 8–107. Central retinal vein occlusion (CRVO) of 24 hours' duration. *A,* Extensive hemorrhages scattered throughout retina. *B,* Section through center of optic nerve head, showing a patent central retinal artery (CRA) (asterisk), diffuse hemorrhage in the retrolaminar portion of the optic nerve nasally (arrows), and a fresh thrombus (arrowhead) in the CRV just posterior to the lamina cribrosa. H and E, ×40.

Illustration continued on opposite page

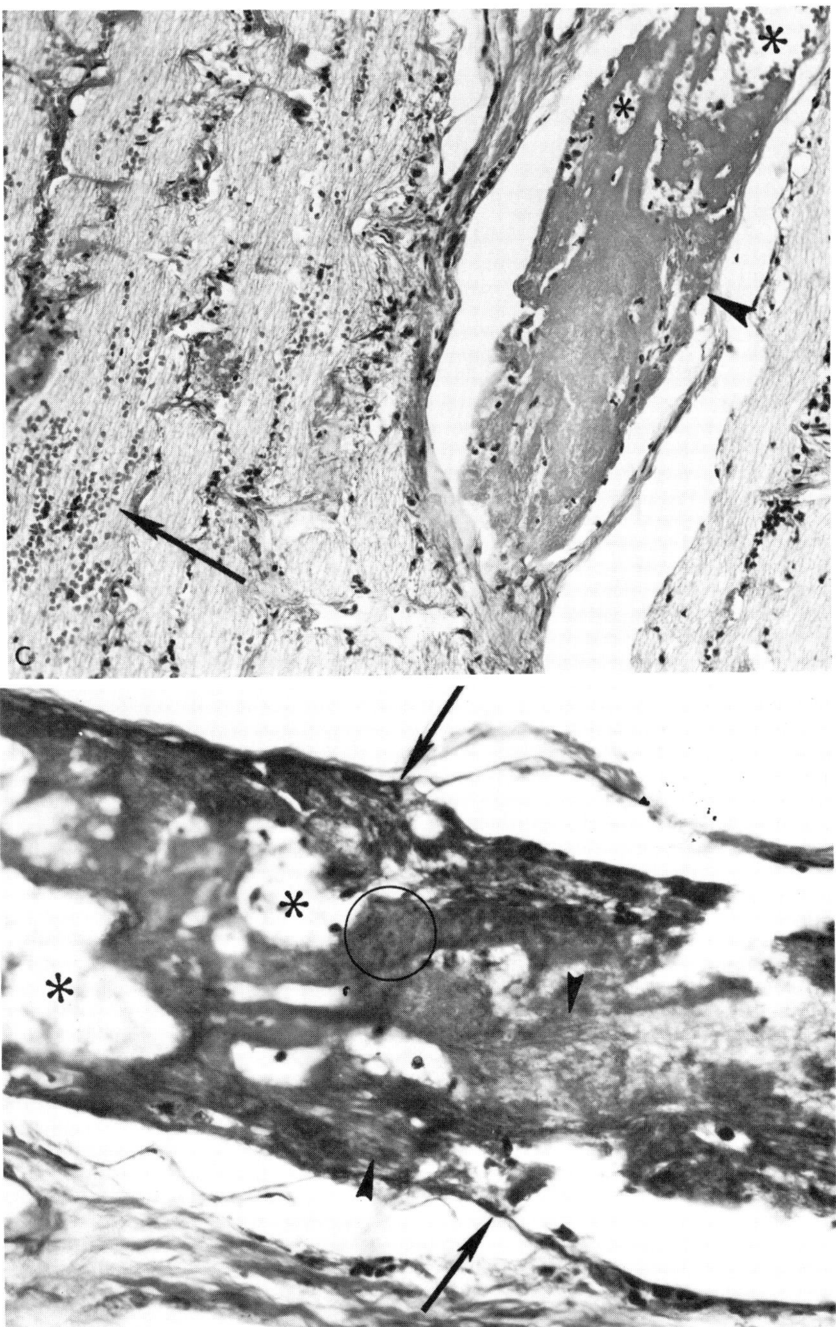

Figure 8–107 *Continued C,* Higher power view, showing thrombus with pockets of erythrocytes anteriorly (asterisks), a light scattering of hemorrhage in the optic nerve nasally (arrow), and adherence of thrombus to the wall of the vein where endothelium is absent (arrowhead). H and E, ×185. *D,* Higher power view of thrombus, showing entrapped pockets of erythrocytes proximally (asterisks), aggregates of platelets (circle), fibrin (arrowheads), and adherence to the wall of the vein where endothelium is absent (arrows). PAS, × 365. EP 45833.

(From Green WR, Chan CC, Hutchins GM, Terry JM: Central retinal vein occlusion. A prospective histopathologic study of 29 eyes in 28 cases. Retina *1*:27–55, 1981, and Trans Am Ophthalmol Soc *79*:371–422, 1981.)

bus (Fig. 8–114) (endophlebitis), in (phlebitis) and surrounding (periphlebitis) the vein wall (Fig. 8–115); and marked sclerosis of the wall of the vein with a single channel of recanalization (phlebosclerosis) (Fig. 8–116).

It is thought that any local or systemic factor that leads to undue turbulence of flow through the constricted area of the lamina cribrosa may lead to CRVO. Green and coworkers (1981) found local diseases associated with CRVO to include glaucoma, papilledema, subdural hemorrhage, optic nerve hemorrhage, and large drusen of the optic nerve head (Fig. 8–117). Associated systemic diseases included hypertension, cardio- and cerebrovascular disease, diabetes mellitus, and leukemia with thrombocytopenia.

Green, Chan, Hutchins, and Terry (1981) observed a fresh CRVO thrombus in 3 of 29 eyes (10.3 per cent) and a recanalized thrombus in 26 eyes (89.7 per cent). Endothelial cell proliferation was a conspicuous feature in 14 (48.3 per cent) of the eyes with older CRV occlusions. Chronic inflammation in the area of the thrombus, the vein wall, or the perivascular area was observed in 14

Text continued on page 705

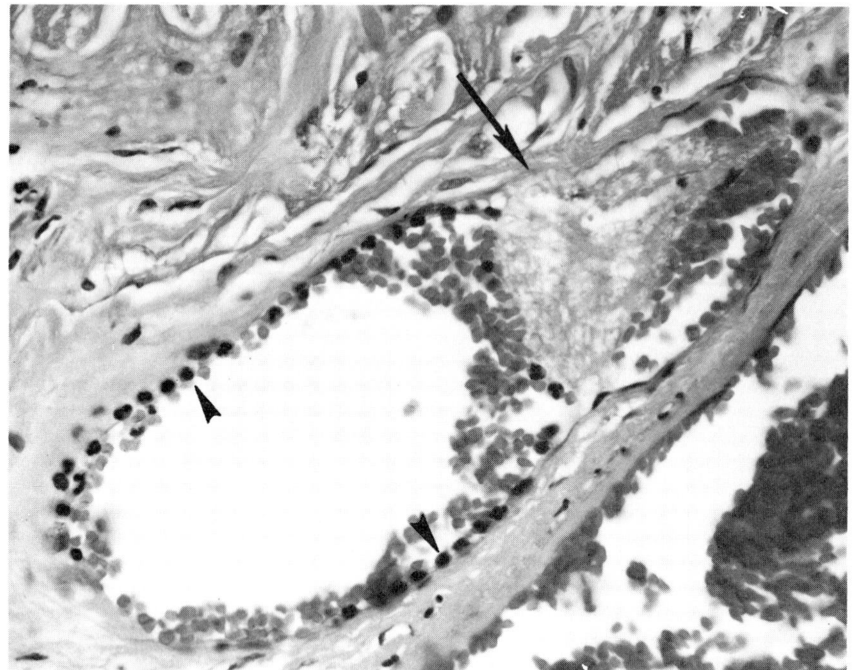

Figure 8–108. Area of fresh thrombus posterior to old recanalized thrombus. The fibrin-containing thrombus is adherent to the wall of the vein (arrow), where endothelium is absent. Neutrophils line the inner aspect of the vein wall and the posterior aspect of the thrombus (arrowheads). H and E, ×400. EP 49053. (From Green WR, Chan CC, Hutchins GM, Terry JM: Central retinal vein occlusion. A prospective histopathologic study of 29 eyes in 28 cases. Retina *1*:27–55, 1981, and Trans Am Ophthalmol Soc *79*:371–422, 1981.)

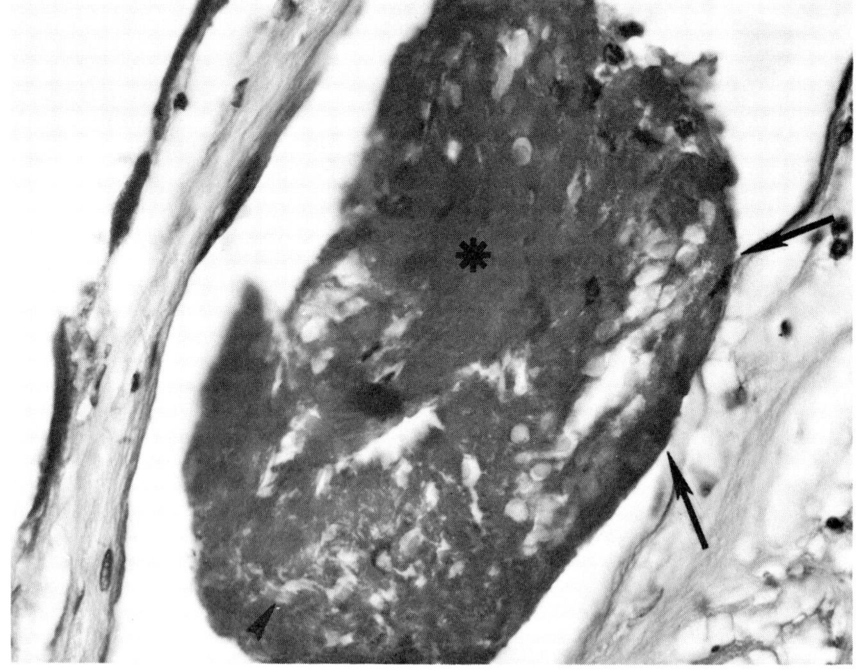

Figure 8–109. Central retinal vein with thrombus containing fibrin (asterisk) and platelet aggregates (arrowhead). Thrombus is adherent to the wall of the vein at the area where endothelium is absent (arrows). PAS, ×550. EP 48994. (From Green WR, Chan CC, Hutchins GM, Terry, JM: Central retinal vein occlusion. A prospective histopathologic study of 29 eyes in 28 cases. Retina *1*:27–55, 1981, and Trans Am Ophthalmol Soc *79*:371–422, 1981.)

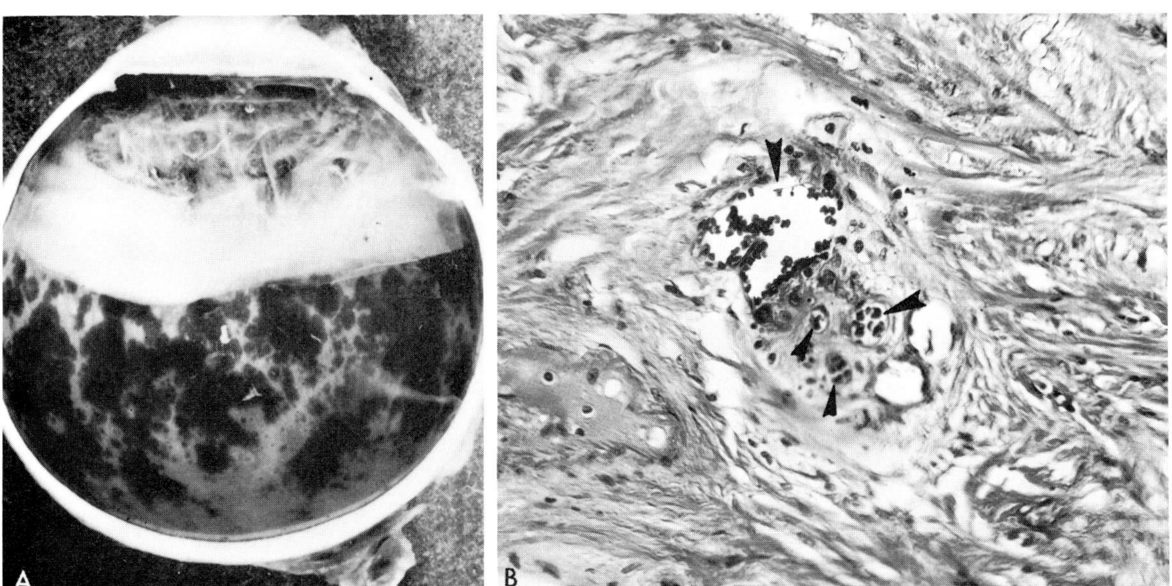

Figure 8–110. *A,* "Blood-and-thunder" gross appearance of **central retinal vein occlusion (CRVO)**. *B,* Recanalized thrombus (arrowheads) in CRV at level of lamina cribrosa. Van de Grift, ×260. EP 46686. (From Green WR, Chan CC, Hutchins GM, Terry JM: Central retinal vein occlusion. A prospective histopathologic study of 29 eyes in 28 cases. Retina 1:27–55, 1981, and Trans Am Ophthalmol Soc *79*:371–422, 1981.)

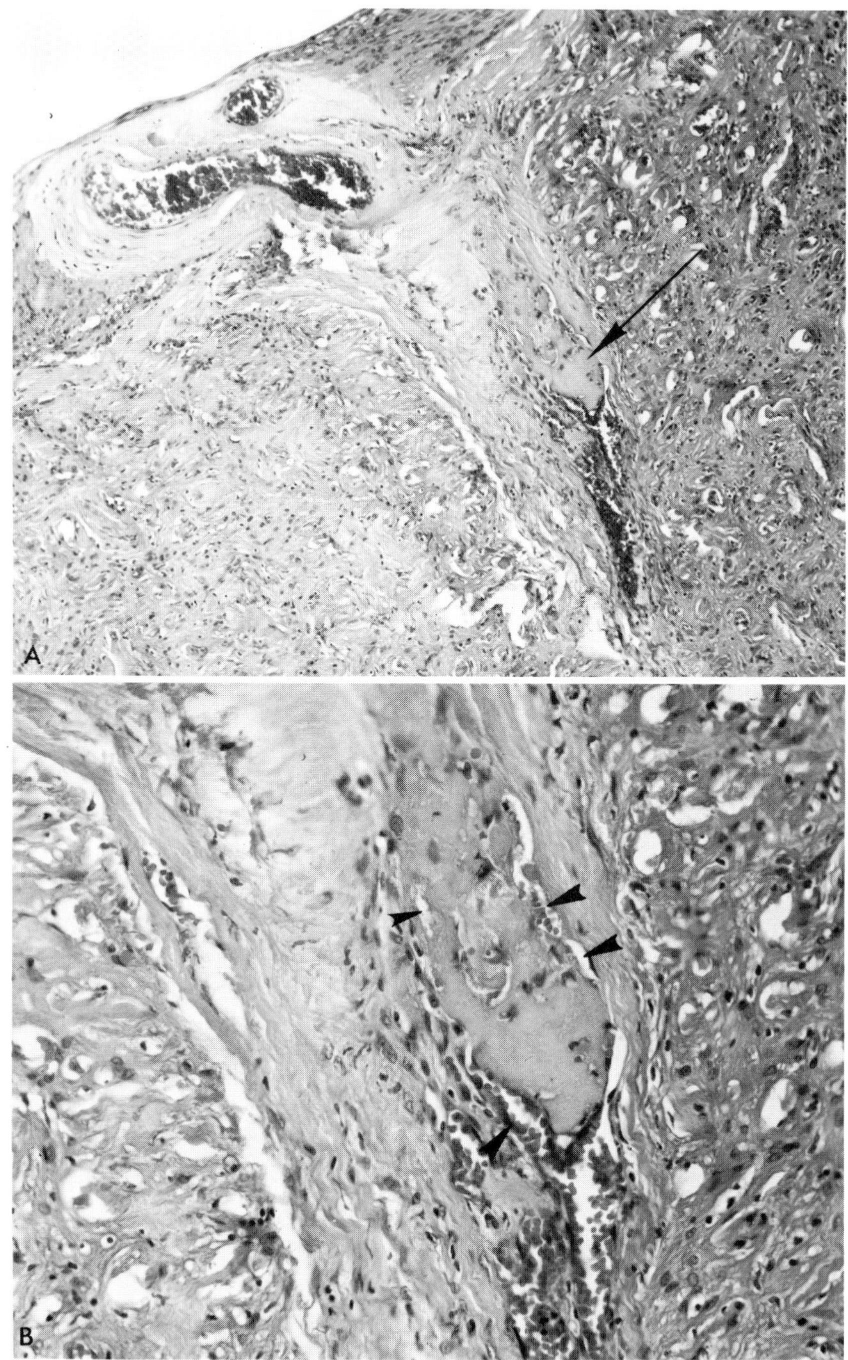

Figure 8–111. *A,* **Recanalized thrombus** (arrow) in central retinal vein just posterior to the lamina cribrosa. H and E, ×100. *B,* Higher power view, showing platelet fibrin thrombus with numerous channels of recanalization (arrowheads). H and E, ×285. EP 38375. (From Green WR, Chan CC, Hutchins GM, Terry JM: Central retinal vein occlusion. A prospective histopathologic study of 29 eyes in 28 cases. Retina *1*:27–55, 1981, and Trans Am Ophthalmol Soc *79*:371–422, 1981.)

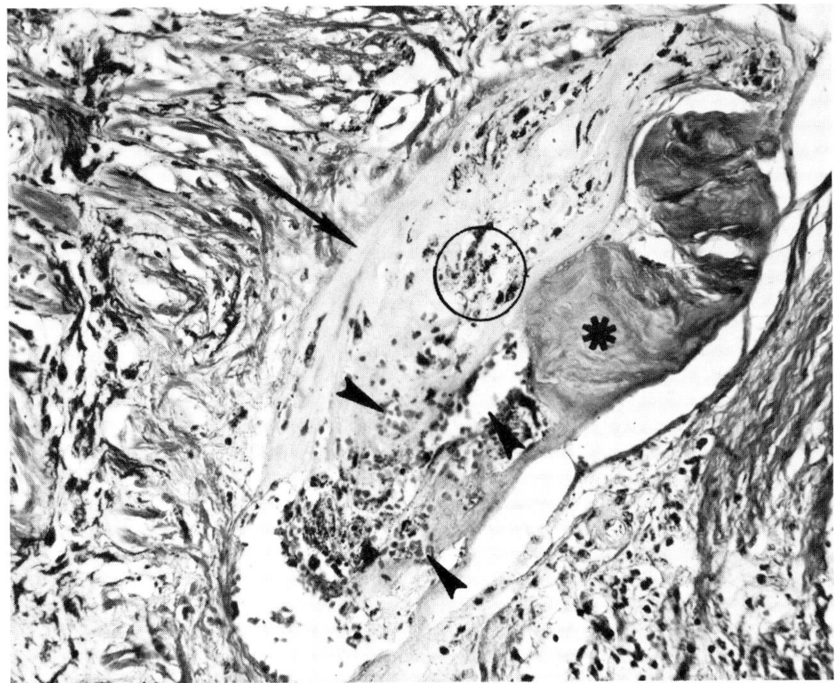

Figure 8–112. Central retinal vein with old thrombus (asterisk) and more recent thrombus (arrow), channels of recanalization (arrowheads), and hemosiderin deposits (circle). H and E, ×285. EP 48267. (From Green WR, Chan CC, Hutchins GM, Terry JM: Central retinal vein occlusion. A prospective histopathologic study of 29 eyes in 28 cases. Retina *1*:27–55, 1981, and Trans Am Ophthalmol Soc *79*:371–422, 1981.)

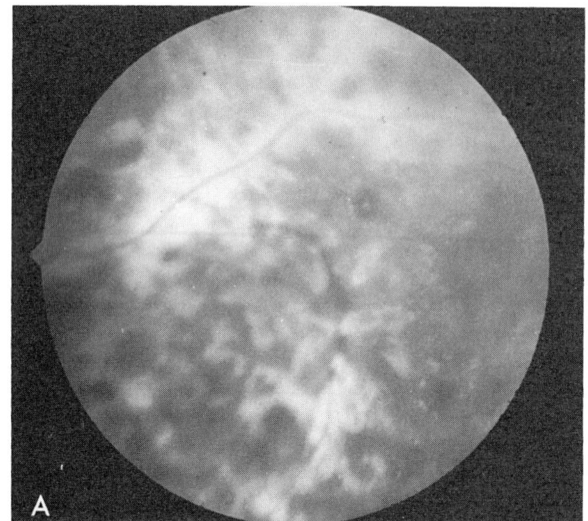

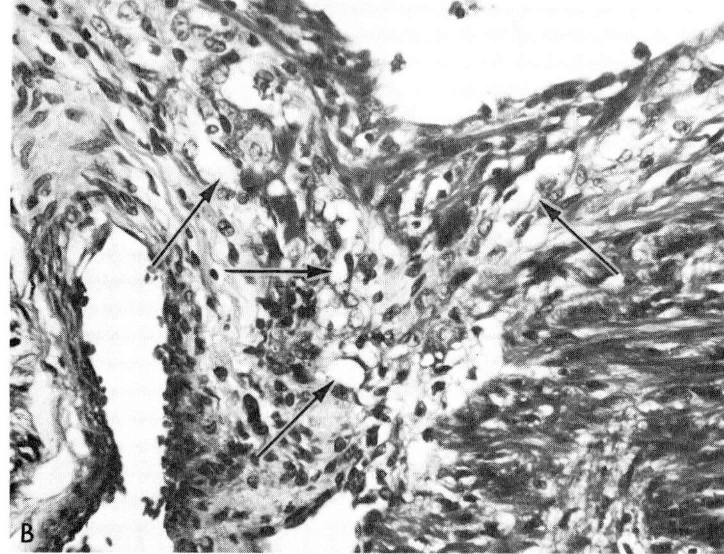

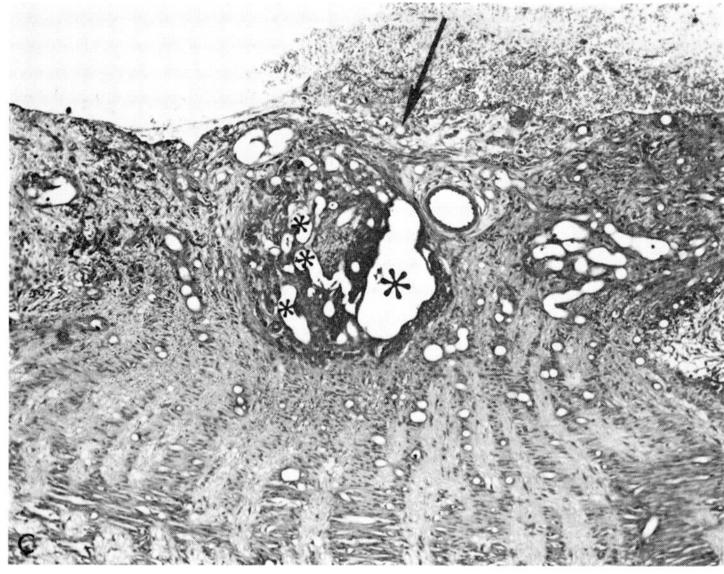

Figure 8–113. Bilateral central retinal vein occlusion (CRVO) in patient with Reyes' syndrome. *A,* Ophthalmoscopic appearance of diffuse retinal hemorrhages in the left eye. *B,* Recanalized thrombus with marked endothelial cell proliferation in prelaminar portion of CRV of right eye (recanalized channels are indicated by arrows). Van de Grift, ×290. *C,* Recanalized thrombus in markedly dilated CRV in optic nerve head of left eye. Numerous channels of recanalization (asterisks) are present, as are disk neovascularization (arrow) and vitreous hemorrhage. PAS, ×90. EP 42767. (From Smith P, Green WR, Miller NR, Terry JM: Central retinal vein occlusion in Reyes' syndrome. Arch Ophthalmol *98*:1256–1260, 1980.)

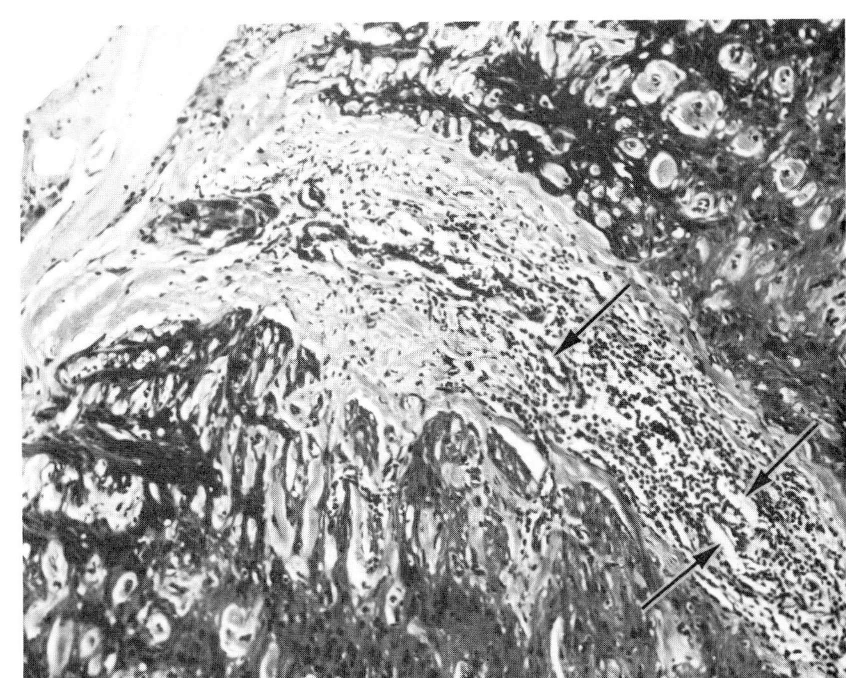

Figure 8–114. Thrombus in retrolaminar portion of central retinal vein, with channels of recanalization (arrows) and marked lymphocytic infiltrations in the area of the thrombus. Van de Grift, ×120. EP 41210. (From Green WR, Chan CC, Hutchins GM, Terry JM: Central retinal vein occlusion. A prospective histopathologic study of 29 eyes in 28 cases. Retina *1*:27–55, 1981, and Trans Am Ophthalmol Soc *79*:371–422, 1981.)

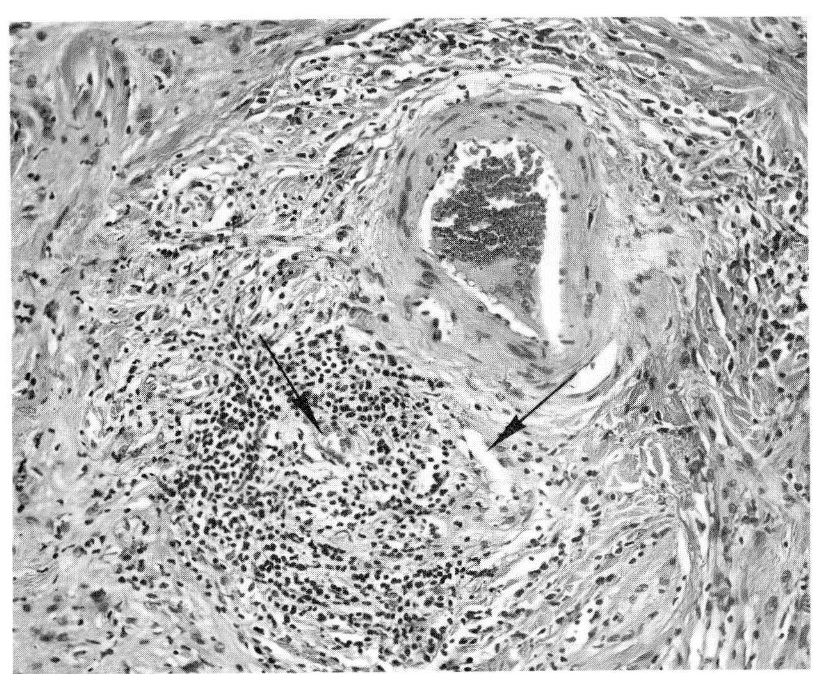

Figure 8–115. Cross-section of optic nerve, showing **channels of recanalization** (arrows) in a central retinal vein thrombus, with intense lymphocytic infiltration. H and E, ×185; Van de Grift, ×285. EP 42480. (From Green WR, Chan CC, Hutchins GM, Terry JM: Central retinal vein occlusion. A prosective histopathologic study of 29 eyes in 28 cases. Retina *1*:27–55, 1981, and Trans Am Opthalmol Soc *79*:371–422, 1981.)

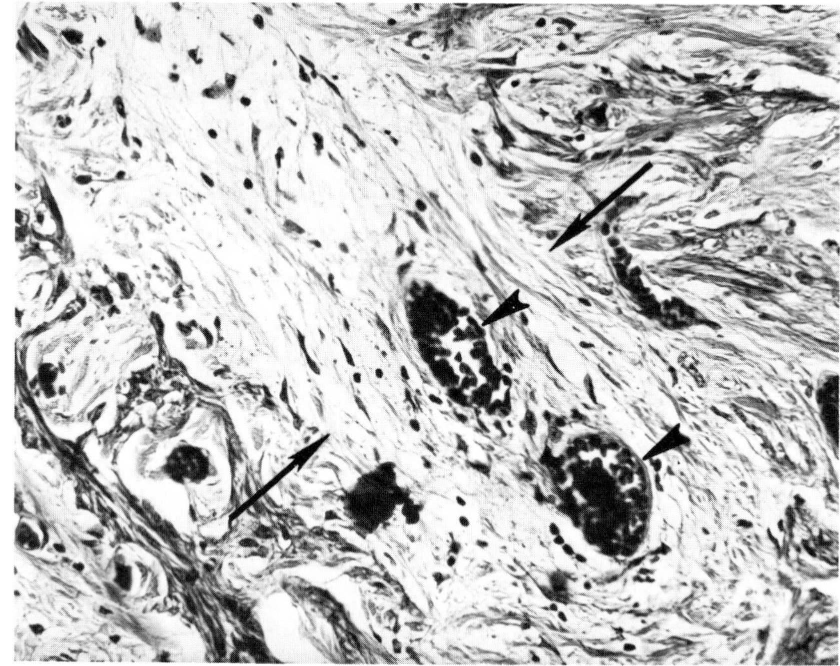

Figure 8–116. Thick-walled central retinal vein (between arrows) with single **channel of recanalization** (arrowheads). Van de Grift, ×160. EP 41898. (From Green WR, Chan CC, Hutchins GM, Terry JM: Central retinal vein occlusion. A prospective histopathologic study of 29 eyes in 28 cases. Retina *1*:27–55, 1981, and Trans Am Ophthalmol Soc *79*:371–422, 1981.)

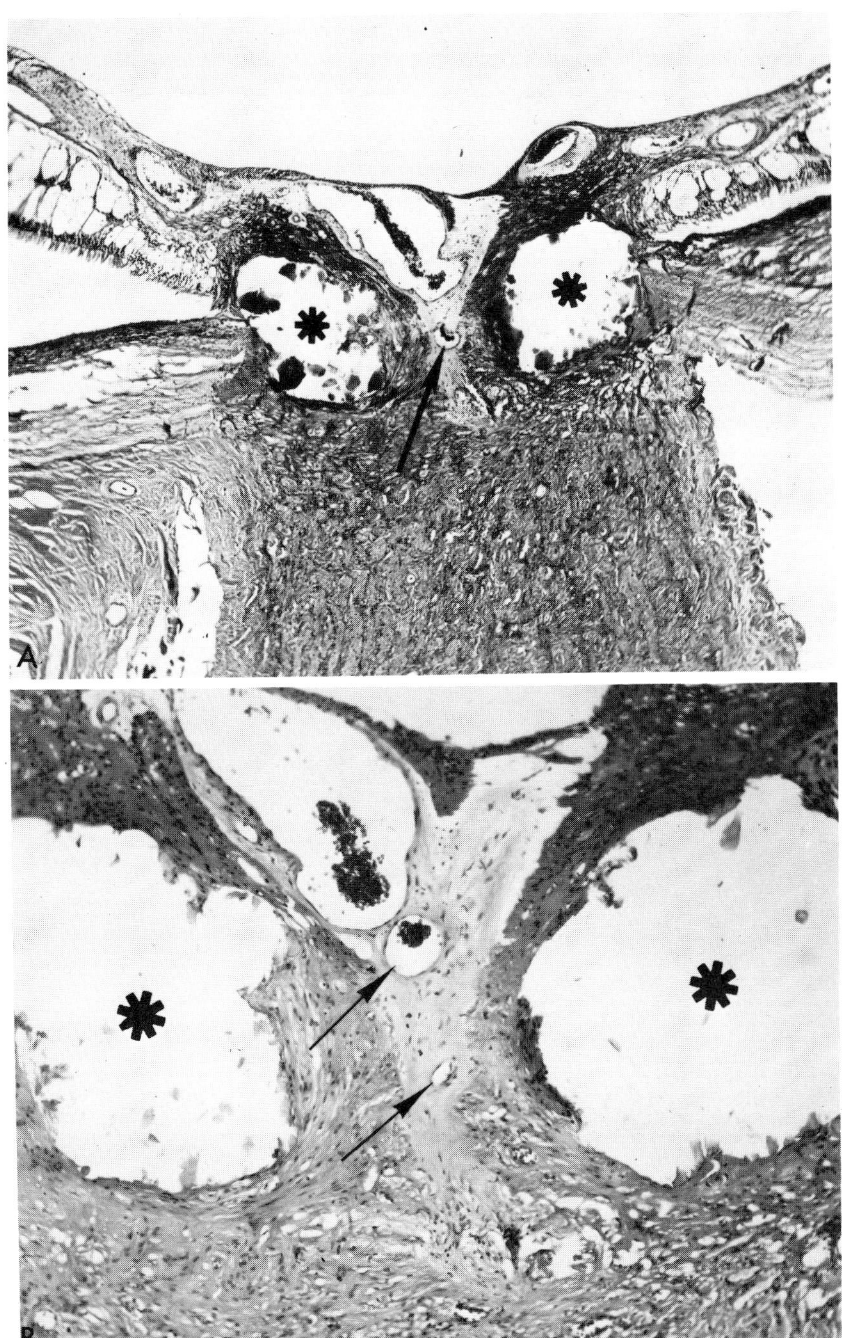

Figure 8–117. Central retinal vein occlusion associated with large drusen of optic nerve head. *A,* Section of center of optic nerve head showing two very large drusen (asterisks) and the thick-walled vein (arrow) going between them. Van de Grift, ×40. *B,* Higher power view showing the single channel (arrows) of a recanalized thrombus between large drusen (asterisks). H and E, ×100. EP 39857. (From Green WR, Chan CC, Hutchins GM, Terry JM: Central retinal vein occlusion. A prospective histopathologic study of 29 eyes in 28 cases. Retina *1*:27–55, 1981, and Trans Am Ophthalmol Soc *79*:371–422, 1981.)

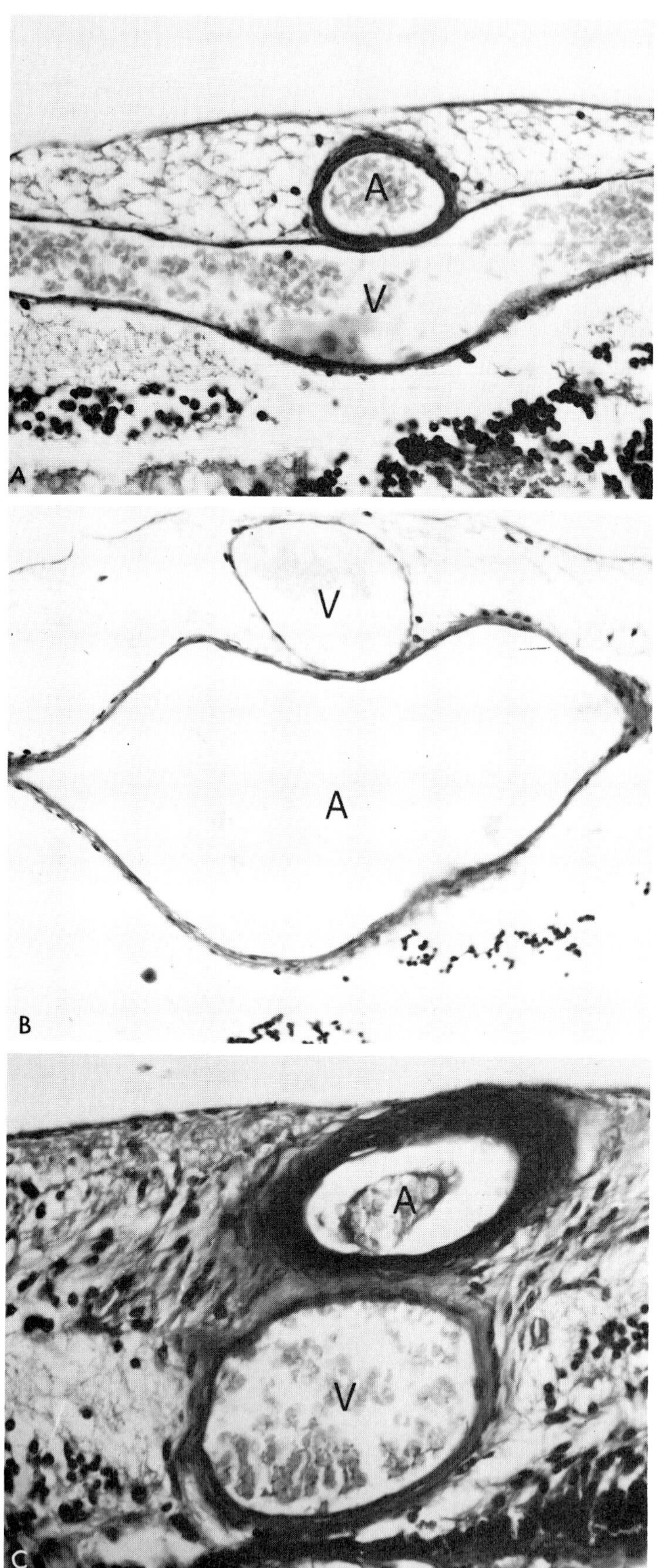

Figure 8–118. Retinal arteriovenous crossings. *A,* Artery *(A)* over vein *(V).* H and E, ×370. EP 49817. *B,* Vein *(V)* over artery *(A).* H and E, ×310. EP 49817. *C,* Sclerotic artery *(A)* over vein *(V).* PAS, ×385. EP 32801.

(48.3 per cent) of the eyes with CRVO, with an interval of 2 or more weeks between the occlusion and histopathologic study. Arterial occlusive disease was observed in only 7 eyes (24.6 per cent). Cystoid macular edema was present in 26 (89.7 per cent) of the eyes.

Neovascularization was a prominent feature in those eyes with CRVO. Iris neovascularization was observed in 24 of the 29 eyes (82.8 per cent). In most of the eyes with rubeosis iridis, the interval between CRVO and histopathologic study was more than 3 months. In cases with good clinical documentation, the interval was 9 and 11 weeks between the CRVO and the observation of rubeosis iridis. Neovascularization was observed at the optic disk in 7 of 29 eyes (24.1 per cent). The interval between CRVO and histopathologic study was 11 days in one eye, 2.5 months in one eye, 5 months in one eye, and more than 1 year in four eyes.

Retinal neovascularization was observed in only one eye, and the interval between CRVO and histopathologic study was 3 years (Fig. 8–104).

Branch Retinal Vein Occlusion. The occlusion usually occurs in a secondary branch of the CRV at the site of an arteriovenous crossing where a portion of the vessel wall is common to both vessels (Fig. 8–118). Distal to the obstruction, the vein becomes distorted and tortuous, and deep and superficial hemorrhages occur in the occluded area. Microinfarctions of the nerve fiber layer also may be observed. The distal portion of the vein usually becomes dilated and tortuous, and the retina becomes edematous. The macula may be directly involved or secondarily involved

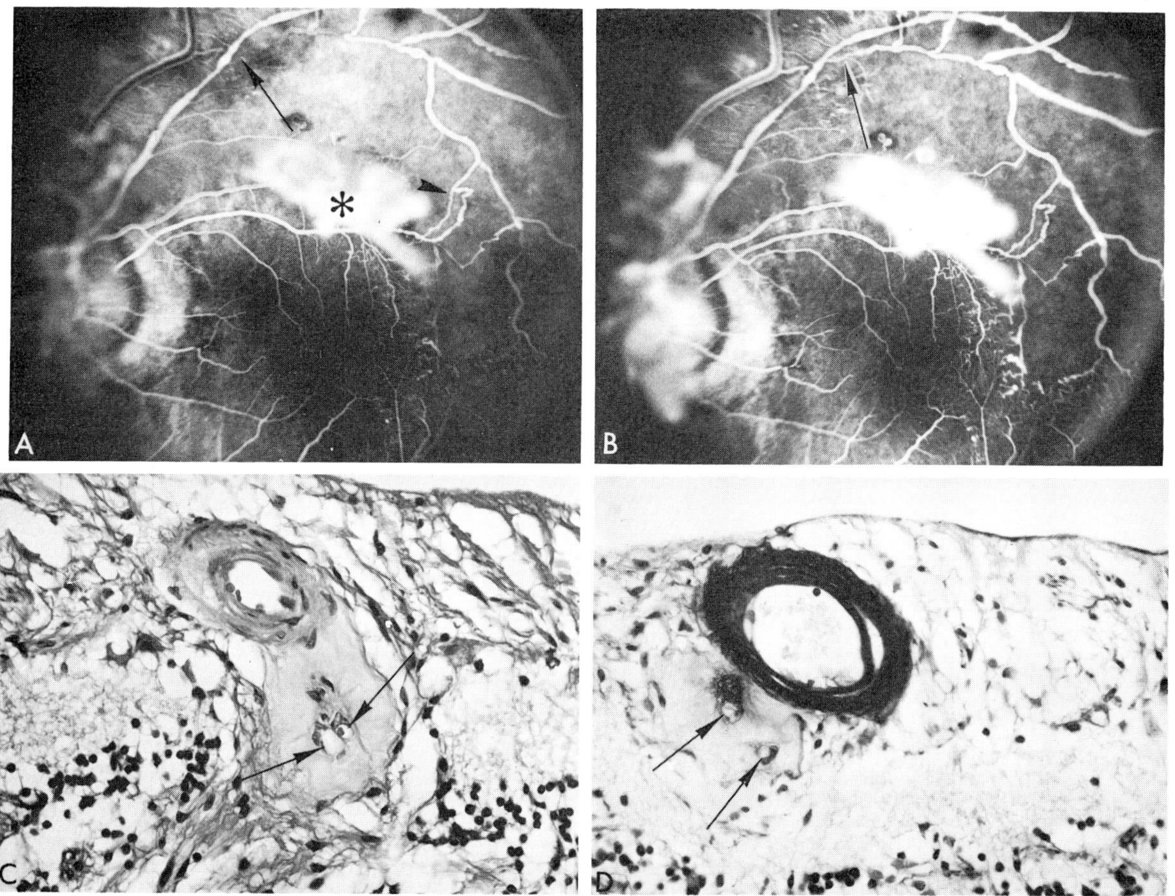

Figure 8–119. Clinicopathologic correlation of branch retinal vein occlusion (BRVO). *A,* Fluorescein angiogram at 20 seconds with a beaded appearance of the superotemporal artery, early laminar flow in the superotemporal vein, occlusion of branch of the superotemporal vein at the first arteriovenous crossing (arrow), vein-to-vein collaterals (arrowhead), and retinal neovascularization just superior to the macula (asterisk). *B,* Later fluorescein angiogram showing a thin line of filling of the partially occluded vein (arrow). *C,* Recanalized thrombus (arrows) of branch of superotemporal vein as it crosses under the arteriosclerotic artery. H and E, ×560. Serial section 560. *D,* Occluded vein on other side of artery shows two channels (arrows) of recanalization. PAS, ×450. Serial section 450. EP 40504. (From Vaghefi HA, Green WR, Kelly JS, et al: Correlation of clinicopathologic findings in a patient. Congenital night blindness, branch retinal vein occlusion, drusen of the optic nerve head, and intraretinal pigmented lesion. Arch Ophthalmol *96*:2097–2104, 1978.)

from edema and exudate. Secondary arterial changes may eventually occur (Wise, 1958). The natural course of the disease (Michels, Gass, 1974; Gutman, Zegarra, 1974) must be taken into consideration when evaluating the effects of photocoagulation therapy.

In a histopathologic study of three cases of branch vein occlusion, Rabinowicz, Litman, and Michaelson (1968) found occlusion of the vein in only one case. In a clinicopathologic study of a case of branch retinal vein occlusion, Vaghefi, Green, Kelley, et al (1978) found that the vein was obstructed as it passed under the arteriole (Fig. 8–119). Inner ischemic atrophy of the retina was observed in the retina peripheral to the vein occlusion.

Figure 8–120 illustrates the clinicopathologic features of a branch retinal vein occlusion of 5 months' duration in a 67 year old woman whose eyes were obtained post mortem.

Frangich, Green, Barraquer-Somers, and Finkelstein (1982) studied occlusions of 9 branch retinal veins in 8 eyes of 7 patients by means of serial sections through the affected areas. A fresh or decanalized thrombus was observed in each instance. Intravitreal neovascularization from the disk, retina, or both was noted in 4 of 8 eyes. Two additional eyes had intraretinal neovascularization (intraretinal microvascular abnormalities). Cystoid macular edema was present in 5 eyes. Inner ischemic atrophy of the retina was found distal to the area of occlusion in 6 of the affected

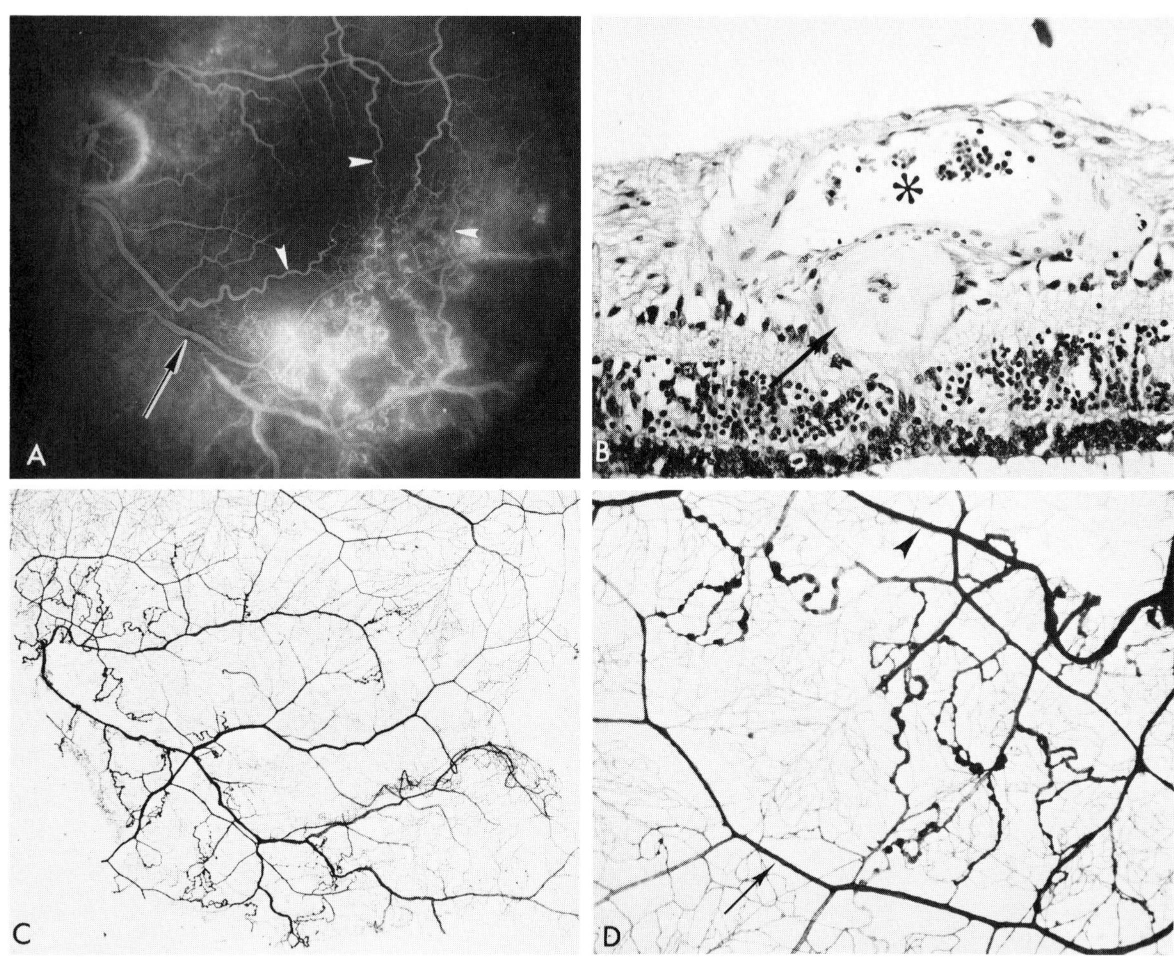

Figure 8–120. Clinicopathologic correlation of branch retinal vein occlusion (BRVO). *A,* Fluorescein angiogram of venous phase, showing obstruction of inferotemporal vein as it crosses under the artery (arrow) and vein-to-vein collaterals (arrowheads). *B,* The vein (arrow) is totally obstructed as it crosses under the artery (asterisk). *C,* Trypsin digestion preparation of retina from inferior cap shows dilation and beading of some interconnecting precapillary arterioles, capillaries, and postcapillary venules. PAS, H and E, ×10. *D,* Higher power showing dilation and beading of some vessels between artery (arrow) and vein (arrowhead). PAS, H and E, ×35. EP 45434. (From Frangieh GT, Green WR, Barraquer-Somer E, Finkelstein D: Histopathologic study of nine branch retinal vein occlusions in eight eyes of seven patients. Arch Ophthalmol *100*:1132–1140, 1982.)

quadrants of the 8 eyes. Although the corresponding branch retinal arteries showed varying degrees of sclerosis (severe, 3 eyes; moderate, 5 eyes; and minimal, 1 eye), no definite thrombus was observed in any of them.

Retinal or optic nerve head neovascularization was observed clinically in 9 of 40 cases (22 per cent) studied by Gutman and Zegarra (1974). Finkelstein, Clarkson, Diddie, et al (1982) reported peripheral retinal neovascularization outside the involved segment in 4 of 366 eyes (0.16 per cent) with branch retinal vein occlusion.

Venous Congestion. In addition to occurring with impending central retinal vein occlusion, venous congestion may be a prominent feature of carbon dioxide retention (as in advanced emphysema, pickwickian syndrome, fibrocystic disease of the pancreas), hyperproteinemic states, papillophlebitis, polycythemia, leukemia, ocular hypotensive retinopathy, carbon monoxide poisoning, and sickle cell retinopathy. Central retinal vein occlusion can occur in some of these conditions. Congenital vascular tortuosity (Goldberg, Pollack, Green, 1972) can be confused with acquired venous congestion.

Papillophlebitis

Papillophlebitis (Lyle, Wybar, 1961; Lonn, Hoyt, 1966; Cogan, 1969b; Hart, Sanders, Miller, 1971; Hayreh, 1972) is characterized by venous congestion and tortuosity, peripheral and sometimes peripapillary retinal hemorrhages, and optic disk edema. The process is usually self-limited, with generally a good visual outcome. The condition is thought to be caused by an inflammatory process of the central retinal vein. No clinically well-documented cases have been studied histopathologically.

Retinal Arterial Macroaneurysms

These macroaneurysms usually involve retinal arterial vessels posterior to the equator. Unlike microaneurysms of the retinal capillary bed, they are rather rare. Occasionally they may be seen in healthy young persons (Pringle, 1917) and in those with angiomatosis retinae, Eales' disease, Leber's miliary aneurysms, and Coats' disease (Nadel, Gupta, 1976). Typically, however, they are found in elderly patients with vascular problems such as hypertension and arteriosclerotic cardiovascular disease (Robertson, 1973).

The major complaint of these patients is blurred vision. This results from retinal edema, exudation, and hemorrhage from a leaking macroaneurysm. If a pulsatile macroaneurysm is present, vitreous or retinal hemorrhage is likely to occur (Shultz, Swan, 1974). Subretinal hemorrhage secondary to a macroaneurysm has resulted in enucleation of the eye from presumed malignant melanoma (Perry, Zimmerman, Benson, 1977).

Fluorescein angiography reveals the aneurysmal dilatation, staining of its wall, and leakage and dilatation of surrounding capillaries.

Retinal macroaneurysms may regress spontaneously as a result of thrombosis, organization, and fibrosis. The retinal exudation and hemorrhage also then may resolve. Because of this spontaneous improvement, the treatment of these lesions is controversial. Although some clinicians prefer not to treat these lesions, disappearance of macroaneurysms and of the attendant exudation after photocoagulation has been reported (Gass, 1972b).

Microscopic examination (Gold, La Piana, Zimmerman, 1976; Perry, Zimmerman, Benson, 1977) shows a greatly distended retinal arteriole with surrounding fibroglial proliferation, dilated capillaries, hemosiderin deposits, lipoidal and proteinaceous exudates, and some extravasated blood (Fig. 8–121). In some instances, excessive bleeding has resulted in confusion of the lesion with a malignant melanoma (Perry, Zimmerman, Benson, 1977; Fichte, Streeten, Friedman, 1978) (Fig. 8–122).

In a large collaborative study of 130 eyes of 120 patients with retinal arterial macroaneurysms, Schatz, Gitter, Yannuzzi, and Irvine (1980) noted that 75 per cent of patients were female and 67 per cent were hypertensive. Hemorrhage around the aneurysm was noted in 43 per cent of the eyes. Hemorrhage occurred only once in all but 1 of the 56 eyes. Impairment of vision due to macular edema was considered an indication for therapy. Of 36 aneurysms treated, vision improved in 26, and there was no improvement in 10 instances.

Retinal Venous Macroaneurysms

Retinal venous macroaneurysms are rarely encountered in proliferative diabetic retinopathy (Fig. 8–123) and central retinal vein occlusion (Fig. 8–124).

Dominantly Inherited Peripheral Retinal Neovascularization

Gitter, Rothschild, Waltman, et al (1978) have described a family with peripheral vascular occlusive disease with associated localized retinal neovascularization and no associated systemic abnormality. No useful information was gained from the histopathologic study of a phthisic eye from a member of this family. See discussion of familial exudative vitreoretinopathy (page 877).

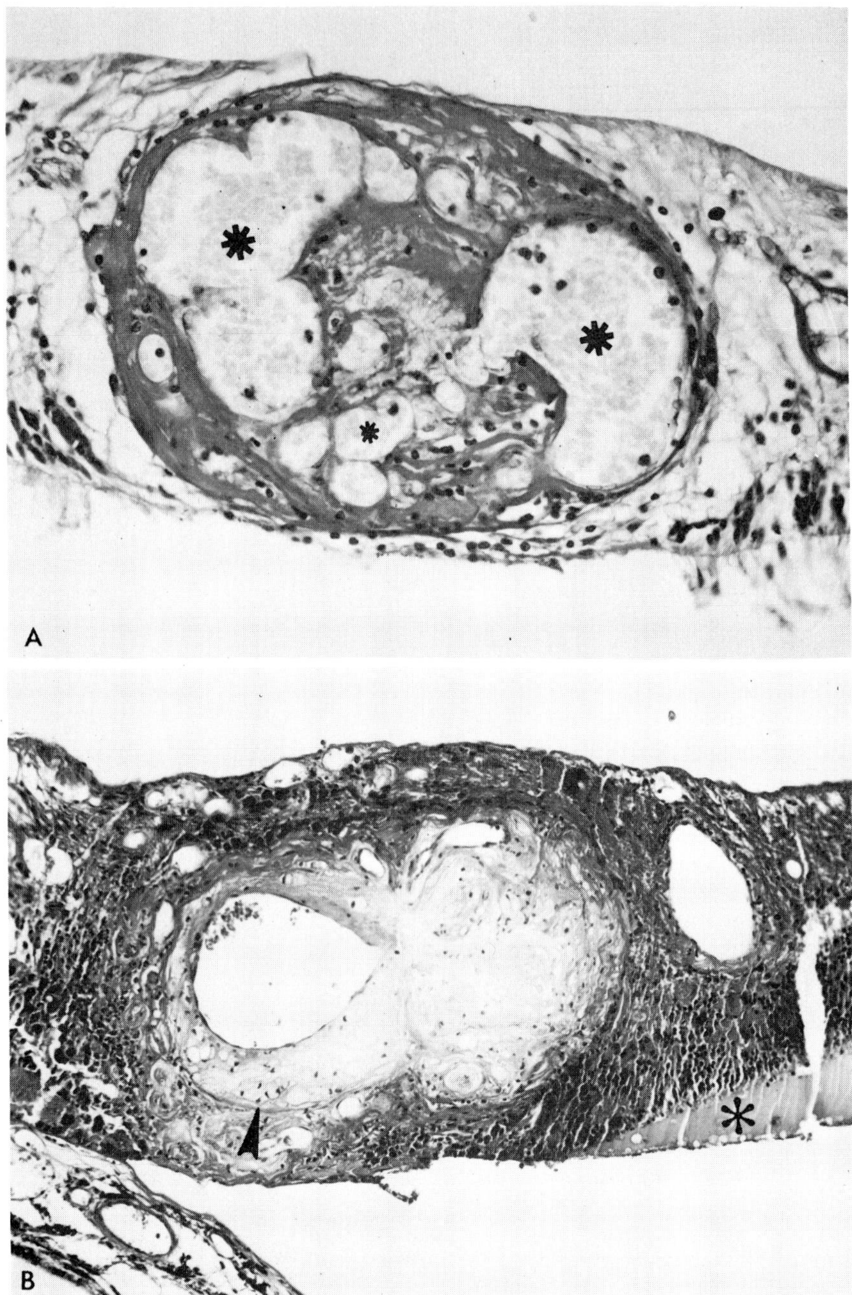

Figure 8–121. Retinal arterial macroaneurysm. *A,* Channels (asterisks) of recanalization in a thrombosed arterial macroaneurysm. PAS, ×310. EP 40103. *B,* Markedly dilated aneurysm with thickened wall (arrowhead). The surrounding retina and subretinal space (asterisk) have a dense proteinaceous exudate. H and E, ×110. EP 42728. (Gold D, LaPiana F, Zimmerman LE: Isolated retinal arterial aneurysms. Am J Ophthalmol *82*:848–857, 1976.)

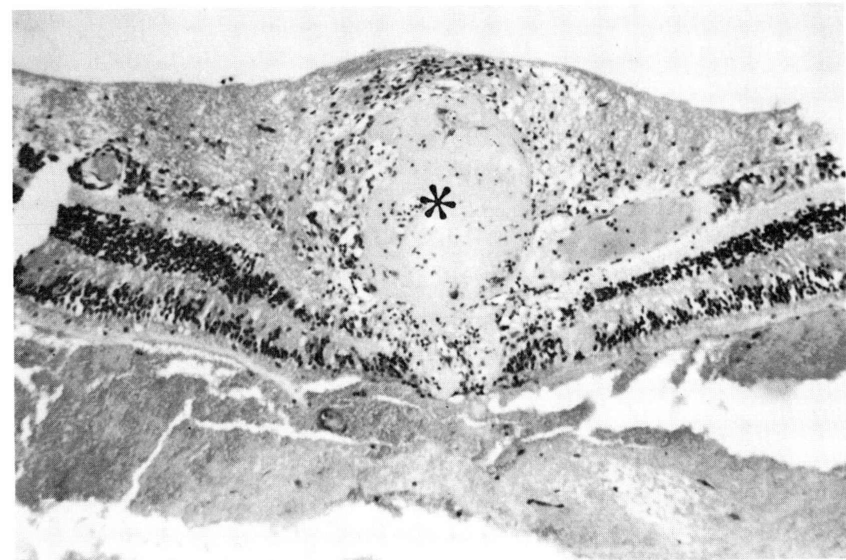

Figure 8–122. Thrombosed retinal arterial macroaneurysm (asterisk) with retinal and subretinal hemorrhage. H and E, ×80. AFIP Neg. 60-6612. (From Perry HD, Zimmerman LE, Berson WE: Hemorrhage from isolated aneurysms of a retinal artery. Arch Ophthalmol *95*:281–283, 1977.)

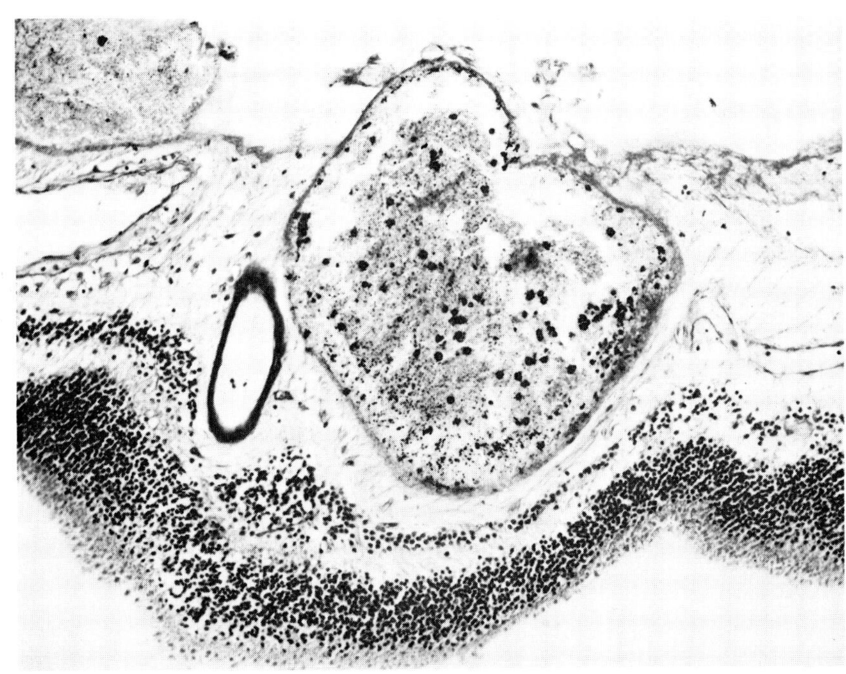

Figure 8–123. Retinal venous macroaneurysm in a diabetic patient. PAS, ×125. EP 48038.

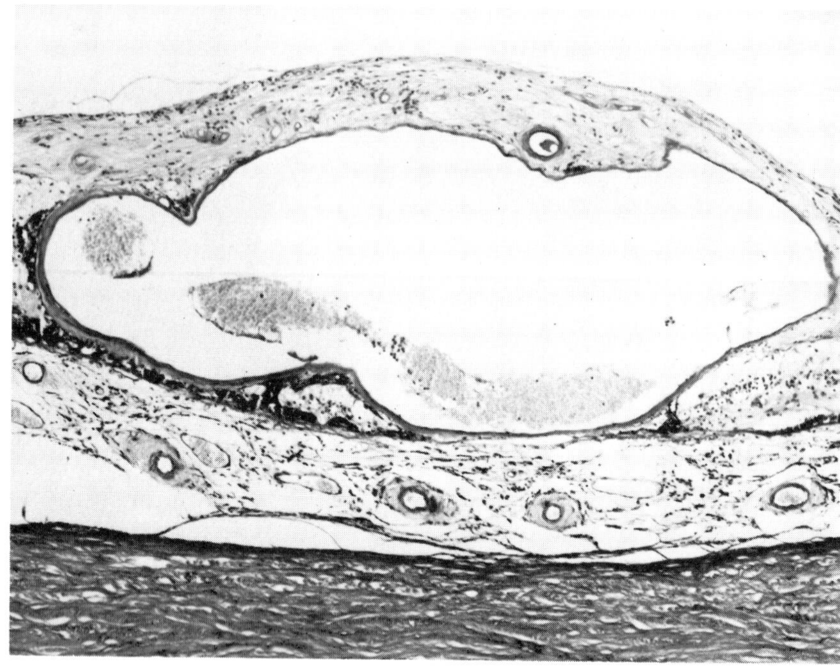

Figure 8–124. Venous macroaneurysm in an eye with central retinal vein occlusion. PAS, ×75. EP 49231.

RETINAL AND PERIRETINAL PROLIFERATIONS

Reparative and Degenerative Processes of the Retina

Glial Proliferation. Glial proliferation of the retina occurs as both a reparative and a degenerative process. Fibroglial proliferation may be observed after some microinfarctions, retinitis, chorioretinitis, central retinal vein occlusion, diabetic retinopathy, and in long-standing processes like pars planitis, retinal detachment, and secondary glaucoma. In most of the foregoing conditions, the glial proliferation is located within the retina.

Massive gliosis of the retina (von Hippel, 1918; Friedenwald, 1926) (Fig. 8–125) is a benign, nonneoplastic proliferation of retinal glia occurring in response to various pathologic states, including congenital malformations, trauma, chronic inflammations, and retinal vascular disorders (Yanoff, Zimmerman, Davis, 1971). These areas of gliosis are composed of groups of spindle-shaped cells, with uniform nuclei and abundant, pale, eosinophilic-staining cytoplasm. Numerous dilated, thick-walled blood vessels are scattered throughout the lesion. Figure 8–126 illustrates a clinicopathologic example of massive gliosis of the retina seen in a patient with old, "burnt-out" Coats' disease (Green, 1967).

Periretinal Proliferations. From both the clinical and pathologic viewpoints, it is increasingly well recognized that various cellular constituents can gain access to the inner surface of the retina and, in this location, can engage in proliferative and secretory activities that result in the fibrocellular tissues broadly termed "epiretinal membranes." Such proliferations can range in severity from the clinically innocuous and incidental "simple epiretinal membrane" to the "surface-wrinkling retinopathy" frequently noted in autopsy eyes (Roth, Foos, 1971) and, further, to the surgically complicated and visually disastrous "massive periretinal proliferation (MPP)." The two latter are most frequently associated with rhegmatogenous retinal detachment (Laqua, Machemer, 1975b; Machemer, Laqua, 1975; Tolentino, Schepens, Freeman, 1967).

The term *proliferative vitreoretinopathy (PVR)* has been recommended to refer to the entity previously known as massive vitreous retraction, massive preretinal retraction, or massive periretinal proliferation (Hilton, 1983). Vitreoretinal membrane shrinkage is subdivided into three major categories, depending on the degree of involvement (Table 8–2).

Recent light and electron microscopic studies of human and experimental epiretinal membranes have implicated various contributing cell types, but the most frequent ones have been glial cells, particularly the fibrous astrocyte, of the retina and optic nerve head in the formation of peripheral retinal membranes (Kenyon, Pederson, Green, Maumenee, 1975), epipapillary membranes, and macular membranes (Roth, Foos, 1972; Bellhorn, Friedman, Wise, Henkind, 1975; Clarkson, Green, Massof, 1977; Hansen, Friedman, Gartner, Henkind, 1977; Foos, 1974b; Kenyon, Michels, 1977; Van Horn, Aaberg, Machemer, Fenzl, 1977). However, in various retinal detachment situations complicated by MPP; the RPE cell is thought to be the major contributor (Laqua,

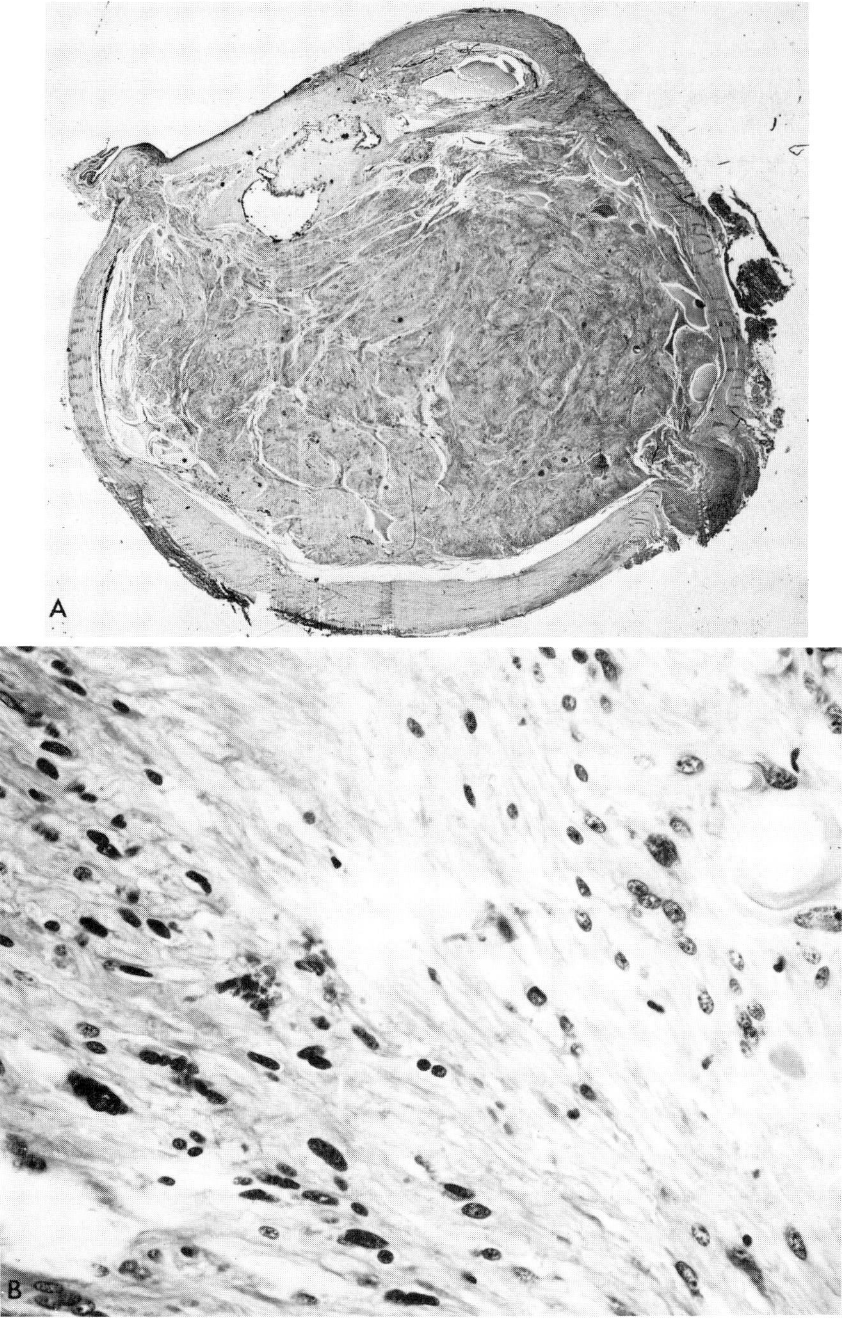

Figure 8–125. *A,* **Massive gliosis** almost filling the entire eye. H and E, ×6.5. *B,* Gliosis with spindle-shaped cells and abundant fibrillary material. H and E, ×300. EP 9715.

Machemer, 1975a; Machemer, Laqua, 1975; Clarkson, Green, Massof, 1977; Machemer, Van Horn, Aaberg, 1978; Wallow, Miller, 1978; Smith, Van Heuven, Streeten, 1976). Other cell types have also been implicated in the proliferative process; these include fibrocytes (Constable, 1975; Constable, Tolentino, Donovan, Schepens, 1974), myofibroblasts, macrophages, inflammatory cells, hyalocytes, and vascular elements.

Fibrous astrocytes are often present in the macular and peripapillary areas, and they have been amply implicated in formation of idiopathic membranes (Roth, Foos, 1971; Roth, Foos, 1972; Bellhorn, Friedman, Wise, Henkind, 1975; Quigley, 1977). The prevalence of idiopathic preretinal membranes with surface-wrinkling retinopathy is about 2 to 3 per cent between the ages of 40 and 60 years, which progresses to about 25 per cent after age 73 years (Roth, Foos, 1971; Foos, 1977).

Astrocytes gain access to the inner retinal surface where the internal limiting membrane (ILM) is disrupted, as in retinal pits and retinal tears (Fig. 8–127) and at points where the ILM is ten-

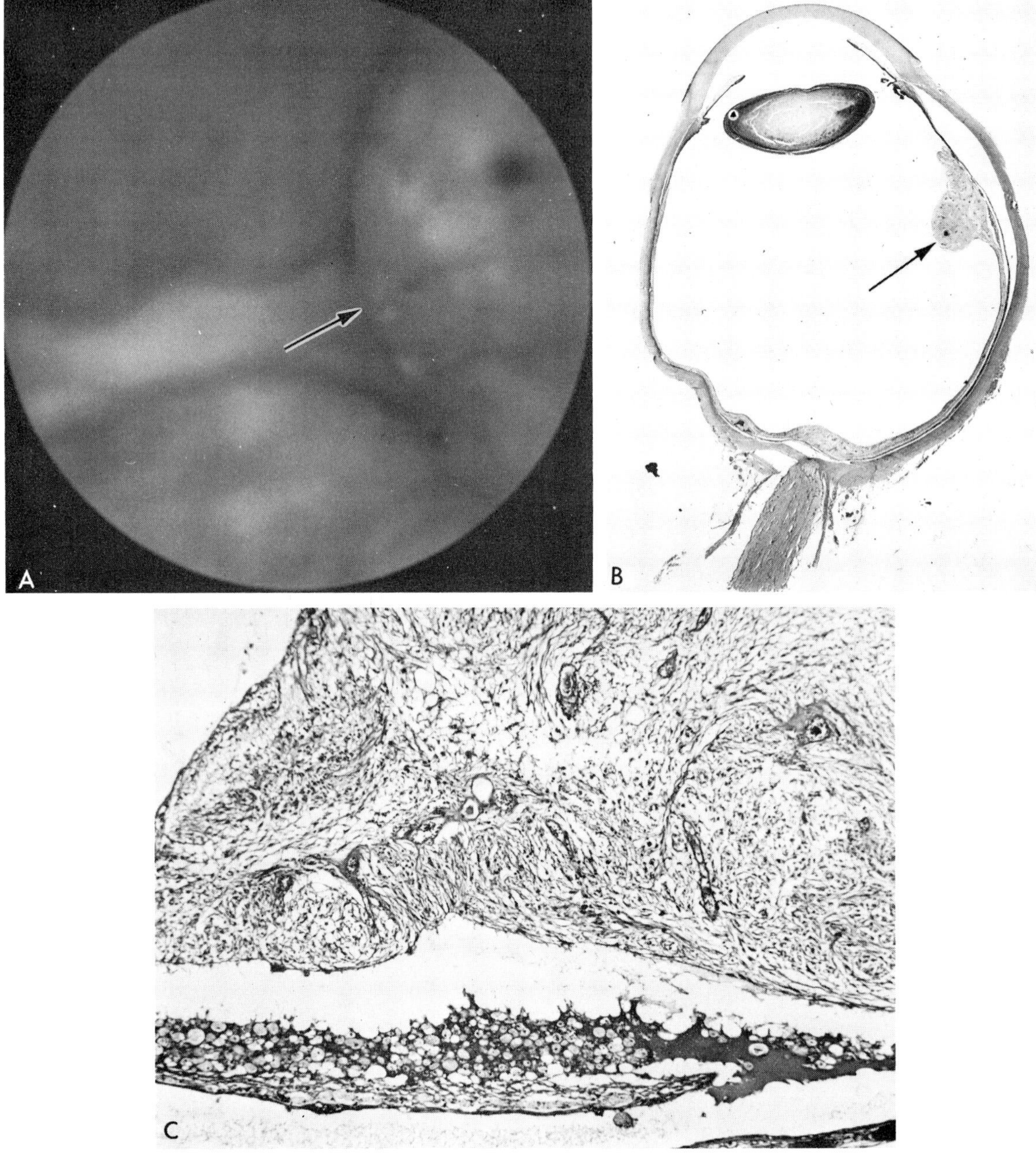

Figure 8–126. *A,* Clinical, *B,* low power, and *C,* higher power view of **massive gliosis** (arrow) in an eye with old Coats' disease. (From Green WR: Bilateral Coats' disease with massive gliosis of the retina. Arch Ophthalmol 77:378–383, 1967.)

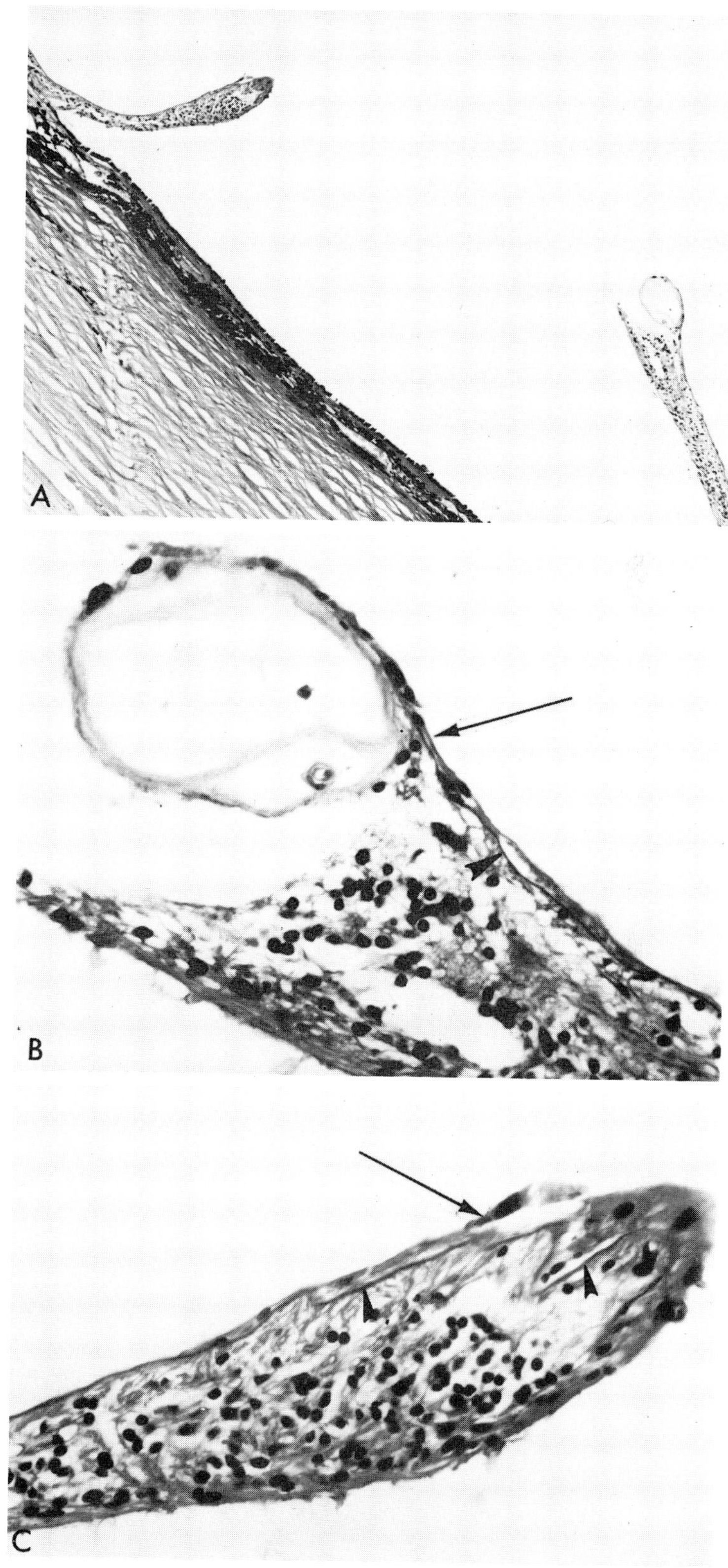

Figure 8–127. *A,* Peripheral retinal hole with glial preretinal membrane extending on the inner surface of the retina anteriorly and posteriorly. PAS, ×65. Higher power view of *B,* anterior and *C,* posterior margins of retinal tear, showing glial preretinal membrane (arrows) extending along the inner surface of the internal limiting membrane (arrows). *B* and *C,* PAS, ×190. EP 30981. (From Clarkson JG, Green WR, Massof D: A histopathologic review of 168 cases of preretinal membrane. Am J Ophthalmol *84*:1–17, 1977.)

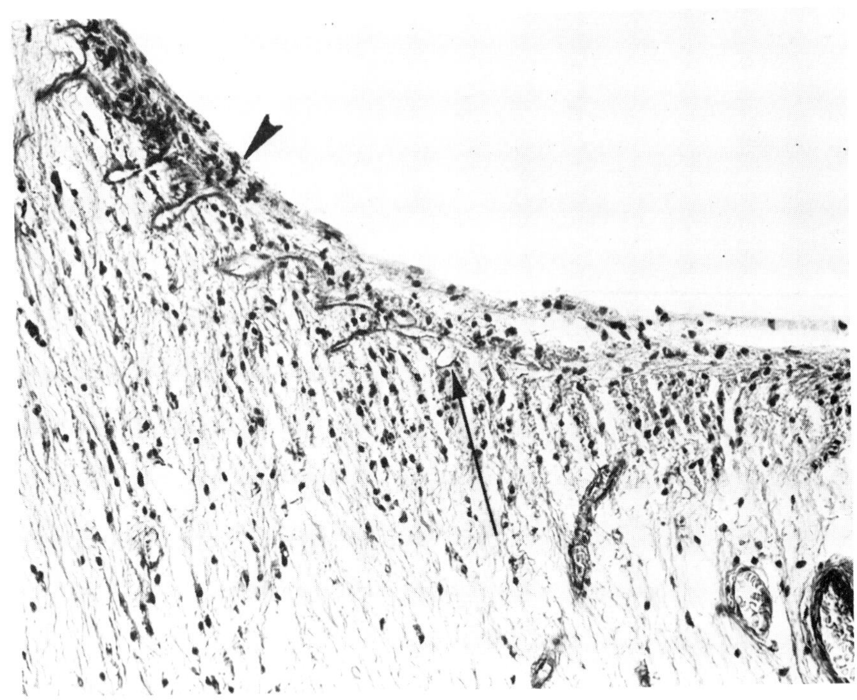

Figure 8–128. Glial preretinal membrane (arrowhead) originating at the optic nerve head at the termination of the internal limiting membrane (arrow) near the center of the optic nerve head. PAS, ×260. EP 27006. (From Clarkson JG, Green WR, Massof D: A histopathologic review of 168 cases of preretinal membrane. Am J Ophthalmol *84*:1–17, 1977.)

uous or absent, as at the optic nerve head (Fig. 8–128), over major retinal vessels (Fig. 8–129), and at the foveola. Idiopathic proliferation may be seen at the macular area (Kampik, Green, Michels, Nase, 1980) and at the optic nerve head (Thomas, Michels, Rice, et al, 1982).

It has been observed also that the prevalence of preretinal membrane increases when there is local ocular disease (Roth, Foos, 1971). It is quite possible that a retinal detachment, and surgery for a retinal detachment with scleral buckling, diathermy, or cryotherapy, can incite or accentuate a pre-existing asymptomatic and unrecognized preretinal membrane of glial origin. However, as Clarkson, Green, and Massof (1977) pointed out, all 16 of their cases of preretinal membranes in which RPE was the principal cell source were in eyes that had been operated on for rhegmatogenous retinal detachment. It is likely that most cases of macular pucker after retinal detachment surgery are due to pre-existing undetected glial membranes, and that the surgery causes the membranes to become manifest, with contractive wrinkling of the ILM and visual impairment. Epiretinal membranes are seen with increased frequency in association with ocular inflammatory disease and trauma and may occur after photocoagulation (Kampik, Green, Michels, Rice, 1981).

Less commonly, the RPE gives rise to new preretinal membrane formation and macular pucker after rhegmatogenous retinal detachment. It is also the principal cell source in MPP with massive vitreous retraction (MVR) after repair of a rhegmatogenous retinal detachment. Radtke, Tano, Chandler, and Machemer (1981) have observed the simulation of massive periretinal proliferation by autotransplantation of RPE cells in rabbits.

A retinal tear thus is one of the predisposing factors to RPE proliferation on the inner surface of the retina and in the vitreous. Figures 8–130 and 8–131 illustrate the direct continuity of RPE through a retinal dialysis and onto the inner surface of the retina.

Judging the identity of cells proliferating in the vitreous and inner retinal surface can be difficult, even with ultrastructural studies. RPE can be

Table 8–2. CLASSIFICATION OF RETINAL DETACHMENT WITH PROLIFERATIVE VITREORETINOPATHY (PVR)

Grade	Name	Clinical Signs
A	Minimal	Vitreous haze, vitreous pigment clumps
B	Moderate	Wrinkling of the inner retinal surface, rolled edge of retinal break, retinal stiffness, vessel tortuosity
C	Marked	Full thickness fixed retinal folds
C–1		One quadrant
C–2		Two quadrants
C–3		Three quadrants
D	Massive	Fixed retinal folds in four quadrants
D–1		Wide funnel shape
D–2		Narrow funnel shape*
D–3		Closed funnel (optic nervehead not visible)

*Narrow funnel shape exists when the anterior end of the funnel can be seen by indirect ophthalmoscopy within the 45° field of a +20 D condensing lens (Nikon or equivalent).

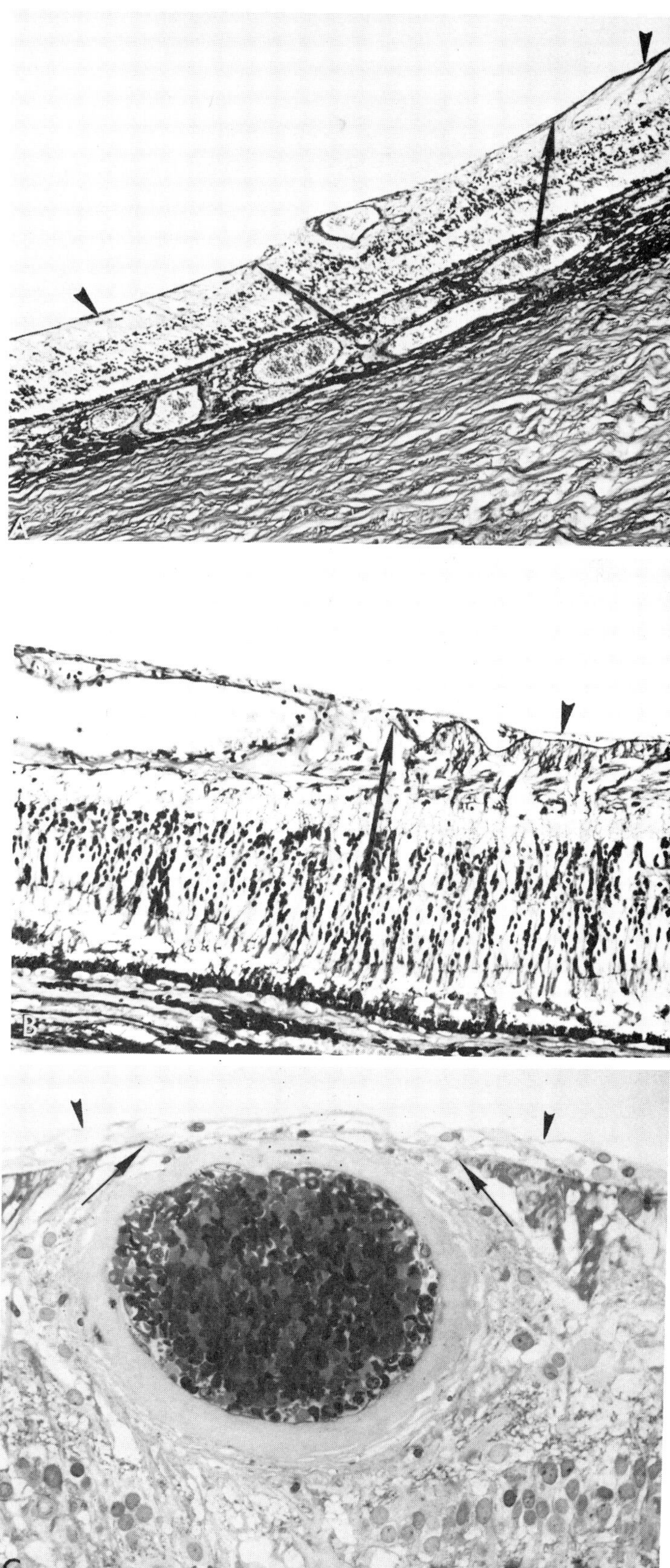

Figure 8–129. *A,* Area of retina temporal to macula, with a broad gap in the internal limiting membrane (ILM) (between arrows). A thin glial preretinal membrane extends to either side (arrowheads). PAS, ×70. EP 38147. *B,* Glial preretinal membrane (arrowhead) originating at a defect in the ILM overlying a retinal vessel. Arrow indicates one end of the discontinuous ILM. PAS, ×170. EP 29182. *C,* Glial preretinal membrane (arrowheads) extending from discontinuity of ILM (arrows) over a retinal artery. Toluidine blue; Epon, ×390. EM 277. (From Clarkson JG, Green WR, Massof D: A histopathologic review of 168 cases of preretinal membrane. Am J Ophthalmol *84*:1–17, 1977.)

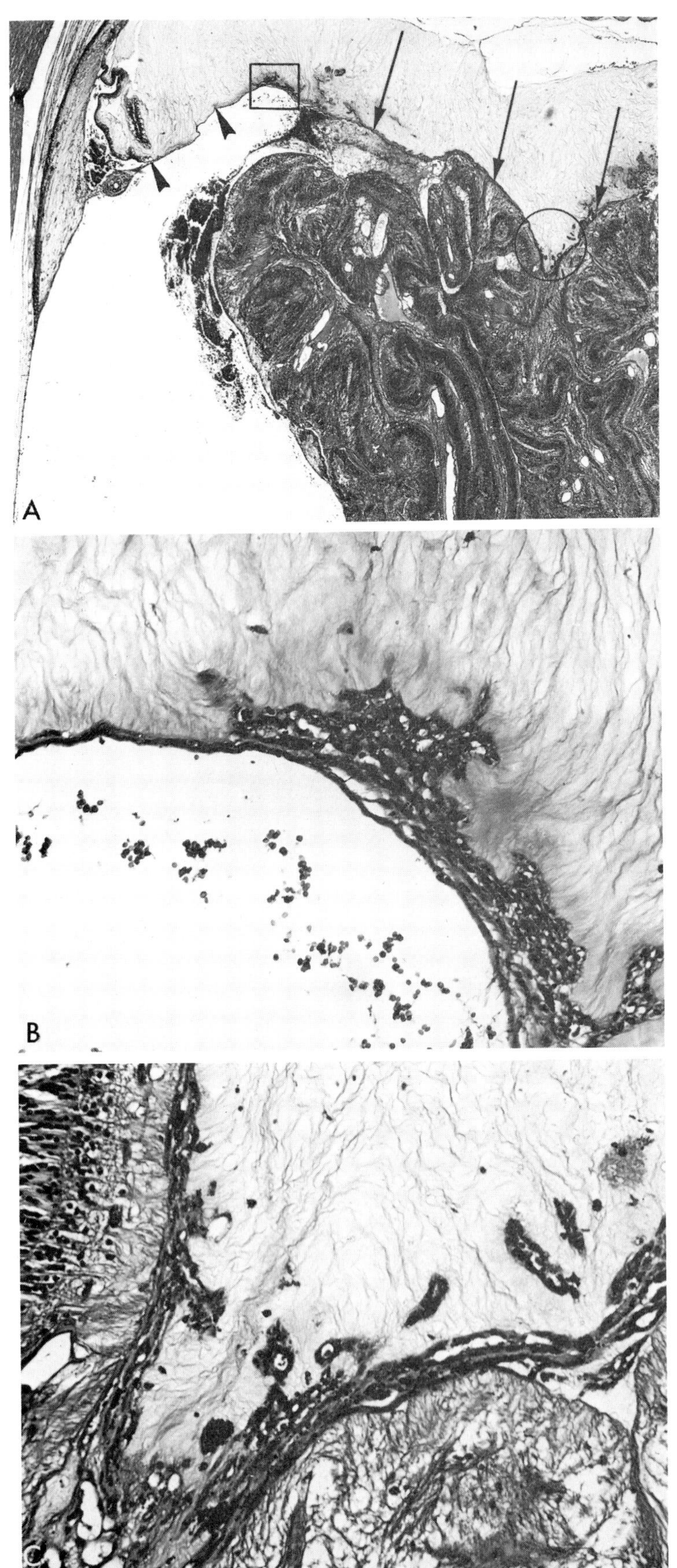

Figure 8–130. *A,* **Retinal dialysis at ora serrata** with retinal pigment epithelium (RPE) extending through the dialysis, along posterior surface of vitreous (arrowheads) and then along anterior surface of retina (arrows). H and E, ×20. *B,* Higher power view of area in *A* in square, showing the RPE membrane along posterior surface of vitreous. H and E, ×200. *C,* Higher power view of area in *A* circle, showing the multilaminated preretinal pigment epithelial membrane and the hyperplastic RPE maintenance of polarity in a laminated or tubuloacinar pattern. H and E, ×180. EP 39434. (From Clarkson JG, Green WR, Massof D: A histopathologic review of 168 cases of preretinal membrane. Am J Ophthalmol *84*:1–17, 1977.)

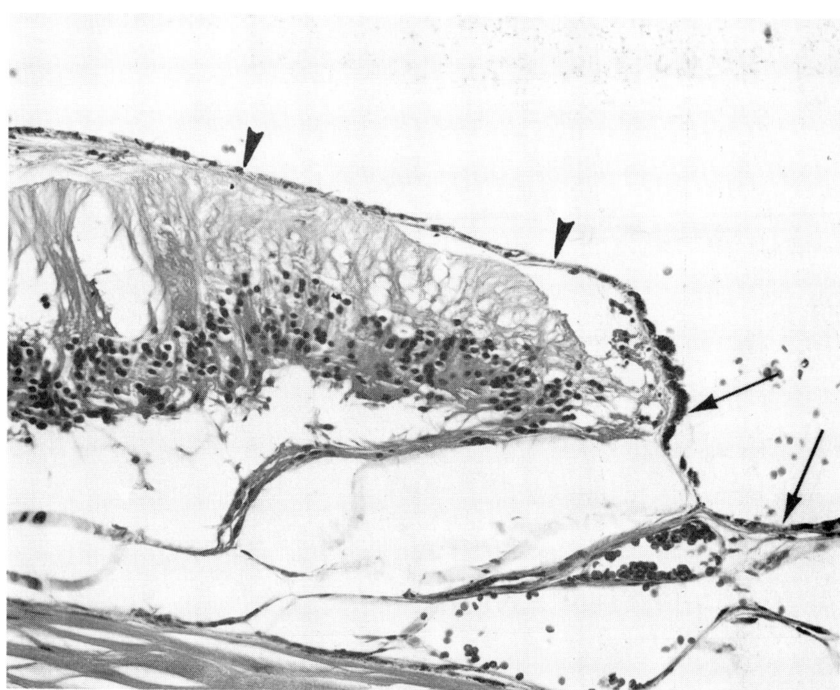

Figure 8–131. Self-healed **retinal dialysis** with direct continuity of retinal pigment epithelium at edge of dialysis (arrows) and extension along the inner surface of retina (arrowheads). H and E, ×230. EP 44485.

identified by its tendency to polarize in a monolayer (Fig. 8–132) or rosette (Fig. 8–133) configuration. In monolayers, the apical (or free) surface of the cells is exposed to the vitreous and shows typical specialization of junctional complexes and fine microvillous processes. Their basal surface is identified by well-developed basement membrane interposed between the cell membrane and collagenous tissue. Numerous single, usually membrane-limited melanosomes are present in the cytoplasm. Intracytoplasmic filaments of the microfilament dimension (about 50 to 75 angstroms), which is consistent with the actin (Gipson, 1977) may be present in RPE-laden cells (Fig. 8–134).

In the rosette-like or acinar configuration, these RPE cells had typical RPE characteristics, despite being embedded within collagenous tissue. Thus, their microvilli-bearing apical surfaces were apposed to form a false lumen, and their basement membrane–invested basal surfaces were directly exposed to the collagenous component. This rosette or acinar configuration had been noted in hyperplastic RPE proliferating over choroidal tumors (Wallow, Tso, 1972) and in vitrectomy specimens from patients with MPP (Machemer, Van Horn, Aaberg, 1978).

Fibrous astrocytes are large and generally fusiform and show a marked tendency to proliferate into a monolayer configuration (Kenyon, Michels, 1977). Interdigitating cytoplasmic processes are especially numerous along the apical and lateral surfaces, and they interconnect by means of junctional complexes of both the adherens and occludens types. The basal surfaces have variable amounts of basement membrane. The most rigorous criterion for this cell type, however, is the presence of masses of intermediate-type filaments of about 100 angstroms' diameter (Gipson, 1977) within the cytoplasm (Fig. 8–135). Myoblastic differentiation of fibrous astrocytes may be observed (Fig. 8–136).

Fibrocytes are usually fusiform and lack polarization with respect to apical processes or basement membrane. Occasional desmosomal attachments are evident wherever these cells are in contact. The cytoplasm often contains numerous cisternae of rough-surfaced endoplasmic reticulum, plus some smooth endoplasmic reticulum and Golgi complexes, occasionally with prominent centrioles (Fig. 8–137). Intermediate filaments are not frequent, and myofibrils (Kenyon, Michels, 1977) seem to be absent.

Myofibroblast-like cells are characterized by lack of polarity, irregularly shaped nuclei, absence of basement membrane, and marginally located microfilaments (Fig. 8–138).

Macrophages are large cells with pleomorphic contents in various stages of degradation within secondary lysosomes or residual bodies (Fig. 8–139). Some of these cells also contain pigment that does not appear to have been phagocytosed. These macrophages may sometimes have been derived from the RPE. Some macrophages have irregularly shaped nuclei and may be derived from hyalocytes (Fig. 8–140).

Variable amounts of fibrillar collagen are present with periretinal proliferative tissue. This collagen consistently measures between 200 and 250 angstroms in diameter, with the usual macroper-

Text continued on page 726

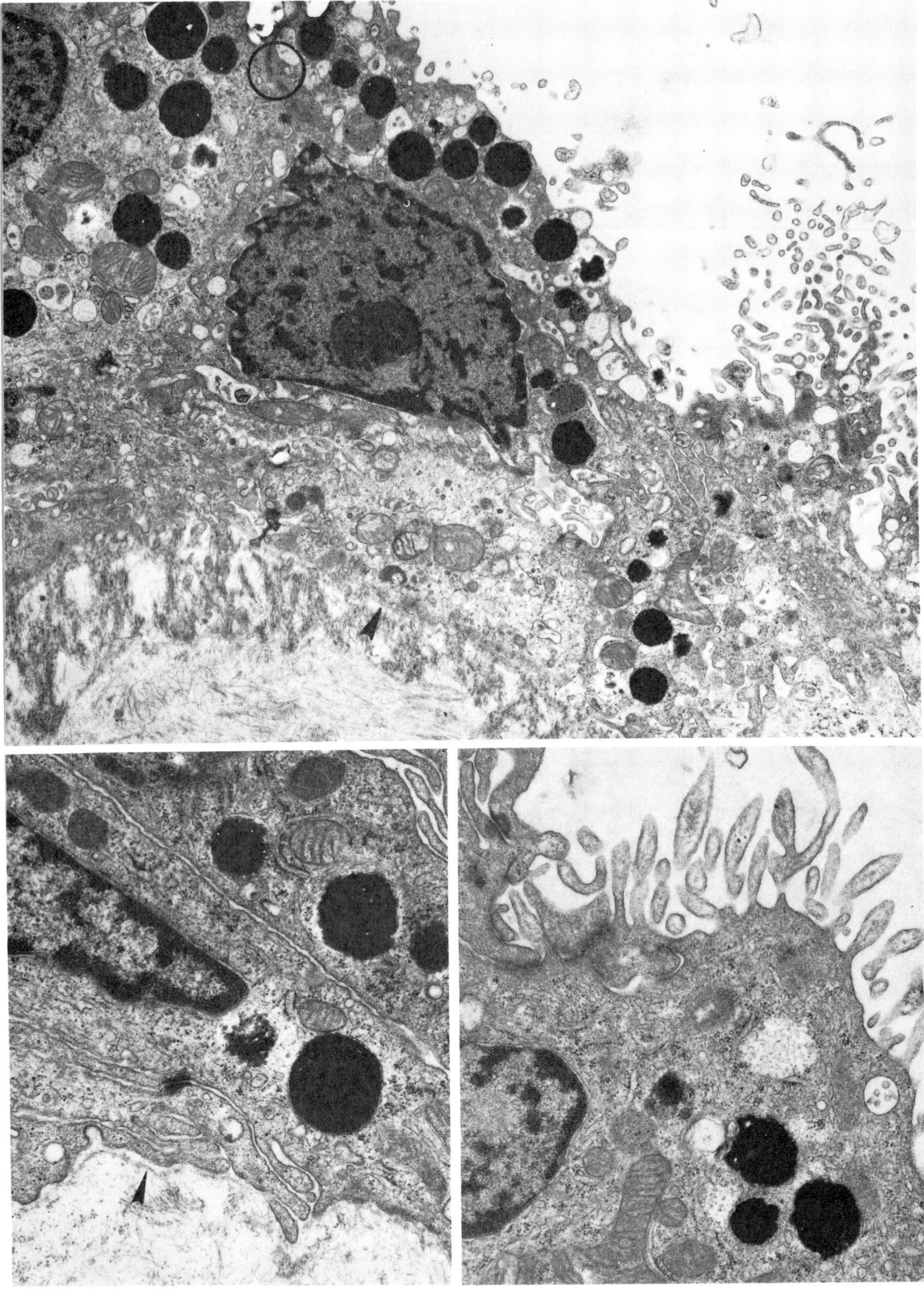

Figure 8–132. Definite retinal pigment epithelium cells of epiretinal membrane occurring after retinal reattachment surgery. Main figure is electron micrograph illustrating polarization of pigment-containing cells with respect to junctional complexes (circled) and numerous fine processes of free-surface apical cell membrane, and nearly continuous basement membrane (arrowhead) closely opposed to basal cell surface. ×8900. Bottom, At higher magnifications, the features of these cells are better seen, including intracytoplasmic melanin granules and extracellular basement membrane (arrowhead) at left (×25,000), and numerous junctional complexes and apical surface processes at right (×22,400).

(From Kampik A, Kenyon KR, Michels, RG, et al: Epiretinal and vitreous membranes: A comparative study of 56 cases. Arch Ophthalmol *99*:1445–1454, 1981.)

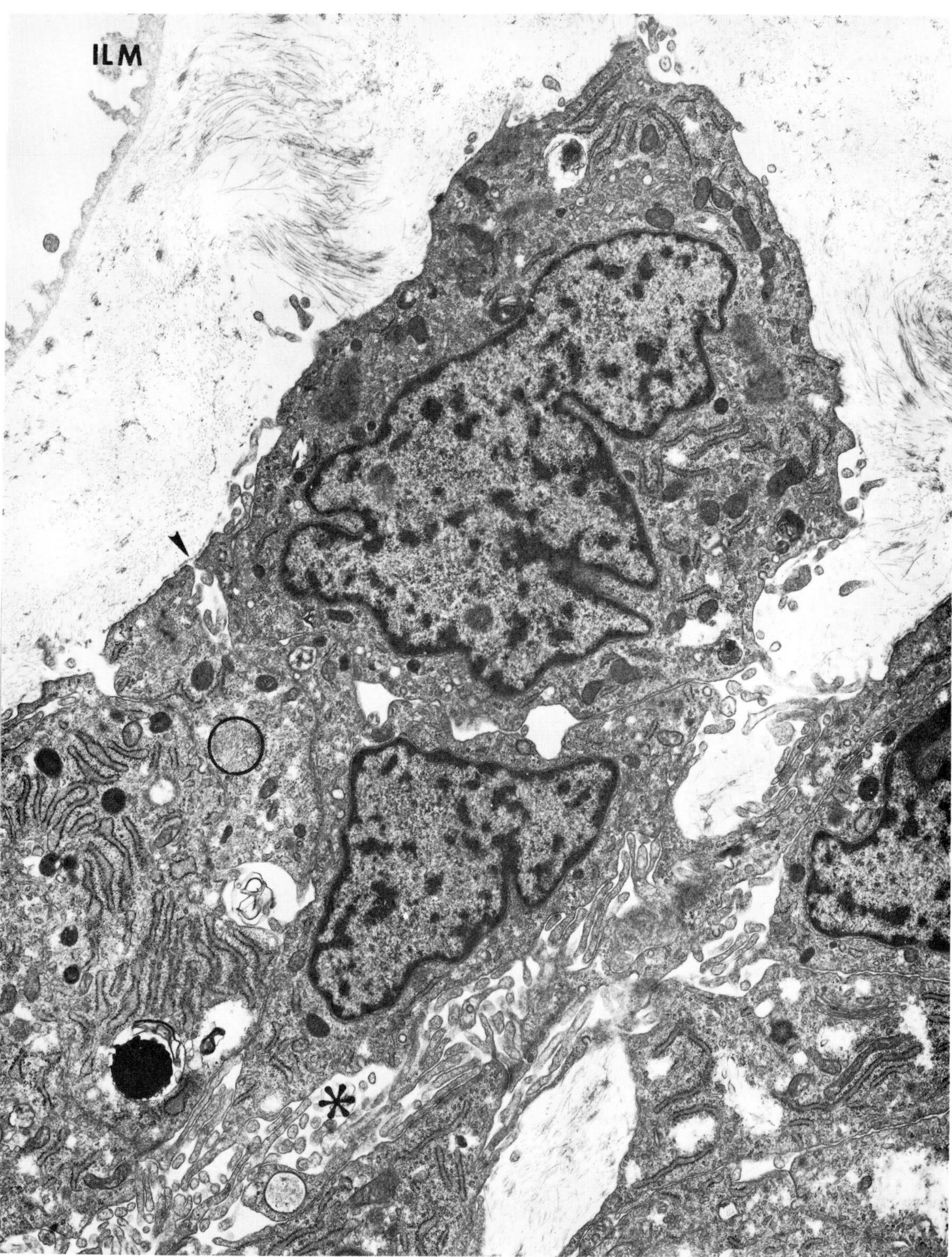

Figure 8–133. Probable retinal pigment epithelium cells of vitreous membrane of massive periretinal proliferation (MPP). Electron micrograph shows segment of internal limiting membrane (ILM) and loose collagenous substance with several epithelioid cells arranged in an acinar configuration, having numerous apical cell processes (asterisk); segments of basement membrane (arrowhead); and small (approximately 50 angstroms in diameter), intracytoplasmic filaments (circle). ×20,000. (From Kampik A, Kenyon KR, Michels RG, et al: Epiretinal and vitreous membranes: A comparative study of 56 cases. Arch. Ophthalmol *99*:1445–1454, 1981.)

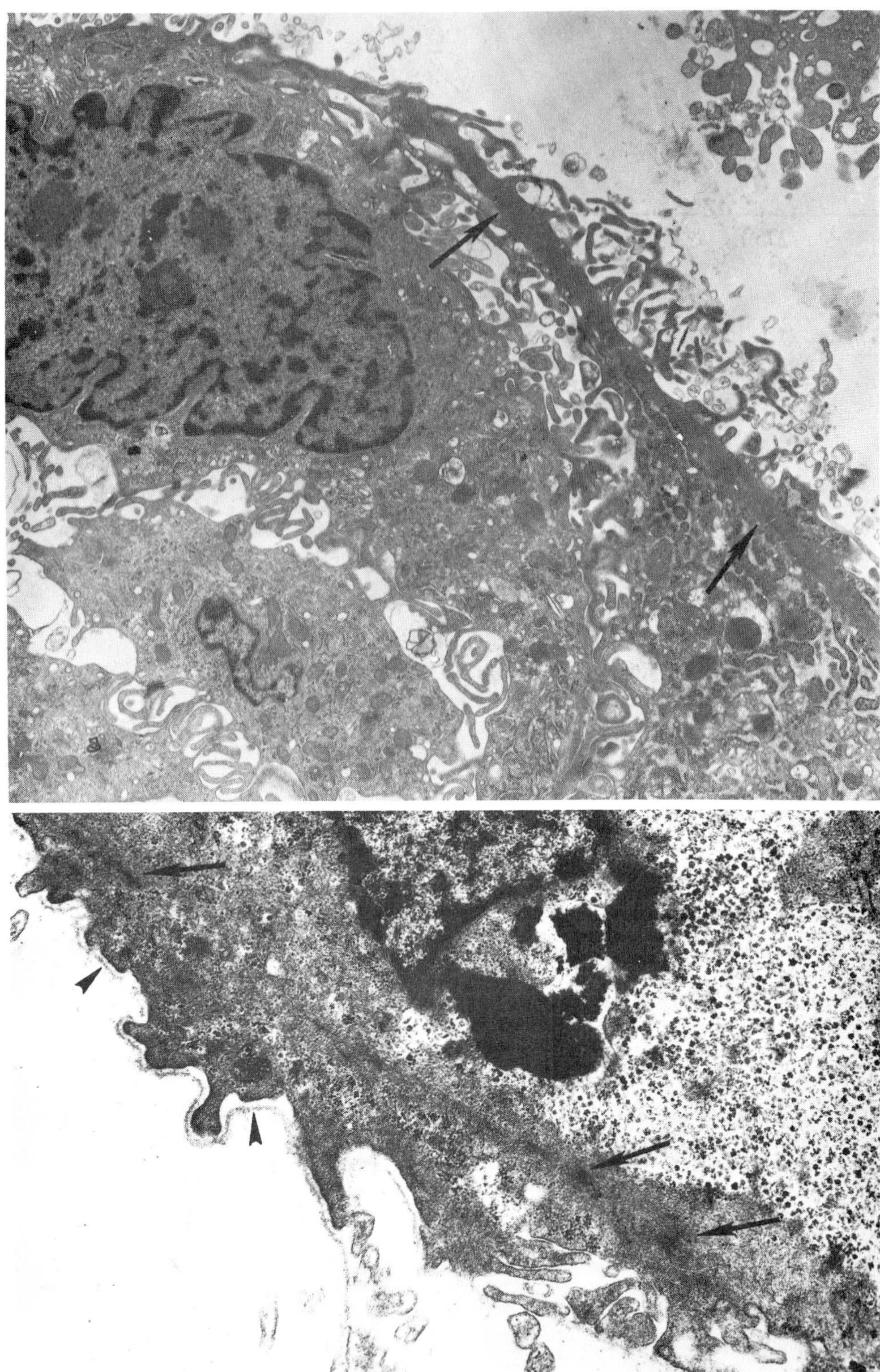

Figure 8–134. Top, **Myofibroblast-like cells** with characteristics of proliferated retinal pigment epithelium cells in massive periretinal proliferation have bands of microfilaments close to their apical surface (arrows). ×10,800. Bottom, Higher magnification of a similar cell shows aggregates of microfilaments with fusiform densities (arrows) close to the basal surface of the cell, which has well-developed basement membrane (arrowheads). ×28,800. (From Kampik A, Kenyon KR, Michels, RG, et al: Epiretinal and vitreous membranes: A comparative study of 56 cases. Arch Ophthalmol *99*:1445–1454, 1981.)

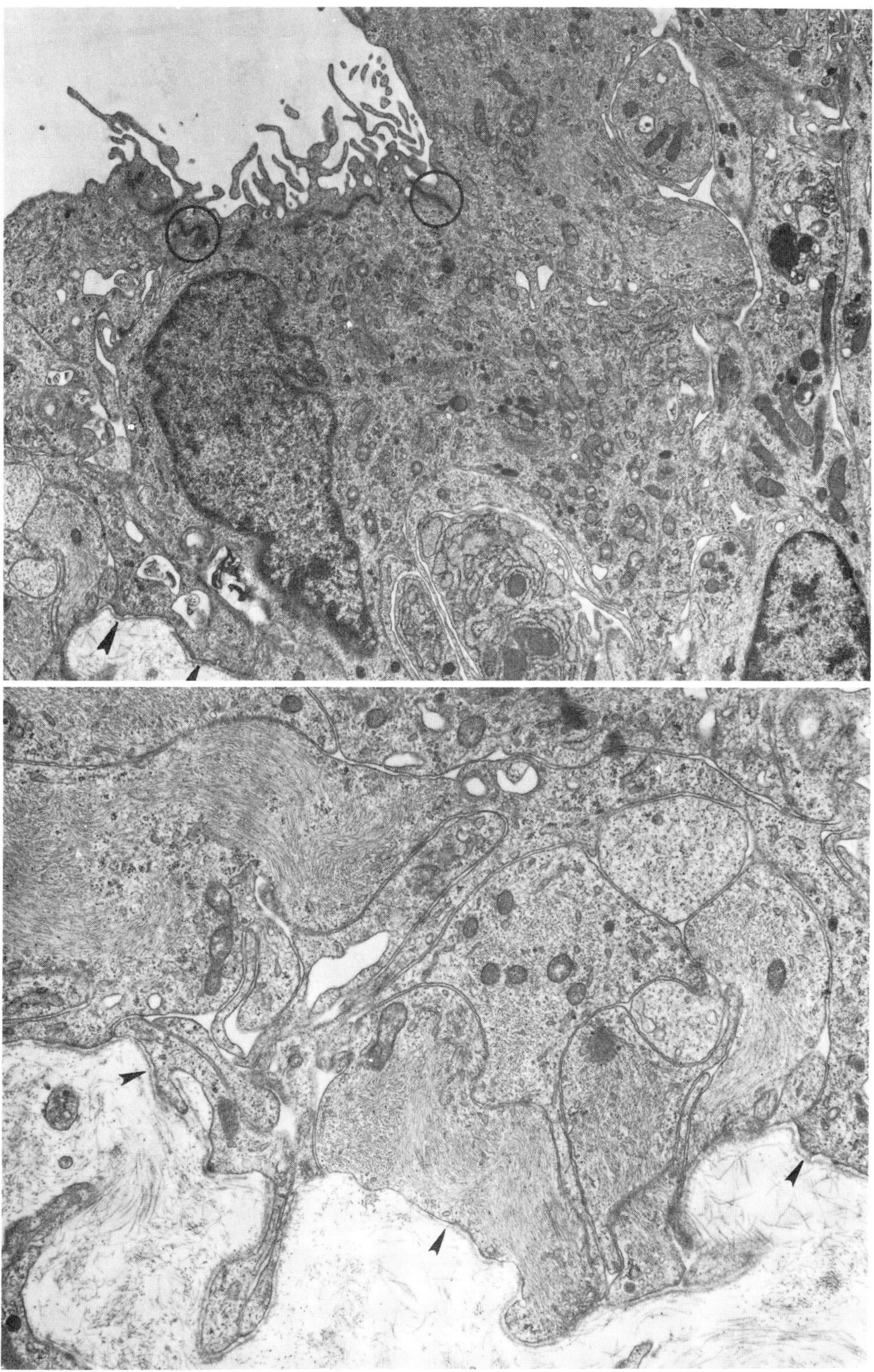

Figure 8–135. Fibrous astrocytes proliferating on the vitreal surface of epiretinal membrane in a case of nonspecific uveitis. Top, Numerous cytoplasmic processes and extracellular basement membrane (arrowheads). Junctional complexes are present (circles). ×7840. Bottom, The distinguishing cytoplasmic feature is the presence of masses of intermediate filaments of approximately 10 nm in diameter and basement membrane (arrowheads). Adjacent collagen fibrils are approximately 23 nm in diameter and therefore represent newly synthesized collagen. ×15,000. (From Kampik A, Kenyon, KR, Michels, RG, et al: Epiretinal and vitreous membranes: A comparative study of 56 cases. Arch Ophthalmol *99*:1445–1454, 1981.)

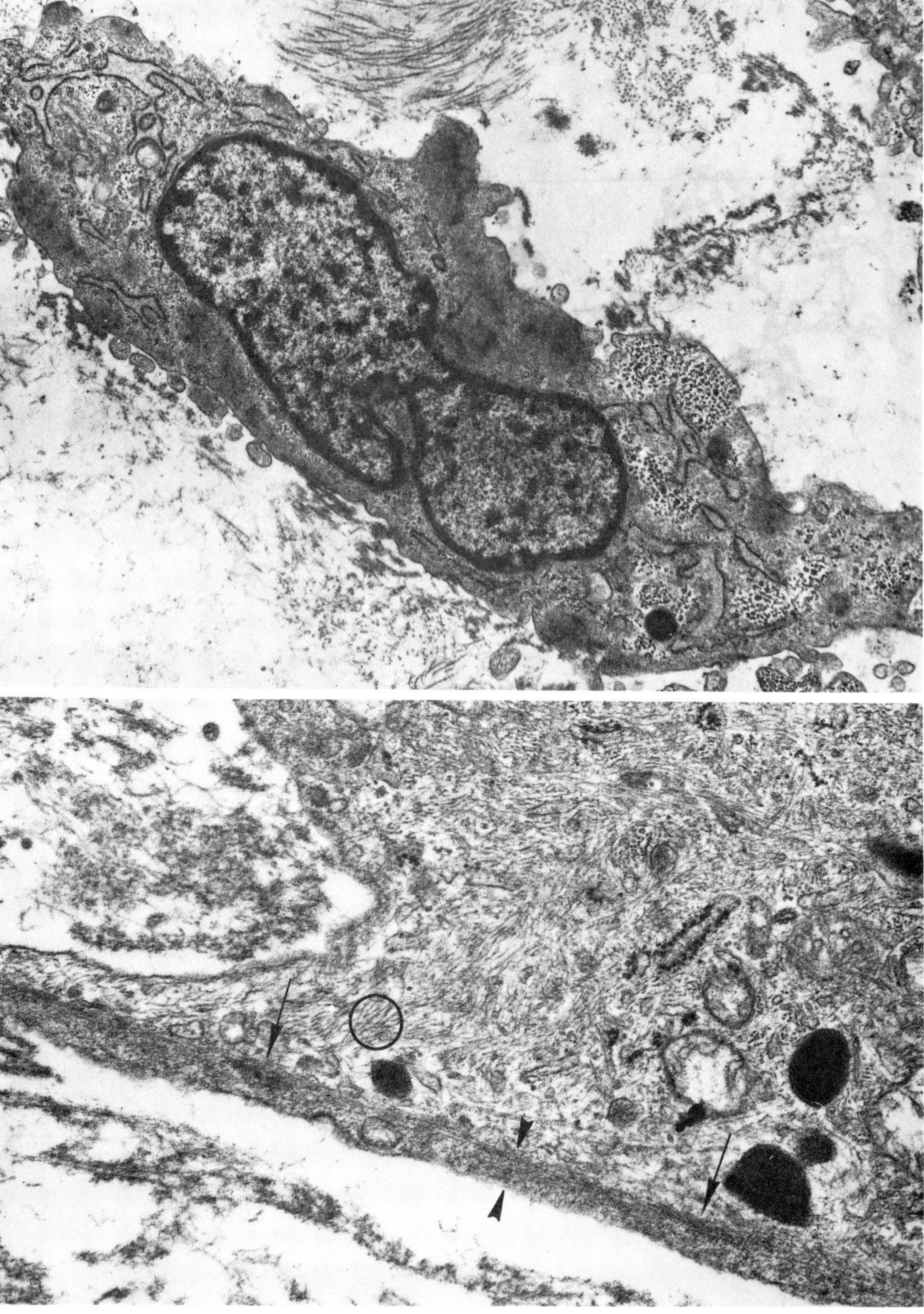

Figure 8–136. Top, **Myofibroblast-like cell in massive periretinal proliferation.** ×12,400. Bottom, Similar cell of same patient, showing myofibroblast-like features with marginally located small filaments (arrowheads) and fusiform density (arrows). The cell also has characteristics of fibrous astrocytes with abundant intracytoplasmic intermediate filaments (circle). ×45,000. (From Kampik A, Kenyon KR, Michels RG, et al: Epiretinal and vitreous membranes: A comparative study of 56 cases. Arch Ophthalmol *99*:1445–1454, 1981.)

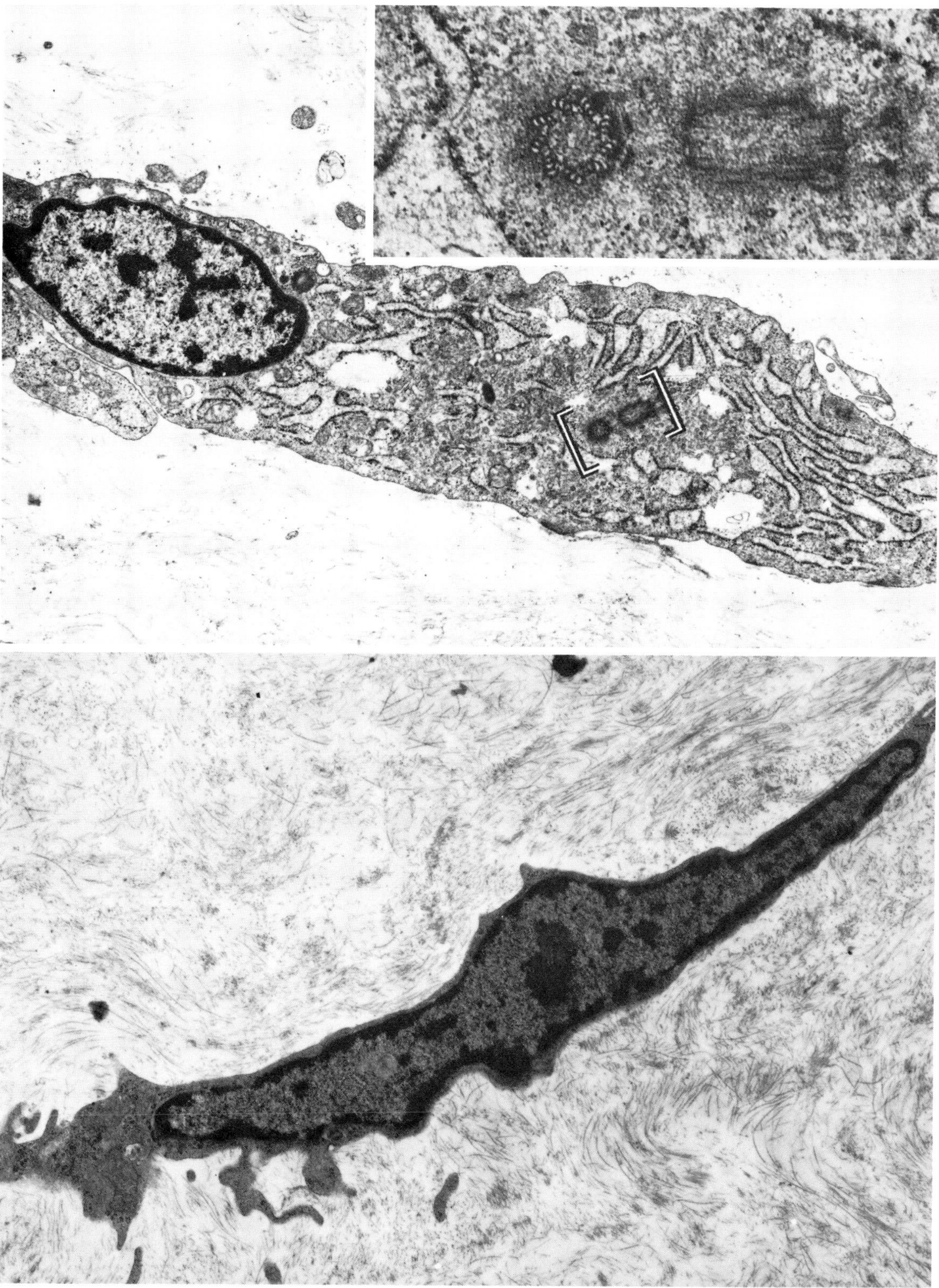

Figure 8–137. Fibrocytes in epiretinal membrane associated with retinal detachment. Top, Identifying characteristics include fusiform configuration of cell, containing numerous profiles of rough-surfaced endoplasmic reticulum and absence of polarity. ×4000. Higher magnification of bracketed area resolves rough and smooth reticulum cisternae, plus prominent centriole (inset, top right, ×45,000). Bottom, Quiescent fibrocyte in collagen matrix. ×11,400. (From Kampik A, Kenyon KR, Michels RG, et al: Epiretinal and vitreous membranes: A comparative study of 56 cases. Arch Ophthalmol *99*:1445–1454, 1981.)

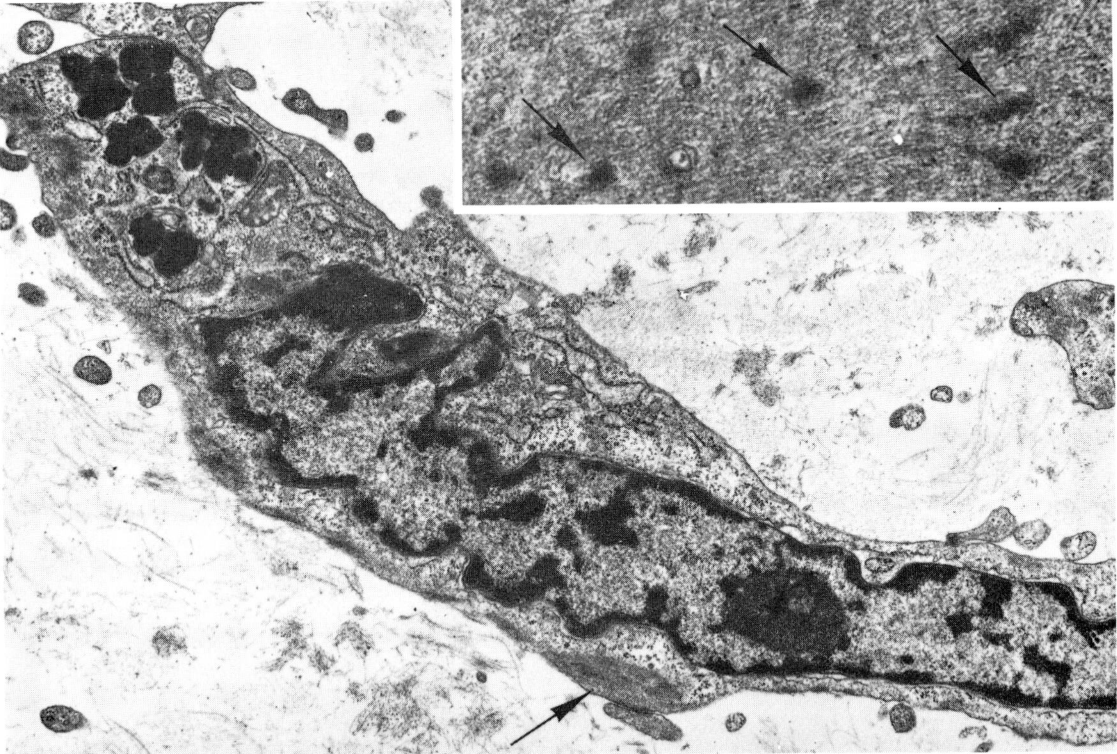

Figure 8–138. Myofibroblast-like cell of vitreous membrane in proliferative diabetic retinopathy. Cell has irregular-shaped nucleus, no polarity, and marginally located aggregates of microfilaments 5 to 7 nm in diameter (arrow). An increased number of lysosomes is observed. Higher magnification of cellular process (inset) shows large aggregations of microfilaments and fusiform densities (arrows) similar to those present in myofibroblasts in granulation tissue. ×12,000; inset, ×41,000. (From Kampik A, Kenyon KR, Michels, RG, et al: Epiretinal and vitreous membranes: A comparative study of 56 cases. Arch Ophthalmol *99*:1445–1454, 1981.)

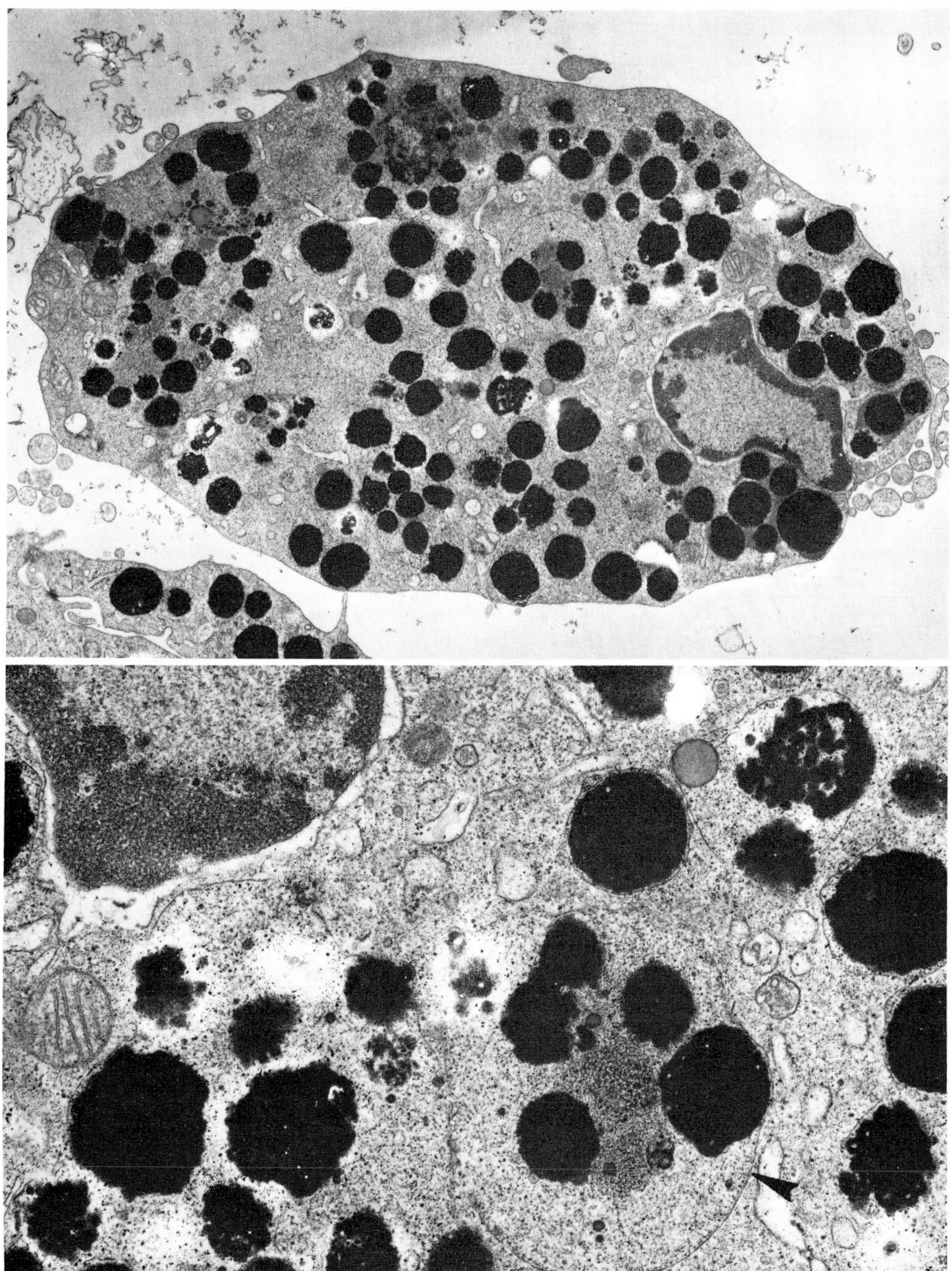

Figure 8–139. Macrophage of epiretinal membrane associated with retinal reattachment surgery. Top, Electron micrograph shows large epithelioid cells containing pigment among other pleomorphic inclusions. ×9350. Bottom, Higher magnification resolves melanin granules, in various stages of degradation, contained within membrane-limited secondary lysosomes (arrowhead) or residual bodies. ×26,500. (From Kampik A, Kenyon, KR, Michels RG, et al: Epiretinal and vitreous membranes: A comparative study of 56 cases. Arch Ophthalmol *99*:1445–1454, 1981.)

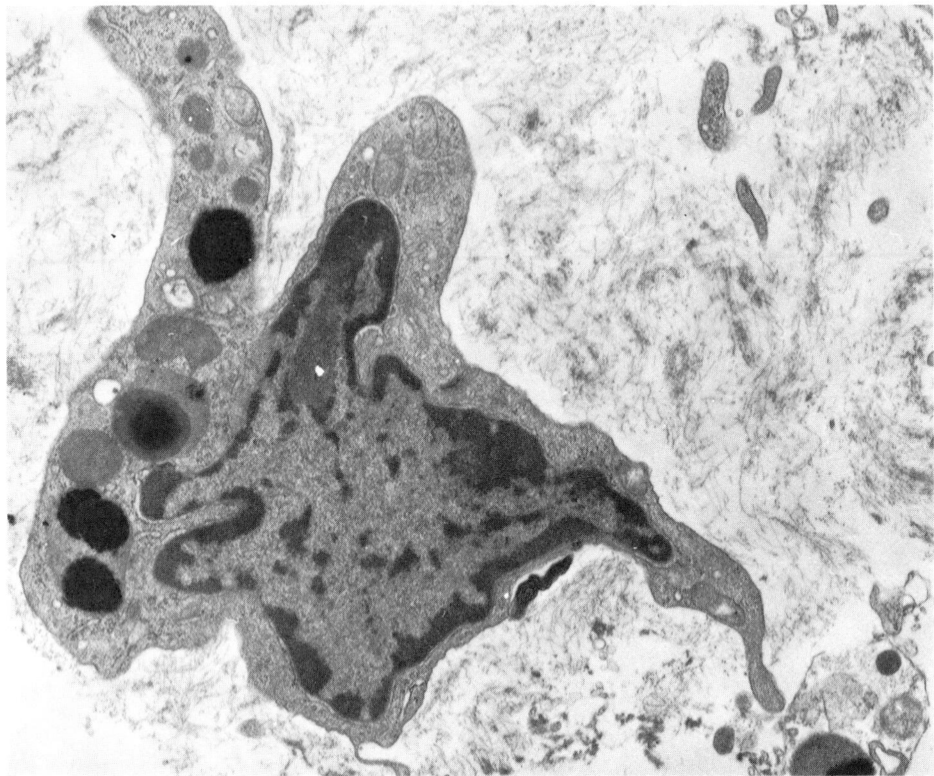

Figure 8–140. Macrophage in massive periretinal proliferation (MPP) with noteworthy irregular shape of cell and nucleus and with membrane-bound granules of varying electron density that may represent a hyalocyte-macrophage. ×7000. (From Kampik A, Kenyon KR, Michels RG, et al: Epiretinal and vitreous membranes: A comparative study of 56 cases. Arch Ophthalmol *99*:1445–1454, 1981.)

iodicity. Since this is nearly twice the diameter of vitreous collagen, it is evident that the cells of these membranes are capable of collagen synthesis, either directly or indirectly.

Kampik, Kenyon, Michels, et al (1980) have presented the ultrastructural findings of 56 epiretinal and vitreous membranes obtained surgically from eyes with various ocular diseases. Five morphologically distinguishable cell types were observed: (1) RPE cells evident only in association with retinal detachment; (2) macrophages; (3) fibrocytes; (4) fibrous astrocytes characteristic

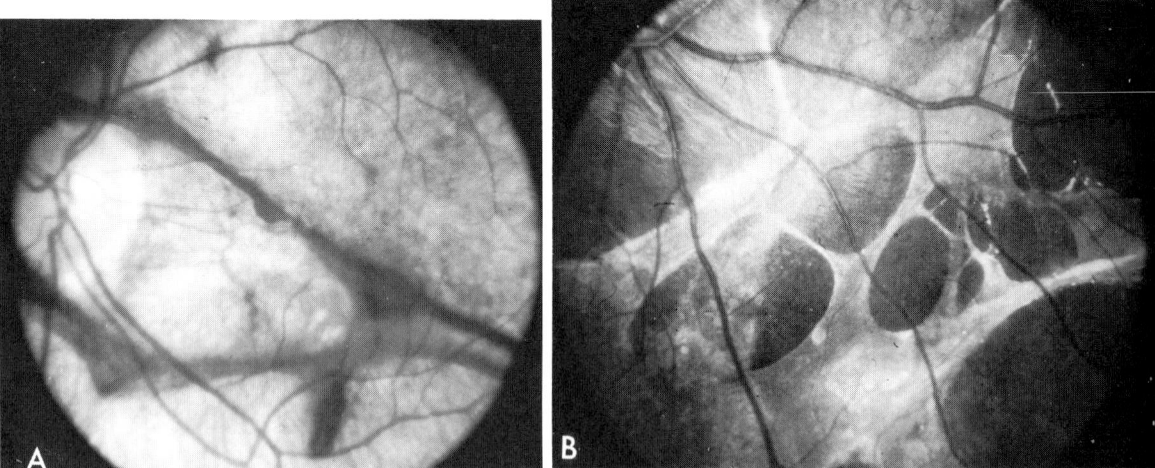

Figure 8–141. *A,* Retroretinal pigmented strands after retinal detachment associated with Harada's disease. *B,* Retroretinal membrane after rhegmatogenous retinal detachment. (From Wallyn RH, Hilton GF: Subretinal fibrosis in retinal detachment. Arch Ophthalmol *97*:2128–2129, 1979.)

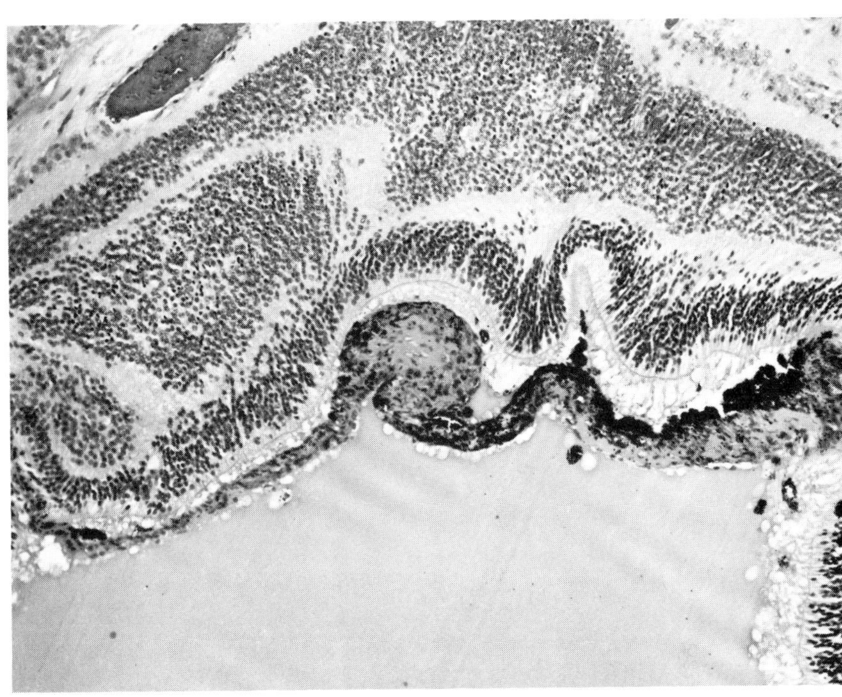

Figure 8–142. Pigmented retroretinal membrane composed of hyperplastic retinal pigment epithelium. H and E, ×110. EP 37591.

of all disease groups; and (5) myofibroblast-like cells that mostly had the characteristics of fibrocytes and occasionally of RPE cells or fibrous astrocytes. The combination of cell types present varies in different types of epiretinal membranes, but the formation of collagen and the development of cells with myofibroblast-like properties are common featues, and they seem to be within the capacity of several cell types. These two common features appear to be the basis for the contractile properties of epiretinal and vitreous membranes.

Retroretinal membranes of both glial and RPE origin may be observed after retinal detachment. At first, the RPE forms a sheet of cells, and then the sheet changes into strands with variable amounts of fibrous tissue (Figs. 8–141 to 8–144). The strands can result in persistent retinal detachment (Fig. 8–145).

Retroretinal membranes have been observed in

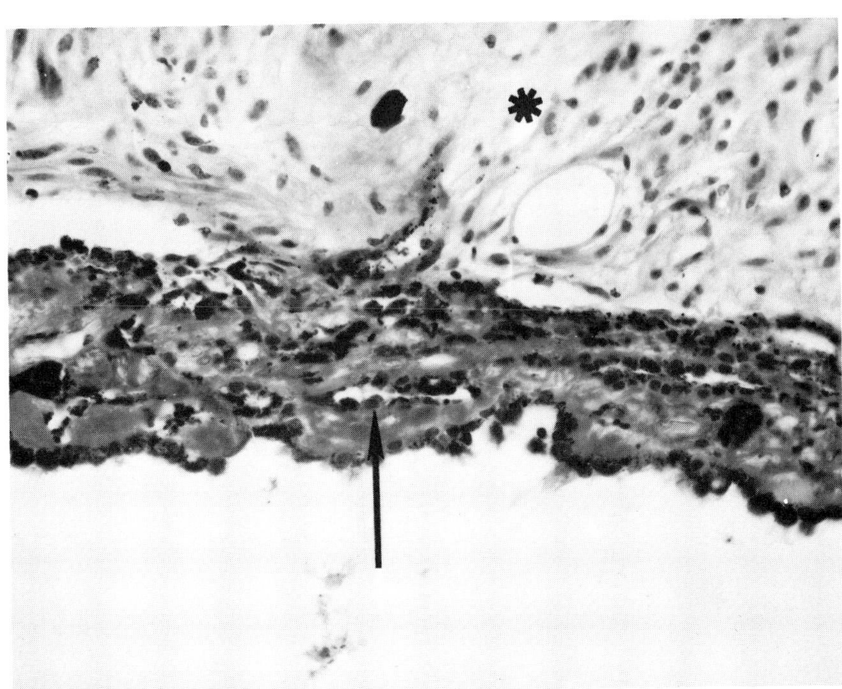

Figure 8–143. Hyperplastic retinal pigment epithelium (arrow) in a characteristic laminated and tubuloacinar pattern on the undersurface of the detached retina (asterisk). Masson, ×310. EP 29082. (From Green WR: Pathology of the Retina, *in* Frayer, WC (ed): Lancaster Course in Ophthalmic Histopathology. Unit 9. Philadelphia, F.A. Davis, 1981.)

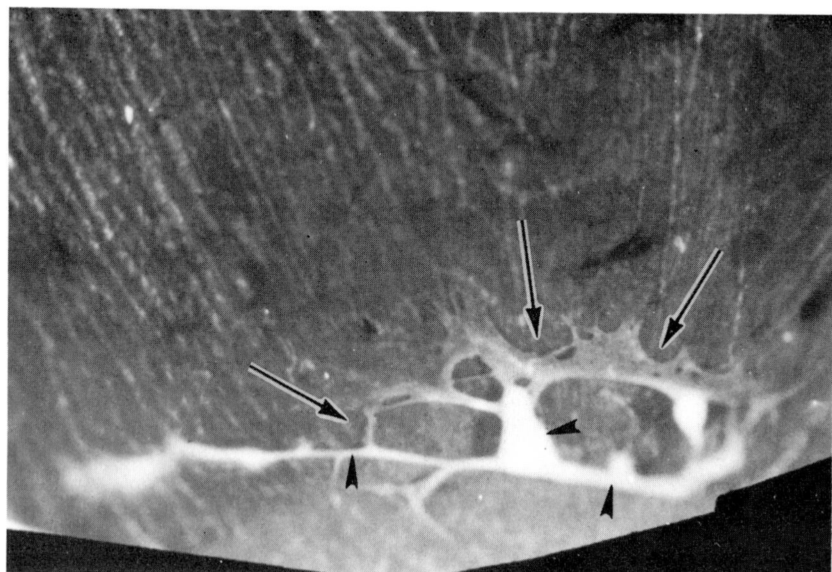

Figure 8–144. View of choroid with retina removed, showing **hyperplastic retinal pigment epithelium (RPE)** in a sheet (arrows) that is continuous with in situ RPE anteriorly and strands of RPE with fibrous tissue (arrowheads) posteriorly. EP 40767.

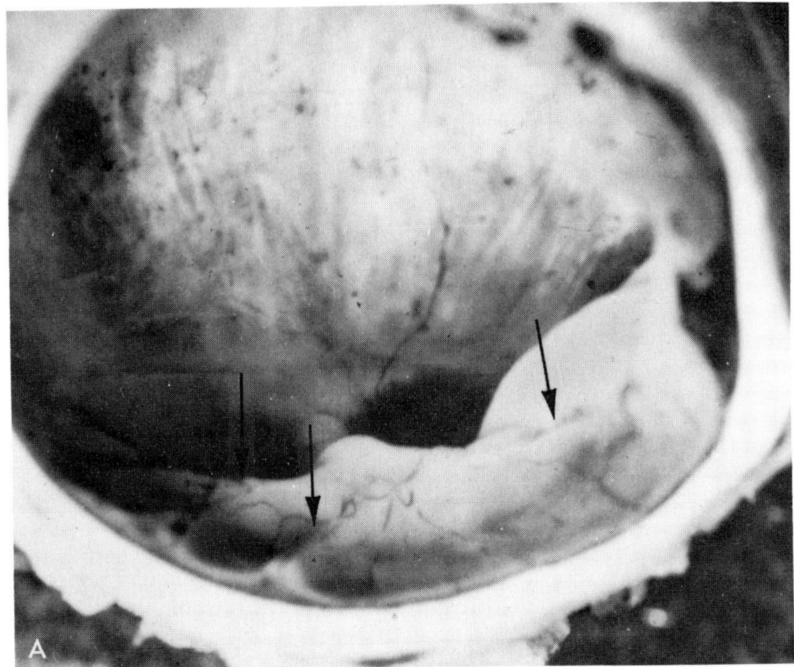

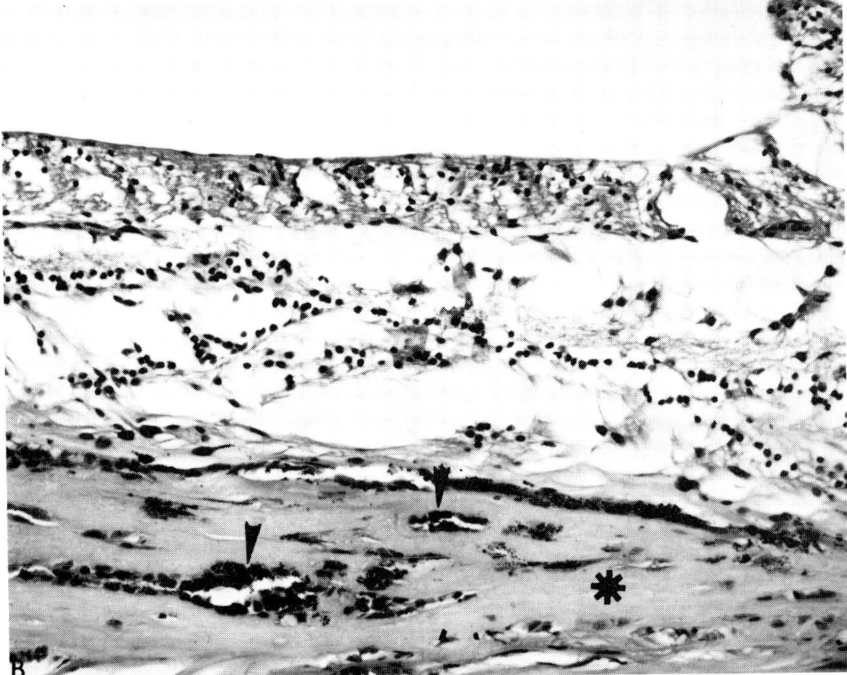

Figure 8–145. *A,* Gross appearance of retina (arrows) being held in a tented-up and detached position by strands of subretinal hyperplastic retinal pigment epithelium (RPE) with a fibrous tissue component in an eye after a perforating injury. *B,* Retroretinal strand of hyperplastic RPE (asterisk) has a laminated and tubuloacinar (arrowheads) pattern and has a rich interspersion of collagenous tissue. H and E, ×180. EP 37590.

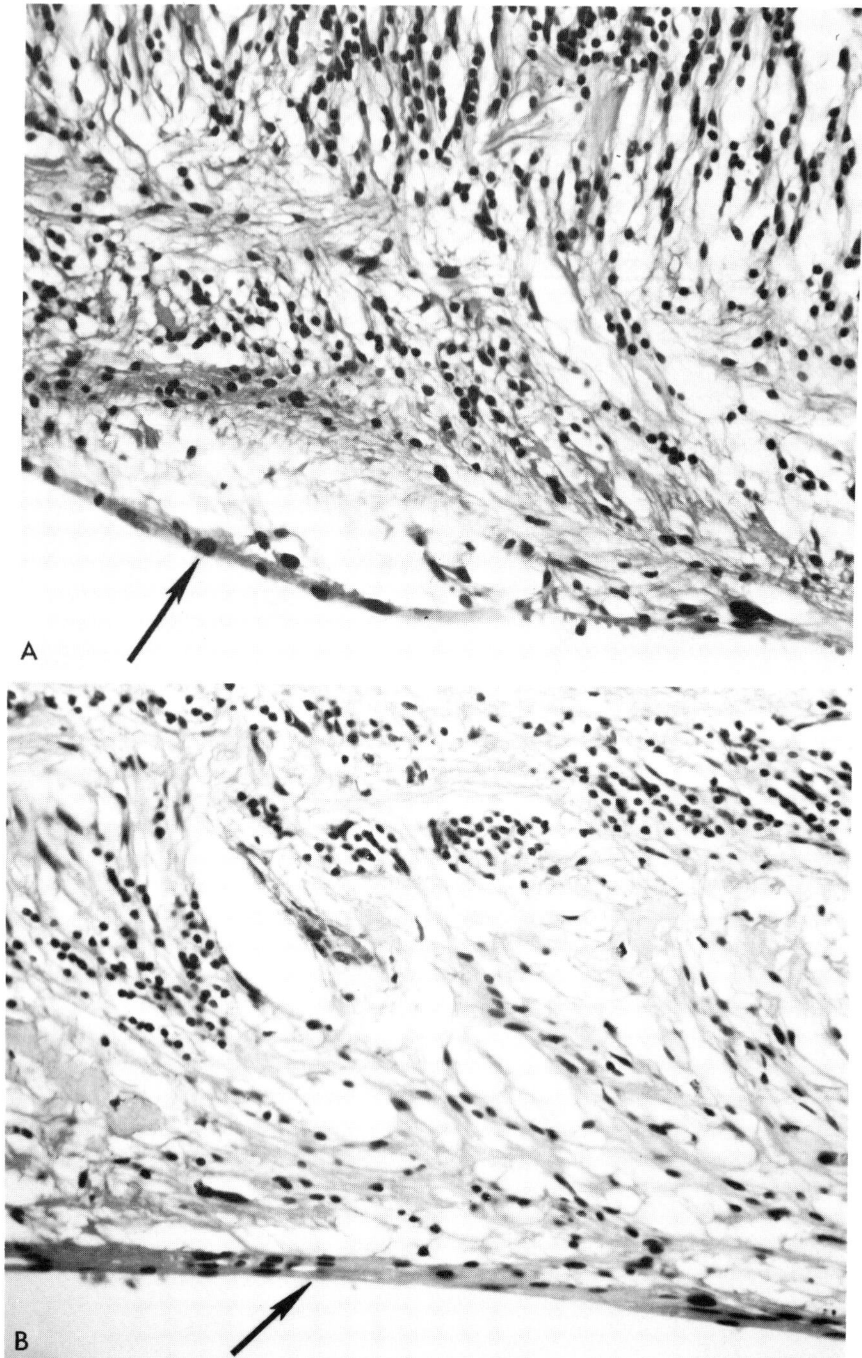

Figure 8–146. Retroretinal membrane of glial cell origin. *A,* Thin layer of glial cells (arrow) lining the undersurface of the detached retina in an eye with numerous sequelae of chronic nongranulomatous uveitis. H and E, ×310. EP 38108. *B,* Multilayered fibroglial retroretinal membrane (arrow) in the eye with end-stage changes of retrolental fibroplasia. H and E, ×300.

3 per cent of 629 consecutive retinal detachment cases (Wallyn, Hilton, 1979). The incidence varied in a linear fashion with the duration of the detachment, varying from 0.8 per cent in cases less than 1 month old to 22 per cent in cases estimated to be more than 2 years old. Retroretinal membranes of glial origin may be seen in long-standing retinal detachment (Fig. 8–146).

INFLAMMATORY DISEASES AND CONDITIONS

This section deals primarily with those inflammatory conditions of the retina that are caused by infectious agents or parasites. These may arise as a primary disease during the course of a systemic infection by endogenous metastasis to the eye or by extension of disease from other parts of the eye or orbit. Those originating in the retina may remain localized to this tissue as a small or large focus that eventually heals after producing more or less destruction of the retinal tissue, or they may spread to involve the vitreous, optic nerve, and uveal tract. This wider spread generally produces an endophthalmitis or a panophthalmitis. If an exogenous inflammation becomes localized in the posterior eye, a vitreous abscess may be formed (metastatic ophthalmia). The etiology and general course of these more widespread inflammations have been discussed in some detail in Chapter 2.

Prior to discussion of specific inflammatory diseases, the general pathology of retinal inflammations is briefly considered.

Most inflammations involve a vascular response similar to that seen in other inflamed tissues (see Chapter 1). The vascular response to the initiating agent produces vasodilation and margination and migration of white blood cells into the tissues. Soon the perivascular area shows an accumulation of white cells that forms sheathlike "cuffs" around the vessels. Fluid also leaks from the lumen of the vessel into the perivascular space, displacing the glial and neuronal tissues and leading to a variable amount of degeneration, depending on the intensity of the response. Edema soon follows, with localization of protein-rich fluid in the tissues around the blood vessels, and fluid gradually diffuses into adjacent nonvascular areas and accumulates in large pools.

With sufficient inflammation, the products of the inflammatory process and pressure exerted by the fluid soon lead to degeneration of retinal elements, producing large spaces containing cellular debris, fibrin, inflammatory cells, and lipid derived from degenerating retinal cells and from the blood. Macrophages from the tissues and blood stream accumulate in the cavities and become filled with debris and lipid from the degenerating retinal cells and serum. These macrophages soon depart from the foci via the blood stream, or they disintegrate in situ. Absorption of fluid from the extravasated material in the tissue spaces leads to coagulation of the solid elements, producing the ophthalmoscopic picture of "hard exudates."

Hemorrhage may occur in the vessel layers. Most often, small linear hemorrhages are in the nerve fiber or inner retinal layers. Larger, round hemorrhages extend into the outer retinal layers or break through the ILM. Persistence or recurrence of such hemorrhages leads to additional necrosis and inflammation, followed by repair, scarring, and deformity.

The neurons respond to the inflammatory process mainly by degeneration of the axons and dendrites and by swelling of the cell bodies followed by disintegration of the cytoplasm and nucleus. Glial cells respond in a similar manner. Some of the macrophages seen in inflammatory processes are derived from pre-existing cells located in the retinal tissues; they are known as microglial phagocytes. Surrounding the affected zones is early and rapid proliferation of the astrocytes, producing the condition known as retinal gliosis. If the inflammatory process is severe, there is usually some occlusion of affected vessels surrounding or within the zone.

If infarction occurs from occlusion of arterioles, necrosis occurs in the axons of the nerve fiber layer, leading to the production of "cotton-wool patches." These cotton-wool patches are composed of swollen nerve fiber axons—the result of obstruction of axoplasmic flow. Histologically, the patches are known as cytoid bodies.

Healing occurs by removal of edema fluid through adjacent vessels and removal of degenerated cells and other debris by the macrophages. Subsequent proliferation of connective tissue elements occurs from around the blood vessels, as well as from the glia from the inner retinal layers, and these elements are incorporated into a fibroglial scar. Organization and contraction of the scar leads to distortion and folding of the retina; and changes may occur in the RPE. If the inflammation is severe, the RPE is destroyed, and the pigment granules are phagocytosed by adjacent cells or by macrophages, which tend to migrate into the retina and localize around the scar and in the perivascular areas. Adjacent RPE cells often undergo hypertrophy and hyperplasia to form clumps, which are commonly seen ophthalmoscopically and microscopically around chorioretinal scars. The proliferation of these cells and alteration of their shape to a spindle form may produce large, heavily pigmented, tumor-like masses between the retina and choroid.

Damage to and loss of the ILM near the focus of inflammation leads to accumulation of cells and fluid on the inner surface of the retina and in the nearby vitreous. New capillaries bud from the retinal vessels and invade this exudate. Eventually, a thin vascular scar may line the retina and extend into the vitreous, producing changes known as retinitis proliferans. Most inflammations that affect the retina involve the adjacent choroid, and the healing process eventually leads to fusion of the outer limiting membrane of the retina to the lamina vitrea of the choroid. In such areas, the RPE is missing centrally but has proliferated toward the periphery of the inflammatory process. If the lamina vitrea has been destroyed, a dense scar unites the choroidal stroma to the retina.

Old chorioretinal scars, therefore, show moderate-to-severe damage in the retina, with loss of neural and supporting cells. The choroid shows a loss of Bruch's membrane and blood vessels. The normal structures are replaced by a dense connective tissue scar containing variable amounts of pigment that unites these two structures. Hyaline and calcareous degeneration is common, especially around the vessels.

Inflammation of the retina can be generally classified into primary and secondary. The primary infections often are endogenous and they lead to an acute suppurative process which either is localized or becomes diffuse. They also can be rather mild and be localized and surrounded by hemorrhage. Such white-centered hemorrhages are due to a septic embolus and are referred to as *Roth spots* (Roth, 1872) (see Fig. 8–90).

Secondary infections most often are of exogenous origin or are endogenous by extension from the anterior portion of the eye or through the optic nerve or uveal tract.

Secondary inflammations also can occur from chorioretinal inflammations in which the primary condition is in the choroid and extends internally to the retina. Frequently, the retinal inflammation is secondary to disease of the anterior eye, especially pars planitis (peripheral uveitis, chronic cyclitis), iridocyclitis associated with joint diseases, or iridocyclitis of unknown origin. In inflammations of the latter types, there is a tendency for macular and peripapillary retinal edema to occur. Chronic cystoid macular edema can lead to macular cyst and lamellar or complete hole formation.

Acute Septic Retinitis

Endogenous purulent retinitis may develop during any systemic bacterial infection, such as puerperal sepsis, meningococcemia, and gonococcal, *Hemophilus,* streptococcal, and other bacterial infections. The process usually leads rapidly to an endophthalmitis. Such ocular complications have been much less frequent since the advent of antibiotic therapy. The inflammatory process may be localized, or it can spread rapidly and lead to severe necrosis of the retina and its blood vessels, with secondary hemorrhage. In the early stages, the retina is edematous. The vessels are congested, and there is intense perivasculitis; a seropurulent exudate forms within and under the sensory retina. The optic nerve and vitreous rapidly become infiltrated with purulent exudate in which organisms can be demonstrated. The eventual outcome of such infections is discussed in Chapter 2.

In a clinical study of patients with septicemia and positive blood cultures, Meyers (1979) found that 18 (20 per cent) had retinal lesions, 12 had cotton-wool lesions, 7 had hemorrhages, and 3 had white-centered hemorrhages.

Embolic retinitis is an embolic infection of the retinal blood vessels occurring in septicemia from various causes. White-centered retinal hemorrhages (Roth's spots) are seen in the retina and represent an area of infarction of the nerve fiber layer, with resulting retinal edema and necrosis. Septic emboli lead to disruption of the vessel walls and hemorrhage, with a central area of bac-

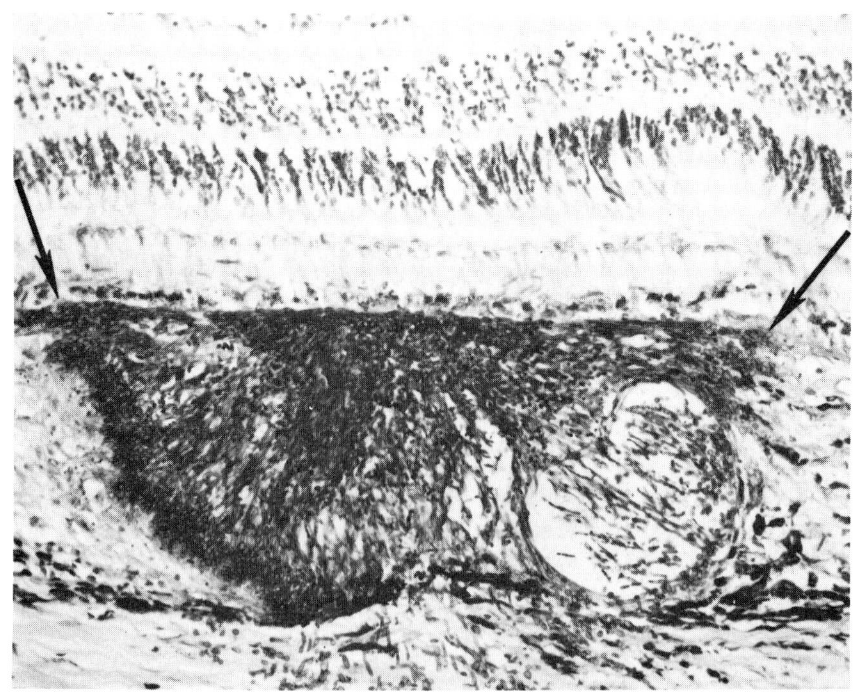

Figure 8–147. *Candida* choroiditis in a 16 year old female who died of acute leukemia. A large cluster of budding yeast with pseudohyphae is present in the choroid (between arrows). PAS, ×200. EP 40937.

terial and neutrophilic infiltration. The lesion may heal without spreading to other areas, or it may extend into the vitreous and produce a suppurative endophthalmitis. Embolic retinitis is seen characteristically in subacute bacterial endocarditis caused by embolization of infected vegetation from one of the cardiac valves.

Candida Retinitis and Vitritis

Septicemia from *Candida albicans* occurs in persons with debilitating diseases who are receiving chemotherapeutic or immunosuppressive drugs and long-term intravenous feeding. It can occur also after gastrointestinal trauma and antibiotic therapy. It is increasingly seen in drug abusers. *Candida* organisms can lodge at almost any point in the uveal tract (Fig. 8–147) and retina (Fig. 8–148). Characteristically, however, patients develop fluffy, whitish-yellow, nondiscrete retinal lesions, which usually extend into the vitreous cavity (Figs. 8–149 through 8–151) (Edwards, Foos, Montgomerie, Guze, 1974; Clarkson, Green, 1976; Thomas, Green, 1979). One or more vitre-

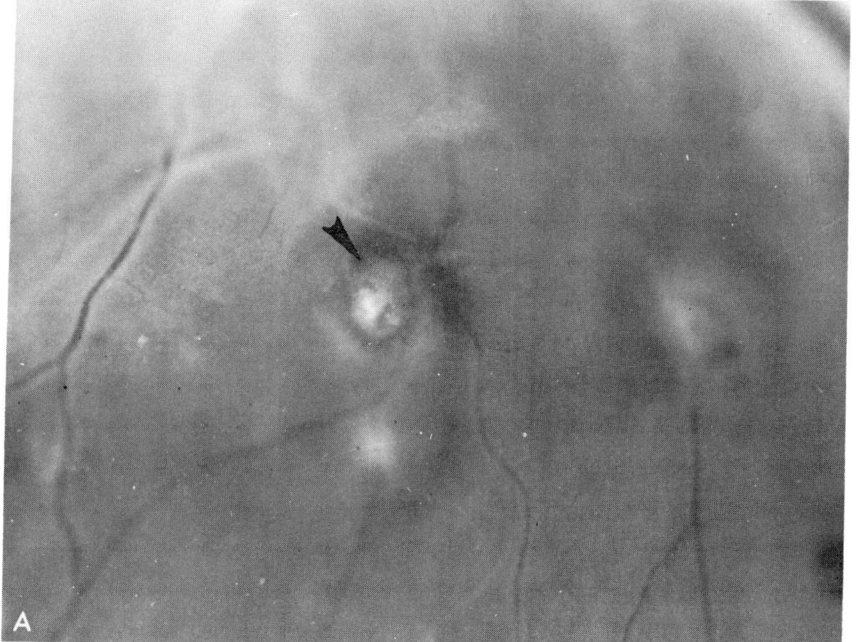

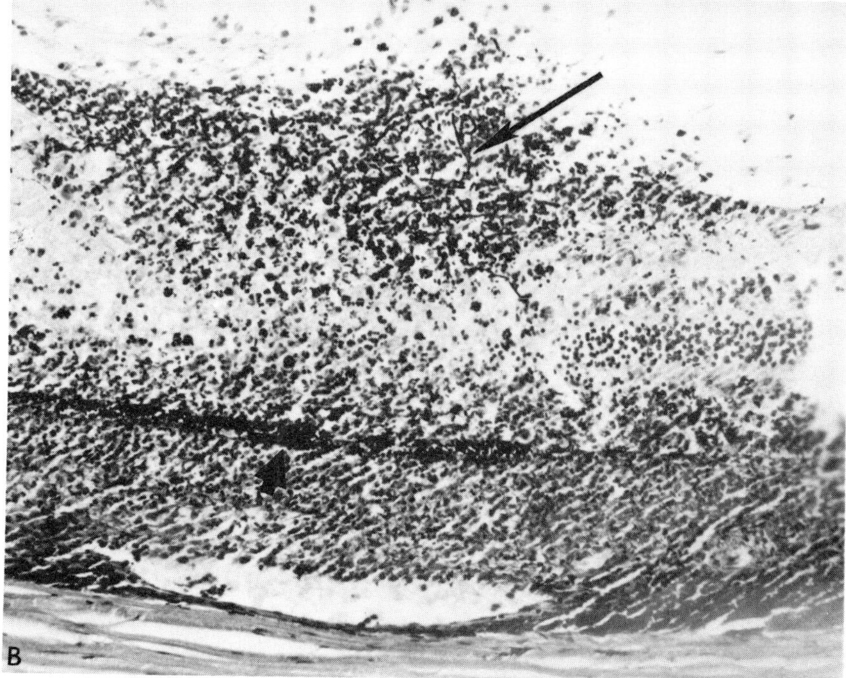

Figure 8–148. *Candida* retinitis in 60 year old man after gastrointestinal surgery. *A,* Gross appearance of three foci of *Candida* retinitis—one is a white-centered hemorrhage (arrowhead). *B,* Section through white-centered hemorrhage shows organisms in the inner aspect of the retina, with extension into vitreous (narrow arrow), and in the region of the choriocapillaris. An intense, acute inflammatory cell infiltration is present in the retina and subjacent choroid (broad arrow). PAS, ×160. EP 29370. (From Michelson PE, Stark WJ, Reeser F, Green WR: Endogenous candida endophthalmitis: Report of 13 cases and review of the literature. Int Ophthalmol Clin 2:125–147, 1971.)

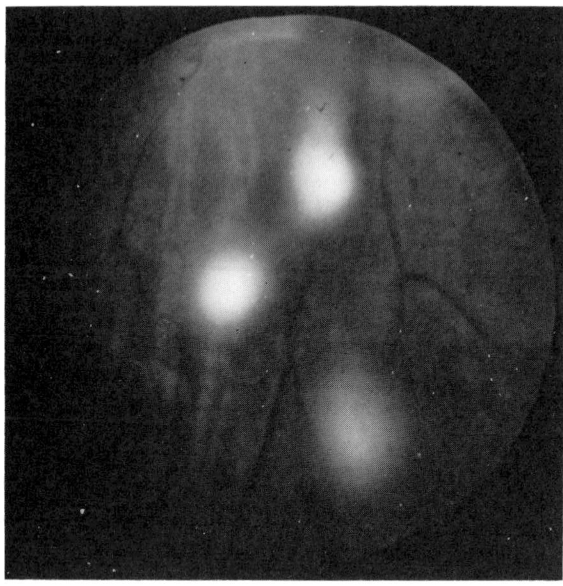

Figure 8–149. ***Candida* vitritis and retinitis** in a 16 year old girl with Crohn's disease. (From Murray HW, Knox DL, Green, WR, Susel RM: Cytomegalovirus retinitis in adults. A manifestation of disseminated viral infections. Am J Med *63*:574–584, 1977.)

ous abscesses at or near the retina may be the main feature. Inflammatory precipitates may be observed along retinal veins. Inflammatory signs in the vitreous and anterior segment of the eye are usually prominent.

Candida endophthalmitis can be successfully treated with amphotericin B (Michelson, Stark, Reeser, Green, 1971). Some cases may resolve with therapy, but with the evolution of fibrous tissue and traction retinal detachment (Fig. 8–150).

Pars plana vitrectomy has been successfully employed in both diagnosis and therapy of *Candida* endophthalmitis (Fig. 8–151) (Snip, Michels, 1976).

Cryptococcus neoformans has an affinity for neural tissues, and the central nervous system is a principal site of infection. Endogenous spread to the eye occurs in some instances and may lead to endophthalmitis (Hiles, Font, 1968; Clarkson, Green, 1976). Localization within the retina has been observed in several instances and may be seen as small, fluffy white lesions or large, fairly discrete infiltrates. The organisms are located in the retina, and the inflammatory reaction may be minimal (Fig. 8–152) (Khodadoust, Payne, 1969), partly because of immunosuppressive agents or chemotherapy. The choroid may also be the site of involvement (Avendano, Tanishima, Kuwabara, 1978).

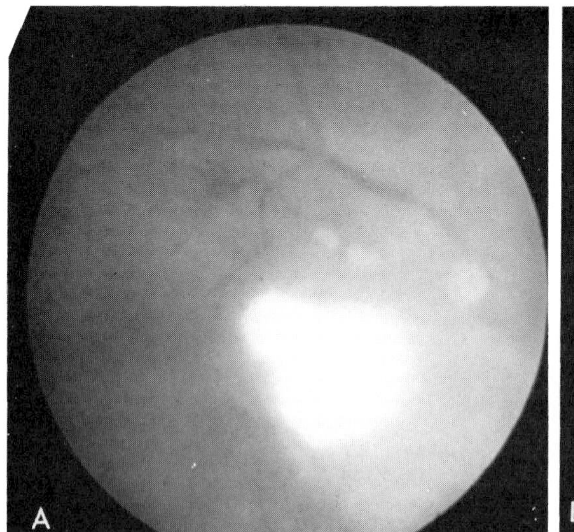

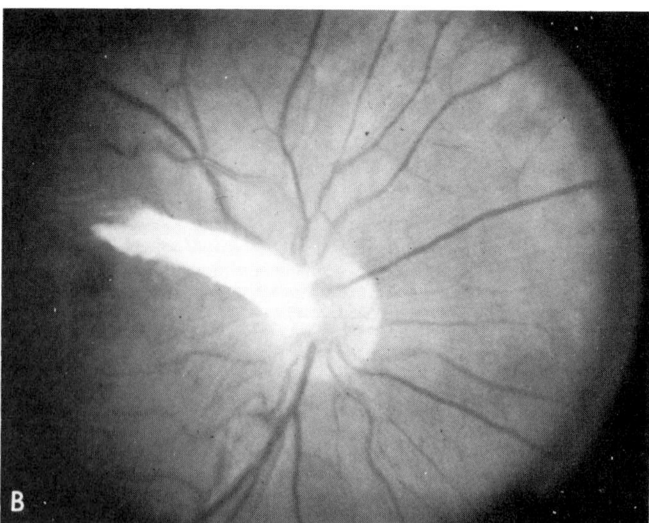

Figure 8–150. ***Candida* retinitis and vitritis** after partial gastrectomy. *A*, Appearance of lesion on presentation. *B*, Resolution of the infection with amphotericin-B therapy, and evolution of a discrete strand of fibrous connective tissue, which is exerting traction on the macular retina. (Courtesy of Dr. R.G. Michels.)

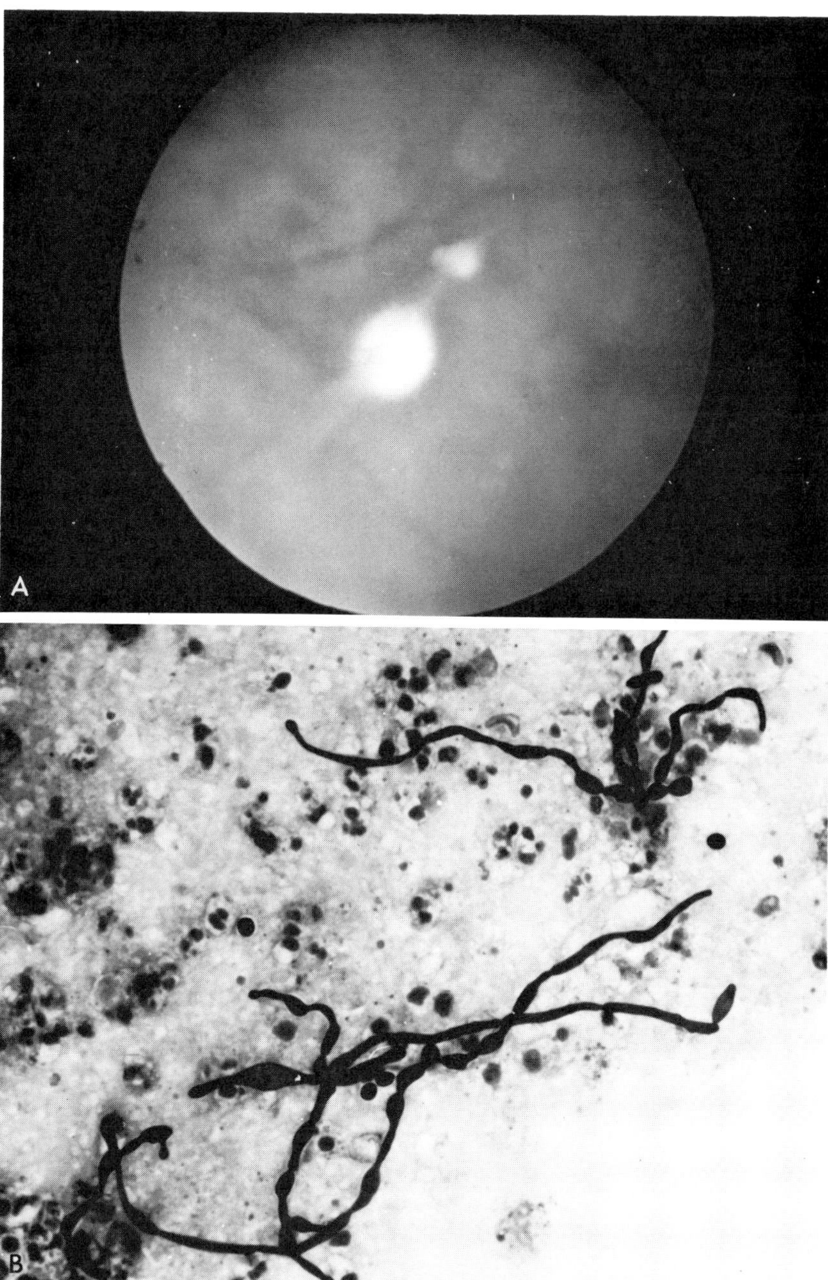

Figure 8–151. ***Candida* endophthalmitis** in a 27 year old drug addict. *A,* Two fluffy white vitreous opacities that taper toward the retina. *B,* Pars plana vitrectomy specimen with pseudohyphae and budding blastospores characteristic of *Candida* species. PAS, ×900. EP 40478. (From Snip RC, Michels RG: Pars plana vitrectomy in the management of endogenous *Candida* endophthalmitis. Am J Ophthalmol *82*:699–704, 1976.)

Other fungi also can produce retinitis, but usually, as in the case of *Aspergillus,* it rapidly evolves to the picture of extensive endophthalmitis. Endogenous *Aspergillus* retinitis and endophthalmitis may occur in immunosuppressed individuals (Figs. 8–153 and 8–154) (Naidoff, Green, 1975) and drug abusers (Doft, Clarkson, Rebell, Forster, 1980; Sugar, Mandell, Shalev, 1971).

The first eye with *Aspergillus* endophthalmitis that was salvaged was treated by pars plana vitrectomy and systemic therapy (Doft and coworkers, 1980). An additional case has been observed (Fig. 8–155).

Chronic Bacterial Retinitis

Tuberculosis. Tuberculosis of the retina may occur from endogenous spread from a primary focus in the lungs or elsewhere in the body. The inflammatory process commences in the vessel layers of the retina. Tuberculosis also may occur in the retina by spreading from the uveal tract. In general, the metastatic lesion in the retina is either of a miliary type, in which there is tubercle formation that remains as a small focus and eventually heals, or it is a massive retinitis, which has the clinical features of heavy vitreous opacification and an extensive gray-white lesion involving

Text continued on page 740

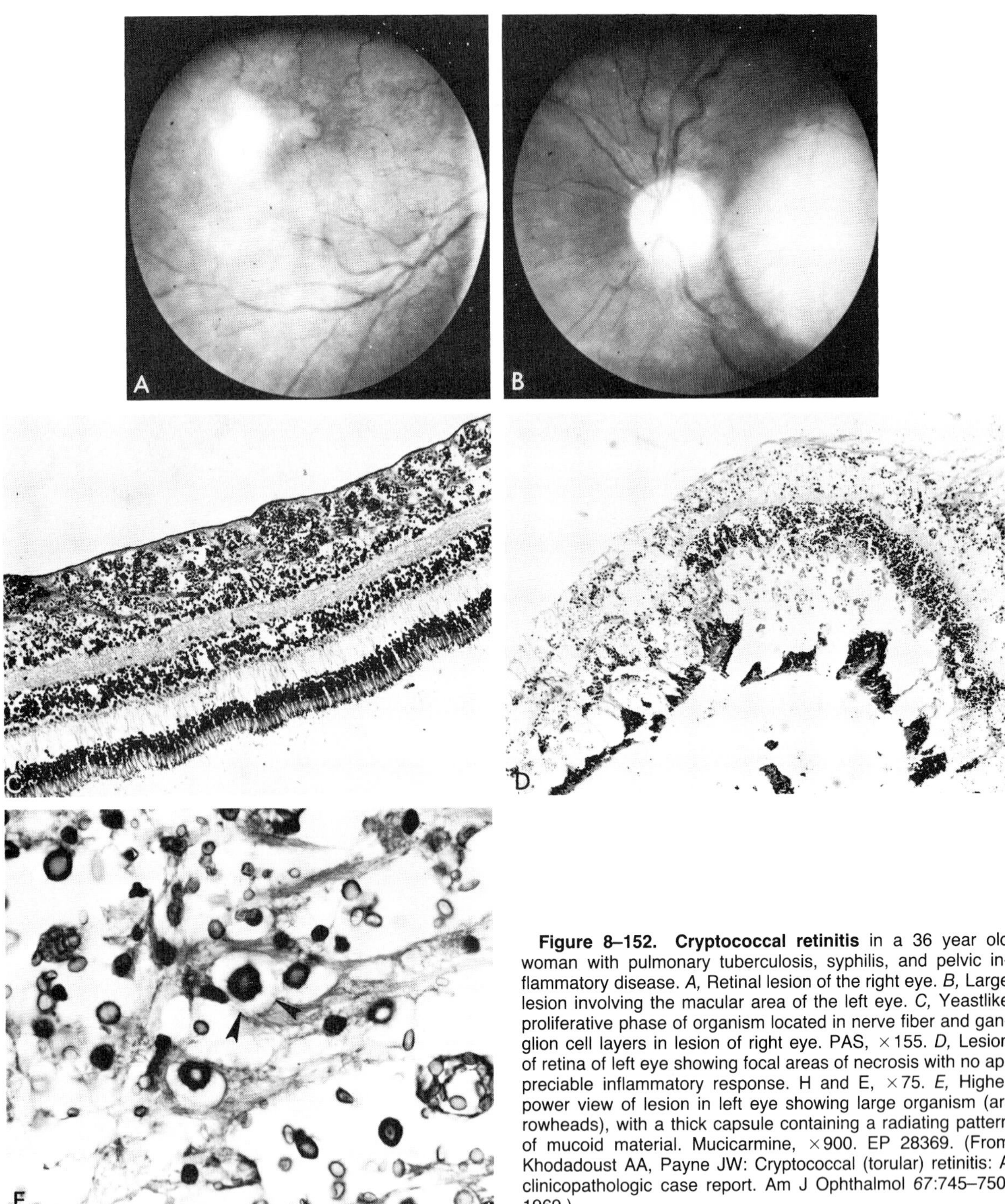

Figure 8–152. Cryptococcal retinitis in a 36 year old woman with pulmonary tuberculosis, syphilis, and pelvic inflammatory disease. *A,* Retinal lesion of the right eye. *B,* Large lesion involving the macular area of the left eye. *C,* Yeastlike proliferative phase of organism located in nerve fiber and ganglion cell layers in lesion of right eye. PAS, ×155. *D,* Lesion of retina of left eye showing focal areas of necrosis with no appreciable inflammatory response. H and E, ×75. *E,* Higher power view of lesion in left eye showing large organism (arrowheads), with a thick capsule containing a radiating pattern of mucoid material. Mucicarmine, ×900. EP 28369. (From Khodadoust AA, Payne JW: Cryptococcal (torular) retinitis: A clinicopathologic case report. Am J Ophthalmol *67*:745–750, 1969.)

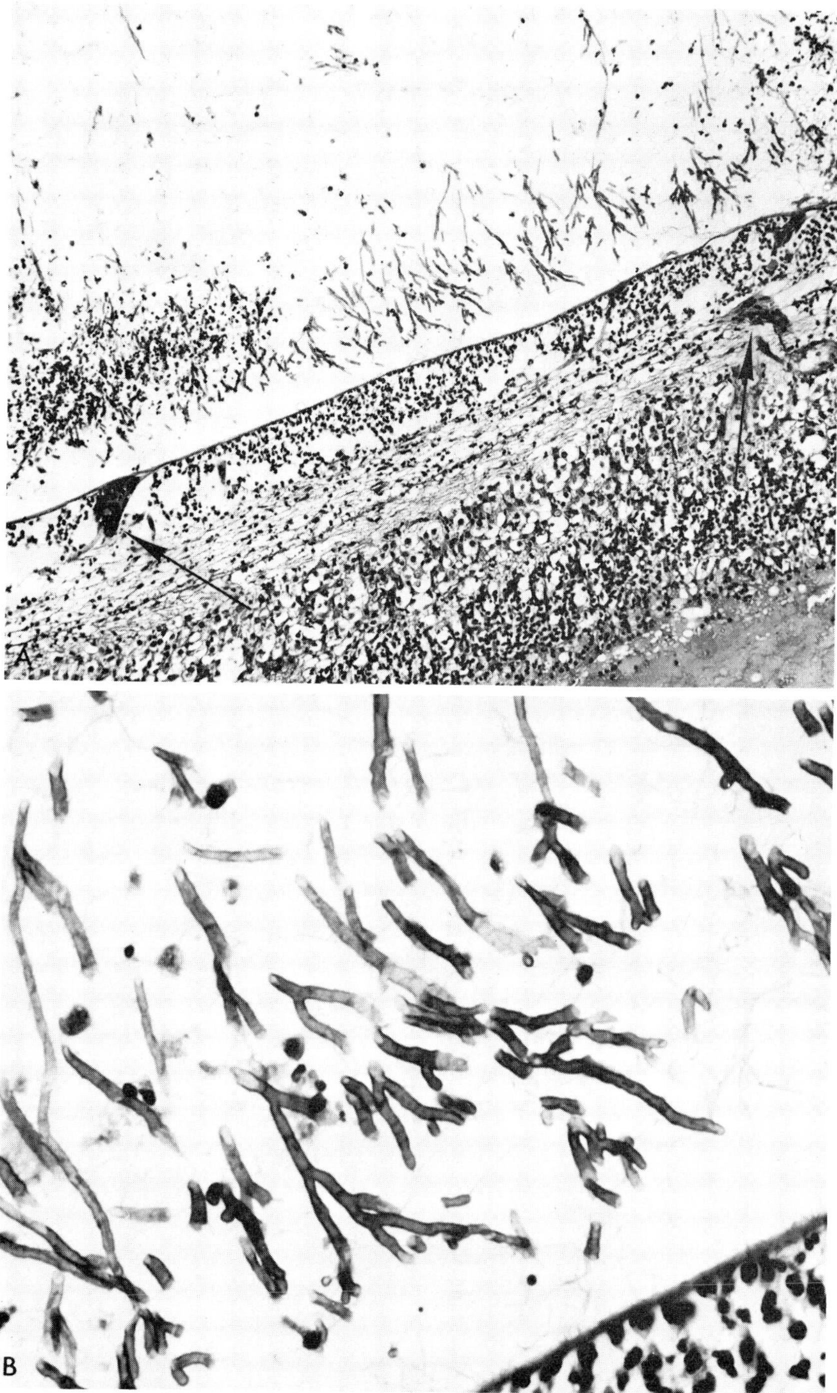

Figure 8–153. ***Aspergillus* endophthalmitis** associated with immunosuppression after renal transplantation. *A,* Cortical area of vitreous with polymorphonuclear leukocytic infiltration and branching septated hyphae. Retina is intensely infiltrated by neutrophils that appear to elevate the internal limiting membrane from the remainder of the retina. Arrows indicate granulomatous inflammatory cellular infiltration with epithelioid and giant cells. PAS, ×100. *B,* Higher power view showing the branching and septated characteristics of the fungus. PAS, ×535. EP 32162. (From Naidoff MA, Green WR: Endogenous *Aspergillus* endophthalmitis occurring after kidney transplantation. Am J Ophthalmol *79*:502–509, 1975.)

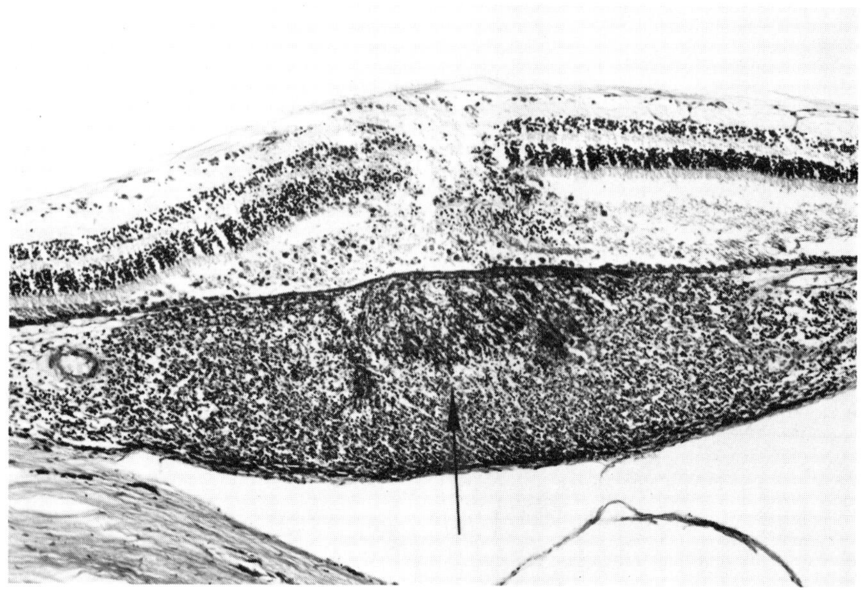

Figure 8–154. Choroiditis with secondary retinitis in eye of an immunosuppressed renal transplant patient. Choroidal abscess with large area of fungal organisms (arrow). Overlying retinal pigment epithelium is disrupted, and retina is detached by blood and inflammatory exudate. Outer retinal layers are also disrupted in one area. PAS, ×75. EP 30361. (From Naidoff MA, Green, WR: Endogenous *Aspergillus* endophthalmitis occurring after kidney transplantation. Am J Ophthalmol *79*:502–509, 1975.)

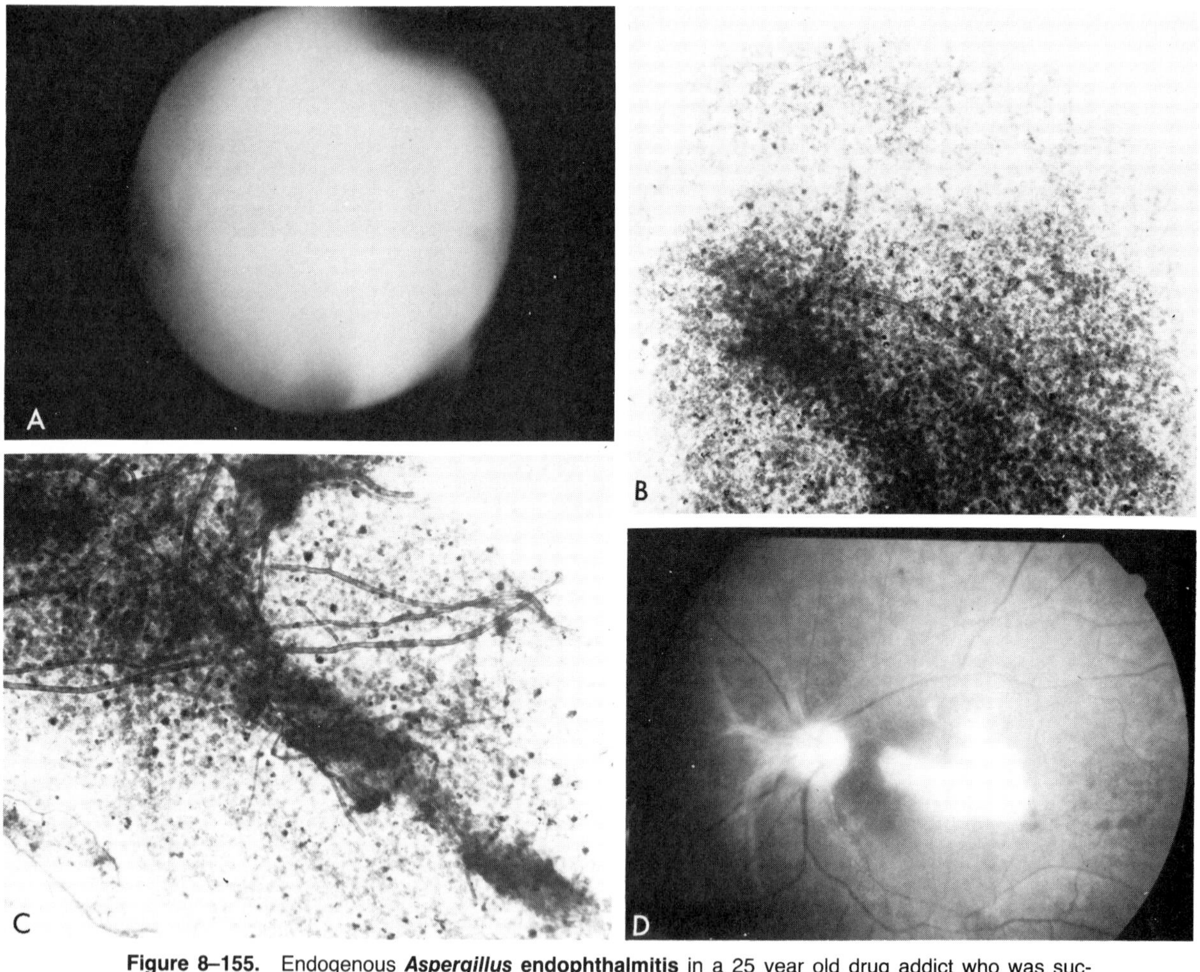

Figure 8–155. Endogenous ***Aspergillus*** **endophthalmitis** in a 25 year old drug addict who was successfully treated by pars plana vitrectomy and systemic antifungal therapy. *A,* External appearance, showing the opaque vitreous. *B* and *C,* Vitreous specimen showing branching, septate hyphae. Millipore filter. *B,* Modified Papanicolaou, ×240; *C,* PAS, ×240. *D,* Post-therapy appearance of chorioretinal scar involving macula. EP 51263. (From Engel HM, Green WR, Michels RG, et al: Diagnostic vitrectomy. Retina *1*:121–149, 1981.)

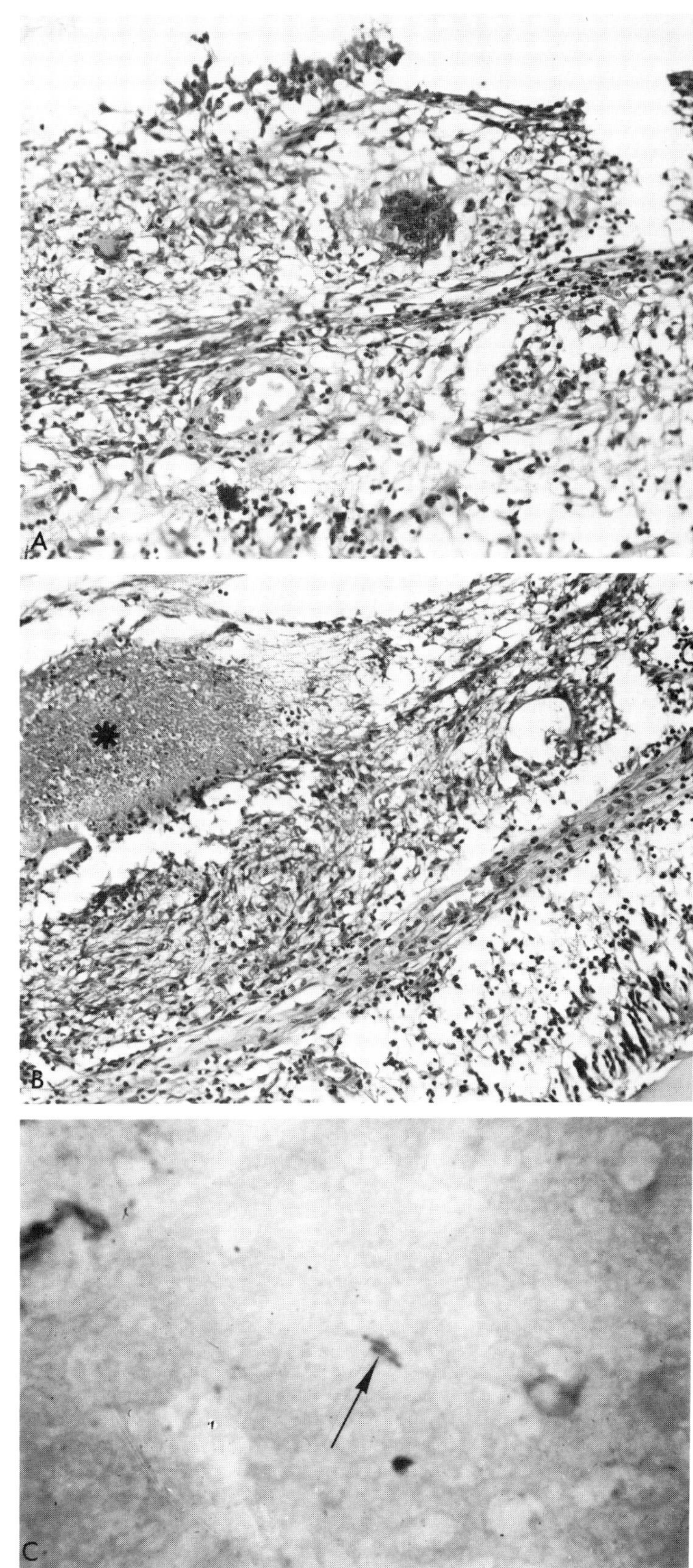

Figure 8–156. Tuberculosis of retina. *A,* Granulomatous inflammatory reaction, with multinucleated giant cells on inner surface of retina. H and E, ×210. *B,* Granuloma with central caseation (asterisk) involving retina and preretinal granuloma. H and E, ×185. *C,* Two acidfast bacilli (arrow) in central necrotic area on a granuloma of retina. Ziehl-Neelsen, ×900. (From Winter F; case presented at Verhoeff Society Meeting, 1974.)

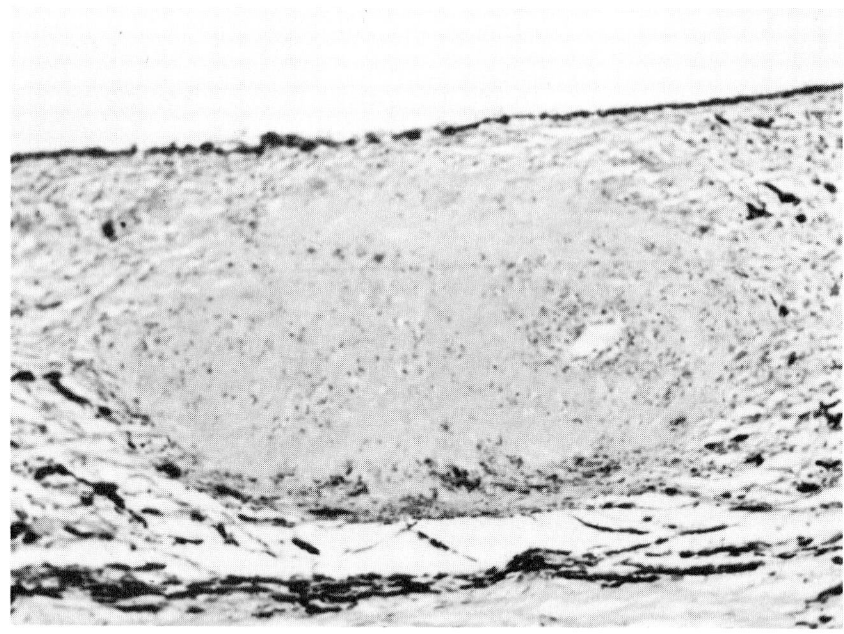

Figure 8–157. Tubercle in choroid of a patient who died of miliary tuberculosis. H and E, ×185.

the retina (Fig. 8–156) in one or another quadrant. Although the retina may be involved in miliary tuberculosis, the original foci of infection are usually in the choroid (Figs. 8–157 and 8–158). A severe endophthalmitis may result from the retinal inflammation, which may lead to loss of the eye (Fig. 8–159). Tubercle bacilli often cannot be demonstrated with special stains, especially in patients who have been treated.

A form of metastatic tuberculosis of the retina occurs in some patients who are under corticosteroid therapy for a systemic illness. Histologically, the tuberculosis lesions are identical with those described in Chapter 1. Typical tubercle formation occurs, with caseation necrosis in the centers, surrounded by a reactive inflammatory infiltration. Usually, heavy involvement of the vitreous with lymphocytes and plasma cells is seen, and also numerous macrophages. There may be a reactive inflammation in the anterior portion of the eye from the retinal lesion, with iritis and formation of "mutton-fat" keratic precipitates (KP) on the back of the cornea.

Leprosy. Retinal lesions have been described in lepromatous leprosy (Somerset, Sen, 1956). The nodules are formed in the inner portion of the retina and result in lesions that have been referred to as "retinal pearls." Histologically, the typical features of a leprous nodule are present, and bacilli are not difficult to demonstrate.

Syphilis. The retina may be a site of early or late syphilitic lesions. A diffuse neuroretinitis with or without retinal vasculitis is a common finding in early lesions occurring in younger persons, and this eventually results in the picture of retinal pigmentary degeneration, or pseudoretinitis pigmentosa. In syphilis of the adult, the initial pathologic picture is one of lymphocytic perivascular infiltration, with extensive edema and destruction of the retinal elements.

Exudative and edematous changes involve the inner retinal layers, and the disk is often affected. The inflammation is usually granulomatous, although it may have a nonspecific character. Organisms may be identified in the acute lesions (Fig. 8–160). The vitreous may be heavily infiltrated with exudate and cells. The rods and cones often degenerate, and the retina and choroid become adherent to each other. The pigment from degenerating RPE cells scatters into the adjacent tissues in the inflammatory exudate. If the disease is severe and chronic, the choroid becomes involved and the late picture resembles retinitis pigmentosa (Fig. 8–161,*A*). A differentiating feature is the formation of chorioretinal scars, with involvement of Bruch's membrane in the postinflammatory pseudopigmentary degeneration, in contrast to the absence of such destruction in primary retinal pigmentary degeneration.

Extensive scarring with gliosis that extends into the choroid (Fig. 8–161) may be prominent (Blodi, Hervouet, 1968). Glial cell extension into the choroid is a nonspecific change and can be seen in chorioretinal scars of numerous and diverse conditions, including the ocular histoplasmosis syndrome (see Fig. 8–278) and as a nonspecific change in a variety of conditions (Fig. 8–162). In postinflammatory pigmentary degeneration, the retinal vessel walls are thickened and their lumina are obliterated. Pigment accumulates about the vascular tree, just as in the primary disease. The optic nerve becomes atrophic.

Ross and Sutton (1980) point out that secondary syphilis should be suspected and investigated

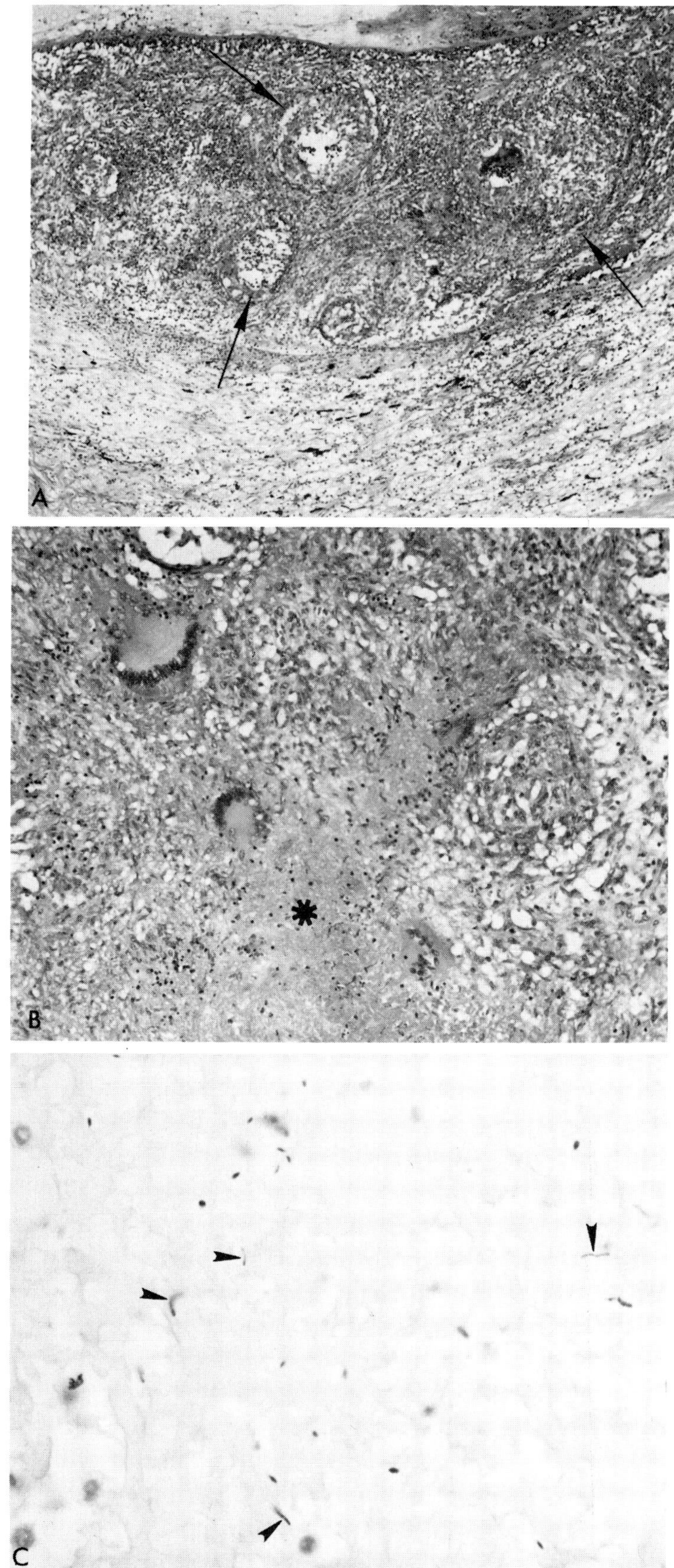

Figure 8–158. Extensive tuberculous chorioretinitis. *A,* Several granulomas (arrows) in retina. H and E, ×55. *B,* Granulomatous inflammation with multinucleated giant cells and necrosis (asterisk) in choroid. H and E, ×150. *C,* Acid-fast bacilli (arrowheads) in granuloma of choroid. Ziehl-Neelsen, ×900. EP 39176.

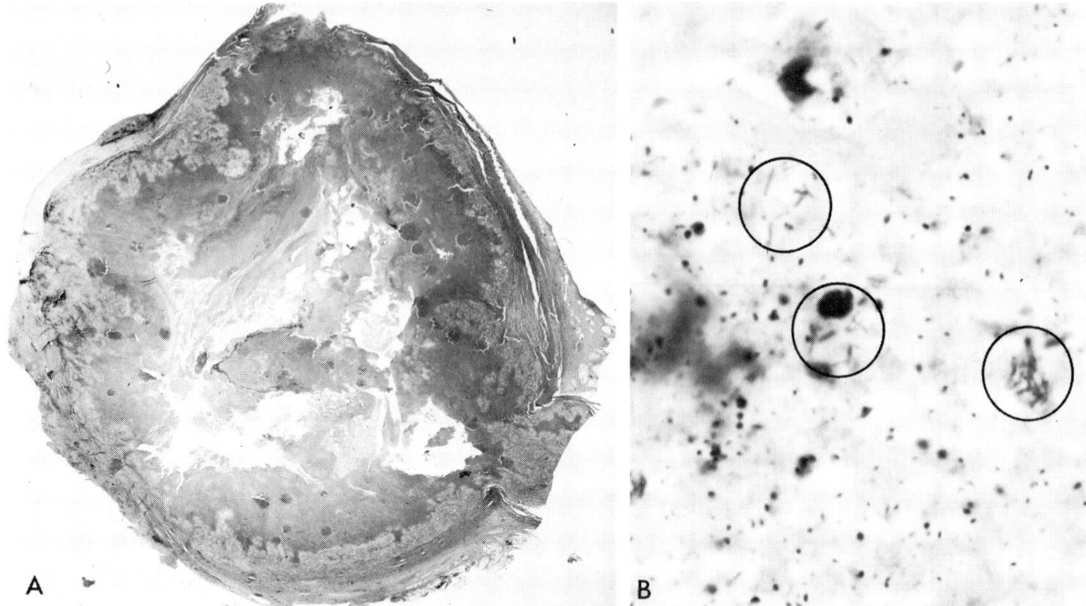

Figure 8–159. Tuberculous panophthalmitis in a 15 year old Ethiopian girl. *A,* The entire eye is filled with an intense, granulomatous, inflammatory cell infiltration. H and E, ×3. *B,* Granuloma showing numerous acidfast bacilli (circles) in interior of eye. Ziehl-Neelsen, ×900. EP 38621.

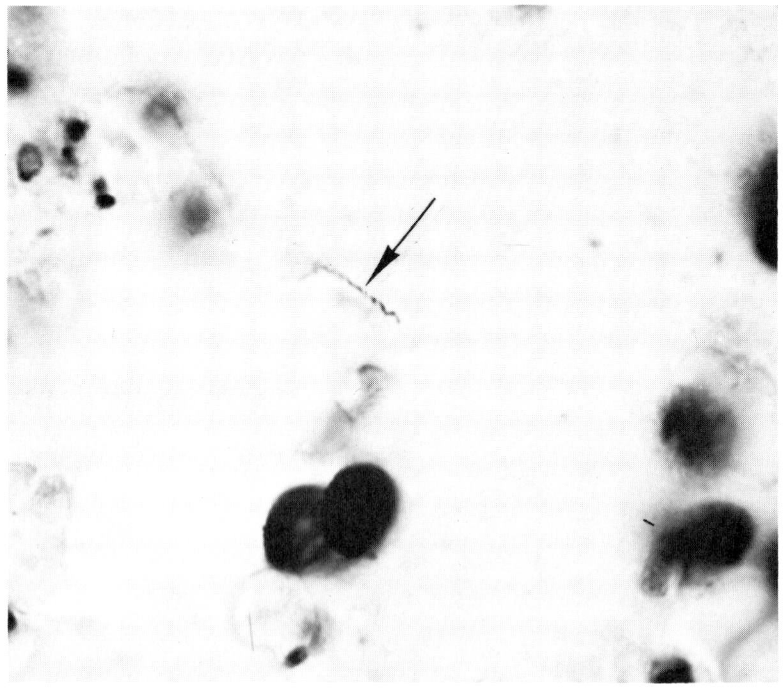

Figure 8–160. Spirochete (arrow) in retina in an eye with **syphilitic retinitis.** Warthin-Starry, ×1900. EP 51823; AFIP Acc. 114775.

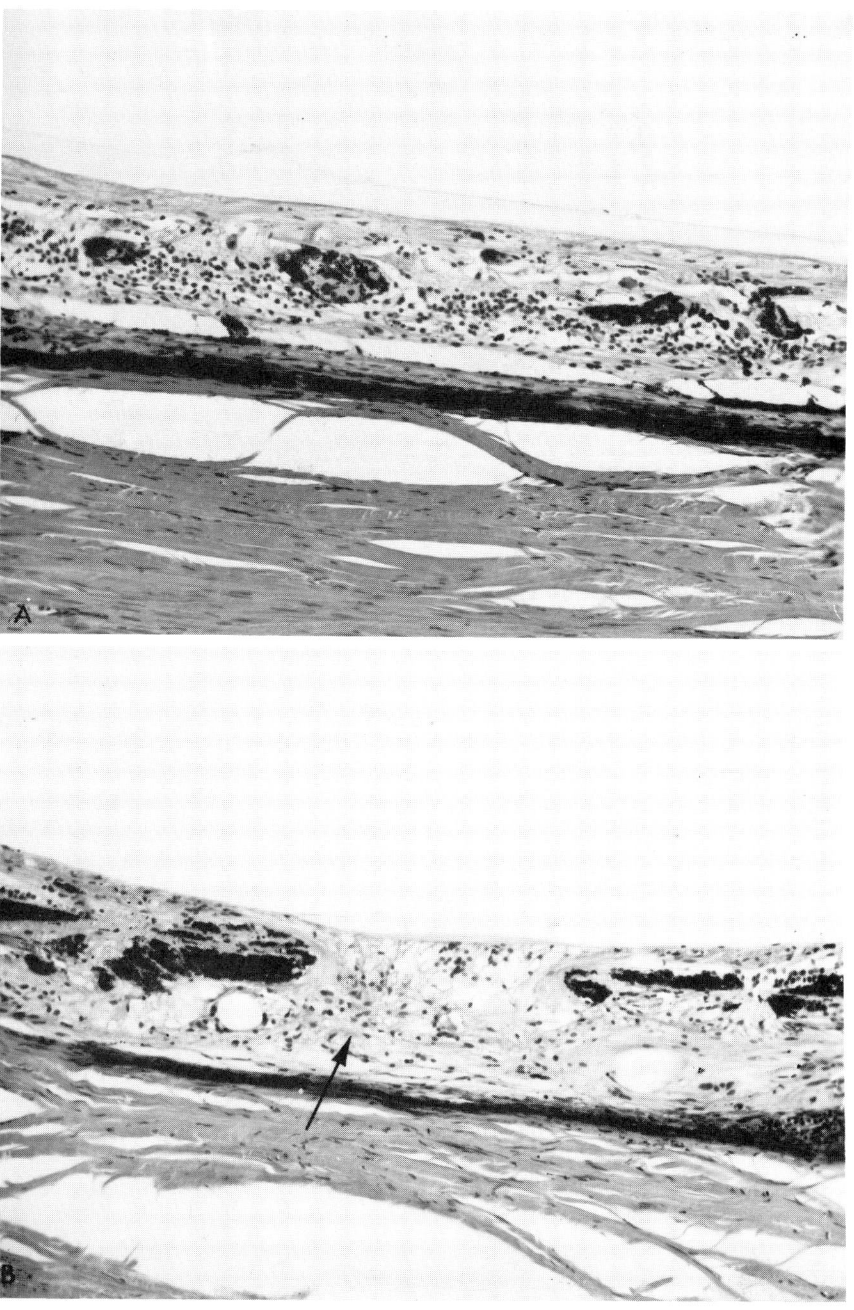

Figure 8–161. *A,* Retinitis pigmentosa–like picture in **congenital syphilis.** There is loss of the photoreceptor cell layer and hyperplasia of the retinal pigment epithelium, with migration into the retina in a perivascular location. H and E, ×130. EP 43913. *B,* Chorioretinal scar in congenital syphilis, with extension of glial cells into the choroid (arrow). H and E, ×130. EP 43913.

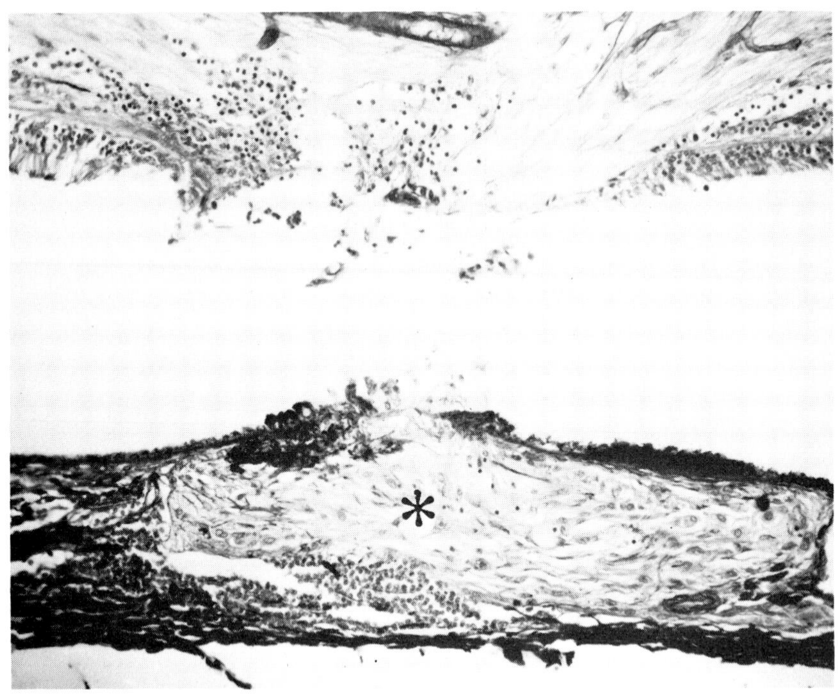

Figure 8–162. Peripapillary chorioretinal scar, with glial cell extension into the choroid (asterisk) in eye with persistent hyperplastic primary vitreous. PAS, ×200. EP 6671.

when a patient has any of the following: an unexplained pupillary abnormality; unexplained optic neuritis or optic atrophy; an apparent retinitis pigmentosa–like picture; any iritis that is unresponsive to topical steroids and mydriatics within a reasonable length of time; and any posterior uveitis that does not respond to oral and periocular steroids but persists or worsens.

Retinal periarteritis secondary to syphilis has been reported by Crouch and Goldberg (1975). Retinitis and phlebitis simulating branch retinal vein occlusion have been observed by Lobes and Folk (1981).

Whipple's Disease. This disease (Whipple, 1907) originally was considered to be an intestinal disorder, but Farnan (1959) showed that it is a multisystem disease. Electron microscopic studies (Yardley, Hendrix, Brown, 1961) and dramatic response to antibiotic therapy (Trier, Phelps, Eidelman, Rubin, 1965) indicate that the disease is

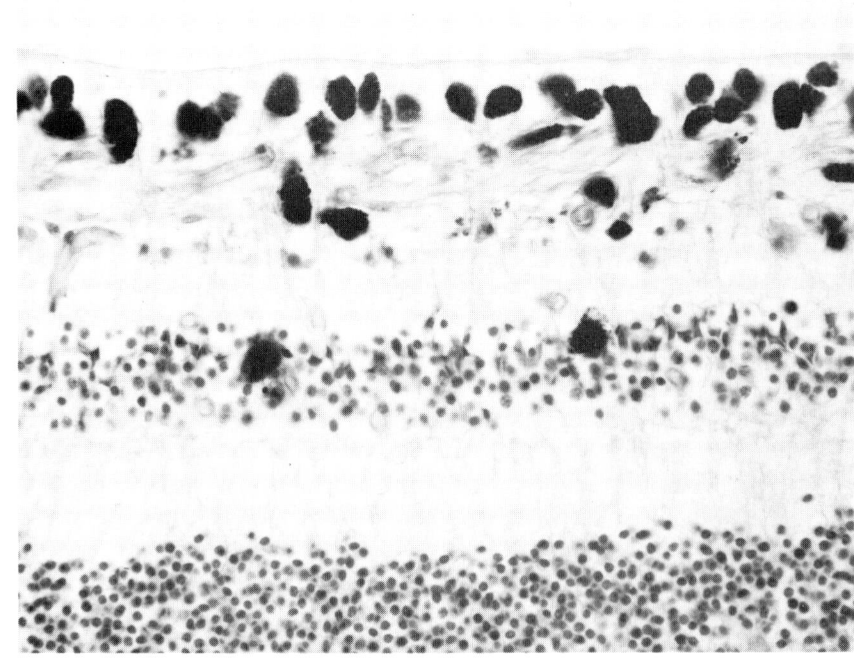

Figure 8–163. Whipple's disease with retinal involvement. Large histiocytes with intense periodic acid–Schiff–positive material are present in the inner layer of retina. PAS, ×350. EP 40864.

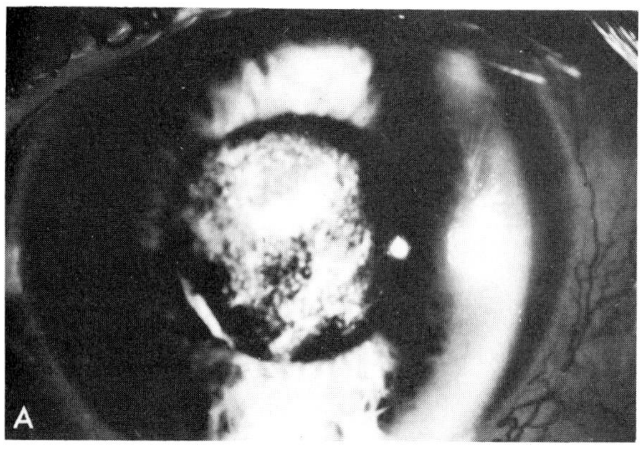

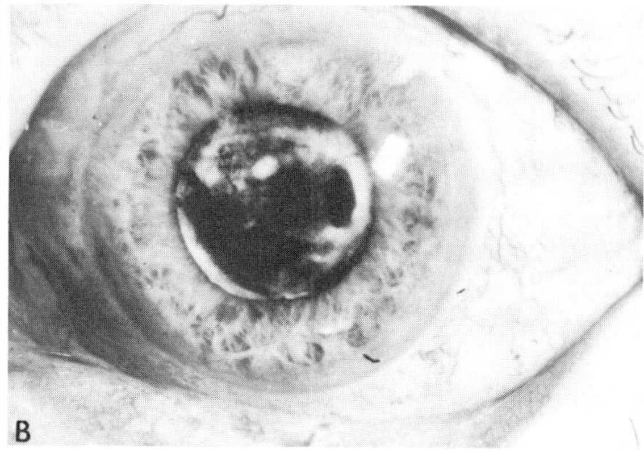

Figure 8–164. Whipple's disease with ocular presentation. Photographs taken about 2 weeks apart show clearing of the vitreous with tetracycline therapy. (From Selsky EJ, Knox DL, Maumenee AE, Green WR: Ocular involvement in Whipple's disease. Retina *4*:103–106, 1984.)

caused in part by an unusual chronic infection with bacteria of uncertain identity.

Ocular involvement was described (Kruecke, Stochdorph, 1962) in a patient who died of Whipple's disease. Histiocytes with cytoplasm that stained positively with the periodic acid–Schiff reaction were observed in the retina (Fig. 8–163). Optic nerve involvement was described in a 49 year old man by Switz, Casey, and Bogaty (1969). In 1968, Knox, Bayless, Yardley, and Chârache described two patients with Whipple's disease who had vitreous opacities that cleared with tetracycline therapy (Fig. 8–164). Systemic antibiotics resulted in improvement of vision and hearing, relief of arthritis and fever, and reduction of PAS-positive macrophages in repeat biopsy specimens of jejunal mucosa.

Histopathologic study of the eyes of a 51 year old man with a history of blurred vision, floaters, and migratory polyarthritis showed histiocytes in the retina and vitreous (Font, Rao, Issarescu, McEntee, 1978). These histiocytes stained positively with the periodic acid–Schiff reaction, and ultrastructural studies showed membranous structures and degenerating bacteria (Fig. 8–165).

Rickettsial Retinitis

The principal retinal lesions in rickettsial infections appear to be vascular in nature, which is to be expected considering the well-known vascular tropism of *Rickettsia*. Vascular lesions include periphlebitis with an Eales' disease–like picture (Morax, Saraux, Moday, Coscas, 1961); central retinal vein occlusion and branch retinal vein occlusion (Thomas, Cordier, Algan, 1959; Fontan, Barbancon, 1960; Morax, Saraux, Moday, Coscas, 1961; Bonamour, Bonnet, 1963); occlusion of central retinal artery (Fontan, Barbancon, 1960; Bonamour, Bonnet, 1963); and retinal vasculitis (Audoueineix, 1960; Morax, Saraux, Moday, Coscas, 1961).

Edema of the retina, perivasculitis, venous thrombosis, and a type of peripapillary chorioretinitis have been described by Thomas, Cordier, and Algan (1959). Scheie (1948) described the ocular findings in scrub typhus fever, characterized by retinal and venous engorgement, hemorrhages, exudates, vitreous opacities, and uveitis (Fig. 8–166). Chamberlain (1952), in a study of 70 patients, found optic nerve and retinal edema to be the most frequent ocular complication.

Several reports of retinal involvement in Rocky Mountain spotted fever have been made. Presley (1969) described the findings in six patients and observed venous engorgement, papilledema, diffuse retinal edema, cotton-wool patches (Fig. 8–167), flame-shaped hemorrhages, Roth spots, and arterial occlusions. Raab, Leopold, and Hodes (1969) and Smith and Burton (1977) have described similar retinopathy in patients with Rocky Mountain spotted fever. François (1968) has presented an excellent review of the ocular manifestations of rickettsial infections.

Rickettsial involvement of the eye is also considered in Chapter 9, Uvea.

Viral Retinitis

Measles Retinitis (measles maculopathy). The retinal lesions of measles are usually located in the macular area and have a degenerative, rather than an inflammatory, appearance (Fig. 8–168). Macular changes occur in the course of subacute sclerosing panencephalitis (SSPE), which is now known to be caused by the measles virus (Horta-Barbosa, Fuccillo, London, et al, 1969; Payne, Baublis, Itabashi, 1969).

SSPE is a progressive central nervous system disorder affecting both gray and white matter. It

Text continued on page 750

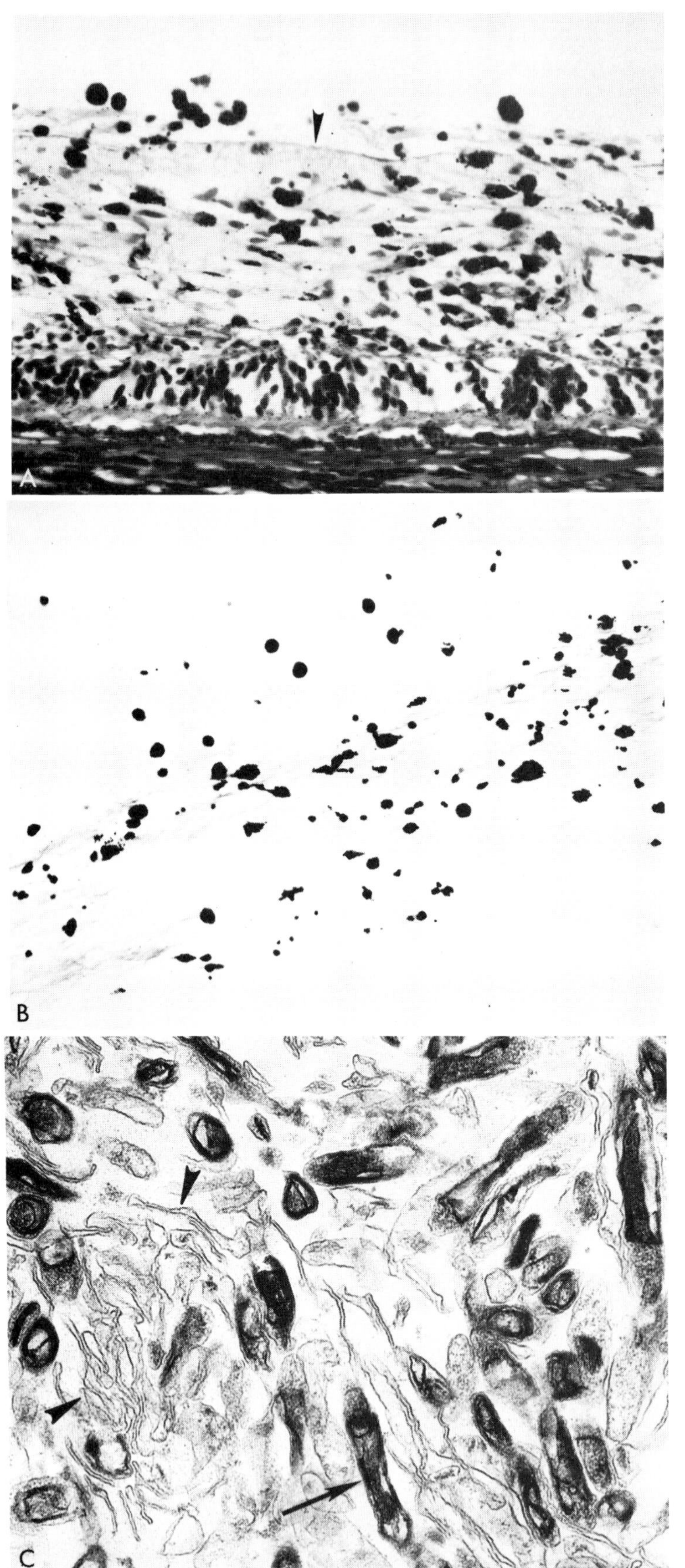

Figure 8–165. **Whipple's disease** in a 52 year old man who had a prolonged history of nondeforming, migratory polyarthritis and an episode of pericarditis that preceded the onset of bilateral vitritis and retinitis. *A,* Histiocytes with periodic acid–Schiff–positive material in retina and vitreous (internal limiting membrane—arrowhead). PAS, ×350. *B,* Similar histiocytes in vitreous. PAS, ×240. *C,* Electron micrograph showing bacteria-derived membranous structures (arrowheads) and degenerating bacteria (arrow). ×90,000. (From Font, RL, Rao, NA, Issarescu S, McEntee, WJ: Ocular involvement in Whipple's disease. Arch Ophthalmol *96*:1431–1436, 1978.)

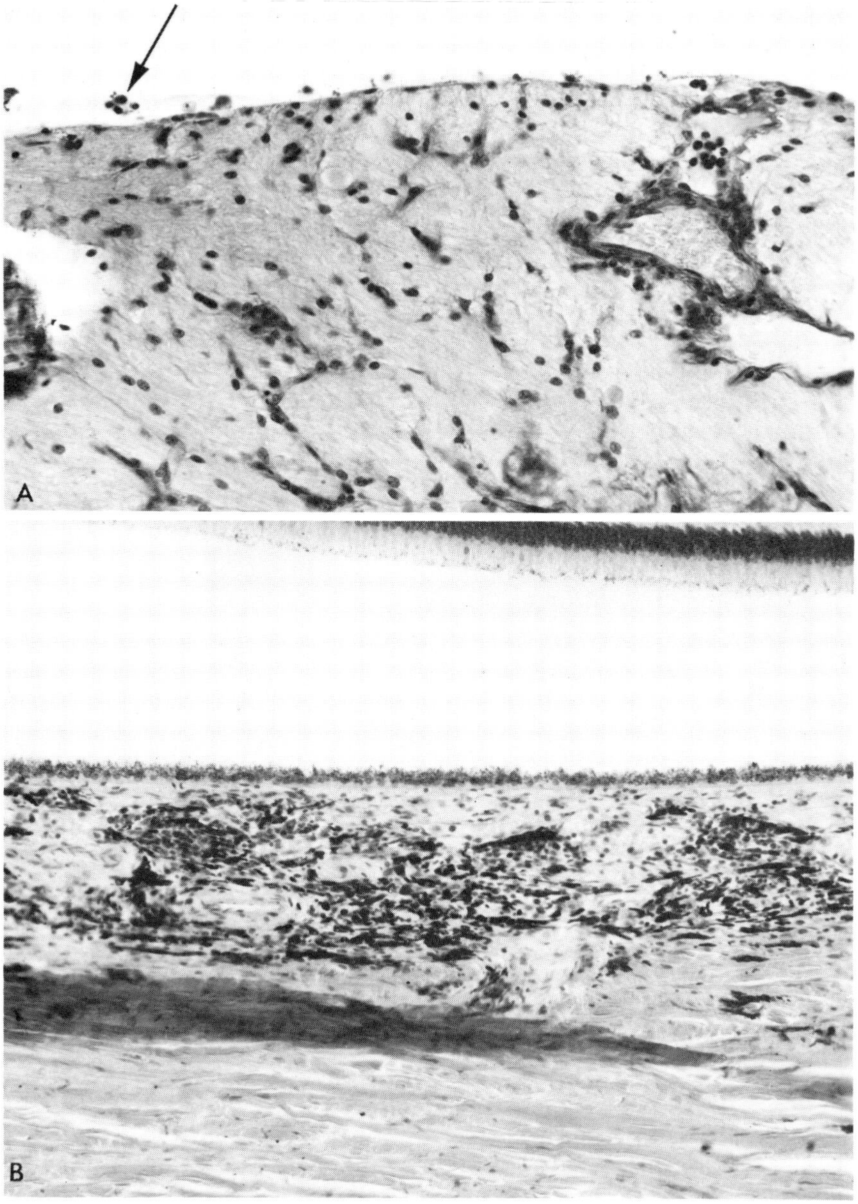

Figure 8–166. Scrub typhus. *A,* Mild, lymphocytic infiltrate in optic nerve head and vitreous (arrow). H and E, ×225. *B,* Moderate, nongranulomatous choroiditis. H and E, ×135. EP 51819.

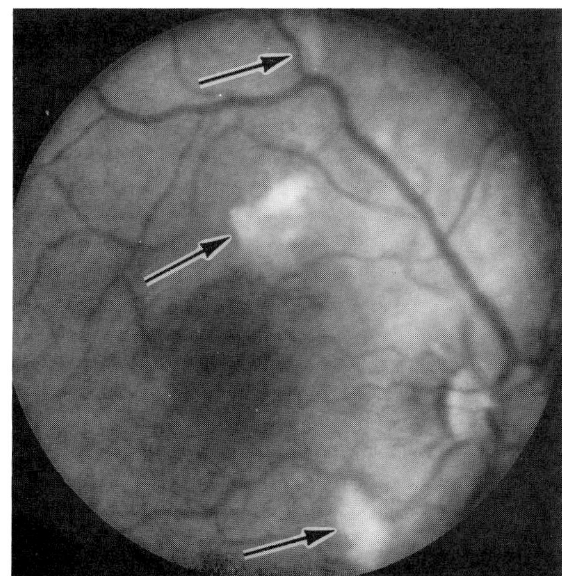

Figure 8–167. Cotton wool spots (arrows) in an 8 year old boy with Rocky Mountain spotted fever. (Courtesy of Dr. J. Ehlers.)

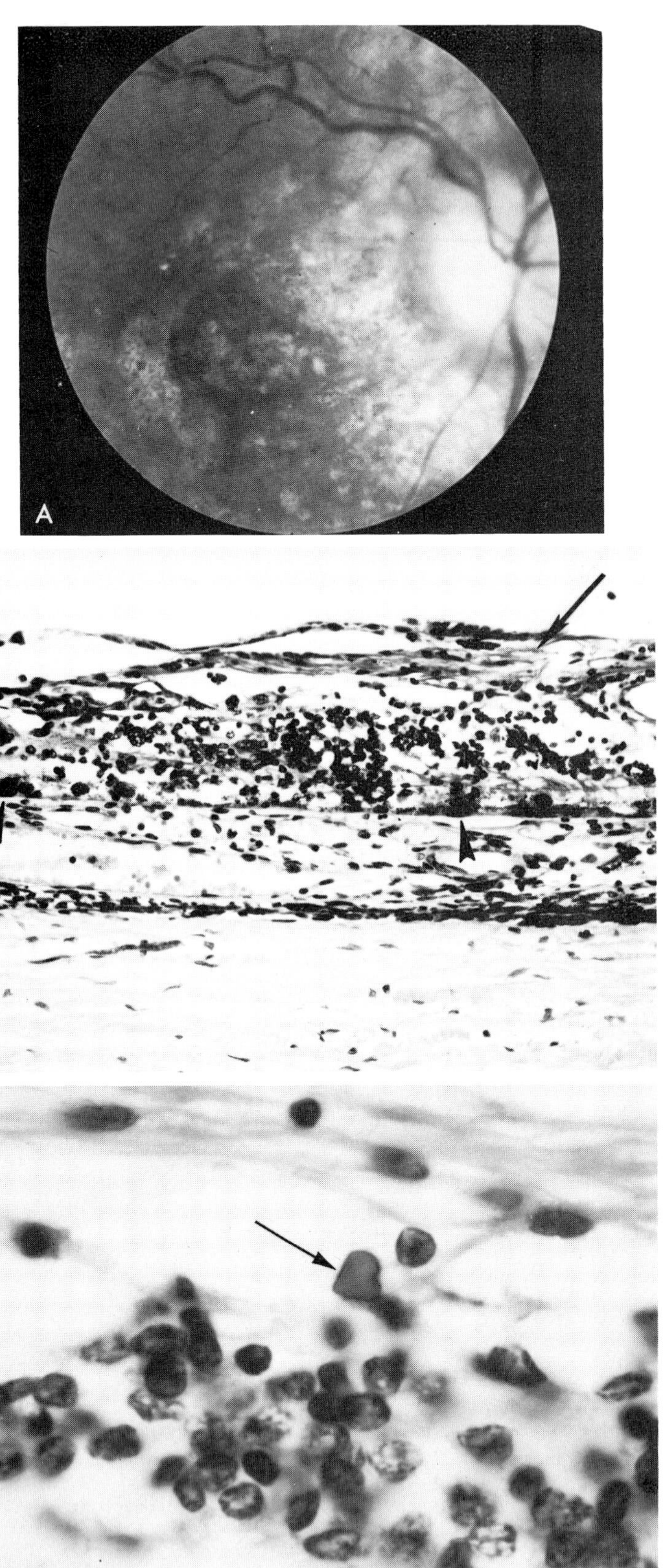

Figure 8–168. Measles maculopathy. *A,* The ophthalmoscopic appearance of the lesion involving the macular area is more degenerative than inflammatory in character. *B,* Area in macula showing total loss of the lamellar architecture and some gliosis (arrow). The retinal pigment epithelium (arrowheads) is discontinuous. H and E, ×270. *C,* Adjacent area of less degenerate retina, showing an intranuclear viral inclusion (arrow). H and E, ×1500. (From Font RL, Janis EH, Tuck RD: Measles maculopathy associated with subacute sclerosing panencephalitis. Arch Pathol *96*:168–174, 1973.)

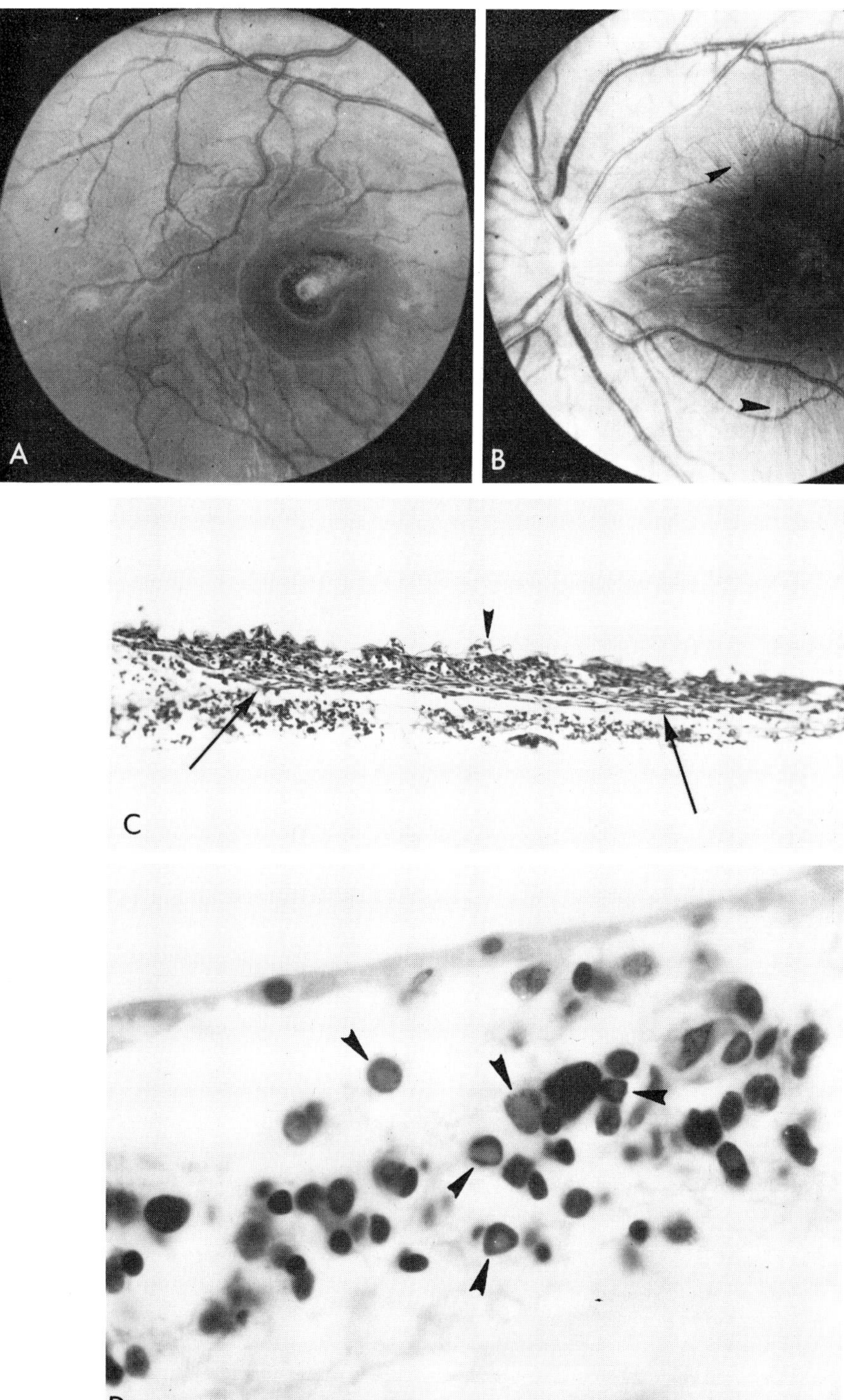

Figure 8–169. Measles maculopathy in a 13 year old girl. She was seen with ocular complaints, had a rapid downhill course, and died about 2 months after onset. *A,* The macular lesion of the right eye was slightly elevated and was at first thought perhaps to be vitelliform dystrophy. Later a hole was thought to be present. *B,* The macular lesion in the left eye was flat and appeared atrophic. Radiating striae of the internal limiting membrane (ILM) (arrowheads) were present. *C,* Section of macular area of left eye shows loss of lamellar architecture with intraretinal gliosis (arrows) and apparent contraction and resultant wrinkling of the ILM (arrowhead). H and E, ×150. *D,* Higher power view showing an area with many viral intranuclear inclusions (arrowheads). H and E, ×1500. (In part, from Nelson DA, Weiner A, Yanoff M, de Peralta J: Retinal lesions in subacute sclerosing panecephalitis. Arch Ophthalmol *84*:613–621, 1970.)

affects children and young adults and, with only occasional exceptions, is fatal. The mean age of onset is about 7 years, and males are affected about three times more often than females. There is a high correlation of SSPE with a preceding rubeola infection, which usually occurs before 2 years of age (Jabbour, Duenas, Sever, et al, 1972). Measles retinopathy and SSPE followed an attack of measles in a 14 year old boy on cytotoxic chemotherapy for a testicular neoplasm (Haltia, Tarkkanen, Vaheri, et al, 1978).

Initially, the ocular lesions have a slightly edematous appearance, then they develop a granular appearance, with hyperpigmentation at the edge. Contraction of the ILM and dragging of retinal blood vessels toward the scar may occur (Fig. 8–169). In the patient presented in Figure 8–169, the wrinkling of the ILM was caused by intraretinal and not epiretinal gliosis. Other lesions have a more punched-out appearance, because of changes in the RPE. There are marked changes in the RPE, with areas of loss and areas of hypertrophy and hyperplasia.

Histopathologic examination shows retinal

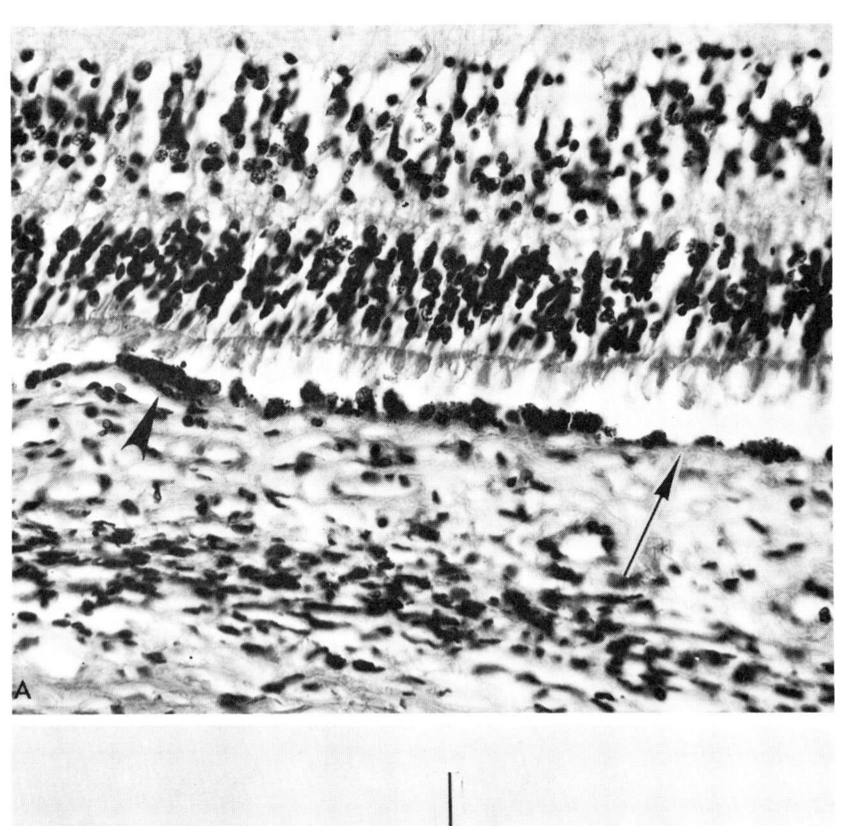

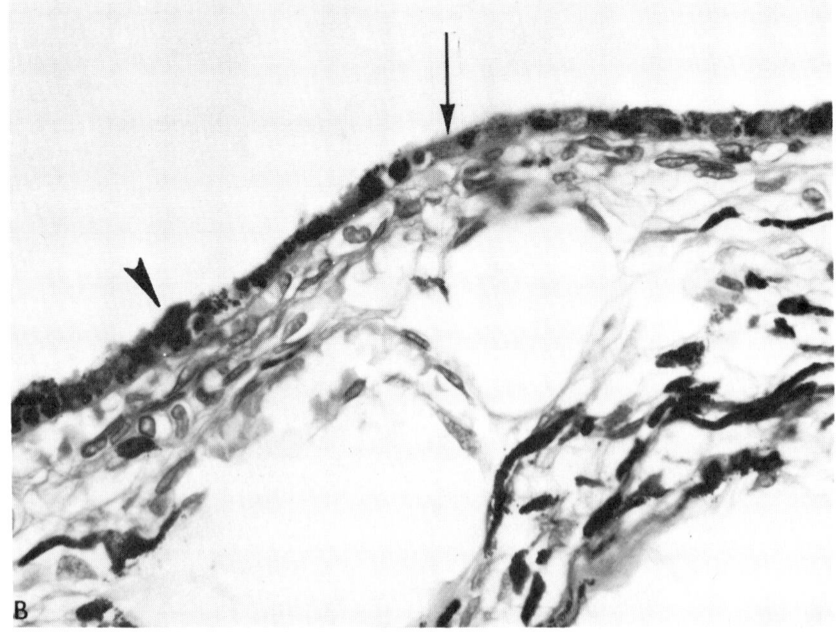

Figure 8–170. Rubella retinopathy. *A,* The retinal pigment epithelium is intact but shows areas of hypopigmentation (arrow) and hyperpigmentation (arrowhead). The outer nuclear layer is intact. The outer segments of the photoreceptor cells have undergone autolysis in the eye, obtained post mortem. H and E, ×330. EP 26027. *B,* Similar changes in a different case. H and E, ×525. AFIP Acc. 1166816.

atrophy and gliosis, and intranuclear inclusions are observed in retinal neurons (Nelson, Weiner, Yanoff, de Peralta, 1970; Landers, Klintworth, 1971) (Figs. 8–168 and 8–169). Immunofluorescent studies have shown the presence of measles antigen in the infected retinal cells, and immunoultrastructural methods using horseradish peroxidase–conjugated antibodies have shown the intranuclear and cytoplasmic viral nucleocapsules in the retina (Font, Lenis, Tuck, 1973).

Rubella Retinopathy. The details of rubella involvement of the eye have been outlined in Chapter 2, but the retinal findings will be described further in this section. Rubella retinitis, congenital cataract, and glaucoma are the three most frequent ocular abnormalities in children who have had congenital rubella. The exact prevalence of the retinal involvement is unknown, since many of these fundi cannot be examined because of congenital cataracts.

The principal finding in this retinopathy is at the level of the RPE. The histology has been described by Bourquin (1948); Boniuk and Zimmerman (1967); Yanoff, Schaffer, Scheie (1968); and Zimmerman (1968).

The changes are confined to the RPE and consist of some areas of increased pigmentation and loss of pigment cells or decrease in pigmentation of existing cells (Fig. 8–170), together with extensive RPE atrophy. The changes may be more prominent posterior to the equator, and in some the macula is more severely affected.

Collis and Cohen (1970) found that the retinopathy of rubella could progress after being first noted; they postulated that the rubella virus may not be completely destructive to the cell and that the virus could remain active in the cells for a considerable period after the birth of an afflicted child. Delayed development of choroidal neovascularization has been observed with rubella retinopathy (Deutman, Grizzard, 1978; Frank, Purnell, 1978; Orth, Fishman, Segall, et al, 1980).

The incidence of severe inflammation leading to phthisis bulbi after surgery on these eyes varies from 5 (Boniuk, Boniuk, 1970) to 24 per cent (Yanoff, Schaffer, Scheie, 1968).

Herpes Simplex. Herpes simplex retinitis appears as small, focal, yellow-white infiltrates. Vascular involvement with venous dilatation and occlusion is usually present (Figs. 8–171 and 8–172). The picture of a necrotizing retinitis ensues. Most cases to date have been associated with primary infections with Type II herpes simplex in neonates with central nervous system involvement (Cogan, Kuwubara, Young, Knox, 1964; Cibis, 1975; Hagler, Walters, Nahmias, 1969; Cibis, Flynn, Davis, 1978). Minckler, McLean, Shaw, and Hendrickson (1976) reported a 44 year old man with herpes simplex retinitis and encephalitis. Diddie, Schanzlin, Mausolf, and associates (1979) have observed the clinical and histopathologic features of necrotizing retinitis in a 33 year old woman with Hodgkins' disease.

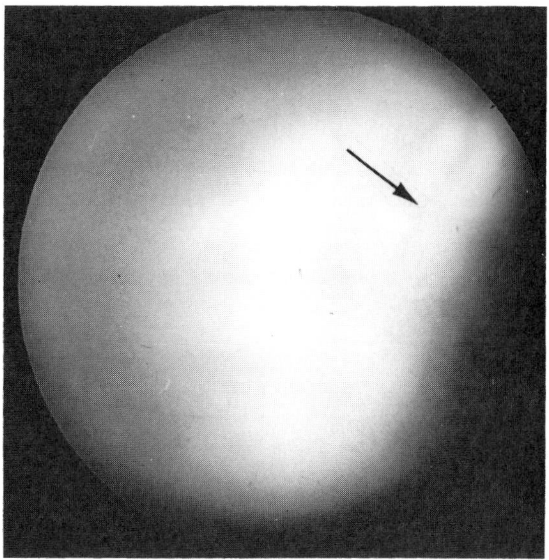

Figure 8–171. Herpes simplex retinitis, especially in a perivascular location, in an infant with the diagnosis established by brain biopsy. Retinal blood vessel (arrow) has a surrounding area of retinal thickening, with a whitish appearance, indiscrete margins, and overlying vitreous haze. (Courtesy of Dr. Daniel Finkelstein.)

Histopathologically, there is retinal necrosis and chronic inflammatory cell infiltration. An intense phlebitis (Fig. 8–172) and venous occlusion (Fig. 8–172) may be present. Typical intranuclear inclusions have been observed in the retina. A marked inflammatory reaction in the vitreous and underlying choroid can occur. In the healed stage, there is extensive chorioretinal scarring (Cogan, Kuwubara, Young, Knox, 1964).

Cytomegalic Inclusion Disease. Cytomegalic inclusion retinitis sometimes occurs in patients undergoing immunosuppressive therapy for connective tissue diseases or after organ transplantation, and in infants. It may occasionally occur in patients with lowered resistance as a result of cancer or other debilitating diseases (Murray, Knox, Green, Susel, 1977).

Cytomegaloviruses are DNA viruses belonging to the group of herpes viruses. The virus may be activated or given an advantage by treatment with immunosuppressive drugs or corticosteroids. The most useful methods for diagnosis are the indirect immunofluorescent test for cytomegalovirus microglobulin, and the complement-fixation test with cytomegalovirus (strain AD-169) antigen. The most sensitive method for detecting the various types of cytomegalovirus infections is isolation of the virus in tissue culture from urine and other body fluids.

The retinitis is usually unilateral, and the le-

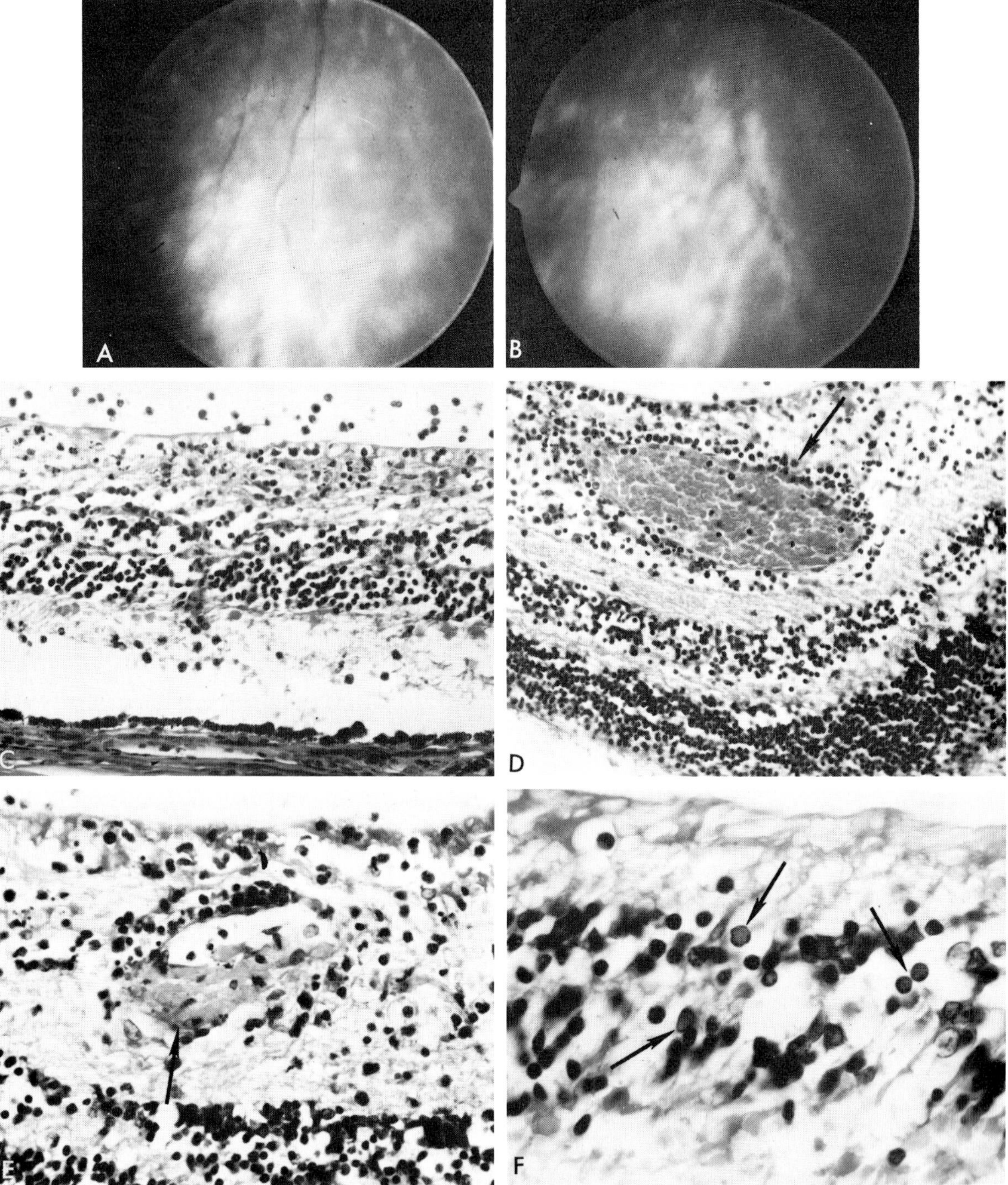

Figure 8–172. Herpes simplex retinitis. *A* and *B,* Gross appearance of multifocal areas of retinitis, with particular involvement along retinal vessels. *C,* Moderate lymphocytic infiltration of retina and overlying vitreous. H and E, ×330. *D,* Intense inflammatory cell infiltration in wall of a large retinal vein (arrow) and surrounding edematous retina. H and E, ×325. *E,* Thrombosed (arrow) vein with inflammatory cells in wall (arrowhead). H and E, ×550. *F,* Higher power view showing viral intraocular inclusions (arrows). H and E, ×1100. (From Curtin V: Herpes simplex retinitis. Presented at the Eastern Ophthalmic Pathology Society, Toronto, September, 1976.)

sions are usually in the posterior fundus. The characteristic clinical finding is an acute necrotizing retinitis with vitreous opacification and vascular involvement. Small-to-large yellowish-white retinal infiltrates with ill-defined margins develop. Perivascular infiltration and small retinal hemorrhages are often present (Fig. 8–173). There are usually minimal signs of vitreous inflammation. Occasionally, small, discrete lesions in the retina or RPE may be present. In the healing stage, scar formation occurs between the retina and vitreous and choroid, with pigmentation and atrophy. Cytomegalic virus infection of the retina in organ transplant patients undergoing immunosuppressive and corticosteroid therapy has been reported (De Venecia, Zu Rhein, Pratt, Kisken, 1971).

Histopathologically, there is necrosis of the retina, which leads to a thin fibroglial scar (Fig. 8–173). In the acute lesion, large cells (neurons) contain eosinophilic intranuclear or cytoplasmic inclusions (Figs. 8–173 and 8–174) (Ashton, Cunha-Vaz, 1966; De Venecia and associates, 1971; Wyhinny, Apple, Guastella, Uygantas, 1973; Chumbley, Robertson, Smith, Campbell, 1975; Cox, Meyer, Hughes, 1975; Johnson, Wisotzkey, 1977; Murray, Knox, Green, Susel, 1977).

Cytomegalovirus disease in congenital infections is probably transmitted to the fetus from the mother and can be detected in the newborn or early neonatal period. Systemic illness consists of jaundice, thrombocytopenia, anemia, hepatosplenomegaly, and neurologic signs. However, many subclinical congenital cases occur that are not associated with the preceding signs. The clinical ocular findings in the newborn infant are similar to those described in the adult eye. Patients have been reported, however, with focal lesions (Burns, 1959; Christensen, Beeman, Allen, 1957; Smith, Zimmerman, Harley, 1966). Lonn (1972) reported a case in which a cytomegalic virus was isolated from tissue fluids and from a liver biopsy; there was also bilateral severe chorioretinitis in the posterior fundus. The patient was followed over a long period of time and eventually the fundus lesions healed, leaving extensive, pigmented, gray-white scars, which in some instances have been interpreted as macular colobomas. The features of infantile cytomegalovirus infections may simulate congenital toxoplasmosis.

Herpes Zoster. Retinal involvement with herpes zoster produces a necrotizing retinitis (Fig. 8–175). Virus particles have been observed in the retina of a 78 year old man with herpes zoster ophthalmicus (Schwartz, Cashwell, Hawkins, et al, 1976). Histopathologic findings in eyes enucleated after herpes zoster ophthalmicus have included perineuritis, diffuse or patchy necrosis of iris and ciliary body (Fig. 8–176,*A*), and retinal vasculitis (Fig. 8–176,*D*); less commonly observed changes have included granulomatous choroiditis and granulomatous arteritis (Figs. 8–176,*B,C*) (Naumann, Gass, Font, 1968) (Figs. 8–175 and 8–176).

Acute Retinal Necrosis Syndrome. The features of this condition include retinal vascular narrowing and obstruction, retinal necrosis with patches of yellow-white to gray-white retinal opacification, anterior and posterior uveitis with mutton-fat keratic precipitates, recalcitrance to therapy, and marked loss of vision in most cases (Willerson, Aaberg, Reeser, 1977; Young, Bird, 1978; Price, Schlaegel, 1980; Sternberg, Knox, Finkelstein, et al, 1982).

Clinical differential diagnoses include Behçet's disease, herpes simplex retinitis, and cytomegalovirus retinitis, but all laboratory investigations have been equivocal or negative.

In a study of 11 cases with review of 30 cases from the literature, Fisher, Lewis, Blumenkranz, et al (1982) found that 50 per cent of affected eyes developed retinal detachment and 64 per cent had a final visual acuity of less than 20/200.

Study of vitreous specimens obtained by pars plana vitrectomy in four cases (Engel, Green, Michels, et al, 1981) has revealed lymphocytes, numerous histiocytes, and occasional multinucleated giant cells and plasma cells. No etiologic agent was observed or cultured.

Histopathologic studies of a surgically enucleated eye from a patient with the acute retinal necrosis syndrome disclosed diffuse uveitis, vitritis, retinal vasculitis, and acute necrotizing retinitis and intranuclear inclusions in retinal cells (Culbertson, Blumenkranz, Haines, et al, 1982). The same investigators observed herpes-like virus particles by electron microscopy. The type of virus was not characterized in culture studies.

Rift Valley Fever (RVF). This viral disease is arthropod-borne and primarily affects domestic animals with occasional involvement in human beings. During an epidemic in Egypt in 1977, Siam, Meegan, and Gharbawi (1980) observed ocular involvement in 7 patients. Ocular lesions were noted in the posterior pole; these included retinal hemorrhages, edema, vasculitis, retinitis, and vascular occlusion. Deutman and Klomp (1981) observed a similar picture (Fig. 8–177) in a 57 year old Dutch woman who lived and worked in Tanzania.

Toxoplasmosis has a worldwide distribution in humans, and it can be found in almost any domestic or wild animal.

Toxoplasma gondii can be classified as belonging to the subphylum Sporozoa and is a coccidian parasite. It exists in two forms in nature: an asexual form, wide-spread among humans, animals, and birds, and a sexual form, found in house cats and other felines. For many years it was speculated that there must also be a sexual cycle, confirmed when Frenkel, Dubey, and

Text continued on page 760

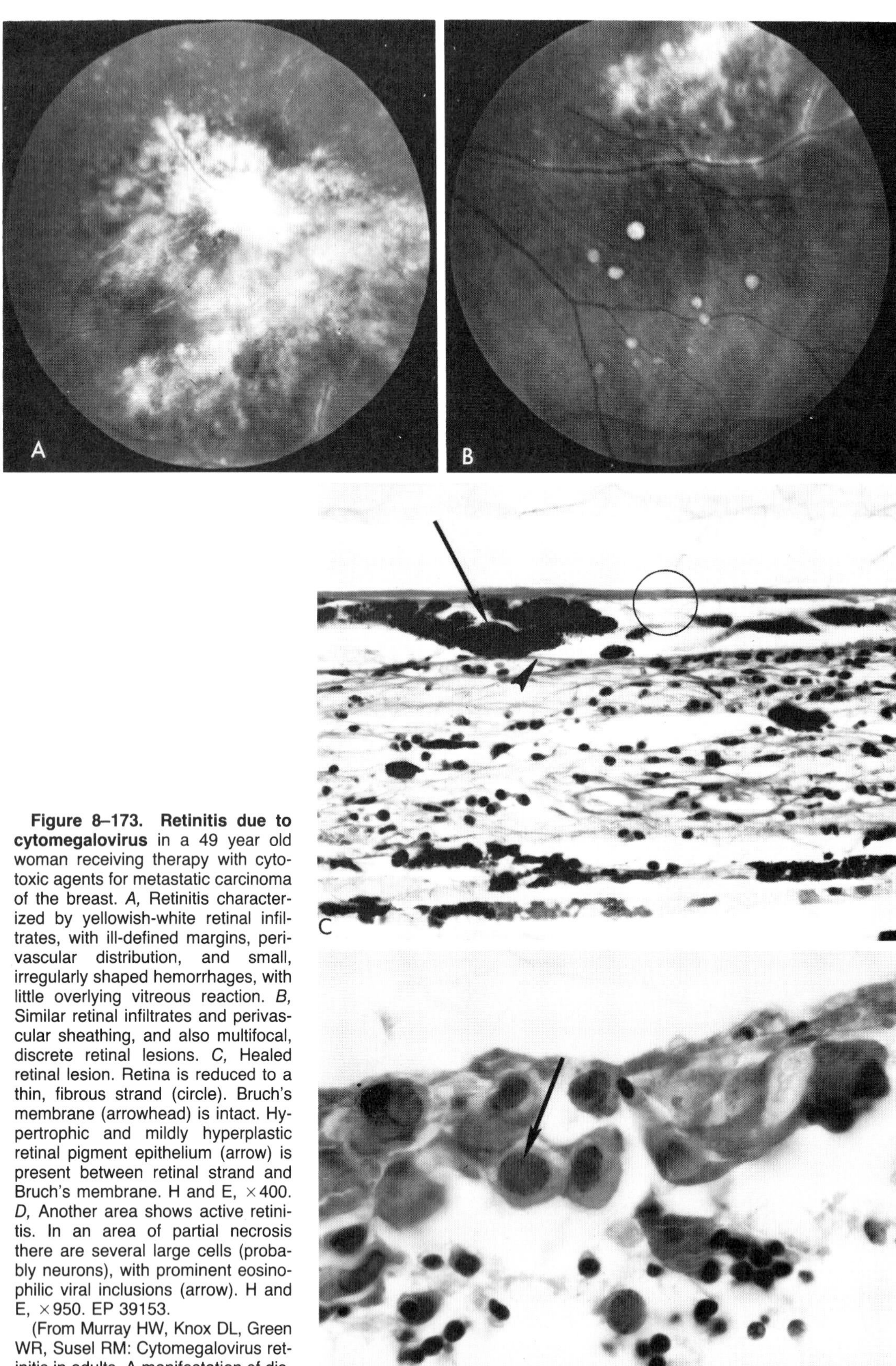

Figure 8–173. Retinitis due to cytomegalovirus in a 49 year old woman receiving therapy with cytotoxic agents for metastatic carcinoma of the breast. *A,* Retinitis characterized by yellowish-white retinal infiltrates, with ill-defined margins, perivascular distribution, and small, irregularly shaped hemorrhages, with little overlying vitreous reaction. *B,* Similar retinal infiltrates and perivascular sheathing, and also multifocal, discrete retinal lesions. *C,* Healed retinal lesion. Retina is reduced to a thin, fibrous strand (circle). Bruch's membrane (arrowhead) is intact. Hypertrophic and mildly hyperplastic retinal pigment epithelium (arrow) is present between retinal strand and Bruch's membrane. H and E, ×400. *D,* Another area shows active retinitis. In an area of partial necrosis there are several large cells (probably neurons), with prominent eosinophilic viral inclusions (arrow). H and E, ×950. EP 39153.

(From Murray HW, Knox DL, Green WR, Susel RM: Cytomegalovirus retinitis in adults. A manifestation of disseminated viral infection. Am J Med *63*:574–584, 1977.)

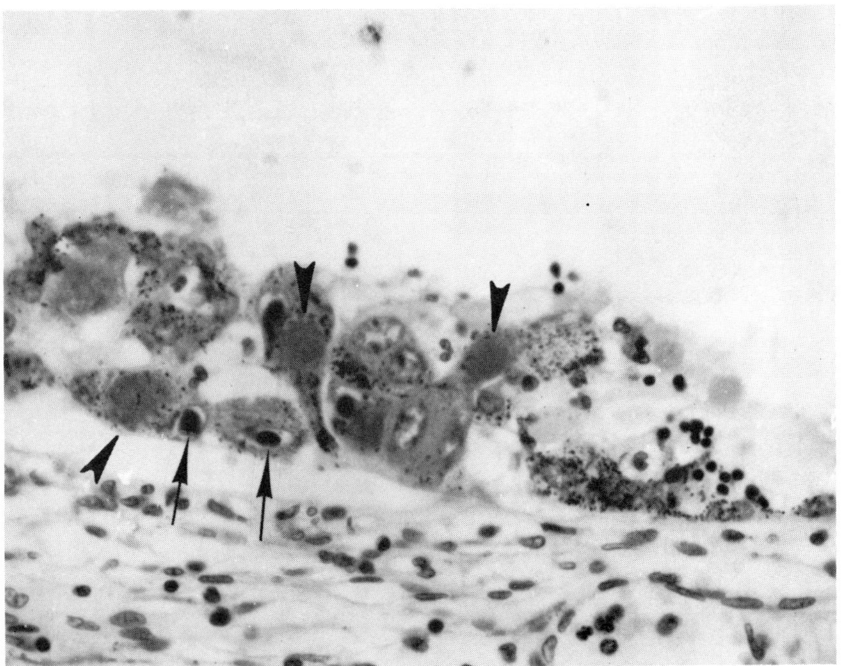

Figure 8–174. Discrete **cytomegalovirus involvement** of retinal pigment epithelium (RPE). The RPE cells are greatly enlarged and contain darker intranuclear (arrows) and lighter-staining cytoplasmic (arrowheads) viral inclusion. H and E, ×550. (From Toussaint D: Cytomegalovirus retinitis. Presented at the combined meeting of the Verhoeff Society and the European Ophthalmic Pathology Society, Washington, DC, April, 1976.)

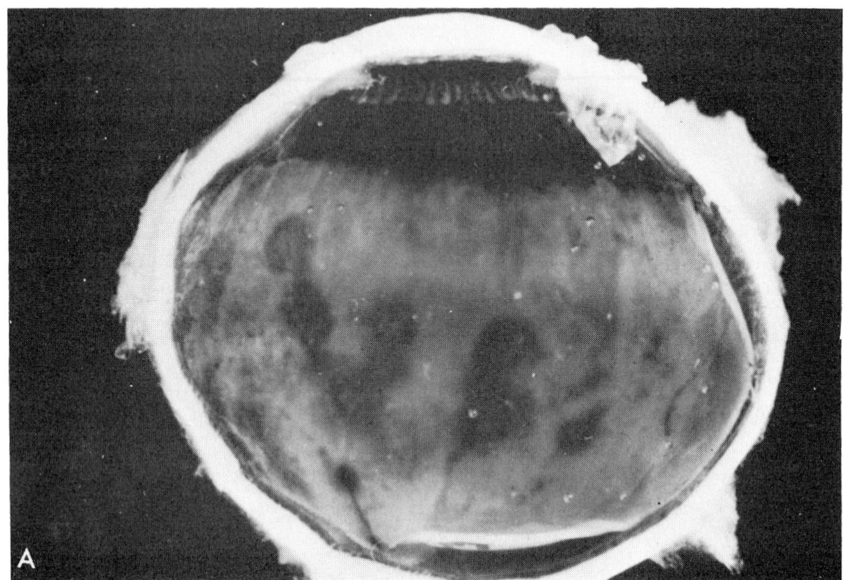

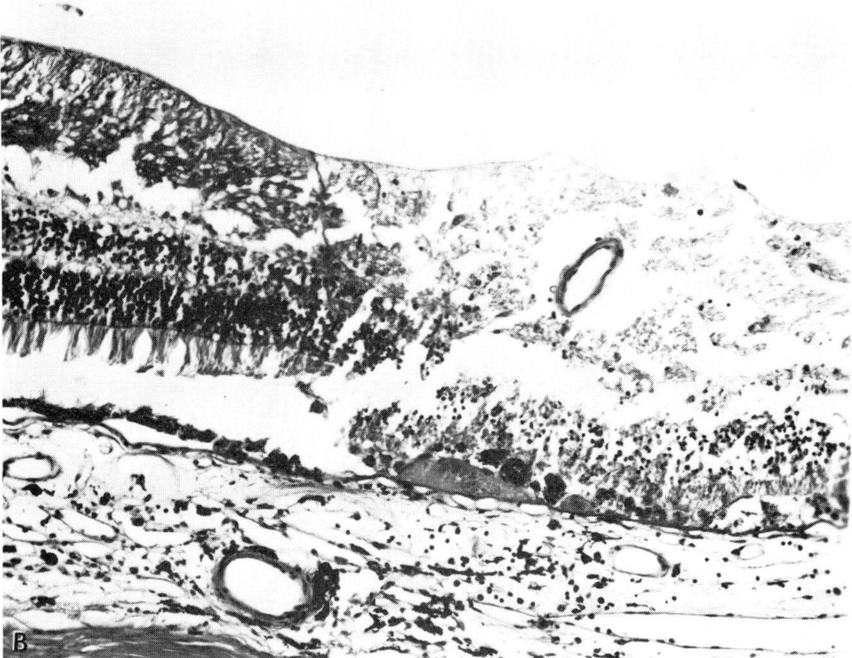

Figure 8–175. Herpes zoster retinitis after a vesicular cutaneous eruption in a 78 year old man. *A,* Gross appearance of dark retinal lesions with irregular margins. *B,* Margin of one lesion, showing relatively intact retina (left) and necrotic retina in lesion (right). H and E, ×146.

Illustration continued on opposite page

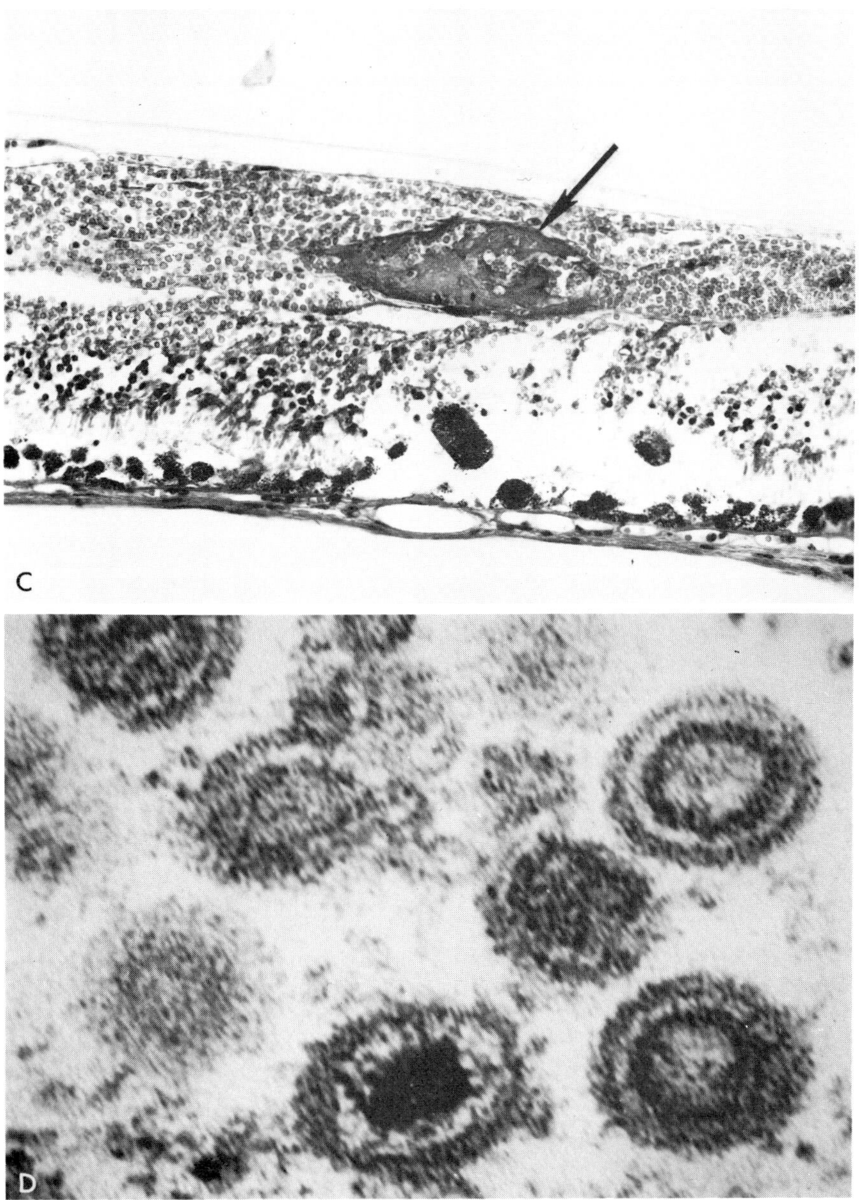

Figure 8–175 *Continued C,* Area of necrotic retina, showing a thrombosed vessel (arrow), hemorrhage, and disrupted retinal pigment epithelium. H and E, ×225. *D,* Viral inclusion in area of retinal necrosis. The viruses are round to ovoid, with double-layered membranous envelopes. Dense macular cores are present in some. ×120,000. (From Schwartz JN, Cashwell F, Hawkins HK, Klintworth GK: Necrotizing retinopathy with herpes zoster ophthalmicus. Arch Pathol Lab Med *100*:386–391, 1976.)

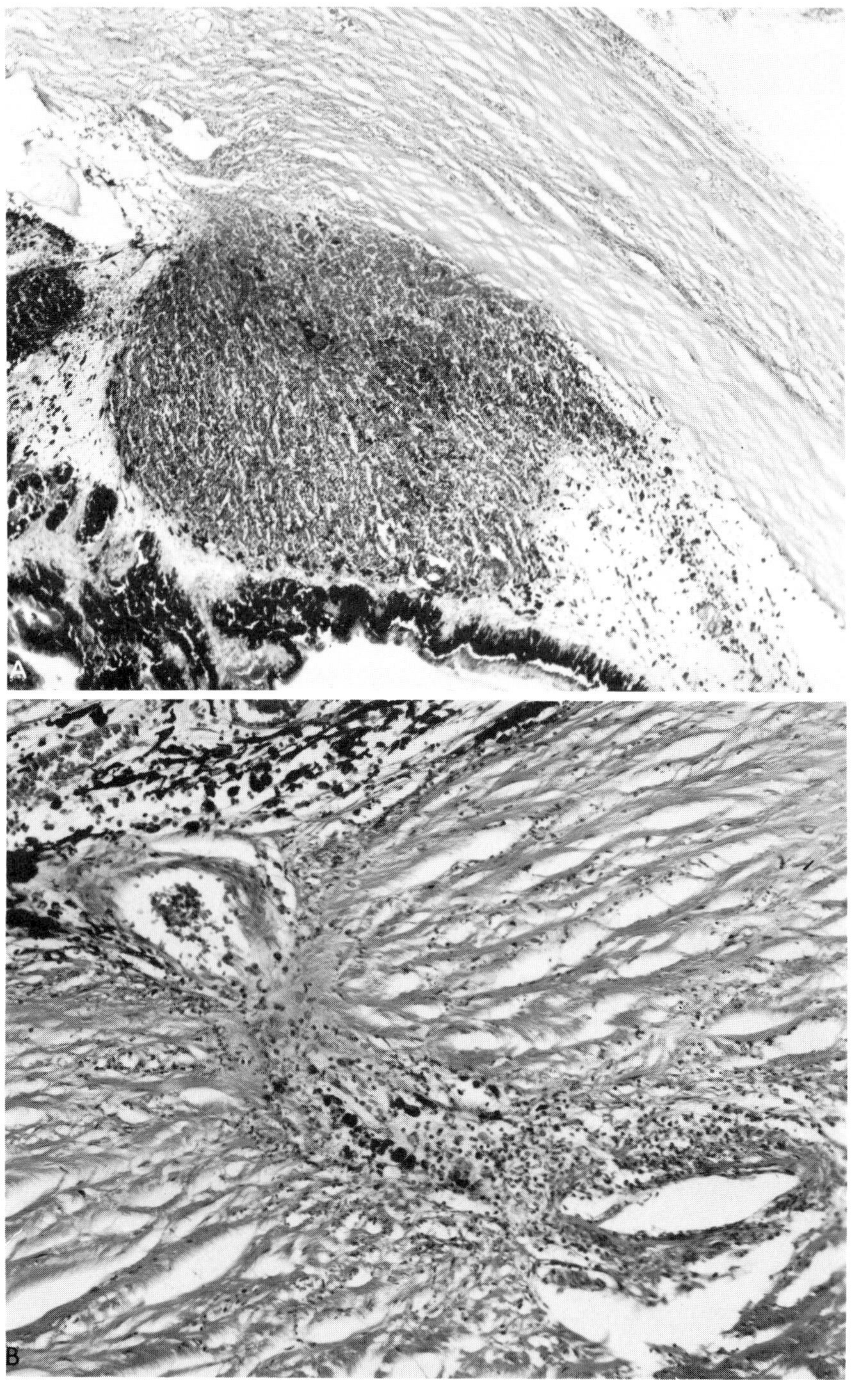

Figure 8–176. Surgically enucleated eye with severe **herpes zoster vasculitis** involving long and short posterior ciliary arteries. *A,* Necrosis of ciliary body, with an intense, neutrophilic infiltration. H and E, ×55. *B,* Short ciliary artery, showing an intense inflammatory cell infiltration in wall and surrounding area. H and E, ×140.

Illustration continued on opposite page

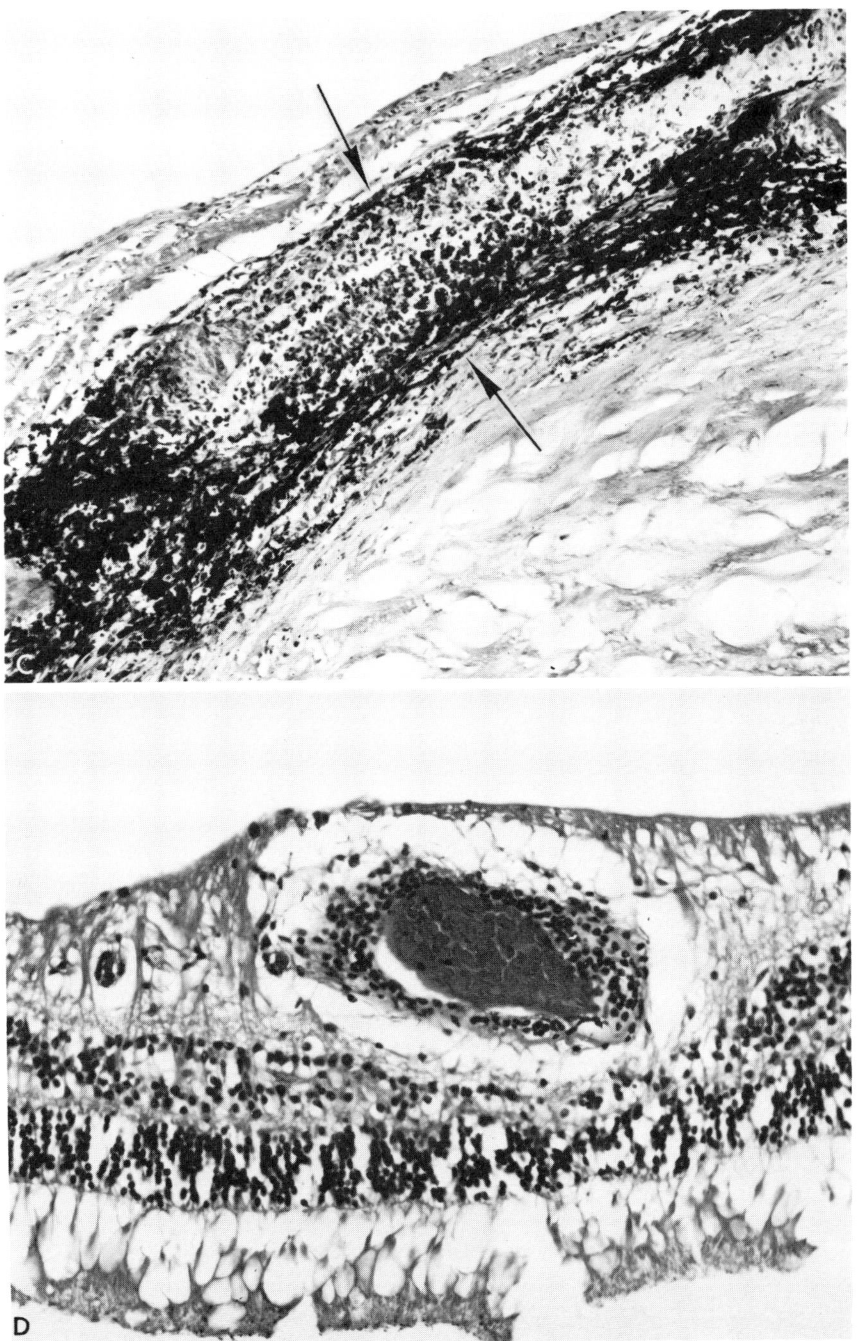

Figure 8–176 *Continued C,* Acute, necrotizing, occlusive vasculitis involving the long posterior ciliary artery (between arrows). H and E, ×135. *D,* Retinal vasculitis. Inflammatory cells are present in the wall of a retinal vessel, which is surrounded by an area of edema. H and E, ×250. EP 48992. (From Chan NR: Herpes zoster ophthalmicus. Presented at the Eastern Ophthalmic Pathology Society Meeting, Baltimore, October, 1978.)

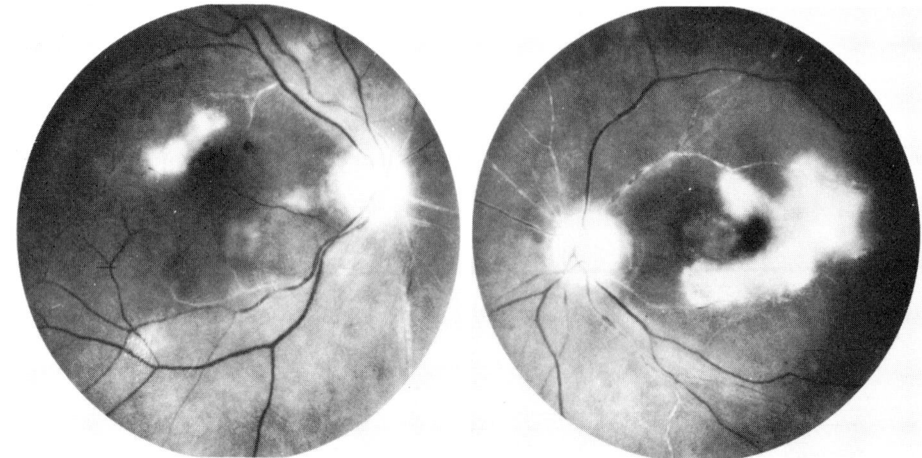

Figure 8–177. Bilateral retinitis and vasculitis of **Rift Valley fever** in a Dutch woman who lived in Tanzania. (From Deutman AF, Klomp HJ: Rift Valley fever retinitis. Am J Ophthalmol *92*:38–43, 1981.)

Miller (1970) and Hutchison, Dunachie, Wock, et al (1971) showed that the sexual cycle occurs in the small intestinal tract of cats. These workers provided evidence of both schizogony and gametogony in the cat intestine. The cyst, which is shed from the cat's intestinal tract, is resistant to drying and other environmental influences and can lie dormant for considerable periods until it is ingested and develops in the bodies of animals and humans, to produce the clinical picture of systemic toxoplasmosis.

Several methods are known for transmission of toxoplasmosis to humans. Epidemics of toxoplasmosis can arise from eating poorly cooked meat. Kean, Kimball, and Christenson (1969) have reported an epidemic in medical students following the ingestion of raw hamburger. Presumably the meat contains the *Toxoplasma* cysts, which, upon ingestion, are dissolved in the intestinal tract, thus leading to a systemic infection. The occurrence of disease would be determined by the number of cysts ingested. Toxoplasmosis is a common, asymptomatic infection, as is indicated by the prevalence of antitoxoplasmic antibodies among the adult population. However, acute toxoplasmosis in normal adults is uncommon. Most reported cases in recent years have occurred in patients who have leukemia, cancer, or other chronic diseases treated with antimetabolites, immunosuppressive agents, or corticosteroids.

In organ transplant patients, there is evidence that the *Toxoplasma* infection sometimes may be induced by actual transplantation of organisms in the donor kidney (Reynolds, Walls, Pfeiffer, 1966). In other instances, the disease may be present in the host before the transplant, and clinical disease may be activated by the postoperative therapy. If toxoplasmosis develops in Hodgkin's disease groups, a predilection for the acute toxoplasmic infection to occur in the central nervous system is noted. Frenkel (1971) has described a number of syndromes in toxoplasmic infections: asymptomatic or inapparent infections; the lymphadenopathic or glandular form; acute febrile toxoplasmosis; encephalitis, especially in immunosuppressed patients or those with cancer; toxoplasmosis during pregnancy; congenital encephalitis and systemic toxoplasmic disease in the neonate; and the ocular form.

Toxoplasmosis

Toxoplasma gondii produces either a congenital or acquired retinitis. In fixed tissue, the extracellular organism appears as circles or small, oval-shaped forms. Rarely, it may have a crescent shape. The intracellular organisms are smaller and somewhat more rounded. Cyst formation often occurs from parasitization of cells. The cyst wall is derived partly from the parasite and partly from the materials contained in the cell wall of the parasitized host cell. The cyst may contain a few or up to several hundred *Toxoplasma* organisms, and they are surrounded by a capsule derived from the parasitized cell.

Congenital Toxoplasmosis. The frequency with which *Toxoplasma* infections derived from the mother during pregnancy cause disease is now fairly well established, as the result of a number of studies, especially those of Desmonts, Couvreur, and Ben Rachid (1965). These investigators studied 64 cases of toxoplasmosis acquired during pregnancy, and 60 of the infants born of these mothers were examined; 22 (36 per cent) had congenital toxoplasmosis. Among the 22 infected children, 16 (73 per cent) presented no clinical evidence of congenital toxoplasmosis, and the follow-up of these children failed to reveal any evidence of disease. Serologic tests on each of these children established the diagnosis of congenital infection, and yet there was no evidence of disease.

Infants may be born with acute toxoplasmosis, or the disease may not become apparent until soon after birth, sometimes 9 to 12 months after birth. If the child does develop the disease, the clinical findings include encephalomyelitis, visceral inflammation, and chorioretinitis. These lesions lead to the classic findings of congenital toxoplasmosis: convulsions, fever, jaundice, paralyses of various types, chorioretinitis, cerebral calcification, and hydrocephalus. The diagnosis most often can be made with the methylene blue dye and complement-fixation tests, which become strongly positive within 3 to 4 weeks after onset of the infection. Remington (1969) has shown that the IgM fluorescent antibody technique is diagnostic for this disease—the IgM antibody being manufactured by the infant in response to *Toxoplasma* antigen.

A maternal history of acute infection is rarely obtained in these cases, and therefore it is believed that the mother has an inapparent or oligosymptomatic infection that is passed to the infant. Remington, Melton, and Jacobs (1960) have isolated *Toxoplasma* organisms from uterine muscle, suggesting that the toxoplasmic cysts within the uterine muscle are liberated and the organisms from the cysts are transmitted to the fetus across the placenta. The studies of Desmonts, Couvreur, and Ben Rachid (1965) in France also indicate that subclinical infections may develop in pregnant women who show no antibody prior to the development of the infection, and that during the course of the acute infection the disease is transmitted to the infant.

In some toxoplasmic infants, the disease is so mild or inapparent that it may be unrecognized for months or even years. A subsequent relapse can call attention to the probable congenital origin of the disease. Infections transmitted from a mother with considerable immunity may explain these milder or less apparent infections in the infant. Also, organisms of lesser virulence may produce less severe infections.

Acute chorioretinitis occurs at birth or soon after birth and is one of the most constant clinical findings in congenital toxoplasmosis. The infection is most often bilateral. The child may have a mild form of chorioretinitis, which is not recognized until later in infancy when mild, generalized signs of infection develop. By this time the chorioretinal lesion may be either active or healed. Late relapses often occur, through the apparent reactivation of dormant organisms in cysts near an old, healed scar.

The disease begins as a retinitis, with severe inflammatory changes in the retina and marked necrosis and exudation into the vitreous (Fig. 8–178). There may be single or multiple foci, and most often the lesions are located in the posterior fundus. The inflammatory process almost always extends into the choroid, and occasionally the sclera is affected. The acute or primary lesion may last for several months, depending on the severity of the infection. Histologically, organisms are almost always found in cysts or are free in the region of the acute lesions (Fig. 8–178). Eventually, the inflammatory process subsides, leaving a pale, atrophic scar surrounded by pigmented margins. Cysts may be found in the relatively normal tissue adjacent to these scars. They contain viable, resting organisms, surrounded by a zone which is argyrophilic and often PAS-positive. Rupture of these cyts may lead to reactivation of the disease.

It is emphasized that at any time, even into late adult life, the organisms within cysts surrounding these scars can be liberated and reactivate the infection. In reported cases, the congenital disease became active again after 40 to 50 years. For this reason, some adults with recurrent retinitis are examples of reactivation of congenital chorioretinal infections.

Adult Toxoplasmic Retinitis. Wilder (1952) first reported the finding of organisms morphologically indistinguishable from *Toxoplasma* in necrotic retina in granulomatous chorioretinal lesions in 53 eyes studied in the Registry of Ophthalmic Pathology of the Armed Forces Institute of Pathology. The patients were from 14 to 83 years of age at the time of enucleation, and, although eye symptoms had been observed for a few weeks to 32 years, the earliest history of onset was at age 12 years. Six patients had a history of onset in the seventh decade of life, and two in the eighth decade. The patients were all free of general symptoms that could be related to the ocular disease, and most had no history of preexisting illness that could have led to the development of chorioretinitis. In only three of these patients was there evidence of bilateral disease, and this suggests that at least these three patient may have had a congenital toxoplasmic infection with later relapse.

In most cases of adult toxoplasmic retinitis evidence of one or more old healed lesions usually exists (Fig. 8–179,*A*). Microscopic examination of the active lesion shows an area of retinal necrosis and acute inflammatory cell infiltration in the retina, vitreous, and subjacent choroid. *Toxoplasma* organisms are present in the necrotic, as well as in the adjacent retina. An immunologically mediated inflammatory reaction also occurs in the anterior segment, with iridocyclitis and mutton-fat keratic precipitates (Fig. 8–179).

Acute acquired ocular toxoplasmosis is rare, and only 2 to 3 per cent of patients with acquired systemic toxoplasmosis have ocular involvement

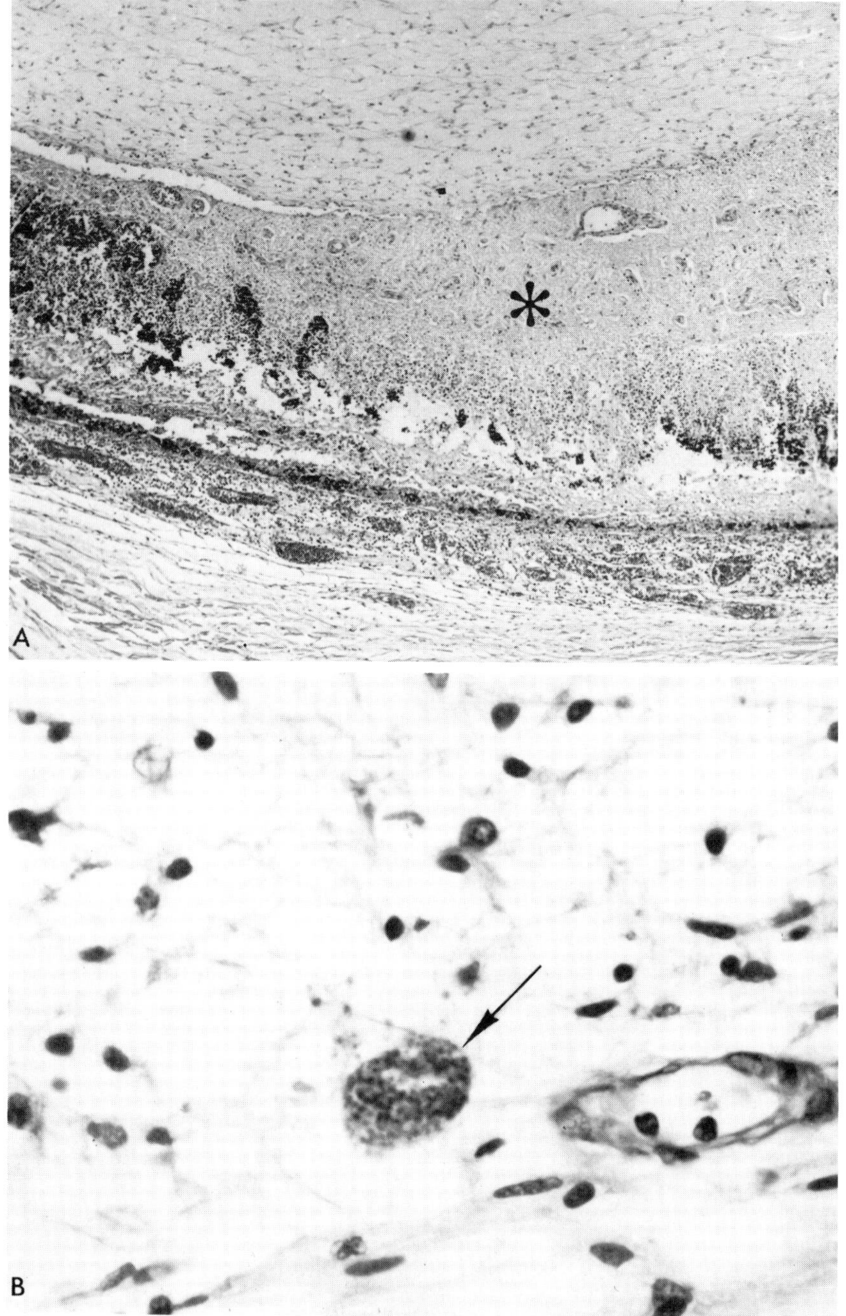

Figure 8–178. Ocular toxoplasmosis in a neonate who died of congenital toxoplasmosis. *A,* Necrotic retina (asterisk) with inflammatory cell reaction in vitreous and subjacent choroid. The retinal pigment epithelium is disrupted. *B,* Margin of necrotic area showing spherical cyst (arrow) containing *Toxoplasma* organisms. PAS, ×750.

Illustration continued on opposite page

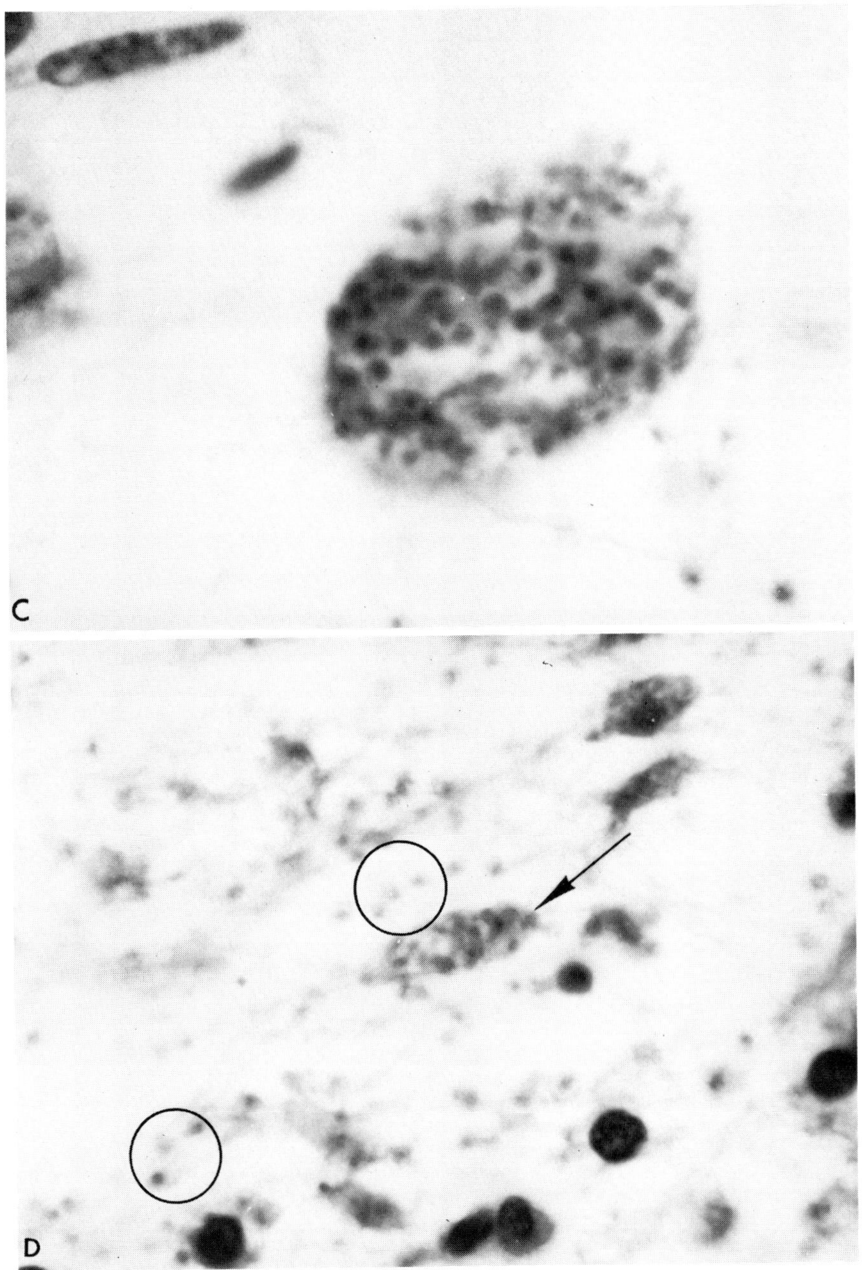

Figure 8–178 *Continued C,* Higher power view of toxoplasmic cyst. PAS, ×2000. *D,* Encysted (arrow) and released (circles) toxoplasmic organisms. PAS, ×1700. EP 32228.

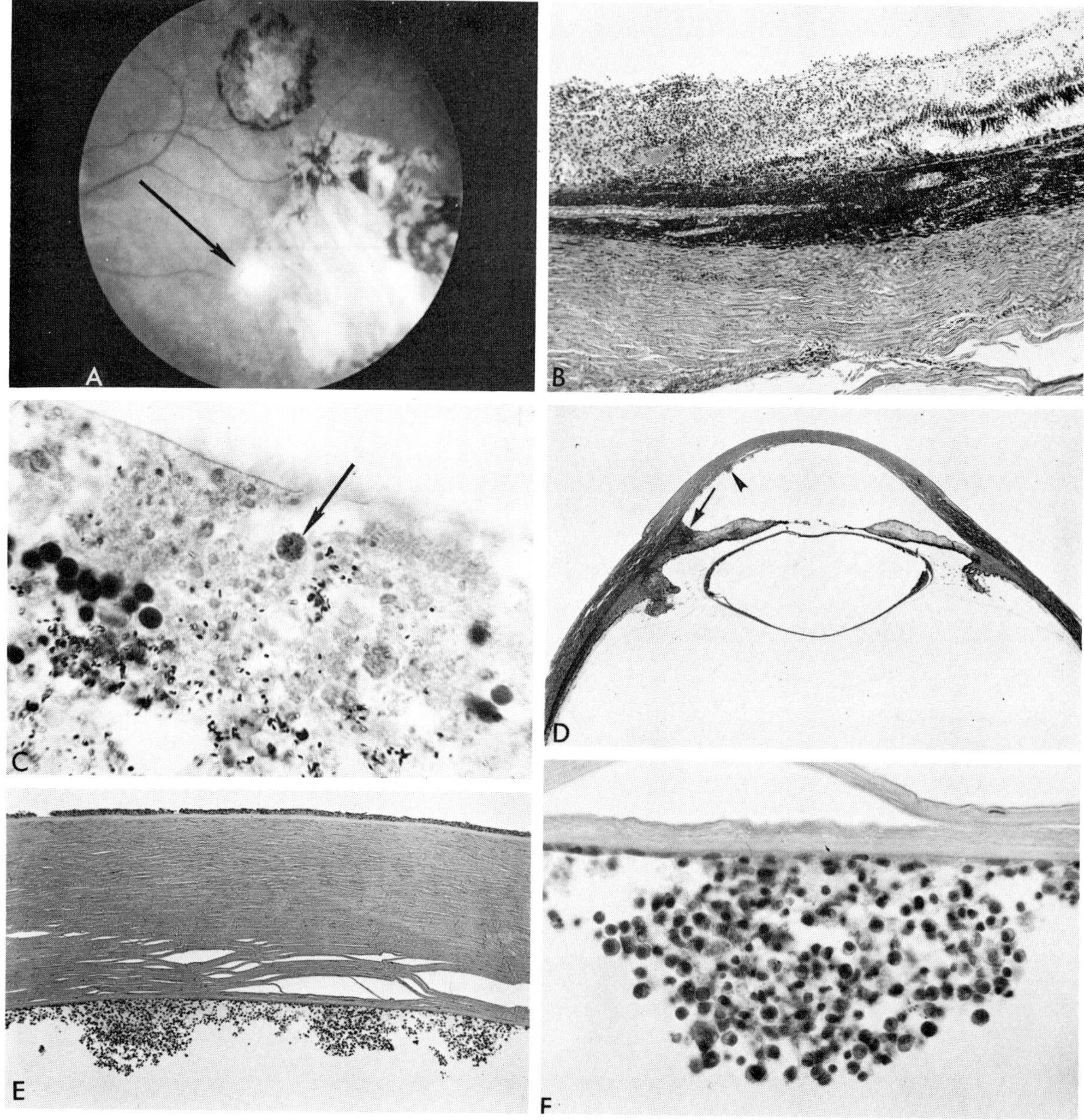

Figure 8–179. Ocular toxoplasmosis. *A,* A recent active area of retinitis (arrow) near areas of healed toxoplasmic retinitis is shown. (From Murray HW, Knox DL, Green WR, Susel RM: Cytomegalovirus in adults. A manifestation of disseminated viral infection. Am J Med *63*:574–584, 1977.) *B,* Acute toxoplasmic retinitis in an adult. Intense inflammatory cell infiltration in the retina, overlying the vitreous, and an intense infiltrate in the subjacent choroid. Retina is partially necrotic, with loss of its lamellar architecture. PAS, × 90. AFIP Neg. 57-1205. *C,* Area of necrotic retina with toxoplasmic cyst (arrow). PAS, ×600.

D, Inflammatory reaction in the anterior segment with iridocyclitis, inflammatory cells occluding the inferior angle (arrow), inflammatory pupillary membrane, and mutton-fat keratic precipitates (arrowhead). *E,* Keratic precipitates. H and E, ×90. AFIP Neg. 57-1207. *F,* Higher power view shows the keratic precipitate to be composed of histiocytes and some mononuclear cells. H and E, ×460. AFIP Neg. 57-1206. AFIP Acc. 754058.

(Perkins, 1973). Schlaegel (1976) reported that less than 1 per cent of patients with acute acquired toxoplasmosis develop retinitis and that most adult ocular disease is of congenital origin. Akstein, Wilson, and Teutsch (1982) studied 37 persons who developed acute systemic toxoplasmosis and were thought to have acquired the disease as the result of aerosolization of oocysts from infected cats in a riding stable. After 4 years of follow up, only one person had developed ocular disease. The investigators suggested that some sporadic cases of toxoplasma retinitis are due to acquired toxoplasmosis.

Occasional cases of ocular toxoplasmosis have

been associated with long-term corticosteroid therapy (Nicholson, Wolchok, 1976) (Fig. 8–180) and an immunosuppressed host (Reeh, 1973). Generalized toxoplasmosis has also been observed after renal transplantation (Reynolds, Walls, Pfeiffer, 1966). The subject of toxoplasmosis in the compromised host has been reviewed by Ruskin and Remington (1976).

The establishment of the exact diagnosis in these adult cases is difficult. Although most patients have positive methylene blue dye tests, the titers are usually low; in fact, one patient with proved infection had a positive dye-test titer only in undiluted serum (Zscheile, 1964). Histologically, organisms can be demonstrated in the lesions in the retina and optic nerve, but up till now they have been found only in the retina and never in the uveal tract. The choroid adjacent to the retinal foci usually shows a granulomatous inflammation, and sometimes the sclera may be thickened and inflamed. After healing, the retina shows severe destruction in the area of the infection, and chorioretinal adhesions are present. Recurrences are common, and most usually occur as satellites near the initial process. Identification of *Toxoplasma* in tissue sections, and its recovery by animal inoculation from the infected ocular tissue, provide the final proof of the diagnosis.

Parasitic Infestation

Nematode Retinitis, Chorioretinitis, and Endophthalmitis. Wilder in 1950 first showed that mi-

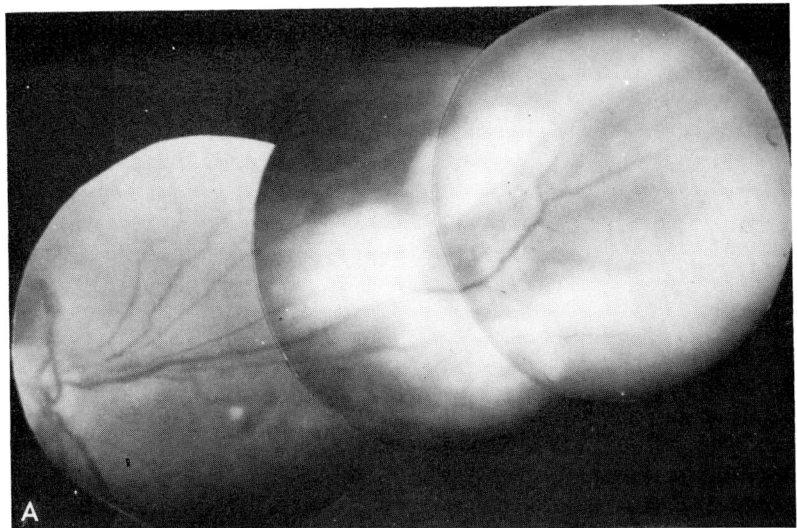

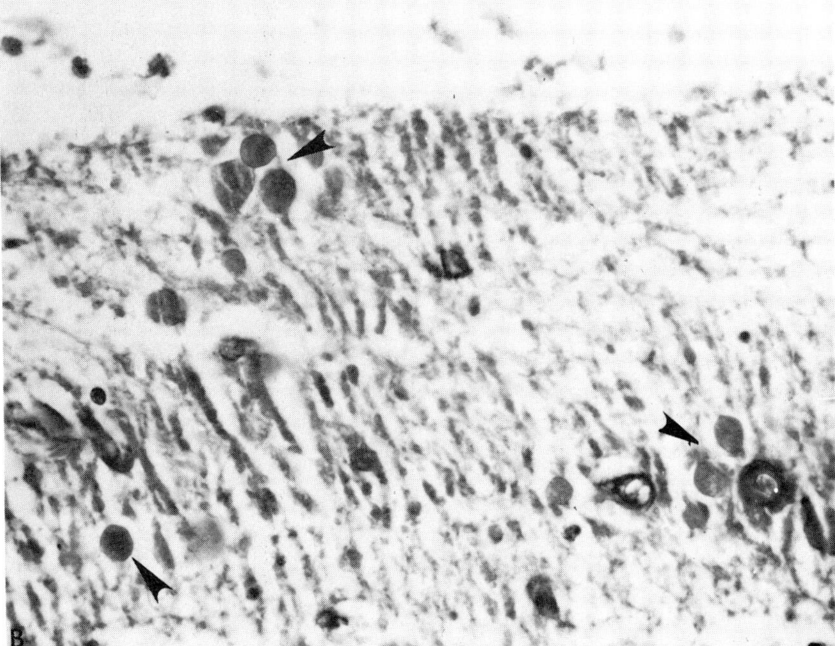

Figure 8–180. Ocular toxoplasmosis in an adult receiving long-term corticosteroid therapy. *A,* Composite fundus photograph showing extensive area of toxoplasmic retinitis. *B,* Necrotic retina showing numerous toxoplasmic cysts (arrowheads), some of which appear necrotic. PAS, ×525.

Illustration continued on following page

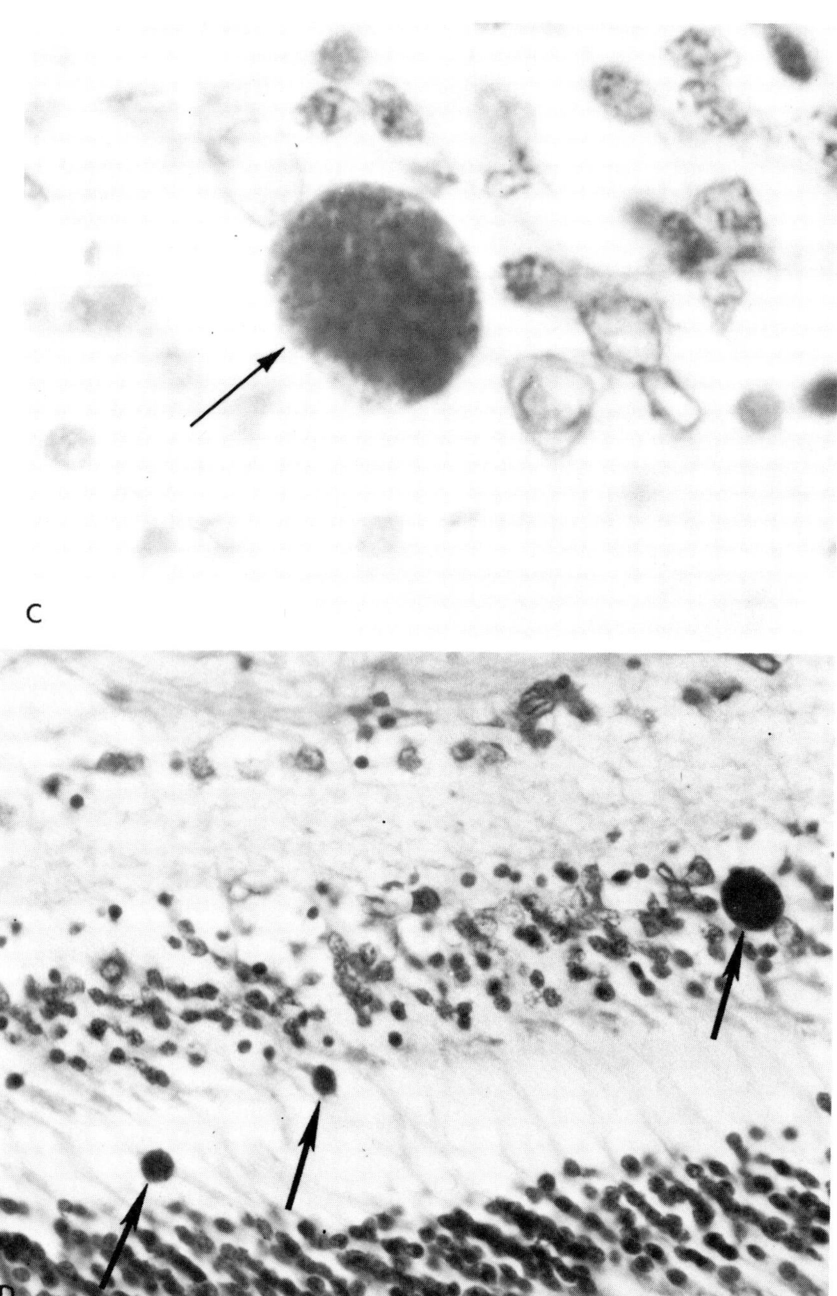

Figure 8–180 *Continued C,* Toxoplasmic cyst (arrow) in area of necrotic retina. PAS, ×1750. *D,* Toxoplasmic cysts (arrows) in adjacent, noninvolved retina. PAS, ×550.
(From Nicholson DH, Wolchok EB: Ocular toxoplasmosis in an adult receiving long-term corticosteroid therapy. Arch Ophthalmol *94*:248–254, 1976.)

gration of nematode larvae of *Toxocara canis* into the eye produced various clinical manifestations, mainly an endophthalmitis, which was often mistaken for a retinoblastoma. Toxocariasis, in fact, proved to be one of the most important etiologic categories in her studies on pseudoglioma and justified the conclusion that nematodiasis was undoubtedly a much more important cause of blindness in children than had been realized. In almost all her patients, the wandering larvae had produced an endophthalmitis that led to massive retinal detachment and formation of a retrolental mass. Within the chronically inflamed and contracted vitreous, there was an abscess or granuloma in which the nematode larva was found (see Chapter 7).

Later, Nichols (1956) identified four of the better-preserved larvae as those of *Toxocara canis,* the cosmopolitan intestinal parasite of the dog. Presumably, the children who developed this endophthalmitis had ingested the ova of Toxocara and developed a systemic infection. The ova, derived from the intestinal tract of the dog or the cat *(Toxocara cati),* can lie dormant under considerable variation in the environment for long periods and, when ingested as a result of eating dirt or playing in sand piles, can produce the human disease.

Ashton (1960) reported four cases of larval granulomatosis of the choroid and retina caused by *Toxocara*. These cases had so much in common, and yet were sufficiently different from the cases of Wilder, that Ashton concluded they formed a new pathologic entity. The patients were children, aged 4, 6, 8, and 16 years. Each had a solitary retinal tumor involving the macula or situated between the disk and the macula (Fig. 8–181). The vitreous was not involved except near the retinal lesion. Microscopically, the retina was elevated, distorted, and partially replaced by an inflammatory mass containing an abundance of dense scar tissue. The subjacent choroid was infiltrated with chronic inflammatory cells and eosinophils. The nematode larvae were buried within the retinal mass, but, judging from the breaks in Bruch's membrane and in the RPE, the *Toxocara* may well have invaded the retina from the choroid.

Since 1960, several reports have been made of a third manifestation of ocular nematodiasis—namely, cases in which the larva had broken through the inner retina into the vitreous, had survived for a variable period, and upon its death had caused an intraocular inflammatory reaction, mainly a retinitis. In a few other cases the larva migrated to the region of the ora serrata, where it produced a retinovitreal inflammatory mass, simulating either a tumor or a focus of toxoplasmosis. Eyes examined histologically with this type of infection show a fibroinflammatory mass, often with eosinophils, inducing extensive destruction of the retina and neovascularization and fibrosis of the vitreous. Within the inflammatory process, the surviving larva could be found (Fig. 8–182). Old nematode lesions are apparently the most common cause of "massive fibrosis" (Fig. 8–183).

In a study of 41 cases, Wilkinson and Welch (1971) found three primary forms of ocular nematodiasis: diffuse, with vitreous involvement and retinal detachment (31.7 per cent); posterior pole lesions (24.4 per cent); and peripheral lesions (43.8 per cent) (Fig. 8–184).

Ocular nematodiasis has presented also as acute uveitis with hypopyon (Smith, Greer, 1971); as peripheral uveitis (Hogan, Kimura, Spencer, 1965); and as diffuse unilateral, subacute neuroretinitis (Gass, Gilbert, Guerly, Scelfo, 1978). The features of 245 published cases up to 1970 have been summarized by Brown (1970).

The nematode has been observed clinically in or under the retina (Rubin, Kaufman, Tierney, Lucas, 1968; Gass and associates, 1978) and has been successfully photocoagulated (Raymond, Gutierrez, Strong, et al, 1978).

The finding of eosinophils in an aqueous aspirate helps support the clinical diagnosis of nematode endophthalmitis (Shields, Lerner, Felberg, 1977).

The development of the enzyme-linked immunosorbent assay (ELISA) test (Cypress, Karol, Zidian, 1977) appears to have some specificity in helping establish the clinical diagnosis (Pollard, Jarrett, Hagler, et al, 1979; Pollard, 1979; Biglan, Glickman, Lobes, 1979).

Cysticercosis. *Cysticercus cellulosae,* the larval form of *Taenia solium* (pork tapeworm) is an important cause of blindness in some areas of the world (Soomsawasdi, Romayananda, Kanchanaranya, 1963).

The normal life cycle of *Taenia solium* starts when the human ingests raw or insufficiently cooked pork containing cysticercus. The larva grows to the adult stage within the small intestine. After larval maturity, ova are discharged in the feces. The pig, the intermediate host, ingests the ovum, which hatches into a larva. The larva penetrates into the circulatory system and invades all tissues of the pig. Human systemic infection occurs when a person accidentally becomes an intermediate host by consuming food or water contaminated by the ova.

Of 807 cases of human systemic cysticercosis, 372 (46 per cent) showed involvement of the eye, eyelids, and/or orbit; 330 (40.8 per cent), the central nervous system; 51, subcutaneous tissues; 28, muscles; and 26, other organs (Vosgien, 1912). The larvae may be located in the aqueous (Fig. 8–185), the vitreous (Figs. 8–186 and 8–187), or under the retina (Figs. 8–188 and 8–189). In the eye, treatment is surgical removal. Many workers have reported successful removal from the eye; some recent ones include: from the vitreous, Ferry, 1980; Hutton, Vaiser, Snyder, 1976; Messner, Kammerer, 1979; Zinn, Guillory, Friedman, 1980; from the subretinal space, Segal, Mrzyglod, Smolarz-Dudarewicz, 1964; Curtin VT, 1970; Bartholomew, 1975; and within the retina, Manschot, 1968b.

If left in the eye, the larva incites an intense fibroinflammatory reaction (Fig. 8–189) with eosinophilic and granulomatous components.

Giardiasis. Knox and King (1982) observed the association of retinal arteritis and iridocyclitis with giardiasis.

Other Parasites. Many different parasites can infect the eye. There are numerous reports of their successful removal from the eye. Some of the parasites that have been reported in or under the retina are

- *Porocephalus armillatus* (Reid and Jones, 1963)
- *Angiostrongylus cantonensis* (Kanchanaranya, Prechanond, Punyagupta, 1972)
- *Cuterebra* larva (ophthalmomyiasis interna) (Dixon, Winkler, Nelson, 1969; Hunt, 1970)
- *Coenurus* (Williams, Templeton, 1971; Manschot, 1976)
- Botfly, subretinal (Fitzgerald, Rubin, 1974)

Text continued on page 777

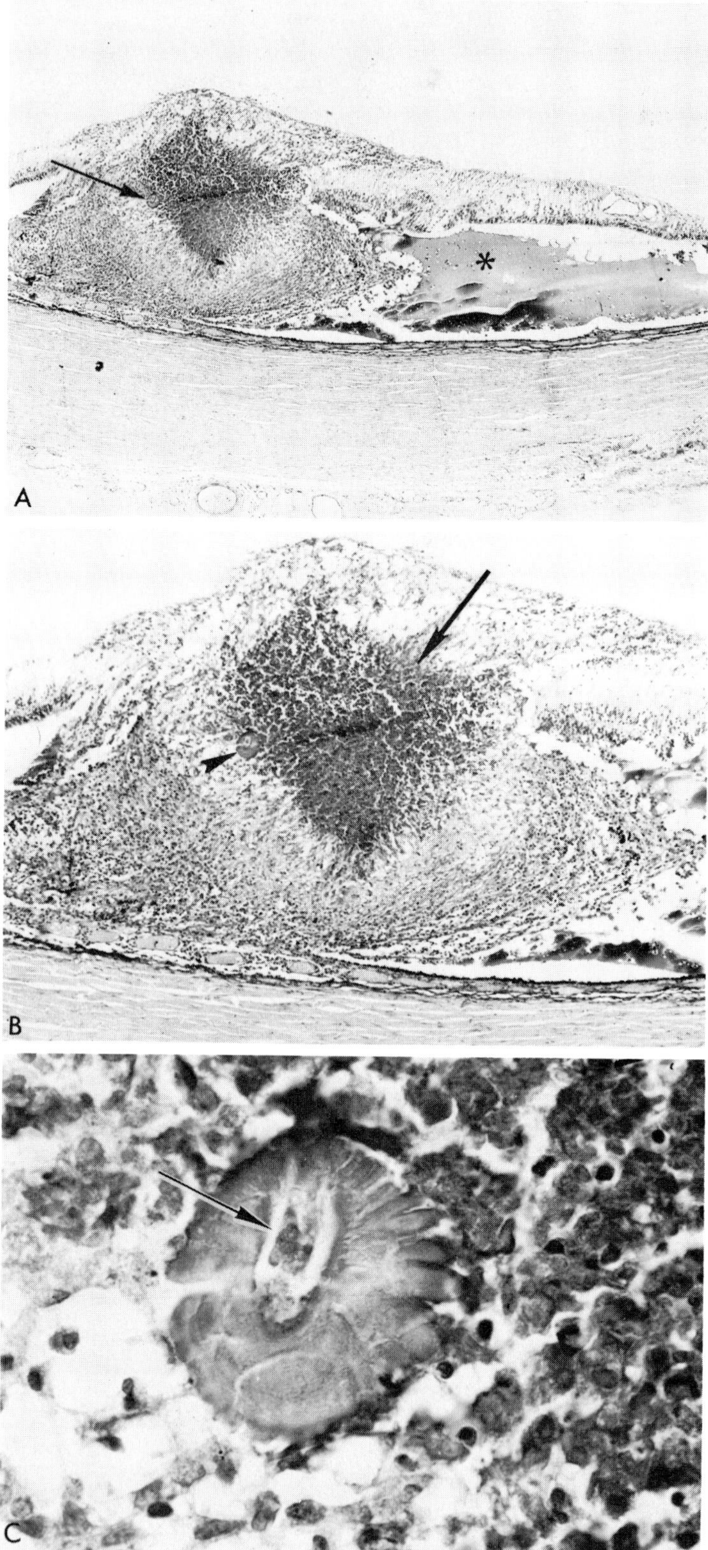

Figure 8–181. *A,* Subretinal fibroinflammatory mass caused by a larva of a nematode (arrow). There is necrosis centrally, a fibroinflammatory tissue beneath the retina internally, and a serous detachment (asterisk) of adjacent retina. H and E, ×35. *B,* Higher power view showing central area of necrosis (arrow) and nematode (arrowhead). H and E, ×60. *C,* Higher power view showing necrotic nematode (arrow) surrounded by an eosinophilic Splendore-Hoeppli precipitate (arrowhead). H and E, ×800. EP 20664. (From Nicholson DH, Green WR: Pediatric Ocular Tumors. New York, Masson, 1981.)

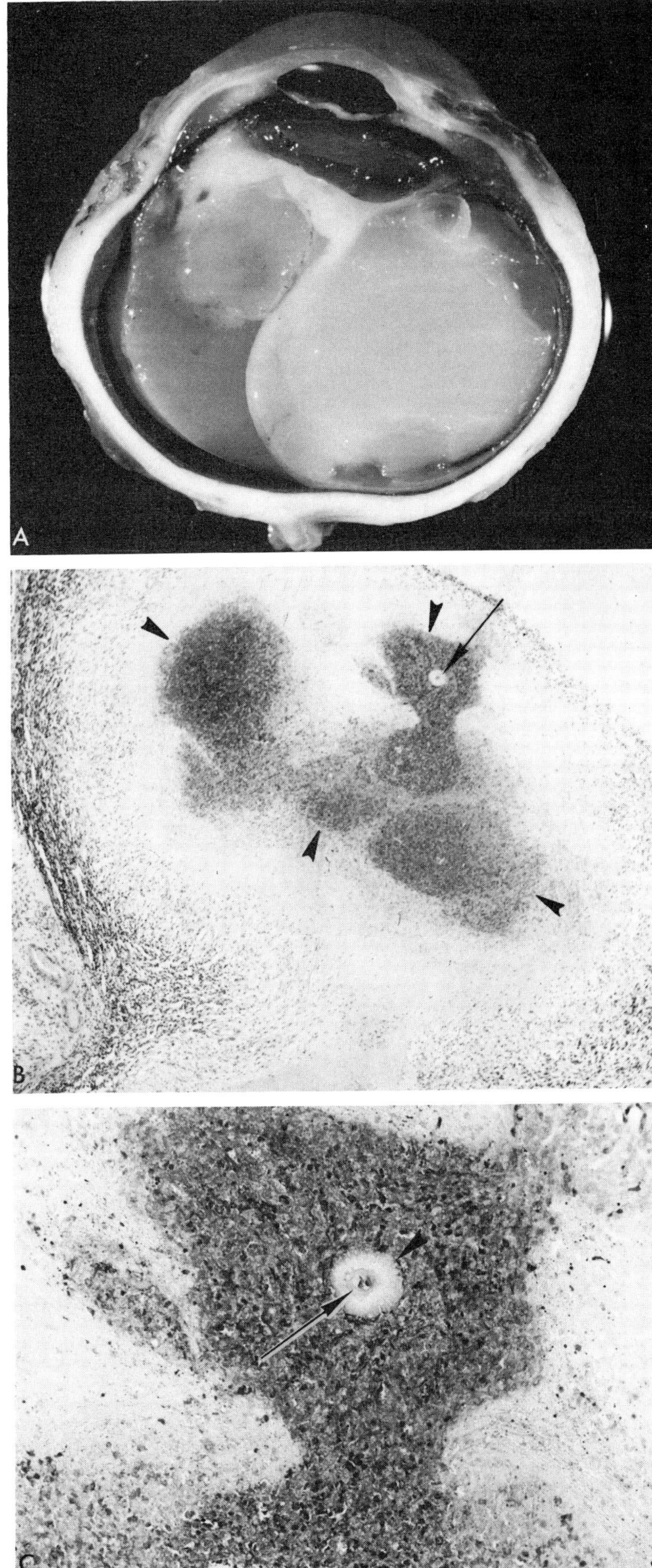

Figure 8–182. Nematode endophthalmitis in a 4 year old child with leukocoria who was considered clinically to have a retinoblastoma. *A,* Gross appearance, showing a total detachment of the retina by a dense, proteinaceous material. *B,* A fibroinflammatory mass is located between the lens and the detached retina. Areas of necrosis (arrowheads) are present within the inflammatory mass; necrotic larva (arrow) is present in one of these. PAS, ×240. *C,* Higher power view, showing necrotic larva (arrow) surrounded by eosinophilic Splendore-Hoeppli precipitate (arrowhead). H and E, ×225. EP 29566.

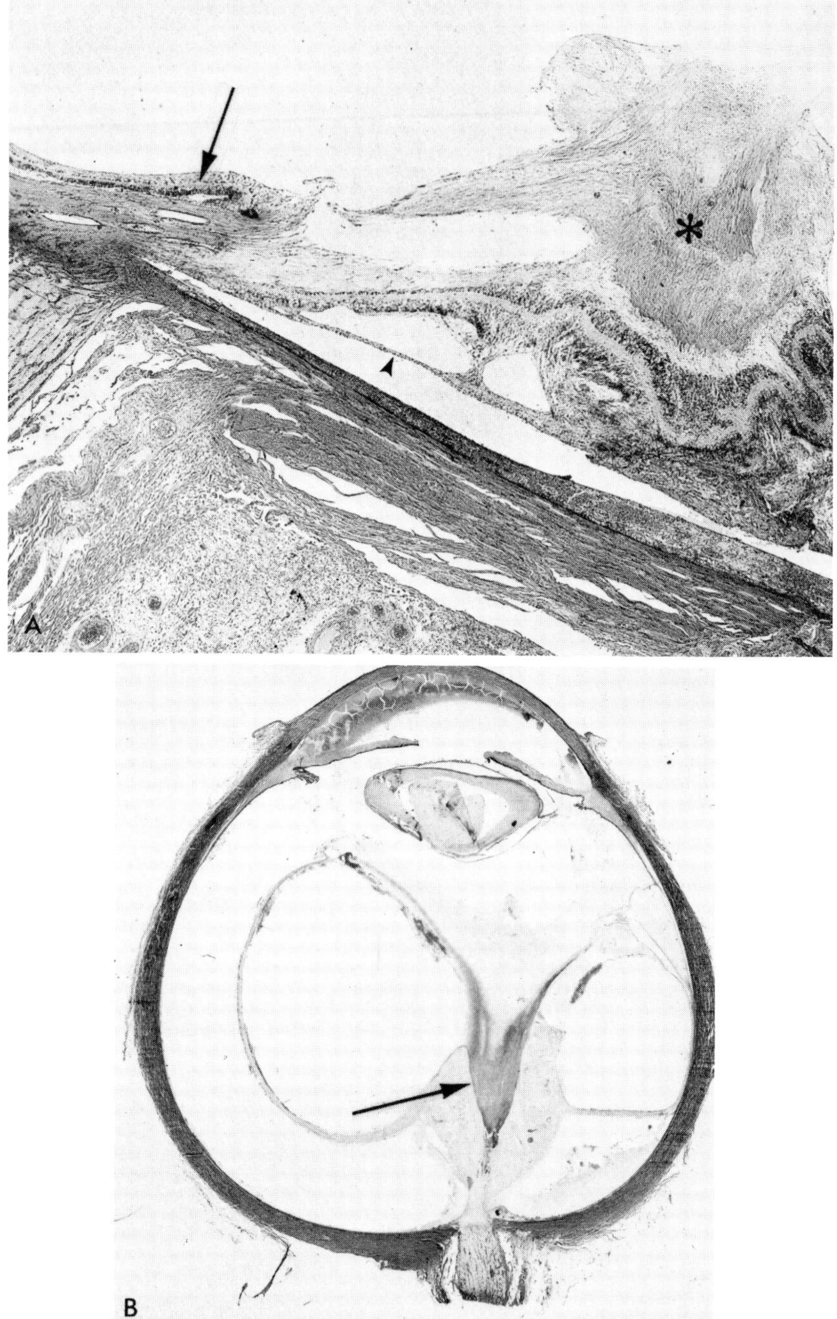

Figure 8–183. "Massive" fibrosis from presumed old nematode endophthalmitis. *A,* Preretinal fibrous tissue mass (asterisk), with distortion and gathering of subjacent retina, traction and dragging of retina over optic nerve head (arrow), and retroretinal membrane formation (arrowhead) in an 8 year old boy. H and E, ×24. EP 44002. *B,* Extensive fibrosis in vitreous (arrow) with traction retinal detachment in a 10 year old child. The patient had been followed for over 3 years with what was clinically considered to be nematode endophthalmitis. Masson, ×4.

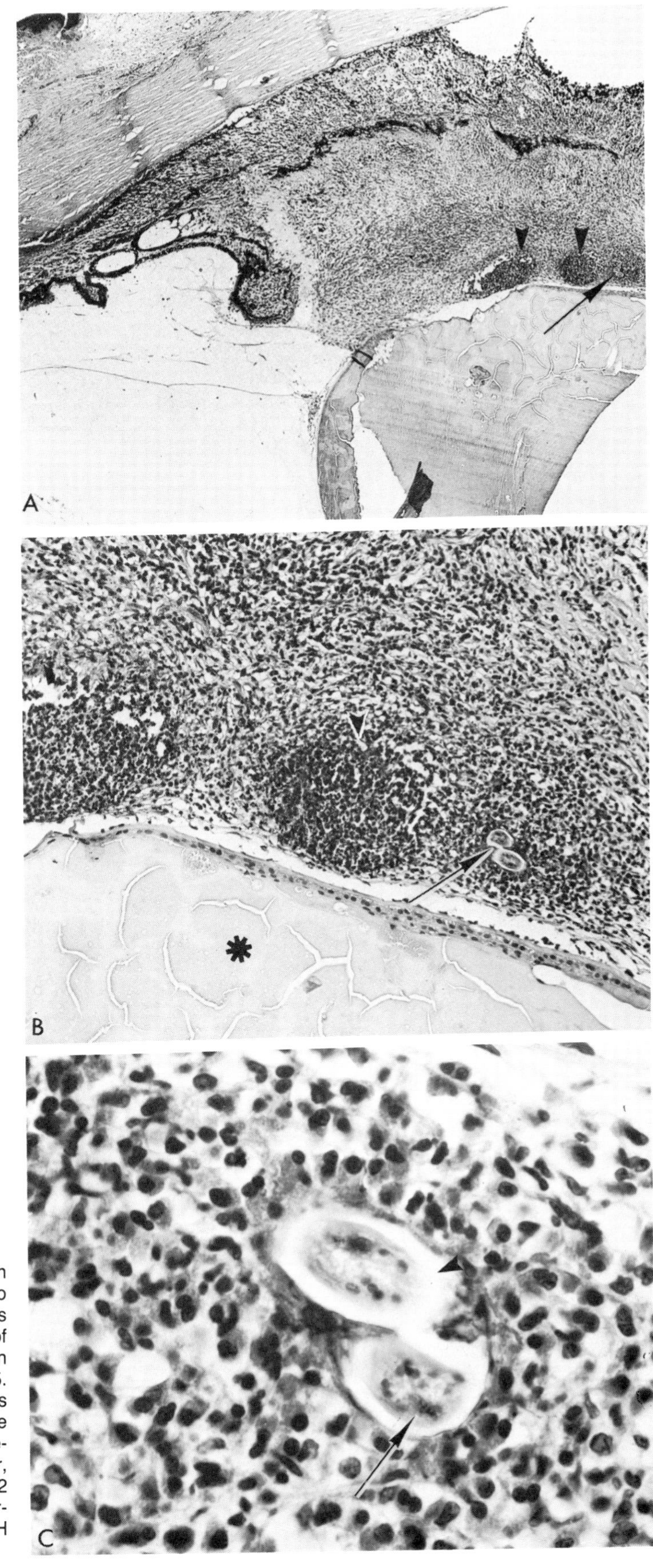

Figure 8–184. Nematode endophthalmitis in a 3 year old child who was thought clinically to have a retinoblastoma. *A,* Fibroinflammatory mass with eosinophilic abscesses (arrowheads), one of which contains a larva (arrow), is located between anteriorly displaced iris and lens. H and E, ×35. *B,* Medium power view of eosinophilic abscesses (arrowhead) and the apparently curved nematode larva cut in two areas (arrow). The asterisk denotes lens. H and E, ×200. *C,* At higher power, the nematode larva is seen to measure about 22 microns in diameter; it has a cuticular border (arrowhead) and some pigment centrally (arrow). H and E, ×900. EP 22892.

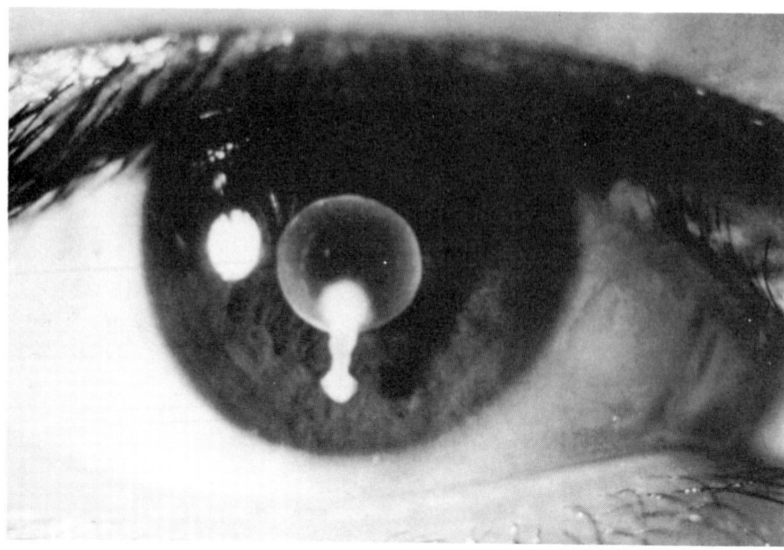

Figure 8–185. Cysticercus with extended scolex in the anterior chamber. (Courtesy of Dr. A.E. Maumenee.)

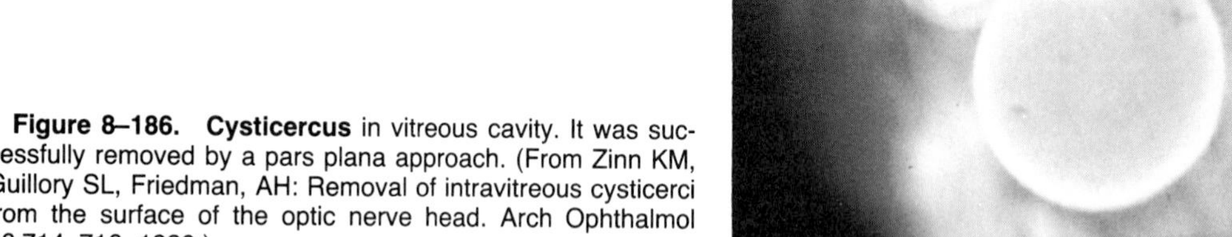

Figure 8–186. Cysticercus in vitreous cavity. It was successfully removed by a pars plana approach. (From Zinn KM, Guillory SL, Friedman, AH: Removal of intravitreous cysticerci from the surface of the optic nerve head. Arch Ophthalmol *98*:714–716, 1980.)

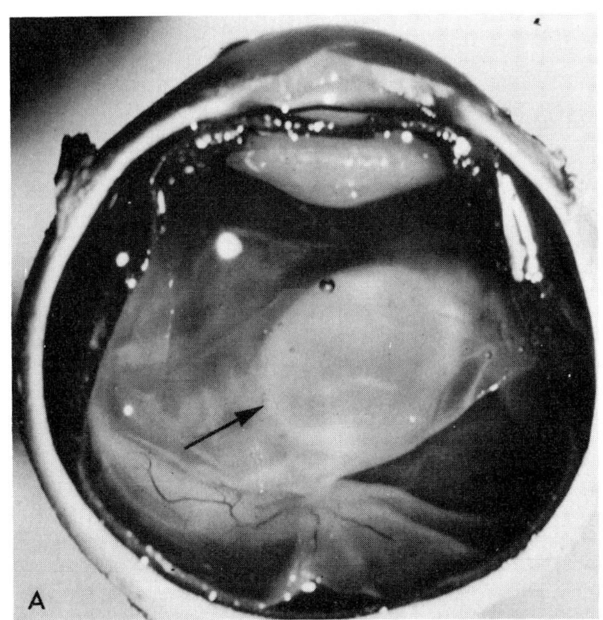

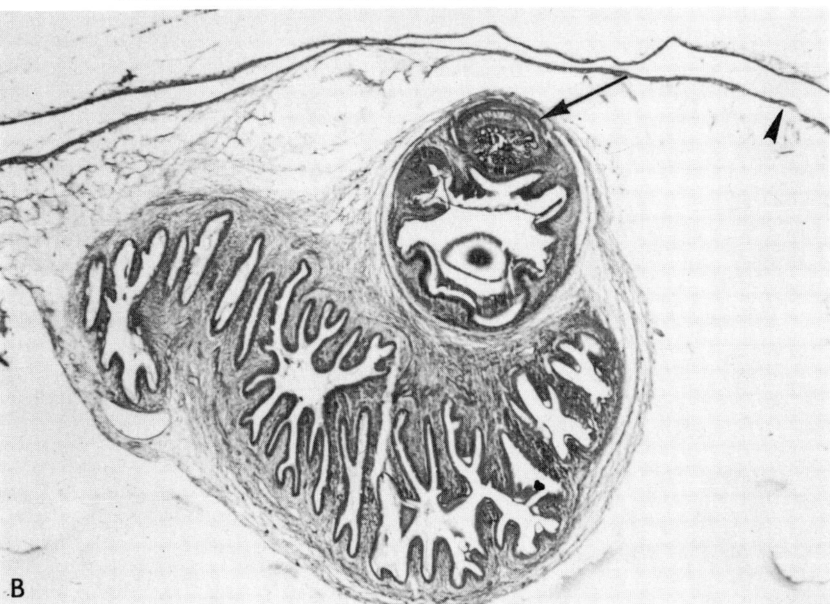

Figure 8–187. *A,* Gross appearance of **cysticercus** (arrow) in vitreous of a 42 year old man. *B,* Section of organism showing cyst wall (arrowhead), scolex (arrow) with approximately 22 hooklets, and body. H and E, ×65. EP 18257.

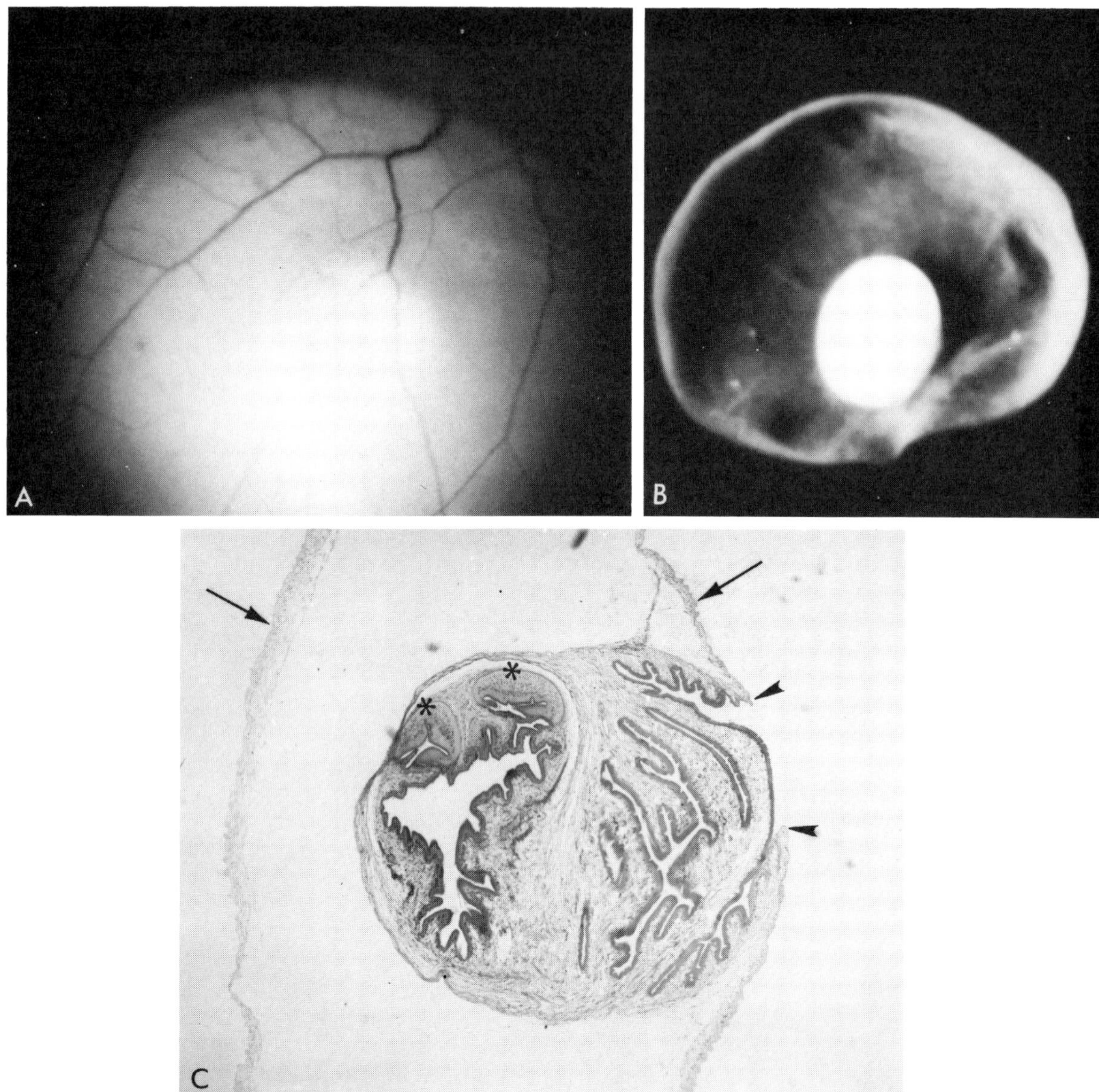

Figure 8–188. Subretinal cysticercus that was successfully removed surgically by Dr. Victor Curtin. *A,* Ophthalmoscopic appearance. *B,* Gross appearance of removed larva. *C,* The intact cyst (arrows), with opening into integument (arrowheads) and scolex (asterisks). H and E, ×70. (Case presented at the Verhoeff Society, Washington, DC, April, 1970.)

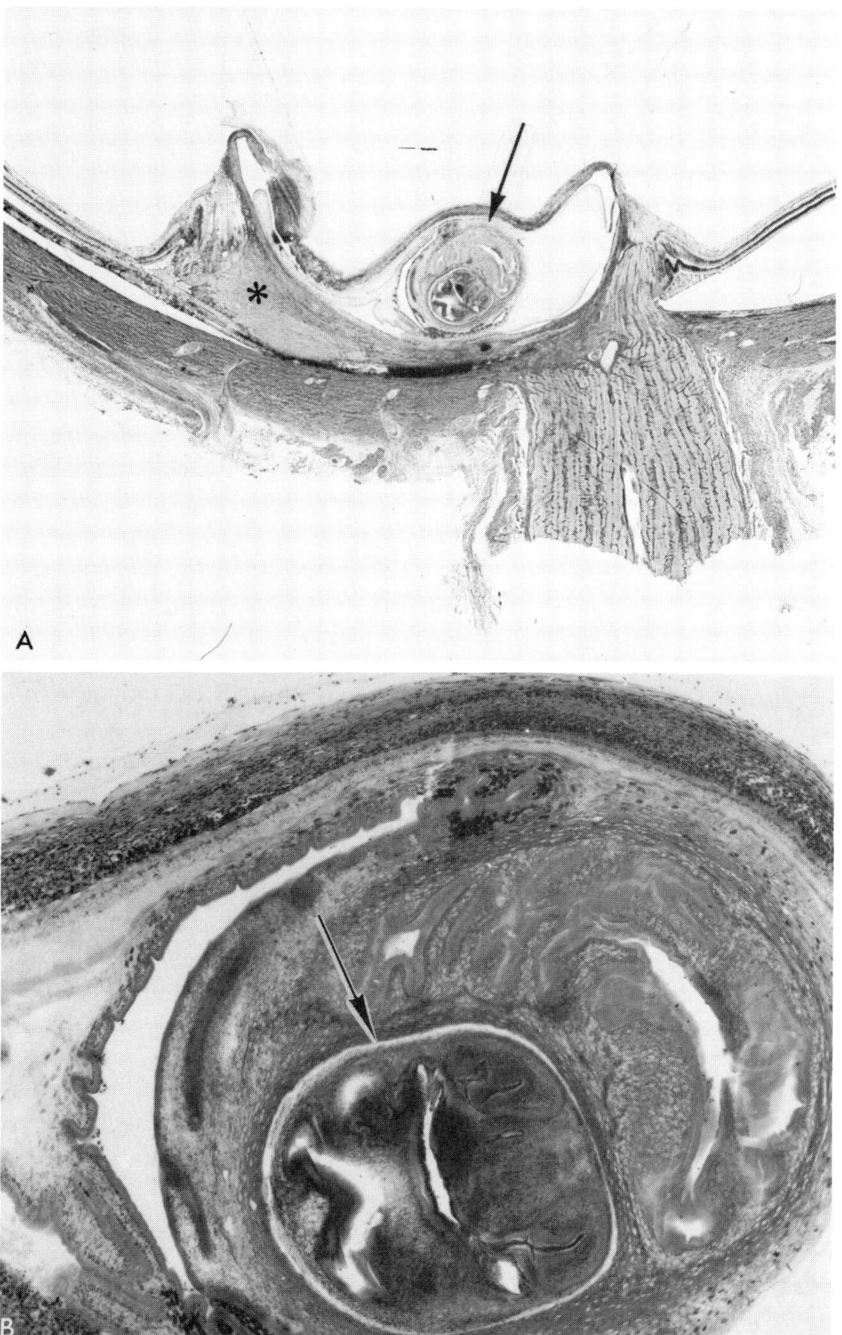

Figure 8–189. *A,* **Subretinal cysticercus** (arrow) with subretinal fibrosis (asterisk). H and E, ×12. *B,* Higher power view, showing scolex (arrow). H and E, ×50. (From Wadsworth J: Ocular cysticercosis. Presented at the Ophthalmic Pathology Club Meeting, Washington, DC, April, 1960.)

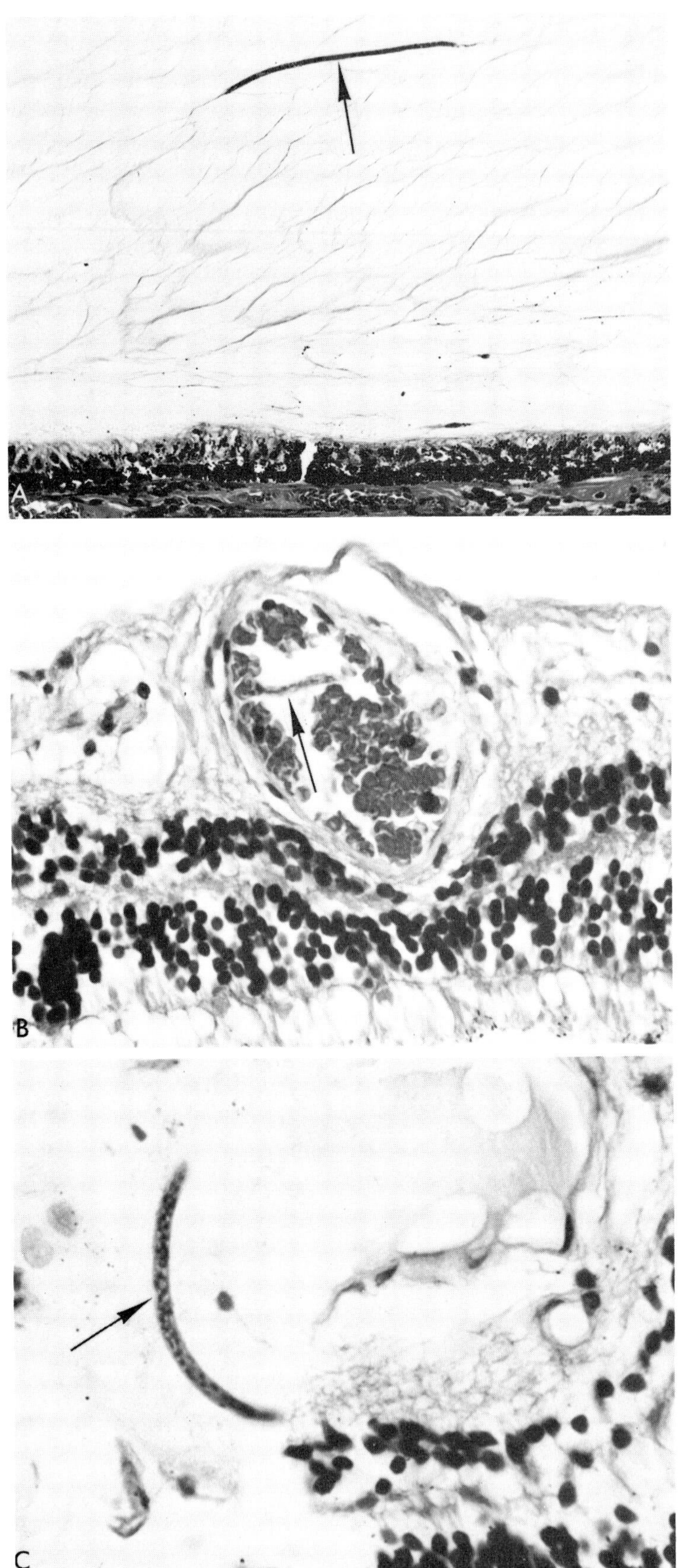

Figure 8–190. Onchocerciasis with microfilariae (arrows) in *A,* vitreous; H and E, ×195; AFIP Neg. 66-7544; *B,* retinal vessel; H and E, ×485; AFIP Neg. 70-6057; and *C,* retina; H and E, ×675; AFIP Neg. 70-2055. (From Paul EV, Zimmerman LE: Some observations on the ocular pathology of onchocerciasis. Hum Pathol *1*:581–594, 1970.)

Gnathostoma spinigerum (Tudor, Blair, 1971)
Larval trematode (Shea, Maberley, Walters, et al, 1973b; Bathrick, Mango, Mueller, 1981)
Taenia crassiceps (Cestoda) (Shea, Maberley, Walters, et al, 1973a)
Intraretinal worm (Price, Wadsworth, 1970)
Larva (Byers, Kimura, 1974)

It is of especial interest that a linear pattern in myiasis interna suggests the tract of larval migration under or in the retina, as was described by Dixon, Winkler, and Nelson (1969). Knox and King (1982) have observed retinal vasculitis in patients with intestinal infection by *Giardia lamblia*.

Onchocerciasis (River Blindness) (Connor, Morrison, Kerdel-Vegas, 1970). This disease deserves special mention, for it is a common cause of blindness in some areas of the world, especially western equatorial Africa and Central America (Taylor, 1981). Blindness may be due to keratitis, nongranulomatous uveitis, and secondary glaucoma (Paul, Zimmerman, 1970). Microfilaria may be seen in virtually any part of the eye (Fig. 8–190).

In a clinical study of 244 selected patients with onchocerciasis from the Sudan Savanna and rain forest areas of the United Cameroon Republic, Bird, Anderson and Fuglsang (1976) found that optic nerve disease, alone or in association with chorioretinal changes, was responsible for 87.6 per cent of the blindness due to posterior segment lesions in onchocerciasis (Fig. 8–191).

The pathogenesis of the chorioretinal lesions is not clear. Clinical and histopathologic studies point to an ischemic process rather than to a direct inflammatory process (Fig. 8–192). Neumann and Gunders (1972, 1973) have observed changes suggesting that the microfilaria gain access to the back of the eye via the scleral canals. Garner (1976) suggests that the marked retinal and choriocapillaris atrophy is attributable to a preceding choroiditis.

Removal of head nodules, combined with micro- and macrofilaricidal therapy, may reduce the developing ocular involvement (Fuglsang, Anderson, 1978).

The microfilariae of the causative parasite, *Onchocerca volvulus,* are sometimes present in the vitreous and elsewhere in the eye, in addition to being in various skin nodules. (See Chapter 9 for a more detailed discussion of onchocerciasis.)

Flubendazole, an injectable benzimidazole, appears to be quite effective in the treatment of onchocerciasis (Dominguez-Vazquez, Taylor, Greene, et al, 1983). The drug apparently sterilizes the adult female parasite.

Miscellaneous Inflammatory Diseases with Retinal Involvement

Acute Retinal Pigment Epitheliitis. See page 1238.

Acute Multifocal Placoid Retinal Epitheliopathy. See page 1238.

Sarcoidosis. Virtually every part of the eye may be involved in this disease (Zimmerman, Maumenee, 1961). Infiltrates may occur in the lid, conjunctiva, lacrimal gland, and orbit, and

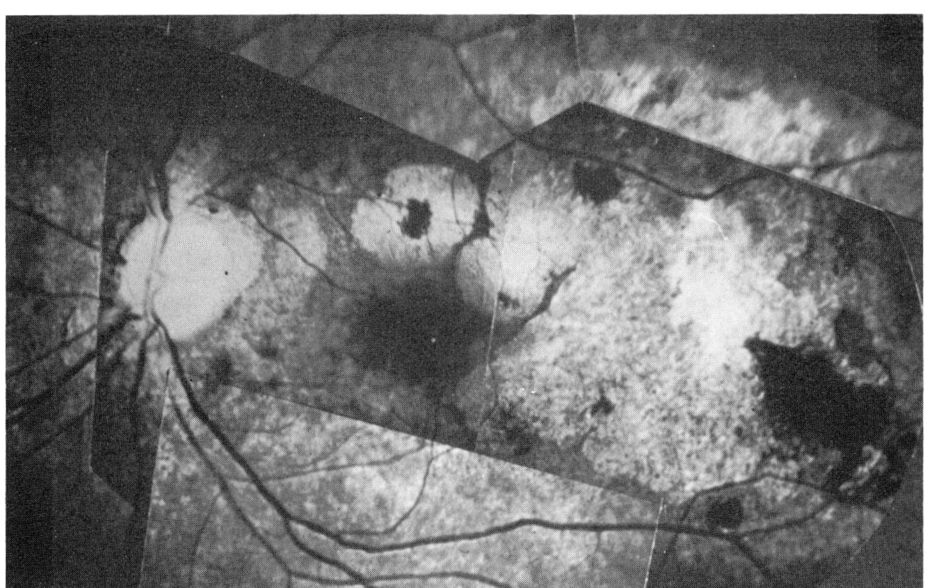

Figure 8–191. Discrete areas of retinal pigment epithelium (RPE) atrophy, with some areas of RPE hypertrophy, in a patient with **onchocerciasis.** (From Bird AC, Anderson J, Fuglsong H: Morphology of posterior segment lesions of the eye in patients with onchocerciasis. Br J Ophthalmol *60*:2–20, 1976.)

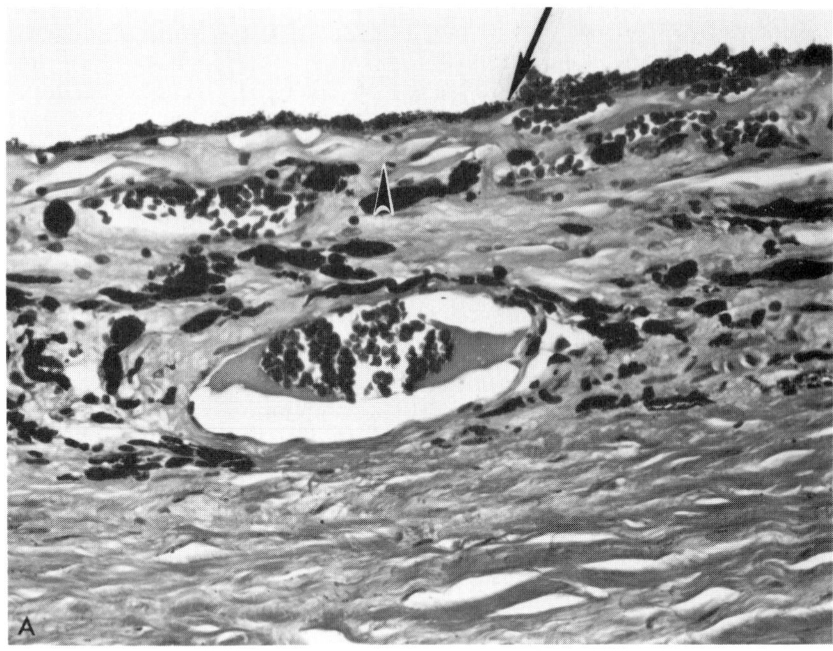

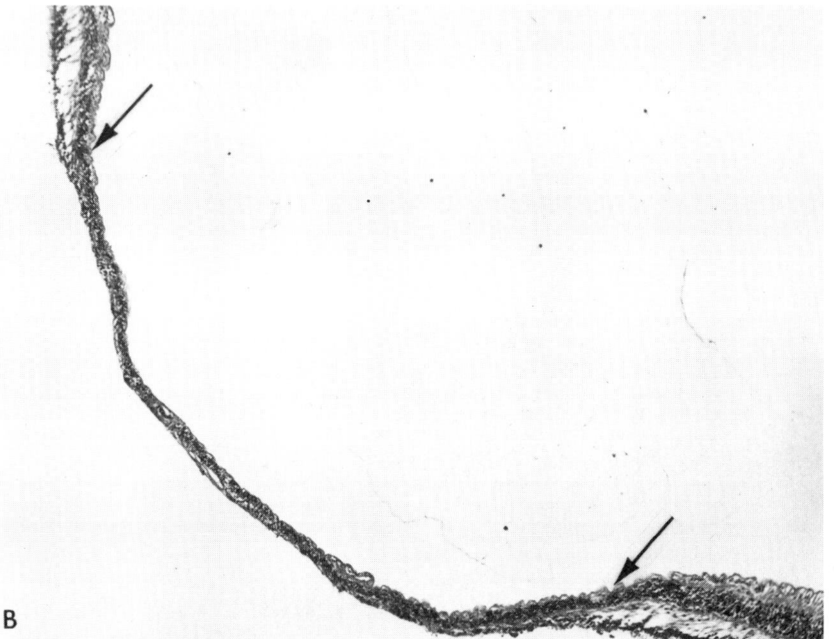

Figure 8–192. Onchocerciasis with retinal involvement. *A,* Area of retinal pigment epithelium thinning and hypopigmentation (left of arrow) associated with partial loss of the choriocapillaris. H and E, ×260. AFIP Neg. 70-6603. *B,* Area of retina showing outer ischemic atrophy (between arrows) and no scarring. H and E, ×50. AFIP Neg. 70-6175. (From Paul EV, Zimmerman LE: Some observations on the ocular pathology of onchocerciasis. Hum Pathol *1*:581–594, 1970.)

also in the uveal tract, retina, vitreous, optic nerve head, and optic nerve.

James and associates made a long, comprehensive study of patients with ocular sarcoidosis in Great Britain and concluded that retinopathy in sarcoidosis was rare and that it was usually overshadowed by a concomitant anterior uveitis (James, Anderson, Langley, Ainslie, 1964; James, Neville, Langley, 1976). Chumbley and Kearns (1972) found the retinal changes to be prominent in their series of patients with sarcoidosis. In their patients, the retinal findings were the exclusive eye manifestations of sarcoidosis. One of the most commonly seen ophthalmoscopic lesions in sarcoidosis is a mild or prominent venous sheathing and associated striae, and flame-shaped or round hemorrhages.

In an extensive review of 532 patients with sarcoidosis, Obenauf, Shaw, Sydnor, and Klintworth (1978) found that ocular manifestations were a prominent feature in 202 (38 per cent). One fifth of those 202 patients reported ocular complaints as the initial manifestation of the disease. Ocular involvement included anterior segment changes in 171 (84.7 per cent) of the patients. Chronic granulomatous uveitis was the most common abnormality in 106 patients (52.5 per cent). Posterior segment disease occurred in

51 (25.3 per cent) and included chorioretinitis or periphlebitis. The incidence of central nervous system sarcoidosis was increased when posterior segment eye involvement was observed. Orbital and adnexal structures, particularly the lacrimal gland, were affected in 53 (27.7 per cent) patients.

The retinal lesions of sarcoidosis may be single or multiple and usually are minute, but large, granulomatous nodules producing retinal detachment may occur. Sarcoid granulomas may be observed in front of, in, and under the retina (Fig. 8–193). Histopathologic studies of eyes with sarcoid lesions of retina and optic nerve head (Fig. 8–194) (Kelley, Green, 1973; Gass, Olson, 1973), retina and optic nerve (Brownstein and Jannotta, 1974), and optic nerve head (Jampol, Woodfin, McLean, 1972; Laties, Scheie, 1970) have been reported. Vascular occlusive disease with peripheral retinal neovascularization has been observed (Asdourian, Goldberg, Bruce, 1975). Other secondary changes include secondary glaucoma and cystoid macular edema (Fig. 8–195).

It is thought by some (Chumbley, Kearns, 1972) that the infiltrates along retinal veins ("en taches de bougie," candle-wax spots) are highly suggestive of sarcoidosis. These lesions are perivenous, scattered, discrete, and gray-white. Some also consider that if a patient has retinal and optic nerve head involvement by sarcoidosis, there is a greater likelihood of central nervous system involvement (Chumbley, Kearns, 1972; Obenauf, Shaw, Sydnor, Klintworth, 1978). Gould and Kaufman (1961) report that 37 per cent of patients with retinal involvement had, or developed, central nervous system sarcoidosis.

Conjunctival biopsies have been reported as helpful in establishing a diagnosis (Bornstein, Frank, Radner, 1962). Noncaseating and non–foreign body granulomas were found in 25 per cent of patients attending a sarcoidosis clinic. Some biopsy specimens were positive even when there was no evidence of conjunctival or intraocular disease.

Nichols, Eagle, Yanoff, and Menocal (1980) reported positive conjunctival biopsies in 55 per cent of patients with biopsy-proved sarcoidosis from other sites. Elliot (1980), in a review of the subject, recommends the following: It is superfluous to do a "blind" conjunctival biopsy in patients with biopsy-proved sarcoid unless one is trying to rule out the advent of a new disease: perform a purposeful biopsy of the conjunctiva in all patients with clinical presumptive sarcoid if a suspicious lesion is discovered; perform a blind biopsy of the conjunctiva in all patients with clinically presumptive sarcoid.

Sarcoid granulomas were observed in biopsy specimens of minor salivary glands in 58 per cent of 75 cases studied (Nessan, Jacoway, 1979).

Lieberman (1975), Nosal, Schleissner, Mishkin, and Lieberman (1979), and Weinreb and Kimura (1980) have observed increased serum angiotensin converting enzyme (ACE) in patients with sarcoidosis. Israel, Park, and Mansfield (1976) found the gallium scan to be helpful in the detection of sarcoidosis. Nosal and associates (1979) and Weinreb, Barth, and Kimura (1980) have observed that combining the ACE assay with gallium scans may be the most sensitive and specific test for sarcoid.

Retinal Vasculitis, Periphlebitis, and Periarteritis. A number of types of phlebitis and arteritis have been observed in the fundus on clinical examination. The most common occurs from uveitis, especially iridocyclitis and other types of anterior uveitis, as described earlier in this section.

Another type of vasculitis occurs with various types of systemic disease, such as sarcoidosis. Other forms are related to allergic states in which the retina acts as a "shock organ" during the course of a systemic allergic reaction. Various other metabolic and hematopoietic diseases have been associated with retinal vasculitis.

Eales' Disease. Apparently there are two forms of Eales' disease: one shows peripheral perivascular striation and sheathing, which slowly extends posteriorly and may or may not be associated with bleeding. There is evidence that this type is related to the development of peripheral arteriolar-venous communications in the retina, and usually it is not associated with exudation of cells into the vitreous or other evidence of ocular inflammation. The second type is a true retinal perivasculitis, more commonly involving the veins, associated with exudation of cells and debris into the vitreous; it is usually found with a mild-to-moderate inflammation in the iris and anterior chamber.

The latter form (considered the classic form) of Eales' disease occurs in healthy young men between the ages of 20 and 30 years and is most often bilateral. A number of reports have implicated tuberculosis, either active or inactive, elsewhere in the body, inducing a hypersensitivity reaction in the retinal vessels to tuberculoprotein. The most convincing report in this respect is that of Elliot (1954). He reported finding peripheral retinal phlebitis in a young man who died of acute fulminating pulmonary tuberculosis. Histopathologic studies have failed to disclose tubercle bacilli in the eye (Kimura, Carriker, Hogan, 1956; Elliot, 1954).

Clinically, there is considerable variation in the severity and manifestations of the vasculitis (Donders, 1958). The process may be quite mild and characterized by only slight peripheral involvement and no tendency for vitreous hemorrhages. It may also be more severe and progressive, with extension toward the posterior fundus and tendency for hemorrhages into the retina and

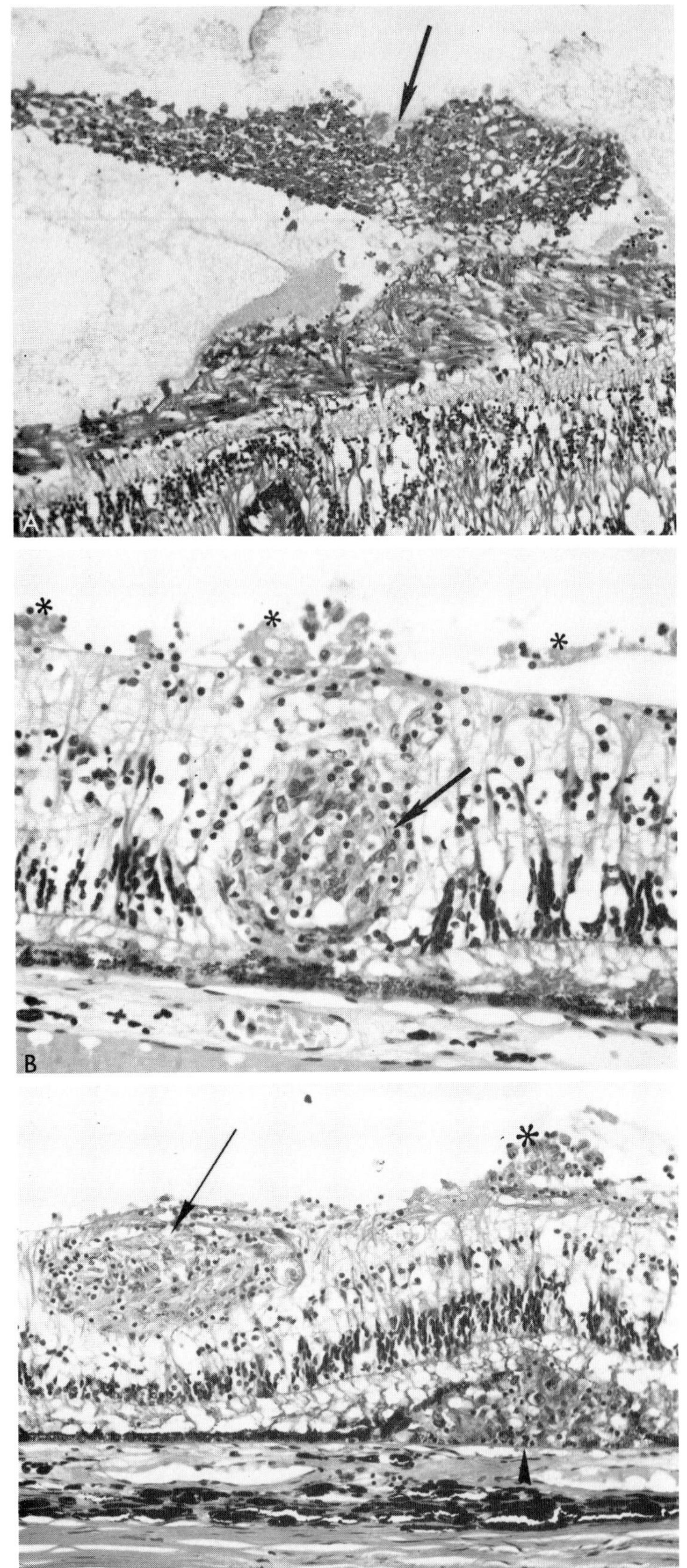

Figure 8–193. Retinal involvement in sarcoidosis. *A,* Granulomatous nodule (arrow) extending into the vitreous from the retinal surface. H and E, ×110. *B,* Intraretinal epithelioid cell nodule (arrow) and inflammatory cell precipitates on the retinal surface (asterisks). H and E, ×290. *C,* Epithelioid cell nodules in retina (arrow), on inner surface of the retina (asterisk), and under the retinal pigment epithelium (arrowhead). The latter resembles the Dalen-Fuchs' nodules seen in sympathetic uveitis. H and E, ×210. EP 43889.

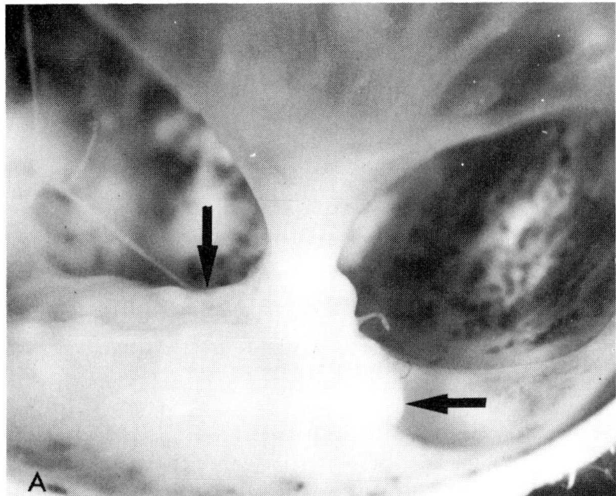

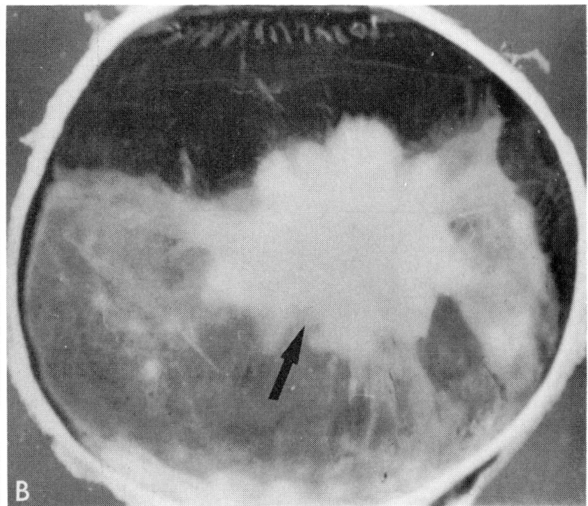

Figure 8–194. **Large sarcoid granulomas** (arrows) involving *A,* the optic nerve head and *B,* The peripheral retina. EP 31023. (From Kelley JS, Green WR: Sarcoidosis involving the optic nerve head. Arch Ophthalmol *89*:486–488, 1973.)

the adjacent vitreous. In the more serious types, there is extensive involvement, with massive recurrent vitreous hemorrhages. In the classic case, the disease mainly affects the veins in the peripheral fundus in one or more sectors.

The cause of retinal periphlebitis/phlebitis is unknown. It is considered to be a local manifestation of systemic disease of inflammatory, vascular, endocrine, or hematologic types (Ashton, 1962; Doden, 1960).

Histologic study of eyes with Eales' disease has always been unsatisfactory because most of the eyes examined have been enucleated in the very late stages of the disease, when the retina was detached and the initial pathology had long been obliterated. In the few eyes examined earlier in the disease, the process is primarily a phlebitis and periphlebitis with some coincident involvement of the smaller arterioles. The vessel walls are inflamed and partly disrupted, and there is perivascular infiltration of white blood cells. Occlusion of these vessels is common. Hemorrhage may be seen within the retina, and often there is damage to the inner limiting membrane, neovascularization, and bleeding into the vitreous, followed by retinal detachment. As the hemorrhage becomes organized and absorbed, wandering cells, fibroblasts, and sprouting capillaries invade the vitreous from the retina and contribute further to the vitreous hemorrhage and retinal detachment.

Elliot (1975) found the prognosis for useful vision to be good in his long-term study of 135 patients with Eales' disease.

Patrinely, Green, and Randolph (1982) have observed clinical and histopathologic features similar to those of Eales' disease in eyes of two patients with multiple calcific emboli (Fig. 8–196).

Retinal Antigen/Rhodopsin Sensitization. To date, this is a purely experimental laboratory animal disease. It is included here briefly because it may have implications for several ocular inflammatory conditions.

Homologous retinal outer segment sensitization (Wong, Green, Kuwabara, et al, 1974) and purified rhodopsin sensitization (Wong, Green, McMaster, Johnson, 1975; Wong, Green, McMaster, 1977) produce a spectrum of inflammatory disease, depending in large part on the dose of antigen. The picture may vary from extreme bullous retinal detachment, as in Vogt-Koyanagi-Harada syndrome (Fig. 8–197), to selective loss of the photoreceptor outer segments with minimal inflammation (Figs. 8–198 and 8–199).

Homologous retina (Wacker, Lipton, 1965) and retinal antigen (Wacker, Donoso, Kalsow, et al, 1977; Rao, Wacker, Marak, 1979) have produced a similar spectrum of dose-related inflammatory ocular disease. The role of retinal antigen in various ocular diseases, including sympathetic ophthalmia, has been suggested (Marak, 1979).

Pars Planitis (Welch, Maumenee, Wahlen, 1960) (Peripheral Uveitis [Schepens, 1950; Brockhurst, Schepens, Okamura, 1961]; Cyclitis with Peripheral Chorioretinitis [Hogan, Kimura, 1961]; Chronic Cyclitis [Kimura, Hogan, 1963]; Basal Uveoretinitis [Bec, Arne, Philippot, 1977]). Because of the prominent retinal involvement in this disease of unknown etiology, it is included in this section on the retina. The disease affects mainly children and young adults, with the insidious onset of vitreous floaters and hazy vision. Edema of the optic disk and macula and dilated,

Text continued on page 791

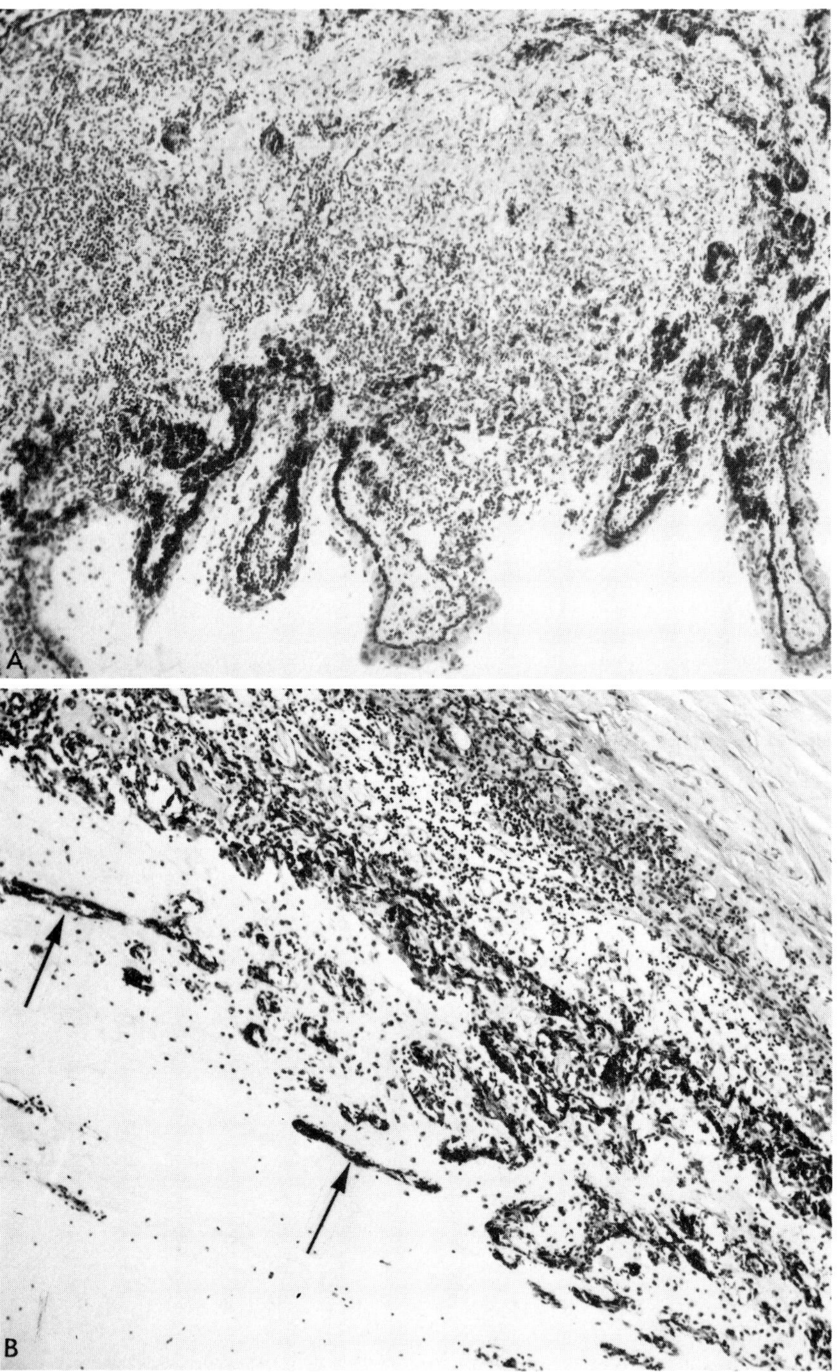

Figure 8–195. Sarcoidosis involving the ciliary body, with retinal phlebitis and cystoid macular edema. *A,* Mixed granulomatous and nongranulomatous inflammatory cell infiltrate of pars plicata. H and E, ×105. *B,* Similar inflammatory process in pars plana, with hyperplasia of ciliary epithelium (arrows) in a "snowbank" configuration. PAS, ×105.

Illustration continued on opposite page

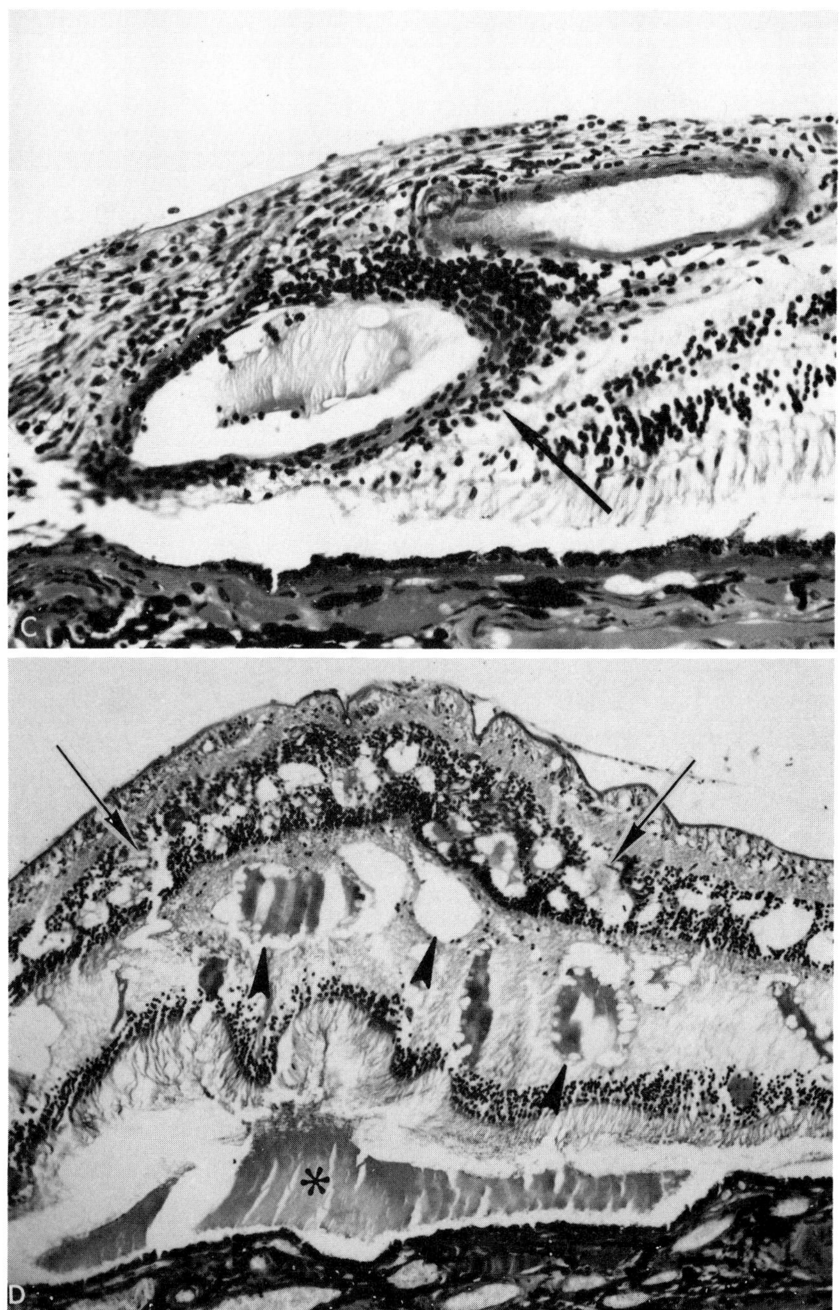

Figure 8–195 *Continued C,* Retinal phlebitis (arrow). PAS, ×225. *D,* Cystoid macular edema, with involvement of the inner nuclear (arrows) and outer plexiform (arrowheads) layers. A small amount of serous material (asterisk) is present under the retina. PAS, ×105. EP 30504.

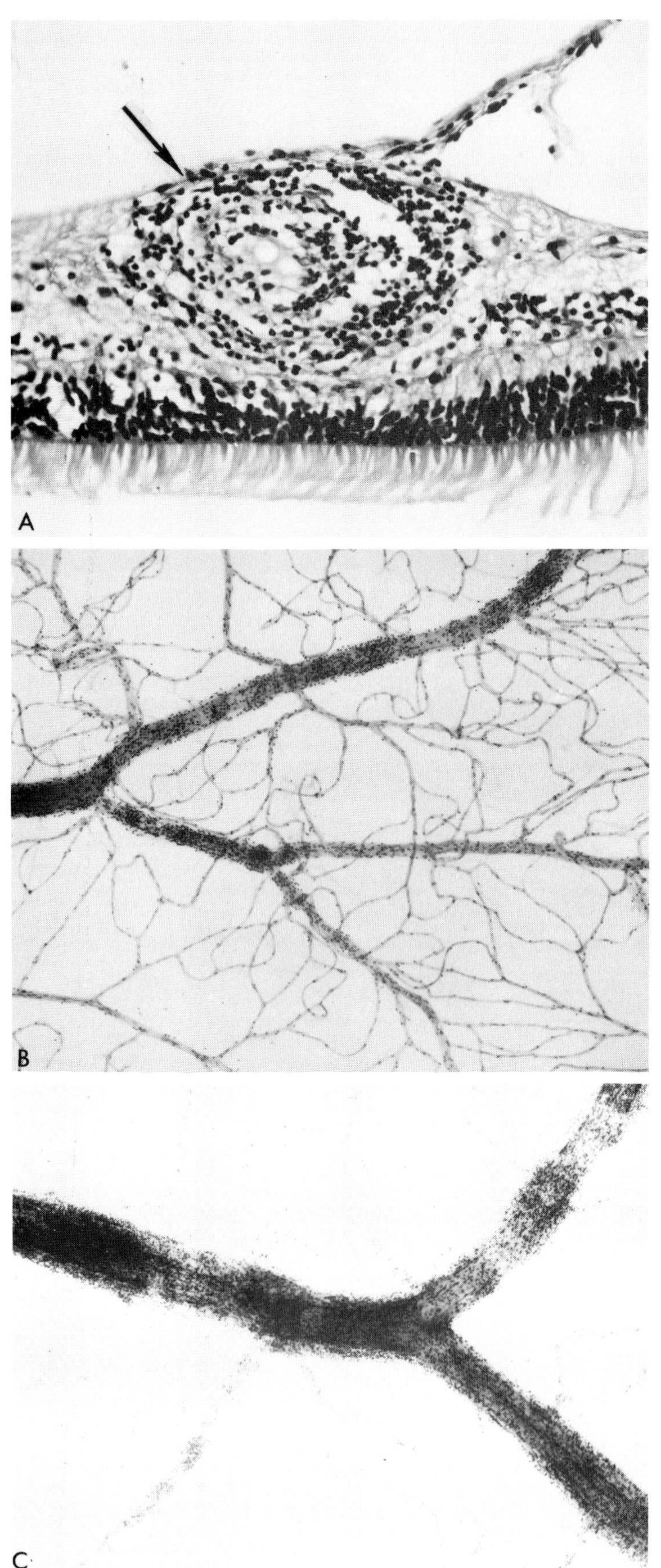

Figure 8–196. Retinal phlebitis associated with several retinal and choroidal calcific emboli. *A,* Intense retinal phlebitis (arrow), with extension into the vitreous. H and E, ×325. *B,* Retinal phlebitis shown by the trypsin digestion technique. PAS, H and E, ×60. *C,* Higher power view showing the vein wall thickened by a lymphocytic infiltrate. PAS, H and E, ×60.

Illustration continued on opposite page

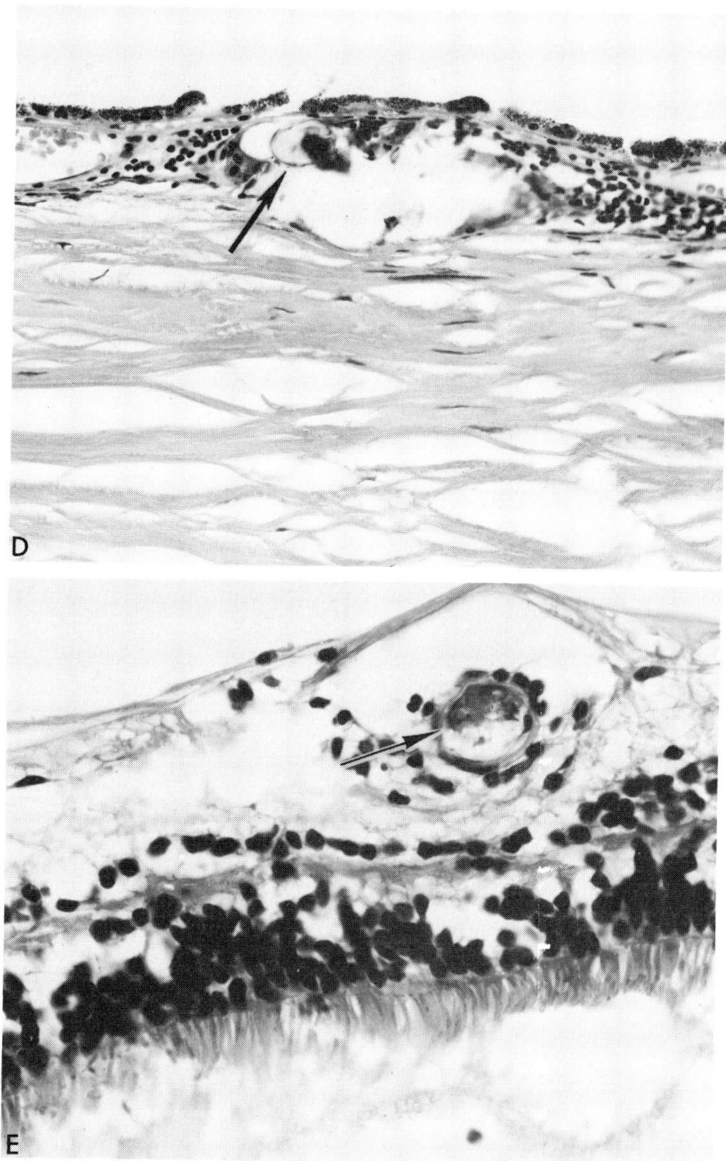

Figure 8–196 *Continued D,* Calcific embolus (arrow) in a choroid vessel. H and E, ×50. *E,* Calcific embolus (arrow) in retinal artery. H and E, ×625. EP 47704.
(From Patrinely JR, Green WR, Randolph ME: Retinal phlebitis with chorioretinal emboli. Am J Ophthalmol *94*:49–57, 1982.)

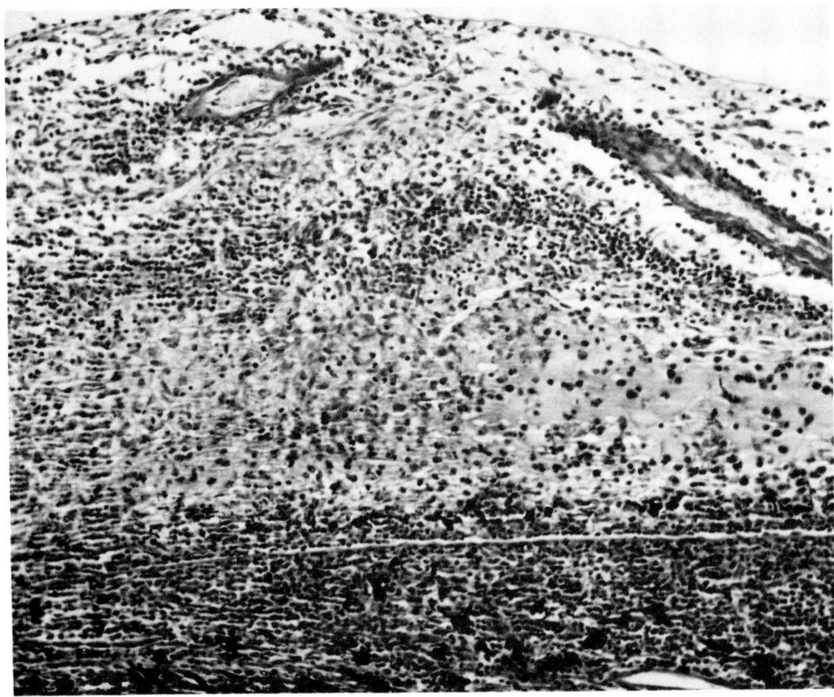

Figure 8–197. Rhodopsin sensitization with large dosage produces an intense inflammatory reaction involving retina and choroid. H and E, ×140. EP 39470.

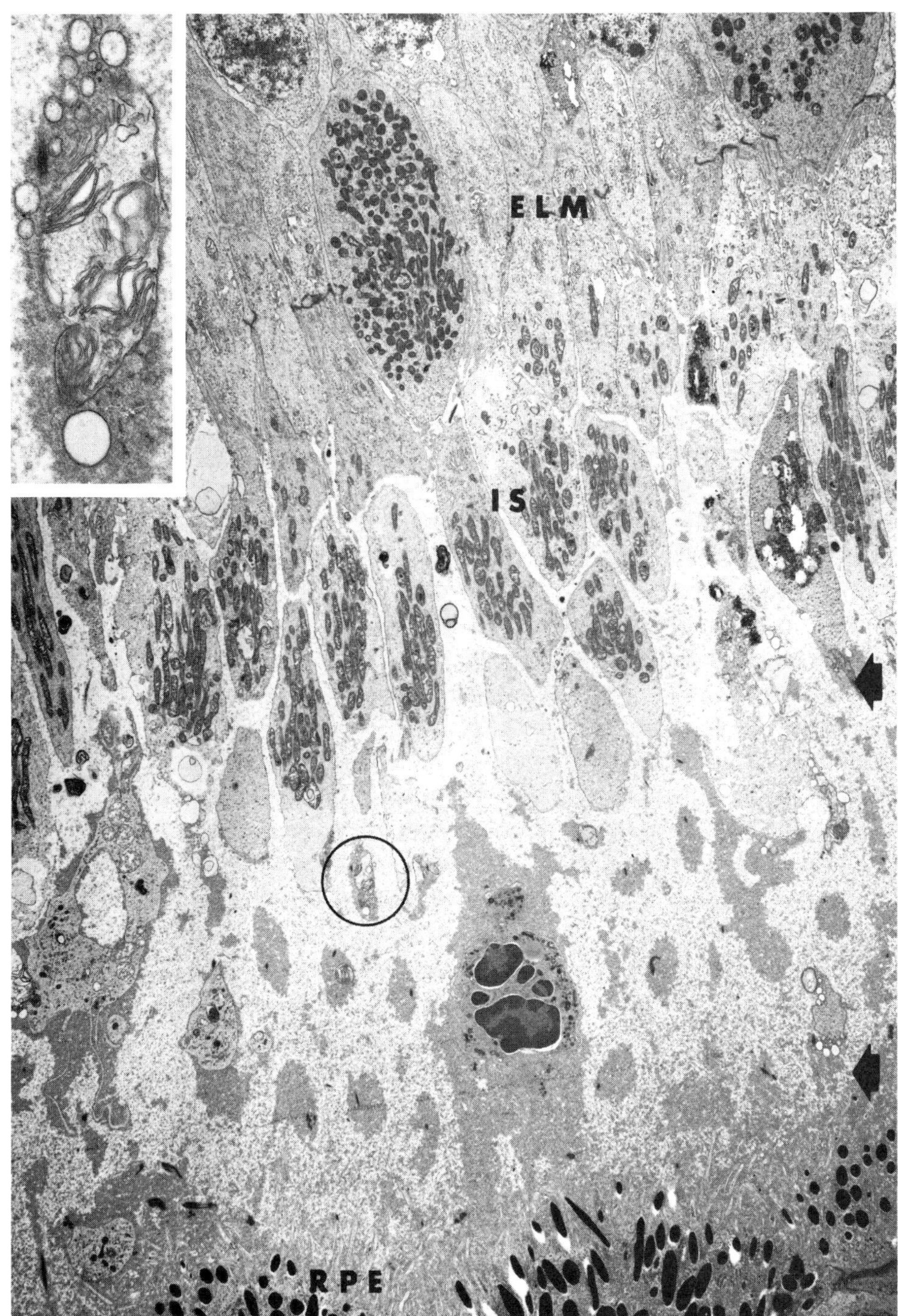

Figure 8–198. Homologous retinal outer segment immunization in monkey. There is almost total destruction of outer segments of rods and cones. The outer segment zone is filled with cellular debris, with occasional fragments of outer segment discs (circle and inset). *ELM,* external limiting membrane; *IS,* inner segments; *RPE,* retinal pigment epithelium. Outer segment zone is indicated by arrows. ×2600; inset, × 14,350. (From Wong VG, Green WR, Kuwabara T, et al: Homologous retinal outer segment immunization in primates: A clinical and histopathologic study. Trans Am Ophthalmol Soc *72*:184–195, 1974.)

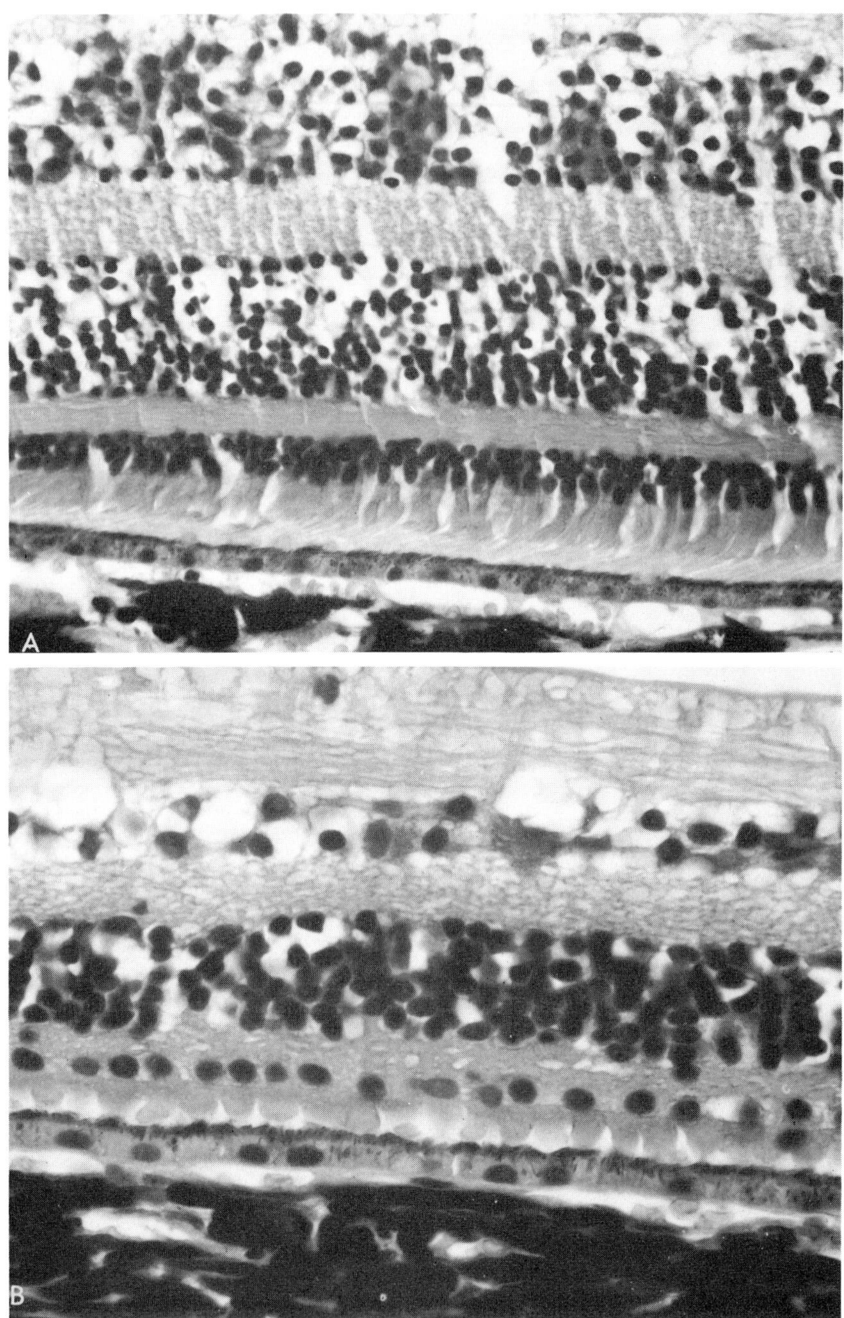

Figure 8–199. Chronic rhodopsin sensitization at low dosage. *A,* Preservation of photoreceptors in macular area. H and E, ×475. *B,* Midperiphery with loss of outer segments, reduction of stubby appearance of inner segments, and thinning of outer nuclear layer. H and E, ×610.

Illustration continued on opposite page

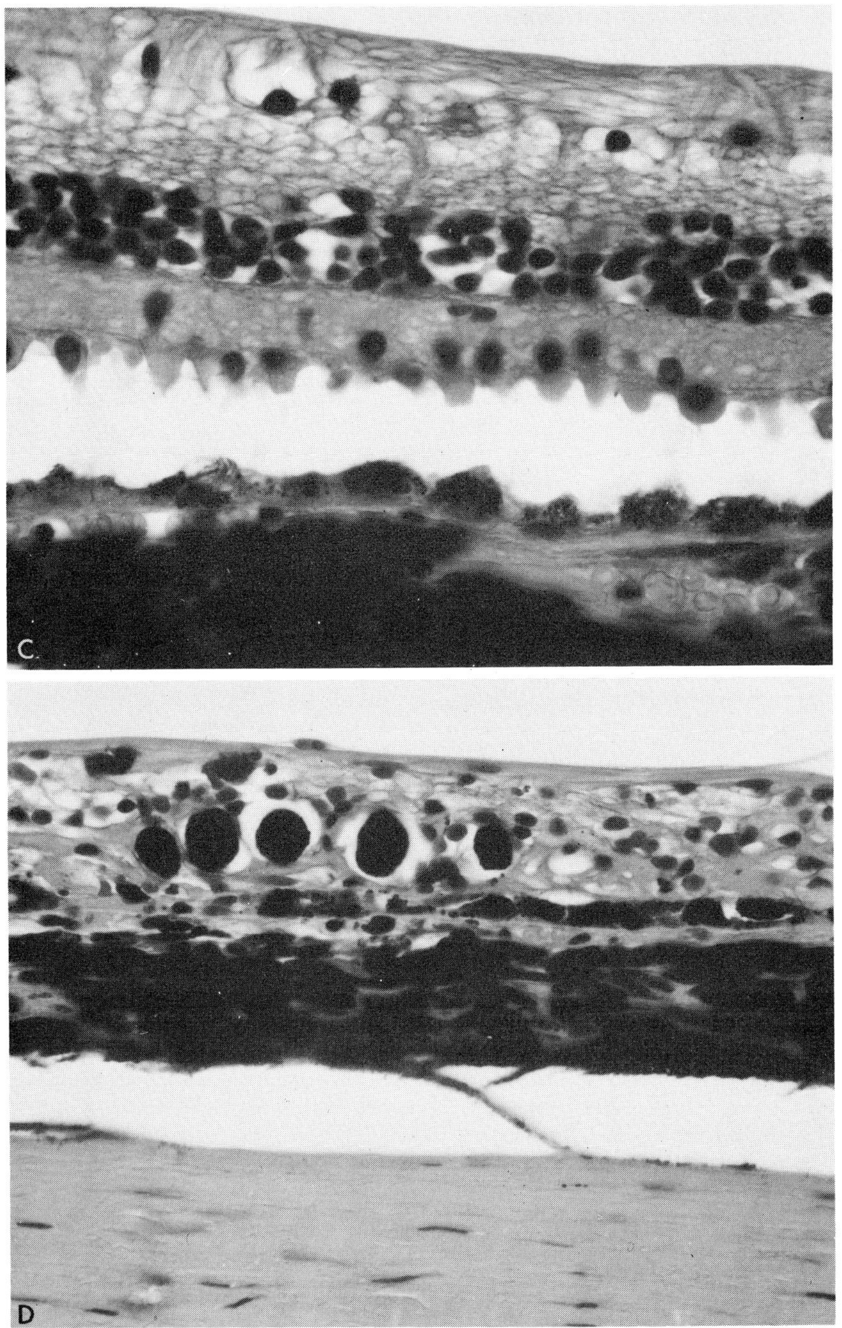

Figure 8–199 *Continued C,* Area just posterior to equator with increased photoreceptor cell loss. H and E, ×475. *D,* Equatorial area showing total loss of photoreceptor cell layer and pigment migration into retina. EP 51460. (Courtesy of Dr. Vernon G. Wong.)

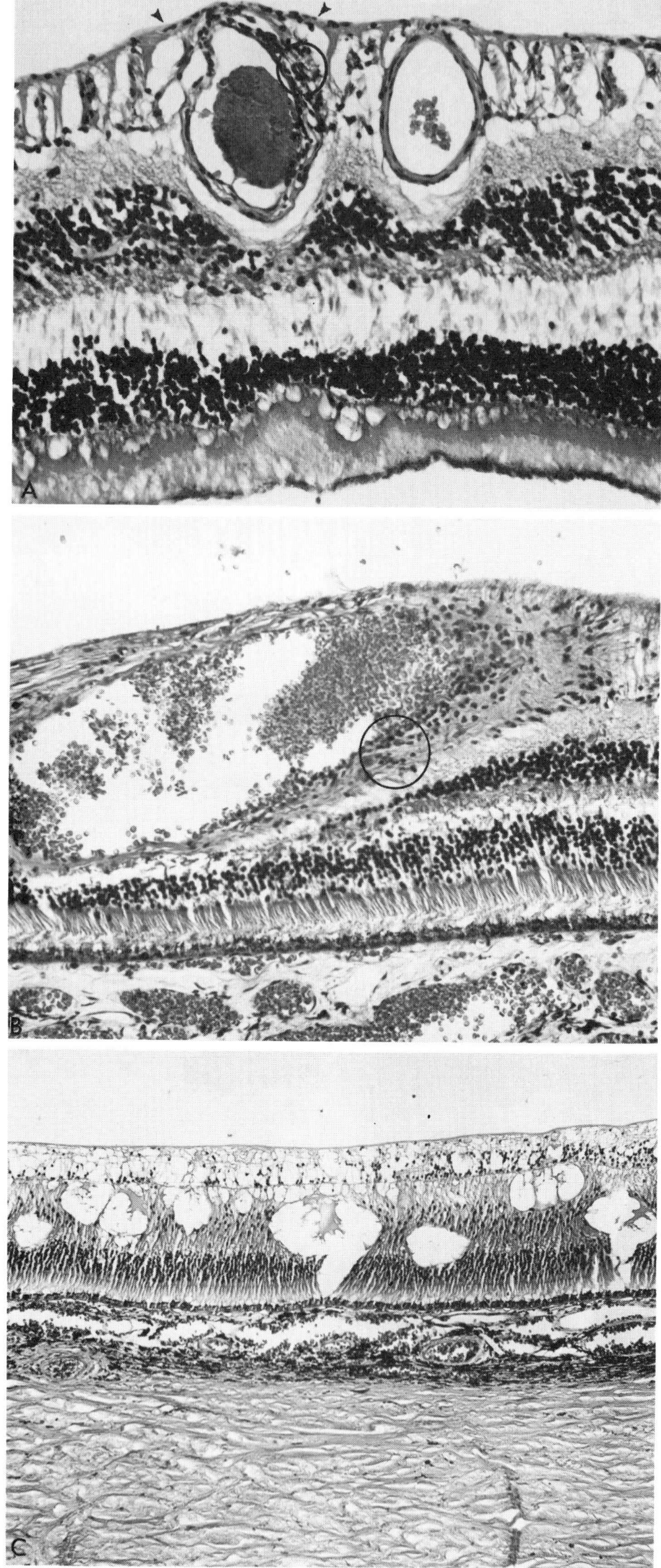

Figure 8–200. Pars planitis. *A,* Posterior retina shows a moderate infiltration of wall of vein by lymphocytes (circled). Adjacent arteriole is not affected. A thin preretinal fibrous layer (arrowheads) overlies the internal limiting membrane. H and E, ×235. EP 37148. *B,* Retinal phlebitis, with lymphocytes (circled) in wall of tertiary branch of central retinal vein. H and E, × 200. EP 31471. *C,* Cystoid macular edema involving nerve fiber, ganglion cell, inner plexiform, inner nuclear, and outer plexiform layers. H and E, ×90. EP 35666.

Illustration continued on opposite page

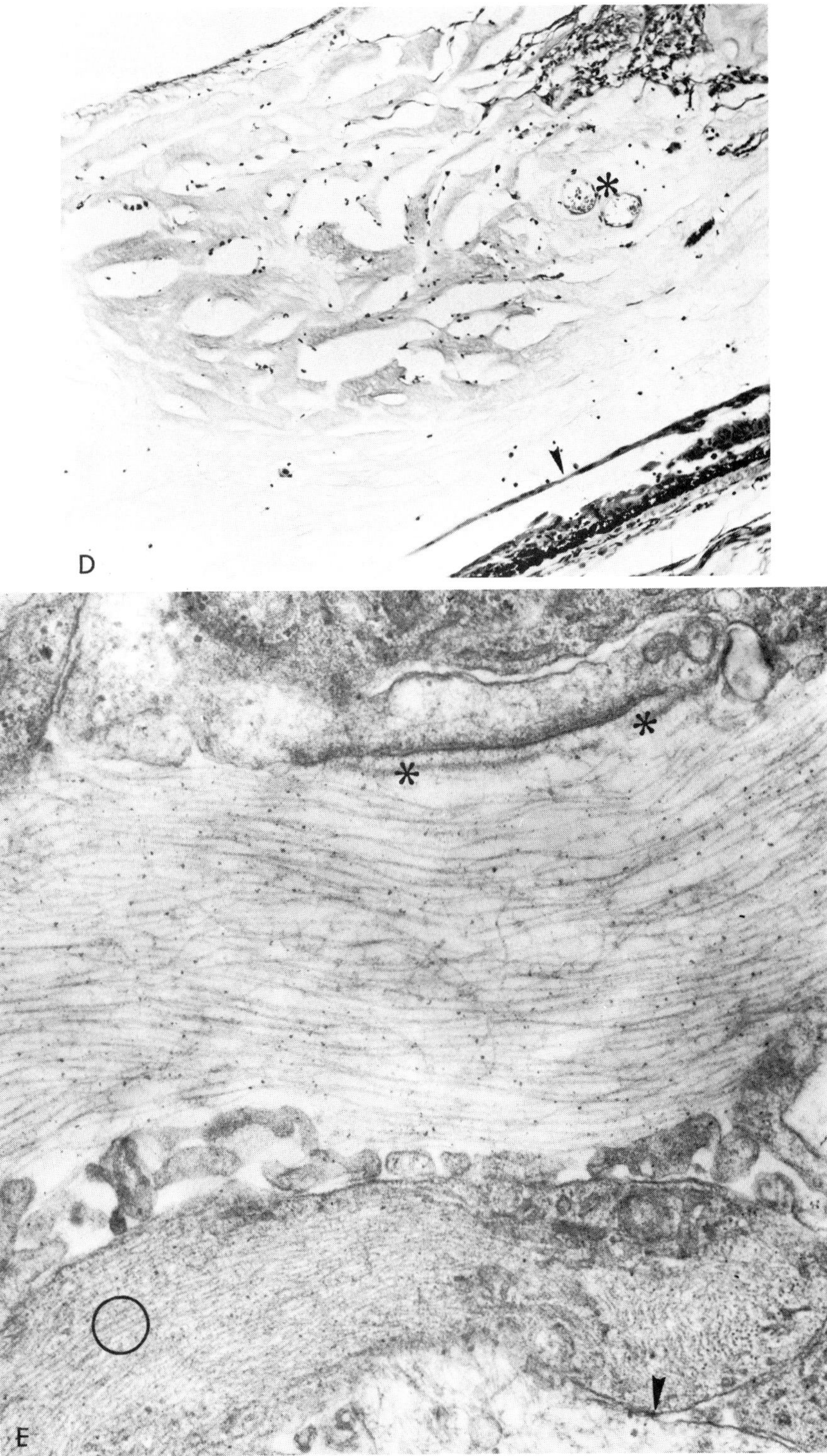

Figure 8–200 *Continued D,* "Snowbank" of pars planitis is composed of vitreous condensate, blood vessels (asterisk), scattered lymphocytes, spindle-shaped cells, and proliferated nonpigmented ciliary epithelium (arrowhead). H and E, ×110. EP 37148. *E,* At higher magnification, these cells show innumerable intracytoplasmic microfilaments, 7 to 8 nm in diameter (circle), intercellular gap and desmosomal junctions (arrowhead), segmental basement membrane (asterisks), and masses of fibrillar collagen, about 24 nm in diameter. ×42,000. EP 42268.
(From Pederson JE, Kenyon KR, Green WR, Maumenee AE: Pathology of pars planitis. Am J Ophthalmol *86*:762–774, 1978.)

sheathed retinal veins occur frequently (Pruett, Brockhurst, Letts, 1974).

Histopathologic studies (Pederson, Kenyon, Green, Maumenee, 1978) disclosed only minor active inflammatory cells in the ciliary body and vitreous. All seven cases in this study showed varying degrees of phlebitis and cystoid macular edema (Fig. 8–200). The snow bank consisted of collapsed and condensed vitreous, with variable components of hyperplastic, nonpigmented ciliary epithelium; retinal neovascularization; fibrous astrocytes; and new collagen (Fig. 8–201).

Study of the vitreous ''fluff balls'' obtained by pars plana vitrectomy in early cases has shown granulomatous inflammatory nodules (Fig. 8–201) (Green, Kincaid, Michels, et al, 1981).

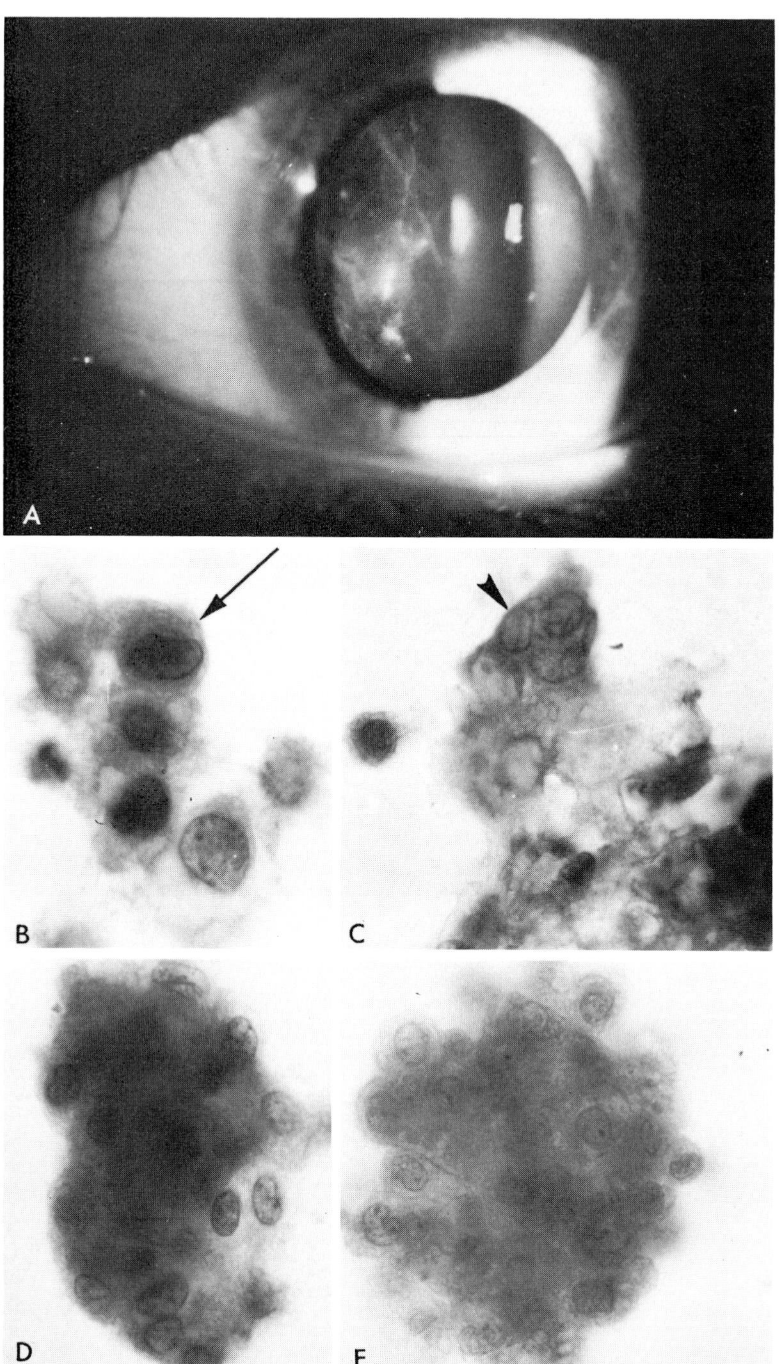

Figure 8–201. Pars planitis. *A,* External appearance of vitreous opacities in a 9 year old girl. Examination of vitreous aspirant using a membrane-filter technique shows large epithelioid cells (*B,* arrow), multinucleated giant cells (*C,* arrowhead), and tight clusters of epithelioid cells (*D* and *E*). *B* throught *E,* Millipore filter, modified Papanicolaou stain, ×1250. EP 42268. (From Green WR, Kincaid MC, Michaels RG, et al: Pars planitis. Trans Ophthalmol Soc UK *101*:361–367, 1981.)

TRAUMATIC LESIONS AND CONDITIONS

Contusion and Concussion. Contusion and concussion injuries in the eye, from blunt trauma or concussion by a bomb or underwater blast, can produce profound disturbances not only in the retinal neural cells, but also in the capillaries and arterioles. The blow or force can distort the globe and alters pressure relations in the tissues so that changes occur in the retinal cells and the walls of retinal vessels. Vasodilatation leads to alteration of vascular pressure, slowing of the blood stream, and leakage of fluid into the tissues. The contusion can cause necrosis of the nerve cells, edema, and hemorrhages. Small retinal lacerations or tears may also occur, especially at the periphery.

Commotio retinae (Berlin's Edema). Ophthalmoscopically, edematous swelling and haziness of the retina surrounding the fovea are seen. After 3 to 4 weeks the edema gradually subsides, and the macular region appears somewhat atrophic and pigmented. Most often there is temporary central visual loss. The damage may extend beyond the macula and may occupy a wide area in the posterior fundus, including the peripapillary region. Microscopically, the edema is most marked in the outer plexiform layer, which is thick and well-developed in the macular area. Considerable fluid collects, however, in the nuclear layers and beneath the retina. As the edema subsides, there is evidence of RPE degeneration and proliferation, formation of large and small cystoid areas in the macular region, and degeneration of the rod and cone fibers. Coalescence of the cystoid areas often produces a large cyst, the walls of which may degenerate and cause a partial or complete macular hole.

Contusions also may produce subretinal, intraretinal, and preretinal hemorrhages, with subsequent hole formation and detachment.

Traumatic Retinopathy. Following severe contusions, there is extensive edema of the retina, even into the periphery. After the edema subsides, the retina may appear atrophic, and a fine or coarse pigmentary stippling of the retina occurs. Histologically, the RPE shows areas of degeneration, exposing the choroid, and there is loss of the photoreceptors and general atrophy of the neuronal and supporting elements. Hyperplasia and migration of the RPE into the retina in a perivascular location produces an ophthalmoscopic picture similar to that of retinitis pigmentosa (Cogan, 1969a) (Fig. 8–202).

Vascular changes in contusion and concussion injuries are common. Clinically, small or large hemorrhages are present in the region of the retinal vessels, and they may be localized or widespread. Histiologically, in the early stages there is degeneration of the cells of the vessel walls, with leakage of plasma into and beyond the vessel walls to contribute to the edema. As healing occurs, gliosis and fibrosis of the perivascular region occur, with occlusions of many vessels by the fibrotic process.

Experimental studies of traumatic retinopathy in primates (Sipperly, Quigley, Gass, 1978) showed that the only abnormality immediately after injury was a disruption of the photoreceptor outer segments. From 1 to 6 days after trauma, many receptor cells undergo degeneration. The RPE cells phagocytose the degenerating outer segments and occasionally migrate into the retina. Sipperly and associates found no retinal edema,

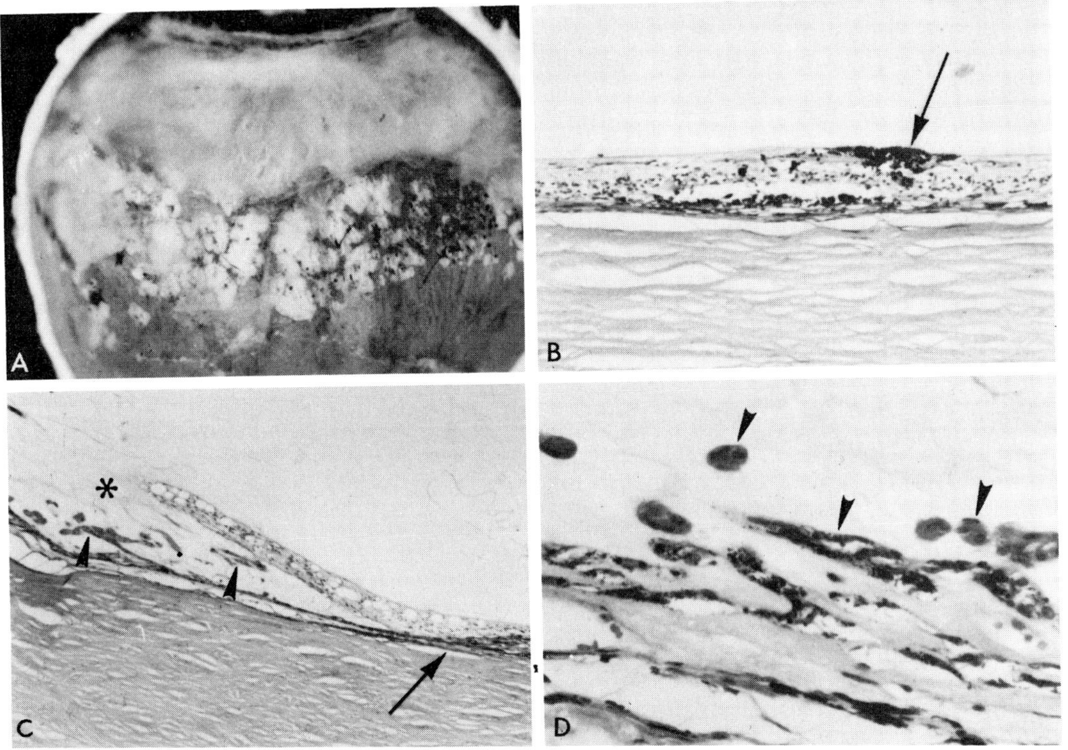

Figure 8–202. Blunt trauma with traumatic retinopathy (*A* and *B*) and a self-healed dialysis at ora serrata. *A*, Gross appearance of traumatic retinopathy. Remaining vitreous obscures underlying oral dialysis. *B*, Traumatic retinopathy showing loss of photoreceptor cell layer and hyperplasia of retinal pigment epithelium, with migration into the retina in a perivascular location (arrow). H and E, ×150. *C*, Oral dialysis with some of vitreous (asterisk) extending under retina, proliferation of ciliary epithelium (arrowheads), and demarcation line (arrow). H and E, ×150. *D*, Higher power of ciliary epithelial hyperplasia (arrowheads) that partially closes the dialysis cleft. H and E, ×300. EP 30799.

(From Smiddy WE, Green WR: Retinal dialysis: Pathology and pathogenesis. Retina 2:94–116, 1982.)

and they suggested that the opacification seen in commotio retinae is due to disrupted receptor cells. They noted that the RPE response to traumatic damage to receptors is similar to that observed in experimental retinal detachment and light-induced retinal damage.

The effects of blunt trauma can be transmitted by the vitreous to the retina in both a direct and a contrecoup fashion. Such changes are documented well in the study by Cox, Schepens, and Freeman (1966). Figure 8–203 (adapted from this study) shows the different types of retinal damage produced by blunt trauma, and some of these problems are directly related to the effect of vitreous on the retina:

A. Dialysis at anterior border of vitreous base
B. Avulsion of vitreous base
C. Macular hole
D. Horseshoe-shaped tear at posterior margin of vitreous base
E. Horseshoe-shaped tear at posterior end of meridional fold
F. Horseshoe-shaped tear at equator
G. Tear with operculum in overlying vitreous
H. Retinal dialysis at posterior border of vitreous base

In an analysis of 196 patients with retinal dialysis, Zion and Burton (1980) observed that most unilateral, nasal, and superior dialyses were produced by trauma. They also noted that trauma was a probable factor in 56 per cent of unilateral inferotemporal dialyses. Bilateral retinal dialyses, which accounted for 14 per cent of the cases, had a much lower incidence of trauma.

Figure 8–204 illustrates a dialysis at the ora serrata in the eye of a 15 year old boy who died 2 weeks after a motorcycle accident. Note the small tag (operculum) of retina that has been avulsed and remains attached to the detached vitreous base. Oral dialysis is also illustrated in Figures 8–202 through 8–207.

Foreign Bodies. A variety of different intraocular foreign bodies is encountered: metallic, vegetable, hair, etc. Copper foreign bodies may lodge in the vitreous near the retina or in the retina itself. The effects depend partly on the copper content of the foreign body. Foreign bodies containing almost pure copper lead to an immediate suppurative reaction with marked destruction and necrosis of the retina, producing all the signs of endophthalmitis. Foreign bodies with a smaller copper content cause little effect except from the mechanical trauma itself, but eventually the copper may diffuse through the retina and into the eye and cause a variable degree of *chalcosis* (Rao, Tso, Rosenthal, 1976). The distribution of copper in the eyes of experimental animals has been studied by Rosenthal, Appleton, and Hopkins (1974, 1975). These investigators have shown also that the inflammatory response to copper can be suppressed by steroid therapy in experimental studies (Rosenthal, Appleton, Zimmerman, Hopkins, 1976).

Delaney (1975) has presented a striking maculopathy that was presumed to be caused by a copper intraocular foreign body and was reversible after extraction of the foreign body. Rosenthal, Marmor, Leuenberger, and Hopkins (1979), in a natural history study, concluded that small intraocular copper foreign bodies can be tolerated

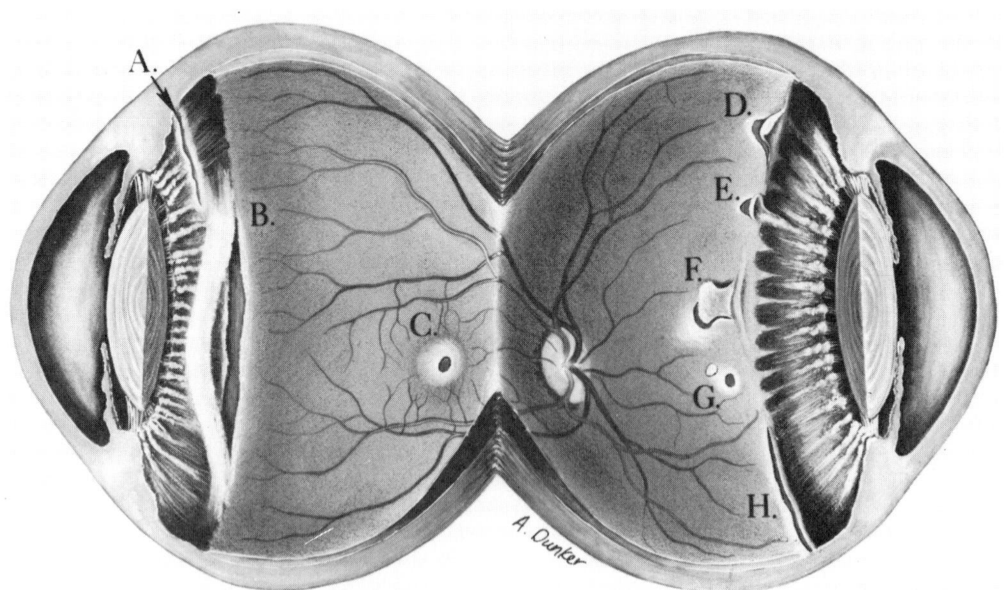

Figure 8–203. Retinal lesions caused by blunt trauma transmitted to the retina by the vitreous (see text for key). (Modified after Cox MS, Schepens CL, Freeman HM: Retinal detachment due to ocular contusion. Arch Ophthalmol *76*:679–685, 1966.)

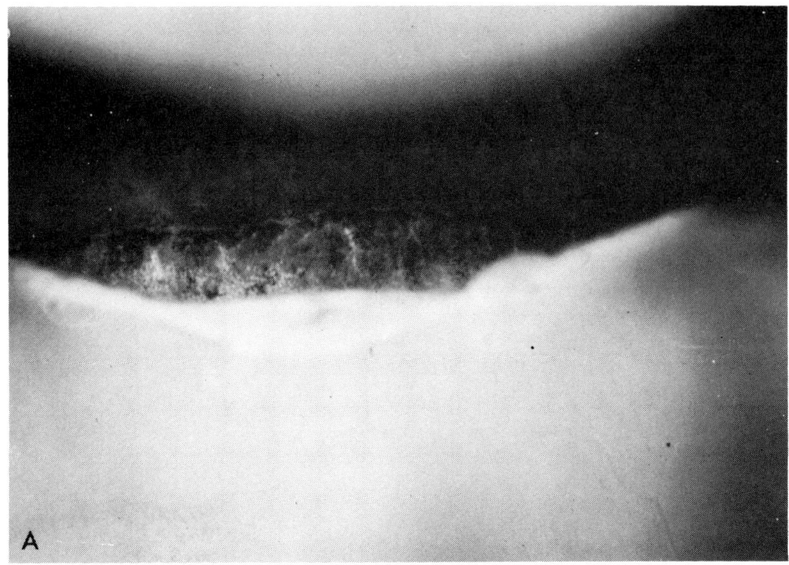

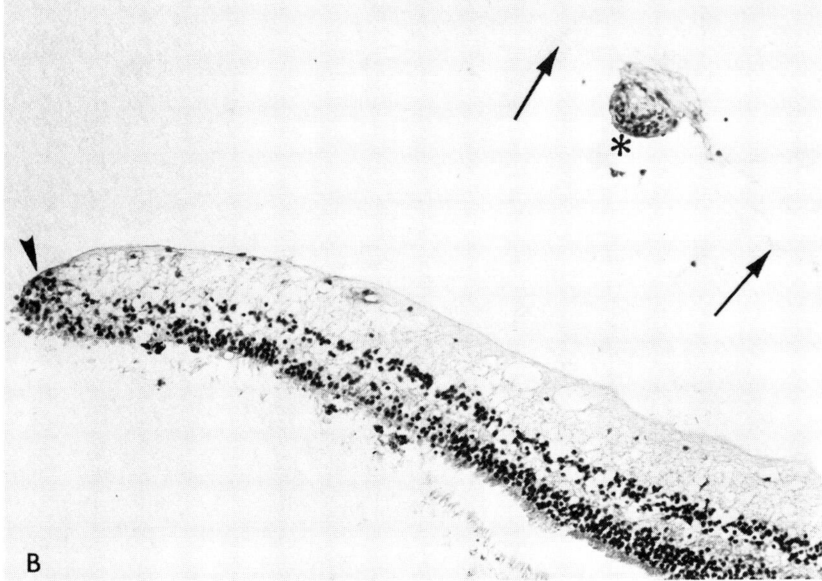

Figure 8–204. Traumatic retinal dialysis in a 15 year old boy. *A,* Gross appearance of superior retinal dialysis. *B,* Section shows margin of dialysis (arrowhead) and detached vitreous base (arrows), with an adherent tag of peripheral retina (asterisk). PAS, ×190. EP 32935. (From Smiddy WE, Green WR: Retinal dialysis: Pathology and pathogenesis. Retina *2*:94–116, 1982.)

for long periods of time without retinal toxicity. They noted that vitreous changes and copper maculopathy may necessitate intervention.

Iron foreign bodies often pass into the eye and lodge in or near the retina. They may pass through the retina and lodge in the sclera; if the iron content is high, localized siderosis then may occur. If the foreign body lodges in the vitreal-retinal region and if the iron content is high, *siderosis bulbi* occurs. More refined iron-containing foreign bodies and high-grade steel are harder and less likely to lead to siderosis.

The retina is seriously affected in siderosis, which can develop within a period of a few months to several years after injury. Clinically, the appearance is one of pigmentary degeneration of the retina, with scattered and pleomorphic clumps of pigment in the retina. Histologically, there is iron staining of the tissues, including the internal limiting membrane (ILM), and an accumulation of iron particles around the neurons and supporting cells, with secondary degeneration. In the early stages, the staining is localized mainly in the ILM and inner retina, where it affects especially the nuclei of the cells. Eventually the iron particles diffuse into the region of the outer limiting membrane, but usually the photoreceptor region is not affected. The RPE cells are affected early. Later, there is degeneration of the cells in the ganglion cell and bipolar layers. They become swollen and eventually atrophy and disappear. The nuclear layers become thinned; eventually, the full thickness of the retina contains particulate iron, and the neuronal tissues are replaced by proliferating glial cells as a reparative process.

The macula may show degenerative changes

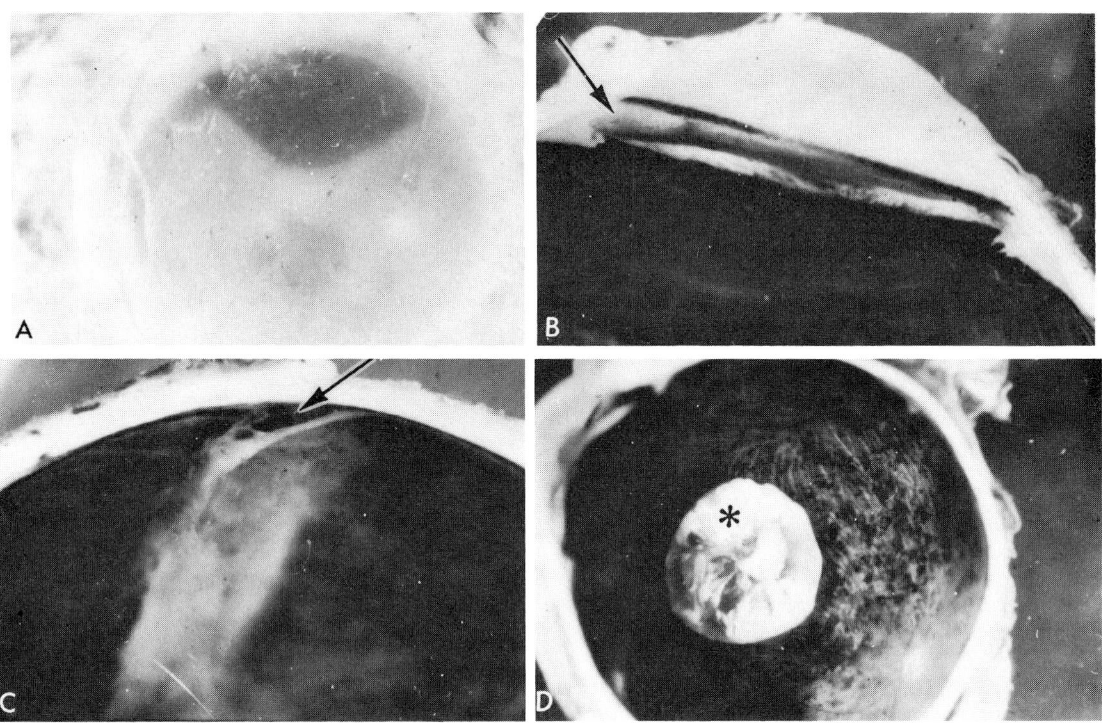

Figure 8–205. Gross appearance of eye with several **effects of trauma**. *A,* Iridodialysis. *B,* Postcontusion deformity (arrow). *C,* Self-healed oral dialysis (arrow). *D,* Traumatic retinopathy and dislocated cataractous lens (asterisk). EP 31369. (From Smiddy WE, Green WR: Retinal dialysis: Pathology and pathogenesis. Retina *2*:94–116, 1982.)

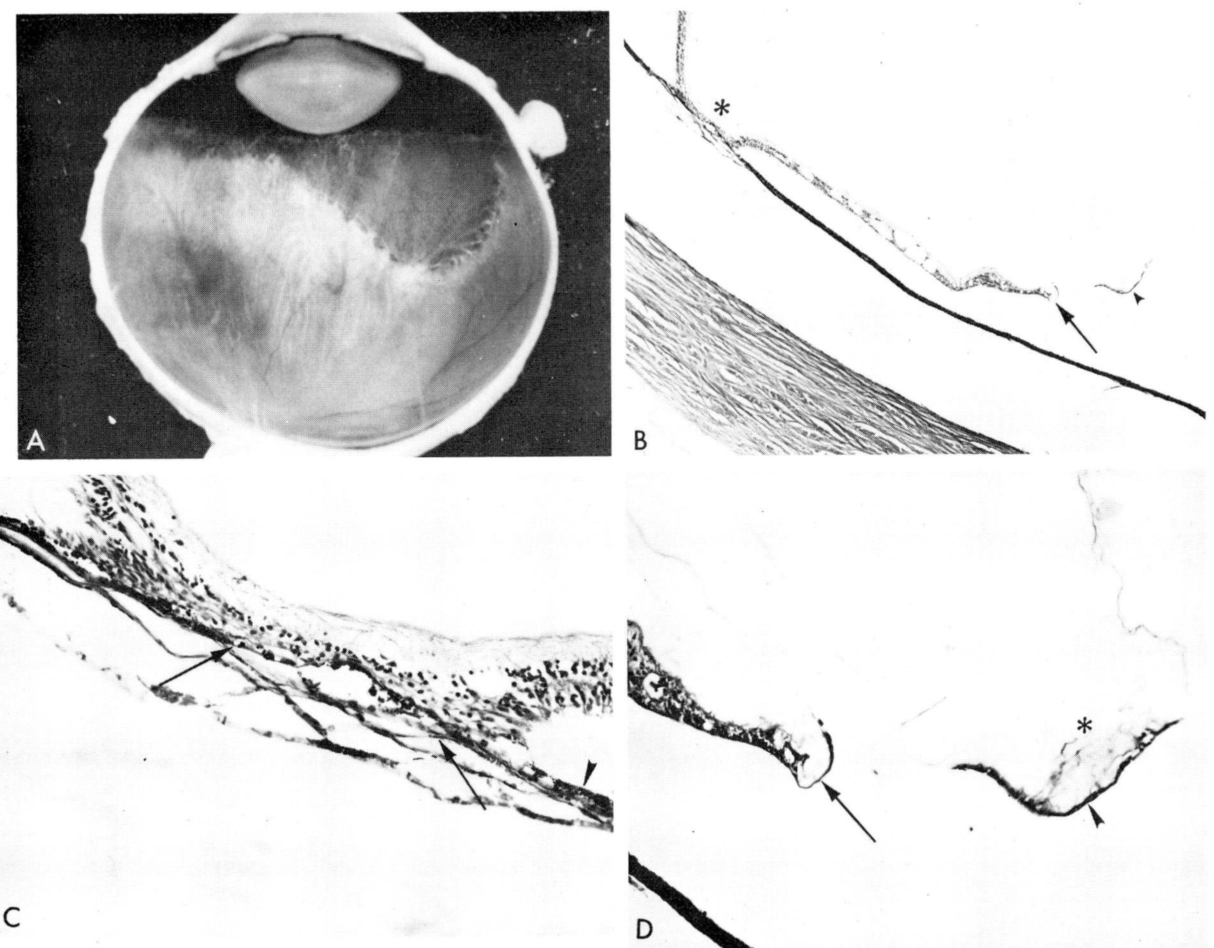

Figure 8–206. Oral dialysis with vitreous base detachment. *A,* Gross appearance of localized retinal detachment, with demarcation line associated with a superonasal oral dialysis. *B,* Features include margin of dialysis (arrow), demarcation line (asterisk), peripheral retinal detachment, and detached vitreous base with adherent portion of ciliary epithelium (arrowhead). PAS, ×30. *C,* Higher power view of demarcation line, showing chorioretinal adhesions with loss of photoreceptor cell layer, partial loss of (RPE) retinal pigment epithelium (between arrows), and chorioretinal adhesion. Adjacent RPE is hypertrophic (arrowhead). PAS, ×220. *D,* Higher power view showing margin of dialysis (arrow) and detached vitreous base (asterisk), with adherent ciliary epithelium (arrowhead). PAS, ×120. EP 32496.

(From Smiddy WE, Green WR: Retinal dialysis: Pathology and pathogenesis. Retina *2*:94–116, 1982.)

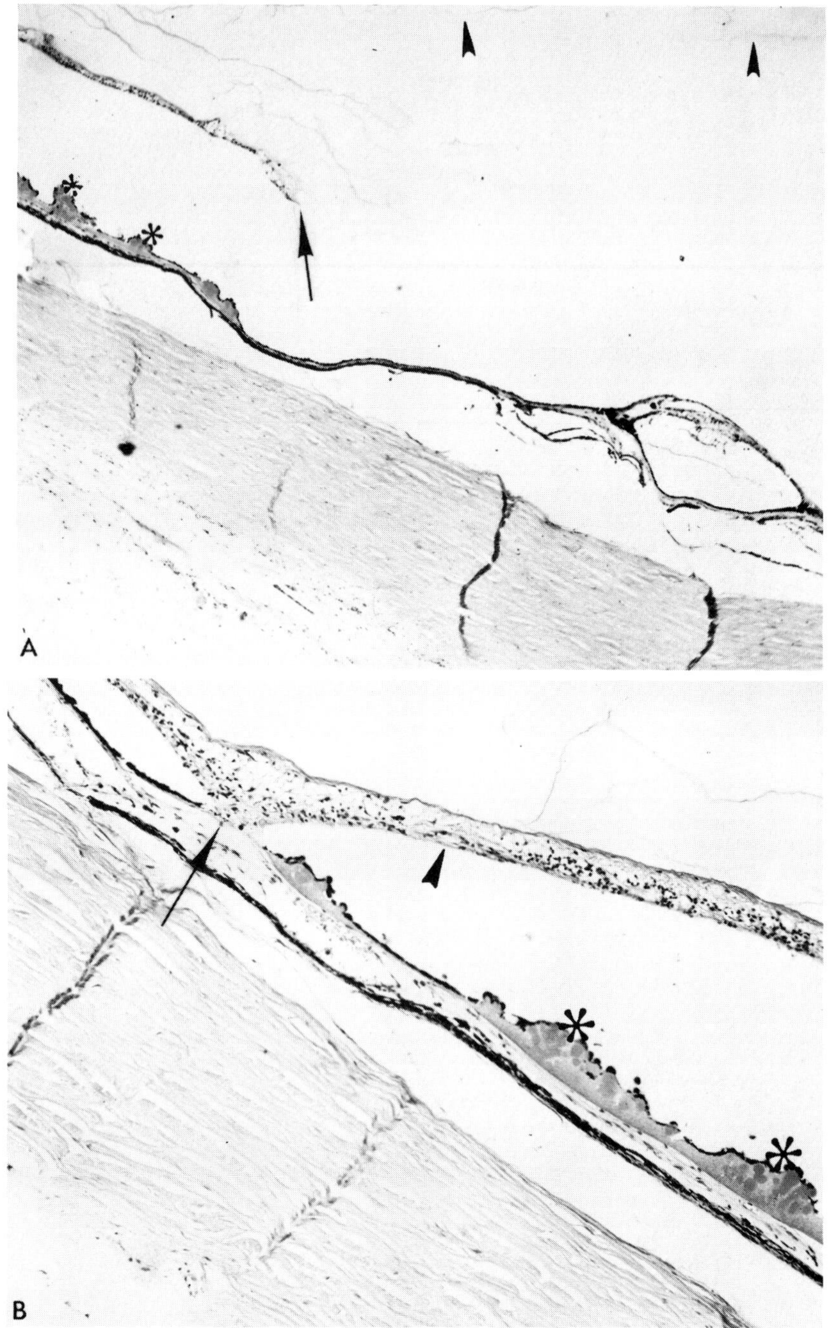

Figure 8–207. Inferotemporal oral dialysis with anterior vitreous detachment. *A,* Features include anterior vitreous detachment (arrowheads), margin of dialysis (arrow), and chronic retinal detachment with extensive drusen (asterisks). Alcian blue, ×35. *B,* More posterior and at higher power, chronic retinal detachment shows loss of photoreceptor cell layer (arrowhead), marked drusen (asterisks), and chorioretinal adhesion (arrow) type of demarcation line. EP 45869. (From Smiddy WE, Green WR: Retinal dialysis: Pathology and pathogenesis. Retina 2:94–116, 1982.)

but no heavy deposition of iron pigment. The retinal vessels show perivascular accumulations of iron pigment. Histologically, the pigment appears to collect in the perivascular space around the vessels. In the final stages, the retina shows diffuse, severe atrophy and both fine and clumped masses of pigment. The eye often sequesters an intraocular foreign body by encasement with fibrous tissue (Fig. 8–208).

Birth Injuries to the Retina. The eyes of newborn infants often show retinal hemorrhages. The flame-shaped hemorrhages are usually located posteriorly. Some may dissect under the internal limiting membrane. Foci of hemorrhage are common in the macular region but also may be observed in the periphery (Fig. 8–209). Large hemorrhages rarely may become organized into elevated scars that resemble tumors, a condition known as massive retinal fibrosis. This type of fibrosis is more often produced by inflammation (especially nematodiasis).

More often the hemorrhages are small, round, or flame-shaped and are confined to the posterior pole. Within 7 to 10 days after birth, they have completely absorbed without causing significant damage.

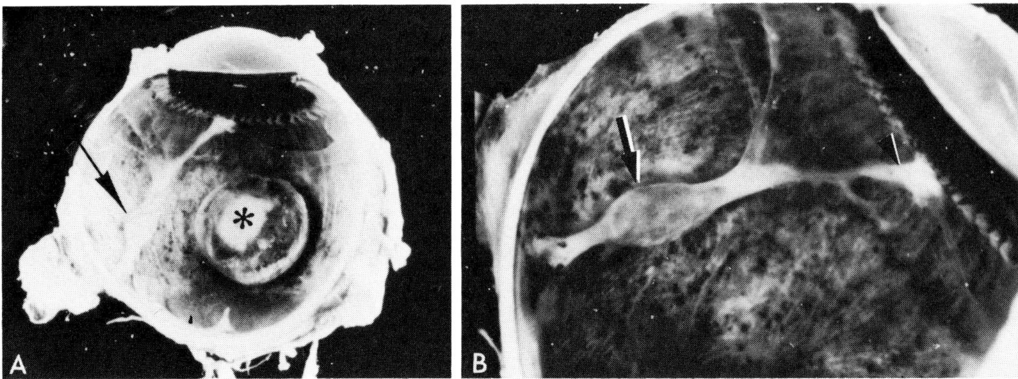

Figure 8–208. Eye with retained intraocular foreign body. *A,* Tract of foreign body is delineated by a strand of fibrous tissue that also encases foreign body (arrow). Cataractous lens with anterior subcapsular fibrous plaque (asterisk) is dislocated in vitreous cavity. *B,* Higher power view more clearly delineates the site of entrance (arrowhead), fibrous tissue strand with encased foreign body (arrow), and traumatic retinopathy. EP 34004.

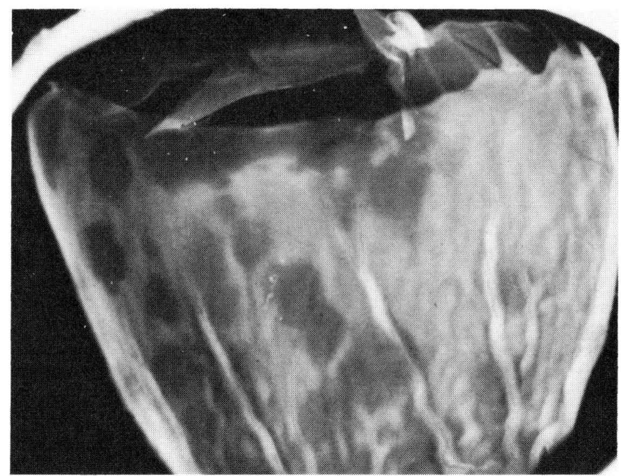

Figure 8–209. Multiple **retinal hemorrhages** present at birth. EP 30868.

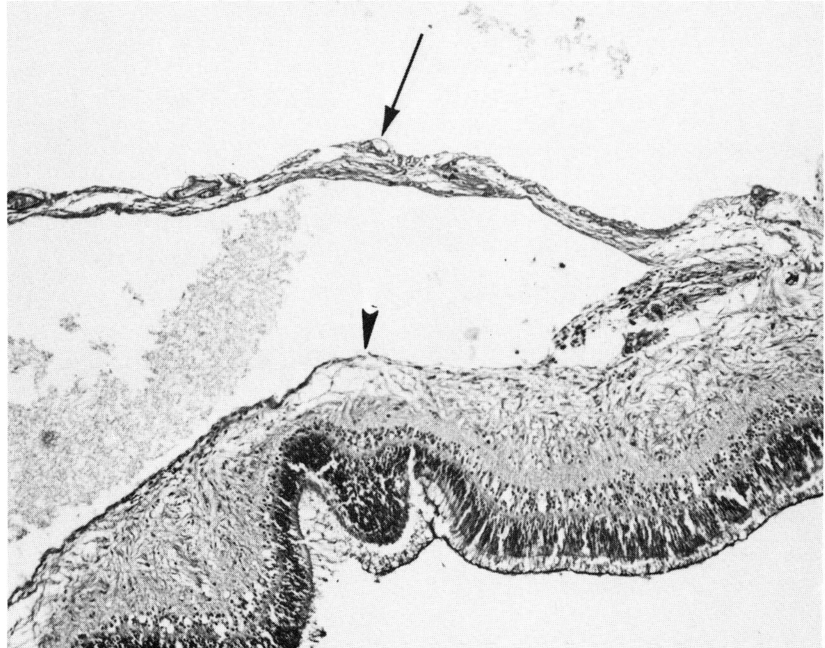

Figure 8–210. Extensive **retinoschisis** from retinal hemorrhage that presumably occurred at birth. The blood has deteriorated, and there is marked hemosiderin staining of both the inner (arrow) and outer (arrowhead) layers of retina. PAS, ×100. EP 14692.

Rarely, hemorrhages may be extensive and produce extensive schisis (Fig. 8–210).

It has been postulated that infantile hemorrhages in the macular region may be a cause of partial amblyopia, but recent studies have indicated that this is probably not so. Von Noorden and Khodadoust (1973) found retinal hemorrhages in 245 of 1000 neonates (24.5 per cent). Eighteen neonates had hemorrhage in the macular area. Follow-up studies in 5 of those 18 patients showed normal visual acuity and ocular motility. The other 13 patients were not available for follow-up.

Purtscher's Traumatic Retinopathy. There are perhaps three forms of Purtscher's retinopathy—one caused by fat emboli, a second caused by rapid increase in the intravascular pressure, and a third from complement-mediated leukostasis.

Fat Emboli. This retinopathy has been seen after trauma in which there is a crushing injury or fractures of long bones. Fat emboli may involve retinal and choroidal vessels (Fig. 8–211). Clinically, the retina shows focal areas of milky white to gray opacification resembling cotton-wool patches. The lesions, which are caused by fat emboli, may lie in front of or behind the retinal vessels, and they are often associated with microinfarction and hemorrhages. They are especially common in the macular region. The opacities gradually disappear over a period of 1 to 2 months, leaving faint mottling and pigmentation of the retina. If there is also impairment of the

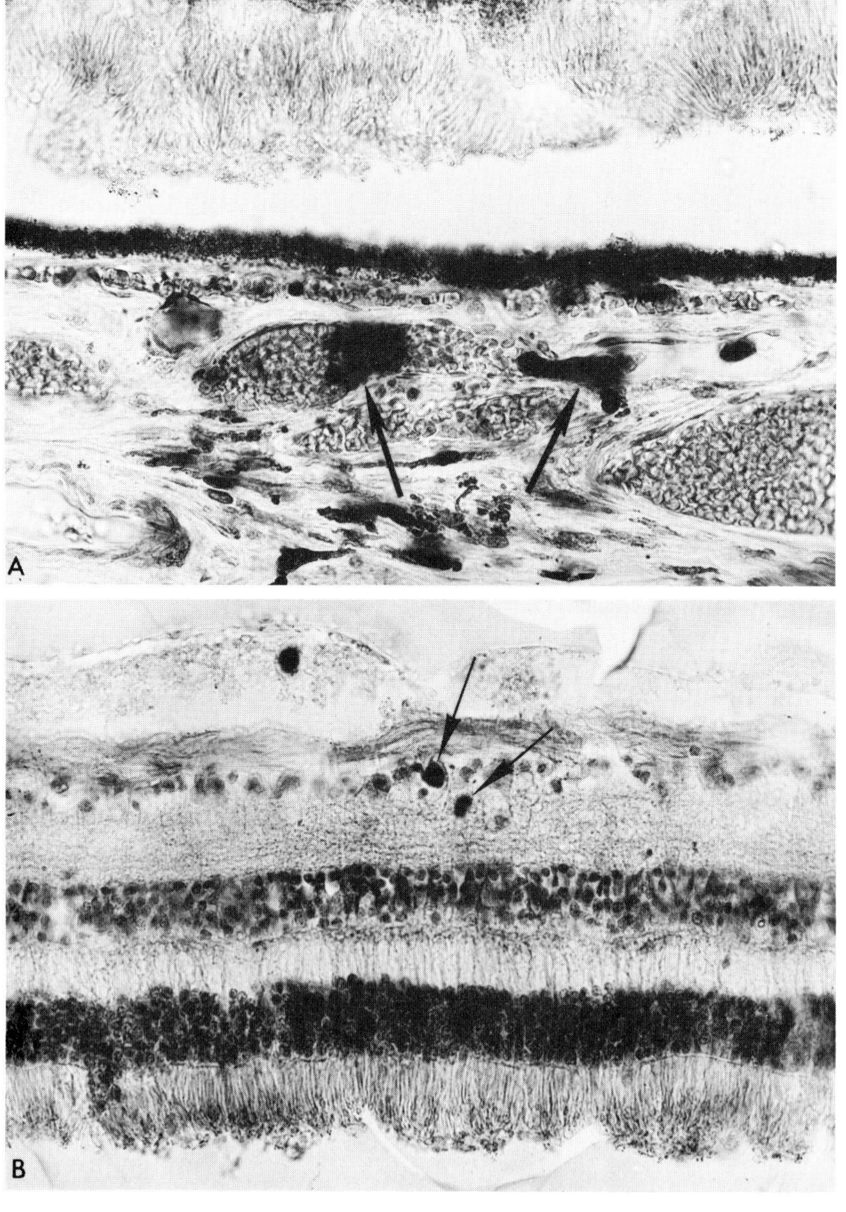

Figure 8–211. Purtscher's retinopathy caused by fat emboli from a crushing injury of leg. Fat emboli (arrows) in *A*, choroidal and *B*, retinal vessels. Oil red O, frozen section. *A*, ×305. AFIP Neg. 59-13910. *B*, ×220. AFIP Neg. 59-13910.

retinal and choroidal vasculature, visual field loss with scotomatous lesions may persist. A patient with fat emboli also can have ocular changes caused by abrupt increase in intravascular pressure (to be discussed).

It was noted early that these fat emboli were soluble in ether. The studies of Urbanek (1933) were the first to show that the presence of fat emboli correlated with the clinical picture. There have been numerous other studies, including those of Fritz and Hogan (1948), Devoe (1949), and Kearns (1956).

Rapid Increase in Intravascular Pressure (Valsalva Hemorrhagic Retinopathy; Duane, 1973) (Hydrostatic Pressure Syndrome; Marr, Marr, 1962). This type of retinopathy is associated with compressing injuries to the thorax (Schmidt, 1968; Hoare, 1970; Kelley, 1972) with an abrupt transmission of pressure to the retinal vasculature, causing focal areas of retinal endothelial damage and hemorrhage (Fig. 8–212).

A similar mechanism appears to be responsible for small, unilateral foveal hemorrhages in young adults after strenuous exercise, such as weight lifting (Pitta, Steimert, Gragoudas, Regan, 1980). Three of 20 patients with microhemorrhages in the macula observed by Pruett, Carvalho, Trempe (1981) were related to Valsalva stress. Abrupt increase in intracranial pressure, as with gas myelography (Oberman, Cohn, Grand, 1979), and intracranial hemorrhage (Terson, 1926; Khan, Frenkel, 1975) also may produce retinal capillary endothelial damage and hemorrhages in the retina, with extension into the vitreous.

Complement-Mediated Leukostasis. The third possible mechanism in the production of a Purtscher's-like retinopathy may be due to complement-mediated leukostasis (see retinopathy of acute pancreatitis, page 1169, Fig. 8–517).

Choroidal Rupture. The discontinuity of the choroid from trauma may be partial or complete, and the overlying retina may be torn or only lose its photoreceptor cell layer (Kaufer, Zimmerman, 1966). Late complications from choroidal ruptures include choroidal neovascularization and serous or serosanguineous retinal detachment (Fuller, Gitter, 1973; Smith, Kelley, Harbin, 1974; Hilton, 1975). (See page 1743 for more complete discussion of choroidal rupture.)

ELECTRICAL AND RADIATION INJURIES

Electrical Injuries

Electrical injuries result from passage of a high-voltage electric current through the body. The effects are similar to those seen in individuals who have been struck by lightning. Retinal edema and hemorrhages and papilledema have been described after such injuries. The effect of passage of electrical current and the resistance of the tissue leads to changes in the vessels and other tissues.

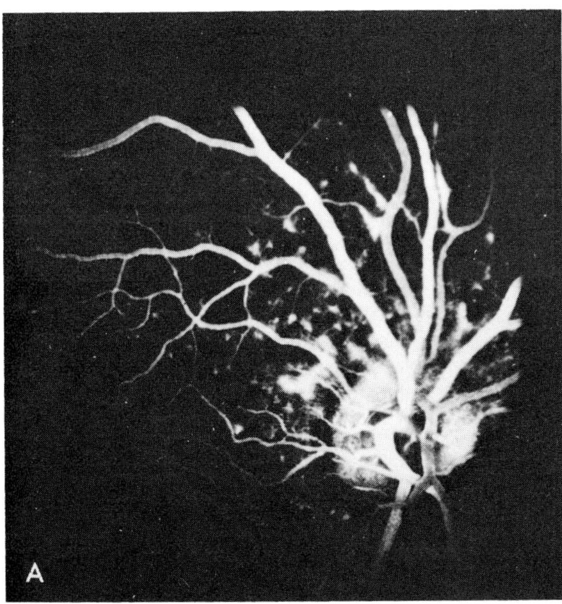

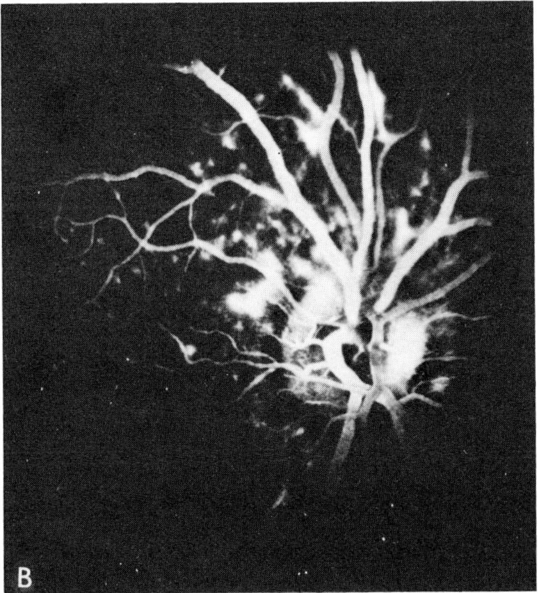

Figure 8–212. Purtscher's retinopathy caused by rapid increase in intravascular pressure in a 24 year old man who was in a minor automobile accident while wearing a lap-and-shoulder seat belt. *A,* Early, and *B,* later fluorescein angiographs, showing staining and leakage of small arterioles and capillaries. (From Kelley JS: Purtscher's retinopathy related to chest compression by safety belts. Am J Ophthalmol *74*:278–283, 1972.)

After a variable period, the retinal edema subsides and there may be diffuse fine and coarse pigmentation of the fundus. The lens is susceptible to electric damage and may show characteristic sequential cataract changes (Fraunfelder, Hanna, 1972).

Radiation Injuries

Abiotic and ionizing radiation injuries to the retina have been observed (MacFaul and Bedford, 1970; Merrian, Szechter, Focht, 1972). Thermal lesions in the retina are caused by direct absorption of energy produced by shorter electromagnetic wavelengths. Among the most important thermal lesions are those involving the infrared band of the electromagnetic spectrum. The effects are pronounced in the retina because of the high absorption of the energy by the RPE. The retinal damage is influenced by the amount of energy transmitted to the retina, and the wavelengths most likely to harm the retina are those between 9000 and 10,000 angstrom units.

Ionizing Irradiation. Ionizing irradiation causes its effects by liberation of ions that encounter cell constituents such as the nucleus and organelles in the cytoplasm. Direct effects may occur from the electrons or nuclei, or secondary radiation may be induced in the tissue itself. The effects of the various types of ionizing irradiation appear to be identical; the difference is related only to the amount of energy available for dissipation, the penetrating power, and the density of the resulting ionization.

Radiation Retinopathy. This complication may be observed after radon seed and external irradiation. It is characterized by the delayed development of capillary microaneurysms, hemorrhages, and cotton-wool patches. Exudates in the posterior region may have a circinate pattern. Telangiectasis of retinal vessels also may be observed (Chee, 1968). These fundus changes are not restricted to the main area of radiation therapy, and they can occur even after treatment of orbital and intracranial lesions (Bagan, Hollenhorst, 1979).

Hayreh (1970) has noted the following features in radiation retinopathy: retinal vascular occlusion, microaneurysms, telangiectasis, neovascularization, cotton-wool exudates, white retinal deposits, hemorrhages, edema, sheathing of larger vessels, perivasculitis, optic atrophy, vitreous hemorrhage, and, rarely, retinal detachment.

In general, the effects of ionizing irradiation on the tissues are twofold: the effect on individual cells, causing functional alterations or death, and an indirect action on the tissues by vascular damage. A most important injury to the cell histologically is the arrest of mitosis, but, if the irradiation effect is severe, the nucleus may degenerate. Cytoplasmic changes include those in the various organelles and also change in the viscosity and permeability of the cell membrane and "sap." Vascular changes include an early swelling of the intima of the small vessels, with degeneration and death of endothelial cells, and degenerative changes in the media and adventitia, with swelling and disappearance of muscular, elastic and collagenous complements.

Clinically, the early changes are characterized by extreme dilatation and engorgement of the vessels and hemorrhage, with increased tortuosity and hyperemia of the tissues (Flick, 1948). Most of these changes develop 3 to 5 weeks after the irradiation injury, but severe sequelae can be seen in the retina as long as 1 to 2 years after the initial treatment for such conditions as retinoblastoma. Subsequent changes include closure of the vessel lumen by thrombus formation or fibrosis. Clinically, vessels of this type have alternate constrictions and dilatations. Histologically, in the retina the neurons and supporting glial cells show disintegration from radiation effects. In the human, however, the neural portion of the retina is rather resistant to effects of irradiation.

In a study of 36 eyes following radiation, Brown, Shields, Sanborn, et al (1982) noted the most common features of radiation retinopathy to be retinal hard exudates, hemorrhages, microaneurysms, cotton-wool exudates, and telangiectasis. Areas of capillary nonperfusion are observed by fluorescein angiography.

Doses greater than 3000 rad are required to produce retinal lesions, by virtue of the ionizing effect on the retinal vasculature. Doses of 10,000 rad are required to cause damage to retinal neural cells and somewhat less than this for rods and cones (Lerman, 1980).

In experimental studies in monkeys (Gragoudas, Zakov, Albert, Constable, 1979), no appreciable effect on the retina outside the chorioretinal lesions was induced by protein irradiation. Gragoudas and associates suggested that proton beam irradiation may reduce markedly the delayed ocular complications that are relatively common in other forms of radiotherapy used in the treatment of intraocular tumors.

Solar Retinopathy. (See also section on Retinal Light Toxicity.) Eclipse blindness or solar retinopathy has been understood for many years. The visible and infrared rays of sunlight are concentrated by the refracting media of the eye onto the macular area in injuries of this type. The clinical condition known as foveal macular retinitis appears now to be related to eclipse blindness but was formerly believed to have other causes. Solar retinopathy usually is bilateral, and is associated with the immediate development of visual dazzling and scotoma. Observation with the opthalmoscope then may show minimal changes or edema with minute hemorrhages. Within 24 hours, one or more yellowish-white spots typically develop, and the burned, edematous areas often is somewhat crescent-shaped. After disappearance of the edema and the hemorrhages, what appears to be a parafoveal hole in the RPE may remain.

Histologically, the light effects involve loss of pigment cells in the burned area and the heaping up of pigment cells at the periphery of the lesion. A coagulation necrosis of the affected retinal elements is present, and often the foveal or parafoveal tissues disappear, with formation of a cyst or hole.

Foveomacular retinitis has been observed in outbreaks in young military personnel. It is not certain whether this condition is solar retinitis. Marlor, Blais, Preston, and Boyden (1973) believed that this condition was probably due to sun gazing.

RETINAL DRUG TOXICITY

Toxic Pigment Epitheliopathies

Chloroquine Retinopathy (Hobbs, Sorsby, Freedman, 1959; Henkind, Rothfield, 1963; Henkind, Carr, Siegel, 1964; François, De Becker, 1965; Babel, 1966; Bernstein, 1967; Böke, Bäumer, Müller-Limmroth, Mludek, 1967). Prior to World War II, it had been shown that chloroquine derivatives were valuable as antimalarial agents. After the war, their use increased greatly, especially for the treatment of systemic lupus erythematosus and rheumatoid arthritis. The use of the synthetic antimalarials has been recognized as a cause of various disorders, including loss of vision from retinal changes.

Ocular side effects are uncommon in patients using the medication in low dosage and for short periods of time, but they become quite common in those receiving it in high doses for prolonged periods (Henkind, Rothfield, 1963; Scherbel, Mackenzie, Nousek, Atdjian, 1965). It was later shown that in the early phases of chloroquine retinal toxicity, macular mottling (with or without loss of the foveal reflex) was the first sign of the disease, and that with continued use of chloroquine a perimacular "bull's-eye" appearance developed.

Clinically, in the well-developed lesion the retinal vessels are narrow and constricted and the disk pale; there are irregular patchy pigmented areas in the retinal periphery and a "bull's-eye" change in RPE pigmentation in the parafoveal area. Visual acuity is usually decreased, and visual field defects in the form of paracentral scotoma and impaired night vision occur.

The electroretinogram (ERG) is either normal or subnormal in the intermediate stages but may be markedly abnormal or extinguished in the later stages. The findings might suggest a type of retinitis pigmentosa, but the dark adaptation remains normal, even though the ERG may be severely affected in chloroquine retinopathy in contrast to retinitis pigmentosa.

Studies on the histopathology of chloroquine retinopathy have been few (Wetterholm, Winter, 1964; Ramsey, Fine, 1972; Monahan, Horns, 1964; Bernstein, Ginsberg, 1964; Bernstein, 1970), and there is some variation in the findings of the investigators. Monahan and Horns (1964), Bernstein and Ginsberg (1964), and Bernstein (1970) found extensive degeneration of the RPE, with migration into the retina. The sensory retina showed extensive degeneration, and it was believed that this degeneration was caused by the retinal vascular sclerosis and occlusion, which was severe in all the retinal vessels and in the iris. Wetterholm and Winter (1964) found changes in the outer nuclear layer and outer plexiform layer, where there were large cells filled with pigment granules and also some loss of the photoreceptor cells (Fig. 8–213). The RPE itself appeared to be normal, however, and the optic disc and optic nerve were normal. With indirect fluorescent technique, the drug was identified in the retinal tissues.

Ramsey and Fine (1972) later restudied with the electron microscope the specimen of Wetterholm and Winter and found multimembranous and curvilinear cytoplasmic inclusions in the retinal ganglion cells (Fig. 8–213), which previously had been thought to be normal. Inclusions also were found in other retinal cells and in the RPE. Chloroquine appears to have its effect primarily on pigmented cells, and a chloroquine affinity for melanin-containing cells has been shown.

Although most experimental studies have shown a primary effect on the RPE (Meier-Ruge, 1965; François, Mandgal, 1967; Babel, Englert, 1969; Nasu, 1960; Smith, Berson, 1971), some have indicated that the retinal ganglion cell is the primary site of toxicity (Gregory, Rutty, Wood, 1970). Rosenthal, Kolb, Bergsma, et al (1978) reported toxic effects on the ganglion cells, then on the photoreceptor cells and on the RPE.

Phenothiazine Derivatives. The phenothiazine derivatives have been responsible for many improvements in the care of mentally ill patients in recent years. The clinical findings following use of some of these drugs reveal pigmentation of the skin of the face, lids, and conjunctiva, and also the cornea and lens. Fine granularity of the fundus from disturbance in the RPE cells has been noted, and occasionally there is fine clumping of the pigment granules. Other patients may have rather heavy pigmentation throughout the fundus.

Patients may begin to have toxic symptoms after receiving 800 mg or more of thioridazine per day for 3 to 8 days (Weekley, Pots, Reboton, May, 1960; Scott, 1963; Connell, Poley, Mc-

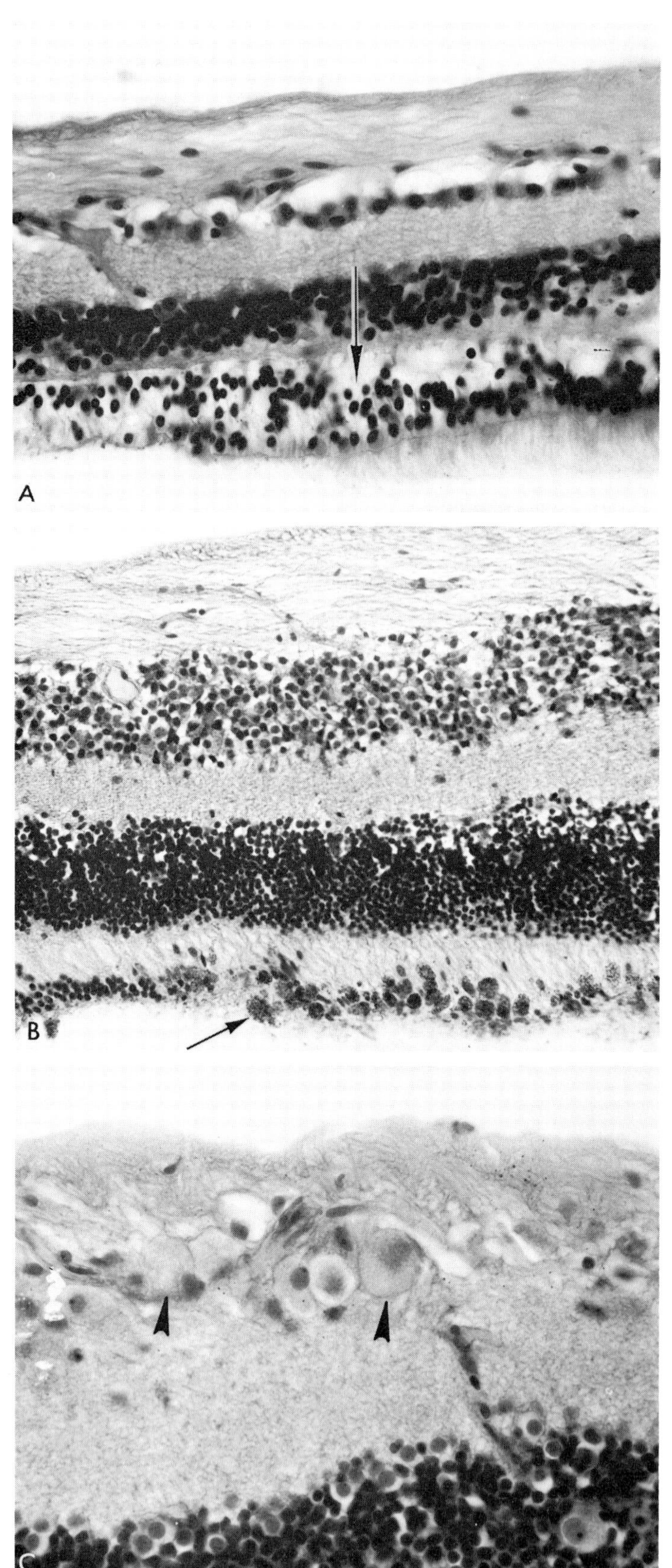

Figure 8–213. Chloroquine retinopathy. *A,* Junction between normal and affected area (arrow). To the right, the photoreceptor cell layer is intact. To the left, there is loss of outer and inner segments and marked thinning of the outer nuclear layer. *B,* Further into the involved area, the outer nuclear layer is absent and large pigmented cells have migrated into the area (arrow). H and E, ×240. *C,* Ganglion cells (arrowheads) are markedly distended. H and E, ×500. EP 38408.

Farlane, 1964). In some instances, toxicity may be observed at lower dosages (Heshe, Engelstoft, Kirk, 1961; Appelbaum, 1963).

Potts (1962) demonstrated in pigmented experimental animals that the uveal pigment granules concentrated the *N*-substituted phenothiazine derivatives. Phenothiazine itself, however, does not concentrate in the uveal tract.

Clinical studies (Davidorf, 1973; Weekley, Potts, Reboton, May, 1960; Delong, Poley, McFarlane, 1965) seem to indicate that widespread atrophy of the RPE and photoreceptor cells may accompany long-term therapy with various phenothiazine drugs.

In clinicopathologic and electron microscopic studies of thioridazine retinopathy, Miller, Bunt-Milan, and Kaline (1982) found widespread atrophy of the RPE and the photoreceptor cell layer (Fig. 8–214,*A*). In areas where the RPE was present, it was hypertrophic (Fig. 8–214,*B*) and showed increased quantities of lipofuscin, melanolysosomes, and curvilinear bodies (Fig. 8–214,*C*). The mechanism of toxicity is unknown, but it seems to take place at the RPE/photoreceptor complex area.

Methoxyflurane

Methoxyflurane (1,1-difluoro-2,2-dichloroethyl methyl ether) is a commonly used, noninflammable, general inhalant anesthetic (Artusio, Van Poznak, Hunt, et al, 1960). This agent can cause postoperative renal failure from renal oxalosis (Crandell, Pappas, McDonald, 1966).

Albert, Bullock, Lahav, and Caine (1975) reported the occurrence of a flecked retina caused by oxalate crystals within the RPE complicating methoxyflurane anesthesia (Fig. 8–215). They were able to produce a similar picture experimentally in rabbits (Caine, Albert, Lahav, Bullock, 1975).

A similar flecked retina can occur with primary hyperoxaluria (Gottlieb, Ritter, 1977) (see page 1164).

Chloromycetin Toxicity in Patients with Cystic Fibrosis of Pancreas

Cystic fibrosis is a genetic disease of Caucasians and is transmitted as an autosomal recessive trait. The disease primarily affects the exocrine glands and is clinically characterized by chronic pulmonary disease, pancreatic insufficiency, and elevated levels of sweat electrolytes (Di Sant'Agnese, Davis, 1976). Retinal vascular dilatation and tortuosity may be present and is related to elevated P_{CO_2}.

In the past, chloramphenicol was given to control the chronic pulmonary infections that often occur in these patients. With chronic use of the antibiotic, some patients developed visual complaints from cecocentral scotomas. Return of vision may be observed with discontinuation of the drug and use of vitamin B. The mechanism of action of the antibiotic on the optic nerve and retina is unknown.

Studies of eyes from several patients with these ocular complications (Wong, Collins, 1965; Harley, Huang, Macri, Green, 1970) showed atrophy of the maculopapillary bundle (Fig. 8–216). There is loss of the nerve fiber and ganglion cell layers in the macula, and atrophy of the temporal aspect of the optic nerve head and optic nerve; these are similar to the changes seen in nutritional amblyopia and subacute necrotizing encephalomyelitis.

Quinine

Quinine is an alkaloid that has been used mainly as an antimalarial agent. Visual problems often occur in patients receiving quinine, but the site of toxicity is controversial.

Histopathologic studies (Casini, 1939) revealed atrophy of the nerve fiber and ganglion cell layers and loss of the photoreceptor cells. (Also see Chapter 9, Uvea, page 1485.)

Tamoxifen

Tamoxifen citrate, a nonsteroid antiestrogen, has been found to have a beneficial effect in the treatment of some metastatic breast cancers (Cole, Jones, Todd, 1971). When used in extremely high dosages for longer than 1 year, an unusual flecklike retinopathy characterized by fine, white, refractile superficial opacities in the retina may be observed (Kaiser-Kupfer, Lippman, 1978). In clinicopathologic studies, Kaiser-Kupfer, Kupfer, and Rodrigues (1981) found deposits in the nerve fiber layer and inner plexiform layers in the paramacular region that measured 30 to 35 microns in diameter.

Histochemical studies suggested that the deposits contained glycosaminoglycans. Electron microscopy disclosed the smaller deposits to be intracellular and the larger ones to be extracellular. The deposits are composed of randomly oriented, branching, electron-dense 6 nm filaments and occasional electron-dense coated vesicles measuring 60 to 70 nm in diameter. The lesions appeared to be occurring in axons and were interpreted as probably representing products of axonal degeneration.

Nicotinic Acid Maculopathy

Gass (1973c) has described the occurrence of an atypical form of cystoid macular edema in a patient receiving large doses of nicotinic acid for

Text continued on page 810

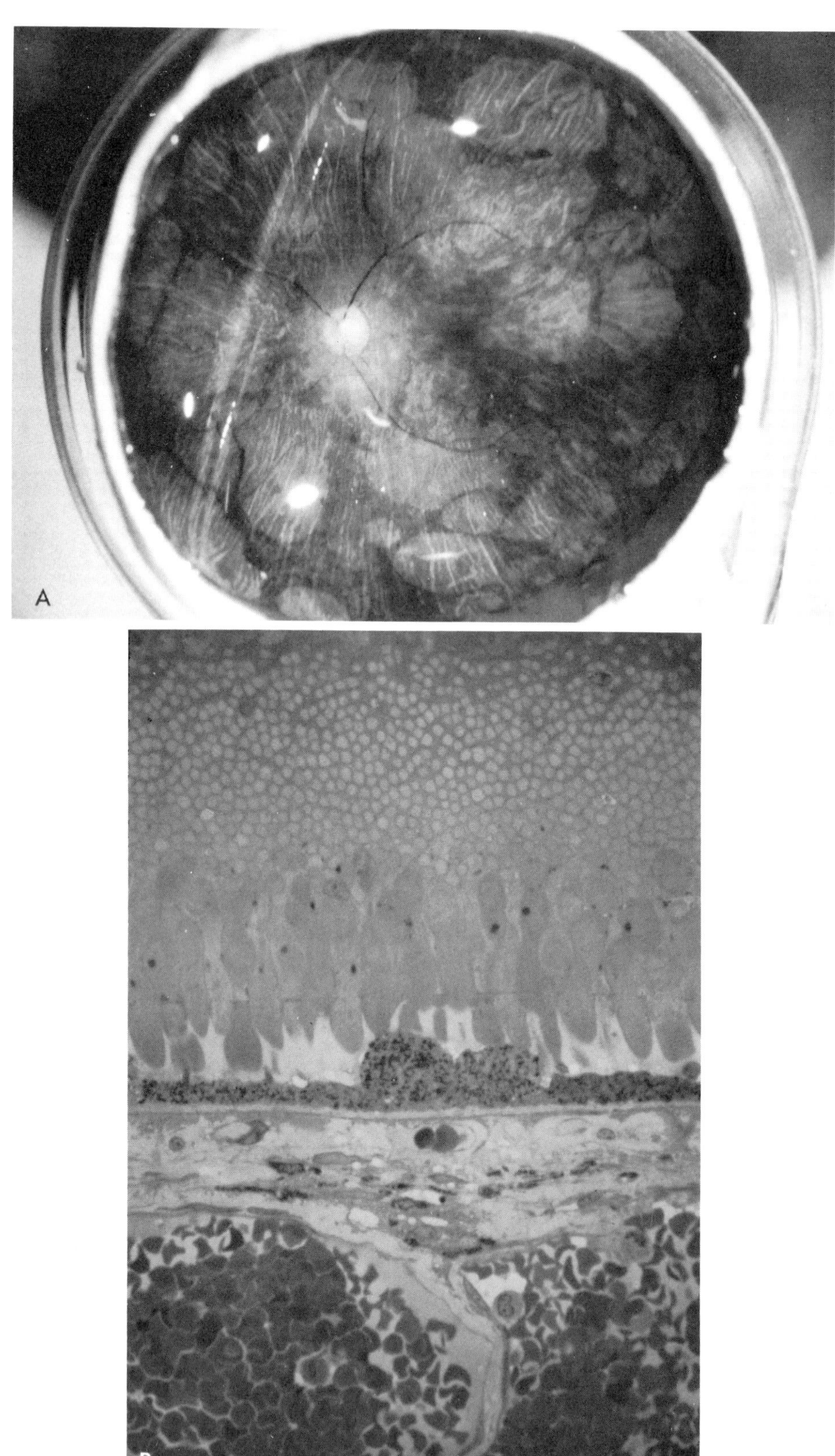

Figure 8–214. Thioridazine retinopathy. *A,* Widespread atrophy of the retinal pigment epithelium (RPE). *B,* Area near macula shows reduced number of cone inner segments and occasional hypertrophied RPE cells.

Illustration continued on opposite page

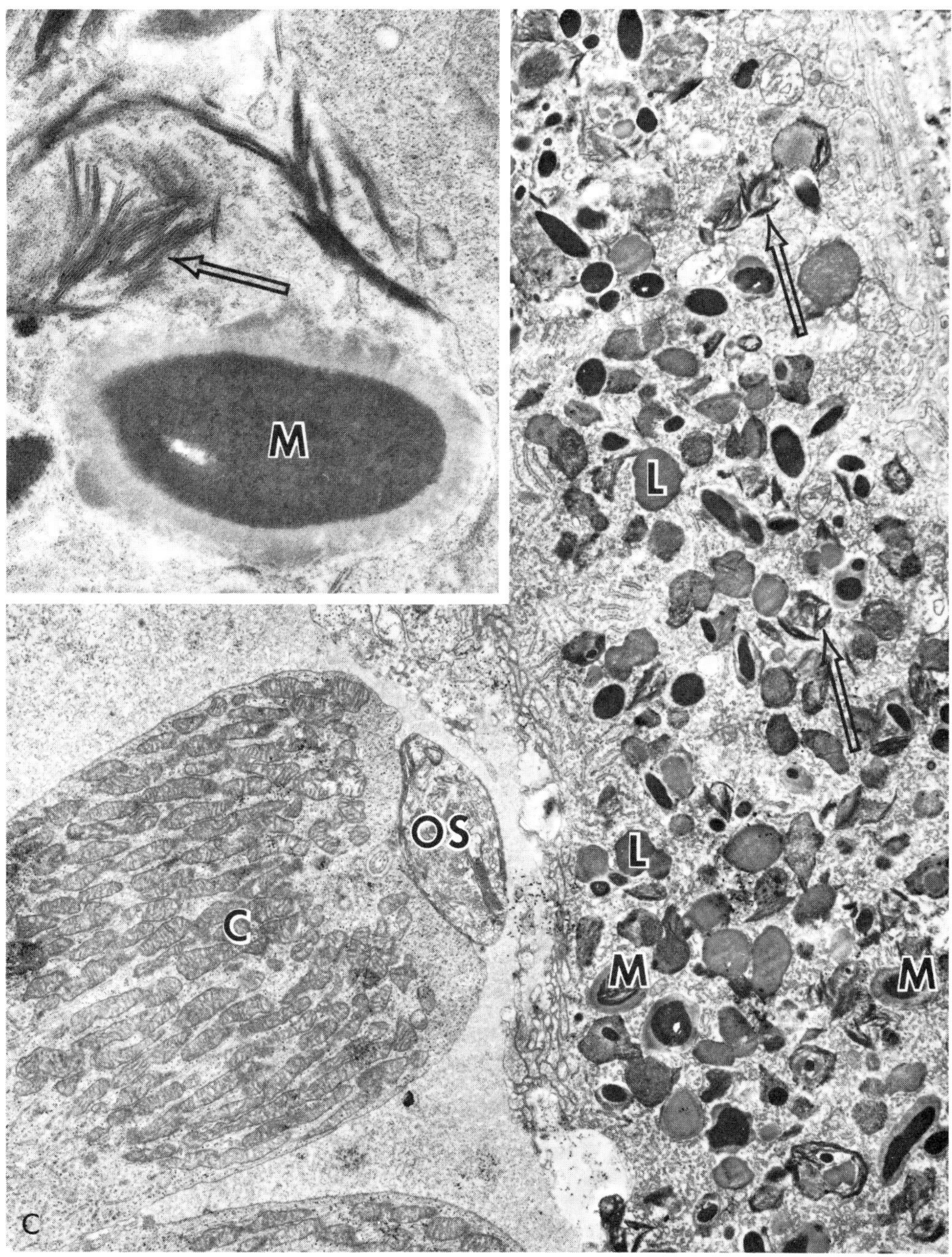

Figure 8–214 *Continued C,* Macula of left eye. Cone inner segments *(C)* are decreased in number with virtually no outer segments *(OS)*. The RPE contains increased quantities of lipofuscin *(L),* melanolysosomes *(M)* and curvilinear bodies (arrows). ×9800. *Inset,* Higher magnification of melanolysosomes *(M)* and curvilinear bodies (arrow). ×51,450. (From Miller FS III, Bunt-Milan AH, Kalina RF: Clinical-ultrastructural study of thioridazine retinopathy. Ophthalmology *89*:1478–1488, 1982.)

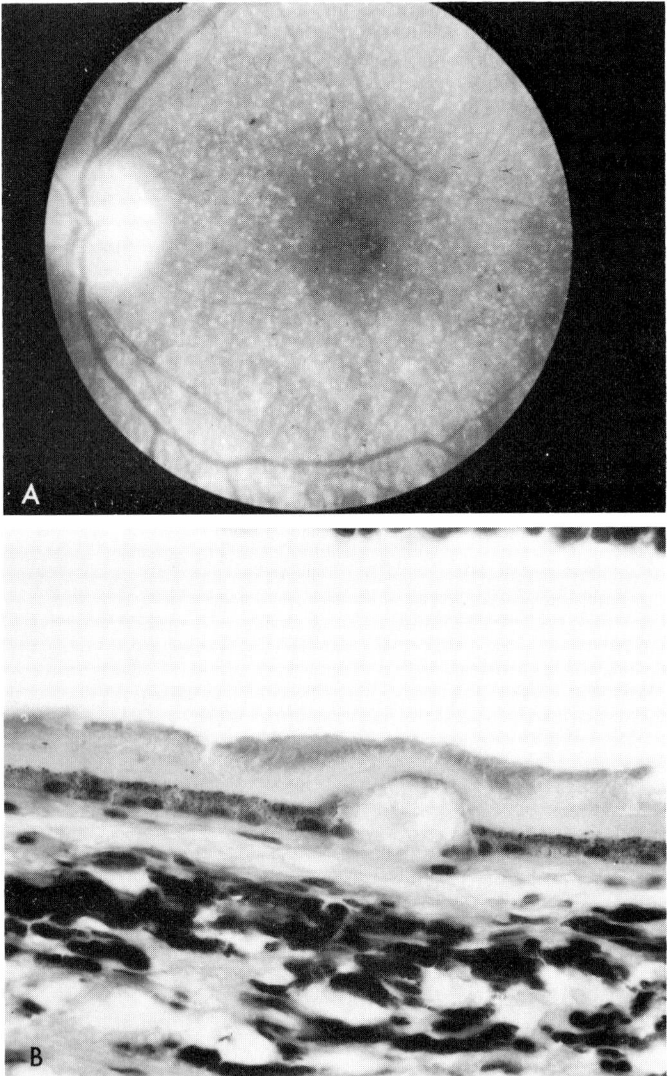

Figure 8–215. *A,* **Flecked retina from oxalate crystals** from methoxyflurane anesthesia. *B,* Birefringent crystal in retinal pigment epithelium area. H and E, ×600. (From Albert DM, Bullock JD, Lahar M, Caine R: Flecked retina secondary to oxalate crystals from methoxyflurane anesthesia: Clinical and experimental studies. Trans Am Acad Ophthalmol Otolaryngol *79*:817–826, 1975.)

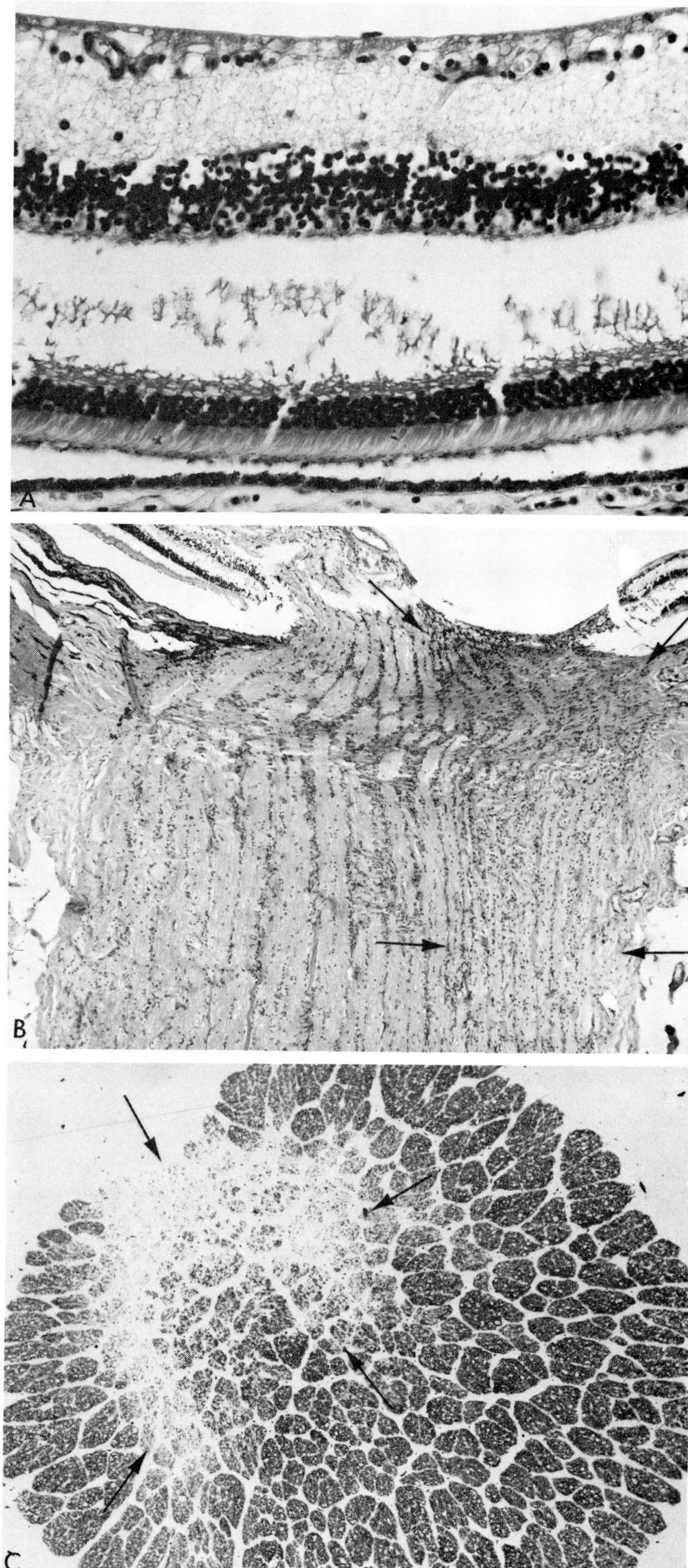

Figure 8–216. Chloramphenicol optic neuropathy with atrophy of maculopapillary bundle in a child with fibrocystic disease of the pancreas. *A,* Section in parafoveal area showing loss of ganglion cell and nerve fiber layers. The defect in the outer plexiform layer is an artifact. H and E, ×300. *B,* Longitudinal and horizontal section of optic nerve head and optic nerve showing atrophy temporally (between arrows). On the temporal side of the optic nerve head there is a reduction in size of the nerve fiber bundles, and columns of astrocytes are closer together, compared with the nasal side. Similarly, in the optic nerve the nerve fiber bundles are narrower and the fibrovascular pial septae are closer together than normal. H and E, ×55. *C,* Cross section of optic nerve shows irregular area of atrophy with demyelinization (arrows). Verhoeff–von Gieson, ×45.

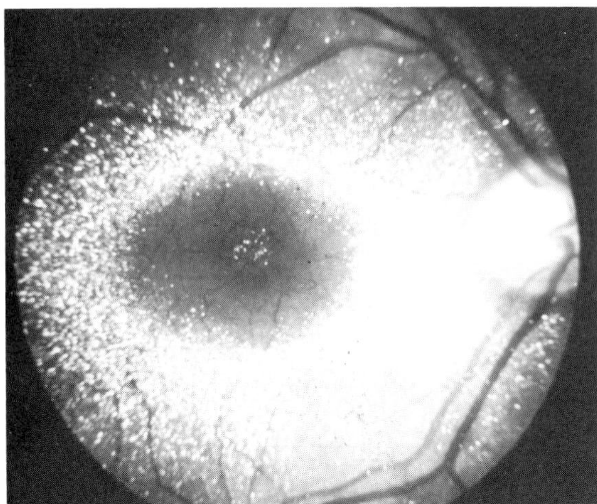

Figure 8–217. Crystalline retinopathy presumably due to use of canthaxanthin. (From Cortin P, Corriveau LA, Rousseau AP, et al: Macuolopathie en paillettes d'or. Can J Ophthalmol *17*:103–106, 1982.)

the treatment of hypercholesterolemia. Flurorescein angiography failed to disclose evidence of leakage from the perifoveal capillaries. Discontinuance of nicotinic acid resulted in improvement of vision and improvement or disappearance of the macular change.

Canthaxanthin Crystallin Retinopathy

Cortin, Corriveau, Rousseau, et al (1982) have observed the occurrence of crystallin deposits arranged in a bull's eye configuration in the macular area (Fig. 8–217) that were presumably due to exposure to canthaxanthin, an oral tanning agent.

Other Drugs

Additional drugs that have or may have retinal or RPE toxicity include the following list from Grant (1974): cephaloridine, chloroquine, chlorpromazine, copper, Cyclyme, diiodohydroxyquin, ethylhydrocupreine, hydroxychloroquine, Iodate, iron, mercuric chloride, oxygen, piperidylchlorophenothiazine, quinine sulfate (Quine), Sparsomycin, and thioridazine.

Stimulated by observation of the development of optic atrophy in a patient receiving large doses of colchicine, Davidson, Green, and Wong (1983) observed retinal atrophy after as little as 1.0 μg of colchicine injected in the vitreous of monkeys.

RETINAL LIGHT TOXICITY

Because of the natural discomfort from staring at the sun, mankind probably always has realized that bright light might harm the eye. However, only since the introduction of artificial sources of intense light, such as arc lamps and lasers—for which natural reflexes and intuitive caution may be absent or suppressed—has retinal hazard from light exposure become a major concern.

The earliest description of a scotoma caused by a solar burn was by Bonetus (1620–1689) who practiced in Geneva (cited by Hamm, 1947). When the opthalmoscope was introduced over 130 years ago, some doctors thought it might be dangerous to admit "naked" light into diseased eyes (Snyder, 1964).

According to Hamm (1947), the first experiments dealing with light damage to the retina were by Czerny in 1867, Deutschmann in 1882, and Widmark in 1893. Czerny in 1867 and Deutschmann (1882) produced ophthalmoscopically visible retinal whitening in rabbits using focused sunlight, and Widmark used a carbon arc source. Deutschmann observed that scarring following intense exposure actually replaced the retina and caused adherence to the choroid. Birch-Hirschfeld (1904) focused ultraviolet light onto a tiny spot on a rabbit retina, producing a lesion much larger than the spot itself, using a retinal exposure much lower than that which could produce a lesion by heating, according to Verhoeff, Bell, and Walker (1916). Birch-Hirschfeld also demonstrated that light that could cause considerable harm to the retina need not necessarily harm the cornea and lens. Widmark (1891) and Fuchs (1896) postulated that erythropsia occurring in aphakic patients was caused by ultraviolet light on the retina. Solar eclipse blindness appears in the literature as far back as Plato's *Phaedo* (Verhoeff, Bell, Walker, 1916). Retinal changes caused by the sun were documented ophthalmoscopically by Deutschmann in 1882. Controversy raged at that time (Verhoeff, Bell, Walker, 1916) about which portion of the spectrum caused the damage.

In 1908, Birch-Hirschfeld found relative scotomas lasting several weeks among workers using mercury vapor illumination (with considerable ultraviolet radiation in the output).

By using photocoagulation, Verhoeff, Bell, and Walker (1916) produced retinal lesions in animals that were mainly of thermal origin. They noted that in near-threshold doses the RPE was the first structure affected histologically. Also, these thermal lesions tended to be sharply demarcated. Maggiore (1933) was the first to study retinal lesions in humans produced experimentally by light prior to enucleation for malignant tumors. Meyer-Schwickerath (1950) and Moron-Salas (1950) were the first to attempt the therapeutic use of photic retinal burns.

Van der Hoeve (1919) (also cited by Fuchs, 1923) suggested a link between senile macular degeneration and repeated exposure to ultraviolet light throughout a person's lifetime. He believed this also partly caused cataracts.

Later (Roggenbau, Wetthauer, 1928), it was discovered that much of the light in the blue-violet end of the spectrum is selectively absorbed by ocular tissues without ever reaching the retina. Wiesinger, Schmidt, Williams, et al (1956) showed that portions of the infrared region are also selectively absorbed by the eyes of rabbits.

Geeraets, Hamm, Williams, et al (1965) studied threshold retinal burns, using ruby lasers and a xenon photocoagulator. They found the RPE to be the first and most severely affected tissue. If a given dose of light was extended over longer periods of time, damage was less likely to occur, but changes extended deeper into the retina. This was consistent with a thermal mode of action, because, with time, heat is conducted further away, lowering the temperature of the primary area. However, for extremely short pulses of light (as from a Q-switched laser) lasting 30 nanoseconds or less, damage thresholds were very much lower than for conventional light sources (0.07 joules/cm^2, or 2.3 mW/cm^2 peak power). This suggested nonthermal and nonlinear effects for these brief pulses; perhaps even acoustic mechanical trauma was partly responsible (Geeraets, Hamm, Williams, et al, 1965).

During the past 30 years, photic retinal changes have been reported with use of astonishingly low levels of light. Brindley (1953), a physiologist, exposed his eye numerous times to small, bright filtered light sources, including green, blue, and violet, for 30 second intervals. Retinal irradiance probably did not exceed 0.1 mW/cm^2 for any of the exposures, yet he experienced an afterimage or relative scotoma that lasted 8 months.

Noell, Walker, Kang, and Berman (1966) exposed unrestrained rats to ordinary fluorescent lights presented through a green filter for 24 hours and found reduction of A- and B-wave amplitudes on electroretinogram that lasted 3 to 4 weeks in many of these eyes. Histologically, all the affected eyes had slight changes in photoreceptor layers. Retinal irradiance undoubtedly did not exceed 0.1 mW/cm^2 at any time in these rats (and was considerably lower than this most of the time). The investigators noted that this retinal light exposure was far too low for a thermal lesion (photocoagulation). Rather, direct light toxicity to the photoreceptors was postulated. They also noted a cumulative effect and a lower damage threshold for lightly pigmented animals. These phenomena suggested quite a different effect than protein coagulation caused by heating.

Evidence that photoreceptor outer segments can regenerate after photic damage in rats was first demonstrated by Gorn and Kuwabara (1967); Kuwabara and Gorn (1968); Kuwabara (1970); and Tso, Fine, and Zimmerman (1972).

That a clinical indirect ophthalmoscope (without an I-R filter) is capable of causing irreversible retinal damage in monkeys after only 15 minutes of exposure was shown by Friedman and Kuwabara (1968).

Further evidence for the existence of a low threshold, direct phototoxic effect came when Harwerth and Sperling (1971) and Sperling (1978) exposed rhesus monkeys to blue and green lights with a retinal irradiance of 1.0 mW/cm^2 for 9 to 28 hours. The blue exposures caused a loss of short wavelength sensitivity lasting 5 months. The green exposure caused a decrease of long wavelength sensitivity for 18 to 30 days.

Tso, Fine, and Zimmerman (1972) and Tso (1973) documented the clinical and histologic features of macular changes in monkeys caused by incandescent light from an indirect ophthalmoscope. The monkeys were exposed for 1 hour with an estimated retinal irradiance of 130 to 250 mW/cm^2. Ophthalmosopic changes did not appear until 1 to 5 days after exposure (in contrast to photocoagulation, in which the effect is almost immediate). Macular gross edema was often present but disappeared by the end of the first week. The RPE showed derangement and pyknosis, and photoreceptor lamellae were broken down into vesicles and tubules during the first week (Fig. 8–218). The next stage involved depigmentation and macrophagic response, sometimes with numerous macrophages in the subretinal space (between the RPE and photoreceptors). As necrotic tissue was removed after the first month, repair began. Proliferation of the RPE and regeneration of the photoreceptor cells continued for up to 5 or more months (Fig. 8–218, *B,C*).

When rats were exposed to fluorescent lights to study possible toxic effects of phototherapy in human neonates, it was discovered that the greater the rat's age, the more susceptible was its retina to damage (Ballowitz and Dämmrich, 1972; O'Steen, Anderson, Shear, 1974). Similar studies in piglets (Sisson, Glauser, Glauser, et al, 1970) and newborn monkeys (Messner, Maisels, Leure-DuPree, 1978) have shown marked damage to photoreceptor cells.

Retinal edema from light exposure has received attention recently (Calkins, Hochheimer, D'Anna, 1980; Tso, Fine, 1979; Henry, Henry, Henry, 1977; Calkins, Hochheimer, 1977) because of the possible relation to cystoid maculopathy after cataract extraction (Irvine-Gass syndrome).

Tso and Fine (1979) exposed monkey foveas to only 1.4 mW/cm^2 from an argon laser (488 nm) for 10 to 15 minutes. Whitening and haze were apparent in the first 24 hours after exposure. Hypopigmentation of the RPE began about 1 week later and lasted as long as 3 years. At 4 years after exposure, *cystoid* changes were present in the Henle fiber layer of the retina (enlargement of

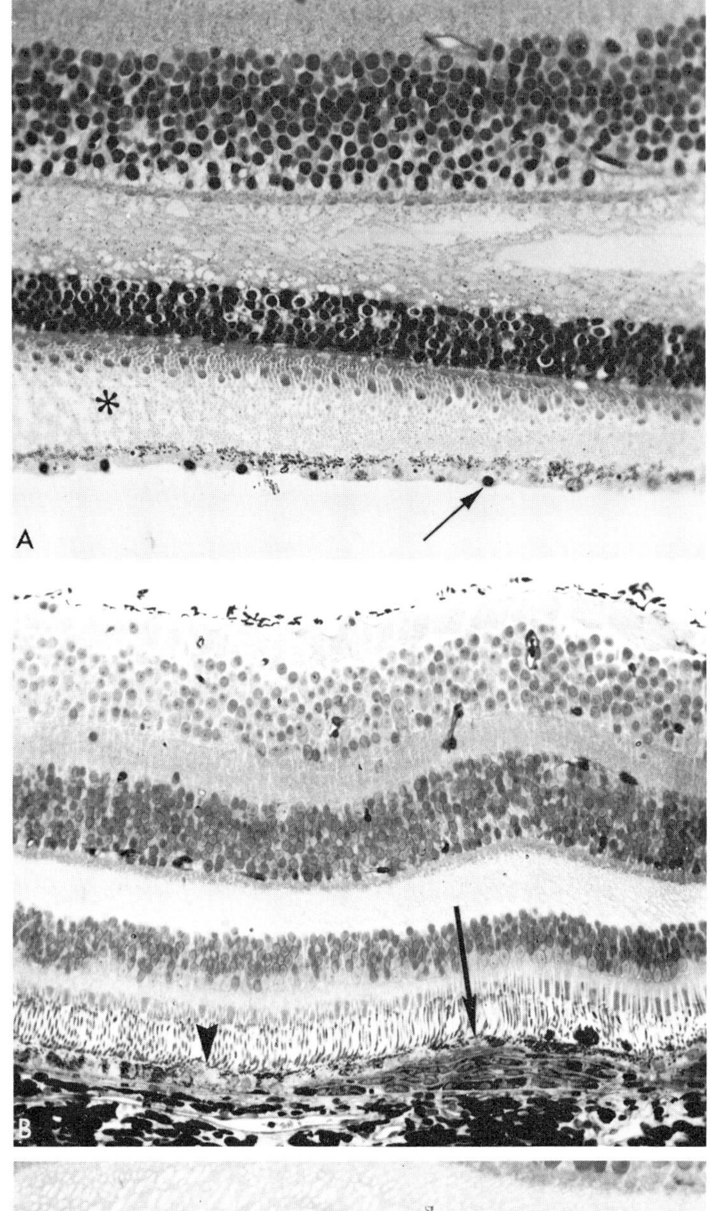

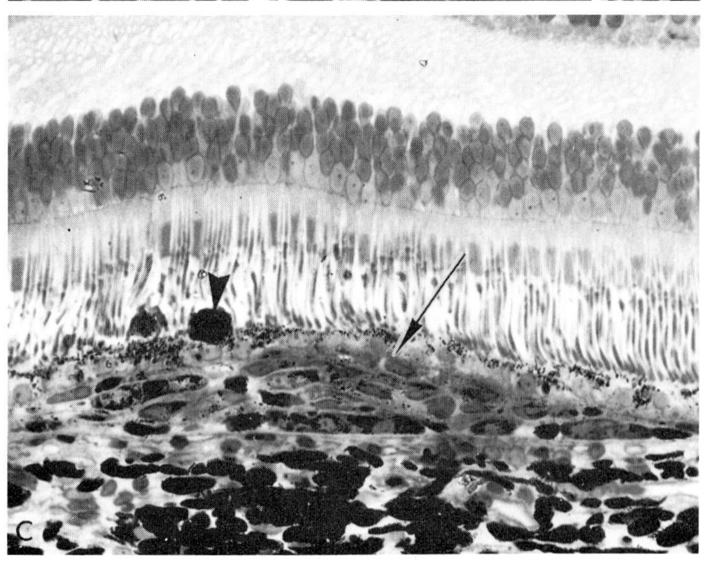

Figure 8–218. Experimental photic maculopathy in a monkey. *A,* Five hours after exposure to the light of an indirect ophthalmoscope for 1 hour. Retinal pigment epithelium (RPE) cells show pyknosis (arrow), and photoreceptors are irregular, granular, and disoriented (asterisk). Toluidine blue, ×300. AFIP Neg. 69-3690. *B,* Fourteen weeks after exposure, plaque of pigmented epithelial cells (arrow) is present between the retina and Bruch's membrane in the macular area. Inner layers of retina and also the outer nuclear layer and the external limiting membrane are intact. Photoreceptor elements are again present but are slightly irregular. RPE (arrowhead) away from the plaque shows irregular depigmentation. Toluidine blue, ×195. AFIP Neg. 69-5362. *C,* At higher magnification, plaque of RPE (arrow) consists of spindle-shaped cells, irregularly pigmented. A layer of cuboidal pavement epithelium has grown over plaque, macrophages (arrowhead) are still present in the subretinal area, and Bruch's membrane appears to be intact. Toluidine blue, ×350. AFIP Neg. 70-3841.

(From T'so MOM, Fine BS, Zimmerman LE: Photic maculopathy produced by the indirect ophthalmoscope. I. Clinical and histopathologic study. Am J Ophthalmol *73*:686–699, 1972.)

the extracellular spaces with watery fluid) and "the foveolar cones appeared malformed, with irregular alignment of the lamellas to form lamellar clusters in disarray. Similar accumulations of extracellular fluid were present between the bases of adjacent pigment epithelial cells . . . and may represent a very early form of serious detachment of the RPE." When the light level was 30 mW/cm^2 (from an argon laser), *cystoid macular changes* were produced in 4 months.

Sunlight was considered the cause of many cases of foveomacular retinitis among sailors on watch duty during World War II (Cordes, 1944).

Henry, Henry, and Henry (1977) were first to suggest that bright lights in the operating room and the internal light source in operation microscopes could be causing or potentiating cystoid maculopathy after surgery. Calkins and associates (1977, 1979, 1979) demonstrated that the internal light source in popular types of surgical microscopes can expose the patient's retina to 100 to 970 mW/cm^2 if the media are clear. Since the microscope may expose the retina for prolonged intervals, retinal light toxicity from routine ocular surgery should not be surprising.

Macular edema has been documented after surprisingly low levels of light exposure. Rothkoff (1978) studied solar eclipse watchers who wore "adequate" eye protection. A 16 year old student using welder's glasses (0.02 per cent transmission measured, with an estimated retinal irradiance of 3 mW/cm^2) (Calkins, Hochheimer, D'Anna, 1979) had a visual acuity of 20/80 the next day, with a "deep exudate" in the macula. Six months later vision was 20/60, with a central scotoma, and macular hyperpigmentation remained. Another 16 year old student viewed the same eclipse through old exposed film (0.8 per cent transmission estimated, with an estimated retinal irradiance of 10 mW/cm^2) (Calkins, Hochheimer, D'Anna, 1979). The next day, bilateral macular edema and "deep macular exudates" were present, with acuity of 20/200 in the right eye and 20/80 in the left eye. After 6 months, vision was 20/30 in each eye, with normal-appearing maculae by ophthalmoscopy.

Recent studies (Sperling, 1978) of retinal light toxicity have shown that functional or histologic damage occurs at amazingly low thresholds for blue light. This supports the concept that damaged retinal components must normally be regenerated and repaired continually, and the ophthalmologist may be largely unaware of previous damage. Otherwise, ordinary daylight exposure and typical industrial light exposure would have produced numerous cases of obvious retinal damage by now.

Sperling (1978) exposed monkeys repeatedly to 10^{-5} to 10^{-4} mW/cm^2 of blue light (463 nm) over several days. This caused a permanent loss of blue cone sensitivity. The ominous implication of this finding is that these doses (each of which presumably were subthreshold) had a *cumulative* effect. This supports the view that repeated doses of light exposure throughout one's life may potentiate or cause senile macular degeneration.

Moon, Clarke, Ruffolo, et al (1978) exposed monkey maculas to 60 mW/cm^2 continuously for 17 minutes, using blue light (441 nm). The monkeys showed reduced visual acuity performance lasting 20 to 30 days. When the dose was 90 mW/cm^2, the visual loss lasted at least 12 months and probably was permanent. This same dose of blue light (90 joules/cm^2) can be received by a human sungazer in less than 1 minute, and this may explain the permanent vision reduction that sometimes occurs. This mechanism also may partly explain why some postoperative cataract patients do not recover 20/20 vision despite clear media, since there is a large proportion of blue light in typical surgical light sources (Calkins, Hochheimer, D'Anna, 1979).

Ham, Mueller, Ruffolo, and Clarke (1979) showed that light toxicity depends very much on wavelength or color, in addition to the known toxic effect of ultraviolet light. Susceptibility to damage increased rapidly in going from the green to blue to violet range. This could not be explained as a thermal effect and must be caused by a direct photochemical effect.

Sperling (1978) indicated that solar retinitis is probably caused almost exclusively by the shorter wavelengths, with only minor toxicity from the red and infrared portions of the sun's spectrum. The longer wavelengths (greater than 580 nm) produce mostly thermal-type lesions, while short wavelengths in the visible spectrum (400 to 580 nm) produce mainly photochemical lesions. Thermal burn lesions tend to be permanent, but moderate photochemical lesions are reparable with time. "Both histopathology and visual-function tests suggest that the melanosomes of the RPE are the initial site of photochemical damage and that only after the supportive functions of the RPE have been impaired do the photoreceptor cells begin to show damage" (Sperling, 1978).

Lanum (1978) provided an extensive review of the damaging effects of light on the retina.

RETINAL PHOTORECEPTOR CELL RENEWAL; LIGHT AND DISEASE
(Young, 1980)

Radioisotope techniques have shown a remarkable metabolic activity of the retinal photoreceptor cells (Young, Droz, 1968). Young (1981, 1982) has developed the concept of retinal *renewal,* and he estimates that the 250 million rods in both eyes produce 7500 trillion rhodopsin molecules daily, throughout life, just for outer segment renewal alone. This extreme degree of metabolic activity is a major biochemical activity of the retinal cells.

A considerable portion of the matabolism of the RPE involves the ingestion and destruction of the membranes shed by the visual cells. This process of shedding, phagocytosis, and renewal follows a daily rhythm. Rods shed membranous disks at dawn and cones shed at the beginning of night.

Light has a damaging effect on the molecules of the visual cells. Restoration of normal structure through continuous renewal is a primary mechanism by which the cells eliminate defective and damaged molecules.

According to Young, the combination of the concept of the damaging effects of light and the molecular renewal system provides a basis for understanding certain retinal degenerative diseases. The basic idea in his theory is that retinal degeneration results when damage from visible radiation and other causes exceeds the capacity of molecular renewal to restore normal structure.

The macular area is especially susceptible to degenerative disease from radiant energy. In addition, if the molecular renewal systems are weakened by genetic defect, drugs, dietary insufficiency, or senescence, the stage is set for macular disease. Light effects on the retinal cells expose any inefficiency of the molecular renewal systems, and, the greater the weakness, the sooner disease will appear.

Young's concept has much appeal and potential implications for many disease processes, including senile macular degenerations, retinitis pigmentosa, genetic/metabolic diseases, drug toxicity, vitamins A and E deficiency, and so on.

PERIPHERAL RETINAL LESIONS, DEGENERATIONS, AND RELATED CONDITIONS

Degenerations—General Considerations

In the section on retinal growth and aging, we covered certain aspects of aging of the retina, including changes in the neurons characterized by accumulation of lipofuscin pigment in the ganglion cells, bipolar layer, outer nuclear layer, and the inner aspects of photoreceptors. To a certain extent, mucoid degeneration occurs in the inner nuclear and outer plexiform layers, with formation of tiny cystoid spaces containing hyaluronic acid. Most of these changes are not visible with the opthalmoscope.

Corpora amylacea (see Figs. 8–17 and 8–18) are considered an aging change and have been found to be derived from nerve fibers.

Vessel changes in the retina are also a common accompaniment of aging. Senescent changes in the arteries and arterioles are those of small vessels generally and include hyaline degeneration of the walls of the vessels and some reduction in the vessel caliber.

Cogan (1963) has described changes in the capillaries and venules. He observed a dropout of endothelial and pericytic cells in areas of the retina, so that eventually the affected vessels had no blood flow. He also found microaneurysms as an apparently normal senile change in the human retina. Studies in experimental animals, however, appear to discount the occurrence of microaneurysms as an aging change (Glatt, Henkind, 1979).

Kornzweig (1965), using flat trypsin-digest preparations of the retina, observed changes in the paramacular capillaries similar to those described by Cogan.

The RPE also shows senile changes, and many of these alterations can be seen clinically as fine, speckling pigmentary changes in the posterior and equatorial fundus. There may be tiny areas of RPE proliferation, to form scattered clumps in the affected areas. More often, there is depigmentation of the RPE, making the choroid more visible. This occurs especially in the peripapillary region and at the equator. Lipid deposits are known to occur in the RPE, commencing in middle age and increasing in older age groups. This lipid is known as lipofuscin and is a wear-and-tear pigment produced as a byproduct of cell metabolism. Vacuoles also have been observed in the cytoplasm of the pigment cells (Garron, 1963).

Bruch's membrane also shows aging changes, commencing at about age 20 years (Hogan, Alvarado, 1967). Lipid and crystalline structures have been identified with the light microscope, and the membrane becomes increasingly sudanophilic and PAS-positive. Changes occur in the RPE basement membrane, causing some thickening, and there is an increased density of the collagenous and elastic layers.

An extensive monograph dealing with the peripheral retina in health and disease has been provided by Bec, Ravault, Arne, and Trepsat (1980).

Cystic Degenerations of Retina and Related Conditions

Peripheral Cystoid Degeneration. Cystic changes in the retinal periphery are a very common degenerative process seen in some degree in virtually all adults. The condition was observed in 86.8 per cent of 500 autopsy cases of all age groups (O'Malley, Allen, 1967). The condition increases in severity until the seventh decade.

There are two types: typical and reticular peripheral cystoid degeneration. Each type has

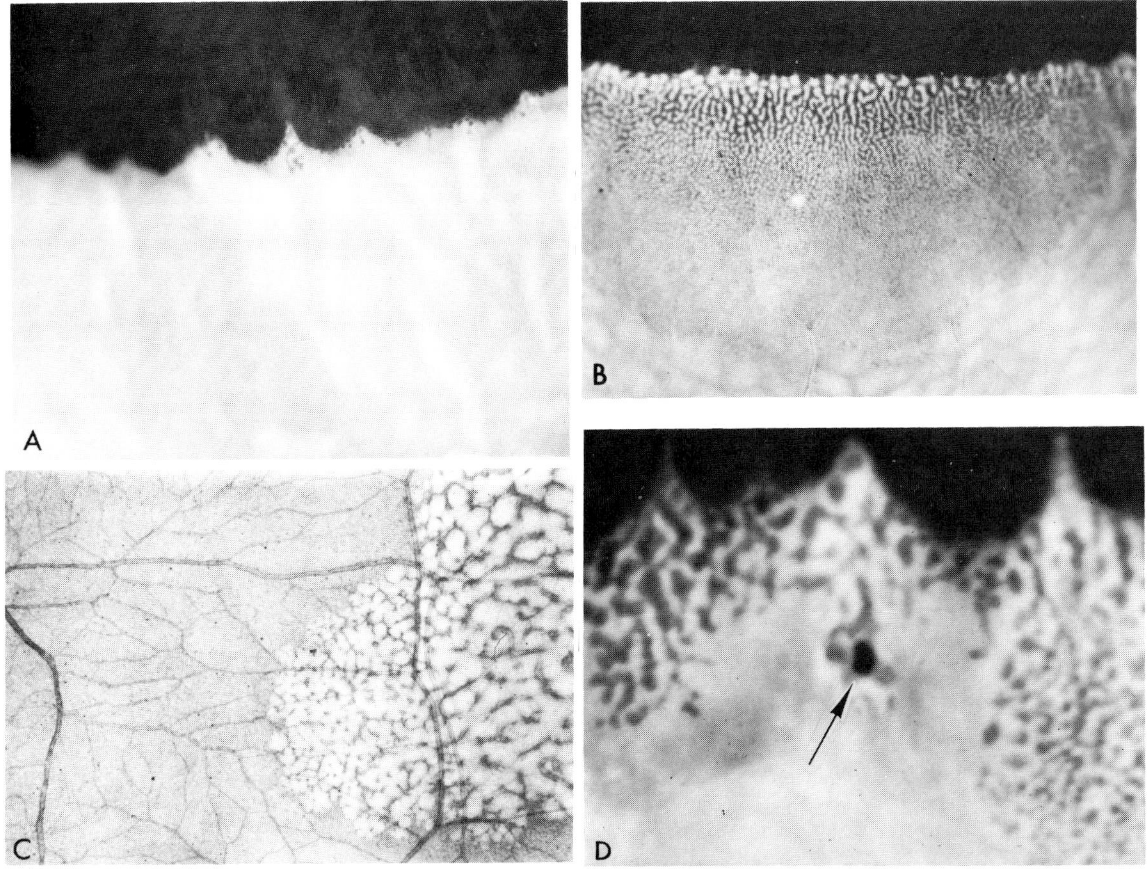

Figure 8–219. Typical peripheral cystoid degeneration (TPCD). *A,* Very early TPCD in a 13 year old boy. EP 30072. *B,* Moderately advanced TPCD in an adult. EP 34376. *C,* Flat preparation of retina showing TPCD. PAS, ×25. *D,* TPCD with hole (arrow) in retina. (*C* and *D* from Green WR: Pathology of the retina, *in* Frayer WC (ed): Lancaster Course in Ophthalmic Histopathology. Unit 9. Philadelphia, F. A. Davis, 1981.)

characteristic ophthalmoscopic, gross, and microscopic features. Differences exist in the prevalence and incidence of complications.

Typical Peripheral Cystoid Degeneration (Blessig-Iwanoff cysts). This type of peripheral cystoid degeneration is characterized by microcysts that often coalesce, giving the appearance of lobulated, irregularly branching, tortuous channels (Fig. 8–219). It may be considered to be a form of mucoid degeneration, since the cystic cavities contain a hyaluronidase-sensitive mucopolysaccharide. This condition is seen in some degree in virtually all adults after the age of 20 years. Some investigators (Straatsma, Foos, Feman, 1976, pages 8–11) have observed the process in infancy.

The cystic cavities typically are present in the outer plexiform layer (Fig. 8–220) and are delineated by the inner and outer nuclear layers, fortified by the middle and external limiting membranes and by the interbridging of neural fibers and Müller's cells coursing between the inner and outer retinal layers. There may be an increased tendency for the process to be present and more markedly developed in association with dentate retinal processes.

Complications occurring from typical peripheral cystoid degeneration (TPCD) are rare. Retinal holes (Fig. 8–219) may occur from rupture of both the inner and outer layers, but such holes do not result in retinal detachment because the vitreous is usually intact over TPCD. Extension posteriorly to the equator is rare. The importance of extensive TPCD is the possibility of its leading to typical degenerative retinoschisis.

Reticular Peripheral Cystoid Degeneration (Foos, Feman, 1970; Foos, 1970). This process is almost always located posterior to and continuous with typical peripheral cystoid degeneration, and it has a predilection for the inferior temporal quadrant. It typically has a linear or reticular pattern that corresponds to the retinal vessels, and a finely stippled internal surface corresponding to points of attachment of residual interbridging pillars of tissue to the inner layer (Fig. 8–221). The cystic spaces in reticular peripheral cystoid degeneration (RPCD) are located in the nerve fiber layer (Fig. 8–221). The inner layer consists of the internal limiting membrane and variable amounts of nerve fibers and blood vessels. This degenerative process is present in about 18 per cent of

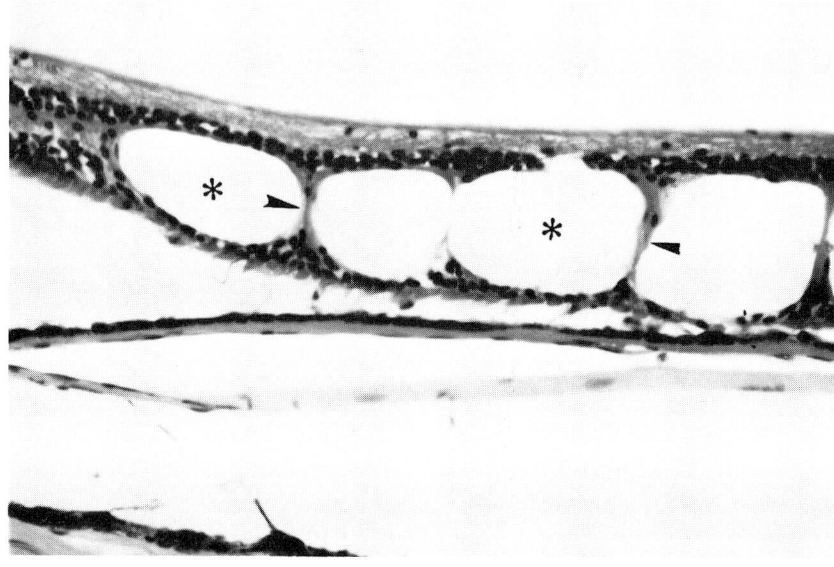

Figure 8–220. Typical peripheral cystoid degeneration. Cystic cavities (asterisks) are located in the outer plexiform layer, delineated by inner and outer nuclear layers and by interbridging of neural fibers and Müller's cells (arrowheads). H and E, ×240. EP 51445.

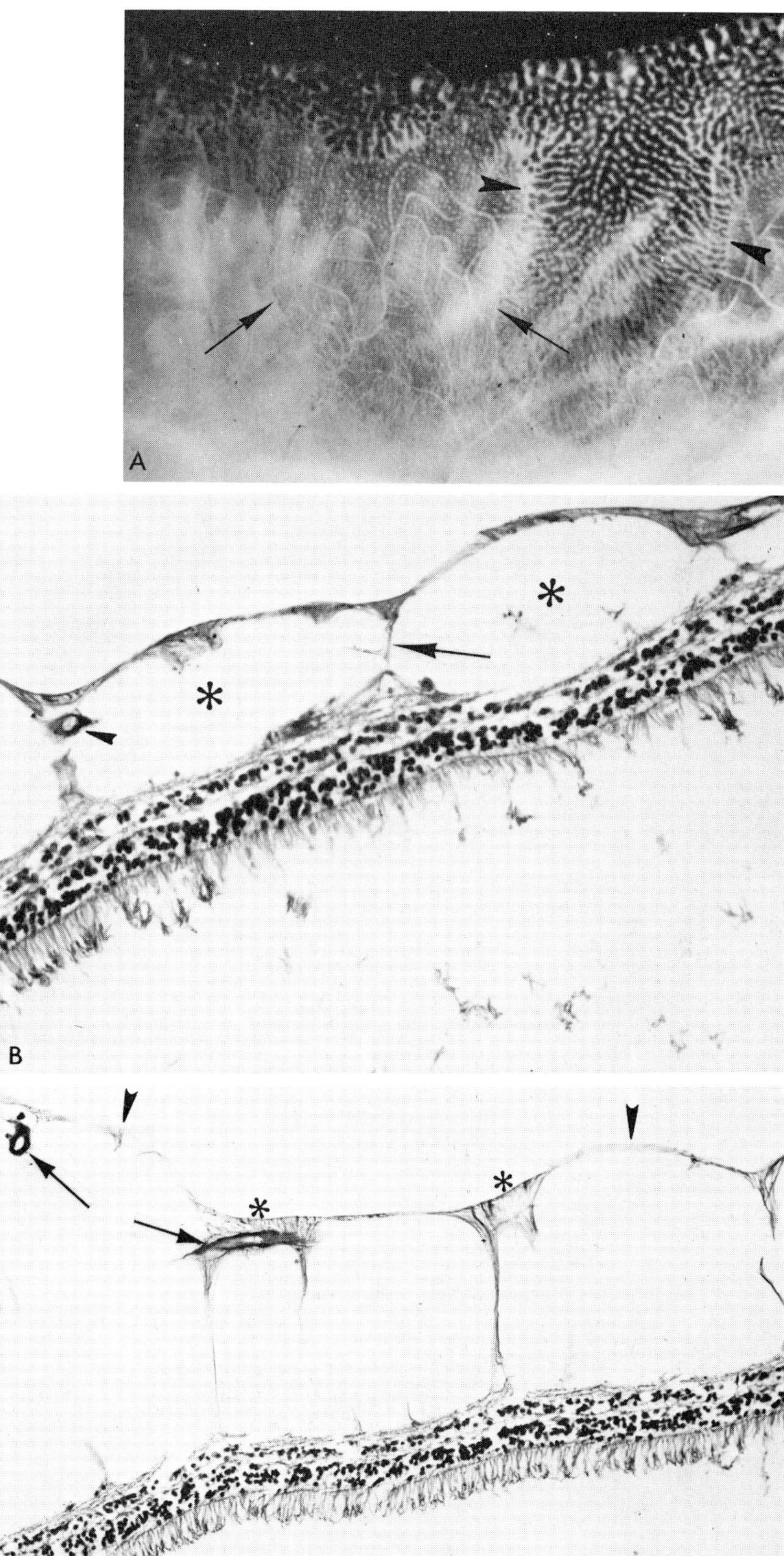

Figure 8–221. Reticular peripheral cystoid degeneration (RPCD). *A,* Gross appearance of RPCD (between arrows) and typical peripheral cystoid degeneration (between arrowheads). RPCD has reticular pattern and finely stippled appearance. (Courtesy of Dr. R.Y. Foos.)

B, Cystic cavities (asterisks) are located in the nerve fiber layer. Thin inner layer consists of the internal limiting membrane (ILM), a few nerve fibers, and some blood vessels (arrowhead). Müller cells and neural processes form inner bridging tissue (arrow). PAS, ×240. *C,* Different area shows the inner layer to consist of only ILM in some areas (arrowheads). Interbridging tissue is on stretch. More tissue is present in inner layer at the point of attachment of inner bridging connections (asterisks). These correspond to the white dots or strippled appearance seen ophthalmoscopically and grossly. Blood vessels (arrows) are present in the inner layer. PAS, ×200.

adults and is bilateral in about 41 per cent of affected patients. The importance of reticular cystoid degeneration is the possibility of development of reticular degenerative retinoschisis (bullous retinoschisis).

Radial Paravascular Rarefaction of the Retina. This degenerative process produces a localized area of retinal thinning with a reticulated appearance, at or posterior to the equator and aligned with a major retinal vessel (Fig. 8–222,*A*) (Spencer, Foos, 1970). Histopathologically, there is cystic degeneration of the retina at the level of the nerve fiber layer (Fig. 8–222,*B*). Vitreous traction is considered to be the cause of radial paravascular rarefaction, but we have observed cases with no evidence of vitreous traction. Other lesions that occur in a radial paravascular distribution include retinal pits and retinal tears, and those are more clearly related to vitreous traction.

Retinoschisis (Splitting of the Retina). Formerly, two types of retinoschisis were recognized: senile and congenital. The senile form (Shea, Schepens, Von Pirquet, 1960; Samuels, Fuchs, 1952) also has been referred to as retinal cysts by some (Teng, Katzin, 1953; François, Rabaez, 1953). Retinoschisis, rarely, has been confused with malignant melanoma (Zimmerman, Spencer, 1960).

Congenital sex-linked recessive retinoschisis is considered elsewhere (see page 646).

Two degenerative forms of retinoschisis are now recognized and are believed to develop from

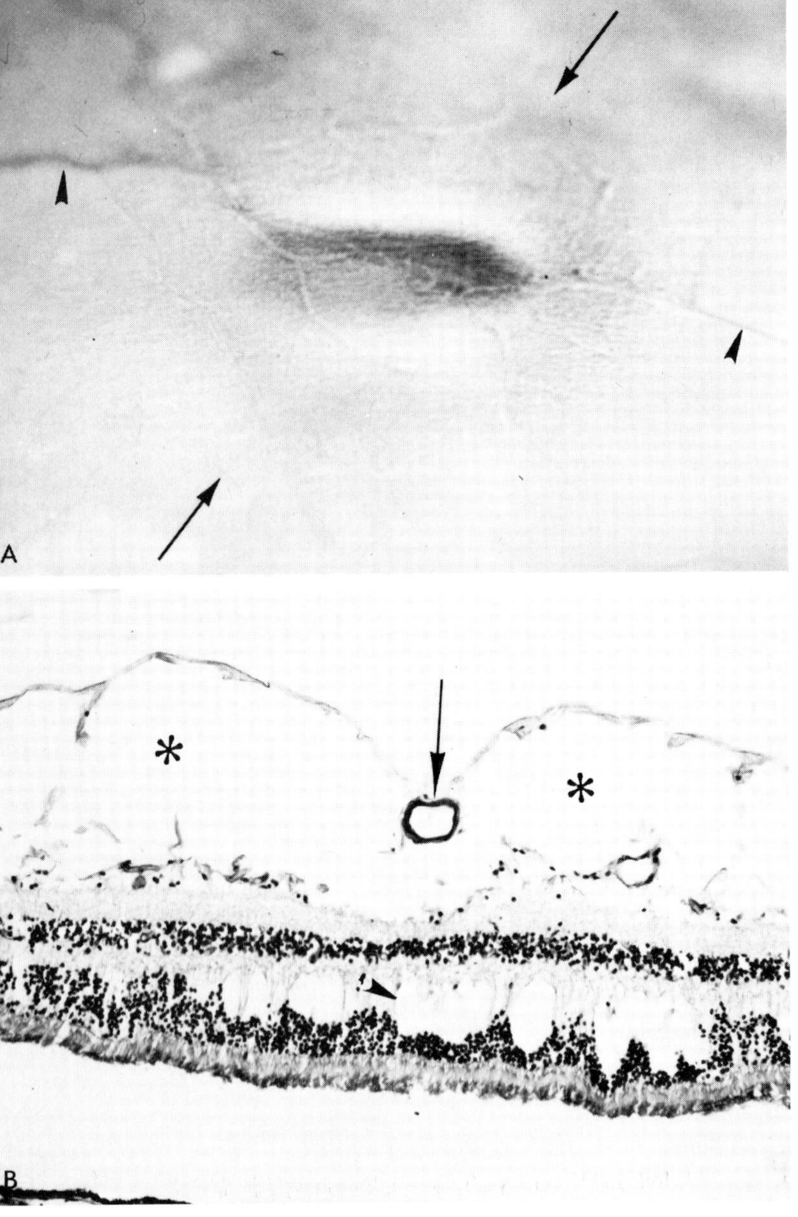

Figure 8–222. Radial paravascular rarefaction. *A,* Gross appearance of lesion (arrows). The retina appears slightly thinned, has a fine reticulated appearance, and is associated with a major retinal vessel (arrowheads). *B,* There is cystic degeneration (asterisks) of the nerve fiber layer near the other side of the retinal vessel (arrow). Cystic degeneration is present also in the outer plexiform layer (arrowhead). PAS, ×120. EP 32972. (From Green WR: Pathology of the retina, *in* Frayer WC (ed): Lancaster Course in Ophthalmic Histopathology. Unit 9. Philadelphia, F.A. Davis, 1981.)

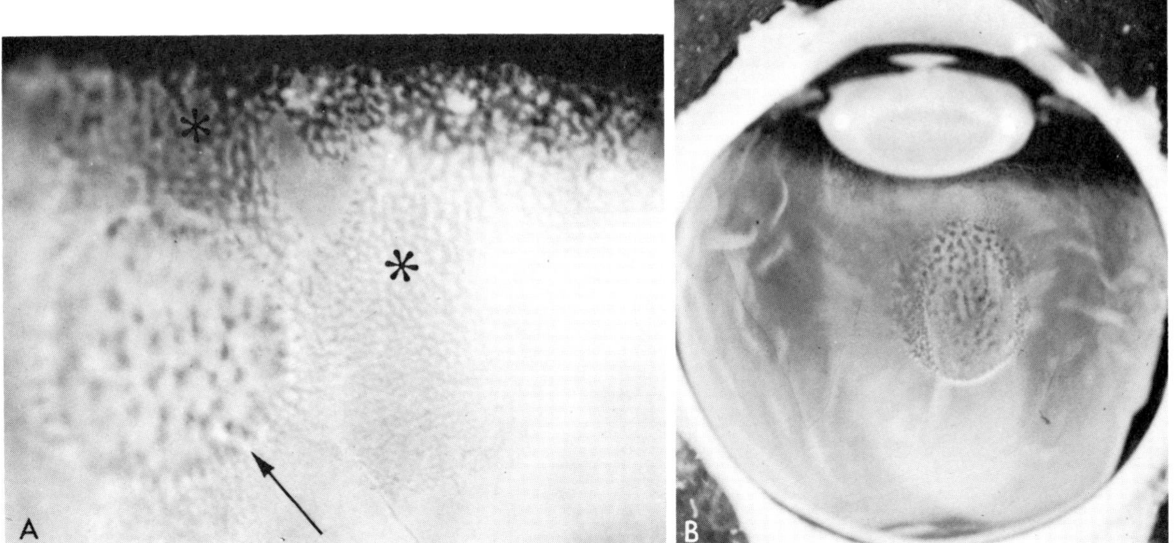

Figure 8–223. *A,* Gross appearance of **tyical degenerative retinoschisis (TDR)** (arrow). Beaten-metal appearance is due to the irregular thickness of the outer layer. Typical peripheral cystoid degeneration (TPCD) (asterisks) is present anterior and to the right of TDR. EP 34278. *B,* Appearance of TDR located at the equator and unassociated with peripheral cystoid degeneration. EP 33487.

pre-existing peripheral cystoid degeneration. Typical peripheral cystoid degeneration can give rise to typical degenerative retinoschisis, and both typical and reticular peripheral cystoid degeneration give rise to reticular degenerative retinoschisis (Foos, 1970). When retinoschisis is extensive enough to produce visual field defects, such defects are typically total, with sharp margins.

Typical Degenerative Retinoschisis. This form of retinoschisis produces a round or oval, smooth, fusiform elevation, typically occurring in the inferotemporal retina in about 1 per cent of adults, 33 per cent of whom have the lesion bilaterally (Straatsma, Foos, 1973). A stippled pattern is present at the periphery, where the schisis blends with typical peripheral cystoid retinoschisis, which often surrounds the lesion (Fig. 8–223). Centrally, the thin inner layer is smooth and contains retinal vessels. The schisis cavity is optically empty. The outer layer is irregular and is responsible for the beaten-metal appearance; it usually turns white on scleral depression. Posterior extension to the equator, or just posterior to the equator, may be observed (Fig. 8–224). Complications, such as hole formation (Figs. 8–225 and 8–226) and marked posterior extension, are very uncommon and rarely require treatment in typical degenerative retinoschisis.

In typical degenerative retinoschisis, the retinal splitting occurs at the outer plexiform layer (Fig. 8–227). The inner layer is thinner and contains the internal limiting membrane (ILM), nerve fiber layer, retinal vessels, and variable portions of the remaining ganglion cells and inner plexiform and inner nuclear layers. Usually, only the ILM, nerve fiber layer, and portions of the inner nuclear layer are evident. The outer layer is thicker and serrated and consists of focal areas of the inner nuclear layer, the outer plexiform and outer nuclear layers, and the layer of rods and cones (Fig. 8–228).

Reticular Degenerative Retinoschisis. (Straatsma, Foos, 1973). This form of retinoschisis is believed to develop from the concurrent presence of typical and reticular cystoid degeneration of the peripheral retina (Foos, 1970). Reticular degenerative retinoschisis is characterized by round or oval areas of retinal splitting in which a bullous elevation of an extremely thin, inner layer occurs (Fig. 8–229), most commonly in the lower temporal quadrant. Blood vessels in the attenuated inner layer may be sclerotic and occluded or, rarely, telangiectatic and may have microaneurysms. The schisis cavity is optically empty, and the outer layer has a pitted, beaten-metal, or honeycomb appearance and turns white with scleral depression. Typical peripheral cystoid degeneration is usually present anterior to this lesion, and reticular cystoid degeneration is usually evident at some site near the lesion.

The lesion is found in about 1.6 per cent of adults, 15 per cent of whom have bilateral involvement. Posterior extension and outer layer hole formation with characteristic rolled edges (Fig. 8–230) are more common than in typical degenerative retinoschisis.

In the reticular form, the splitting usually occurs in the nerve fiber layer, with the thin inner layer containing only ILM, some retinal vessels, and variable portions of the nerve fiber layer. The

Text continued on page 824

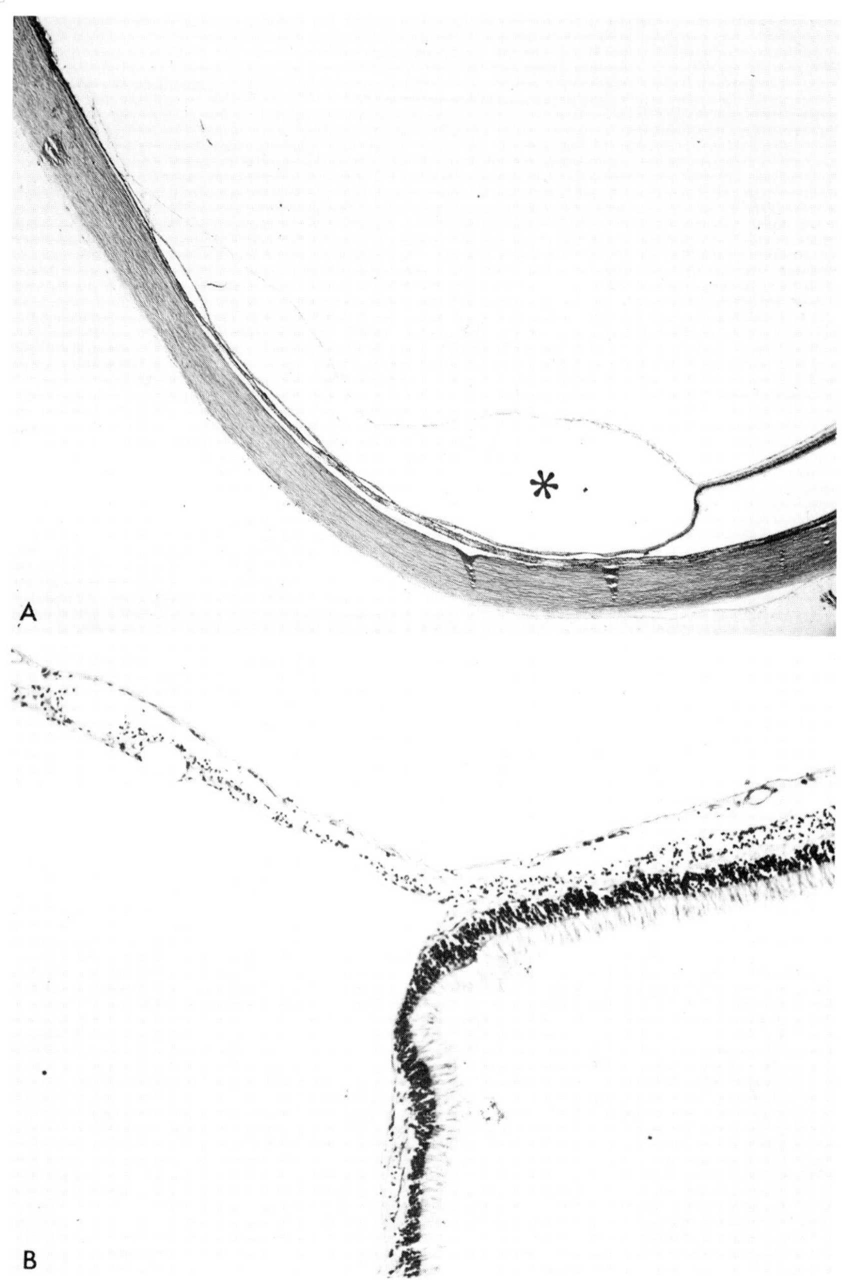

Figure 8–224. *A,* **Typical degenerative retinoschisis (TDR)** (asterisk) with extension posterior to equator. PAS, ×10. *B,* Higher power view of posterior extent of TDR, showing the split to have occurred in the outer plexiform layer. PAS, ×100. EP 44892.

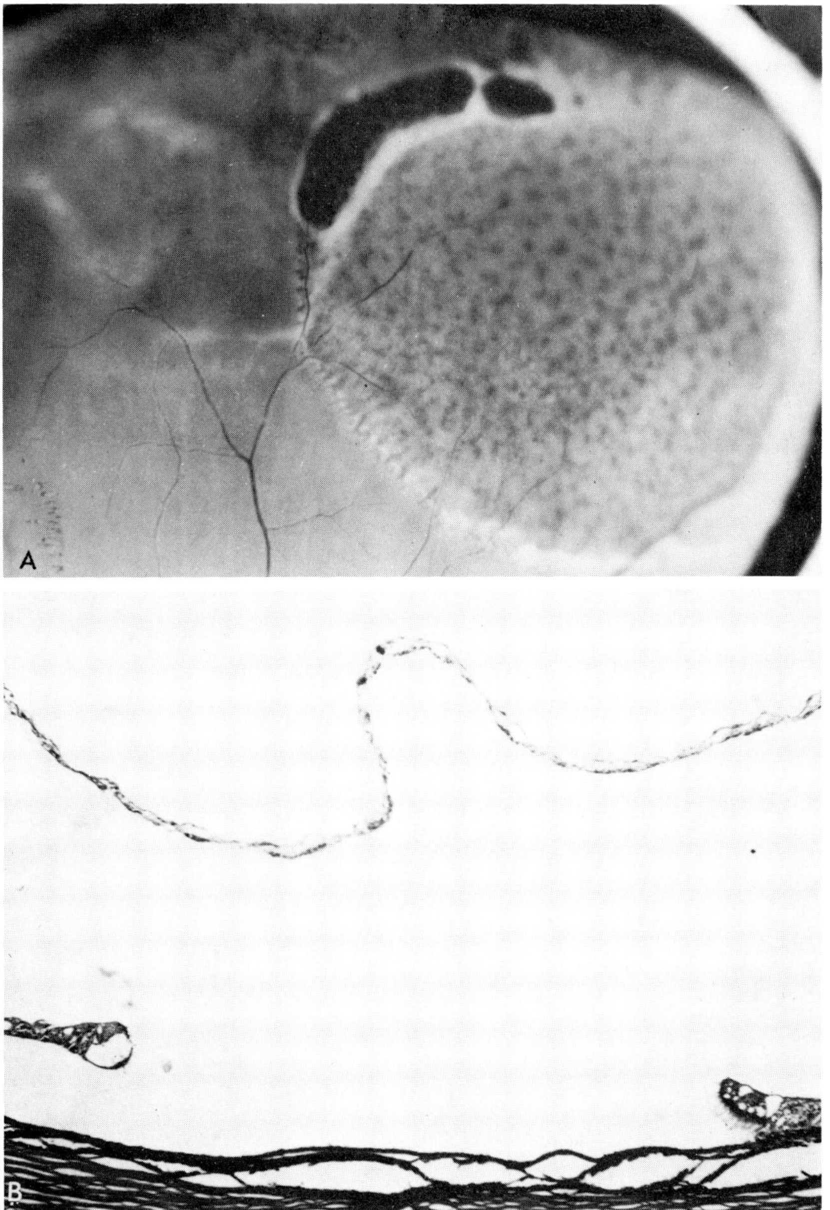

Figure 8–225. *A,* Gross appearance of **typical degenerative retinoschisis,** with hole in outer layer at periphery of lesion. *B,* Section of same lesion showing area of hole. H and E, ×35. EP 39197.

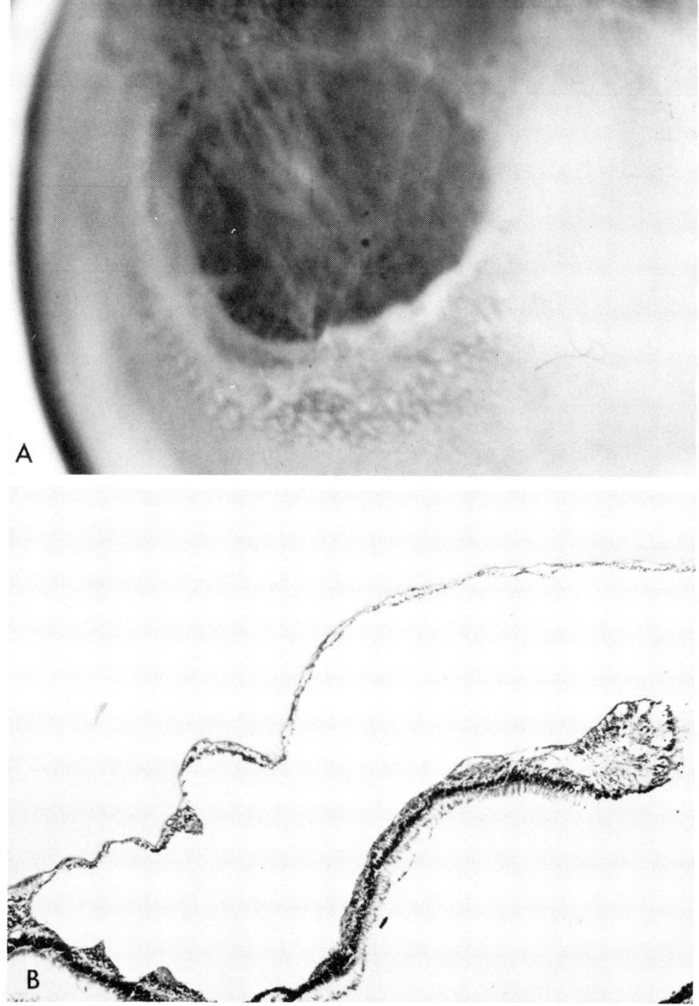

Figure 8–226. *A,* Gross appearance of **typical degenerative retinoschisis,** with large central hole in outer layer. Margin of hole has a denser appearance. *B,* Section of same lesion showing margin of hole in outer layer, which has a rolled margin. Margin of hole is everted internally and is responsible for the denser appearance seen ophthalmoscopically and grossly. PAS, ×45. EP 44372.

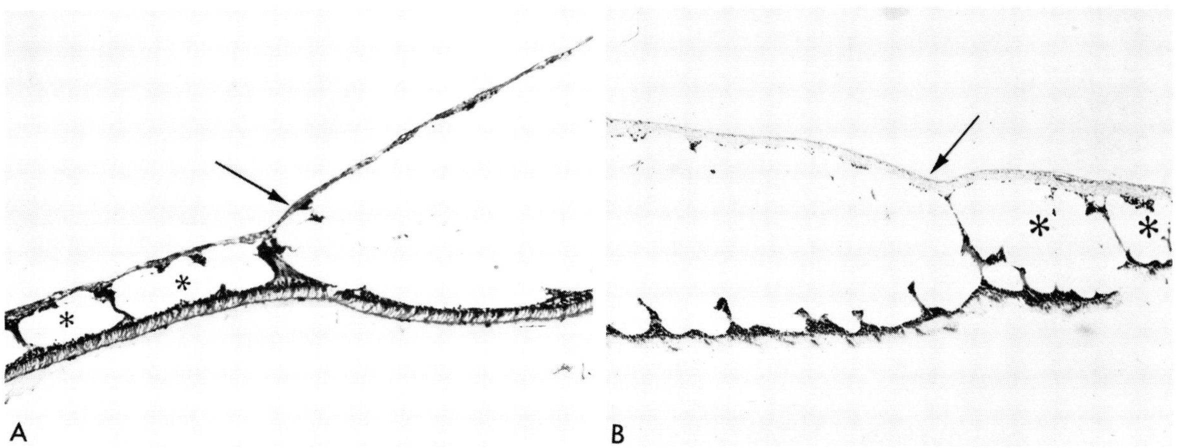

Figure 8–227. Typical degenerative retinoschisis (arrow) continuous with typical peripheral cystoid degeneration (asterisks). *A,* H and E, ×100. EP 30768. *B,* H and E, ×130. EP 43146.

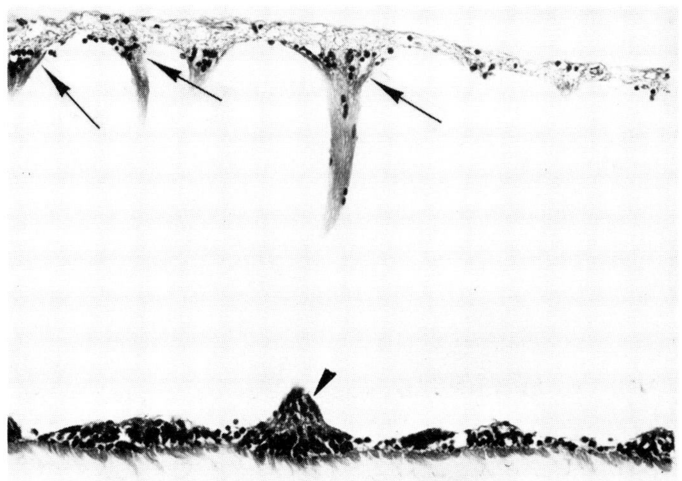

Figure 8–228. Higher power view of **typical degenerative retinoschisis**. Residual inner nuclear layer is present in the inner layer of schisis (arrows) and in one area of the outer layer of schisis (arrowhead). The outer layer is composed mostly of outer nuclear layer. H and E, ×225. EP 23102.

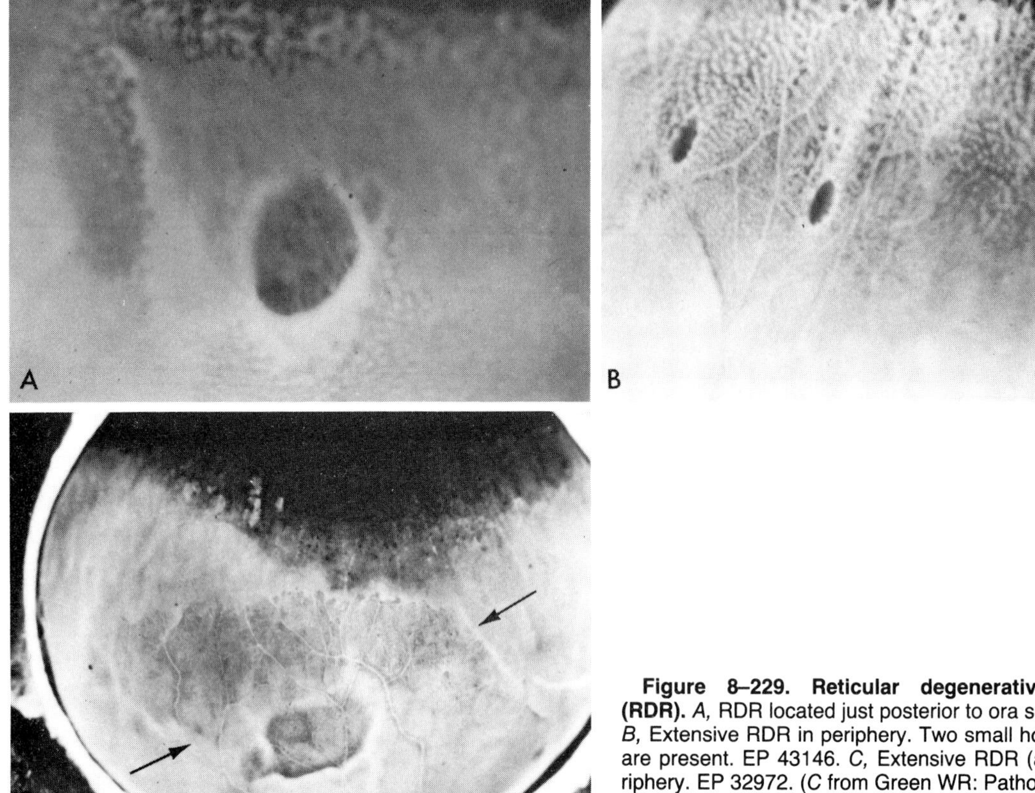

Figure 8–229. Reticular degenerative retinoschisis (RDR). *A,* RDR located just posterior to ora serrata. EP 42397. *B,* Extensive RDR in periphery. Two small holes in outer layer are present. EP 43146. *C,* Extensive RDR (arrows) in midperiphery. EP 32972. (*C* from Green WR: Pathology of the retina, *in* Frayer WC (ed): Lancaster Course in Ophthalmic Histopathology. Unit 9. Philadelphia, F.A. Davis, 1981.)

outer layer contains the relatively intact remaining retinal layers. In some instances, glial cells or cells of the inner nuclear layer may be present in the inner layer. Holes in the outer layer are observed in up to 23 per cent of the lesions and usually have a rolled margin (Figs. 8–229 and 8–230). Rarely, holes may be in the inner layer of the schisis (Fig. 8–231).

Occasionally, typical and reticular degenerative retinoschisis may occur together.

Treatment of reticular degenerative retinoschisis may be indicated if (1) progression threatens the macular area; (2) there is an associated nonrhegmatogenous retinal detachment, and both are progressive and threaten the macula; (3) there are breaks in both layers; and (4) there are breaks

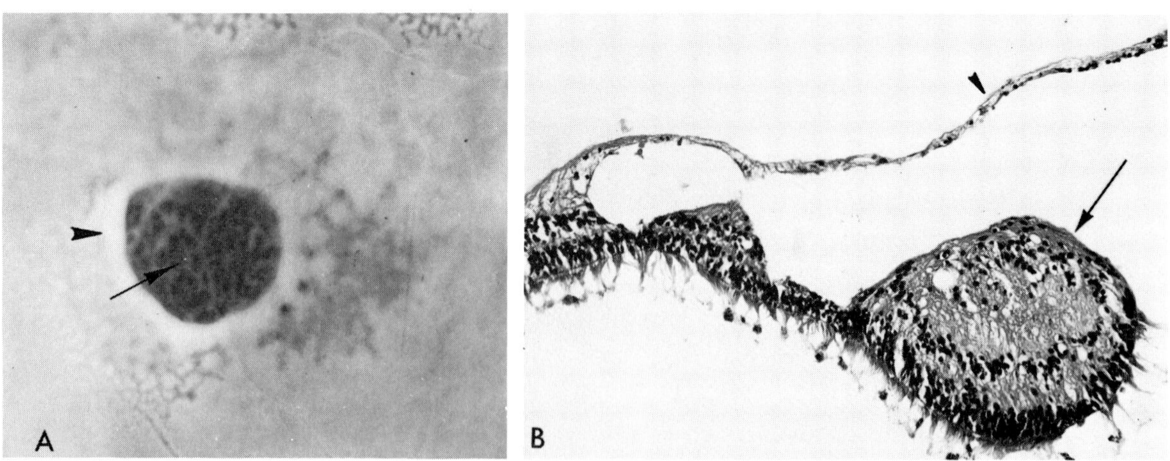

Figure 8–230. *A,* Gross appearance of **reticular degenerative retinoschisis,** with a hole with rolled margins in outer layer (arrowhead). Thin reticulated inner layer (arrow) is more apparent over area of hole. *B,* Hole in outer layer with eversion of margin (arrow). Thin inner layer of schisis (arrowhead) is intact. H and E, ×210. EP 33510.

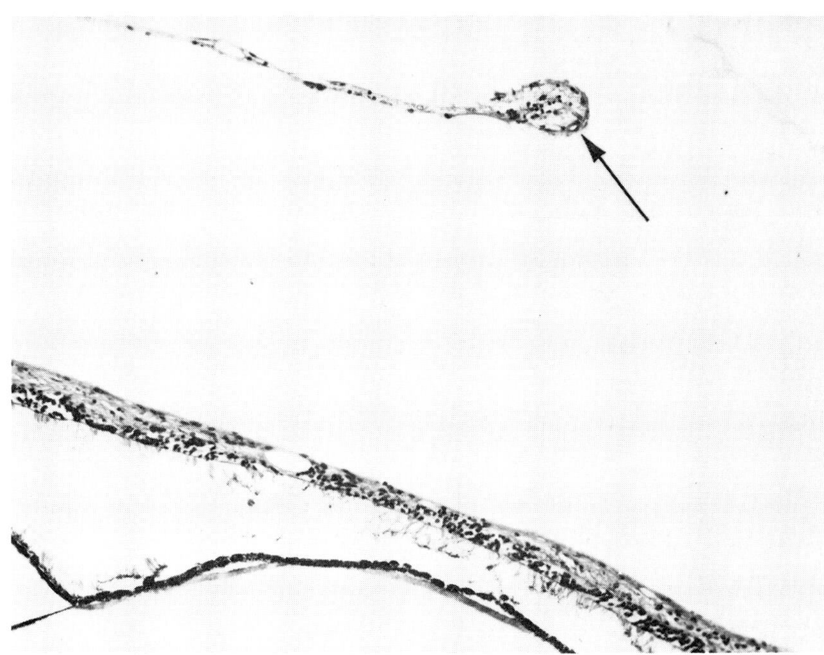

Figure 8–231. Reticular degenerative retinoschisis layer (arrow). PAS, ×130. EP 48825.

in both layers and an associated rhegmatogenous retinal detachment (Straatsma, Foos, Feman, 1976, page 13).

Secondary Cystic Degeneration and Retinoschisis. Cystic degeneration of the retina and coalescence of cystic areas to form retinoschisis may be observed with vitreous traction, retinal edema from trauma, retinal vascular lesions, ocular inflammatory conditions, choroidal lesions, resolving retinal hemorrhages, and others.

Vitreous Traction. Localized vitreous traction of the retina may induce cystic degeneration and retinoschisis. This process may be observed in the macula (Figs. 8–232 through 8–234), in the peripapillary area (Fig. 8–235), and the midperiphery (Figs. 8–236 through 8–239).

Inflammatory Conditions. Chronic ocular inflammatory disease with subsequent cystoid macular edema can, with time, lead to coalescence of cystoid spaces and produce schisis. Figure 8–240 is an example of early retinoschisis in cystoid macular edema in an eye with chronic iridocyclitis. An extreme example of retinoschisis in the posterior pole in an eye with chronic uveitis is shown in Figure 8–241.

Retinal Vascular Lesions. Leaky vascular retinal lesions can lead to cystic degeneration and splitting of the retina. Histopathologic examples

Text continued on page 832

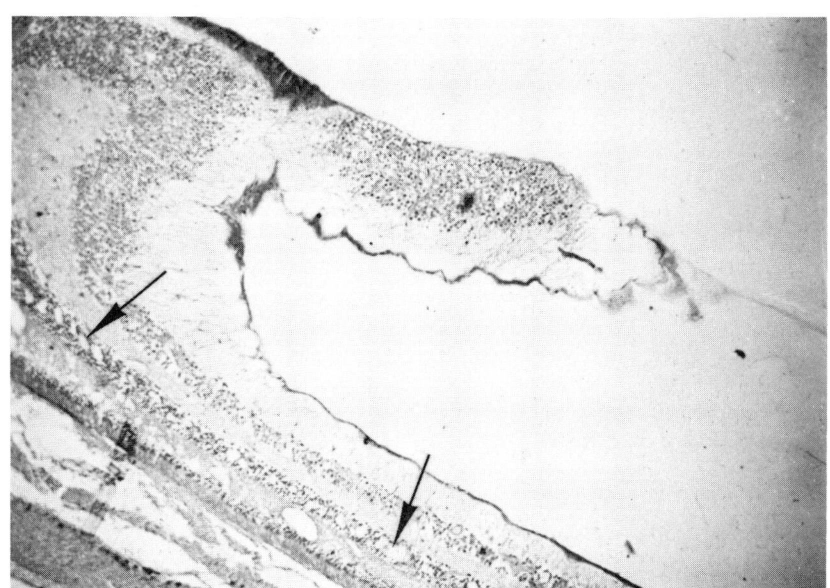

Figure 8–232. Cystoid macular edema (arrows) associated with vitreous traction. Masson, ×130. AFIP Acc. 121995. (From Reese AB, Jones IS, Cooper WC: Macular changes secondary to vitreous traction. Am J Ophthalmol *64*:(Suppl) 544–549, 1966.)

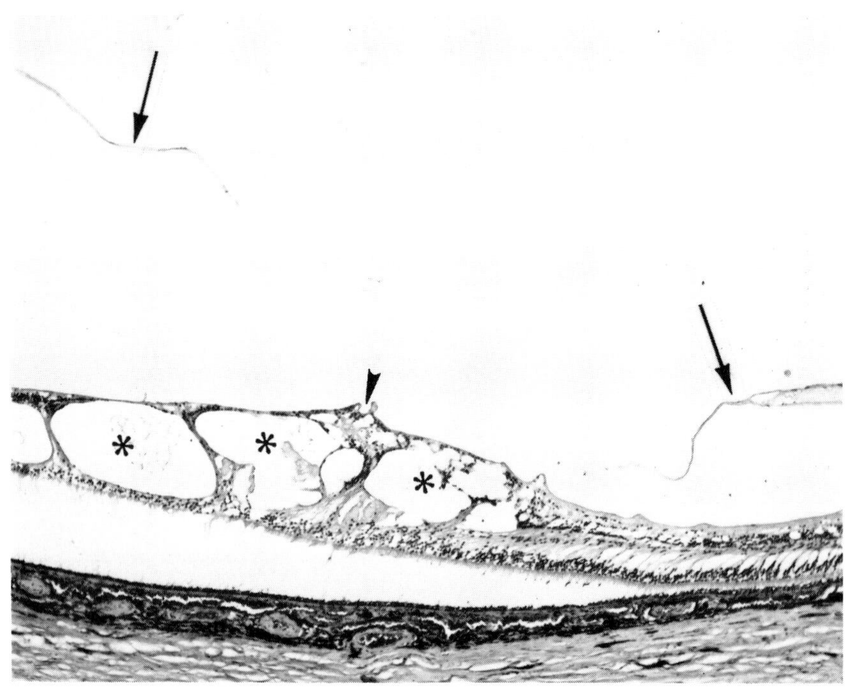

Figure 8–233. Traction-induced cystic degeneration in macular area (asterisks) with proliferative diabetic retinopathy. Strands of vitreous (arrows) are artifactitiously broken from their attachment to tented-up area of retina (arrowhead). H and E, ×45. EP 38109. (From Green WR: Pathology of the retina, *in* Frayer WC (ed): Lancaster Course in Ophthalmic Histopathology. Unit 9. Philadelphia, F.A. Davis, 1981.)

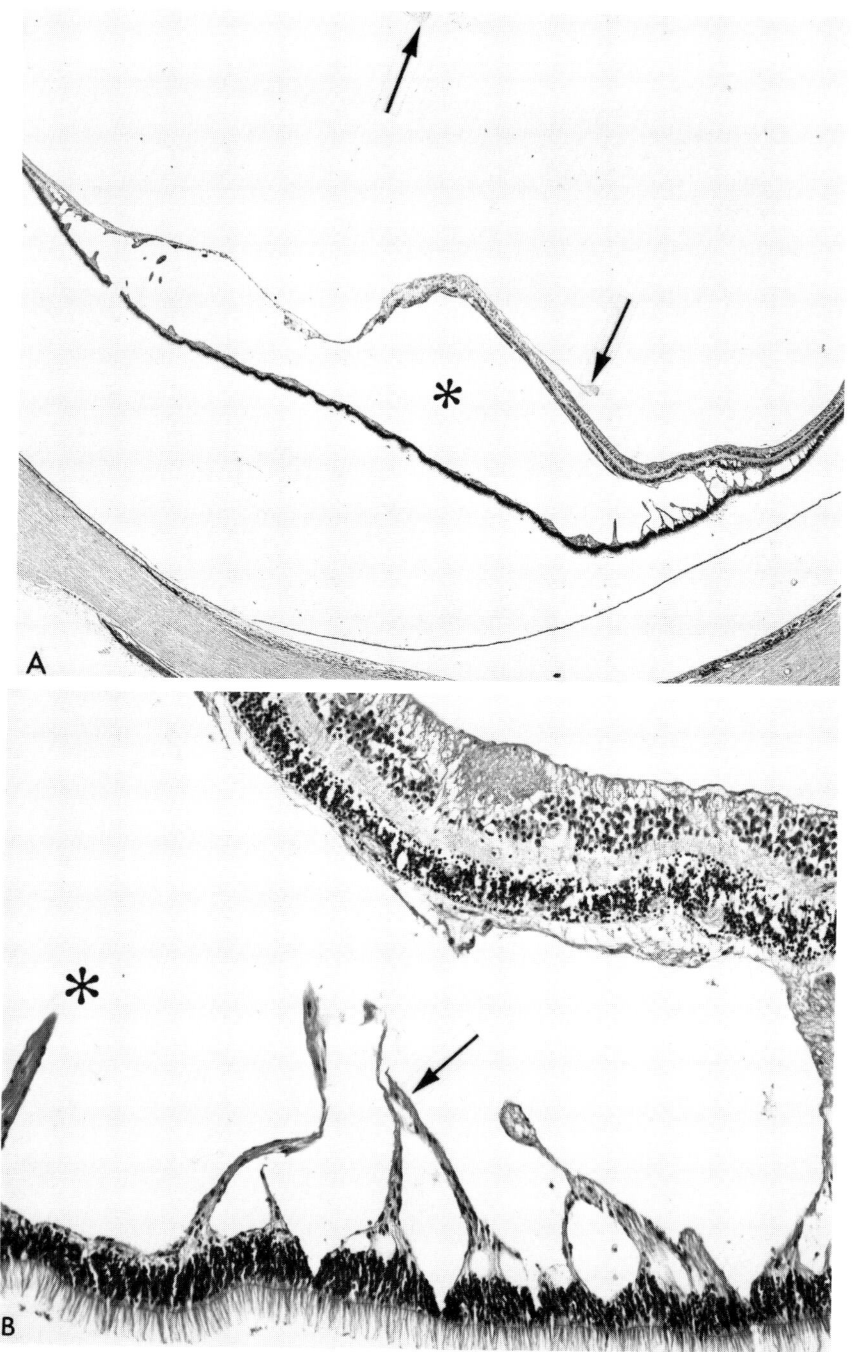

Figure 8–234. *A,* Extensive area of vitreous **traction-induced retinoschisis** (asterisk) in midperiphery, with extension into macular area. Dense strand of vitreous (arrows) is artifactitiously disrupted during processing. H and E, ×12. *B,* Higher power view of macular area, showing retinoschisis (asterisk). Some remaining interbridging strands of tissue (arrow) are present. H and E, ×100. EP 24284.

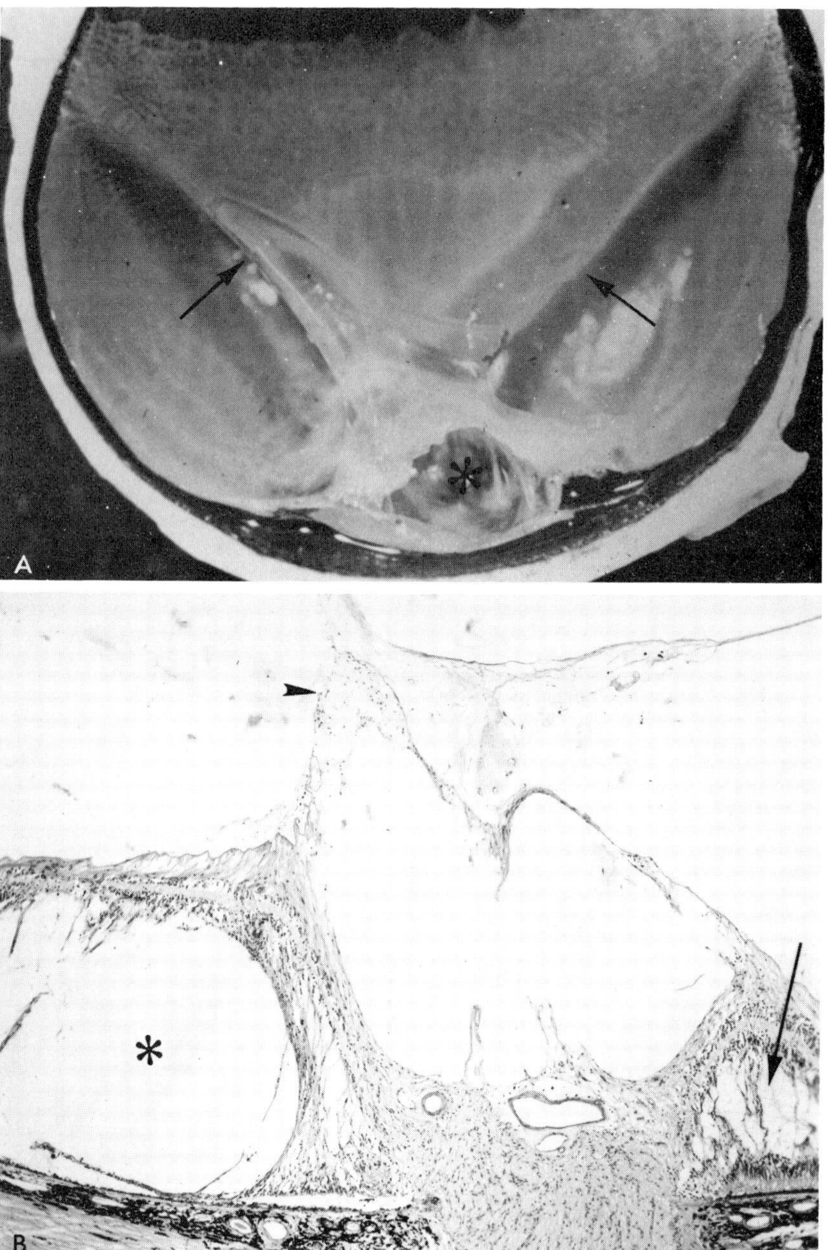

Figure 8–235. *A,* Gross appearance of **retinoschisis** (asterisk) **from vitreous traction** (arrows) in eye with proliferative diabetic retinopathy. *B,* Cystic degeneration (arrow) and retinoschisis (asterisk) of peripapillary retina from vitreous traction (arrowhead). PAS, ×30. EP 37625.

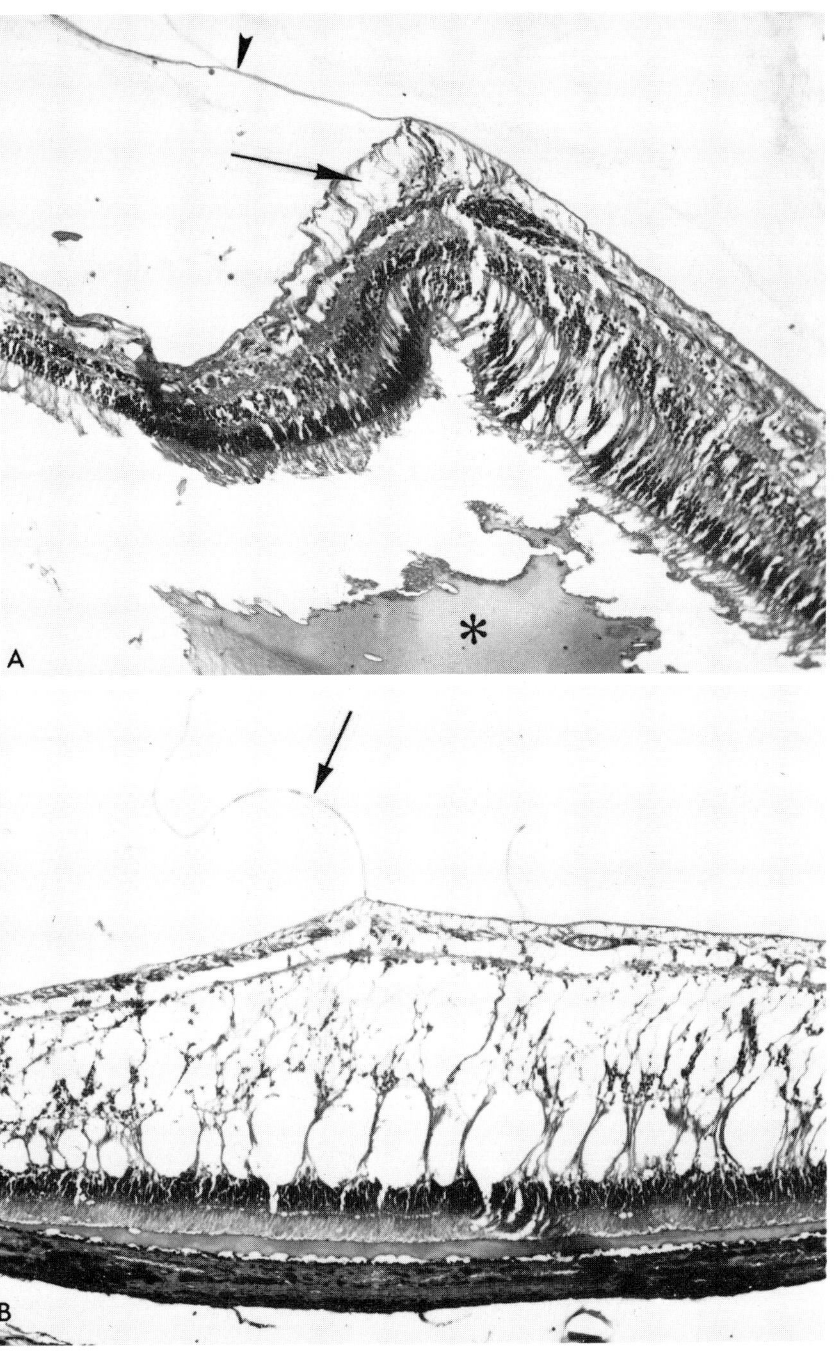

Figure 8–236. *A,* **Mild cystic change** (arrow) **and retinal detachment** (asterisk) **from vitreous traction** (arrowhead). H and E, ×100. *B,* More marked area of cystic degeneration associated with vitreous traction (arrow). H and E, ×75. (Courtesy of Dr. Harold Kirk; case presented at Ophthalmic Pathology Club, Washington, DC, April, 1965.)

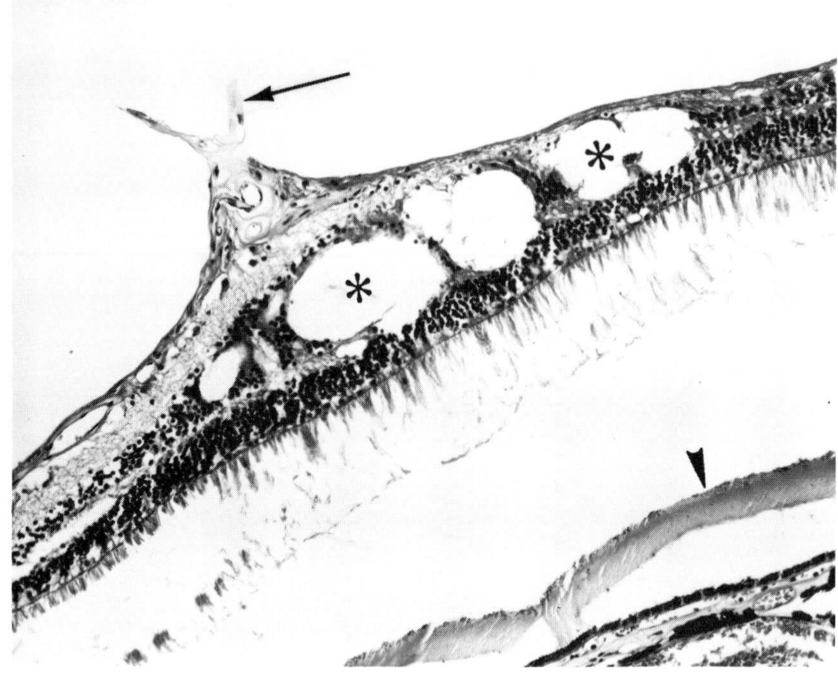

Figure 8–237. Cystic degeneration of retina (asterisks) **and flat serous retinal detachment** (arrowhead) **from vitreous traction** (arrow) in eye with proliferative sickle cell retinopathy. H and E, × 120. EP 30356.

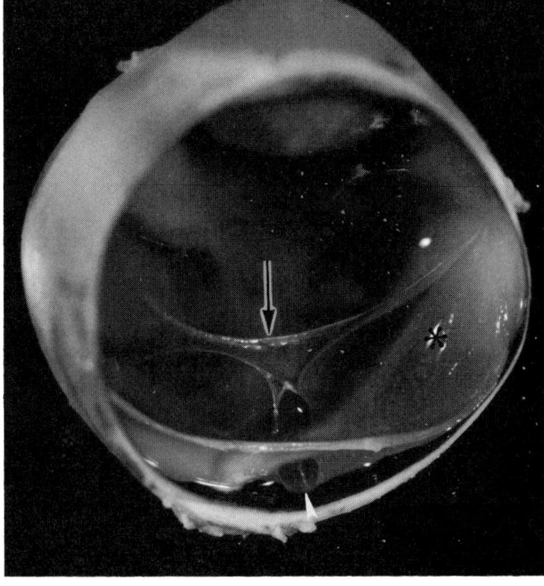

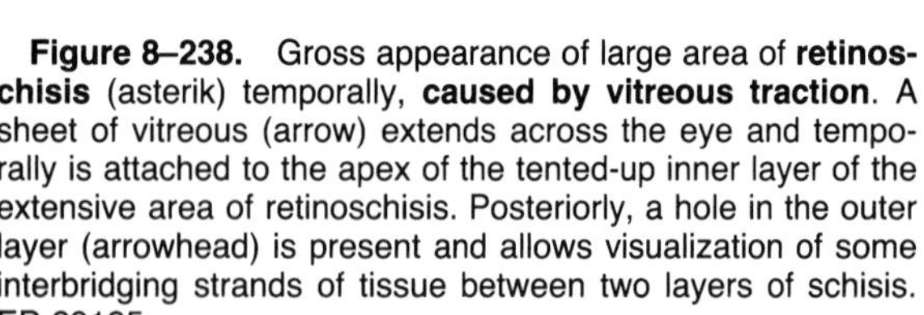

Figure 8–238. Gross appearance of large area of **retinoschisis** (asterik) temporally, **caused by vitreous traction**. A sheet of vitreous (arrow) extends across the eye and temporally is attached to the apex of the tented-up inner layer of the extensive area of retinoschisis. Posteriorly, a hole in the outer layer (arrowhead) is present and allows visualization of some interbridging strands of tissue between two layers of schisis. EP 29185.

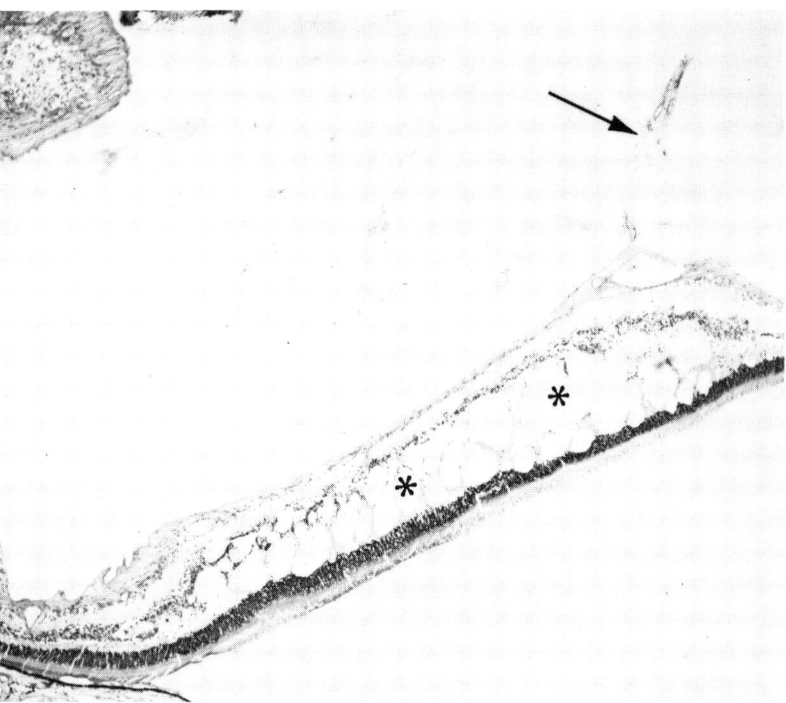

Figure 8–239. Traction-induced cystic degeneration (asterisks) in macular area in proliferative diabetic retinopathy. A fibrovascular membrane (arrow) is attached to tented-up retina. PAS, ×35. EP 39400.

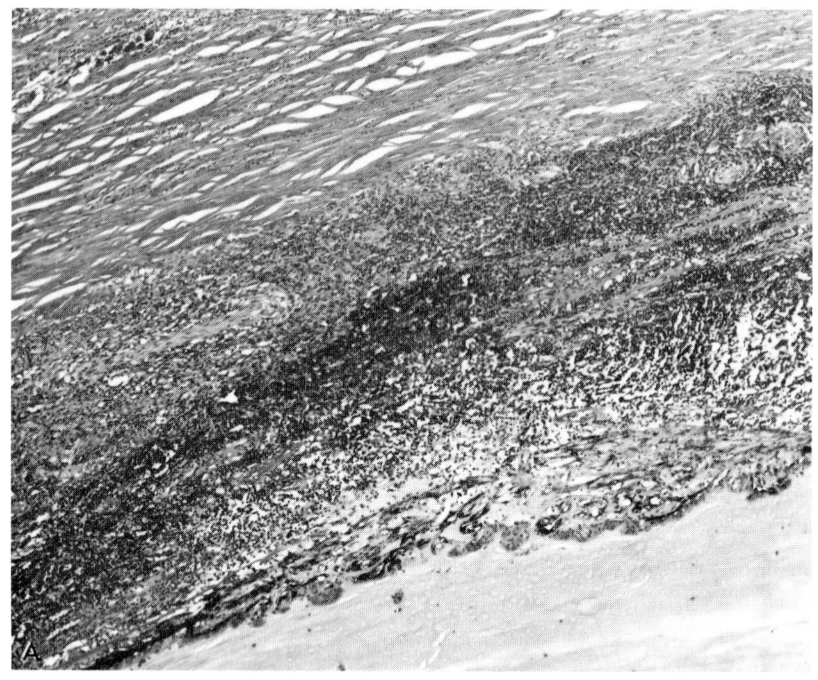

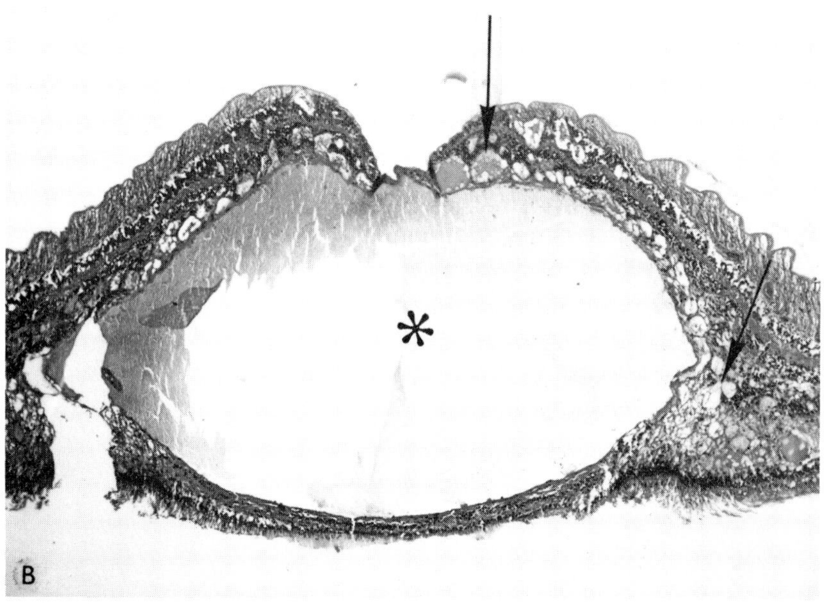

Figure 8–240. Chronic iridocyclitis with secondary cystic degeneration and retinoschisis involving the macula. *A,* Dense lymphocytic and plasmacytic infiltration is present in the ciliary body. Adjacent vitreous has proteinaceous material with a few inflammatory cells present. H and E, ×55. *B,* Cystic edema (arrows) and a large area of retinoschisis or a macrocyst (asterisk) are present in the macula. H and E, ×40. EP 43852.

of retinoschisis occurring in association with Coats' disease are illustrated in Figures 8–40 and 8–41 (see page 629).

Cystic Degeneration in the Macula. This may be observed in association with branch and central retinal vein occlusion (see Fig. 8–102). Figure 8–242 illustrates extensive cystic degeneration in the macular area associated with a central retinal artery occlusion.

Choroidal Lesions. Choroidal lesions, such as melanoma and hemangioma, may lead to cystic degeneration and retinoschisis of the overlying retina. Note the discrete cystic degeneration of the retina overlying the small choroidal malignant melanoma in Figure 8–243. The late retinal staining of cystoid spaces with fluorescein is usually seen with choroidal hemangiomas.

Trauma. Edema in the macular area after trauma may lead to cystic degeneration, retinoschisis, and hole formation. Cystic degeneration and, rarely, retinoschisis may occur elsewhere in the retina after blunt ocular trauma (Fig. 8–244).

Retinal Hemorrhage. Retinal hemorrhage, especially when located just beneath the ILM, may leave a schisis cavity as the hemorrhage absorbs. In sickle cell retinopathy, such hemorrhages lead to a characteristic lesion called an iridescent spot (see Figs. 8–80 and 8–81) (Romayananda, Gold-

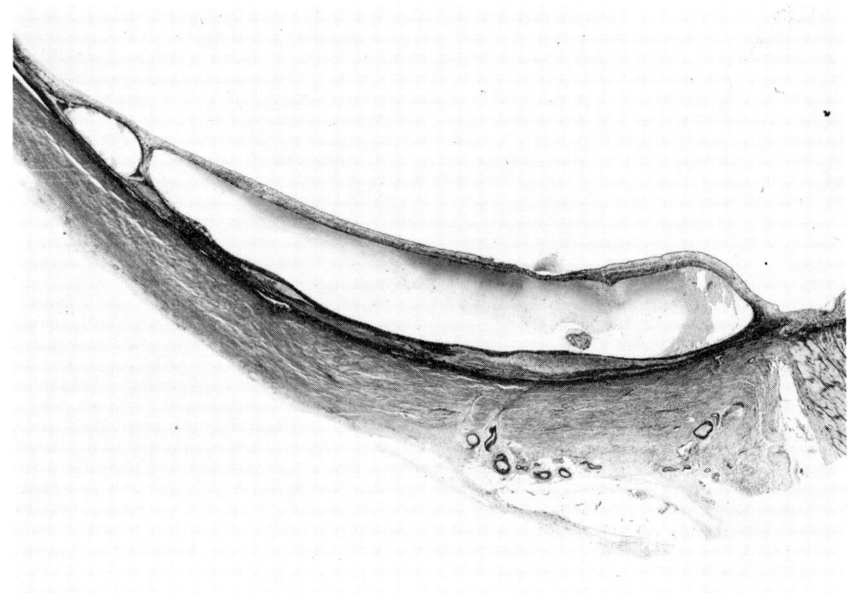

Figure 8–241. Extensive retinoschisis in posterior pole in eye with chronic uveitis. H and E, × 11. AFIP Neg. 65-4379.

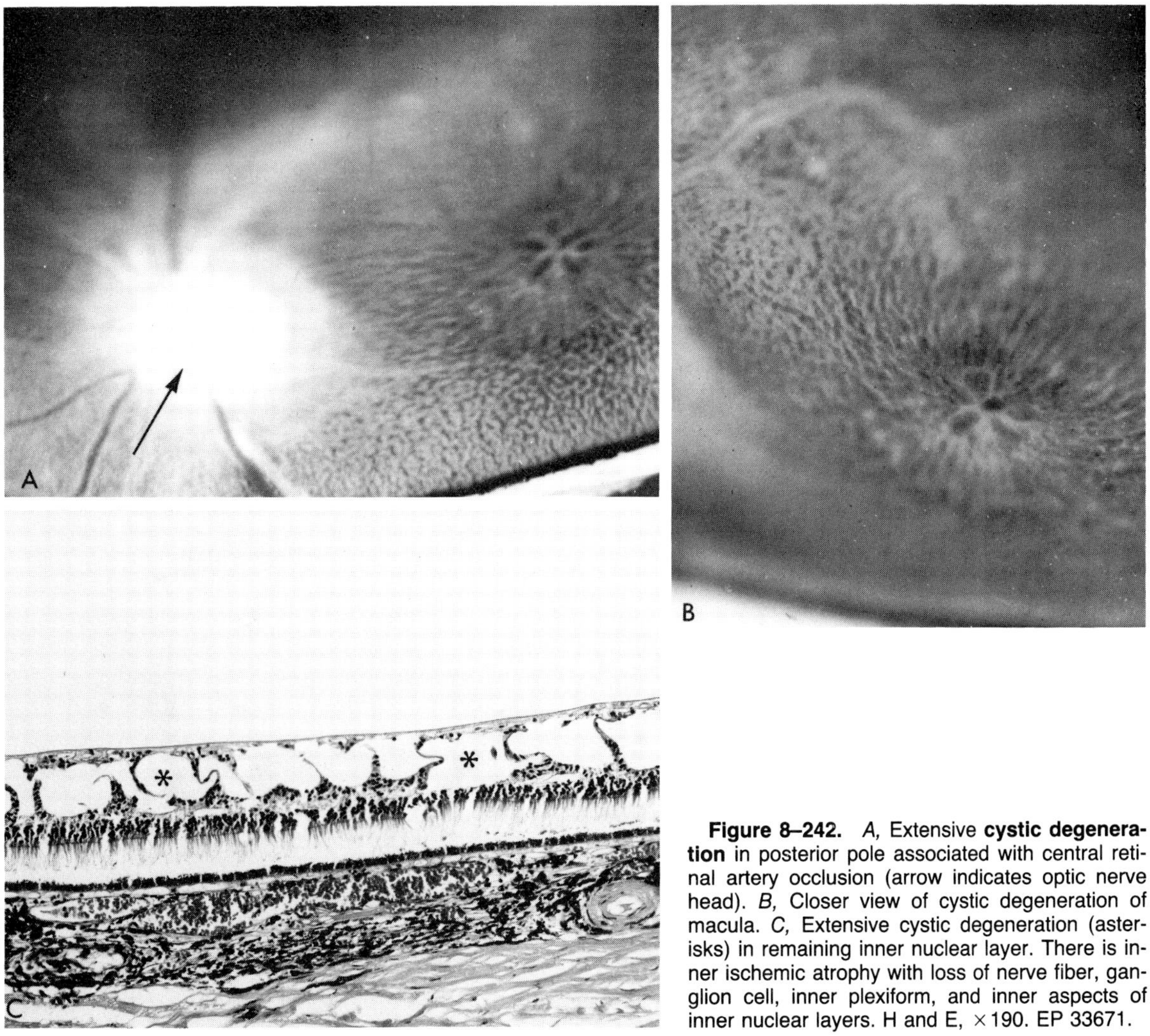

Figure 8–242. *A,* Extensive **cystic degeneration** in posterior pole associated with central retinal artery occlusion (arrow indicates optic nerve head). *B,* Closer view of cystic degeneration of macula. *C,* Extensive cystic degeneration (asterisks) in remaining inner nuclear layer. There is inner ischemic atrophy with loss of nerve fiber, ganglion cell, inner plexiform, and inner aspects of inner nuclear layers. H and E, ×190. EP 33671.

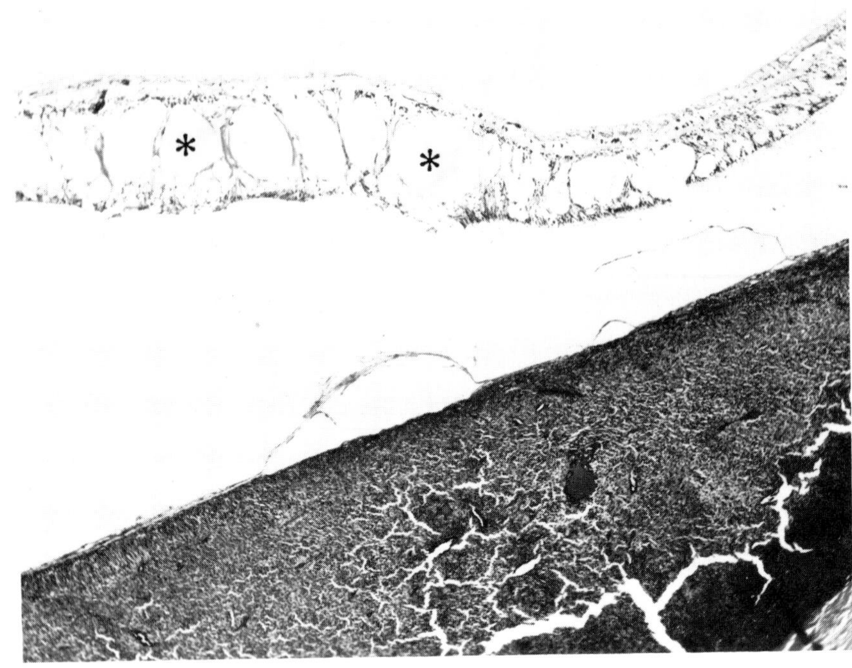

Figure 8–243. Cystic degeneration of retina (asterisks) overlying a choroidal melanoma. H and E, ×30. EP 31371.

berg, Green, 1973). Clinically, an iridescent spot appears as an oval or round, discrete lesion with a yellowish-orange refractile appearance; spots also may be observed in diabetic retinopathy, leukemia, and other conditions. Histopathologically, there is a flat schisis of the retina beneath the ILM. Hemosiderin staining of the surrounding tissue and hemosiderin-laden macrophages indicate a resolving hemorrhage and give the lesion its yellowish-orange and refractile appearance.

Figure 8–210 shows the appearance of the eye of a 9 month old boy with what was considered to be a retinal detachment with possible tumor, detected shortly after birth. There is an extensive retinoschisis with much hemosiderin deposition that was interpreted as being the result of massive retinal hemorrhage occurring at birth, leading to the clinical picture of retinal detachment.

Pars Plana Cysts. These cysts (Fig. 8–245) are observed in up to 16 per cent of all persons and,

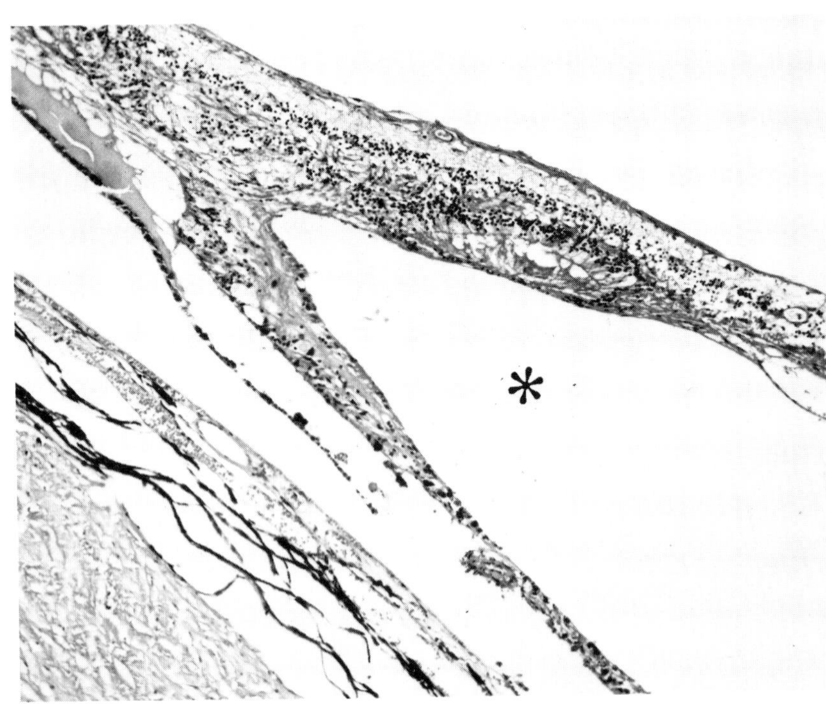

Figure 8–244. Retinoschisis (asterisk) in midperiphery in eye with severe blunt trauma. H and E, × 100. EP 31868.

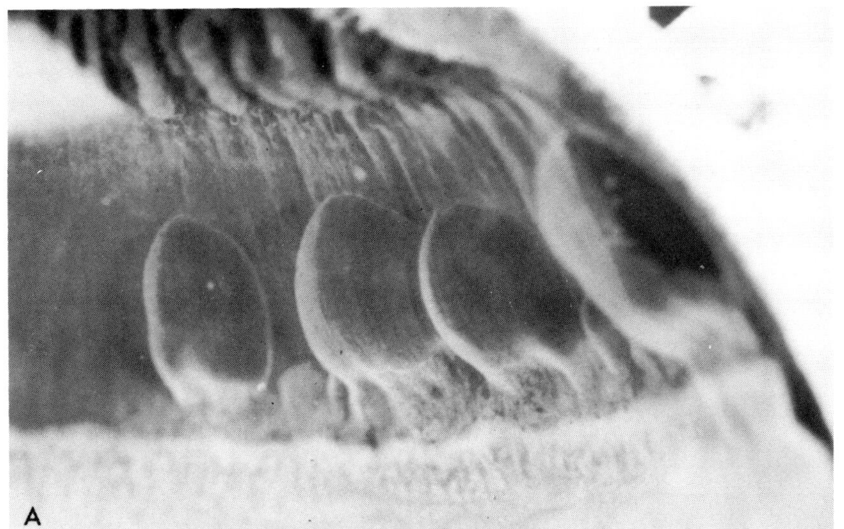

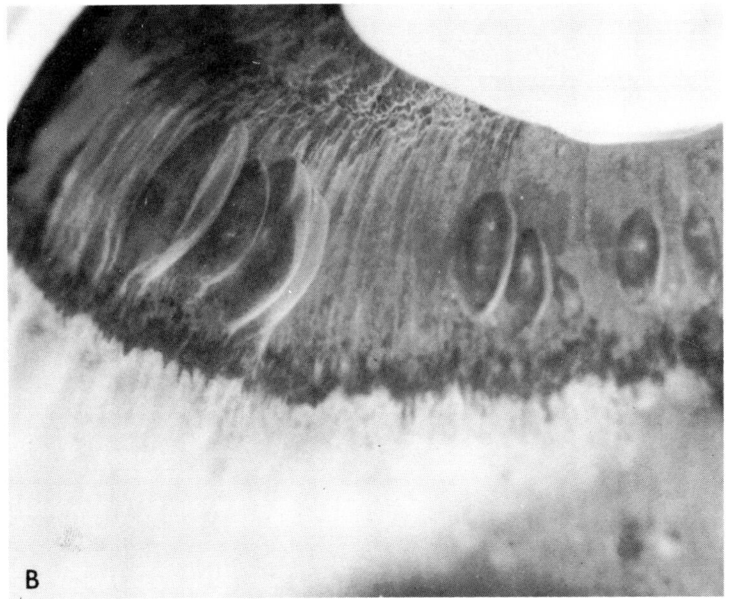

Figure 8–245. Gross appearance of large **pars plana cysts.** *A,* EP 31671. *B,* EP 44840. (*A* from Green WR: Pathology of the retina, *in* Frayer WC (ed): Lancaster Course in Ophthalmic Histopathology. Unit 9. Philadelphia, F.A. Davis, 1981.)

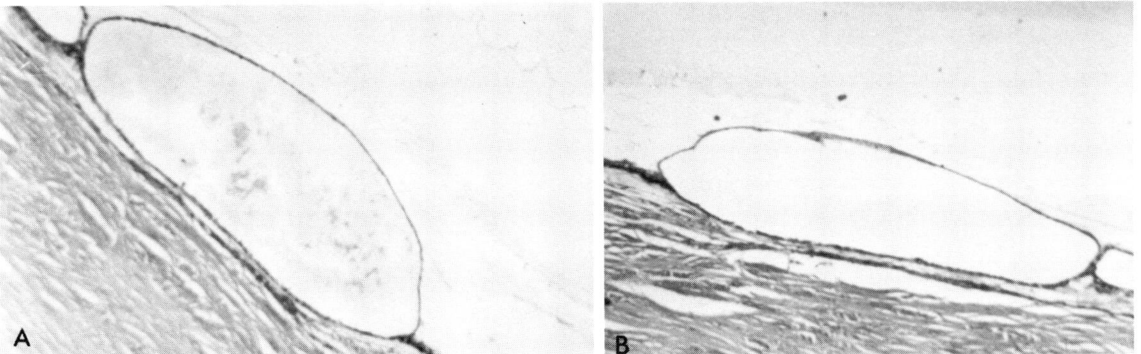

Figure 8–246. Histochemical test to show **pars plana cyst** containing hyaluronic acid. Both *A* and *B* are stained with Alcian blue for acid mucopolysaccharide. Specimen *B* was pretreated with enzyme hyaluronidase and shows no staining reaction in the cyst. *A* and *B,* Alcian blue, ×100. EP 31671. (From Green WR: Pathlogy of the retina, *in* Frayer WC (ed): Lancaster Course in Ophthalmic Histopathology. Unit 9. Philadelphia, F.A. Davis, 1981.)

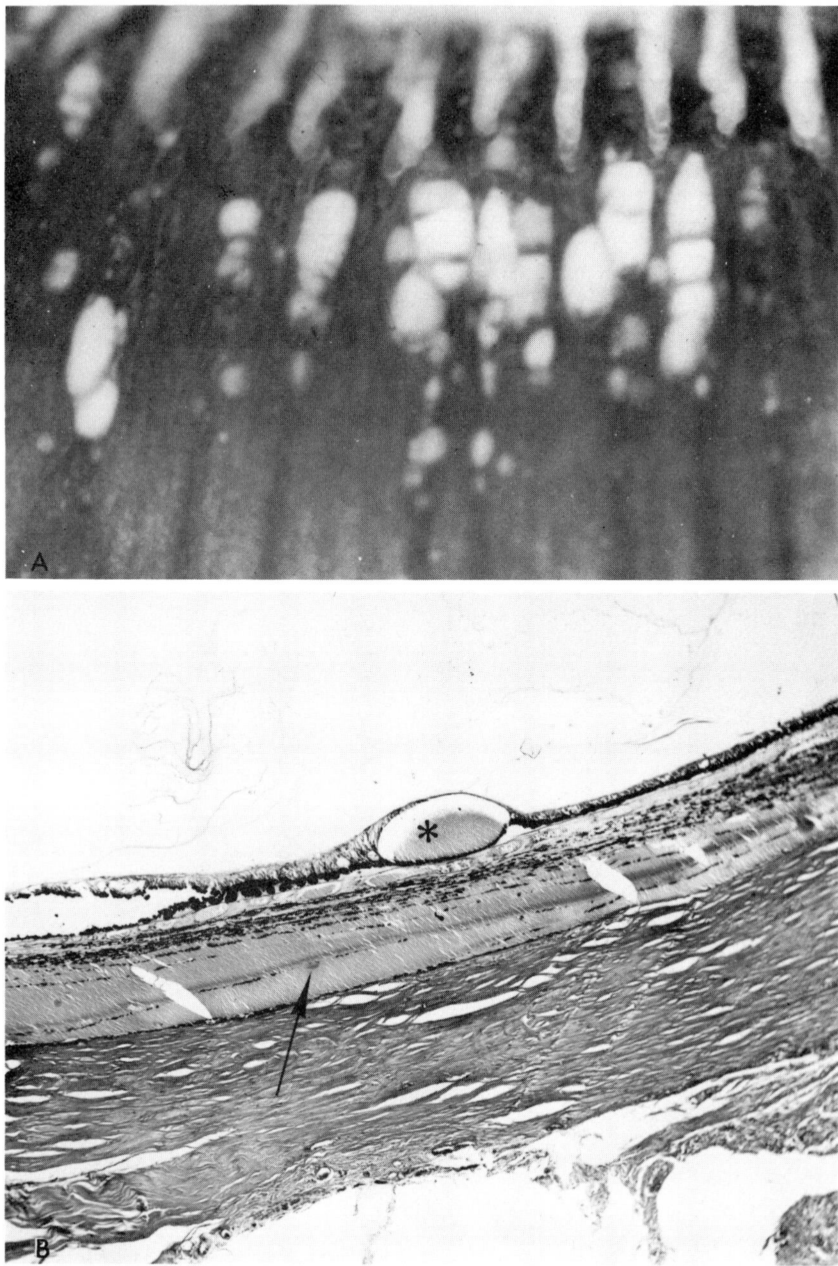

Figure 8–247. *A,* Gross appearance of opaque **pars plana cyst** in eye of a patient with hyperproteinemia. *B,* Cysts contain a dense proteinaceous material (asterisk). Ciliochoroidal effusion (arrow) with similar material is present. H and E, ×40. EP 30763. (From Green WR: Pathology of the retina, *in* Frayer WC (ed): Lancaster Course in Ophthalmic Histopathology. Unit 9. Philadelphia, F.A. Davis, 1981.)

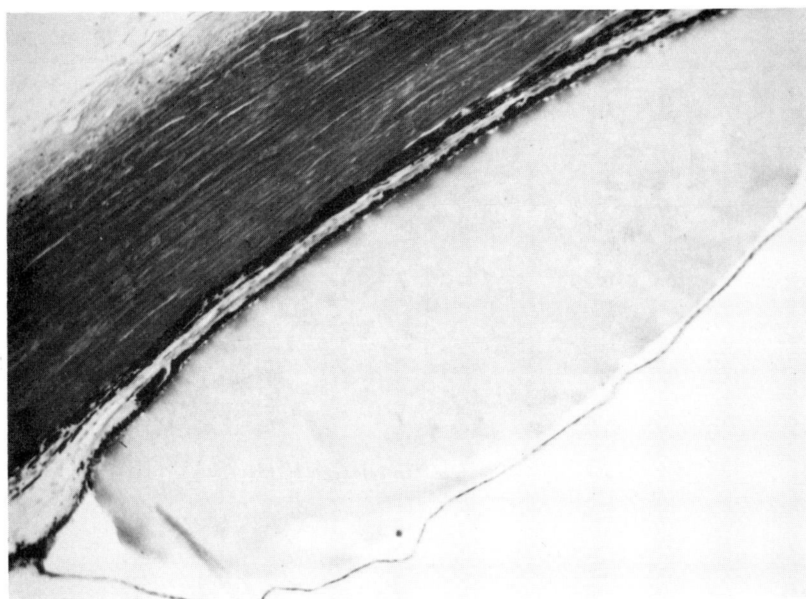

Figure 8–248. Large, opaque **pars plana cyst** in eye of a patient who had multiple myeloma. H and E, ×140.

according to Okun (1961b), increase with age—affecting about 24 per cent of persons over the age of 40 years and 34 per cent of those over the age of 70 years. The cysts contain hyaluronic acid (Fig. 8–246), as in typical peripheral cystoid degeneration of the retina. Pars plana cysts are of no pathologic importance except that in hyperproteinemic states they may be more common and more numerous and may contain proteinaceous material (Figs. 8–247 and 8–248) (Johnson, Storey, 1970). With fixation, these cysts appear opaque. A ciliochoroidal effusion with similar material also may be present (Fig. 8–247). Gärtner (1972) has shown that gaps are present in the epithelium of pars plana cysts, through which capillary-like vessels from the ciliary body extend into the cyst.

Occasionally, pars plana cysts may have a dense base (Snell's plaque) as a result of proliferation of the ciliary epithelium, vascularization from subjacent ciliary body, and collagen production (Fig. 8–249).

Clinically evident giant cysts of the pars plana also have been observed (Ruiz, 1971).

Retinal Pigment Epithelial Hypertrophy

This is an aging and degenerative change that commonly occurs in the periphery and in association with numerous disease and degenerative processes. In this condition the RPE cells may be somewhat thicker than normal, but the distinguishing histologic feature is the appearance of the melanin pigment granules that become large and spherical. Normally, RPE melanin granules are small and oval or lancet-shaped. This change in the melanin pigment granules gives the hypertrophic RPE a much darker brown or even blackish appearance. Hypertrophy of the RPE may occur as a localized lesion (Fig. 8–250), as a diffuse, bandlike change just posterior to the ora serrata (Figs. 8–251 through 8–254), and in the equatorial area (Figs. 8–255 and 8–256), and often forms a dark crescent in the peripapillary area (Fig. 8–257). Hypertrophy of the RPE may be seen following trauma (Fig. 8–258).

The hypertrophy we have discussed here is an aging process and is to be contrasted with grouped pigmentation or "bear tracks," which are congenital. Solitary lesions of RPE hypertrophy are possibly congenital and have the following typical features: flat, densely pigmented, central lacunae of depigmentation, and a halo zone with relatively less or absent pigmentation. Solitary hypertrophy of the RPE is discussed in more detail elsewhere (see page 1227).

Retinal Pigment Epithelial Hyperplasia

The RPE is one of the most reactive tissues in the eye. It reacts by undergoing atrophy, hypertrophy, hyperplasia, migration, and metaplasia. It is rarely involved in neoplasia (see page 1244). One of the most important clinical signs of hyperplasia is migration into the retina in a perivascular location, giving the lesion a spiculate appearance. Hyperplasia of the RPE may occur as a localized, multifocal, or diffuse change (also see page 1231).

Multifocal. This is a relatively common change observed in older persons.

Ora Serrata. In some instances, this spiculate-appearing hyperplastic pigment epithelium may extend anteriorly onto the pars plana or posteriorly onto the retina, denoting the variation of the vitreous base attachment (Figs. 8–259 and

Text continued on page 848

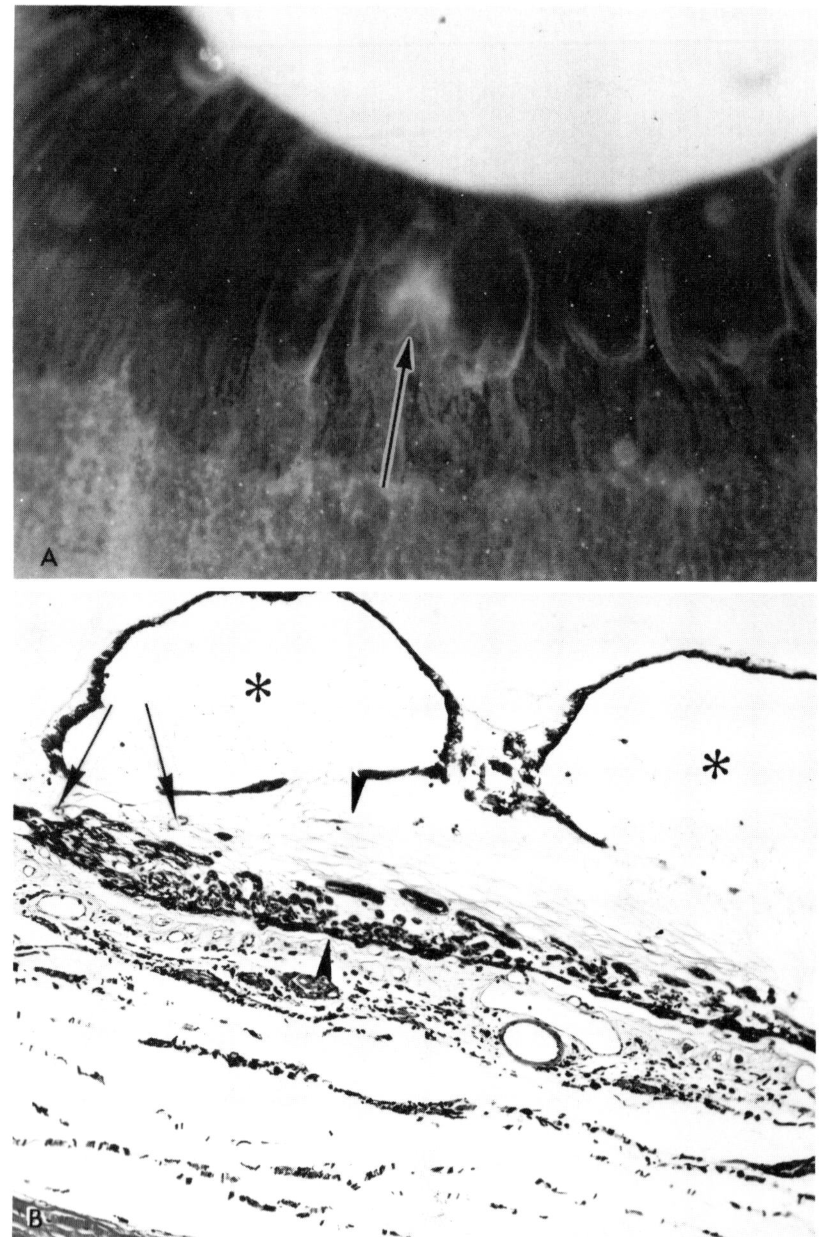

Figure 8–249. *A*, Gross appearance of **pars plana cysts**—one with a Snell's plaque (arrow). *B*, Section through Snell's plaque shows pars plana cysts (asterisks), an area of collagen and ciliary epithelial hyperplasia (between arrowheads), and blood vessels (arrows) from vessel tract. H and E, ×100. EP 49727.

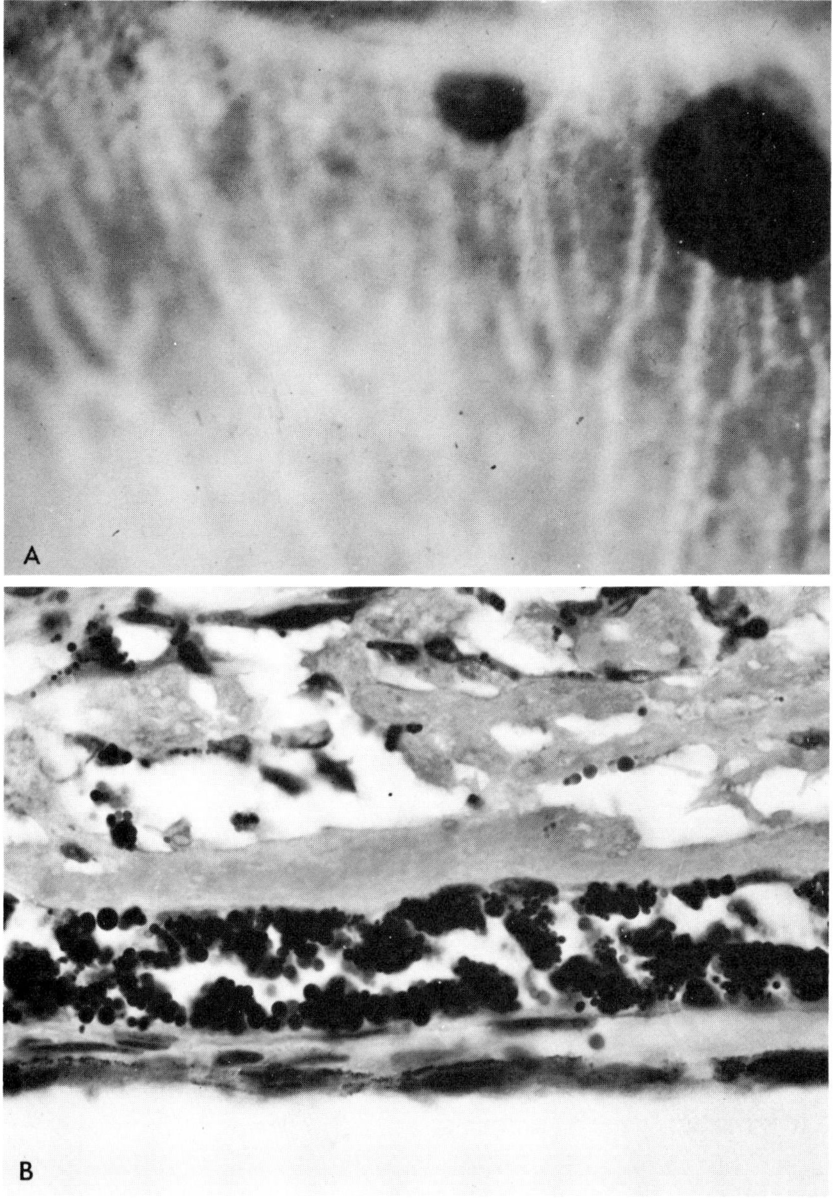

Figure 8–250. *A,* Gross appearance of two focal areas of **retinal pigment epithelium (RPE) hypertrophy**. *B,* Section of one of these lesions shows larger than usual RPE cells that contain large spherical granules. H and E, ×900. EP 30966. (From Green WR: Pathology of the retina, *in* Frayer WC (ed): Lancaster Course in Ophthalmic Histopathology. Unit 9. Philadelphia, F.A. Davis, 1981.)

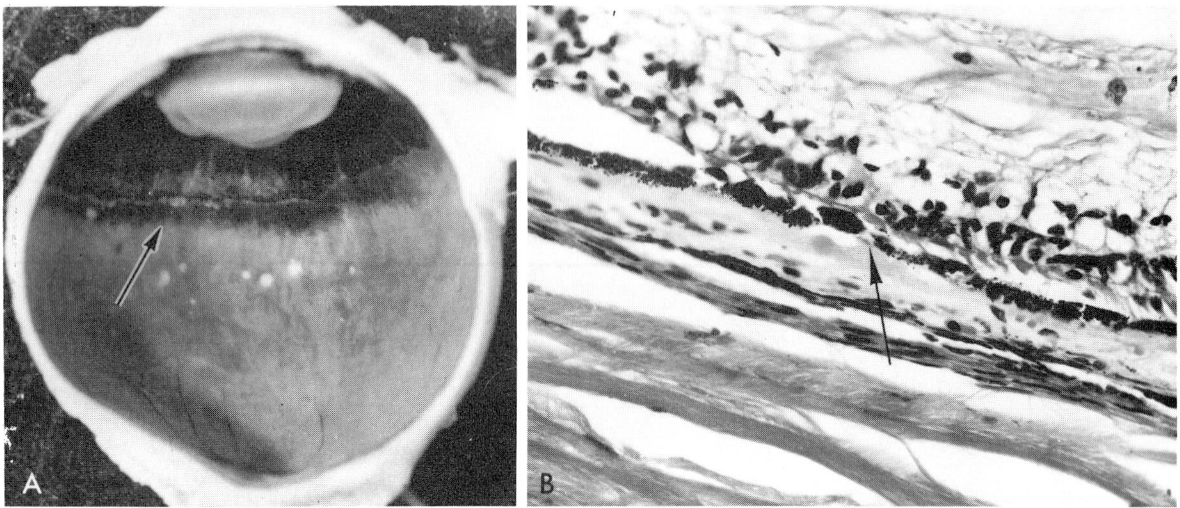

Figure 8–251. *A,* Gross appearance of peripheral **retinal pigment epithelium (RPE) hypertrophy** (arrow). *B,* Hypertrophic RPE has large, spherical granules (left of arrow). H and E, ×400. EP 33867. (From Green WR: Pathology of the retina, *in* Frayer WC (ed): Lancaster Course in Ophthalmic Histopathology. Unit 9. Philadelphia, F.A. Davis, 1981.)

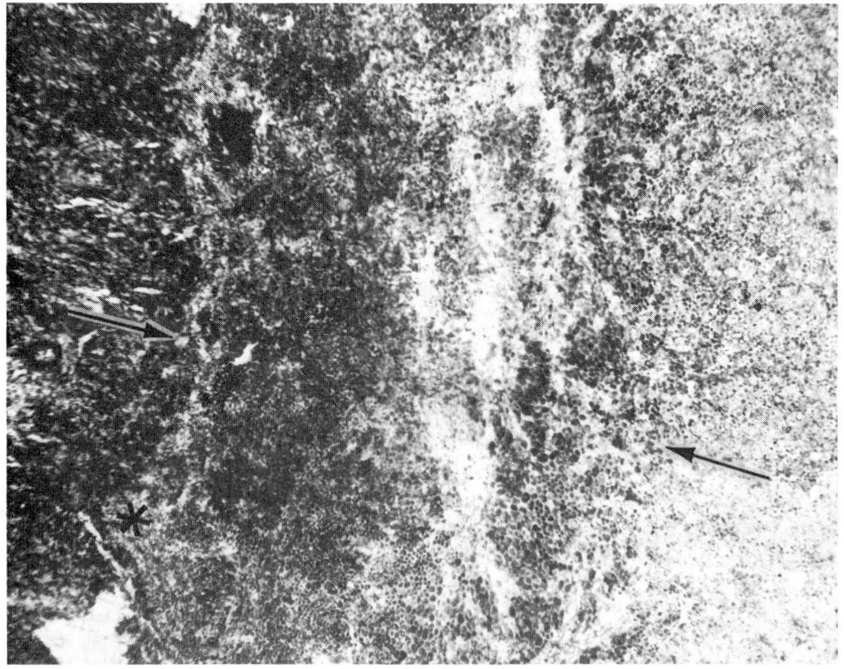

Figure 8–252. Flat preparation of **peripheral retinal pigment epithelium (RPE) (hypertrophy** (between arrows). Asterisk marks junction between ciliary epithelium and RPE. Unstained, ×30. EP 466601.

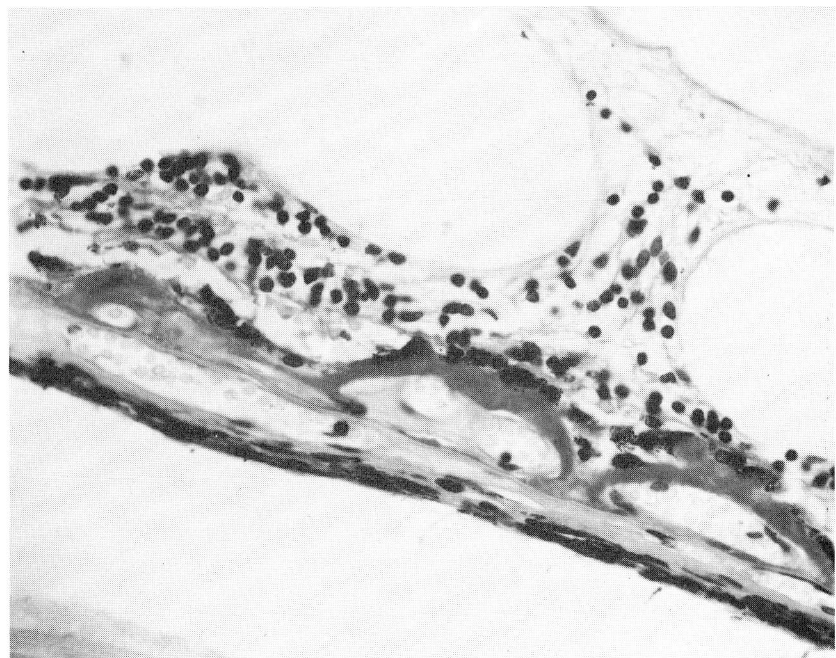

Figure 8–253. Peripheral retinal pigment epithelium (RPE) hypertrophy associated with sub-RPE (intra-Bruch's membrane) neovascularization. PAS, ×525. EP 31313.

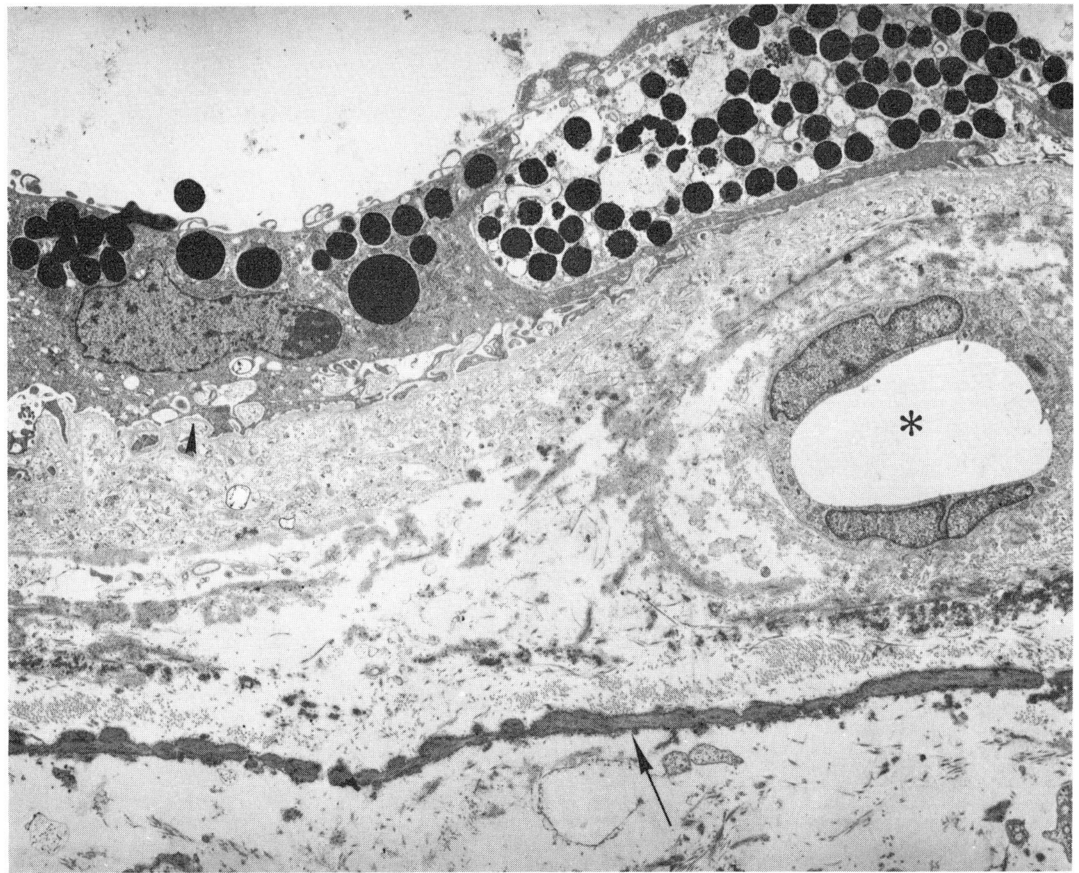

Figure 8–254. Electron micrograph showing **hypertrophic retinal pigment epithelium (RPE)** with large spherical pigment granules associated with vascularization (asterisk), located between basement membrane of RPE (arrowhead) and remainder of Bruch's membrane (arrow). EP 48154.

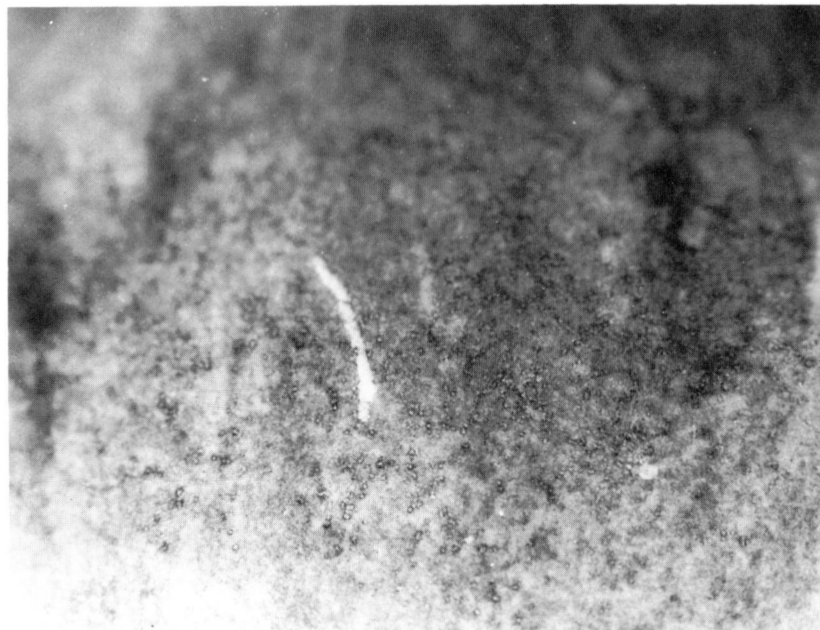

Figure 8–255. Drusen with surrounding area of hypertrophic retinal pigment epithelium in equatorial area. H and E, ×35. AFIP Neg. 69–2894.

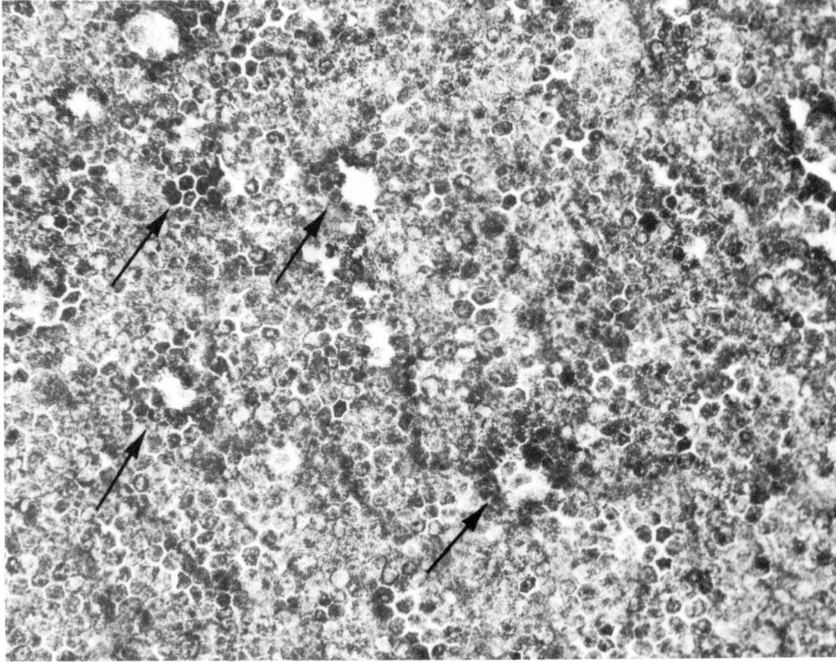

Figure 8–256. Flat preparation of retinal pigment epithelium (RPE) from equatorial area showing **drusen** with surrounding area of hypertrophic RPE (arrows). H and E, ×145.

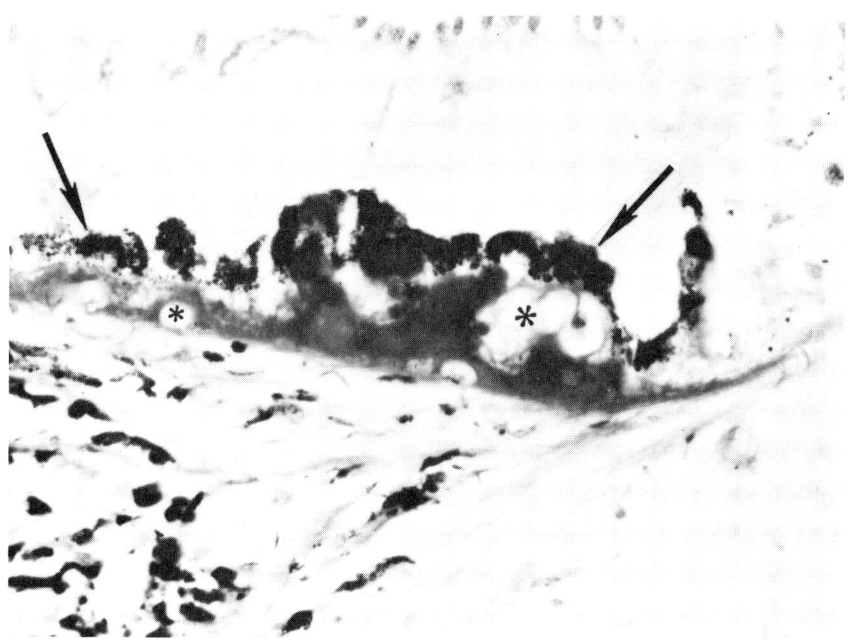

Figure 8–257. Peripapillary retinal pigment epithelium, associated with vascularized (asterisks) drusen. H and E, ×250. EP 37369.

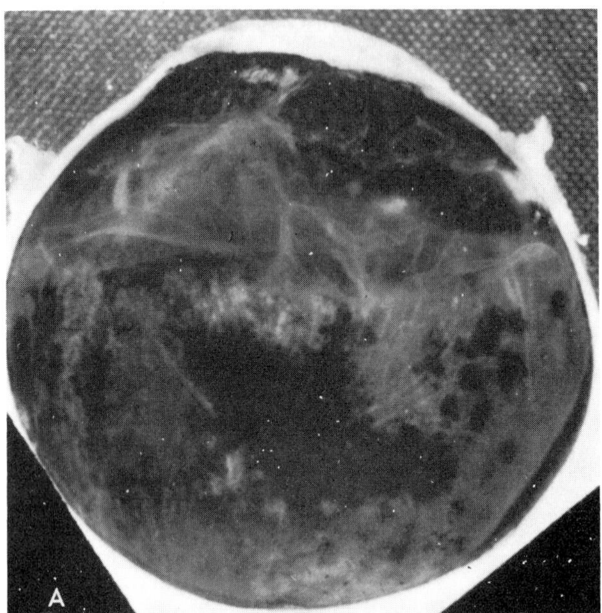

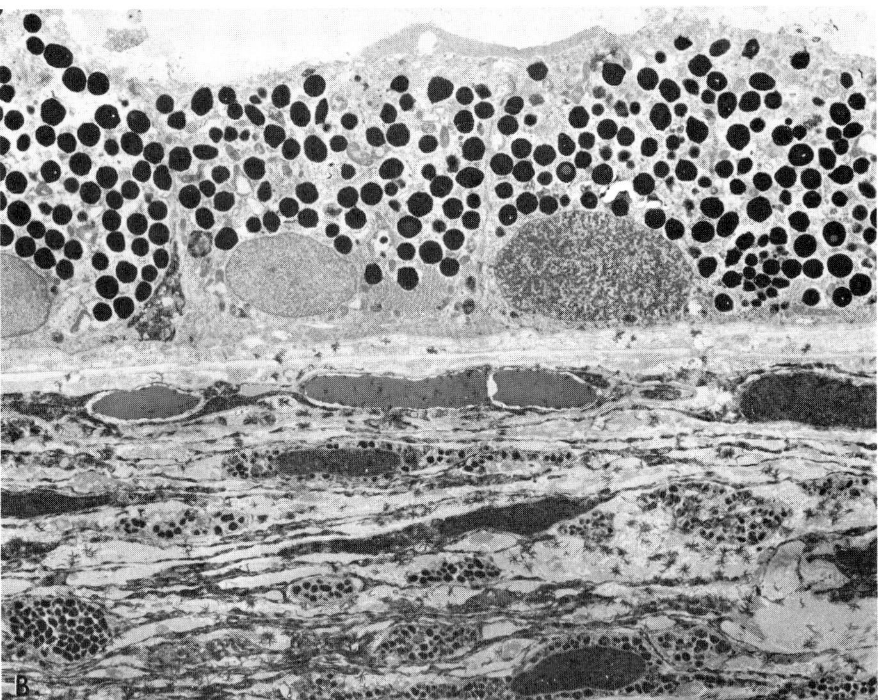

Figure 8–258. *A*, Acquired **hypertrophy of retinal pigment epithelium (RPE)** in an eye after blunt trauma. On one side of the eye there was choroidal rupture; this side shows numerous areas where the RPE has a black appearance. *B*, Electron micrograph shows choroid, choriocapillaris, Bruch's membrane, and RPE to be intact. RPE cells are enlarged, with cytoplasm distended by large spherical pigment granules. ×4000. EP 42434.

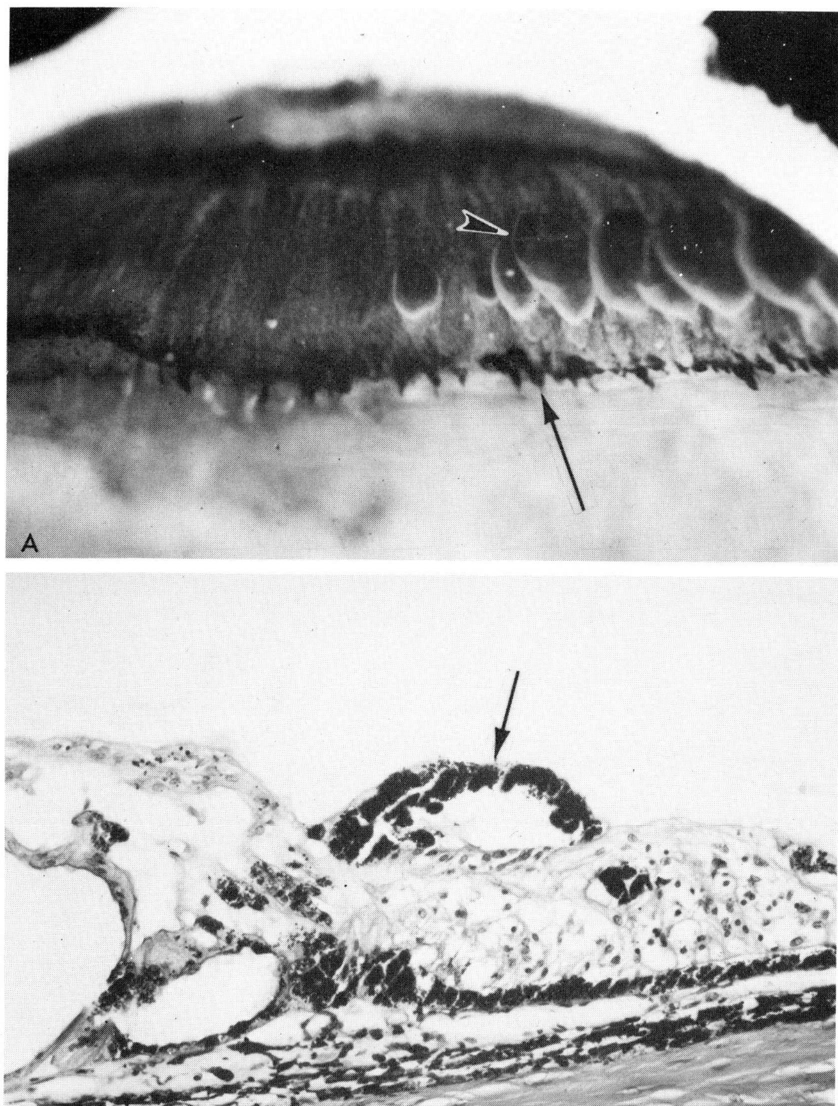

Figure 8–259. Hyperplasia of pigment epithelium at ora serrata. *A*, Hyperplastic epithelium has a spiculate appearance and is located at ora serrata (arrow). Arrowhead indicates pars plana cysts. *B*, Appearance of hyperplastic pigment epithelium (arrow) as it extends into the vitreous cavity at the ora serrata. PAS, ×220. DP 31929. (From Green WR: Pathology of the retina, *in* Frayer WC (ed): Lancaster Course in Ophthalmic Histopathology. Unit 9. Philadelphia, F.A. Davis, 1981.)

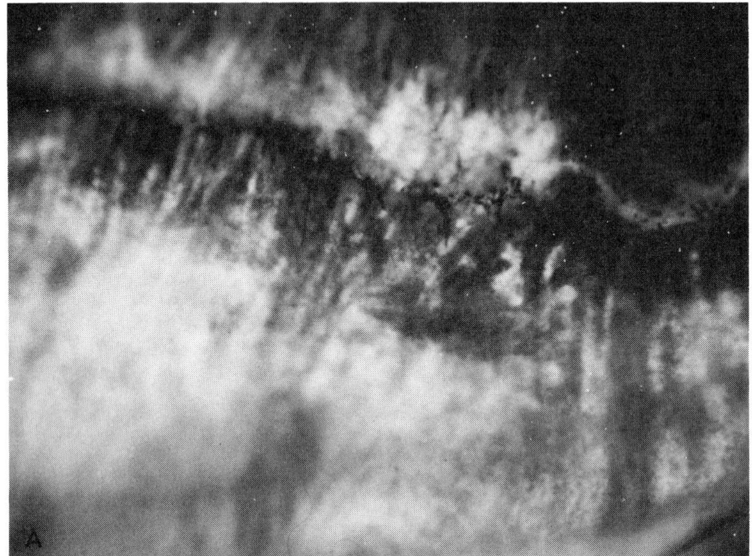

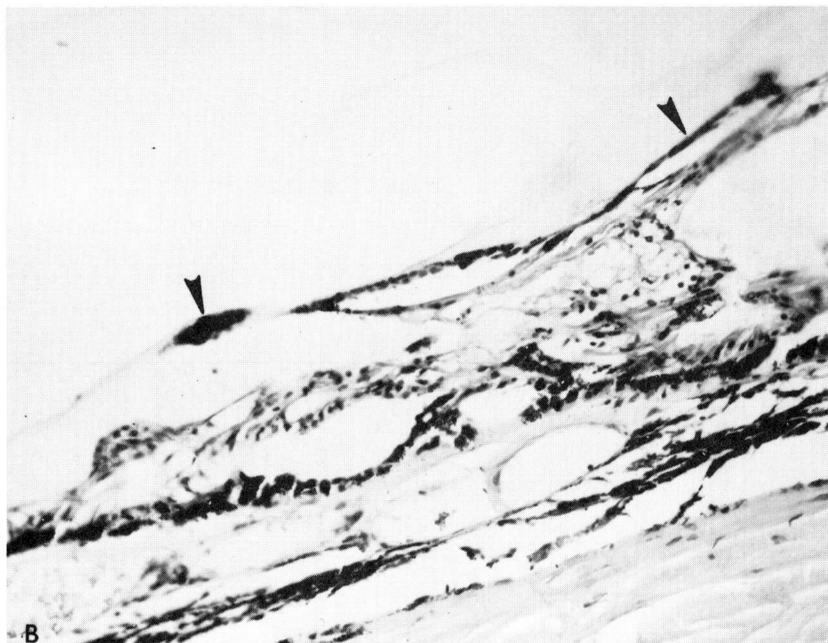

Figure 8–260. *A*, Gross appearance of **hyperplastic pigment epithelium** at ora serrata. *B*, Hyperplastic pigment epithelium (arrowheads) in vitreous base at ora serrata. H and E, ×220. EP 31468.

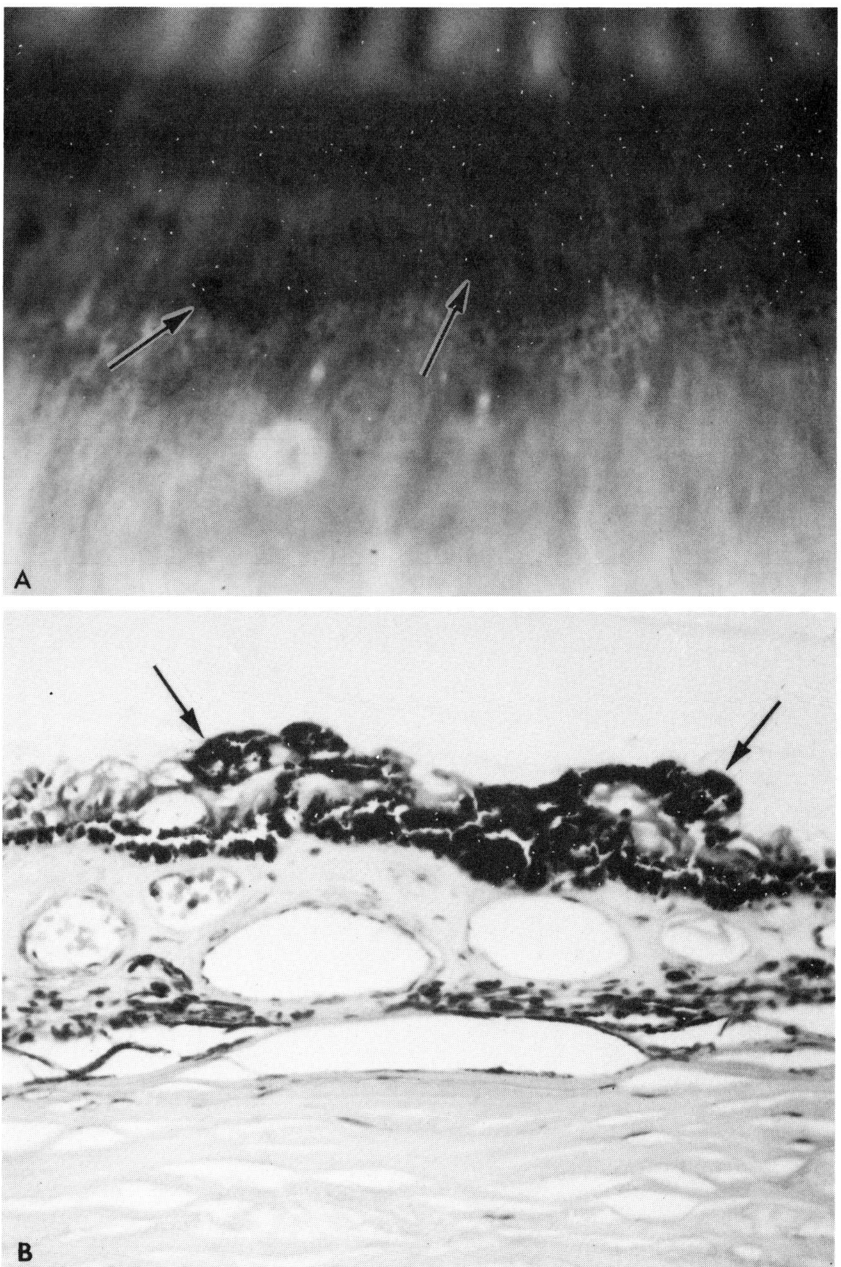

Figure 8–261. Nodular hyperplasia of pigment epithelium in pars plana. *A,* Gross appearance of nodules (arrows). *B,* Hyperplastic pigment epithelium (arrows) is present at inner surface of pars plana. H and E, ×250. EP 30655.

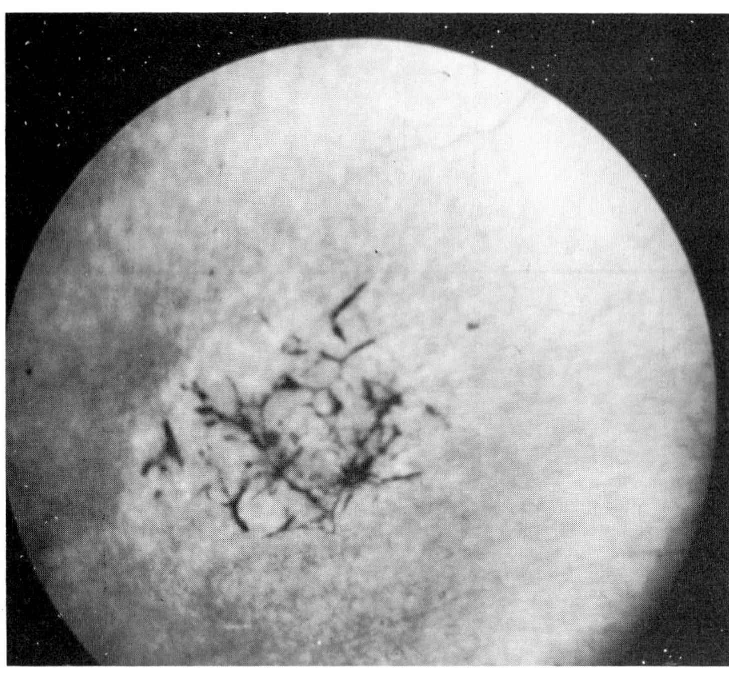

Figure 8–262. The "black sunburst" sign of sickle cell retinopathy is characterized by a round area with hyperplasia of the retinal pigment epithelium, with migration into the retina in a perivascular location, giving the lesion a spiculate appearance.

8–260). These findings suggest that chronic vitreous base traction may be responsible for this change seen in many adult eyes.

Pars Plana. These discrete nodules of proliferated pigmented epithelium (Fig. 8–261) and those seen at the ora serrata may be related to chronic vitreous base and zonular traction.

Localized. Some of these lesions may be caused by old healed choroiditis and others by subretinal hemorrhage (Fig. 8–262), but most are nonspecific and unassociated with any known cause. The important features are the dark appearance and the presence of pigment in the retina in association with retinal vessels. In some instances the hyperplastic epithelium may remain under the retina (Figs. 8–263 and 8–264), where it has a characteristic laminated appearance, with alternate layers of RPE and new basement membrane production. The hyperplastic RPE may disappear and leave only the laminated basement membrane (Fig. 8–264); this process may be quite marked. The hyperplasia resembles adenomatous tissue. Such proliferations are referred to as pseudoadenomatous hyperplasia of the RPE (Fig. 8–265).

The RPE has this feature because of its remarkable capacity to maintain polarity of the cells. It proliferates, forming two layers, with the apex of the cell toward the lumen and the base of the cell with variable basement membrane toward the outside of the lumen. Repetition of this arrangement leads to a laminated appearance. The size of the luminal units and the way they are sectioned result in a tubuloacinar pattern (Fig. 8–265,*D,E*). The localized hyperplasia of the RPE at the ora serrata, associated with chronic retinal detachment, has been referred to as ringschwiele.

Diffuse. Hyperplasia of the RPE occurs throughout the retina in a perivascular location. This is most often a sequela of traumatic retinopathy (Figs. 8–266 and 8–267) and is present in retinitis pigmentosa.

Pigmentary Patterns of the Peripheral Fundus. Various combinations and intensities of atrophy, hypertrophy, and hyperplasia of the RPE account for seven pigmentary patterns of the peripheral fundus, as described by Bastek, Siegel, Straatsma, Foos (1982). These patterns are linear, dusting, spicular, granular, clumping, reticular, and tapetochoroidal hypopigmentation.

Peripheral Chorioretinal Atrophy
(Cobblestone or Pavingstone Degeneration)

This rather common chorioretinal degenerative process is present in up to 27 per cent of persons over the age of 20 years (O'Malley, Allen, Straatsma, O'Malley, 1965). It is typically located between the ora serrata and the posterior aspect of the equator. Ophthalmoscopically, it appears as a small, discrete, yellowish-white area with prominently visible choroidal vessels, and it may be highlighted by dark, hypertrophic RPE at the margin. These lesions may occur singly or in groups (Fig. 8–268) and may become confluent, producing a band of depigmentation just posterior to the ora serrata.

Histopathologic studies show an attenuation or absence of the choriocapillaris, loss of the RPE and outer retinal layers, and some degree of chorioretinal adhesion (Figs. 8–269 and 8–270). No

Text continued on page 854

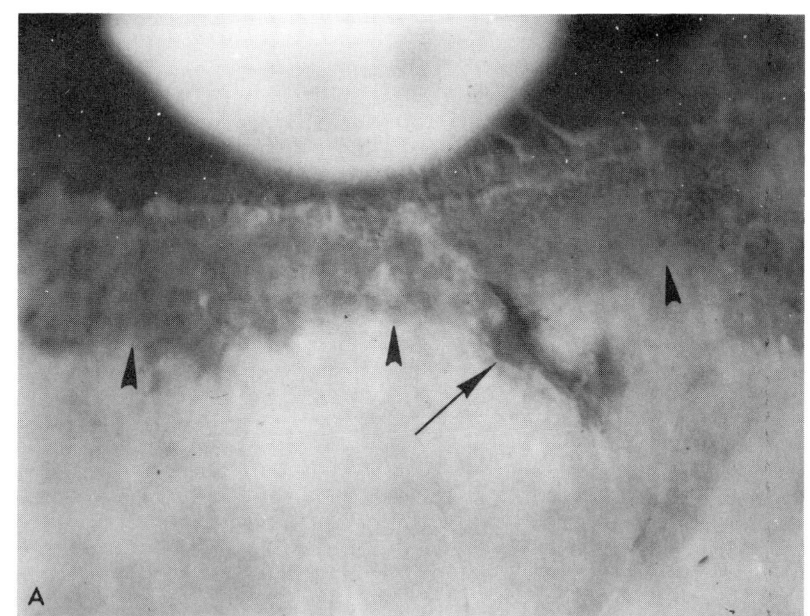

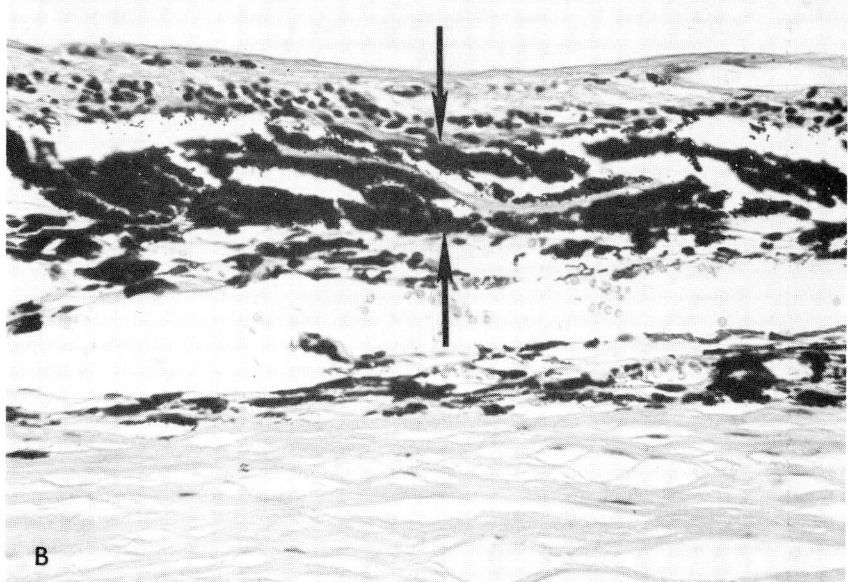

Figure 8–263. *A*, Gross appearance of **retinal pigment epithelium (RPE) hyperplasia** that remains under retina (arrow). A peripheral band of RPE hypertrophy (arrowheads) is also evident. *B*, Section through subretinal hyperplastic RPE shows laminated configuration (between arrows). H and E, ×290. EP 34753. (From Green WR: Pathology of the retina, *in* Frayer WC (ed): Lancaster Course in Ophthalmic Histopathology. Unit 9. Philadelphia, F.A. Davis, 1981.

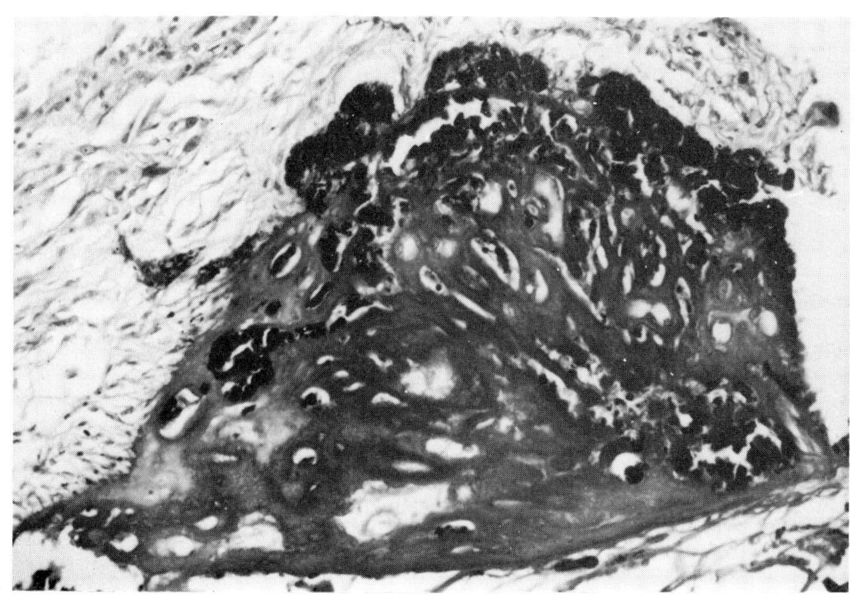

Figure 8–264. Peripapillary nodule of hyperplastic retinal pigment epithelium (RPE) in an eye with persistent hyperplastic primary vitreous. RPE in mid and deeper portions of nodule has degenerated, leaving only laminated basement membrane. PAS, ×230. EP 6671.

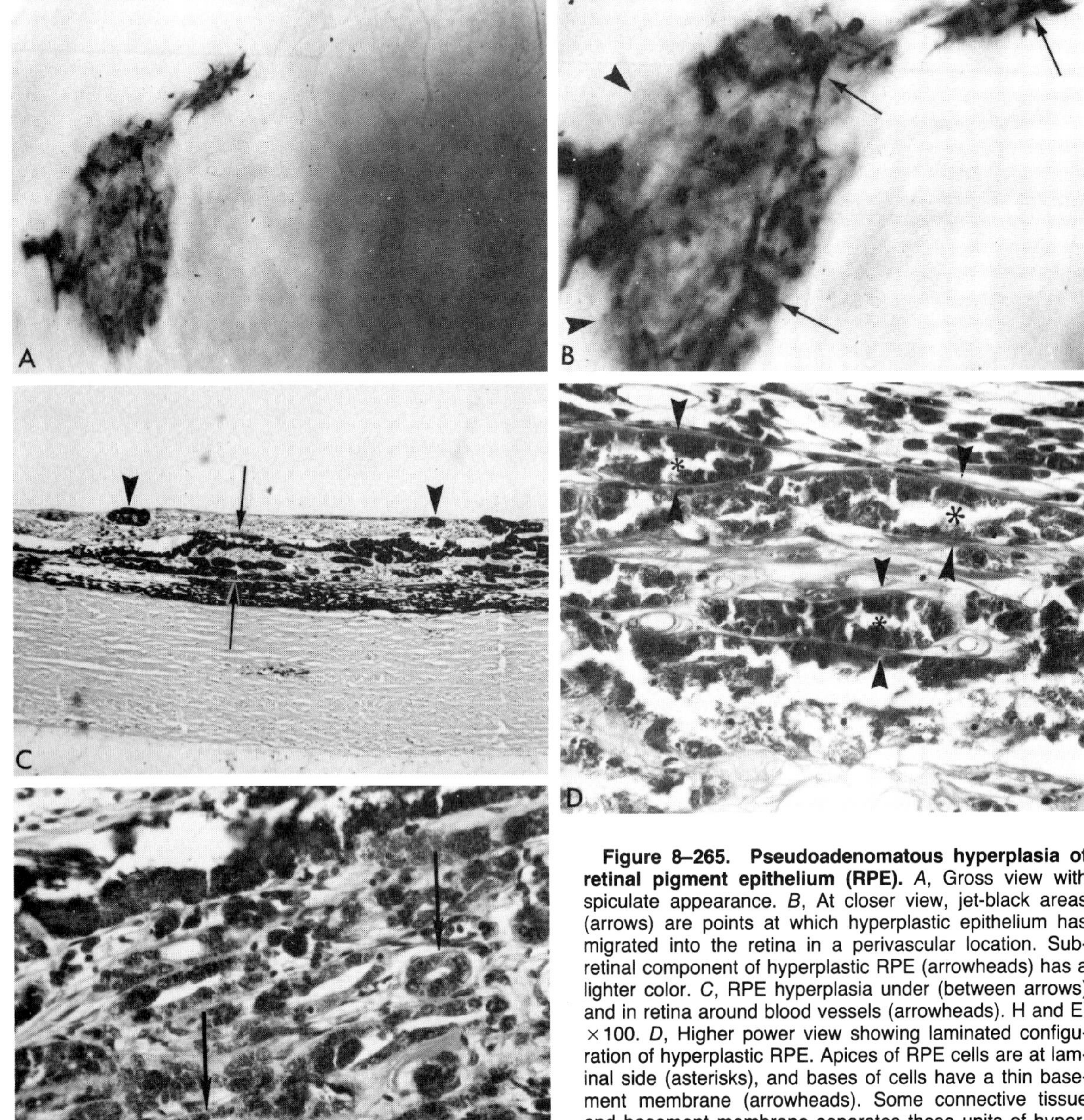

Figure 8–265. Pseudoadenomatous hyperplasia of retinal pigment epithelium (RPE). *A*, Gross view with spiculate appearance. *B*, At closer view, jet-black areas (arrows) are points at which hyperplastic epithelium has migrated into the retina in a perivascular location. Subretinal component of hyperplastic RPE (arrowheads) has a lighter color. *C*, RPE hyperplasia under (between arrows) and in retina around blood vessels (arrowheads). H and E, ×100. *D*, Higher power view showing laminated configuration of hyperplastic RPE. Apices of RPE cells are at laminal side (asterisks), and bases of cells have a thin basement membrane (arrowheads). Some connective tissue and basement membrane separates these units of hyperplastic RPE. Partially bleached, PAS, ×450. *E*, Same features are noted here. Some areas have a more acinar-like configuration (arrows). Partially bleached, PAS, ×450. EP 30575. (From Green WR: Pathology of the retina, *in* Frayer WC (ed): Lancaster Course in Ophthalmic Histopathology. Unit 9. Philadelphia, F.A. Davis, 1981.)

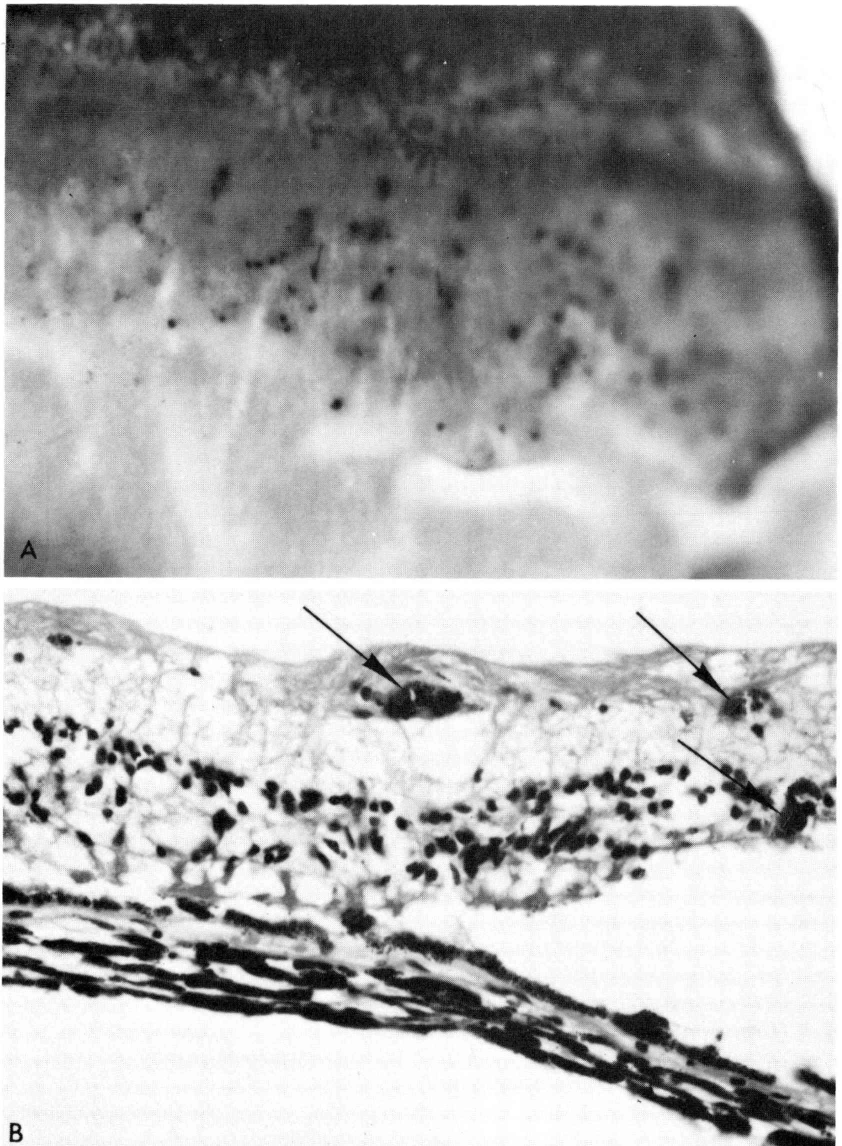

Figure 8–266. Traumatic retinopathy. *A*, Gross appearance of diffuse multifocal hyperplasia of retinal pigment epithelium (RPE), with some migration into retina. *B*, Hyperplastic RPE in retina (arrows). There is loss of photoreceptor cell layer. H and E, ×360. EP 31661.

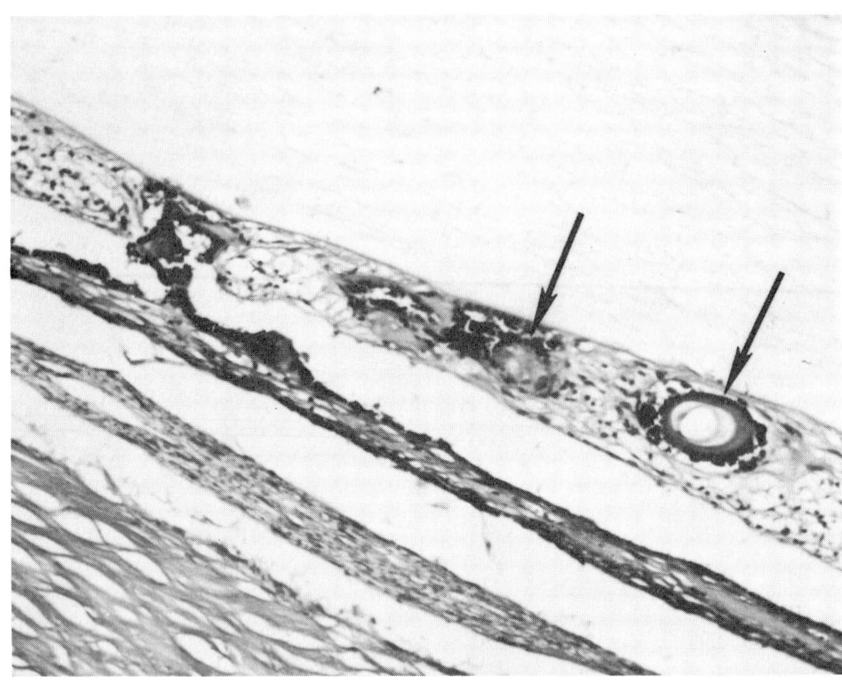

Figure 8–267. Extensive traumatic retinopathy. Hyperplastic retinal pigment epithelium has migrated into the retina in a perivascular location (arrows), and there is loss of photorecepter cell layer. H and E, ×145. EP 32733.

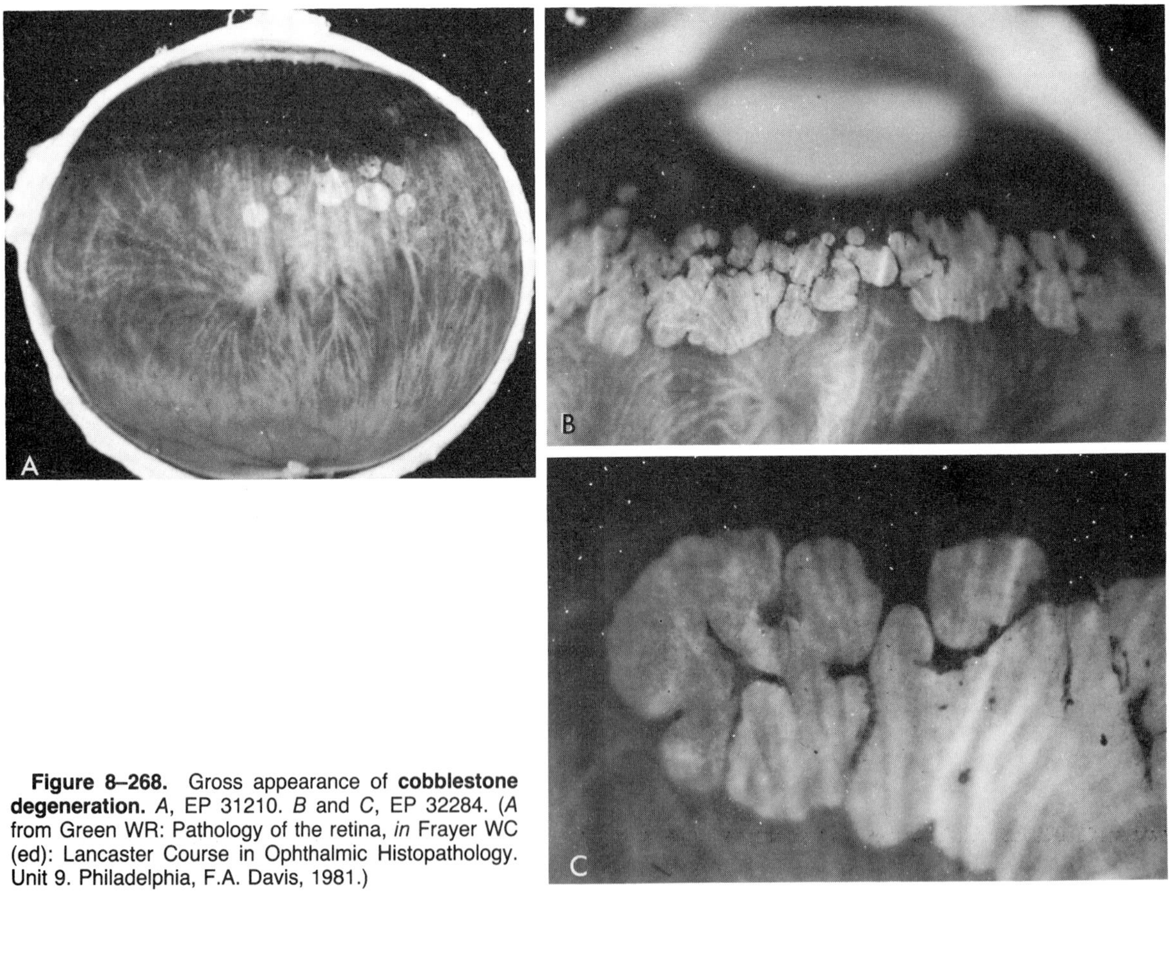

Figure 8–268. Gross appearance of **cobblestone degeneration.** *A*, EP 31210. *B* and *C*, EP 32284. (*A* from Green WR: Pathology of the retina, *in* Frayer WC (ed): Lancaster Course in Ophthalmic Histopathology. Unit 9. Philadelphia, F.A. Davis, 1981.)

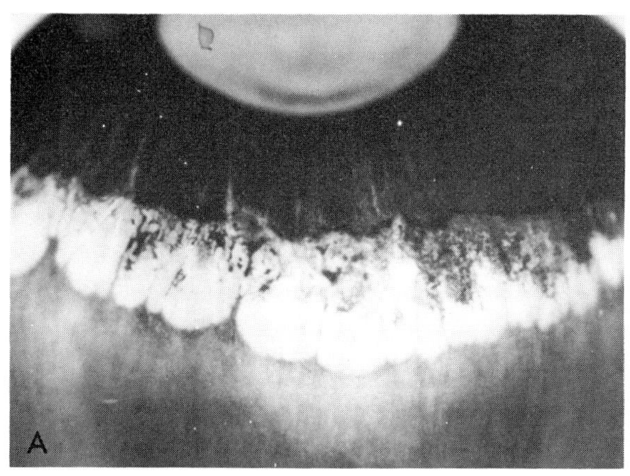

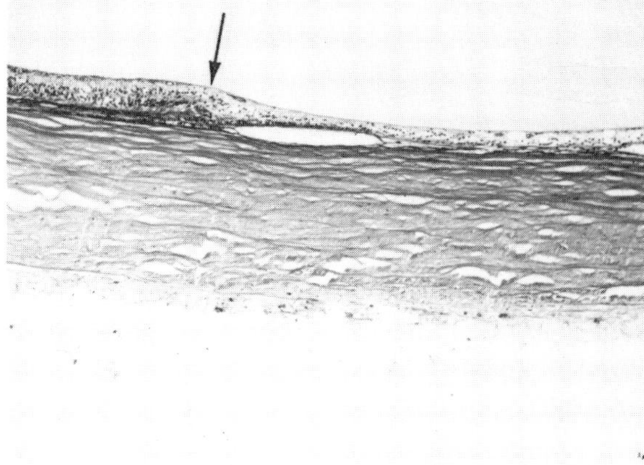

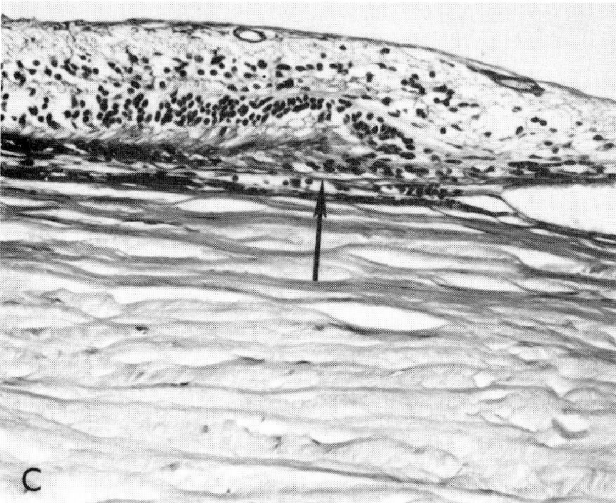

Figure 8–269. *A*, Gross appearance of extensive, confluent **cobblestone degeneration** just posterior to ora serrata. *B*, Abrupt transition (arrow) between normal and affected area. Pattern of atrophy is that of outer ischemic atrophy of retina, with loss of retinal pigment epithelium, outer nuclear and outer plexiform layers, and outer portion of inner nuclear layers. Remaining inner retina is adherent to Bruch's membrane. No scarring or other reparative processes are present. PAS, ×60. *C*, Higher power view showing junction (arrow) between normal retina and that affected by outer ischemic atrophy. PAS, ×235. EP 31031.

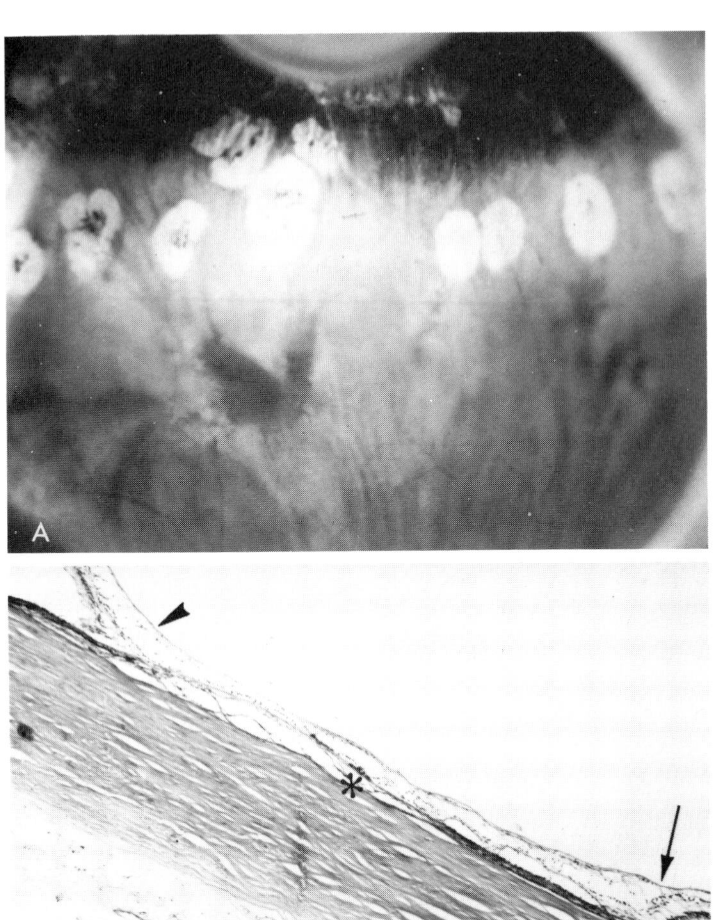

Figure 8–270. *A*, Numerous medium-sized areas of **cobblestone degeneration.** *B*, Section through one of these shows intact retina anteriorly (arrowhead) and posteriorly (arrow). In between, remaining portion of inner nuclear layer is adherent to Bruch's membrane. A small island of hypertrophic retinal pigment epithelium is present in the center of the lesion (asterisk). PAS, ×50. EP 42503.

reparative processes, such as fibrovascular scarring or proliferation of the RPE, are observed. Thus, the changes are those of outer retinal ischemic atrophy. There may be a small area of surrounding dark-appearing hypertrophic RPE.

Choroidal vascular insufficiency is thought to be the cause of cobblestone degeneration, because the changes are limited to that portion of the retina supplied by the choriocapillaris. No reparative processes are associated, and a similar lesion can be produced in rabbits by ligation of a portion of the choroidal blood supply (Nicholls, 1938).

Also implicating vascular ischemia is the observation of this process in hypotensive retinopathy. In one case studied clinically and histopathologically, extensive cobblestone degeneration extending posterior to the equator was observed in the ischemic eye, while in the fellow eye the degenerative process was absent (Fig. 8–271) (Michelson, Knox, Green, 1971) (see page 1046).

The presence of cobblestone degeneration is not of great pathologic significance. However, it may be a sign of peripheral vascular disease. If a retinal detachment occurs in an eye with more posterior lesions, a secondary retinal tear may occur because of chorioretinal adhesion at the site of a cobblestone lesion.

Peripheral Punched-Out Lesions

Solitary or multiple lesions in the midperiphery may be caused by a choroidal vascular insufficiency or may be the sequelae of focal healed choroiditis.

Choroidal Ischemia (discussed in more detail in Chapter 9, Uvea, page 1502). ***Small Ischemic Punched-Out Lesions.*** The lesions are identical to solitary cobblestone lesions but are located at or posterior to the equator (Figs. 8–272 and 8–273). The lesion may be surrounded by hypertrophic RPE (Fig. 8–273). Histopathologic find-

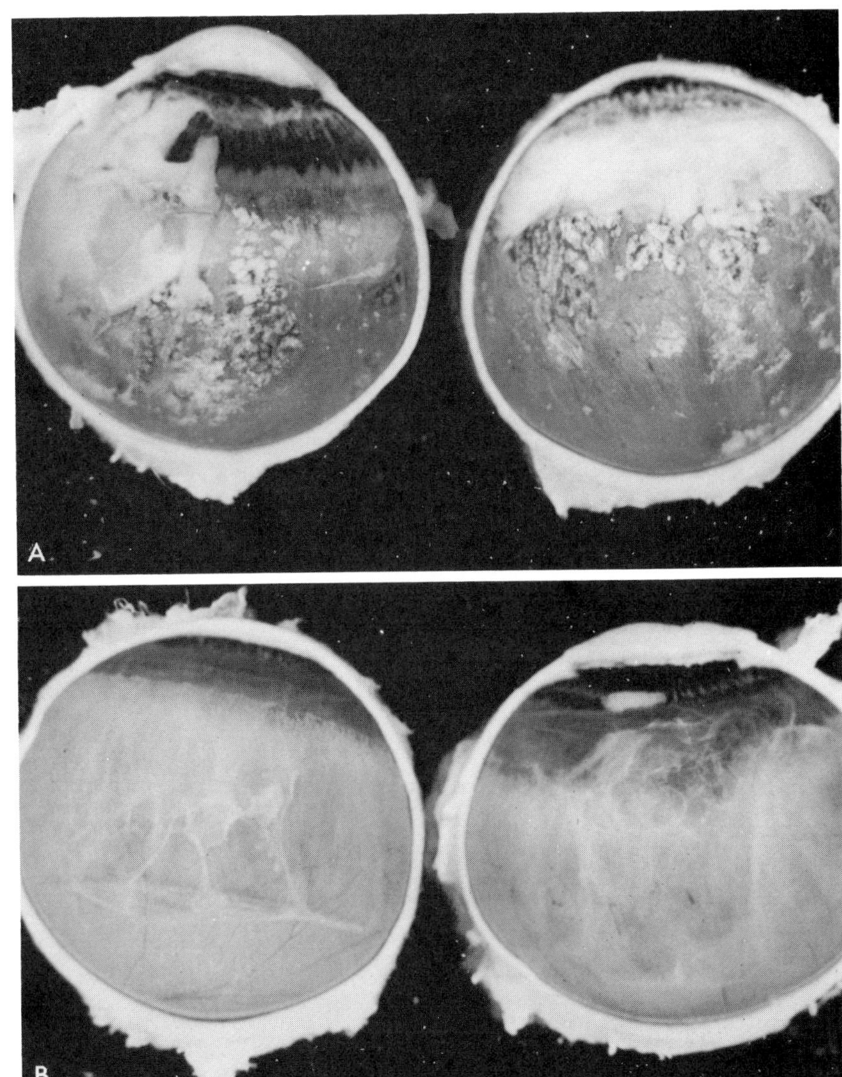

Figure 8–271. Hypotensive retinopathy (ocular ischemic inflammatory syndrome). *A*, Ischemic eye has extensive cobblestone degeneration extending posterior to equator, whereas *B*, the fellow, nonischemic eye has none. (From Michelson, PE, Knox, DL, Green WR: Ischemic ocular inflammation: A clinicopathologic case report. Arch Opthalmol *86*:274–280, 1971.)

ings are identical to those seen with cobblestone degeneration (Figs. 8–272 and 8–273).

Elschnig Spots. Larger choroidal ischemic lesions have been referred to as Elschnig spots (Figs. 8–274 through 8–276) (Klien, 1968; Morse, 1968). Residual hypertrophic and, sometimes, hyperplastic RPE may be present in the central and/or peripheral areas of the lesion.

Focal Healed Choroiditis. This type of lesion is characteristically seen in healed choroidal lesions of coccidioidomycosis (Fig. 8–277), histoplasmosis (Fig. 8–278), and other pathogenic mycotic organisms, unassociated with any known infection (Fig. 8–279). This type of punched-out lesion has a variable amount of scarring in the choroid and adjacent outer layers of retina. Chorioretinal adhesion is evident. Retinal pigment epithelium is usually absent centrally but may show hypertrophy, hyperplasia, and migration in the retina. In some instances, hyperplastic RPE and retinal glial cells may migrate into the choroidal scar. There is usually a discontinuity of Bruch's membrane, but choroidal neovascularization does not usually occur in lesions outside the area centralis. Retinochoroidal vascular anastomosis in a midperipheral lesion in the presumed ocular histoplasmosis syndrome has been observed rarely (Fig. 8–280).

Peripheral Albinotic Spots

This curious lesion occurs in the midperiphery and is a discrete area of loss of pigment, allowing choroidal vessels to be seen well (Fig. 8–281). Histopathologic studies (Schlernitzauer, Green, 1971) have shown the choriocapillaris, RPE, and photoreceptor cells to be normal, but there is a reduction or absence of melanin pigment granules in the RPE (Fig. 8–282).

In a survey of a Maryland community, 6 per cent of the general population was found to have peripheral albinotic spots (Smith, Ganley, 1972).

Text continued on page 867

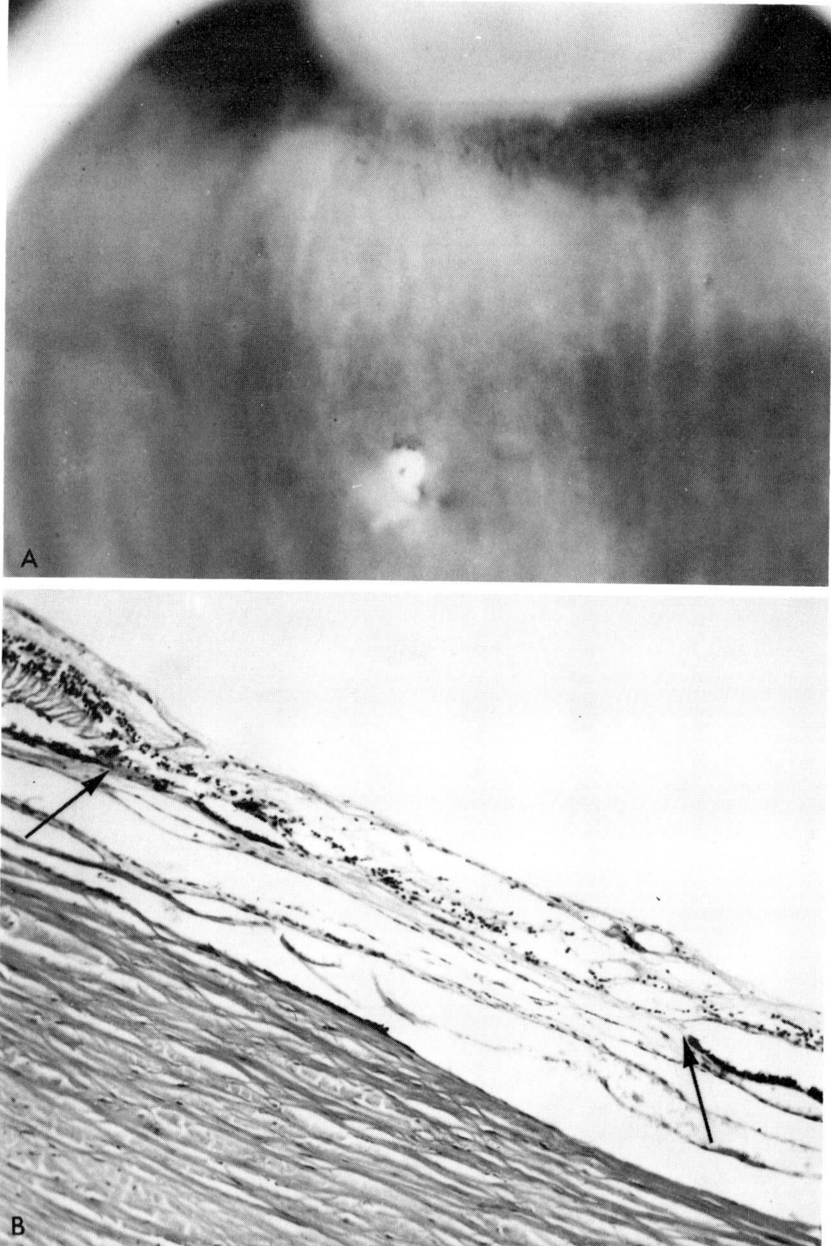

Figure 8–272. A peripheral punched-out lesion caused by a small choroidal infarction, with outer ischemic atrophy of retina. *A*, Gross appearance of a small, discrete lesion with loss of retinal pigment epithelium (RPE). *B*, Lesion shows absence of choriocapillaris and loss of RPE, outer nuclear and outer plexiform layers, and outer portion of inner nuclear layer (between arrows). Remaining inner portion of inner nuclear layer is adherent to Bruch's membrane. There is no scarring or other reparative processes. PAS, ×105. EP 30330.

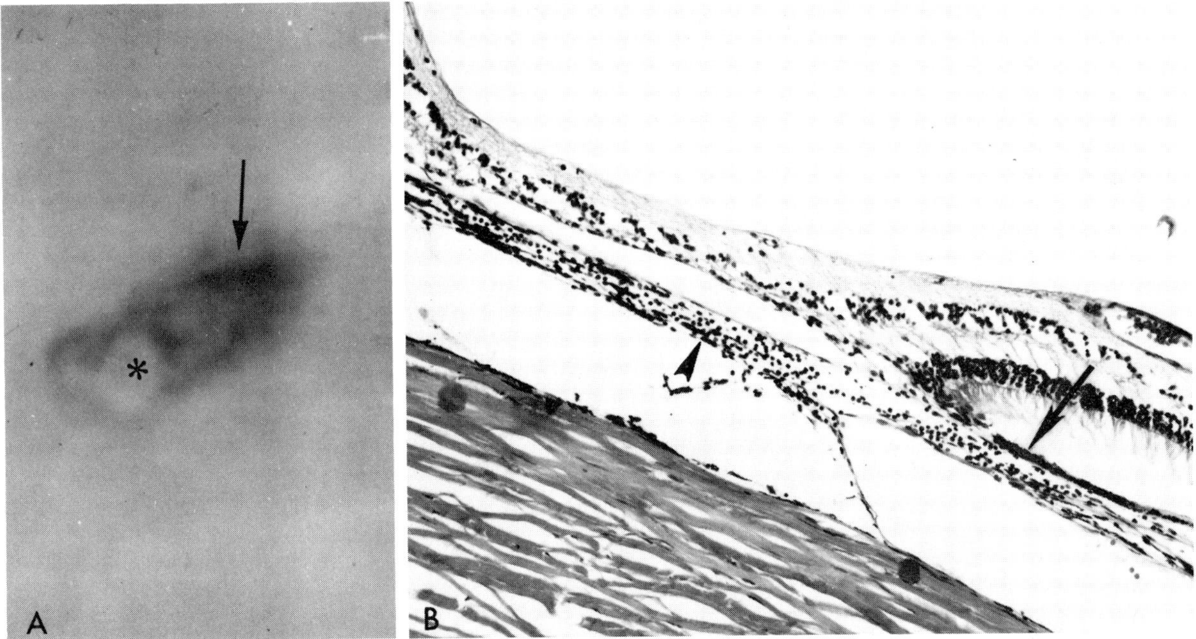

Figure 8–273. Peripheral punched-out lesion resulting from small choroidal infarction. *A*, Retinal pigment epithelium (RPE) is lost centrally (asterisk), and the lesion is partially surrounded by hypertrophic RPE (arrow). *B*, Lesion is discrete, with loss of outer retinal layers. Hypertrophic RPE (arrow) is present on anterior margin. There is no scarring or other reparative processes. Mild lymphocytic infiltrate is present in subjacent choroid (arrowhead). H and E, ×130. EP 34241.

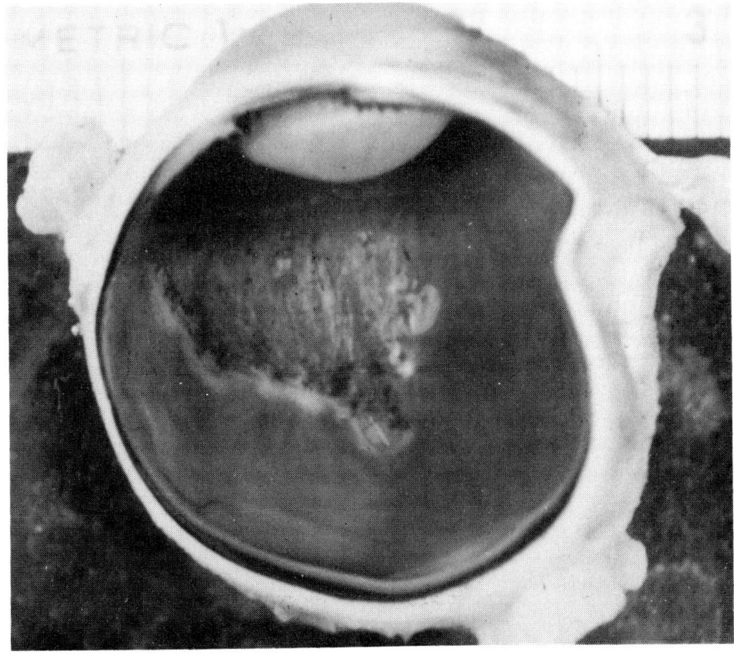

Figure 8–274. Gross appearance of a wedge-shaped **choroidal infarction**. EP 37765.

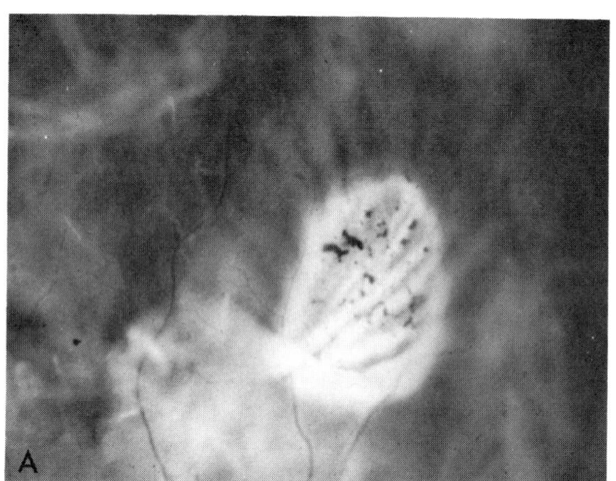

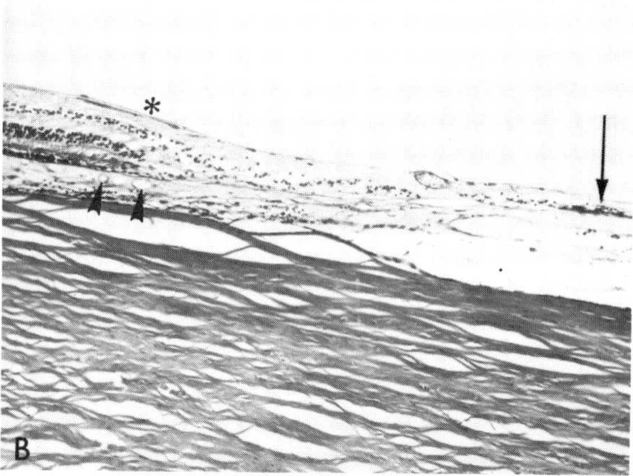

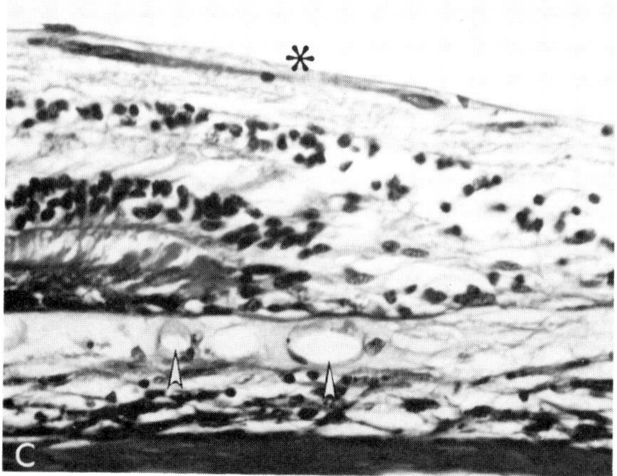

Figure 8–275. Elschnig spot. *A*, Lesion is round and discrete, with loss of retinal pigment epithelium (RPE). A few specks of hypertrophic RPE are present. *B*, Margin of lesion (asterisk) shows abruptness of transition. Choriocapillaris (arrowheads) is intact outside lesion and is absent within lesion. There is outer ischemic atrophy of the retina, with loss of RPE and all outer layers, including the outer portion of the inner nuclear layer. No scarring is present. A small island of hypertrophic RPE (arrow) is present in the center of the lesion. PAS, ×105. *C*, Higher power view of junction (asterisk), showing abrupt loss of choriocapillaris (arrowheads), RPE, and outer retinal layers. PAS, ×400. EP 30785.

From Green WR: Pathology of the retina, *in* Frayer WC (ed): Lancaster Course in Ophthalmic Histopathology. Unit 9. Philadelphia, F.A. Davis, 1981.)

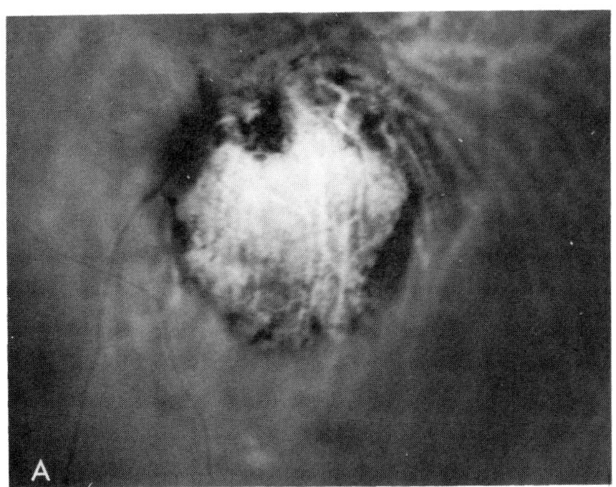

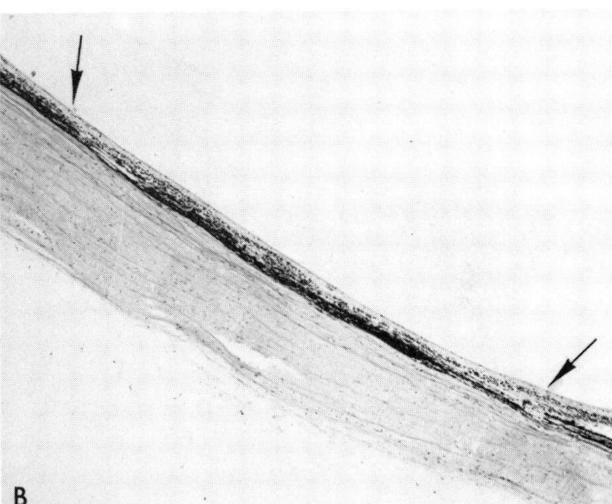

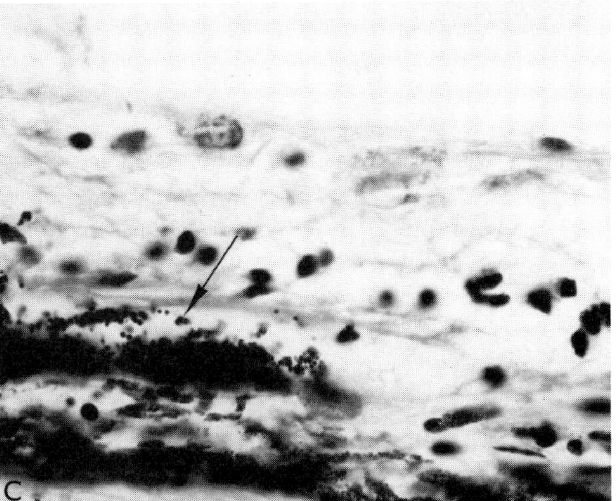

Figure 8–276. *A,* **Elschnig spot** with hypertrophic retinal pigment epithelium (RPE) at margin. *B*, Low power view showing abrupt margin (arrows). H and E, ×40. *C*, Margin of lesion, showing hypertrophic RPE with large spherical pigment granules (arrow). H and E, ×900. EP 30455.

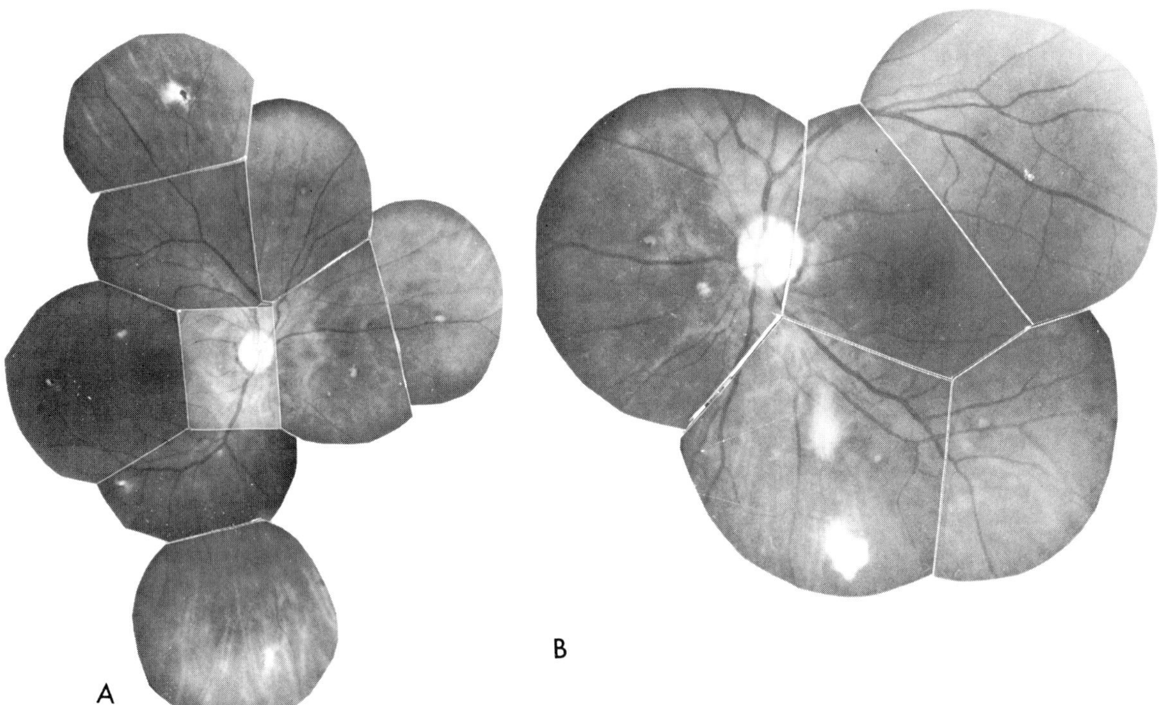

Figure 8–277. Chorioretinal scars in patient with disseminated coccidioidomycosis. *A*, Composite photograph of right eye showing 13 healed chorioretinal scars. *B*, Left eye had 8 healed scars. (From Green WR, Bennett JE: Coccidioidomycosis: Report of a case with clinical evidence of ocular involvement. Arch Opthalmol. *77*:337–340, 1967.)

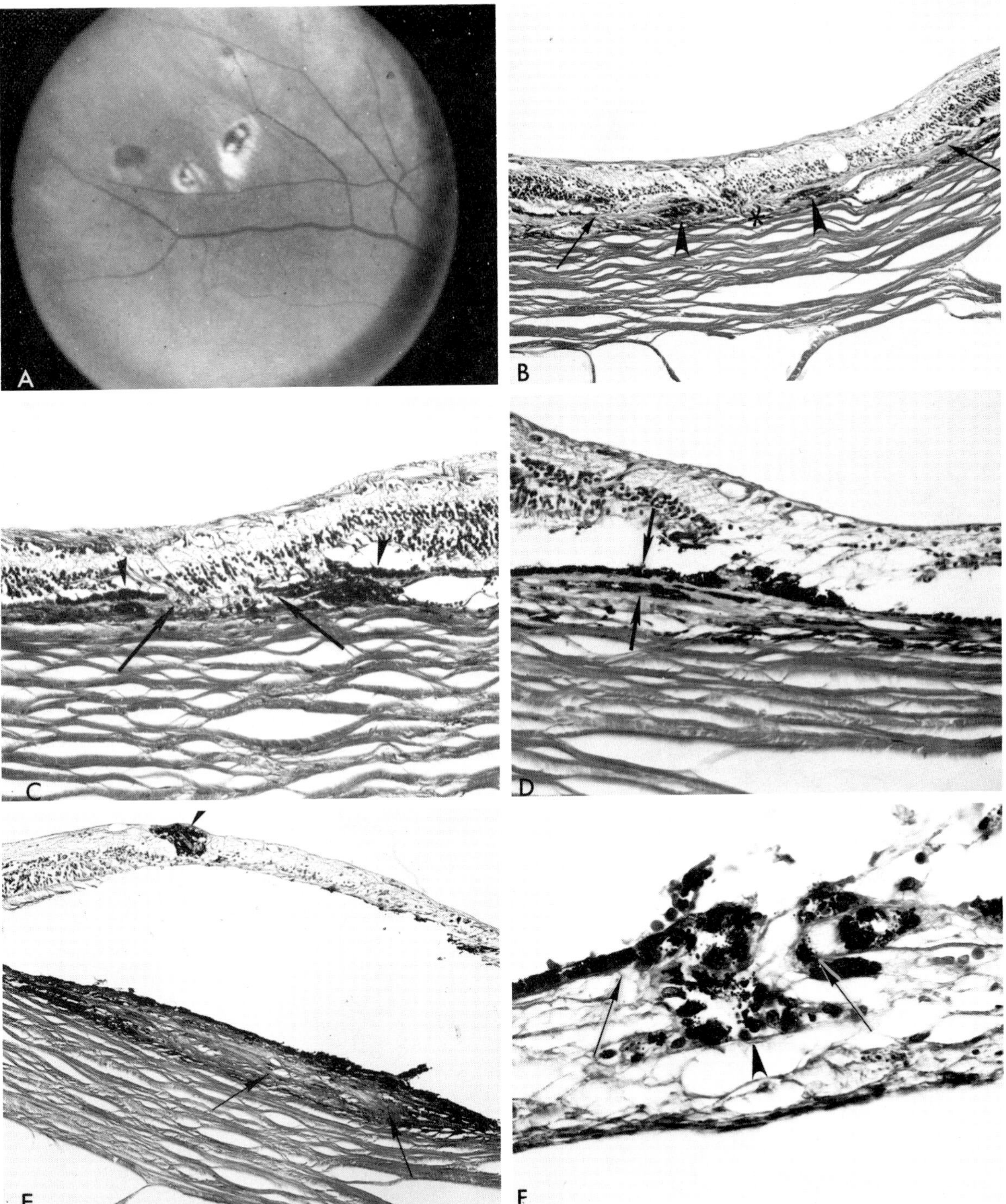

Figure 8–278. Peripheral punched-out lesions in ocular histoplasmosis. EP 43070. *A*, Ophthalmoscopic appearance of cluster of chorioretinal scars. *B*, Chorioretinal scar (between arrows). There is loss of retinal pigment epithelium (RPE) and photoreceptor cells. Centrally, there is a discontinuity in Bruch's membrane, with extension of glial cells (asterisk) and RPE (arrowheads) into scarred choroid. Firm chorioretinal adhesion is apparent. INS 23; Van de Grift. ×100. *C*, Small chorioretinal scar, with discontinuity of Bruch's membrane centrally and minor extension of glial cells into choroid (between arrows). Hypertrophic RPE (arrowheads) is present at either margin. INS 68. Van de Grift, ×275. *D*, Chorioretinal scar with slightly laminated, hypertrophic, and hyperplastic RPE (between arrows) and loss of retinal layers. Bruch's membrane is intact. Van de Grift, ×240. *E*, Larger chorioretinal scar, with discontinuity of Bruch's membrane (between arrows) and hyperplasia of RPE with migration into retina (arrowhead).PAS, ×120. *F*, Chorioretinal scar with discontinuity of Bruch's membrane (between arrows), and hypertrophy and hyperplasia of RPE with migration into choroidal scar (arrowhead). EP 41434. Van de Grift, ×490. (*F* is from Meredith, TA, Green, WR, Key, SN III, et al: Ocular histoplasmosis: Clinicopathologic correlation of three cases. Surv Opthalmol. 22:189–205, 1977.)

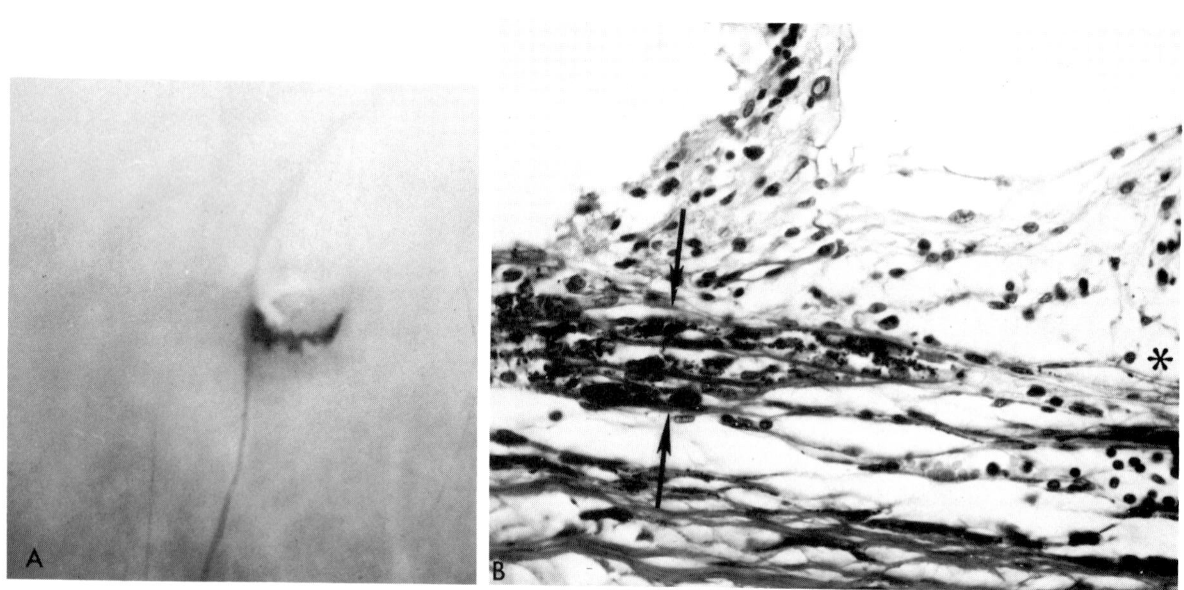

Figure 8–279. *A,* **Peripheral punched-out lesion** with pigmented margin. *B,* There is chorioretinal adhesion with loss of retinal pigment epithelium (RPE) anteriorly (asterisk) and an area of laminated hyperplastic RPE posteriorly (between arrows). PAS, ×450. EP 31325.

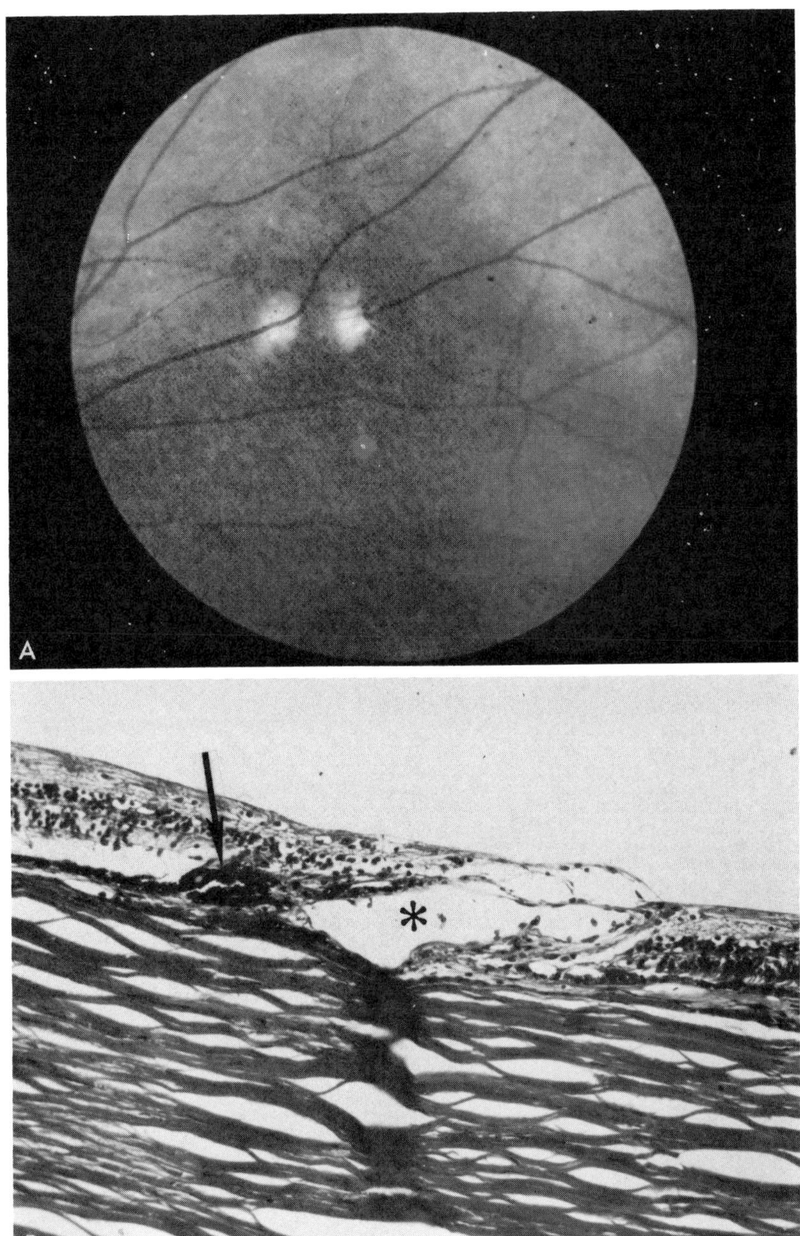

Figure 8–280. *A*, Ophthalmoscopic appearance of a **chorioretinal vascular anastomosis** at a chorioretinal scar in ocular histoplasmosis. (Courtesy of Dr. D.L. Knox.) *B*, Chorioretinal scar in ocular histoplasmosis, showing a blood vessel (asterisk) extending through a discontinuity in Bruch's membrane. Hypertrophic and hyperplastic retinal pigment epithelium is present at one margin (arrow). SNS 54. Van de Grift, ×300. EP 43070.

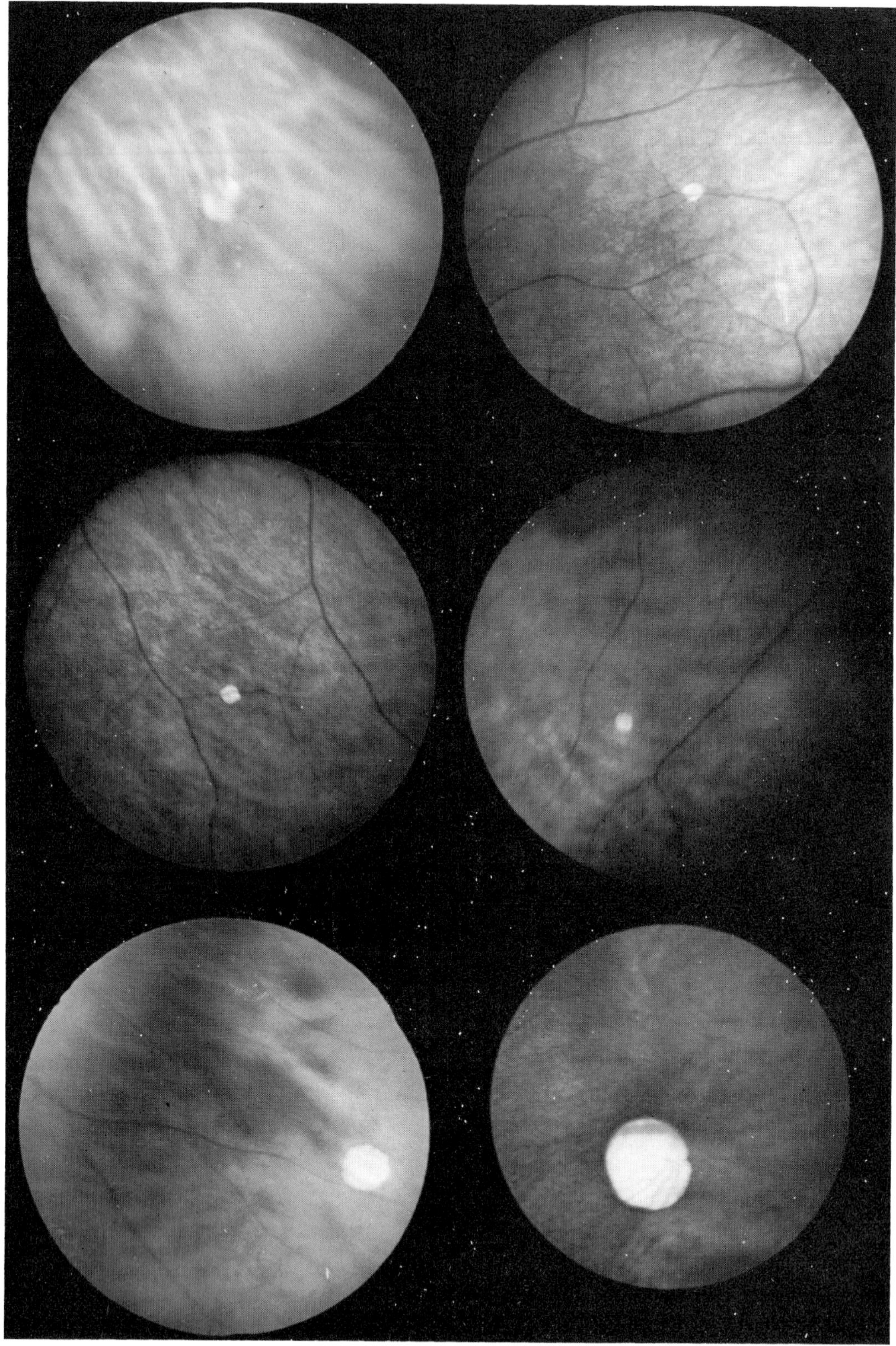

Figure 8–281. Ophthalmoscopic appearance of **peripheral albinotic spots.**

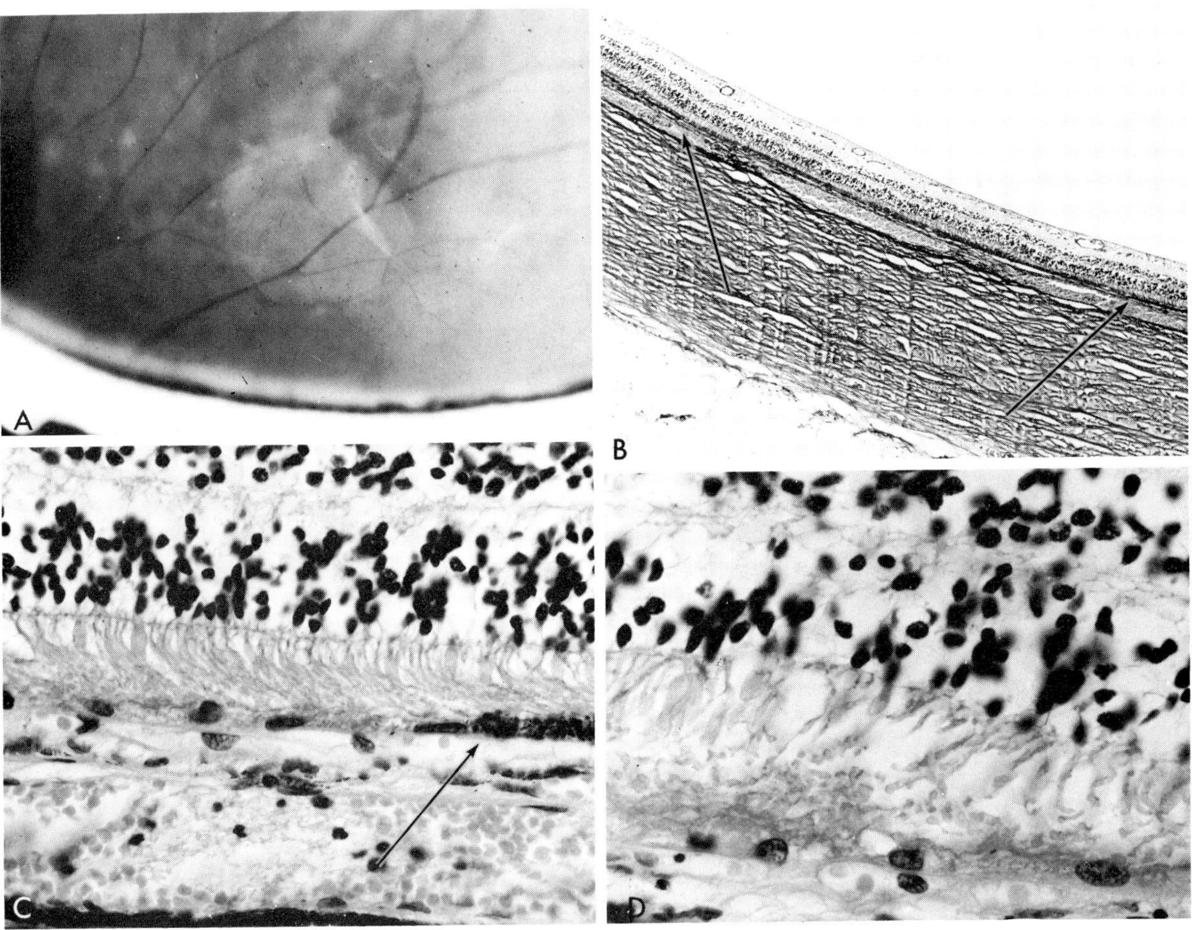

Figure 8–282. *A,* Gross appearance of **peripheral albinotic spot.** *B,* Overall view shows discrete round area of depigmentation (arrows). PAS, ×45. *C,* Higher power view of border of lesion (arrow), showing abrupt transition from normal-appearing retinal pigment epithelium (RPE) to abnormal RPE with absence of pigment. H and E, ×575. *D,* Center of lesion shows RPE to be slightly flattened, elongated, and amelanotic. Choriocapillaris and outer nuclear layer are normal. Post mortem autolysis of photoreceptors is present. H and E, ×800. EP 30967.
From Schlernitzauer DA, Green WR: Peripheral retinal albinotic spots. Am J Ophthalmol *72*:729–732, 1971.)

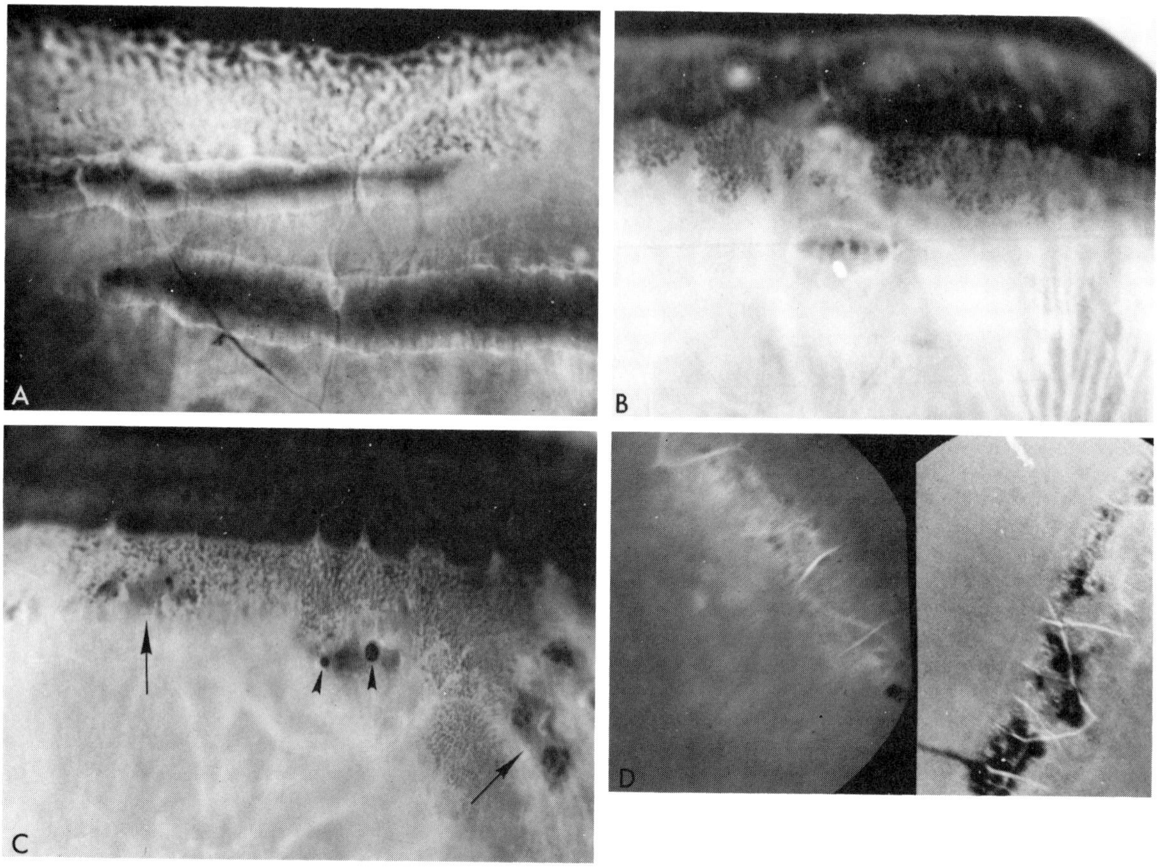

Figure 8–283. Various appearances of **lattice degeneration of retina.** *A,* Overlapping linear areas of retinal thinning. Condensed vitreous at margin is apparent. EP 31974. *B,* Small area of retinal thinning, with vitreous condensation at margin and pocket of fluid vitreous centrally. EP 30295. *C,* Several areas of retinal thinning (arrows). One area has two holes (arrowheads) within area of thinning. EP 30979. *D,* Ophthalmoscopic appearance of lattice degeneration (left) with a linear area of lattice "wicker" caused by sclerotic blood vessels. In addition, photo on right shows secondary retinal pigment epithelium hyperplasia, with migration into retina.

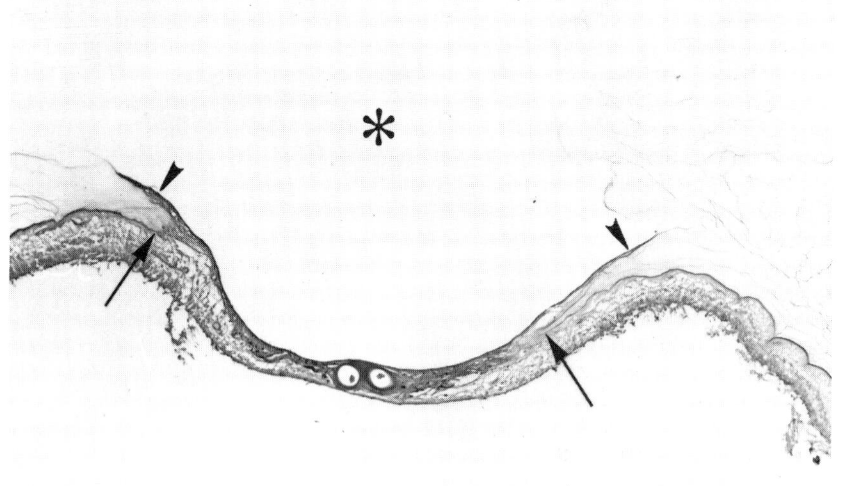

Figure 8–284. Changes include a pocket of fluid vitreous (asterisk), discontinuity of internal limiting membrane (arrows), retinal thinning, sclerosis of vessels, and condensation and adherence of vitreous at margin (arrowheads). Alcian blue, ×55. EP 43287.

Similar lesions have been observed in the dog by Herrmann and coworkers (1973).

Lattice Degeneration

Lattice degeneration is a vitreoretinal degenerative process characterized by sharply demarcated, circumferentially oriented areas of retinal thinning located anterior to the equator, most commonly in the vertical meridians (Fig. 8–283). Secondary RPE hypertrophy, hyperplasia, and migration into the retina may occur and bring attention to the lesion. In only 9 per cent of the lesions is a lattice-wicker appearance evident on initial examination (Byer, 1965). With long-term studies, however, Byer (1974a) observed that 12.3 per cent of lattice lesions had white lines. Of patients with lattice degeneration, 30 per cent have at least one lesion with white lines. He also noted with a 3 to 10 year follow-up that 5 per cent of patients develop new areas of lattice. Familial transmission has been observed (Cambiaggi, 1969; Lewkonia, Davies, Salmon, 1973; Everett, 1967).

The prevalence of lattice degeneration of the retina is between 6 and 11 per cent of the population, judging from the reports of Straatsma and Allen (1962, autopsy study): 6 per cent; Byer (1965, clinical study): 7.1 per cent; and Straatsma, Zeegan, Foos, et al (1974, autopsy study): 10.7 per cent.

Histopathologically, lattice degeneration is characterized (Fig. 8–284) by (1) discontinuity in the internal limiting membrane; (2) variable thinning of the retina with loss of the inner layers, sometimes with holes (Fig. 8–285); (3) a variable degree of vitreous condensation at the margin of the lattice—sometimes fortified by glial cell proliferation (Fig. 8–286); (4) a pocket of degenerated liquefied vitreous overlying the area of lattice (Fig. 8–287); (5) sclerosis and occlusion of capillary bed in the area of lattice (Fig. 8–288) (best seen by trypsin digestion [Streeten, Bert, 1972]);

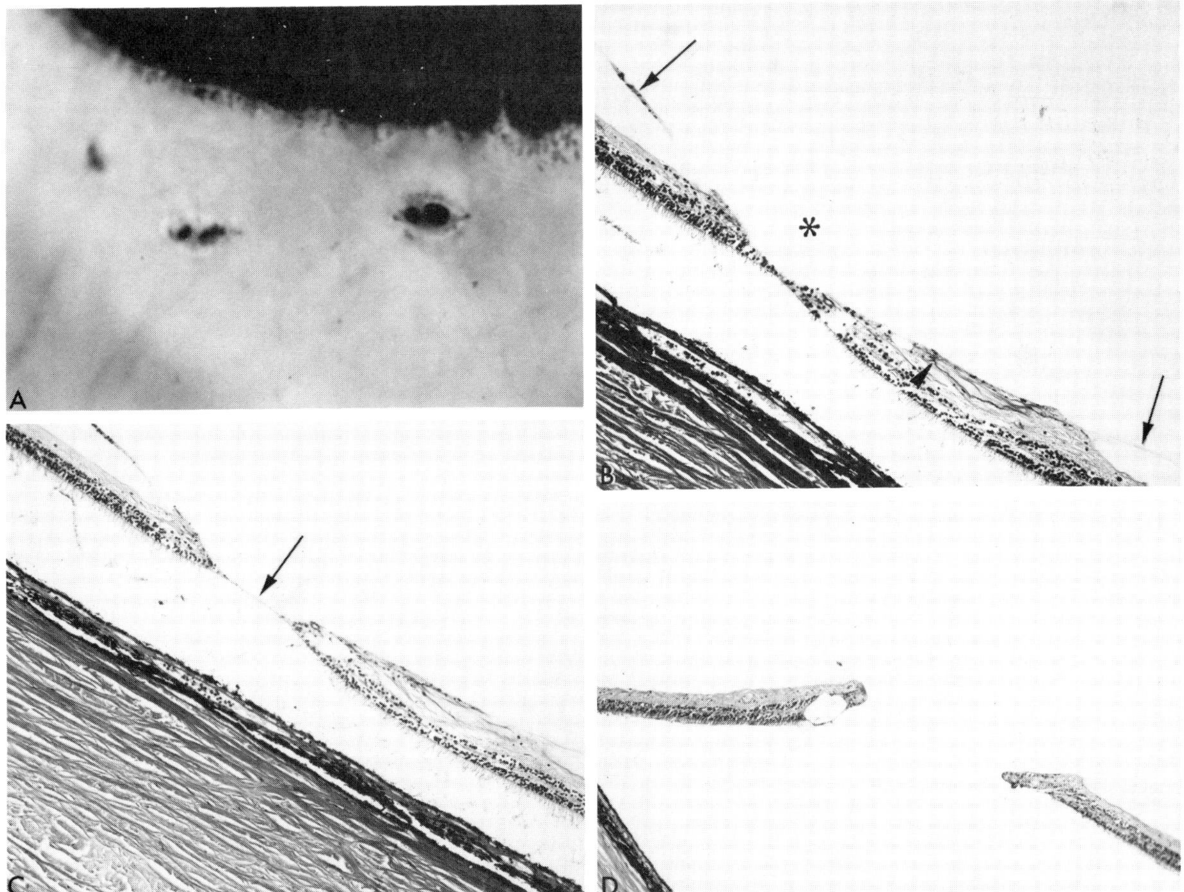

Figure 8–285. *A*, Gross appearance of two small areas of **lattice degeneration with hole formation.** *B*, Features include overlying vitreous degeneration (asterisk), retinal thinning, vitreous adherence to margin with cellular proliferation at one margin (arrows), discontinuity of internal limiting membrane (arrowhead). PAS, ×110. *C*, Different level, showing same features but more thinning, and only external limiting membrane area persists (arrow). PAS, ×100. *D*, Different level, showing hole in area of lattice changes. H and E, ×50. EP 30544.

From Green WR: Pathology of the vitreous, *in* Frayer WC (ed): Lancaster Course in Ophthalmic Histopathology. Unit 8. Philadelphia, F.A. Davis, 1981.)

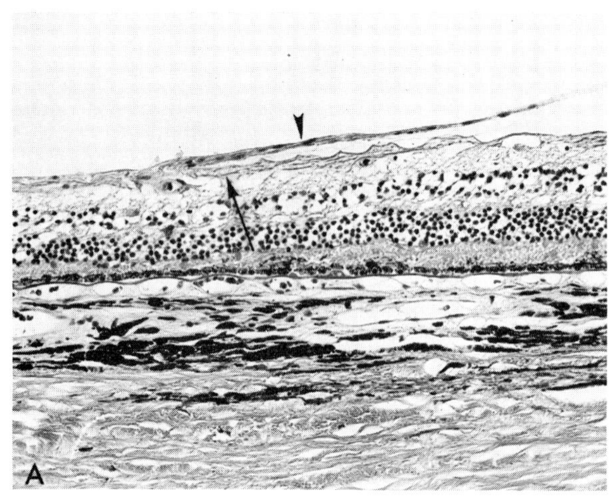

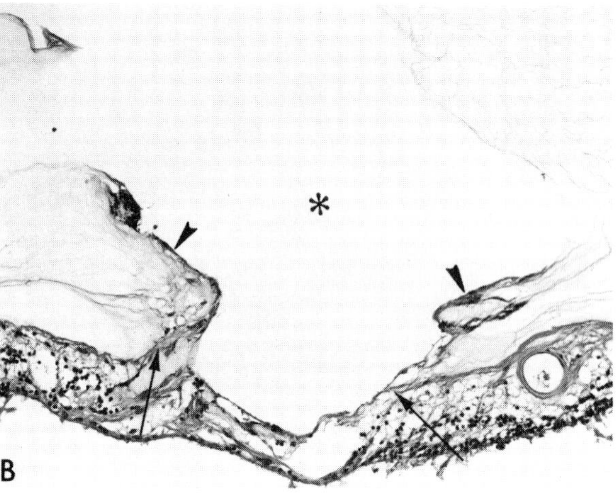

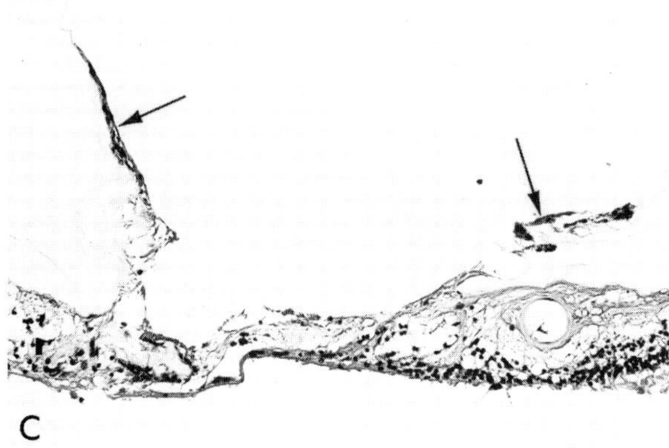

Figure 8–286. Glial cell proliferation in vitreous condensation at margins of lattice degeneration. *A*, Internal limiting membrane (ILM) (arrow) is discontinuous. Vitreous adherent at margin has glial cell proliferation (arrowhead). Van de Grift, ×185. *B*, Features include retinal thinning, discontinuity of ILM (arrows), pocket of fluid vitreous (asterisk), and glial cell proliferation in vitreous at margin (arrowheads). (Alcian blue, ×145). *C*, Glial cell fortification (arrows) of vitreous adherent at margins of lattice degeneration, Van de Grift, ×145. EP 43287.

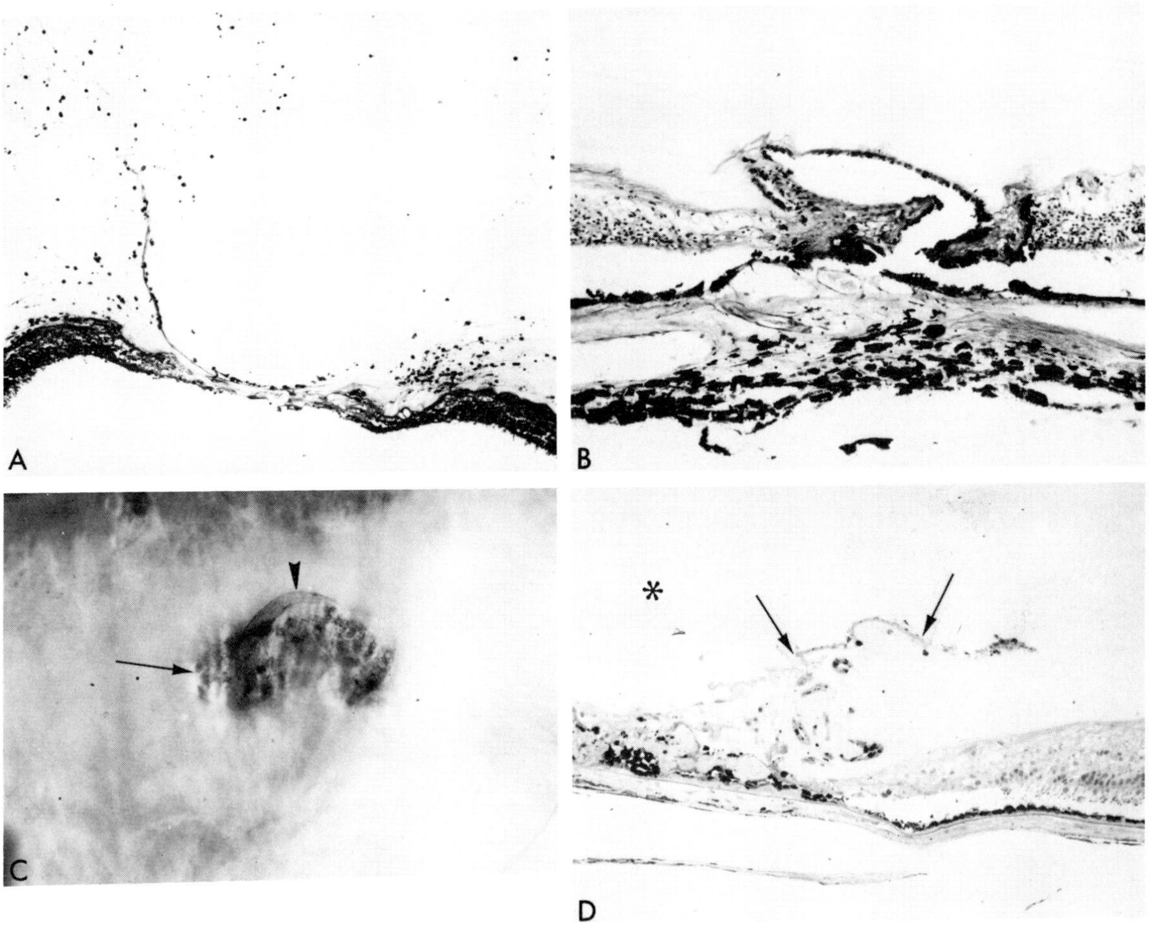

Figure 8–287. Pocket of fluid vitreous in lattice degeneration of retina. *A*, This pocket of degenerated vitreous is delineated by the presence of neoplastic and inflammatory cells in the remaining formed vitreous, in an eye with reticulum cell sarcoma. EP 48454. *B*, Small pocket of fluid vitreous is outlined by hyperplastic retinal pigment epithelium (RPE) in this lesion. PAS ×115. EP 50433. *C*, Gross appearance of lattice degeneration. *D*, Hyperplastic RPE (arrows) partially lining the inner aspect of the pocket of fluid vitreous (asterisk) at the anterior margin of the area of lattice degeneration (arrowhead). Epon, paraphenylenediamine, ×130. EP 52801.

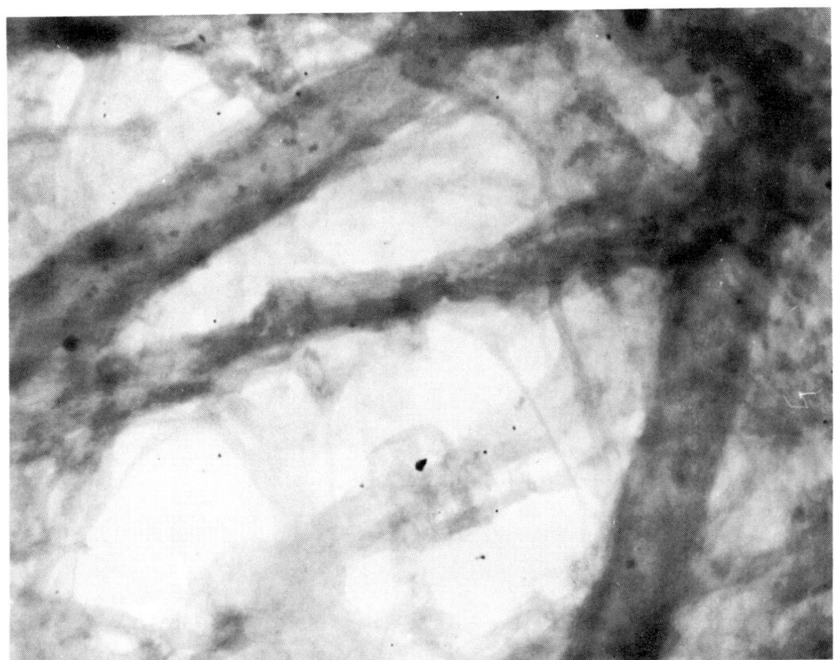

Figure 8–288. Thick-walled and acellular capillaries in area of **lattice degeneration**. Trypsin digestion preparation; PAS, H and E, ×900. EP 43287.

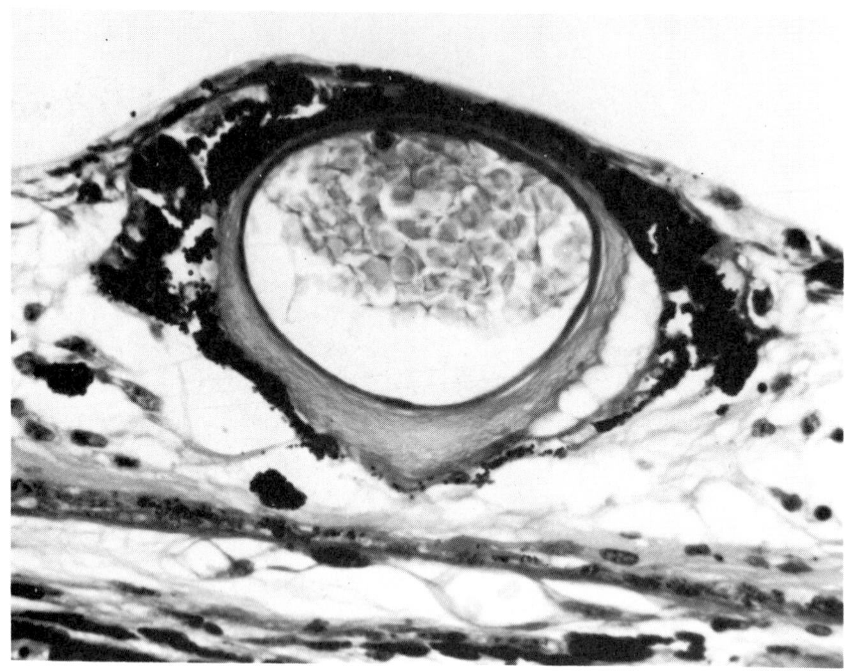

Figure 8–289. Center of **lattice degeneration of retina**, showing sclerotic retinal artery surrounded by hyperplastic retinal pigment epithelium. PAS, ×500. EP 43287.

(6) a variable degree of sclerosis of the larger retinal vessels that traverse the area of lattice (Fig. 8–289); and (7) a variable degree of RPE hypertrophy, hyperplasia, and migration into the retina (Figs. 8–289 and 8–290). The underlying choroid, and especially the choriocapillaris, is not remarkable. This is a *vitreoretinal* degenerative process and *not* a chorioretinal degenerative process. Occasionally lattice degeneration can be very small and have the appearance of retinal pits (Fig. 8–291).

The holes that may occur within an area of lattice degeneration are not important from the standpoint of retinal detachment. However, some investigators (Tillery, Lucier, 1976) have reported this association. Such a detachment theoretically can occur if the pocket of fluid vitreous over the area of lattice degeneration is in communication with a central area of vitreous syneresis.

The importance of lattice degeneration is its occurrence in association with posterior vitreous detachment. Because of the somewhat firmer attachment of the vitreous at the margin of lattice degeneration, a retinal tear is likely to occur at the posterior margin when the vitreous detaches to this point (Fig. 8–292). This is why one often sees lattice degeneration in the operculum of horseshoe-shaped tears (Fig. 8–292,*C*). This mechanism is thought to account for about 30 per cent of retinal tears.

Lattice degeneration with hole formation in the far periphery may simulate an oral dialysis (Fig. 8–293).

Radial Perivascular Lattice Degeneration. This has the same histopathologic features (Parelhoff, Wood, Green, Kenyon, 1980) as lattice degeneration but is usually more extensive, more posterior, and radially oriented, and it may be responsible for a more severe form of retinal detachment. The latter is true because of the association of large retinal tears with posterior locations. There is also more likelihood of RPE changes, with hypertrophy, hyperplasia, and migration into the retina in a perivascular location. Radial perivascular lattice degeneration is probably the same lesion reported as "radial perivascular chorioretinal degeneration" by Hagler, Crosswell (1968).

Figures 8–294 and 8–295 illustrate the gross appearance of radial perivascular lattice degeneration, with retinal thinning, posterior and perivascular location, prominent RPE hypertrophy, hyperplasia, and migration into the retina. Histopathologically, there is inner retinal atrophy, vascular sclerosis, RPE migration, and vitreous attachment at the margin. Trypsin digestion shows sclerosis of the capillary bed and larger vessels and also adherent migrated RPE with excessive basement membrane production (Fig. 8–294,*D,E*). An abrupt transition occurs between the normal capillary bed and the sclerosed capillary bed of the radial perivascular lattice degeneration.

Vitreoretinal Degenerations

In addition to typical and radial perivascular lattice degeneration and congenital retinoschisis

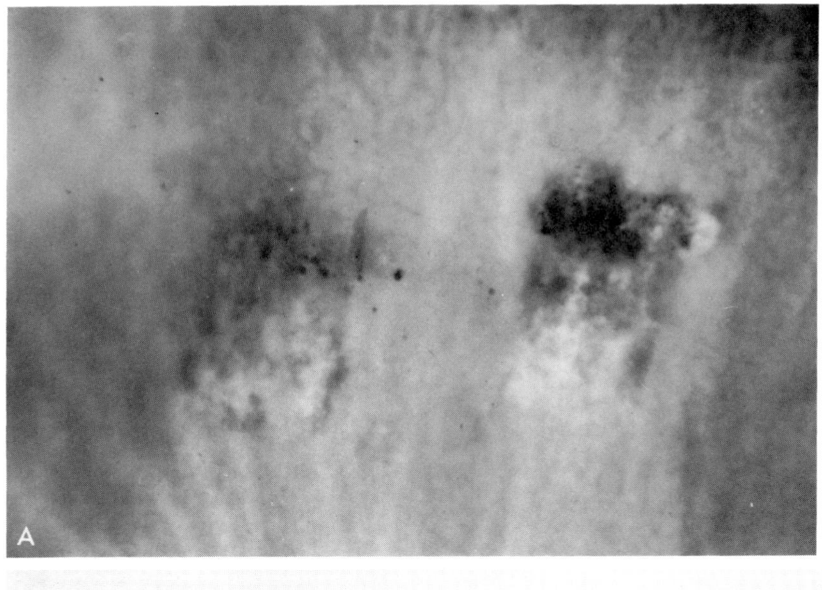

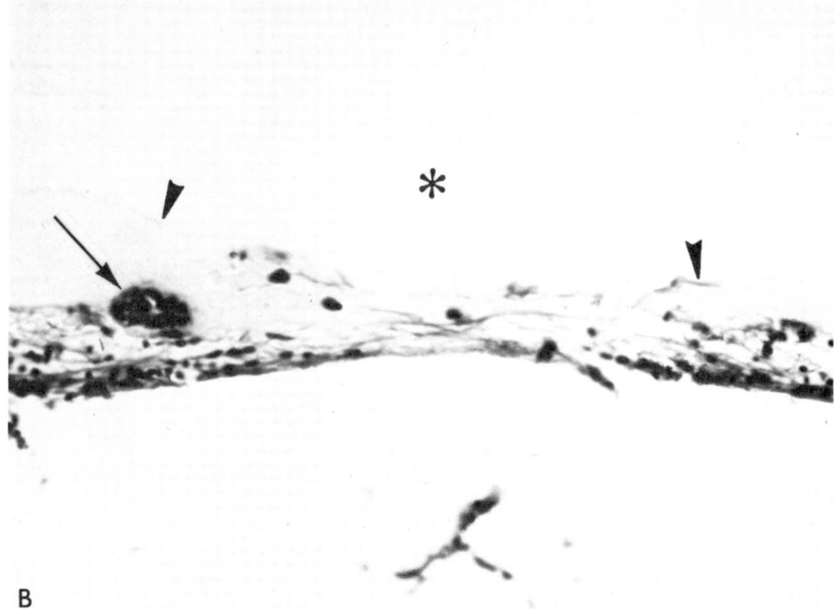

Figure 8–290. *A*, The main gross feature of this area of lattice change is pigmentation. *B*, Features include hyperplastic retinal pigment epithelium in retina (arrow), pocket of fluid vitreous (asterisk), and condensation of vitreous at margins (arrowheads). H and E, ×240. EP 30851.

(discussed elsewhere), there are a number of other vitreoretinal degenerations, some of which have important hereditary features. Histopathologic studies of some of these conditions have not been conducted or have not been done early in the course of the process. As a result, our understanding of the morphologic features is limited.

Snail-Track Degeneration. This is probably a variant of lattice degeneration, but histopathologic studies have not been conducted. The lesions have sharp margins; are white, crinkled, or frosted in appearance; and resemble tracks made by a snail (Gonin, 1904, 1934). Cibis (1965) noted vitreous condensation and adhesion at the margins of the lesion. Aaberg and Stevens (1972) noted the possible hereditary tendency and observed the linear lesions to be parallel to the ora serrata and to be located at the anterior or mid-equatorial area of the superior quadrants, particularly the superotemporal quadrant. Holes that occur within the lesions, as well as holes at the posterior margin of the lesion, and their predisposition to retinal detachment have been observed by all investigators dealing with the subject.

Snowflake Degeneration of the Retina. In 1974, Hirose, Lee, and Schepens described a hereditary vitreoretinal degeneration in 15 members of a family, 5 of whom had retinal detachment. The progressive and probable autosomal dominantly transmitted disease evolved through four stages: extensive white-with-pressure, snowflake degeneration, sheathing of retinal vessels and pigmen-

Text continued on page 876

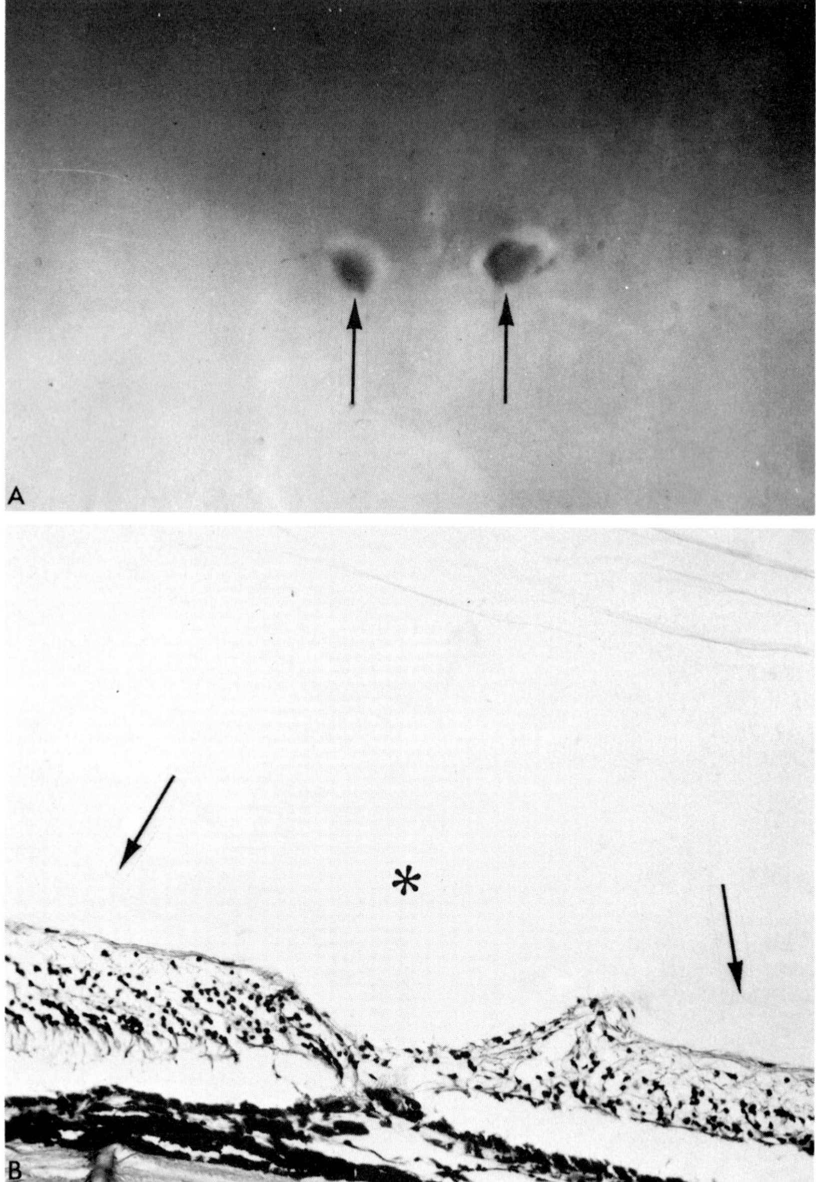

Figure 8–291. *A*, Small areas of lattice degeneration resembling retinal pits (arrows). *B*, Small localized area of retinal thinning and a pocket of fluid vitreous (asterisk). Vitreous at margins of lesion (arrows) is faint. H and E, ×205. EP 30819.

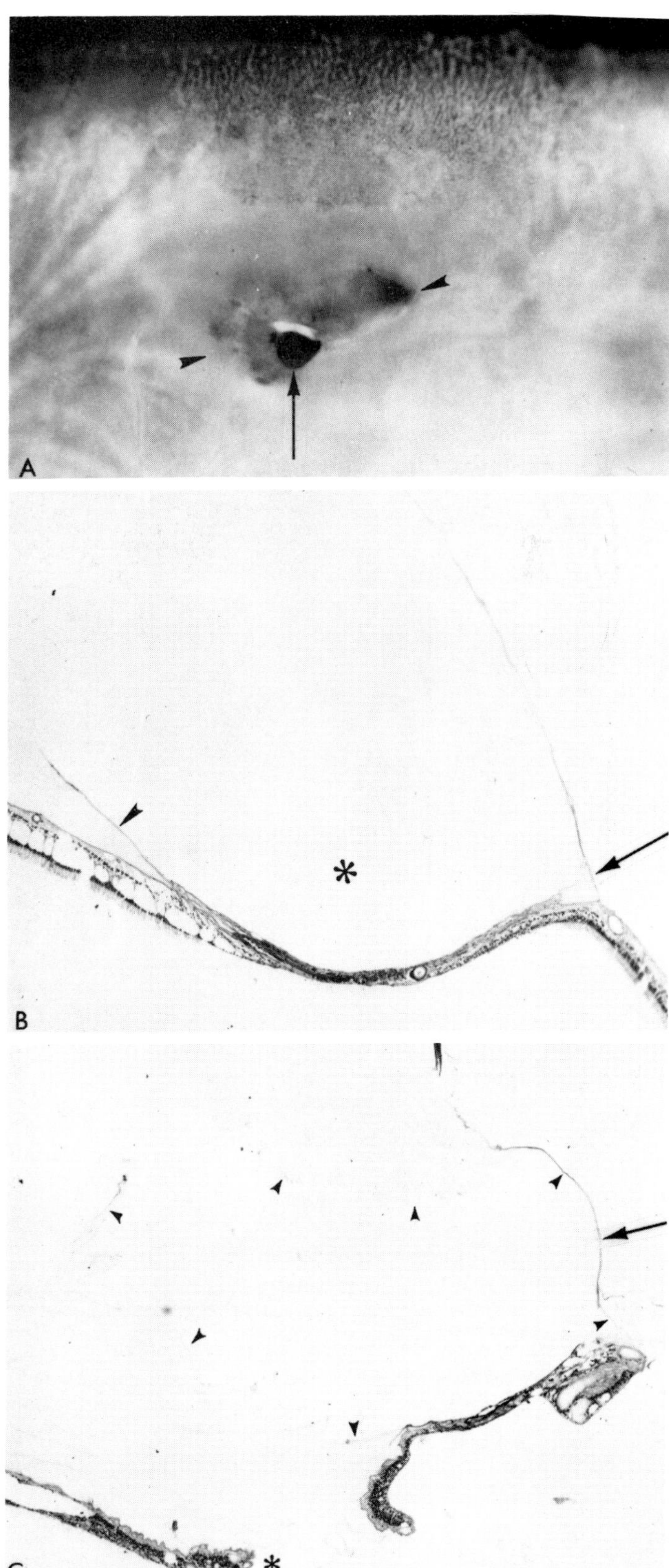

Figure 8–292. Vitreous traction at areas of lattice degeneration. *A*, Gross appearance of retinal tear (arrow) at posterior margin of lattice degeneration (between arrowheads). EP 30775. *B*, Posterior vitreous detachment and traction at posterior margin (arrow) of an area of lattice degeneration. Within area of lattice there is retinal thinning, an overlying pocket of fluid vitreous (asterisk), and condensed vitreous adherent to anterior margin (arrowhead). PAS, ×50. EP 43198. *C*, Lattice degeneration in detached operculum of a retinal tear. There is posterior vitreous detachment (arrow). Features of lattice degeneration in detached operculum include retinal thinning and a pocket of fluid vitreous (outlined by arrowheads). Posterior margin of hole is not included. Anterior margin of hole (asterisk) has rounded margin. PAS, ×45. EP 51566.

A, from Green WR: Pathology of the vitreous, *in* Frayer WC (ed): Lancaster Course in Ophthalmic Histopathology. Unit 8. Philadelphia, F.A. Davis, 1981.)

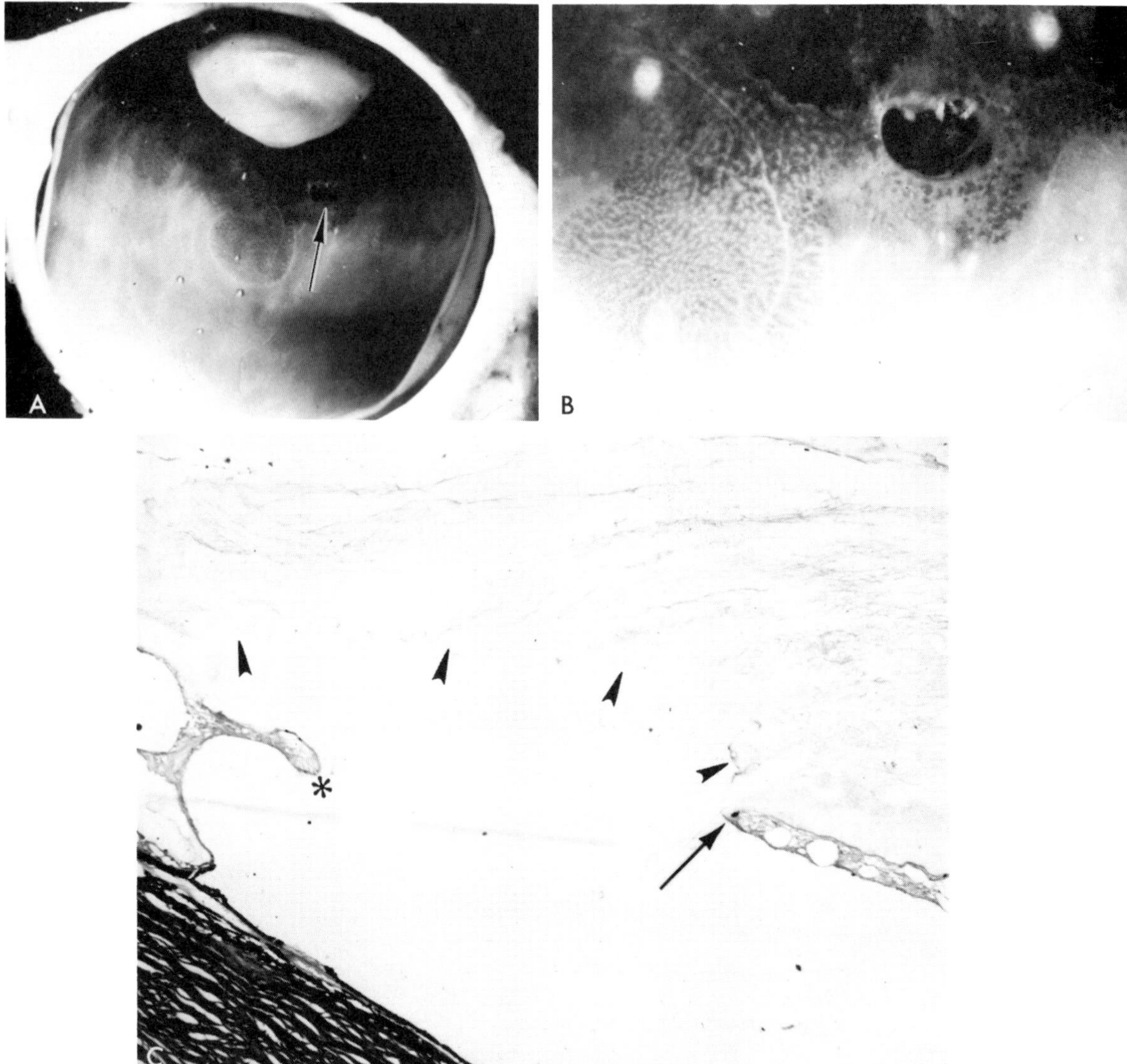

Figure 8–293. *A*, Gross appearance of **hole in lattice degeneration** just posterior to ora serrata, simulating a retinal dialysis (arrow). *B*, Higher power view showing same features. *C*, Anterior (asterisk) and posterior (arrow) margins of hole in lattice degeneration. Pocket of fluid vitreous (outlined by arrowheads) is evident. Colloidal iron, ×35. EP 48037. (From Smiddy WE, Green WR: Retinal dialysis: Pathology and pathogenesis. Retina *2*:94–116, 1982.)

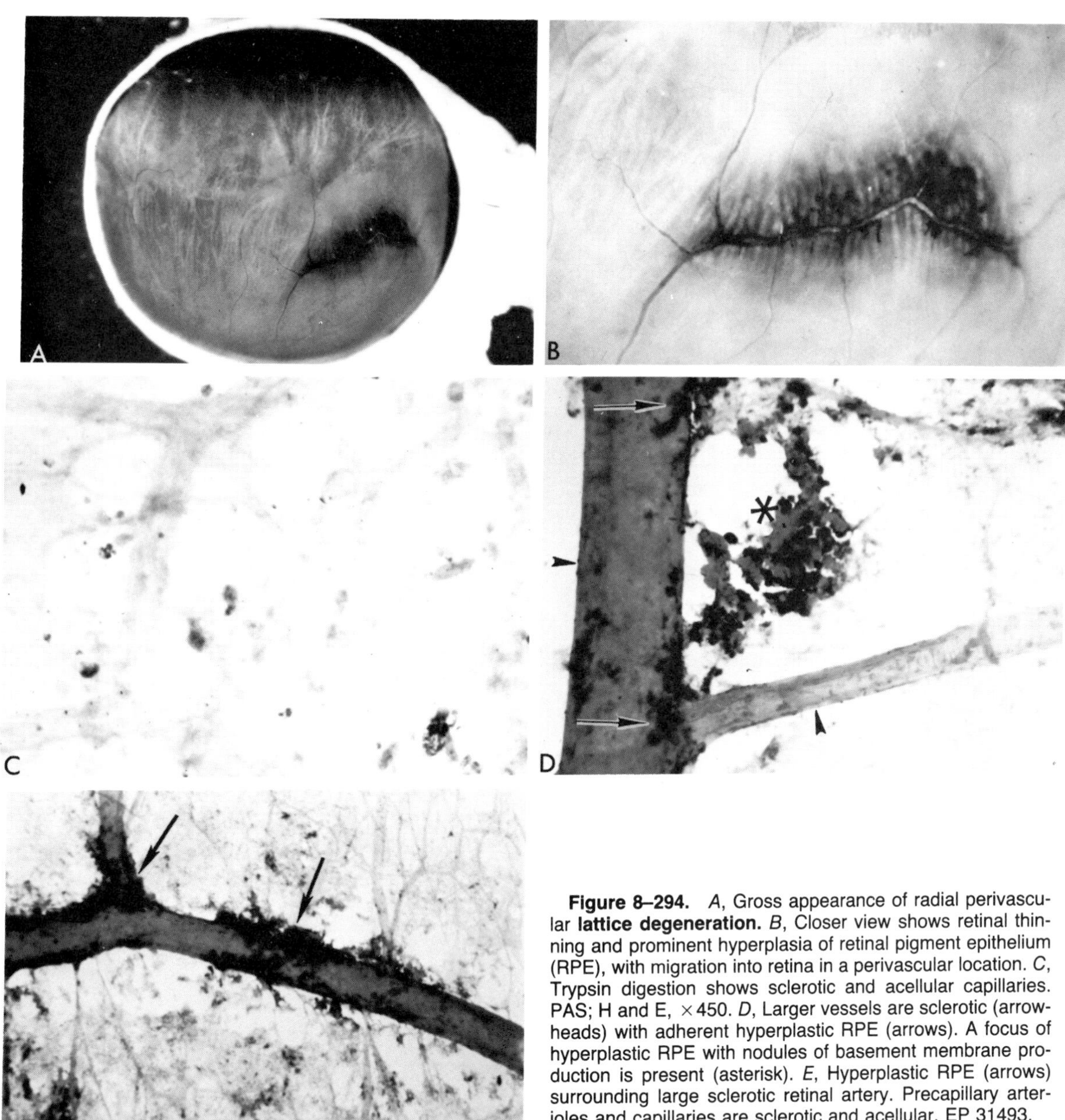

Figure 8–294. *A*, Gross appearance of radial perivascular **lattice degeneration.** *B*, Closer view shows retinal thinning and prominent hyperplasia of retinal pigment epithelium (RPE), with migration into retina in a perivascular location. *C*, Trypsin digestion shows sclerotic and acellular capillaries. PAS; H and E, ×450. *D*, Larger vessels are sclerotic (arrowheads) with adherent hyperplastic RPE (arrows). A focus of hyperplastic RPE with nodules of basement membrane production is present (asterisk). *E*, Hyperplastic RPE (arrows) surrounding large sclerotic retinal artery. Precapillary arterioles and capillaries are sclerotic and acellular. EP 31493.

(From Parelhoff ES, Wood WJ, Green WR, Kenyon KR: Radial perivascular lattice degeneration of retina. Ann Ophthalmol *12*:25–32, 1980.)

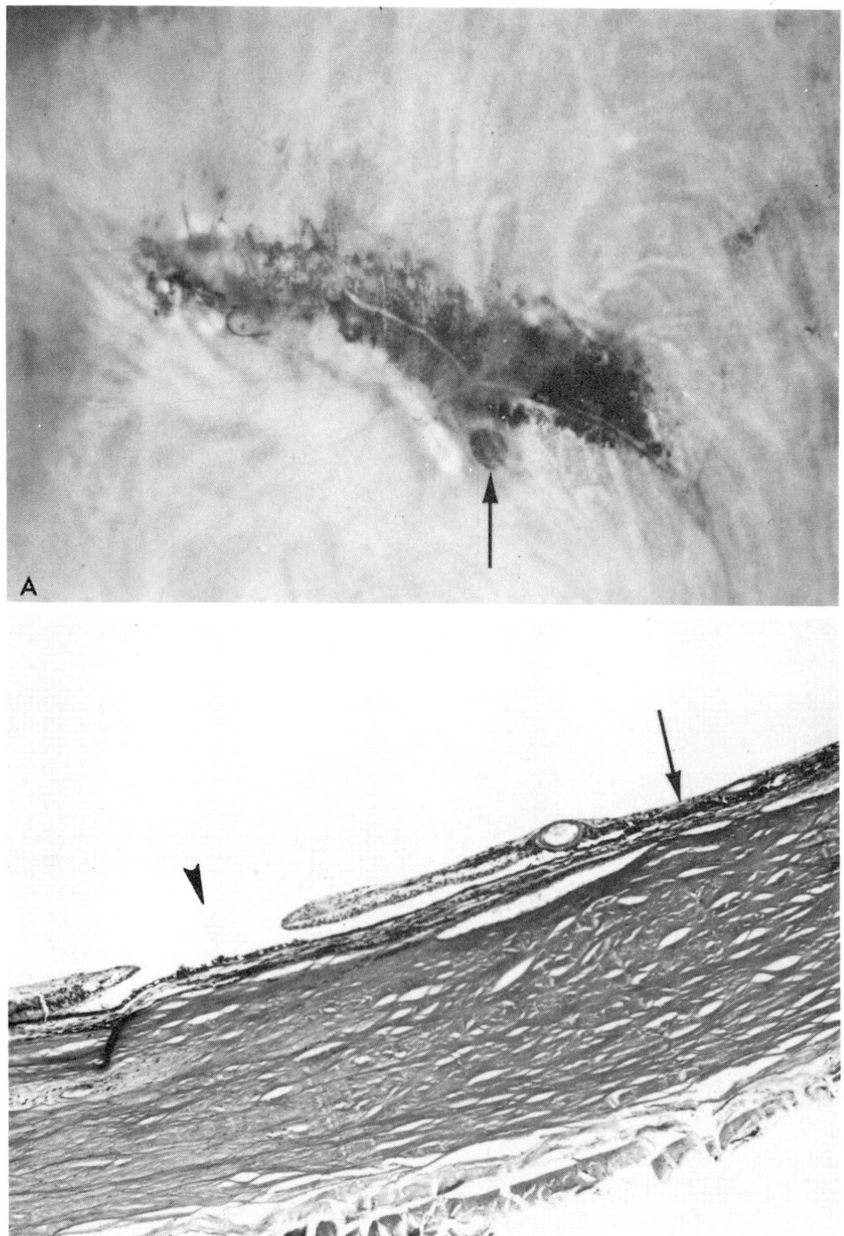

Figure 8–295. *A*, Radial perivascular **lattice with hole at posterior margin** (arrow). *B*, Section of hole (arrowhead) posterior to area of lattice (arrow). Vitreous has apparently detached further anteriorly with no other effects than a small hole. EP 51566.

tation, and increased pigmentation and disappearance of retinal vessels. Fibrillar degeneration of the vitreous was also progressive.

Robertson, Link, and Rostvold (1982) described ten patients in four families with granular-like white or yellow-white deposits that measure 100 to 200 microns in size, are located circumferentially near the equator, and focally thicken the retina. Vitreous liquefaction, vitreoretinal traction, retinal breaks, and retinal pigmentation were not always associated with the lesions. The investigators noted that, in its pure form, snowflake degeneration may be an innocent, dominantly inherited finding. When associated with lattice degeneration, it may be of clinical significance.

No histopathologic studies of this condition have been conducted.

Wagner Disease. Wagner vitreoretinal degeneration is transmitted as an autosomal dominant trait and is characterized by an optically empty vitreous cavity that has occasional vitreous fibers or membranes, narrow and sheathed retinal vessels, pigmented spots in the periphery or along retinal vessels, atrophy of the choroid, cataract, myopia, concentric contraction of the visual fields, reduction of electroretinogram, and optic atrophy in the late stages (Wagner, 1938). Maumenee (1979) and Maumenee, Stoll, and Mets (in press) have pointed out that in the original study by Wagner and in a follow-up study of the same family with additional members, Bohringer, Dieterle and Landolt (1960) found no retinal detachments.

Jansen Disease. Jansen (1962) described 30 affected members of two families that he thought had the vitreoretinal degeneration of Wagner. The appearance of the fundus and vitreous was indistinguishable from that reported by Wagner. Retinal detachment occurred in many patients at an early age and was often bilateral. He also found subnormal responses in the dark-adapted and dark- and light-adapted states. All affected patients had mild-to-moderate myopia, astigmatism, and lens opacities after the age of 10 years. Glaucoma was often present after the age of 30 years. No systemic abnormalities were described. Maumenee (1979) pointed out that similar features, including vitreoretinal degeneration and familial retinal detachments, have been described by others (Alexander, Shea, 1965; Hagler, Crosswell, 1968; Opitz, 1972; Hirose, Lee, Schepens, 1973).

Stickler Syndrome. Stickler, Belau, Farrell, et al (1965) described a progressive, hereditary arthro-ophthalmopathy with autosomal dominant transmission and hereditary retinal detachments. Cleft palate and sensorineural deafness were also present (Stickler, Pugh, 1967). Opitz (1972) and Opitz, France, Hermann, and Spranger (1972) reported additional cases and proposed the eponymic designation.

Additional ocular abnormalities include myopia, chronic simple glaucoma, lens opacities, vitreoretinal degeneration, perivascular pigmentary retinopathy, and retinal detachment. Orofacial abnormalities include midfacial flattening, cleft palate, and the Pierre Robin malformation complex (micrognathia, cleft palate, and glossoptosis).

Skeletal abnormalities include joint hyperextensibility and enlargement, arthritis, and spondyloepiphyseal dysplasia (Schreiner, McAlister, Marshall, et al, 1973; Turner, 1974; Hermann, France, Spranger, et al, 1975; Blair, Albert, Liberfarb, Hirose, 1979; Young, Hitchings, Sehmi, Bird, 1979; Regenbogen, Godel, 1980). Blair, Albert, Liberfarb, and Hirose (1979) also pointed out that some previously reported cases of Wagner disease, familial retinal detachment, hyaloideoretinopathy with cleft palate, and Pierre Robin syndrome probably had the Stickler syndrome.

Ocular histopathologic findings in three patients with advanced Stickler syndrome showed total retinal detachment, disorganization of retina, and periretinal proliferation (Blair, Albert, Liberfarb, Hirose, 1979).

Maumenee (1979) recognized two forms of hereditary arthro-ophthalmopathy: a marfanoid variety (Stickler syndrome) (Popkin, Polomeno, 1974) and the Weil-Marchesani–like variety (Frandsen, 1966).

Goldmann-Favre Disease (Vitreotapetoretinal Dystrophy of Goldmann-Favre). This condition is transmitted as an autosomal recessive trait and is characterized by vitreous degeneration, central and peripheral retinoschisis, lattice-like degeneration, preretinal proliferation, and peripheral pigmentation. There is progressive loss of vision, severe night-blindness, and a depressed or unrecordable electroretinagram (ERG). Complicated cataract occurs, and the dystrophic retinal process progresses to blindness (Goldmann, 1957; Favre, 1958; Ricci, 1960; François, DeRouck, Cambie, 1974). MacVicar and Wilbrandt (1970) observed an unusual angioma-like tumor in an affected man and a possible heterozygous trait in the form of gro·.plike pigmentation in two women.

Fishman, Jampol, and Goldberg (1976) observed peripheral vascular occlusion, retinal vascular imcompetence, and cystoid macular edema in three patients from two families with the Goldmann-Favre syndrome. Two patients also showed a discrepancy on ERG between single-flash photopic amplitudes and flicker-fusion frequency.

In a histopathologic study of an eye-wall biopsy from a patient with the Goldmann-Favre syndrome, Peyman, Fishman, Sanders, et al (1977) observed diffuse degenerative changes of the sensory retinal layers, relatively normal RPE and choroid, sclerosis and occlusion of retinal vessels, and a preretinal membrane.

Familial Exudative Vitreoretinopathy. Criswick and Schepens (1969) described a disease that resembled retrolental fibroplasia, with a familial incidence, and characterized by a slowly progressive vitreoretinal process with exudation and retinal detachment. Gow and Oliver (1971) noted an autosomal dominant inheritance and identified three stages. Stage 1 was notable for posterior vitreous detachment, vitreous traction on the retina, and vitreous membranes. Stage 2 was characterized by abnormal, tortuous retinal veins in the temporal periphery. These tortuous veins were continuous with large caliber veins that extended to, and ran parallel to, the ora serrata. There was subretinal lipid-rich exudation and subretinal and intraretinal fibrovascular proliferation. Condensation of the overlying vitreous was present. There appeared to be organization of the exudate and fibrovascular tissue, with traction on the retina that resulted in dragging of the disk and macula. The third stage was characterized by long-standing retinal detachment, secondary cataract, band keratopathy, iris atrophy, posterior synechiae, secondary glaucoma, and blindness.

Fluorescein angiography has demonstrated closure of peripheral retinal vasculature and elevated temporal fibrovascular tissue (Canny, Oliver, 1976). Ober, Bird, Hamilton, et al (1980) noted that there is great variability in the phenotypic expression of the defect and that patients with mild disease may be detected with certainty only by fluorescein angiography (Swanson, Rush, Bird, 1982).

Slusher and Hutton (1979) noted that an advanced stage of the disease can occur at an early age.

Gitter, Rothschild, Waltman, et al (1978) described a similar familial condition. These investigators observed dominantly inherited peripheral retinal neovascularization. The condition was characterized by arteriolar ischemia, retinal neovascularization in the periphery, hemorrhage, and retinal detachment. A wide spectrum of the disease process was noted.

Brockhurst, Albert, and Zakov (1981) studied the histopathologic features of two eyes from two patients with end-stage disease. They observed total retinal detachment, periretinal proliferation, and dense vitreous bands.

Autosomal Dominant Vitreoretinochoroidopathy. Kaufmann, Goldberg, Orth, et al (1982) have described an autosomal dominant vitreoretinochoroidopathy that is apparently distinct from previously described vitreoretinopathies. This condition is characterized by abnormal chorioretinal hypopigmentation and hyperpigmentation, usually between the vortex veins and the ora serrata for 360 degrees. The posterior border of this zone is discrete. Preretinal punctate opacities, retinal arteriolar narrowing and occlusion, and (in some cases) choroidal atrophy are present in this zone. Most of the affected patients have diffuse retinal vascular leakage, cystoid macular edema, and presenile cataracts. The vitreous shows fibrillar condensation and a moderate number of cells. The ERG is normal in younger affected persons and is only moderately abnormal in older patients. Retinal neovascularization was present in the proband. None of the patients had systemic or skeletal abnormalities, high myopia, optically empty vitreous, lattice degeneration, areas of white-without-pressure, retinal breaks, or retinal detachments.

Autosomal Recessive Vitreoretinopathy and Encephaloceles. Knobloch and Layer (1971) and Cook and Knobloch (1982) have described 5 affected individuals of a 26 member pedigree with recessively inherited encephaloceles, severe myopia, and vitreoretinal degeneration. This syndrome apears to be distinct from the other vitreoretinopathies reported.

Maumenee (1979) has stressed vitreoretinal degeneration as a sign of generalized connective tissue disease. She has proposed a classification based on two groups. Group I consists of only ocular lesions and no systemic manifestations. There are two types in Group I: Type 1, with no associated retinal detachment (Wagner disease); and Type 2, with a high incidence of retinal detachment (Jansen disease).

Group II includes those cases of vitreoretinopathy with associated systemic anomalies. These include Type 1, hereditary arthro-ophthalmopathy, marfanoid variety (Stickler disease); Type 2, hereditary arthro-ophthalmopathy with stiff joints (Weill-Marchesani–like variety); Type 3, spondyloepiphyseal dysplasia variant; Type 4, Kniest syndrome; Type 5, diastrophic variant; and Type 6, spondyloepiphyseal dysplasia congenita (Hamidi-Toosi, Maumenee, 1982).

Retinal Pits

In the process of detaching posteriorly, the vitreous may pull small areas of the inner retinal

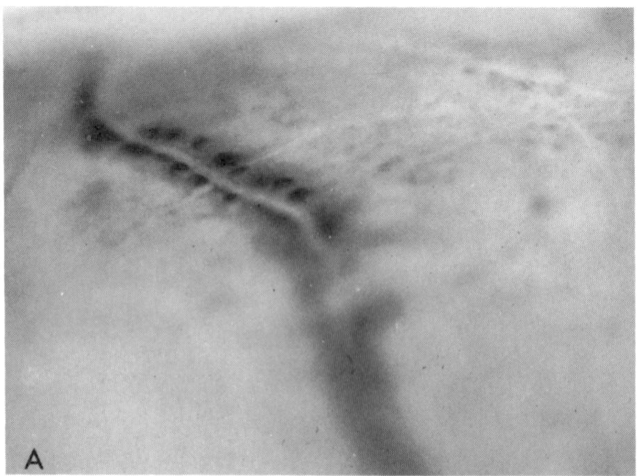

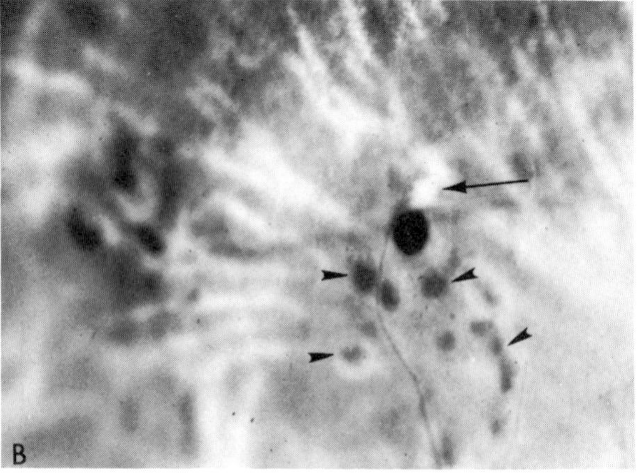

Figure 8–296. *A*, **Retinal pits** along either side of a major retinal vessel. EP 31030. *B*, As vitreous detached in this eye, it apparently produced retinal pits along the retinal vessel (arrowheads) and, more anteriorly, a horseshoe-shaped retinal tear (arrow). EP 30448. (From Green WR: Pathology of the vitreous, *in* Frayer WC (ed): Lancaster Course in Ophthalmic Histopathology. Unit 8. Philadelphia, F.A. Davis, 1981.)

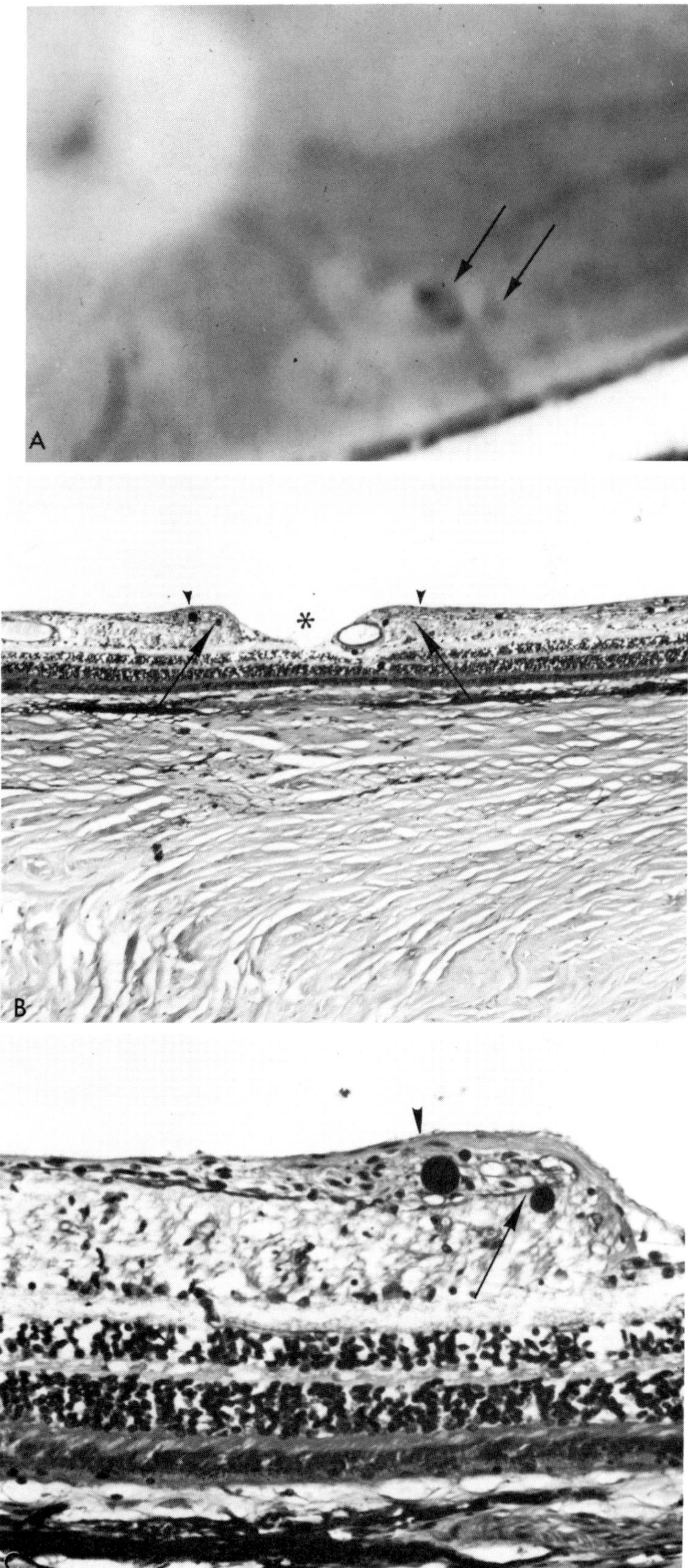

Figure 8–297. *A,* **Retinal pits** (arrows) near optic nerve head. *B,* Pit (asterisk) is adjacent to a retinal artery. The internal limiting membrane (ILM) is absent (between arrows) along with inner retinal layers. Glial cells extend onto the inner surface of the retina to form a preretinal membrane. PAS, ×75. *C,* Margin of pit showing discontinuity of the ILM (arrow) and a glial cell preretinal membrane (arrowhead). PAS, ×185. EP 30738. (From Clarkson JG, Green WR, Massof D: A histopathologic review of 168 cases of preretinal membrane. Am J Ophthalmol *84*:1–17, 1977.)

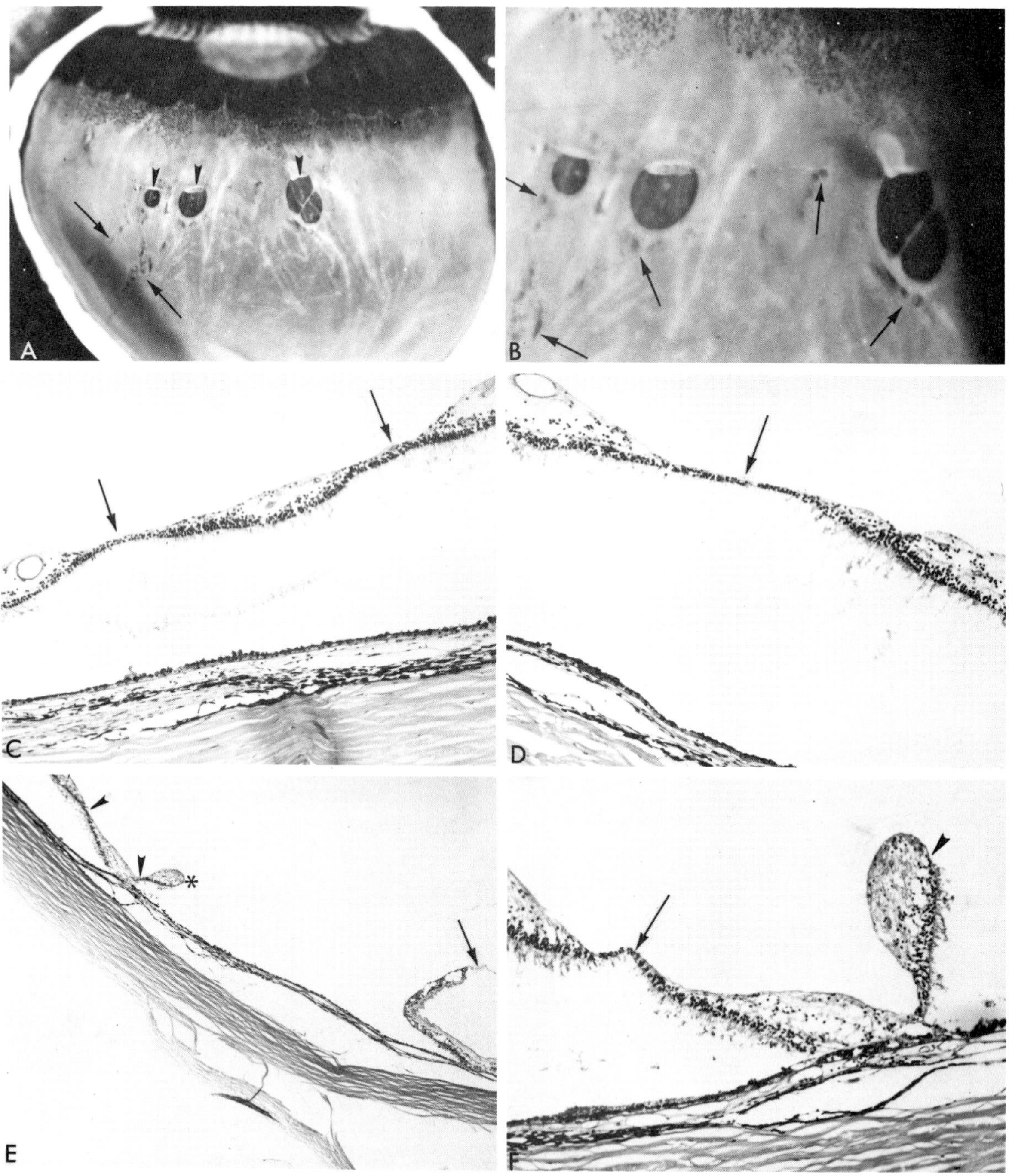

Figure 8–298. Retinal pits and tears. *A*, Gross appearance of eye with posterior vitreous detachment, a string of retinal pits along vessels (arrows), and three horseshoe-shaped retinal tears (arrowheads). *B*, Closer view shows pits (arrows) and horseshoe tears. *C*, Appearance of two pits (arrows). PAS, ×120. *D*, Higher power view shows only remnants of the outer nuclear layer in the area of a pit (arrows), PAS, ×115. *E*, Area of a horseshoe tear. Posteriorly detached vitreous is adherent to the posterior margin of the retinal flap (arrow). The posterior margin of the hole has a rounded margin (asterisk), and two pits (arrowheads) are just posterior to the hole. PAS, ×35. *F*, Higher power view of the posterior margin of the hole (arrowhead) and retinal pit (arrow). PAS, ×130. EP 42238.

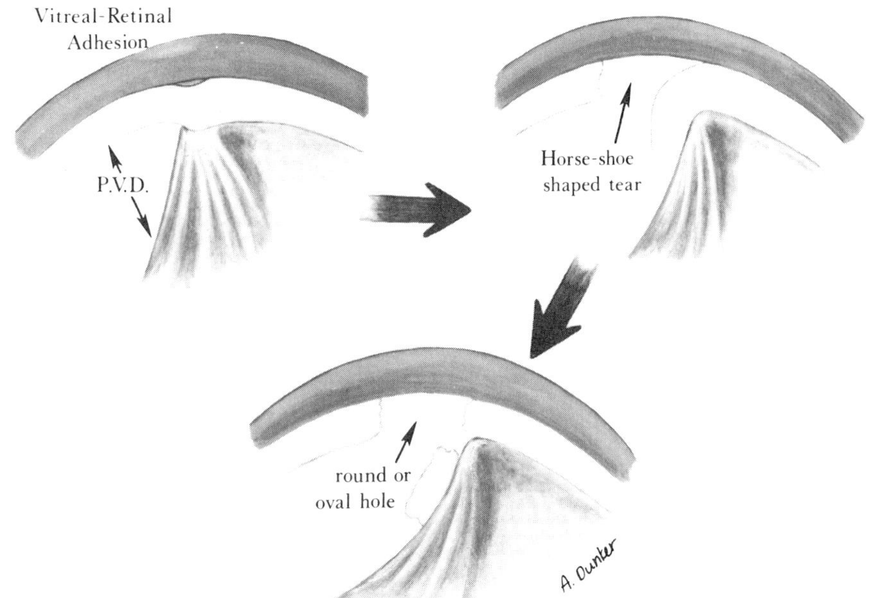

Figure 8–299. Mechanism of retinal tear formation with posterior vitreous detachment (PVD); retinal traction occurs at a point of firmer vitreoretinal attachment, causing a tenting-up of retina. With further traction, a horseshoe tear occurs. With still further traction, the operculum may be detached, leaving a round or oval hole. (Modified after Okun E: Retinal detachment. JAMA *174*:2218–2220, 1960.)

layers away, leaving one or more pits (Fig. 8–296) (Meyer, Kurz, 1963). These may occur at any point but usually are present along the major retinal vessels, which suggests that the vitreoretinal attachment is somewhat firmer here than elsewhere. The clinical importance of retinal pits is that they are a sign of posterior vitreous detachment and vitreous traction, and they can be the site at which glial cells grow internally and form preretinal membranes (Fig. 8–297) (Clarkson, Green, Massof, 1977). Figures 8–296,*B* and 8–298 illustrate eyes with posterior vitreous detachment, a series of retinal pits, and one or more horseshoe-shaped retinal tears.

Wolter (1964) and Foos (1974b) have shown naturally occurring areas of attenuation or discontinuity of the retinal internal limiting membrane over major retinal vessels. Spencer and Foos (1970) have observed further that vitreous herniation and incarceration may occur at those points of discontinuity. These findings explain why, with posterior vitreous detachment, pinpoint traction can occur and thus predispose to the development of retinal pits and retinal tears (Foos, 1978).

Retinal Holes and Tears

Most retinal tears occur from vitreous traction. The mechanism of retinal tear formation is illustrated by the drawings in Figure 8–299, modified from Okun (1960). When an area of vitreous detaches posteriorly and reaches a point of firmer vitreoretinal attachment, the following may occur: (a) it may pull on the retina, producing a tear; if the pulled-out portion of the retina re-

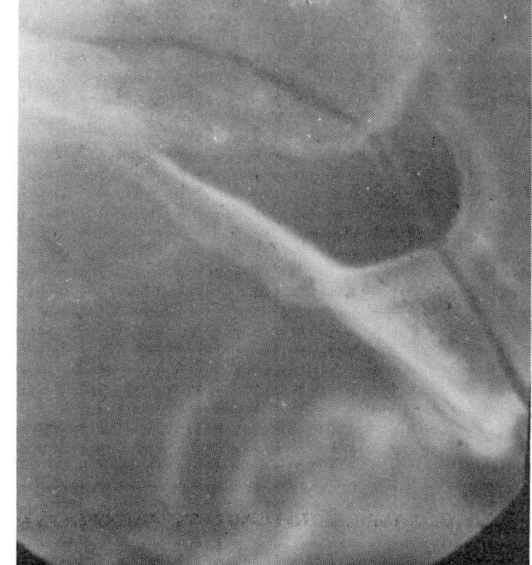

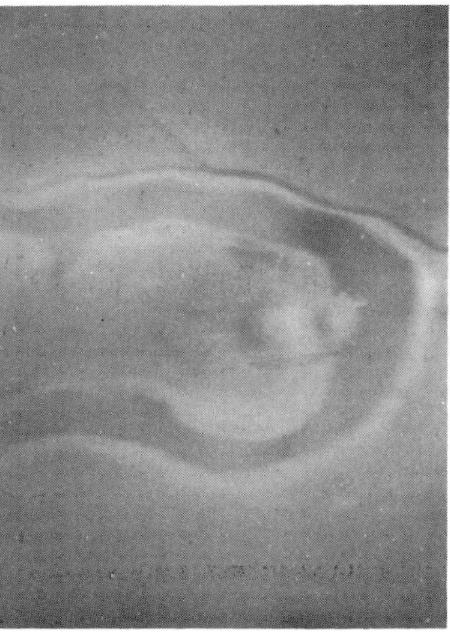

Figure 8–300. Horseshoe-shaped tears associated with retinal vessels. A retinal vessel bridges the tear on the left. Horseshoe tear on right is near a major retinal vessel. With such features, it is understandable how vitreous hemorrhage may occur with retinal tears. (Left photo, courtesy of Dr. Edward W.D. Norton.)

mains partially attached, the hole has a "horseshoe" configuration, with the open end of the horseshoe located anteriorly (Figs. 8–300 and 8–301); (b) if a full-thickness portion of retina is pulled entirely away, a round or oval hole is left; or (c) the detached operculum may sometimes be visible clinically, attached to the posterior aspect of the detached vitreous (Figs. 8–302 and 8–303). With time, the operculum may disappear (Fig. 8–304). Some retinal tears have a small area of surrounding retinal detachment delineated by a demarcation line (Figs. 8–305 and 8–306).

The occurrence of retinal tears varies among reported studies. In a study of eyes obtained post mortem, Okun (1961a) found an overall prevalence of 4.8 per cent for all ages combined. Seven per cent of eyes from persons over the age of 40 years had retinal breaks. Most of these breaks were either horseshoe-shaped or were round without an operculum. Round holes with an operculum and holes in cases of "retinal degeneration," were less frequently observed.

In another study of autopsy eyes, Foos and Allen (1967) found that 10.5 per cent had either retinal tears or holes, as distinguished by the shape of the retinal discontinuity.

Clinical investigators also have reported a variable prevalence of retinal breaks. Byer (1967) found an occurrence of retinal breaks in 5.8 per cent of 1700 patients. Rutnin and Schepens (1967b) reported a 13.73 per cent prevalence of retinal breaks in normal subjects. Friedman, Neumann and Hyams (1973) reported a 13.5 per cent incidence of retinal holes in a study of 200 nonmyopic aphakic eyes. In a survey of an entire Maryland community, retinal breaks were seen in fewer than 1 per cent of the population (Smith, Ganley, 1972).

Although the role of retinal breaks as a factor in the pathogenesis of retinal detachment is undisputed, the significance of finding a retinal break in a patient may not always be entirely clear. However, some information is available. Byer (1974b) observed a series of 162 retinal breaks in 125 phakic, non-"fellow" eyes in patients without treatment for from 3 to 9 years. None of the breaks progressed to clinical retinal detachment. He concluded that the presence or absence of symptoms in association with the retinal break is the most important prognostic criterion. He recommended prophylactic therapy only in cases of symptomatic breaks.

In another clinical study, Davis (1974) observed 166 eyes with retinal breaks, with follow-up for from 6 months to 16 years. He noted progression was greater under certain circum-

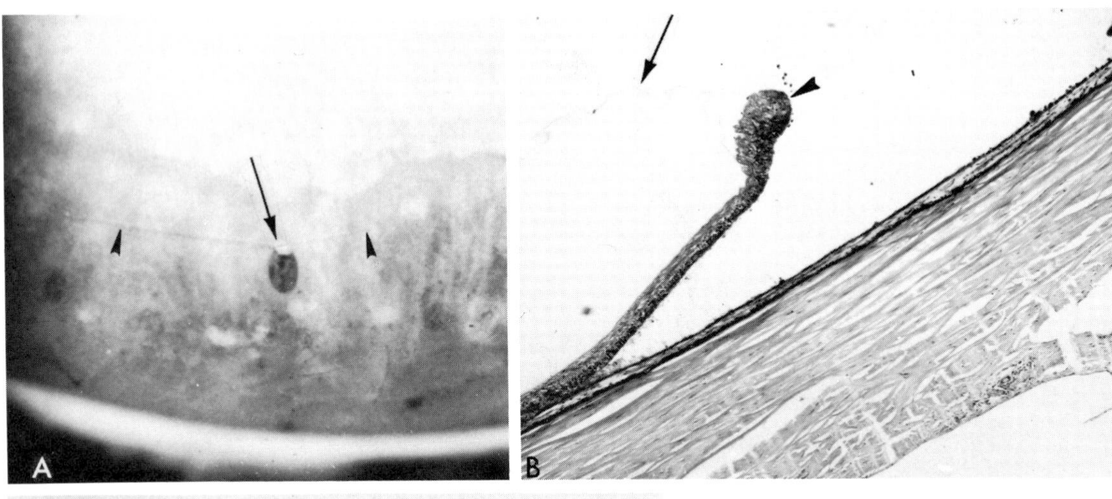

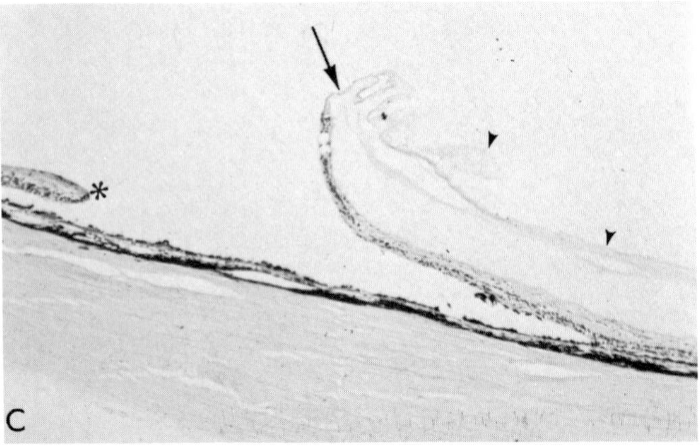

Figure 8–301. *A*, Posterior vitreous detachment (arrowheads) with attachment to and traction on operculum (arrow) of a **horseshoe-shaped retinal tear.** *B*, Section of same case shows vitreous (arrow) attached to posterior aspect of operculum (arrowhead). H and E, ×60. EP 51857. Horseshoe-shaped retinal tear with vitreous (arrowheads) attached to posterior margin of operculum (arrow) and a rounded edge of posterior margin of tear (asterisk). H and E, ×35. EP 30448.

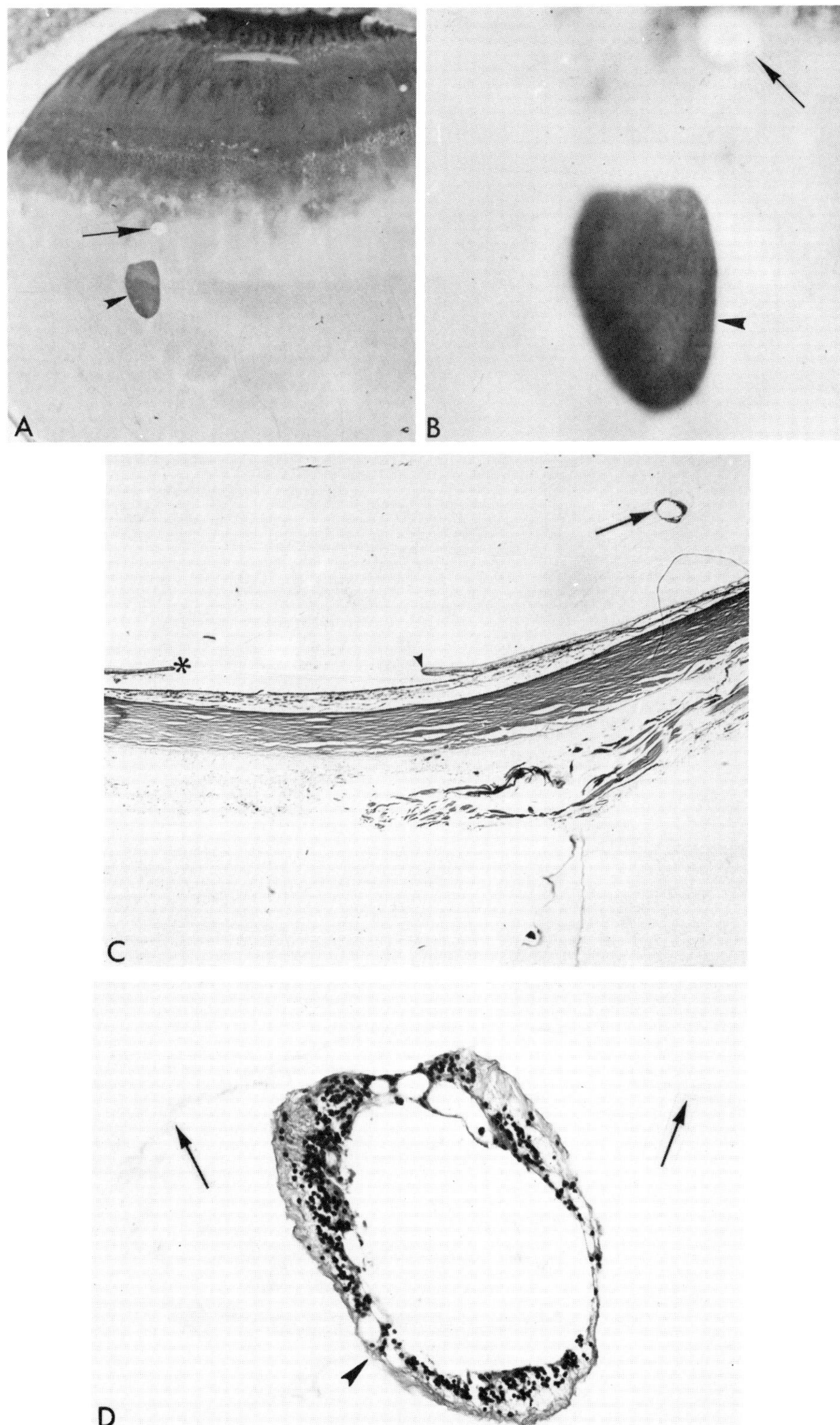

Figure 8–302. *A*, Gross appearance of a **retinal tear** (arrowhead) **with a detached operculum** (arrow). *B*, Higher power view showing retinal tear (arrowhead) and detached operculum (arrowhead). *C*, Microscopic features include rounded anterior (arrowhead) and posterior (asterisk) margins of the hole and coiled-up, detached operculum (arrow) that remains attached to the posterior surface of the detached vitreous. PAS, ×16. *D*, Coiled-up fragment of detached operculum (arrowhead) attached to the posterior surface (arrows) of detached vitreous. PAS, ×210. EP 34238. From Green WR: Pathology of the vitreous, *in* Frayer WC (ed): Lancaster Course in Ophthalmic Histopathology. Unit 8. Philadelphia, F.A. Davis, 1981.)

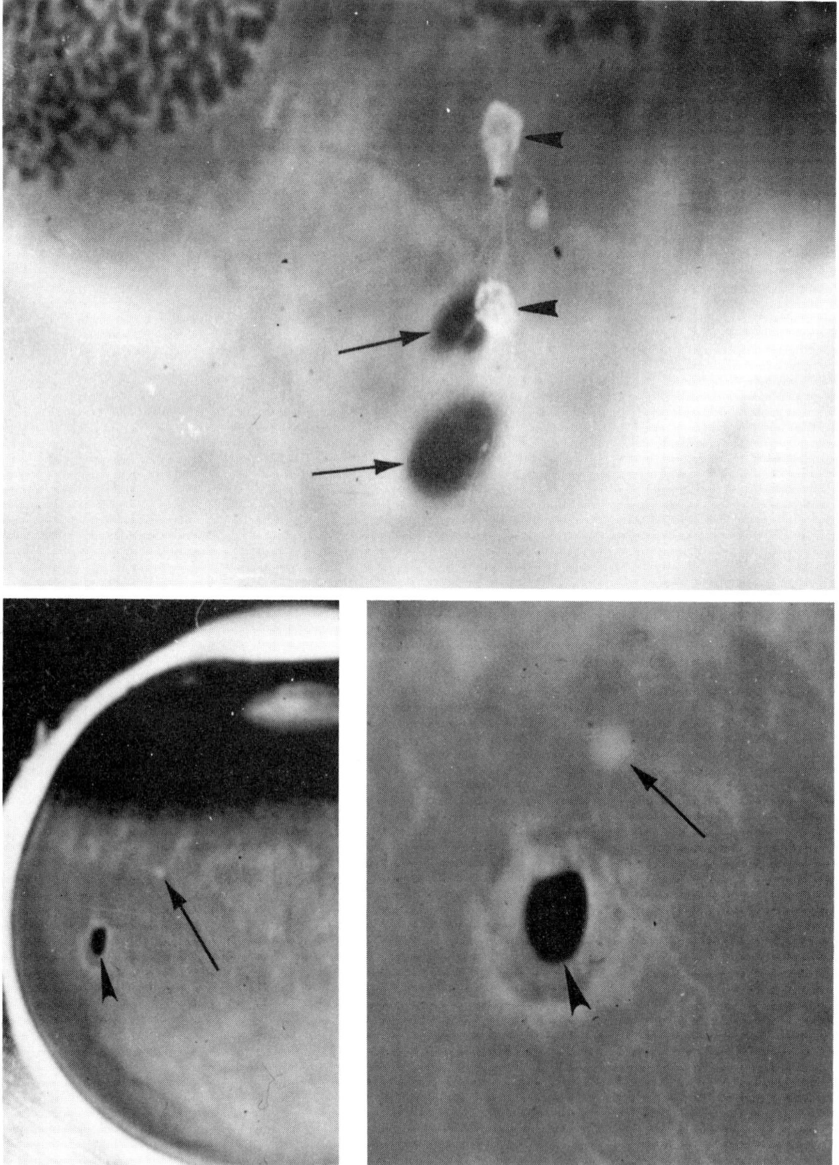

Figure 8–303. *A*, Two **retinal tears** (arrows) almost in same meridian with detached operculum (arrowheads). EP 31736. *B*, Oval retinal tear (arrowhead) with detached operculum (arrow). EP 34584.

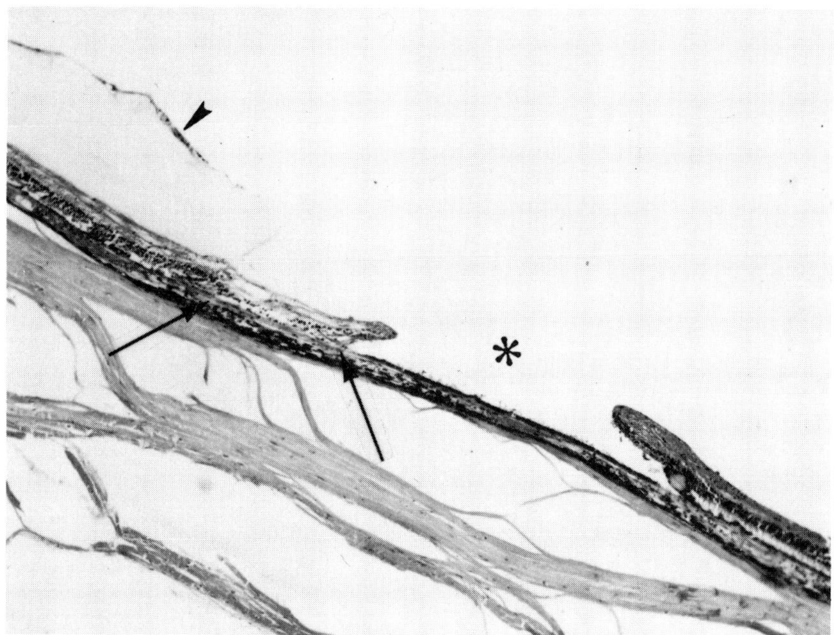

Figure 8–304. Retinal tear (asterisk) with rounded margins. Vitreous is detached anterior to the tear and has residual tissue of operculum (arrowhead) adherent to the posterior surface of vitreous. Cobblestone lesion (arrows) at the anterior margin of the tear possibly prevented formation of a larger tear. H and E, × 45. EP 30448.

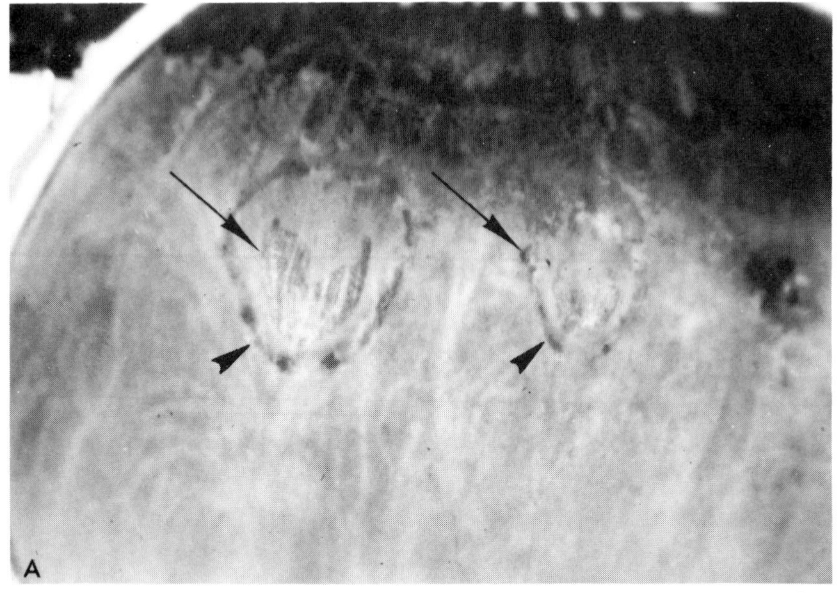

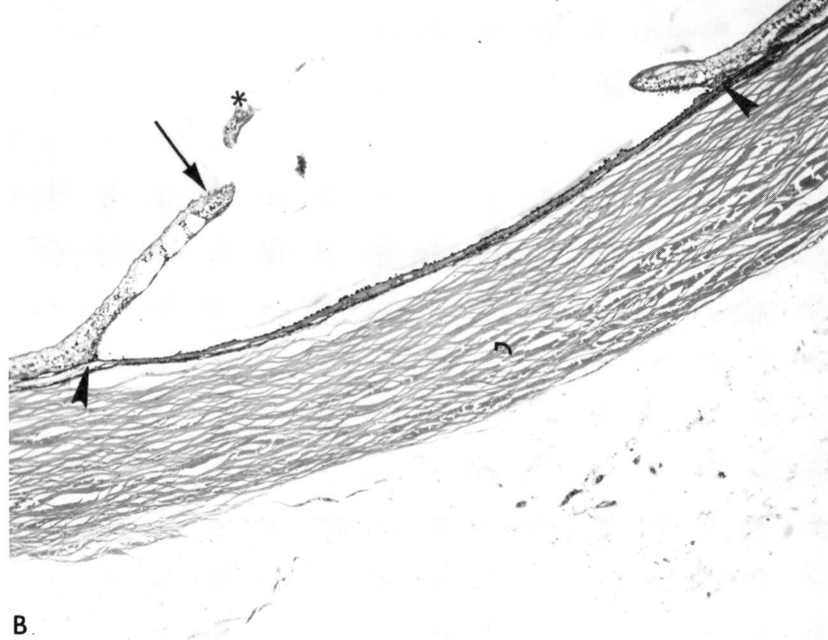

Figure 8–305. *A,* Two **horseshoe-shaped retinal tears** (arrows), with a small area of surrounding retinal detachment delineated by a pigmented demarcation line (arrowheads). *B,* Section through one of these tears shows posterior margin of hole, anterior flap (arrow), demarcation line (arrowheads), and a small fragment of torn-away operculum (asterisk). H and E, ×30. EP 42112.

stances: (1) fresh, symptomatic horseshoe-shaped tear; (2) breaks with subclinical detachment; and (3) aphakic eyes. Progression in eyes containing asymptomatic horseshoe-shaped tears was unusual (5 to 10 per cent).

Retinal holes in the far retinal periphery (between the anterior aspect of the equator and the ora serrata) were observed in 2.4 per cent of a large autopsy series (Foos, 1978). Of these, 0.1 per cent were holes with no apparent cause or associated features. The remaining 2.3 per cent were associated with lattice degeneration most commonly, then zonular traction tufts, chorioretinitis, meridional folds, and pavingstone degeneration.

Macular holes are discussed elsewhere (page 991).

Retinal Dialysis. Retinal dialysis is a tear of the retina from its insertion at the ora serrata. Microscopically, the key features are a separation of the retina from its attachments to the RPE and nonpigmented ciliary epithelium (see Fig. 8–204). Retinal dialysis is part of a dynamic process, as there are several features that appear to be secondary to the dialysis. A demarcation, recognized clinically as representing a reparative process, represents hyperplastic RPE cells and some degree of chorioretinal adhesion delimiting the posterior detachment margin (Fig. 8–307,*A*). Other secondary changes may include photore-

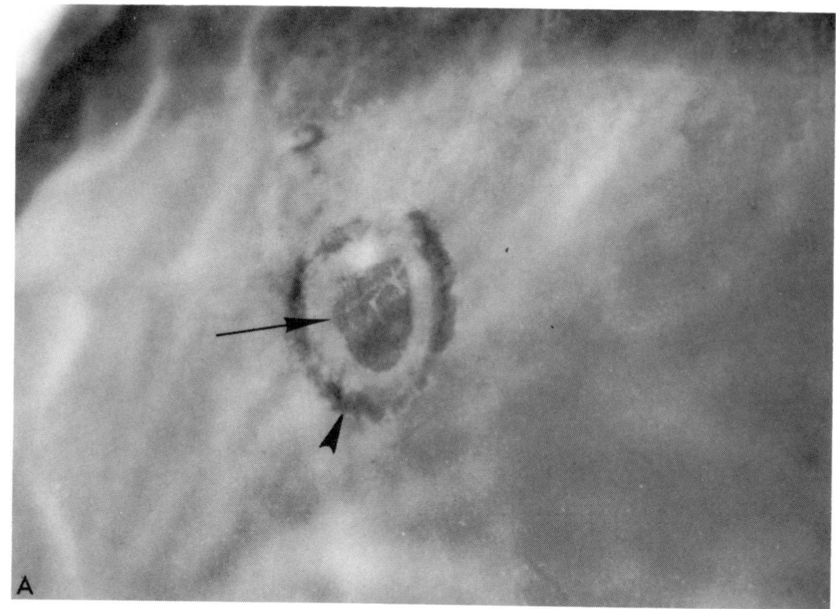

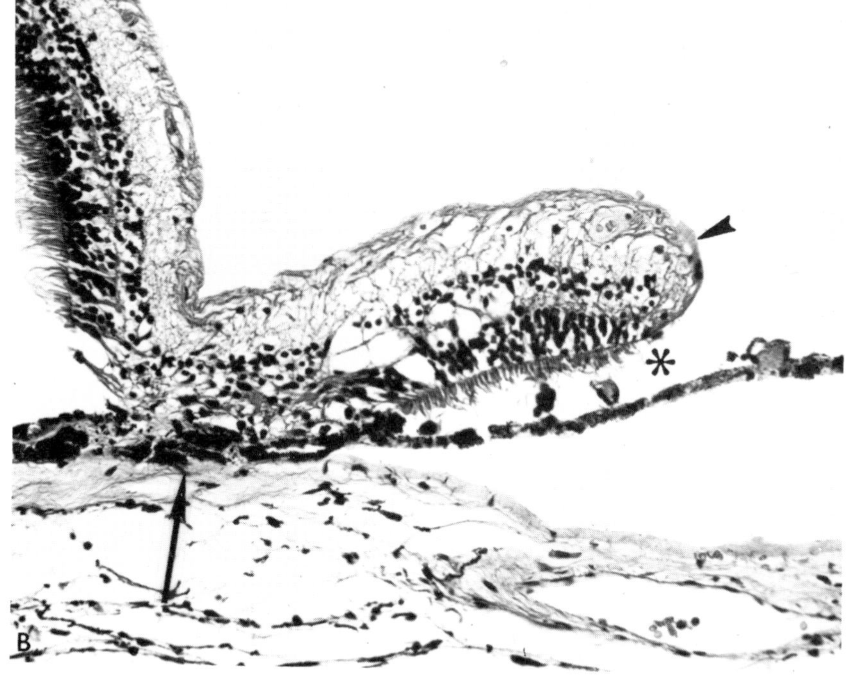

Figure 8–306. *A,* **Horseshoe-shaped retinal tear** (arrow), with small, surrounding area of retinal detachment delineated by a pigmented demarcation line (arrowhead). *B,* Section shows rounded posterior margin of tear (arrowhead) and area of retinal detachment (asterisk); demarcation line (arrow) is a point of chorioretinal adhesion with retinal pigment epithelium hyperplasia. H and E, ×220. EP 49625.

ceptor cell degeneration, RPE migration onto the inner retinal surface, vitreous herniation under the dialysis margin, hyperplastic ciliary epithelium, minor choroidal neovascularization, and drusen formation (Figs. 8–307,*A* and 8–307,*B*).

In a histopathologic review of 103 cases of retinal dialysis, Smiddy and Green (1982) defined five major etiologic groups: penetrating trauma, blunt trauma, idiopathic, inflammatory induced, and surgically induced. Penetrating trauma was the most common cause. The dialysis was frequently a secondary feature in these cases (Fig. 8–307,*C*). In the second group of cases, there was blunt trauma without ocular rupture or penetration (see Fig. 8–204). The third group of cases had no history or histopathologic evidence of trauma (Fig. 8–307,*A*), was occasionally bilateral (Fig. 8–307,*D* and *E,* and, in two cases, was associated with lattice degeneration in the far periphery of the retina (Fig. 8–307,*F*). In the fourth group of ases, the dialysis followed ocular inflammation (Fig. 8–307,*G*). The final group included those with dialyses that occurred after intraocular surgery (Fig. 8–307,*H*). In the surgical group, trauma may also be a factor. The findings suggest that although trauma is the most common cause

Text continued on page 893

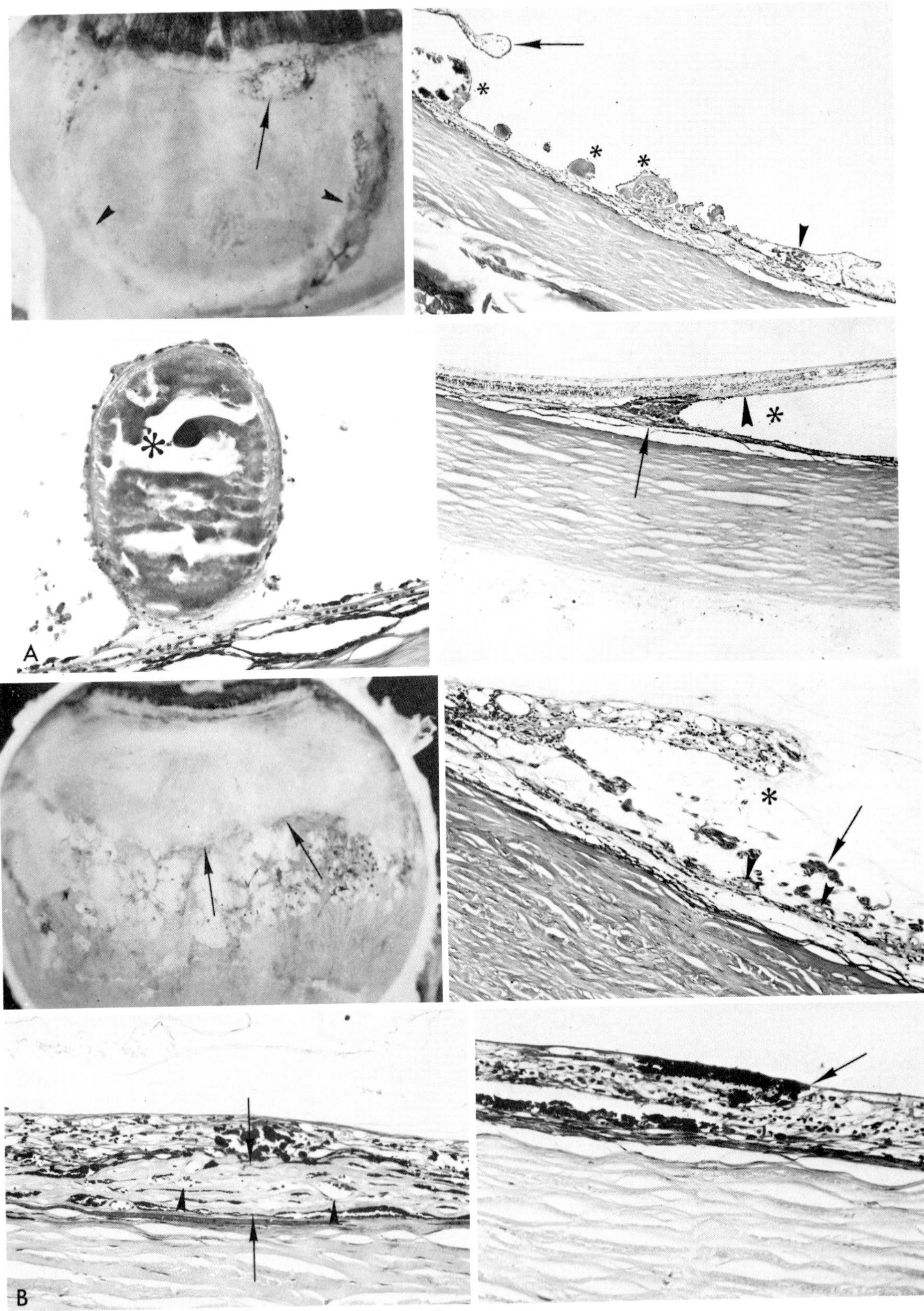

Figure 8–307 *See legend on opposite page*

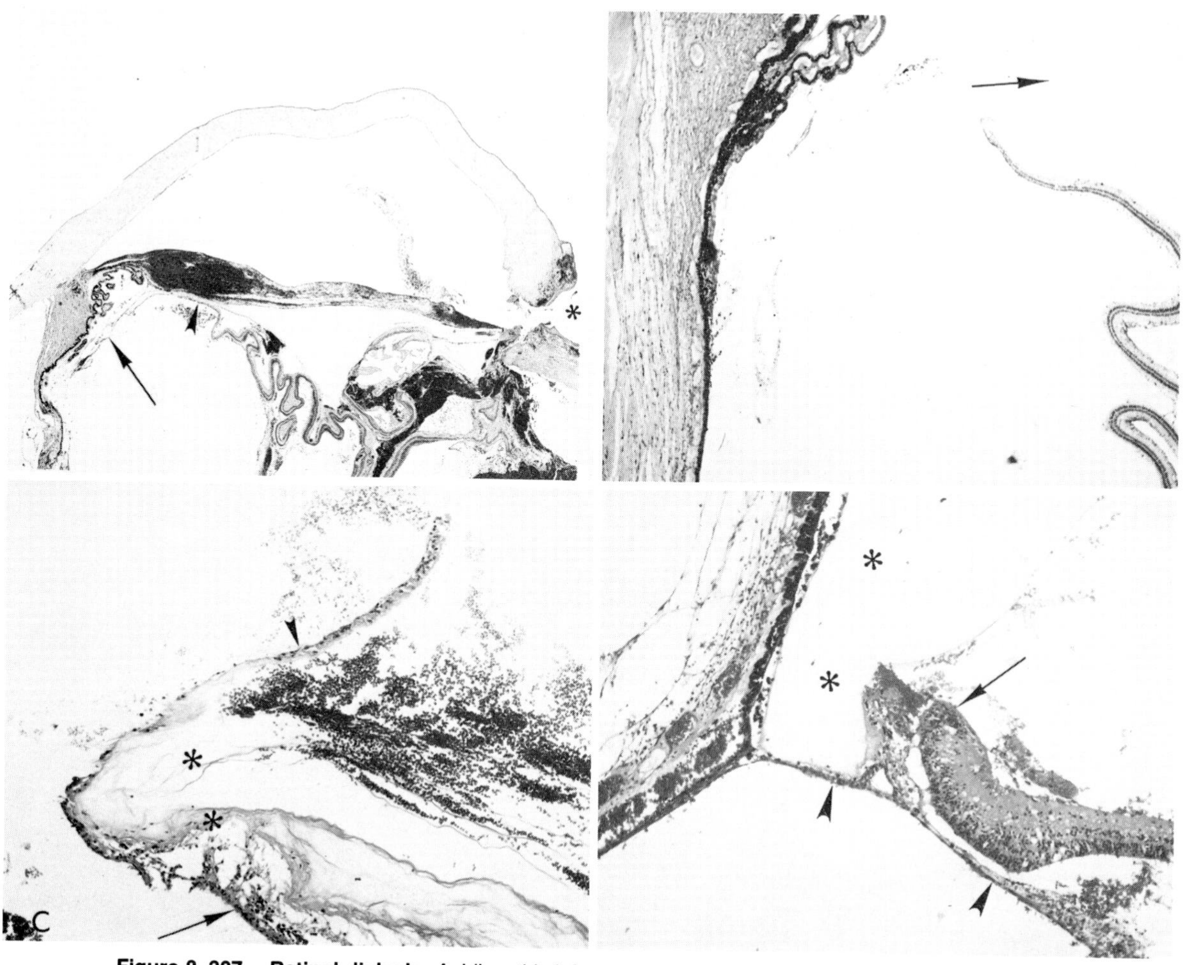

Figure 8–307. Retinal dialysis. *A,* Idiopathic inferotemporal retinal dialysis with chronic localized retinal detachment with demarcation line in post-mortem eye of a 66 year old man. Top left, gross appearance of dialysis (arrow) and demarcation line (arrowheads). Top right, area showing margin of dialyzed retina (arrow), large drusen formation (asterisks), and hyperplasia of nonpigmented ciliary epithelium (arrowhead). H and E, ×35. Bottom left, higher power view of large druse (asterisk) that has a laminated appearance and is covered by attenuated and depigmented retinal pigment epithelium (RPE). PAS, ×280. Bottom right, area of demarcation line (arrow), with local hyperplasia of the RPE and adhesion of the retina. Anteriorly, retina is detached (asterisk) and shows degeneration of photoreceptor cell layer (arrowhead). PAS, ×45. EP 30427.

B, Self-heated traumatic retinal dialysis in post-mortem eye of a 65 year old woman. Top left, gross appearance showing posterior vitreous detachment (arrows) and traumatic retinopathy. The vitreous base is dense and obscures the area of dialysis. Top right, area of dialysis showing rounded margin of retina, vitreous herniation under the edge of the dialysis (asterisk), hyperplasia of nonpigmented ciliary epithelium (arrow), and peripheral choroidal–pars plana neovascularization (arrowheads) extending into vitreous. Bottom left, area posterior to dialysis showing a demarcation area with laminated hyperplastic pigment epithelium (between arrows) and neovascularization (arrowheads). H and E, ×170. Bottom right, equatorial retina showing changes of traumatic retinopathy with photoreceptor cell degeneration and hyperplasia of RPE with migration into retina (arrow). H and E, ×190. EP 30799.

C, Examples of penetrating trauma mechanism of retinal dialysis. Top left, inferotemporal limbal perforation with vitreous incarceration (asterisk). Inferior vitreous base has avulsed retina (arrowhead) and nonpigmented ciliary epithelium (arrow) from attachment. H and E, ×7. Top right, traumatic perforation temporally, with dialysis of retina nasally. Vitreous base (arrow) remains attached to dialyzed retina. PAS, ×35. Bottom left, traumatic dialysis. Vitreous base (asterisks) remains attached to the separated retina (arrow) and nonpigmented ciliary epithelium (arrowhead). H and E, ×115. Bottom right, traumatic dialysis (arrow). A strand of tissue extends along the posterior margin of the vitreous base and to the undersurface of the retina (arrowheads). The vitreous base (asterisks) remains attached to the pars plana area. H and E, × 100. EP 41038.

Illustration continued on following page

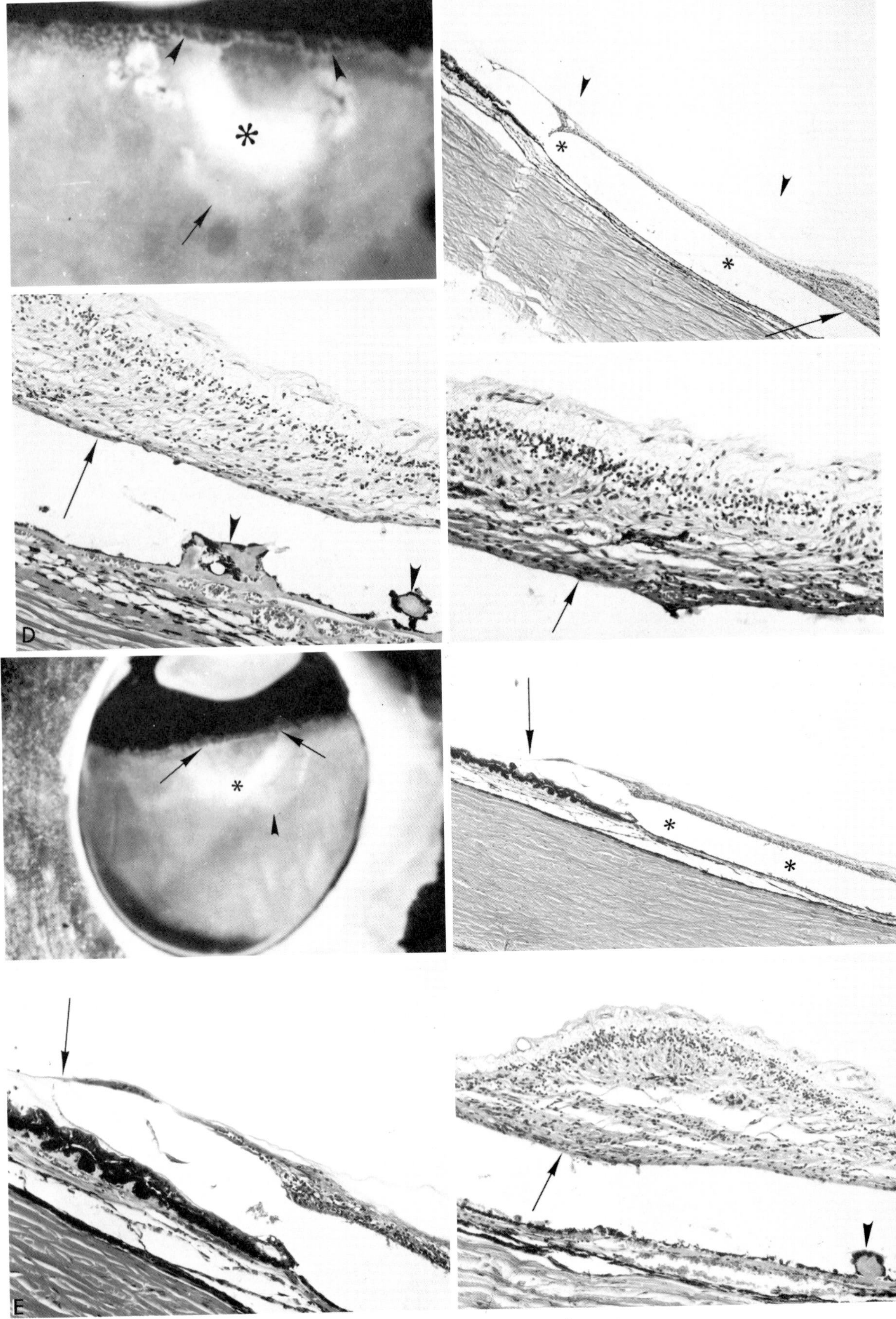

Figure 8–307 *See legend on opposite page*

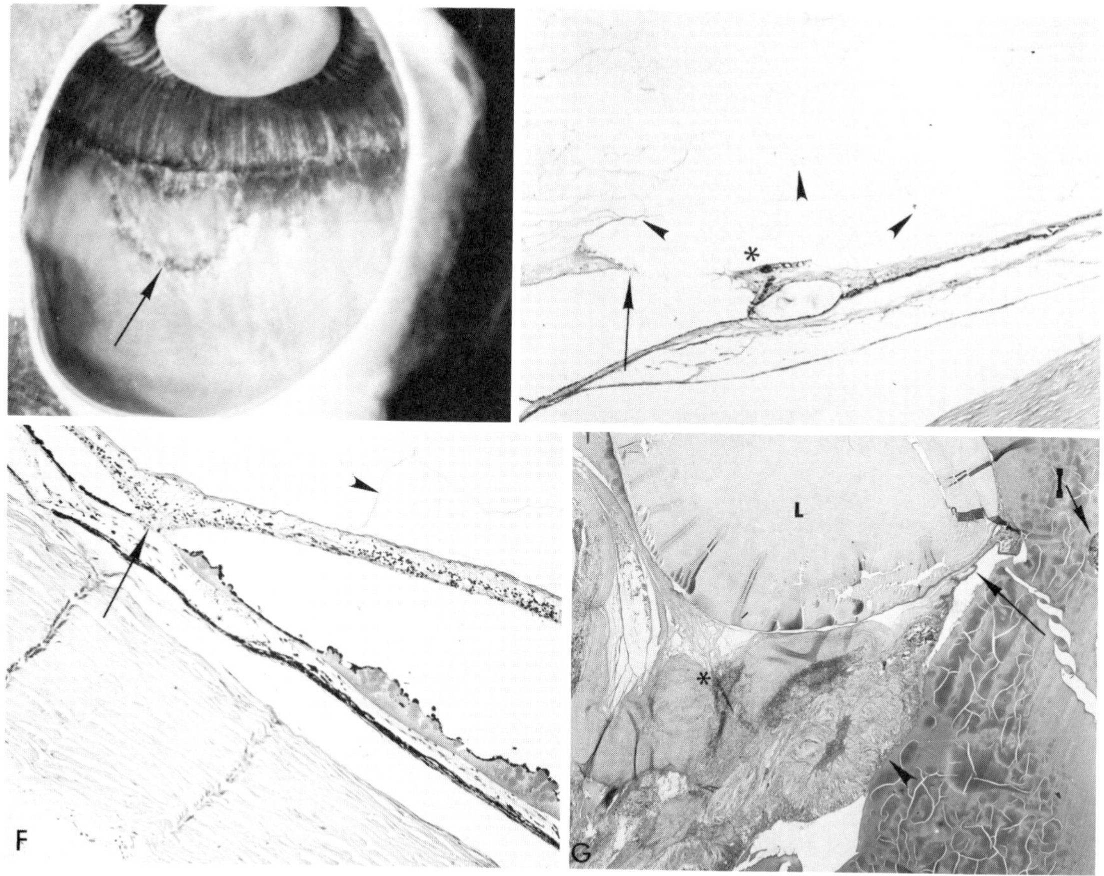

Figure 8–307. *Continued D,* Right eye with idiopathic inferotemporal dialysis and localized chronic retinal detachment in post-mortem eye of a 40 year old man. Top left, gross appearance of small area of chronic retinal detachment (arrow) and slitlike areas of dialysis of the retina at the ora serrata (between arrowheads). A portion of detached retina has a thickened, opaque appearance (asterisk). Top right, area of chronic retinal detachment (asterisks) with photoreceptor cell degeneration and area of extensive gliosis (arrow) on posterior surface of detached retina. The vitreous (arrowheads) is intact and remains normally attached to peripheral retina and pars plana. H and E, ×35. Bottom left, higher power view of chronic retinal detachment, showing loss of photoreceptor cell layer, marked gliosis (arrow), and drusen (arrowheads). H and E, ×155. Bottom right, higher power view of area of thick fibroglial membrane (arrow) involving the posterior surface of the retina in an area of chronic detachment. H and E, ×185. EP 45854.

E, Left eye of patient illustrated in *D.* Top left, gross appearance of slitlike area of retinal dialysis (between arrows), chronic localized retinal detachment (arrowhead), and thickening of portion of detached retina (asterisk). Top right, area showing dialysis (arrow), chronic retinal detachment (asterisks), numerous drusen, photoreceptor cell degeneration, and extensive retroretinal fibroglial cell proliferation. Vitreous remains attached to retina and nonpigmented ciliary epithelium. H and E, ×55. Bottom left, higher power view of area of dialysis, showing minimal inward separation of retina and intact overlying vitreous. Only a thin strand of vitreous (arrow) holds the retina at the ora serrata. H and E, ×155. Bottom right, higher power view of retroretinal fibroglial membrane (arrow), with apparent slight contraction resulting in a mild buckling appearance of the suprajacent retina. Druse in area of chronic retinal detachment (arrowhead). H and E, ×135. EP 45854.

F, Top left, nontraumatic inferotemporal retinal dialysis with area of chronic retinal detachment delineated by demarcation line (arrow). Top right, low-power view showing pocket of liquefied vitreous (arrowheads). Formed vitreous remains attached to the posterior margin of the hole-dialysis (arrow) and to residual retinal tissue at the ora serrata (asterisk). Alcian blue, ×40. Bottom left, area of chronic retinal detachment with photoreceptor cell degeneration, posterior chorioretinal demarcation-adhesion (arrow) and numerous large drusen (asterisks). Posterior vitreous detachment (arrowhead) is present. Alcian blue, ×100. EP 45869. *G,* Surgically enucleated eye from a 7 year old girl with nematode endophthalmitis. A dense, fibroinflammatory tissue (asterisk) is adherent to the internal surface of the detached and folded retina (arrowhead). The peripheral retina and fragment of nonpigmented ciliary epithelium (arrow) have been detached. A dense proteinaceous material occupies the subretinal space and is directly continuous with similar material in the anterior chamber. *L,* lens; *I,* iris. PAS, ×16. EP 47226.

Illustration continued on following page

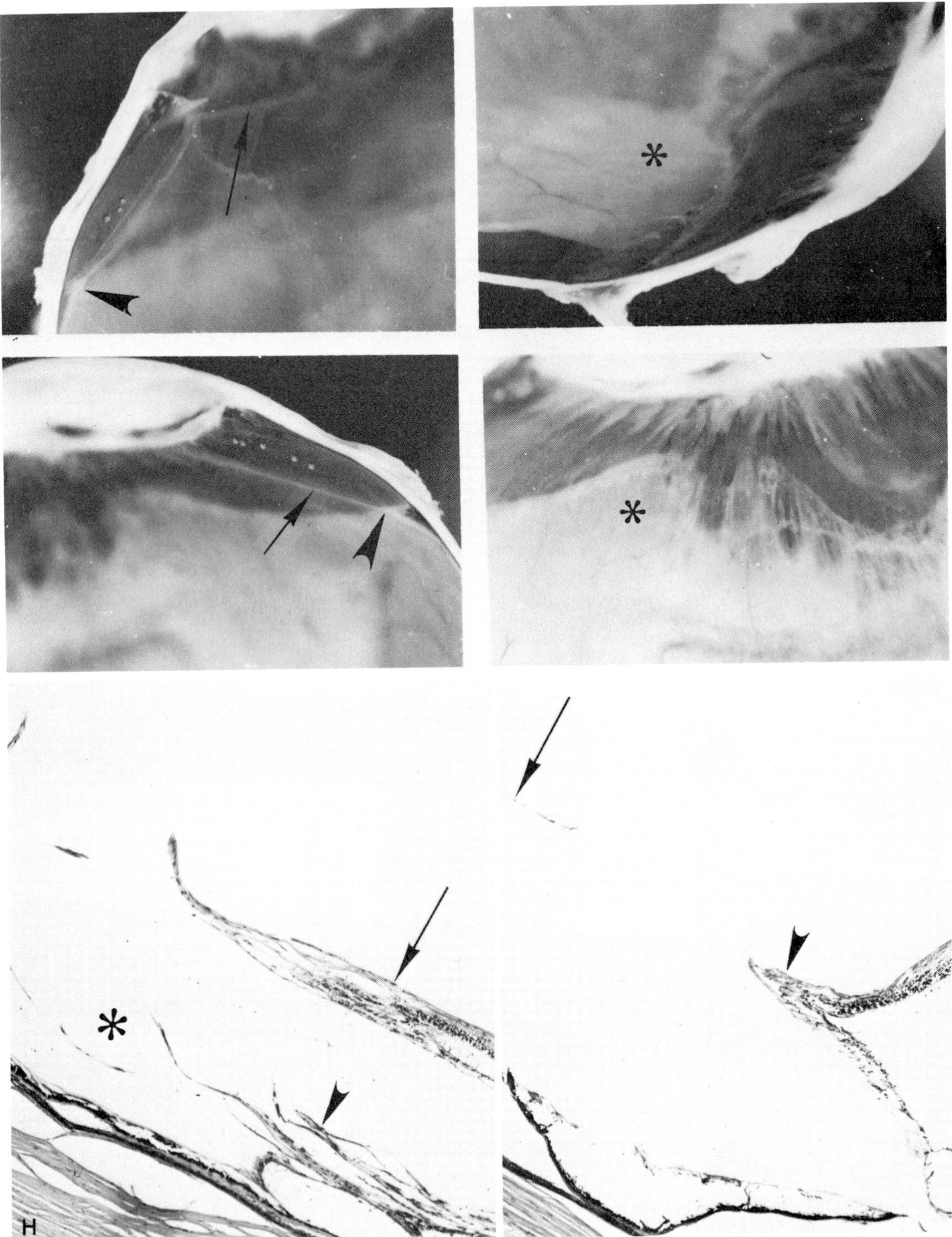

Figure 8–307 *Continued H,* Retinal dialysis in eye of a 23 year old man with a previous history of traumatic cataract that was extracted, complicated by vitreous incarceration in the wound. Top left and right and center left and right, gross appearance showing vitreous strand (arrows) from corneal wound exerting traction on peripheral retina. The peripheral retina is tented-up (arrowheads) and drawn over the pars plana in some areas (asterisks). Bottom left, inferior area showing dialyzed retina (arrow) having been pulled anteriorly over the pars plana. Vitreous base (asterisk) remains attached anterior to the dialysis. Hyperplastic ciliary epithelium (arrowhead) extends into the vitreous base. H and E, ×60. Bottom right, different areas showing vitreous strand (arrow) attached to an anterior, tented-up area of retina (arrowhead). PAS, ×60. EP 32421.

(All figures from Smiddy WE, Green WR: Retinal dialysis. Pathology and pathogenesis. Retina 2:94–116, 1982.)

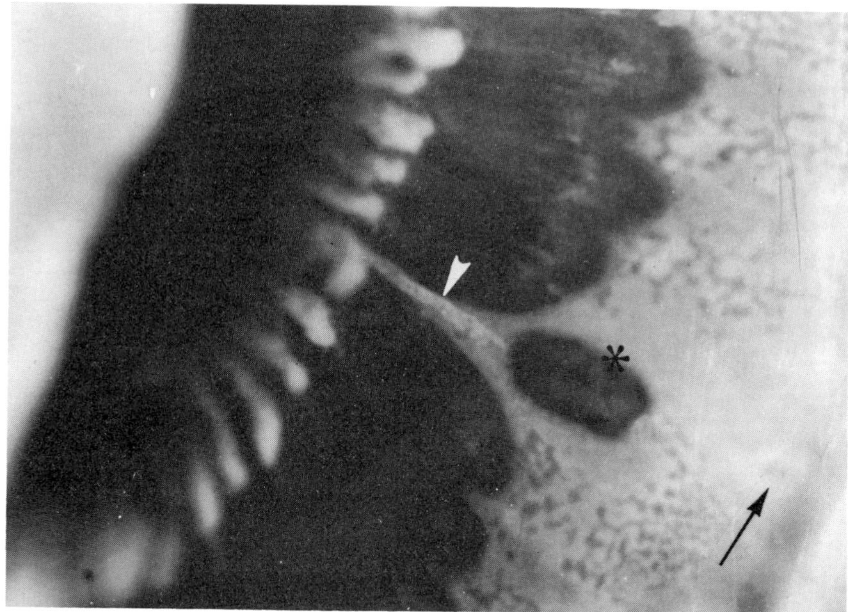

Figure 8–308. Peripheral retinal excavation (arrow) posterior to and aligned with a meridional complex, consisting of a dentate process (arrowhead) that is continuous with pars plicata and an area of entrapped pars plana (asterisk). EP 39305. (From Green WR: Pathology of the retina, *in* Frayer WC (ed): Lancaster Course in Ophthalmic Histopathology. Unit 9. Philadelphia, F.A. Davis, 1981.)

of dialysis, a distinct class of nontrauma-induced cases exists, which in some cases may represent a primary vitreoretinal degeneration.

Peripheral Retinal Excavations

These lesions, described by Foos and Allen (1967), are small oval depressions posterior to and aligned with a retinal meridional fold or complex (Fig. 8–308). The depression or excavation is due to the loss of inner retinal layers. The lesion was seen in 10 per cent of autopsy cases, and 43 per cent of the cases were bilateral. There is a predilection for the superotemporal quadrant (Straatsma, Foos, Feman, 1976, pages 7–8).

Retinal Tufts (Tags)

Peripheral retinal tufts, or tags, have been classified by Foos and Allen (1967) into noncystic, cystic, and zonular traction types.

Noncystic Retinal Tufts. These are formed by a thin strand of retina and glial tissue that extends internally within the zone of the vitreous base in adults (Fig. 8–309). These innocuous lesions were present in 72 per cent of adult autopsy cases, were bilateral in 50 per cent of cases, and were most common in the inferonasal quadrant (Foos, Allen, 1967; Straatsma, Foos, Feman, 1976, pages 21–23).

Cystic Retinal Tufts. This type of internal projection from the retina is larger than the noncystic type, is located at the posterior portion of the vitreous base or just posterior to the vitreous base, and is surrounded by cystic degeneration of the retina (Fig. 8–310). The incidence and location of this lesion vary (Foos, Allen, 1967; Straatsma, Foos, Feman, 1976, pages 23–24).

Zonular Traction Retinal Tufts. (Foos, 1969). This type of retinal tuft projects internally and anteriorly from the peripheral retina and often overhangs the pars plana (Figs. 8–311 through 8–314). Zonular attachment may be present at the apex of the lesion on histopathological examination. The strand of tissue is composed of fibroglial tissue (Figs. 8–311 and 8–312). In some instances, an embryonal type of epithelium is present, suggesting the embryologic derivation of some of these lesions (Fig. 8–313). Rarely, these tufts may be composed of pigmented epithelial cells (Fig. 8–314).

The lesion is observed with equal frequency at all ages; it was seen in 15 per cent of patients, of whom 15 per cent had bilateral lesions (Straatsma, Foos, Feman, 1976, page 24). Zonular traction tufts are significant because of the possibility of the development of small, round peripheral retinal holes from direct traction at the time of intracapsular cataract extraction.

Localized retinal tufts at and posterior to the equator are due to posterior vitreous detachment and vitreous traction (Fig. 8–315).

Meridional Folds

(Spencer, Foos, Straatsma, 1970)

Meridional folds are radially oriented, linear elevations of the peripheral retina (Figs. 8–316 and 8–317) and have been observed in 26 per cent of autopsy cases. In 55 per cent of cases, the lesions were bilateral. The lesion has a predilection for the superonasal quadrant. The incidence of meridional folds is the same in all age groups. Al-

Text continued on page 900

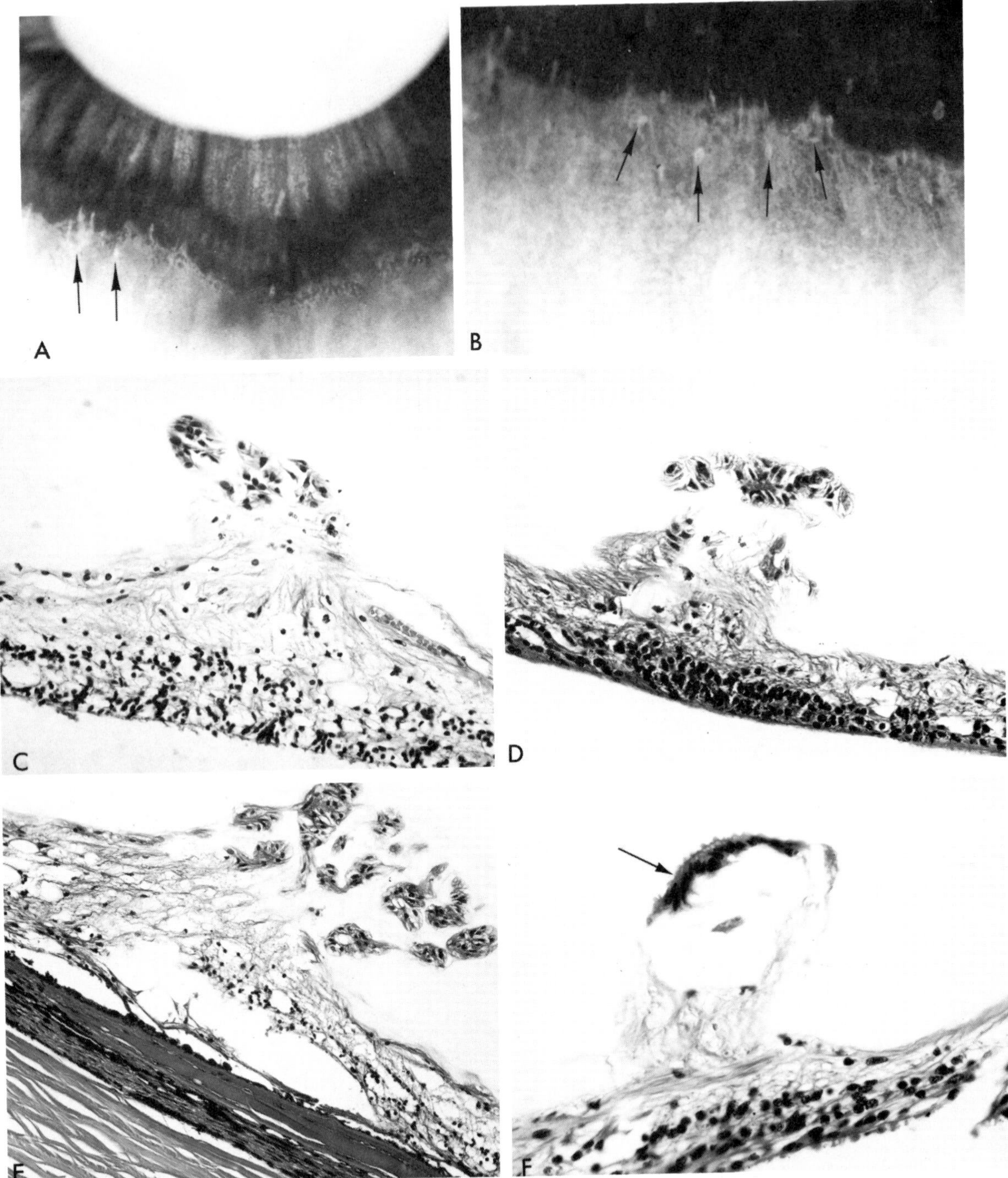

Figure 8–309. Gross and microscopic appearances of **peripheral noncystic retinal tufts**. *A,* EP 48448. *B,* EP 47981. *C,* Tuft composed of probable glial cells. H and E, ×310. EP 30600. *D,* Tuft composed of probable glial cells. H and E, ×310 EP 46986. *E,* Tuft composed of numerous small lobules of probable glial cells. H and E, ×215. EP 39420. *F,* Tuft with a single layer of cuboidal, epithelium-like cells (arrow). H and E, ×450. EP 31743.

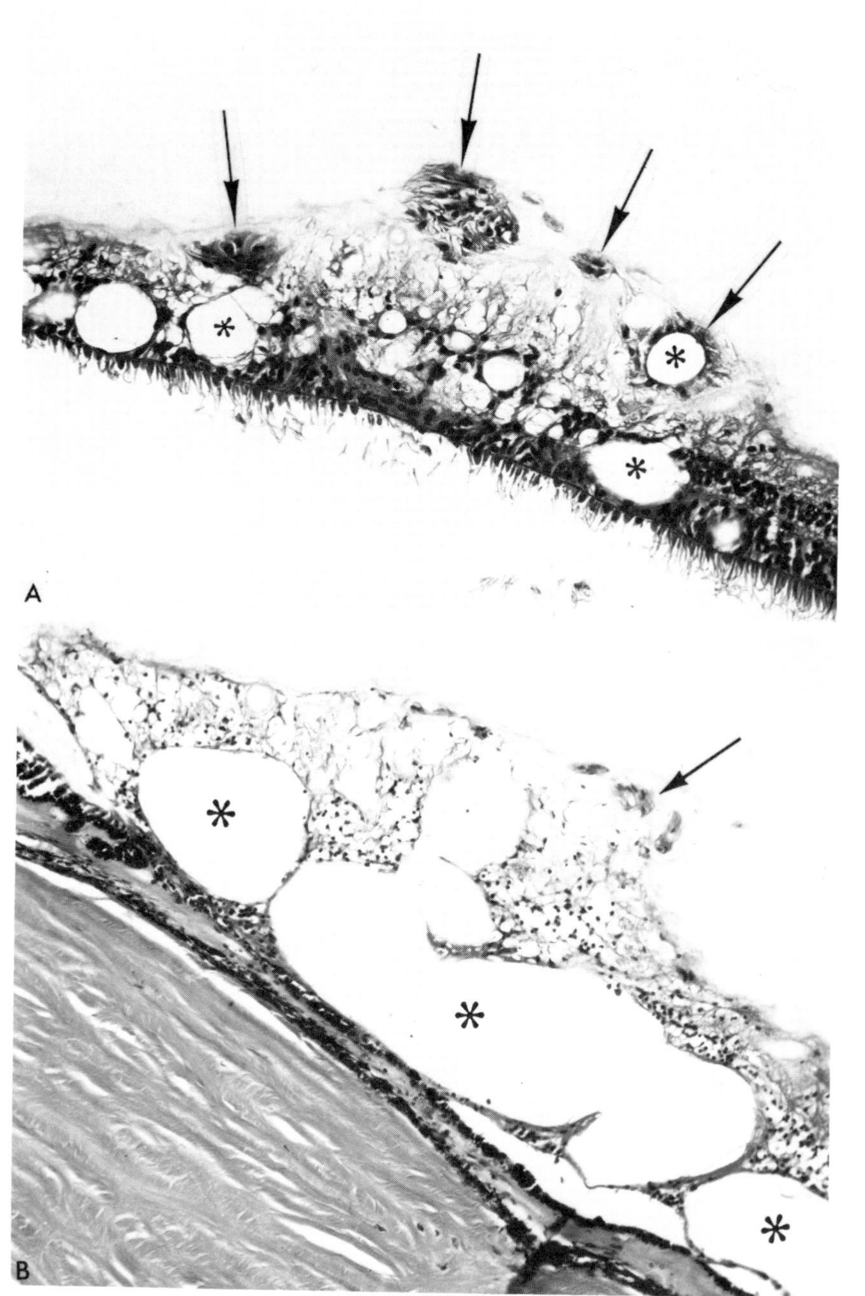

Figure 8–310. Cystic retinal tuft. A, Lesion consists of an area of retinal thickening caused by cystic changes (asterisk) and probable glial cell proliferation (arrows). H and E, ×220. EP 48822. *B*, Retina tuft has cysts (asterisks) and minor glial cell proliferation (arrow). H and E, ×110. EP 42112.

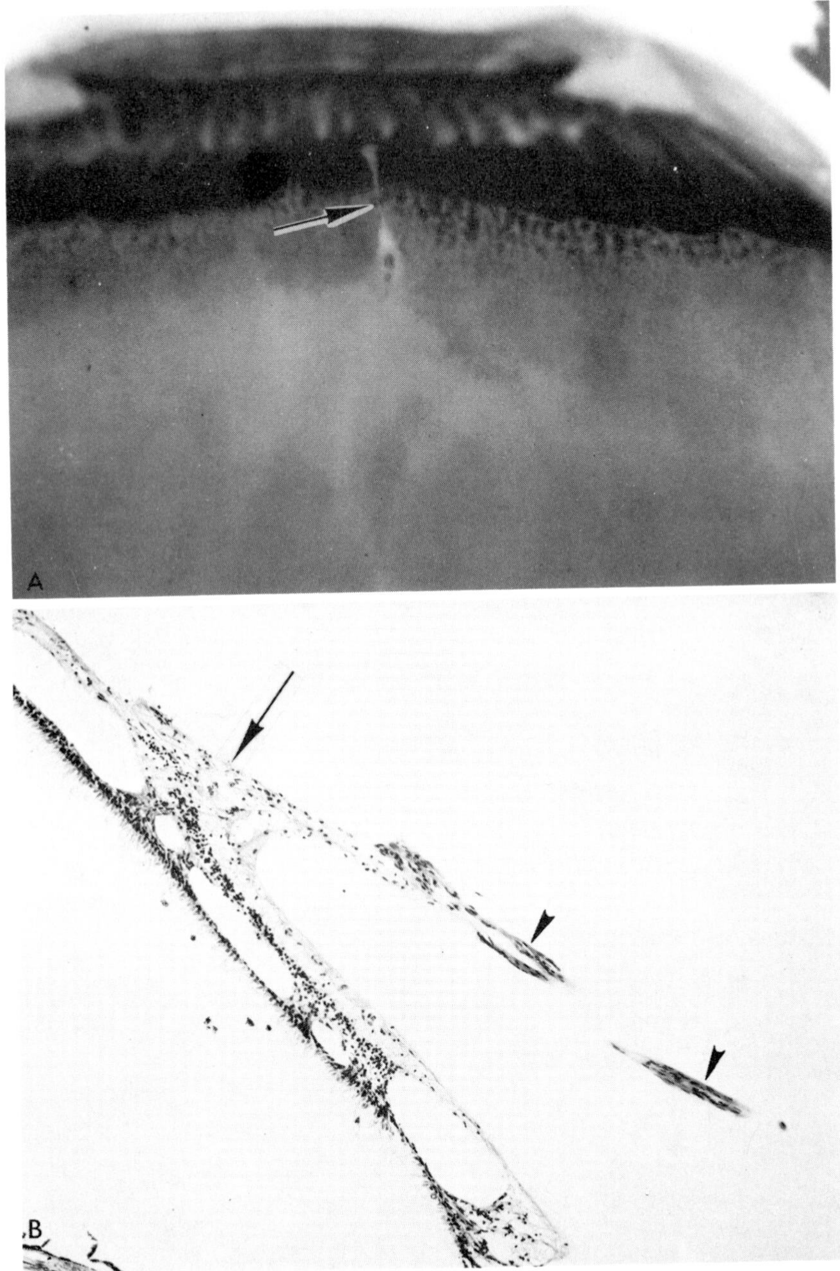

Figure 8–311. *A,* Gross appearance of **zonular tractional tuft** (arrow). *B,* Tented-up area of retina (arrow) with strand of glial cell proliferation (arrowheads) extending anteriorly over peripheral retina and pars plana. H and E, ×100. EP 34471. (From Green WR: Pathology of the retina, *in* Frayer WC (ed): Lancaster Course in Ophthalmic Histopathology. Unit 9. Philadelphia, F.A. Davis, 1981.)

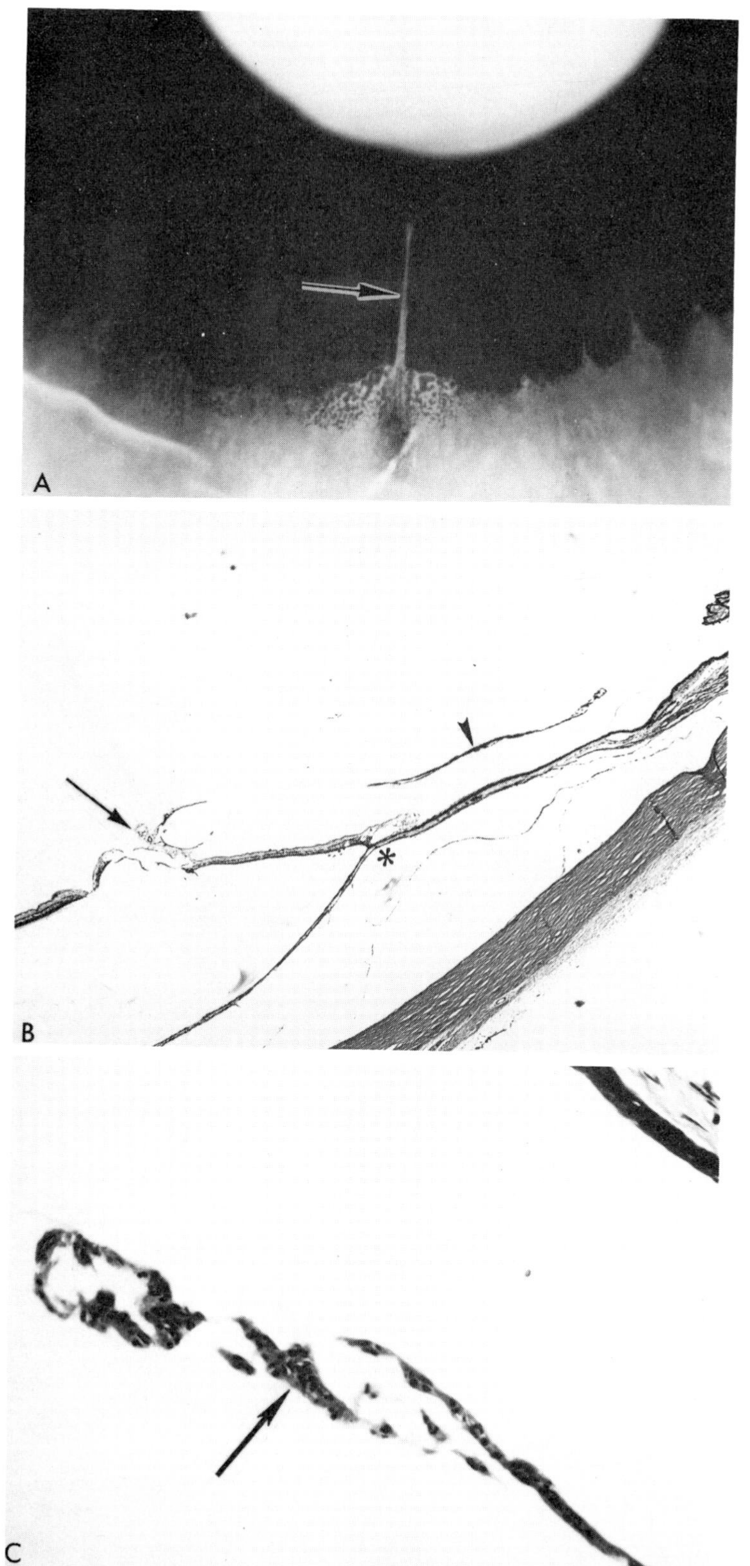

Figure 8–312. *A,* **Zonular tractional tuft** (arrow) extending over pars plana from peripheral retina. *B,* Tuft is attached to peripheral retina (arrow) and extends (arrowheads) over entire pars plana. Asterisk indicates ora serrata. H and E, ×18. C. Tuft (arrow) is composed of probable glial cells. H and E, ×300. EP 42224.

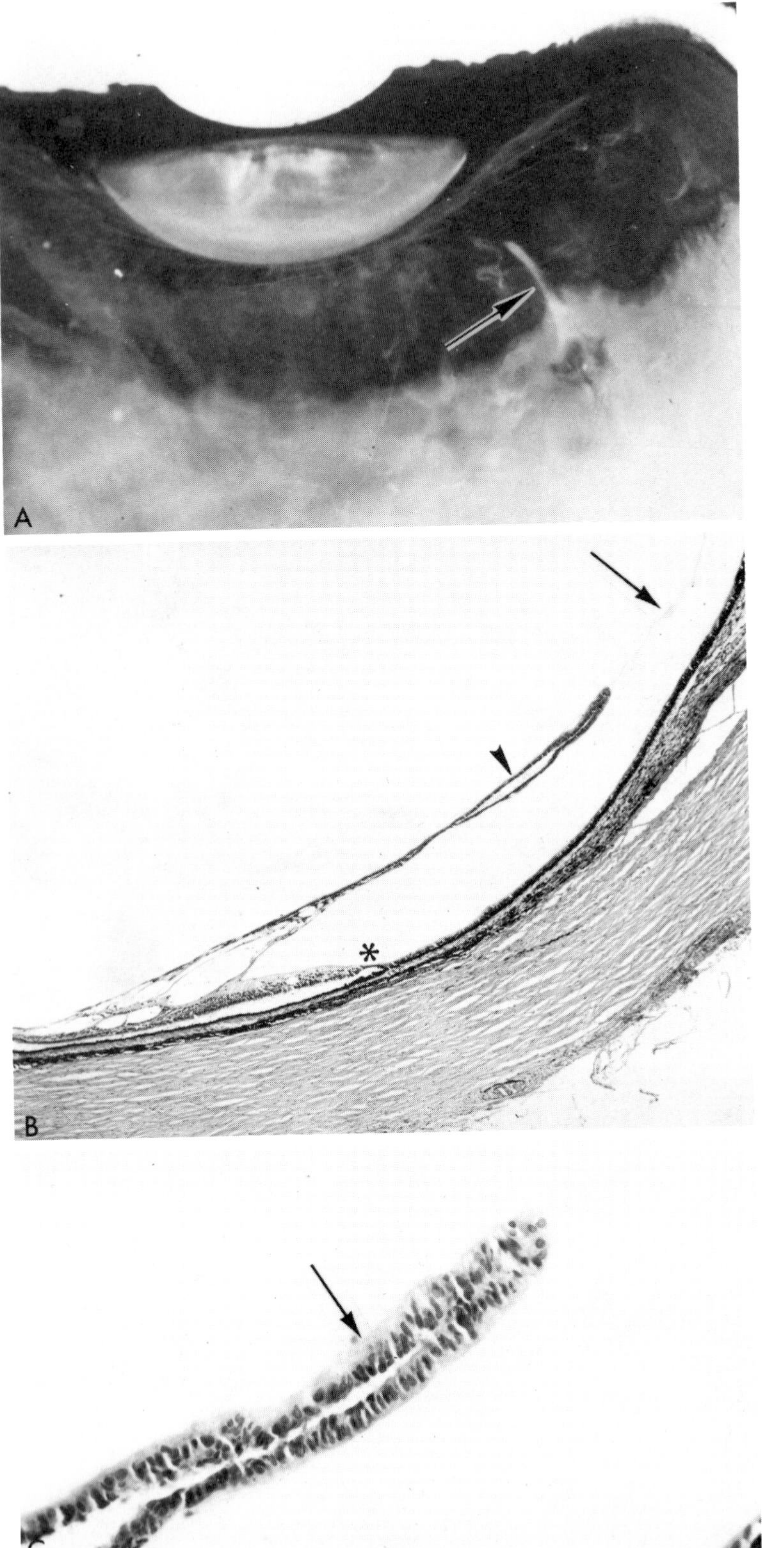

Figure 8–313. *A,* Gross appearance of **zonular tractional tuft** (arrow). *B,* Tuft extends from peripheral retina, overhangs pars plana, and is continuous with a zonular fiber (arrow). Anterior part is composed of two layers of epithelium-like cells (arrowhead). Asterisk indicates ora serrata. H and E, ×30. *C,* Higher power view shows anterior portion of tuft composed of two layers of embryonal-like epithelium (arrow). H and E, ×290. EP 30711.

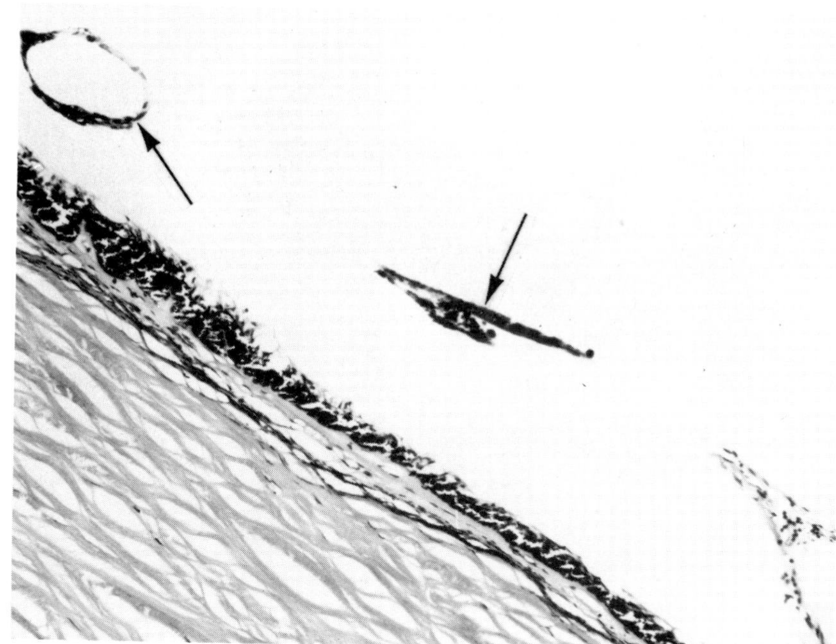

Figure 8–314. Zonular traction tuft composed of pigmented epithelial cells (arrows). H and E, ×120. EP 30917.

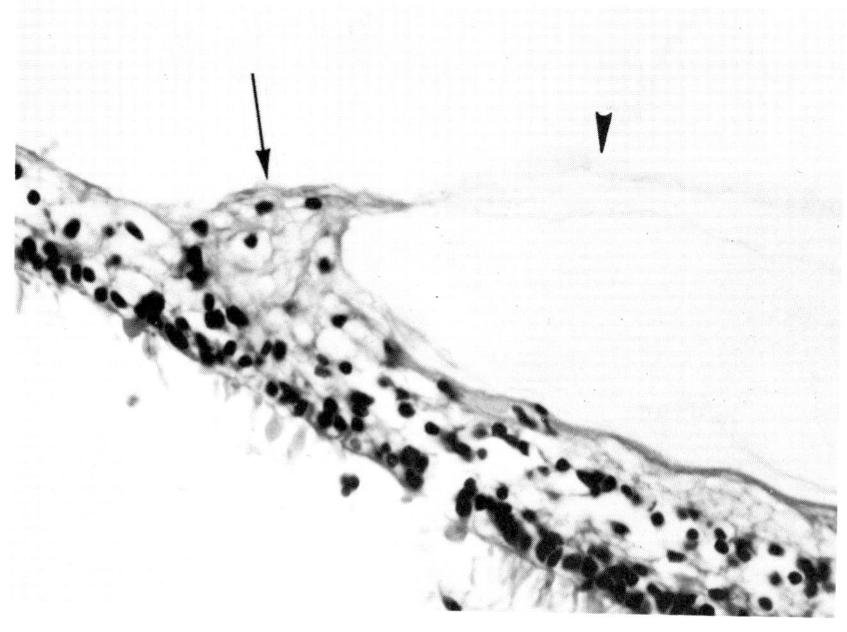

Figure 8–315. More posterior **retinal tufts** (arrow) are due to vitreous traction (arrowhead). H and E, ×460.

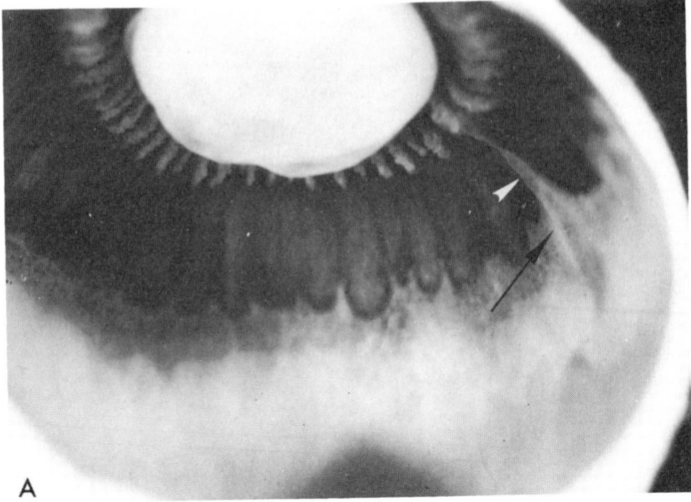

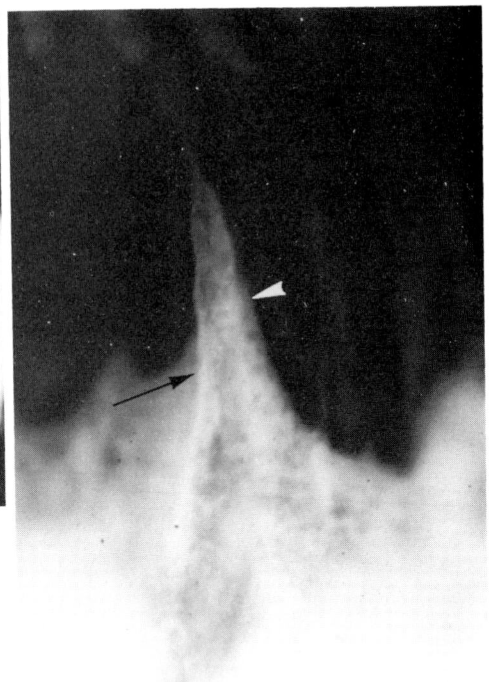

Figure 8–316. *A,* **Meridional fold** (arrow) in line with a prominent dentate process (arrowhead). *B,* Closer view shows tented-up area of retina (arrow), meridionally oriented and in line with a dentate process (arrowhead). EP 30600. (From Green WR: Pathology of the vitreous, *in* Frayer WC (ed): Lancaster Course in Ophthalmic Histopathology. Unit 8. Philadelphia, F.A. Davis, 1981.)

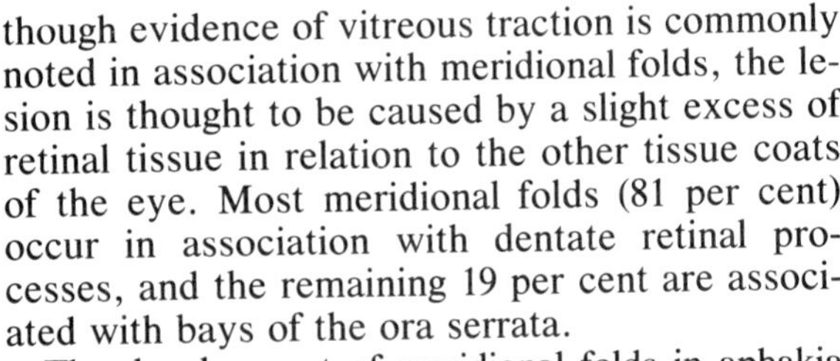
though evidence of vitreous traction is commonly noted in association with meridional folds, the lesion is thought to be caused by a slight excess of retinal tissue in relation to the other tissue coats of the eye. Most meridional folds (81 per cent) occur in association with dentate retinal processes, and the remaining 19 per cent are associated with bays of the ora serrata.

The development of meridional folds in aphakia may be a sign of vitreous traction.

Meridional Complexes

(Spencer, Foos, Straatsma, 1970)

A meridional complex is the configuration, usually in the nasal periphery, in which a dentate retinal process is in meridional alignment with a ciliary body process (Figs. 8–308, 8–317, and 8–318). A meridional retinal fold is usually present on the dentate process, and a retinal excavation is located posteriorly in the same meridian. This

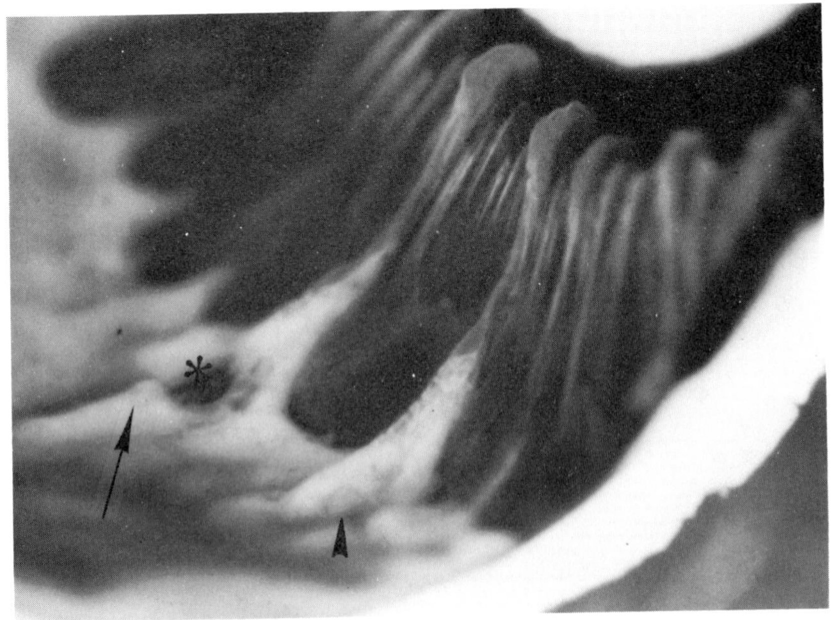

Figure 8–317. Meridional folds—one in line with a meridional complex (arrow) and another (arrowhead) in line with a dentate process. The meridional complex consists of a dentate process that is continuous with the pars plicata; it has an area of entrapped pars plana posteriorly (asterisk). EP 37408. (From Green WR: Pathology of the retina, *in* Frayer WC (ed): Lancaster Course in Ophthalmic Histopathology. Unit 9. Philadelphia, F.A. Davis, 1981.)

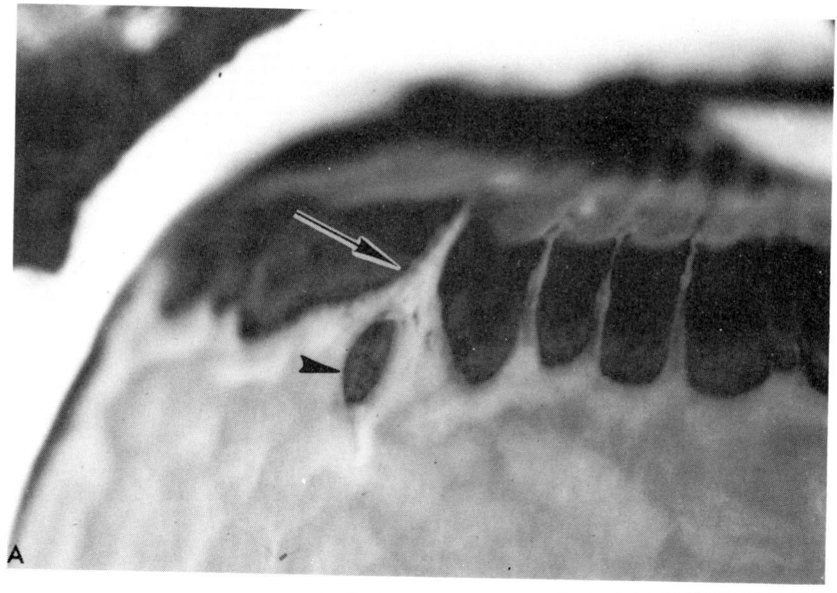

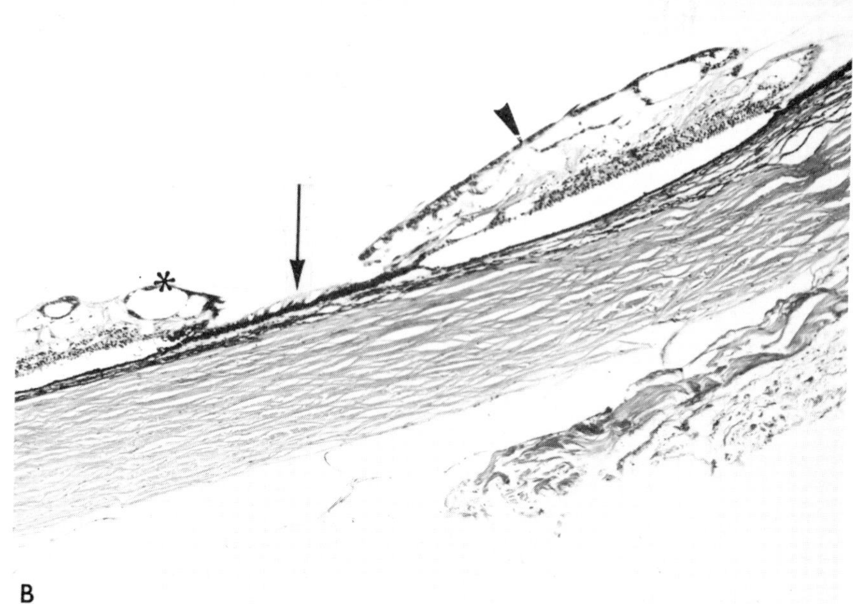

Figure 8–318. *A,* **Meridional complex** with dentate process (arrow) and entrapped area of ora serrata (arrowhead). Three dentate processes are also present. *B,* Features include a dentate process area of entrapped pars plana, with nonpigmented and pigmented ciliary epithelium (arrow). Glial and epithelial cell proliferation is present on the inner surface of the retina of the dentate process (arrowhead) and retina posteriorly (asterisk). PAS, ×50. EP 37408.

anatomic arrangement was observed in 16 per cent of autopsy cases, and in 58 per cent of cases they were bilateral.

Enclosed oral bays may be seen in association with meridional complexes (Figs. 8–308, 8–317, and 8–318) (Straatsma, Foos, Feman, 1976, page 7).

Ora Pearls

Ora pearls appear as darkly pigmented or glistening small white nodules in the retina, within a dentate process, extending over the pars plana. In a series of 700 consecutive eyes studied, 20 per cent had ora pearls (Lonn, Smith, 1967). Ora pearls were observed in 10 of 50 patients (20 per cent) examined with the Goldmann indentation contact lens (Daicker, Eisner, 1968). Some pearls are dark brown or black in appearance because of overlying hypertrophic, and in some instances hyperplastic, RPE. This curious structure is periodic acid–Schiff positive and may have a laminated appearance with calcification (Fig. 8–319). Some pearls are surrounded by pigment epithelium. This finding, along with the appearance of elaborated basement membrane, suggests that ora pearls are derived from the RPE (Fig. 8–320).

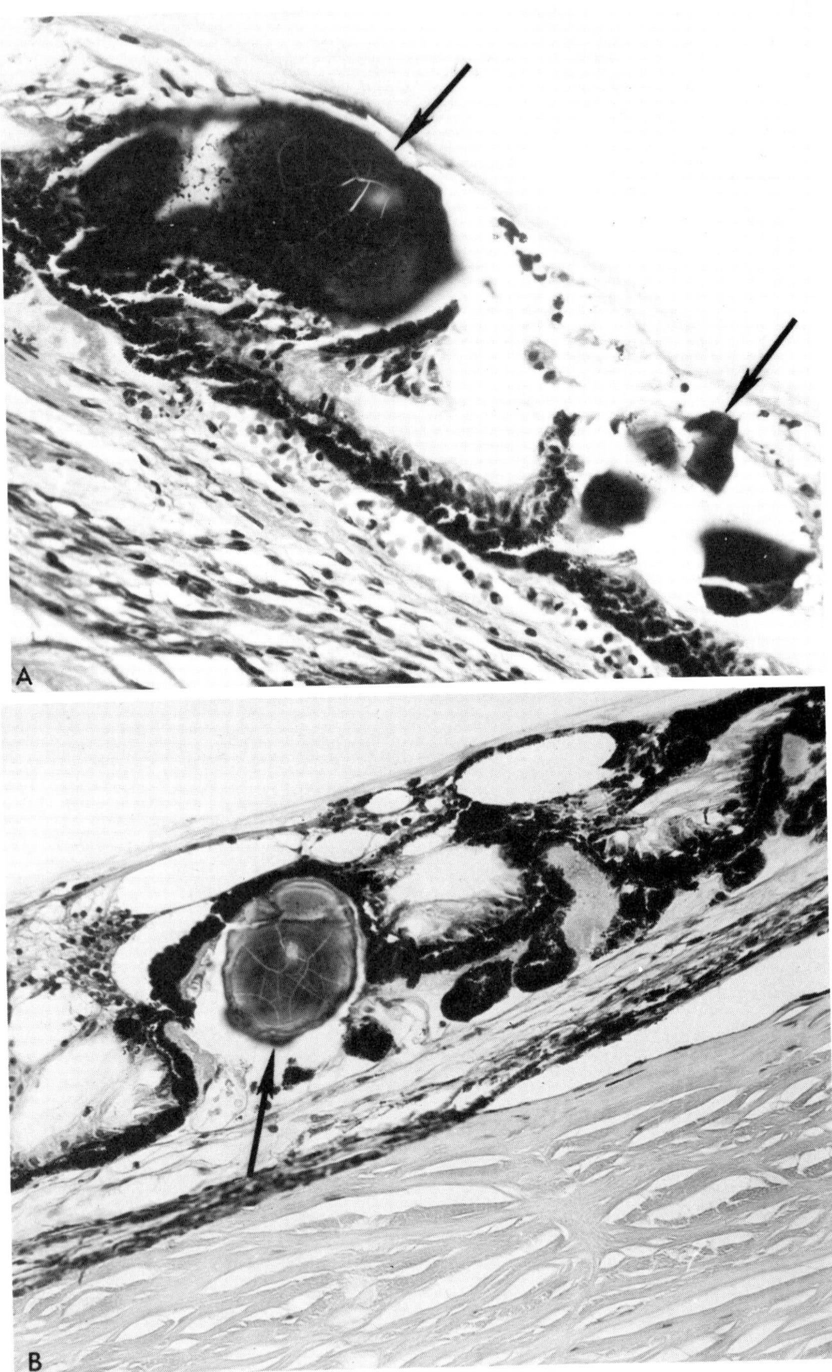

Figure 8–319. *A,* Homogeneous **ora pearl** (arrows) that stains intensely with periodic acid–Schiff. × 300. EP 38206. *B,* Ora pearl (arrow) with a concentric laminated configuration and calcific stippling. H and E, ×210. EP 29759.

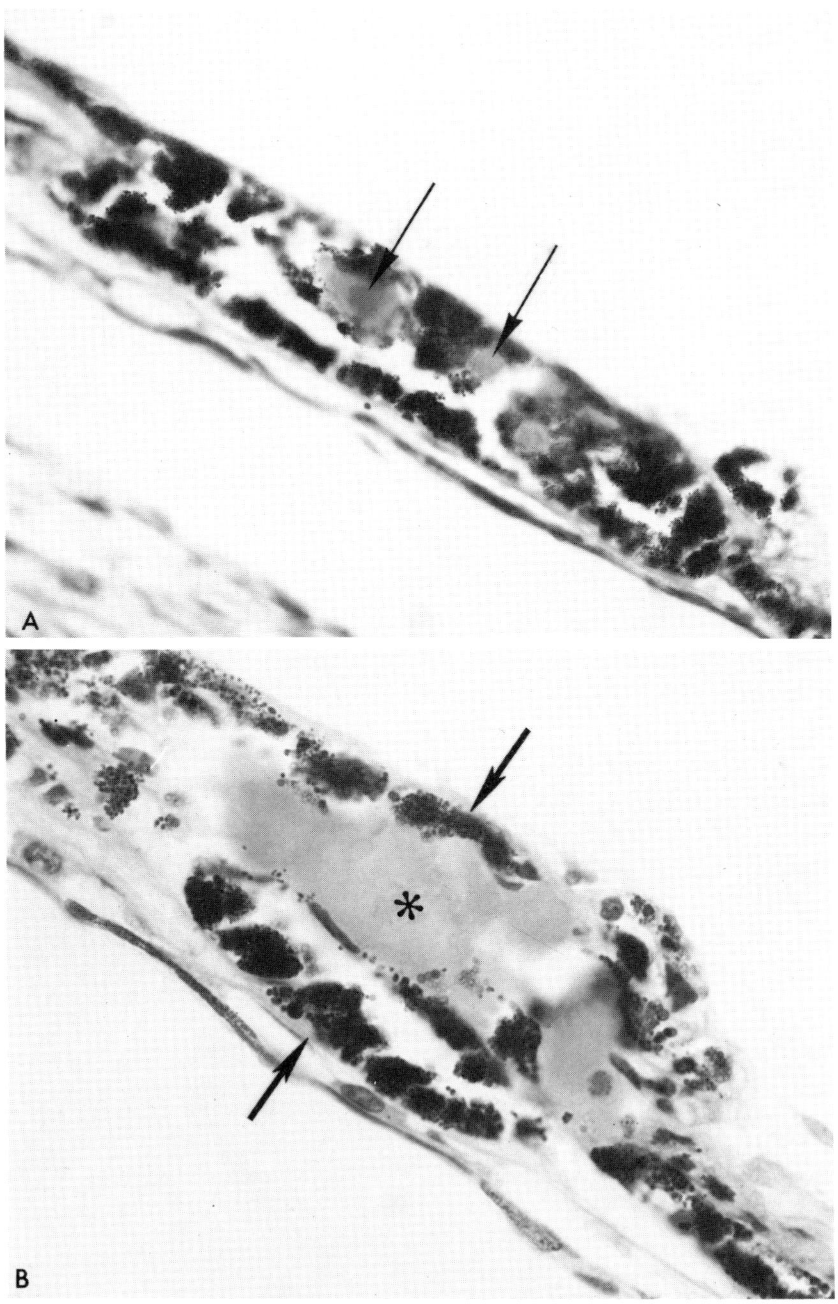

Figure 8–320. *A,* Small **ora pearls** (arrows) surrounded by pigment epithelium. PAS, ×525. *B,* Higher power view of a different area, showing ora pearl (asterisk) surrounded by pigment epithelium (arrows). H and E, ×750. EP 31908.

RETINAL DETACHMENT

From the optic disc to the ora serrata the anatomic attachment of the sensory retina to the pigment epithelium is weak. A potential space exists here, the vestige of the central cavity of the optic vesicle in the early embryo. Accumulation of fluid in this potential space constitutes a separation of the retina. Strictly speaking, detachment of the retina would be a detachment of the RPE from Bruch's membrane of the choroid. Usage, however, allows us to speak of a separation of the rods and cones from the RPE as a detachment of the sensory retina.

The photoreceptors are surrounded by a mucopolysaccharide ground substance that stabilizes them and also probably tends to hold the sensory retina to the pigment epithelium. The outer segments of the photoreceptors are intimately related to the extensive villus processes of the RPE, and this also tends to keep the retina in contact with the pigment epithelium. There are no strong junctional attachments between the outer segments and the villus processes of the RPE. On the inner side of the retina, the internal limiting membrane is intimately related to the vitreous, especially up to the age of 45 or 50 years. The cortical collagen fibrils of the vitreous blend with the basement membrane of the retinal Müller cells to provide a rather firm bond; in fact, the attachments here are stronger than those between the photoreceptors and the RPE.

Changes in the vitreous, therefore, can lead to alterations in the vitreoretinal relations and, at times, can initiate retinal detachment because of traction. Disease of the retina in the region of the inner limiting membrane can lead to vitreoretinal adhesions, and, if there is a detachment of the vitreous from the retina in other areas, traction on these adhesions can produce tears in the retina.

Mechanisms of Retinal Detachment

Retinal detachments occur by three principal mechanisms.

1. The first is by *accumulation of fluid beneath the retina,* with the fluid being derived from blood vessels of the retina or choroid or both. Examples of this type of retinal detachment include those associated with choroidal tumors, such as malignant melanoma, leukemia, hemangioma, and metastatic carcinoma; vascular lesions of the retina, such as Coats' disease or angiomatosis retinae; inflammatory processes, such as sympathetic uveitis, Harada's disease, uveal effusion, scleritis, and so on; and in hypertension, malignant hypertension, and eclampsia. In papilledema, slight peripapillary detachment of the retina is often present; the subretinal fluid comes from the optic nerve head or the peripapillary retina or both.

2. The second mechanism is *vitreous traction,* or pulling, on the retina. This can result from vitreous condensation and fibrosis after accidental or surgical trauma. With incarceration of vitreous in a cataract wound, traction may be transmitted to the retina inferiorly and may lead to retinal detachment (see Fig. 8–307,*H*). The development of vitreous fibrous and fibrovascular bands in various proliferative retinopathies also can lead to traction on the retina, as in sickle cell disease, diabetic retinopathy, and retrolental fibroplasia.

3. The third and most common mechanism of retinal detachment is the *accumulation of subretinal fluid via a retinal hole,* plus vitreous traction.

Not all retinal holes, however, lead to detachment (Foos, 1974a). In a study of 2406 pairs of autopsy eyes, tears were present in 1.9 per cent of the eyes and were uniformly distributed in all quadrants. In the affected eyes, they were present in the equatorial zone in 95 per cent, were related to vitreal retinal traction in 94 per cent, were of the flap type in 64 per cent, and were accompanied by posterior vitreous detachment in 79 per cent. They were significantly more prevalent in eyes with lattice degeneration (17 per cent). Macular holes may lead to detachments rarely.

The causes of retinal holes are most often degenerative changes in the retina that are associated with alterations in the vitreous. Most frequent of all these degenerations are those that are equatorial and of the lattice type. It has been established that in degenerative retinal lesions of this type, there are vitreoretinal adhesions to the internal limiting membrane (ILM) and that traction is produced by the vitreous on the ILM. This eventually can lead to hole formation in the weakened retina. Also, additional traction is likely to be produced as a result of vitreous degeneration (syneresis). Syneresis is a common finding in individuals beyond age 50 years, the period when retinal hole formation and retinal detachment are most common. If syneresis occurs with detachment of the vitreous, and if there are adhesions of areas of vitreous to weakened portions of the retina, hole formation and detachment can occur.

Vitreous degeneration, lattice degeneration, retinal holes, and retinal detachment are more common in myopic than nonmyopic eyes. Presumably, the thinning and stretching of the retinal tissue in myopic eyes predisposes the retina to hole formation. Minor and major traumas also predispose the retina to degeneration and hole formation. The role of indirect trauma in these retinal changes has always been debated, but, in a retina that has previously been damaged by degenerative changes, minor trauma of an indirect type can lead to sudden movements of the vitreous and traction on pre-existing adhesions. Also, it is not uncommon for retinal detachment to occur after removal of cataract; presumably the trauma produced by extraction of the lens, causing traction on pre-existing adhesions at weakened points in the retina, can lead to hole formation. However, the frequency of spontaneous retinal holes without retinal detachments in many eyes suggests that the trauma of cataract extraction can aggravate a pre-existing condition and lead to detachment. Uveitis also can be a factor in production of retinal holes, by formation of vitreoretinal adhesions.

As noted, retinal holes are classified as either round or horseshoe-shaped in type. A round hole frequently has an operculum in the vitreous adjacent to one edge of the hole. Horseshoe-shaped tears have a flap at the posterior edge, to which vitreous membranes adhere. Holes are most often found in the equatorial region of the eye (45 per cent), and about 27 per cent are found in the peripheral region. A smaller number (12 per cent) are found peripherally. Only 15 per cent occur in the postequatorial region, and macular holes comprise about 1 per cent. Holes are much more frequent in the superior and inferior temporal fundus, presumably because the long temporal side of the retina is more vulnerable because of its greater area. Holes are frequently found bilaterally in eyes, and bilateral retinal detachment is not uncommon.

Classification of Retinal Detachment

Retinal detachment is classified into two types, depending on whether a retinal tear is present or not. Schepens introduced the term "rhegmatogenous" retinal detachment to designate those detachments due to a retinal hole or tear. *Rhegma* is derived from a Greek word meaning rent or break. The two basic types of retinal detachment, then, are rhegmatogenous and nonrhegmatogenous. Rhegmatogenous retinal detachment can be classified on the basis of the location of the essential pathology:

1. Rhegmatogenous Retinal Detachment

Equatorial: as in myopia and associated with lattice degeneration and horseshoe-type or round retinal holes.

Oral type: as in surgical aphakia, inferior temporal dialysis in young men, traumatic dialysis (usually superonasal), and some giant retinal breaks.

Macular type: as in high myopia, post-traumatic holes, and senile macular holes.

2. Nonrhegmatogenous Retinal Detachment This type of retinal detachment occurs without a retinal hole or tear and is a result of accumulation of blood, exudate or transudate beneath the retina. This type occurs in various ocular inflammatory diseases, tumors of the choroid, retinal vascular lesions, hypertension, and vitreous traction, and from proliferative retinopathy as noted earlier.

Predisposing Factors to Rhegmatogenous Retinal Detachment

All factors already have been discussed in detail and illustrated elsewhere. The following factors are among the more important: surgical aphakia, myopia with vitreous detachment, trauma, vitreoretinal adhesion, retinal holes and tears, retinal pits (as a sign of areas of vitreous detachment and traction), lattice degeneration, and retinoschisis, especially reticular degenerative.

Pathologic Changes Following Retinal Detachment

With separation of the retina from the RPE, the biochemical interplay between the photoreceptor cells and the RPE is impaired, as is also the choroidal blood supply to the outer retinal layers. This leads first to a loss of the outer segments of the photoreceptor cells. With long-standing detachment, the entire photoreceptor cell layer atrophies (see Fig. 8–307,*A*). Monkey retina outer segments degenerate after detachment and rapidly regenerate after surgical reattachment (Kroll, Machemer, 1969; Machemer, Kroll, 1971). Rods recovered more rapidly and more completely than cones during a period of up to 1 month following retinal reattachment.

When the macula detaches, the visual acuity may never return to predetachment levels even with successful reattachment. This suggests that some alteration persists.

Other pathologic changes that may occur in long-standing retinal detachment include cystic degeneration and macrocyst formation, demarcation lines (see Figs. 8–305, 8–306, 8–307,*A*), rubeosis iridis, and extensive, large drusen formation.

As with hypoxic retinal vascular conditions, a vasoproliferative factor is postulated to be elaborated by the hypoxic and chronically detached retina, and this factor is presumed responsible for the iris neovascularization.

Pathologic Changes in Eyes after Surgery for Retinal Detachments

Diathermy. Diathermy by various methods produces localized areas of inflammation in the retina and choroid, with destruction of the neural and connective tissue elements and the blood vessels and eventual formation of a fibrotic scar that binds the retina to the choroid at the site of the degenerative process or the hole.

Cryopexy. Cryopexy (cryotherapy) has been used extensively for the treatment of retinal detachment and sealing of retinal holes. The effects are mechanical disruption of the cells by formation of intracellular ice crystals (Archambeau, Henderson, 1965; Curtin, Fujino, Norton, 1966; Lincoff, Kreissig, 1971). Histologically, there is damage to the smaller blood vessels by the freezing, but the larger ones appear to be unaffected. The RPE shows extensive degeneration, with migration of pigment and accumulation of macrophages at the site of the pre-existing epithelium. There may be proliferation of the surrounding undamaged epithelial cells, thus contributing to the scar. The photoreceptors and outer nuclear layer are usually destroyed, and the outer portion of the retina becomes gliotic and adherent to the choroid.

Light Coagulation. Xenon light was shown by Meyer-Schwickerath to be effective in closing pre-existing retinal holes or for closure of holes over retinal buckles where the hole was not quite in contact with the buckled wall of the eye. The principle is that light is absorbed by the retinal pigment epithelium and that destruction of the cells occurs. The photoreceptors and outer portion of the retina are also damaged by the absorption of light and by the heat produced. The result is a chorioretinal scar, much like that seen after diathermy.

Laser Light Coagulation. This also has been used extensively for closure of retinal holes and also for sealing holes after retinopexy. The changes are similar to those with diathermy and xenon coagulation. The effects of laser treatment

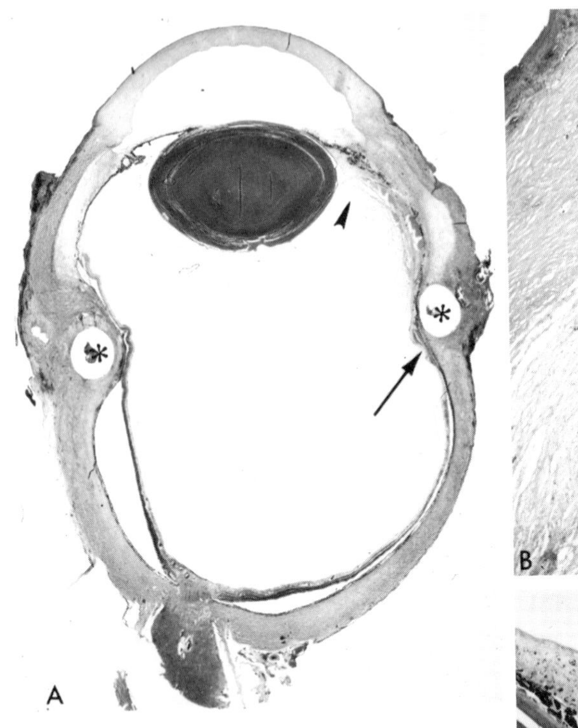

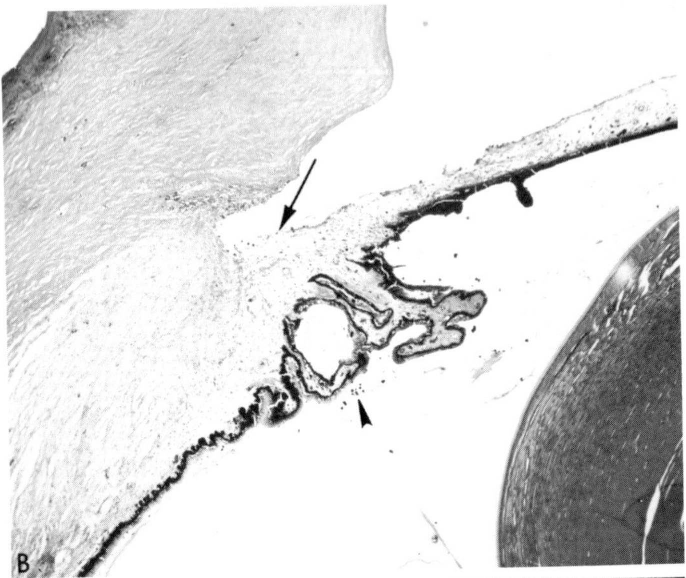

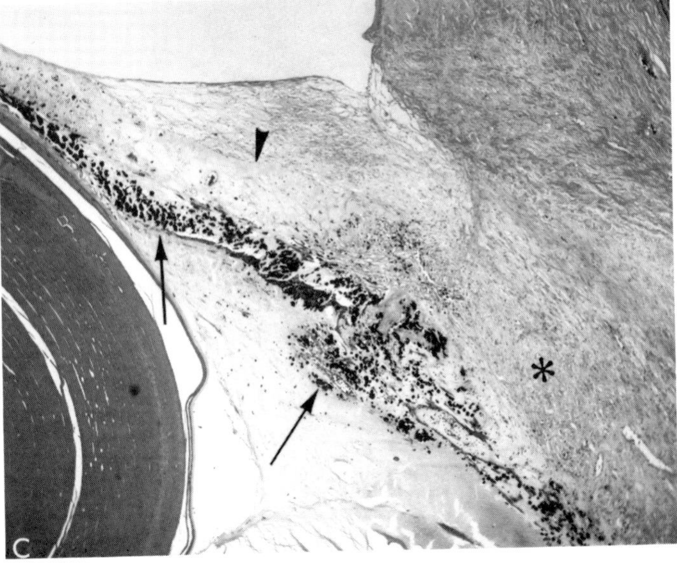

Figure 8–321. *A,* **Anterior segment necrosis** after retinal reattachment surgery. Iris and ciliary body on left are normal and those on right are necrotic (arrowhead). An intrascleral polyethylene tube is present (asterisk) and has eroded through sclera (arrow) on the side of necrosis of iris and ciliary body. H and E, ×5. *B,* Higher power view of normal iris and ciliary body on left side. A few pigmented macrophages are present in anterior (arrow) and posterior (arrowhead) chambers. H and E, ×35. *C,* Iris and ciliary body on right side show postischemic changes, with loss of cellularity (arrowhead), fibrosis (asterisk), peripheral anterior and posterior synechiae, pigment rounding-up and dispersion (arrows), and loss of ciliary epithelium. H and E, ×35. EP 52240.

are on the RPE, and the heat absorbed by the pigment cells is radiated to adjacent structures. The result is to cause destruction of RPE, choriocapillaris, and the photoreceptor system. A firm chorioretinal scar results from this treatment.

The greatest application of laser therapy has been in the treatment of leaky vascular lesions and the proliferative retinopathies.

Numerous histopathologic studies in experimental animals and humans have documented the ocular morphologic features of xenon arc and laser photocoagulation (Marshall, Mellerio, 1967; Apple, Goldberg, Wyhinny, 1973; Wallow, Tso, Fine, 1973; Wallow, Tso, 1973a and b; Wallow, Lund, Gable, et al, 1974; Apple, Wyhinny, Goldberg, et al, 1976; Tso, Wallow, Elgin, 1977; Wallow, Tso, Elgin, 1977; Wallow, Davis, 1979).

Boniuk and Zimmerman (1962) reported the histopathologic features of 204 eyes that came to enucleation after retinal detachment surgery. A striking finding was that 60 of the 204 eyes (30 per cent) had unsuspected tumors (56 melanomas, 2 metastatic tumors, and 1 hemangioma and 1 neurofibroma). The investigators obtained clinical information about the presence of retinal holes in 26 of the 60 tumor cases, but in 22 of the 26 cases no retinal break was observed histologically. An additional 14 of the 204 eyes had been enucleated for the suspicion of tumor, but none was found.

Another striking finding was the evidence of anterior segment necrosis in 47 eyes (23 per cent). This complication relates to surgical detachment of the rectus muscles, the placement of diathermy or a buckle or both in the region of the long ciliary arteries, and perhaps elevated intraocular pressure from the buckle. One of these eyes is illustrated in Figure 8–321. The scleral buckle from the encircling polyethylene tube is evident. Compare the intact ciliary body on the left with the necrotic area on the right in the same eye.

Patients with sickle cell hemoglobinopathy have an increased risk of development of anterior segment necrosis if adequate measures are not taken for the maintenance of blood oxygenation (Ryan, Goldberg, 1971).

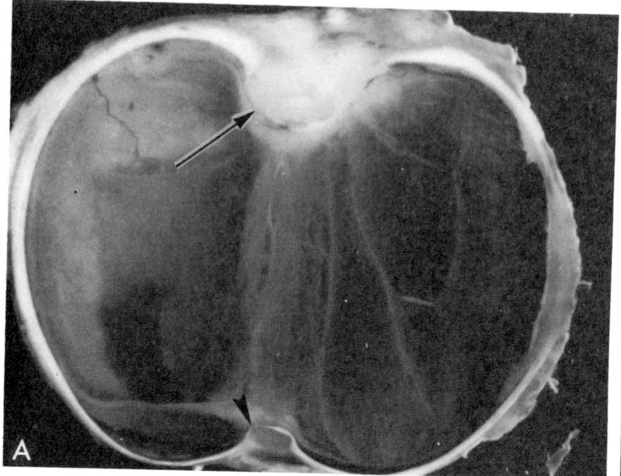

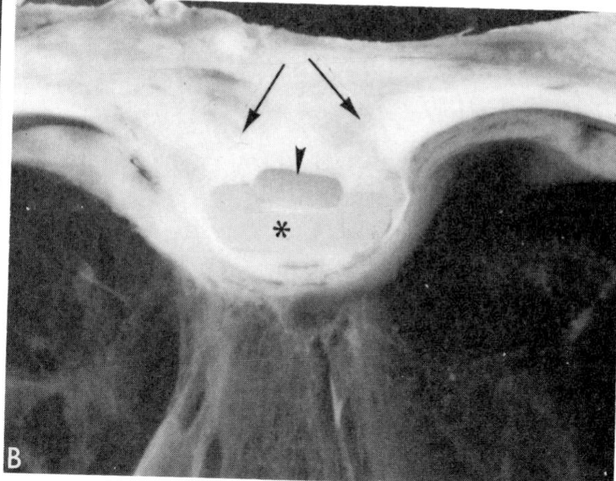

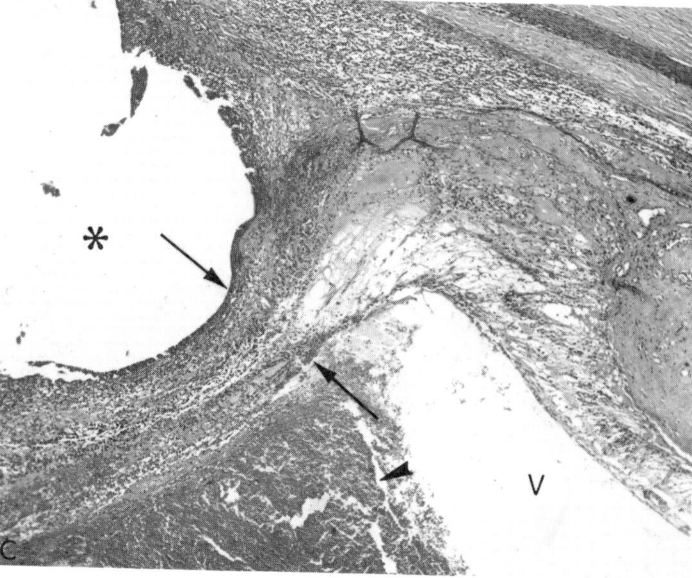

Figure 8–322. *A,* Gross appearance of eye after **scleral buckling procedure,** with erosion of silicone plate (arrow) and Silastic band (arrowhead). *B,* Closer view of eroded silicone plate (asterisk). Silastic band (arrowhead) is in place in groove of plate. Sclera is discontinuous (arrows), and plate is located internal to sclera. *C,* Section shows space (asterisk) where plate was located. Only a thin layer of inflammatory tissue (between arrows) and blood (arrowhead) separates plate from vitreous cavity *(V).* H and E, ×35. EP 31808. (From Green WR: Pathology of the retina, *in* Frayer WC (ed): Lancaster Course in Ophthalmic Histopathology. Unit 9. Philadelphia, F.A. Davis, 1981.)

Glaucoma was a conspicuous feature in most of the eyes studied by Boniuk and Zimmerman (1965). Other less frequent features were lens-induced endophthalmitis, sympathetic uveitis, granulomatous uveitis, keratitis, inflammatory reaction to sutures and implants, internal erosion of implants (Fig. 8–322) and tubes, and infected tubes.

Even with successful retinal reattachment surgery, vision may be severely reduced. In a series of 2000 eyes, 11 had unexplained blindness (Jarrett, Brockhurst, 1965). Complications observed after successful reattachment surgery may include central retinal artery occlusion, pigmentary changes in the macula, macular edema, macular cyst, and macular pucker (Sarin, McDonald, 1970).

Macular pucker (also see page 710) is a complication that is now commonly recognized; some of these cases are being treated surgically by stripping off the preretinal membrane. An example of untreated macular pucker after successful retinal detachment surgery is a 71 year old man who had a bilateral uncomplicated cataract extraction in both eyes in 1967. In April, 1968, he developed a retinal detachment that was successfully repaired. Postoperatively, he developed a macular pucker, with visual acuity of 20/200. A retinal detachment subsequently developed in the right eye in June, 1969. Vision 3 months postoperatively was 20/200, which was attributed to a macular hole.

Both eyes were obtained post mortem in February, 1974; microscopic examination showed similar findings in both eyes. In the right eye, a thin, hypocellular preretinal membrane was present in the macular area that apparently had contracted, producing wrinkling of the ILM (Fig. 8–323,*A*). In one area the contracted preretinal membrane had detached and had gathered the ILM in a coiled-up configuration (Fig. 8–323,*B*). The apparent glial cell preretinal membrane could be traced to discontinuities in the ILM (Fig. 8–323,*C*). A similar thin, hypocellular preretinal membrane with wrinkling of the ILM was also present in the left eye. There was also an area

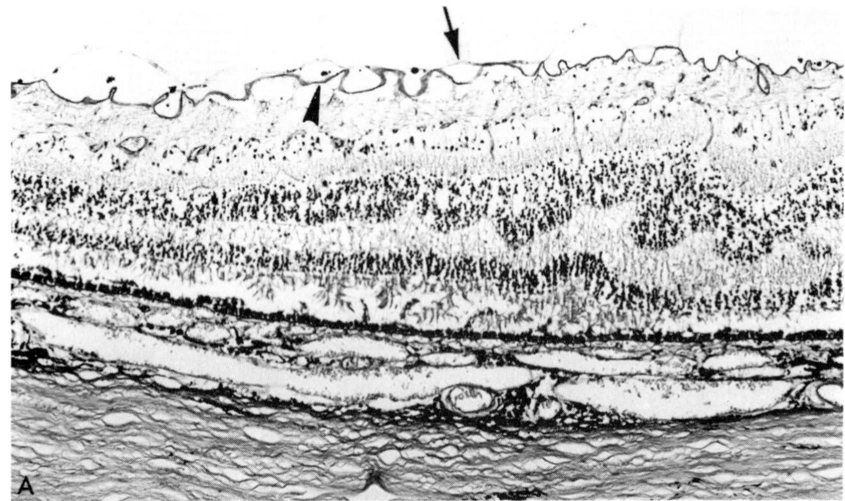

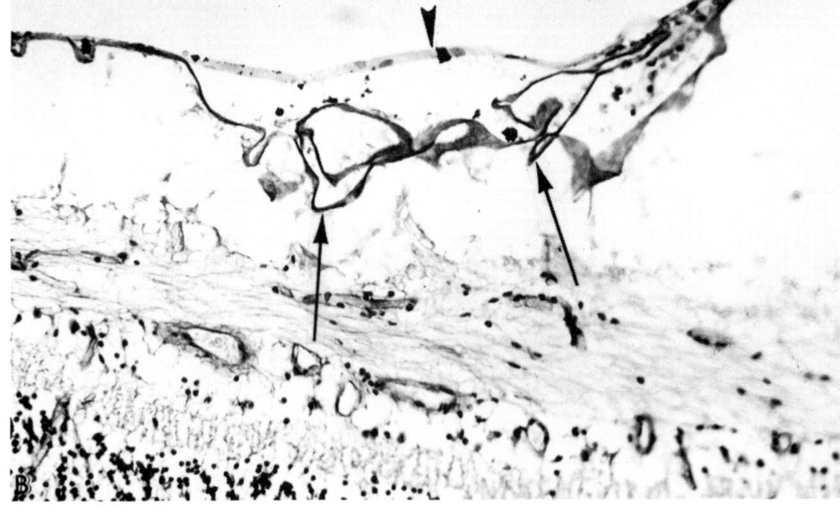

Figure 8–323. Bilateral macular pucker after retinal reattachment surgery. *A*, Right eye. Thin, hypocellular, preretinal membrane (arrow) with wrinkling of internal limiting membrane (ILM) (arrowhead). PAS, ×70. *B*, Right eye. Adjacent area showing marked gathering of ILM (arrows) by contracted preretinal membrane (arrowhead). PAS, ×185.

Illustration continued on opposite page

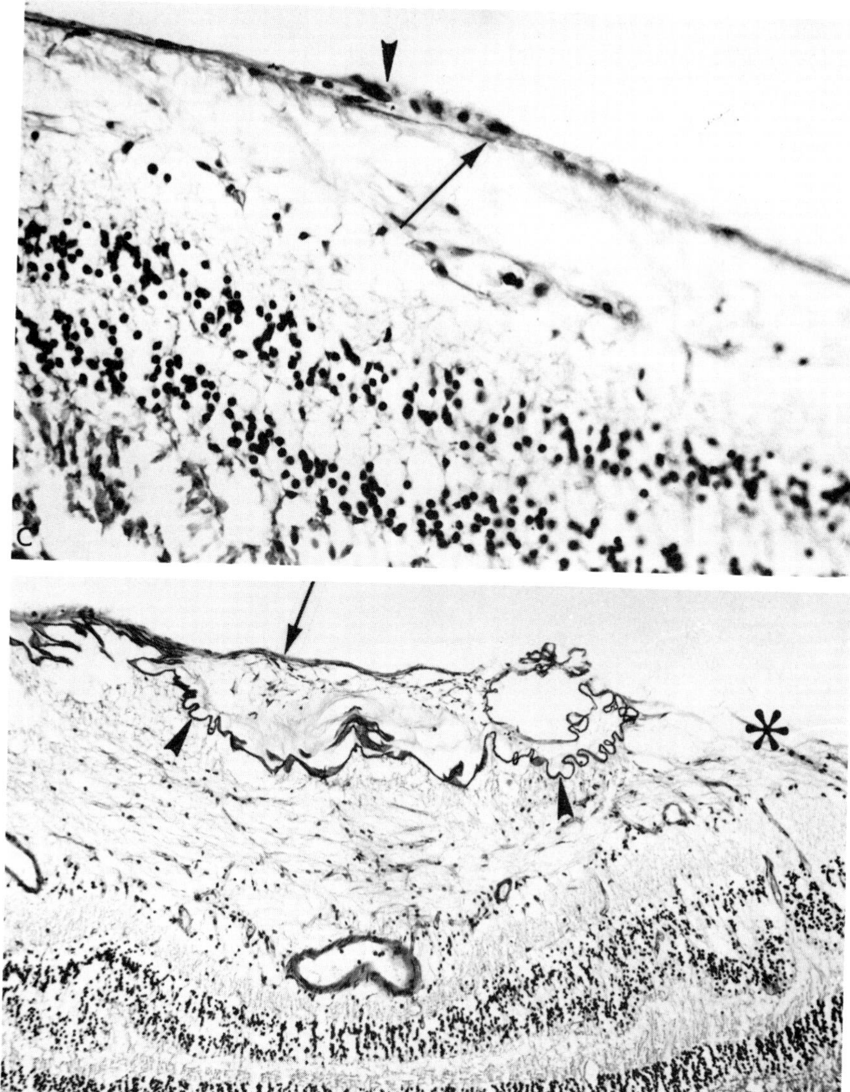

Figure 8–323 *Continued C,* Right eye. Additional area showing continuity of preretinal membrane (arrowhead) with discontinuity in the ILM (arrow). PAS, × 270. *D,* Left eye. Contraction of preretinal membrane (arrow) with marked wrinkling of ILM (arrowheads). Large area of retina has been stripped of ILM (asterisk) by contraction of preretinal membrane. PAS, ×90. EP 38147. (Courtesy of Dr. R.B. Welch. From Green WR, Kenyon KR, Michels RG, et al: Ultrastructure of epiretinal membranes causing macular pucker after retinal reattachment surgery. Trans Ophthalmol Soc UK *99*:63–77, 1979.)

where the membrane was thicker and had contracted to the point of avulsion and gathering of a large portion of the ILM (Fig. 8–323,*D*).

A second example is a 63 year old man who had an uncomplicated intracapsular cataract extraction with good visual results in 1971. Bilateral retinal detachment procedures were performed in 1973, after which he was noted to develop macular pucker in both eyes, with vision of 20/50 in the right eye and 20/400 in the left. Both eyes were obtained post mortem in 1975.

Microscopic examination of the right eye disclosed an extensive, thin, hypocellular preretinal membrane that was partially detached and had induced marked wrinkling of the ILM (Fig. 8–324,*A*). In another area, a strand of vitreous was attached to a thickened, partially detached area of preretinal membrane, with a large component of detached and coiled ILM (Fig. 8–324,*B*). A large adjacent area had no ILM. Microscopic examination of the macular area in the left eye showed even more marked changes. The contracted preretinal membrane had produced extreme folding of the macular retina and eversion at the point of an apparent hole (Fig. 8–324,*C–E*). The ILM was markedly folded and distorted.

Ultrastructural studies (Green, Kenyon, Michels, et al, 1979) have shown the principal cells of origin of these epiretinal membranes to be astrocytes.

Proliferative vitreoretinopathy (PVR) is a devastating complication of retinal detachment. Such proliferations in the vitreous and inner retinal surface then occur with great rapidity and lead to a fixed, folded, and detached retina. The princi-

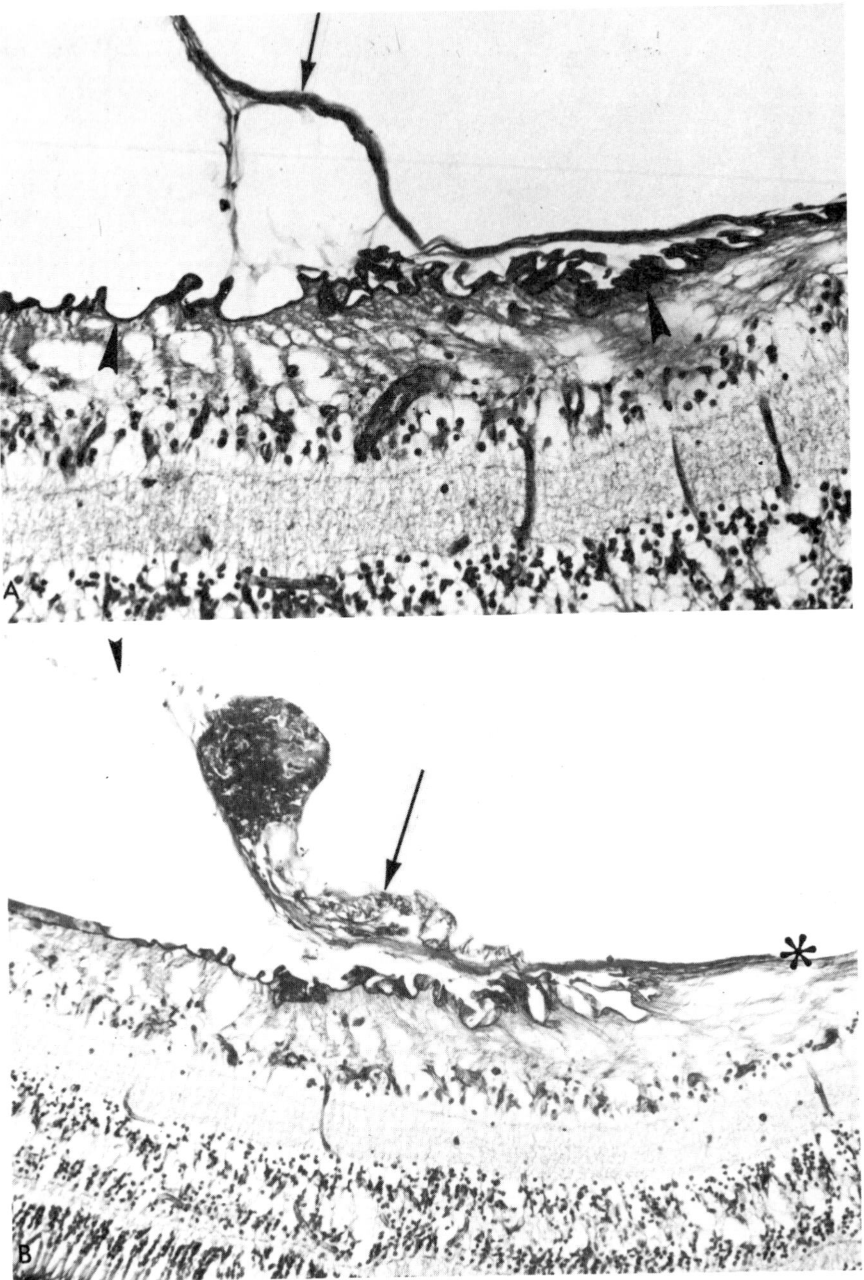

Figure 8–324. Bilateral macular pucker after retinal reattachment surgery. *A,* Right eye. Partially detached, hypocellular preretinal membrane (arrow), with marked wrinkling of internal limiting membrane (ILM) (arrowheads). PAS, ×200. *B,* Right eye. Another area, showing a partially detached, thickened area of preretinal membrane with a large segment of coiled ILM (arrow). A strand of vitreous is attached (arrowhead), and an adjacent area of retina has been stripped of its ILM (asterisk). Adjacent ILM is wrinkled. PAS, ×135.

Illustration continued on opposite page

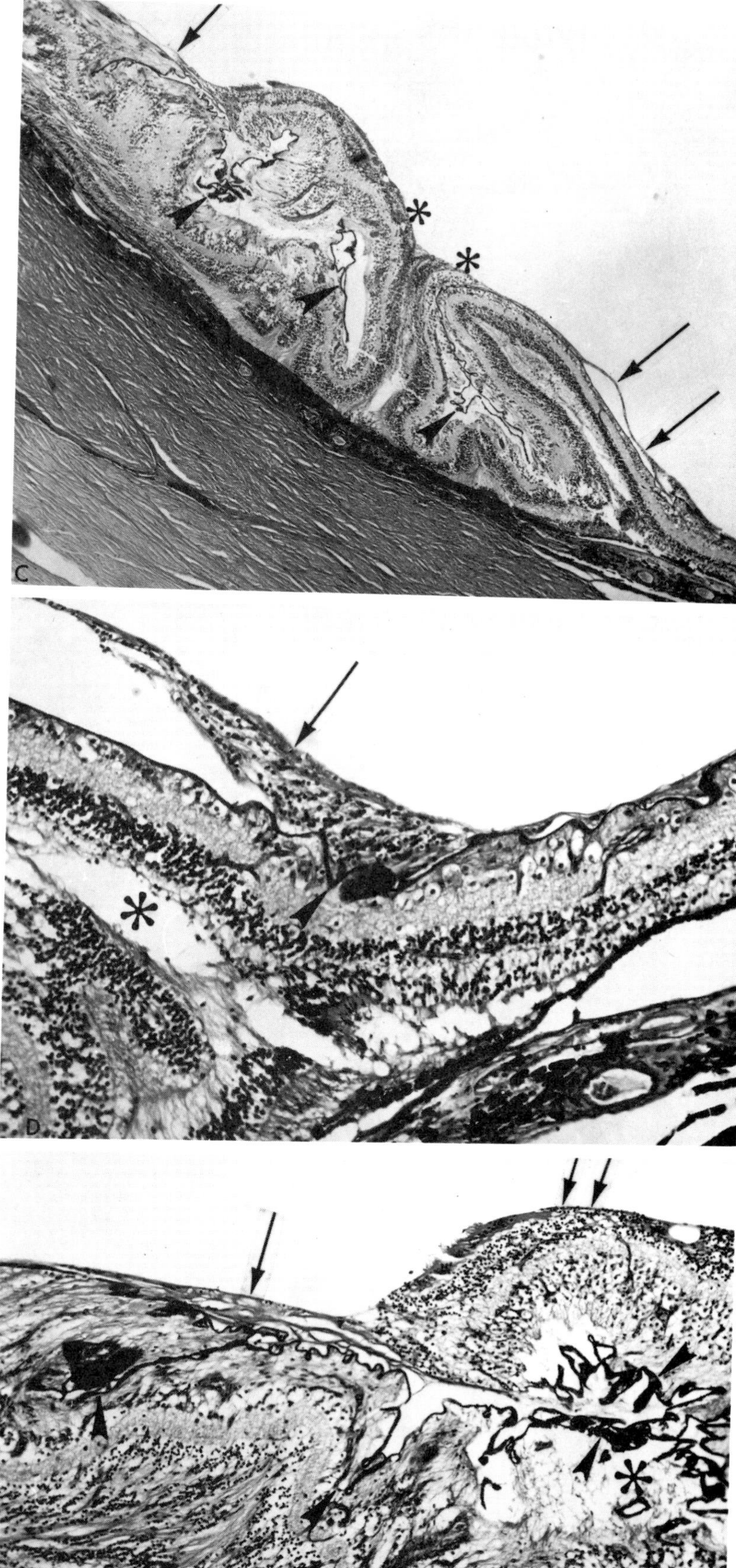

Figure 8–324 *Continued C,* Left eye. Extreme distortion of macular area from contraction of preretinal membrane (single arrow: nasal, two arrows: temporal). ILM (arrowheads) is contorted, and retina has been everted (asterisks) at site of an apparent hole. PAS, ×30.

D, Left eye. Higher power view of preretinal membrane (arrow) at temporal margin of extreme macular pucker. Retina is folded (asterisk), and ILM (arrowhead) is wrinkled. PAS, × 185. *E,* Left eye. Higher power view of nasal aspect of macular pucker, showing preretinal membrane (arrow), extreme wrinkling and gathering of ILM (arrowheads), separation of ILM (asterisk), and eversion of retina (two arrows). PAS, ×100. EP 40748.

(From Green WR, Kenyon KR, Michels RG, et al: Ultrastructure of epiretinal membranes causing macular pucker after retinal reattachment surgery. Trans Ophthalmol Soc UK *99*:63–77, 1979.)

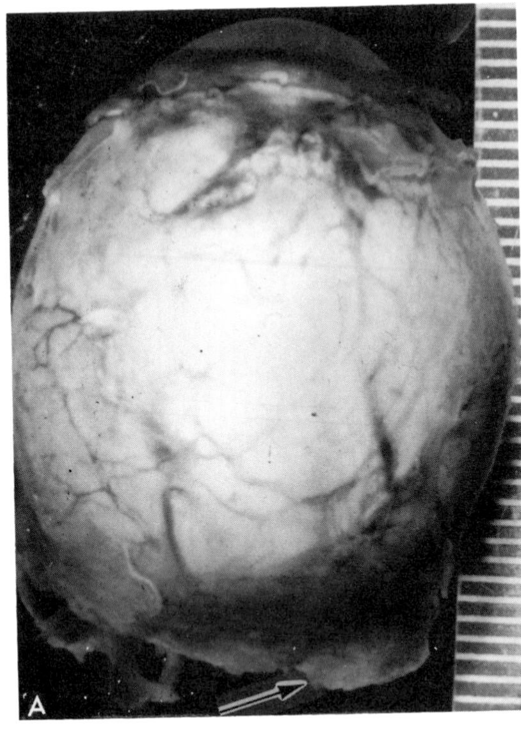

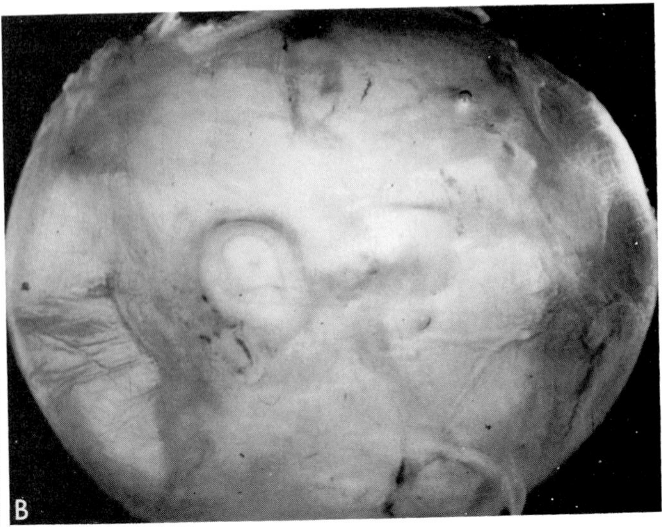

Figure 8–325. *A,* **Myopia.** View from above of left eye that measured 34 mm anteroposteriorly, 27 mm horizontally, and 27 mm vertically from a patient who had −14 diopters of correction. Arrow indicates optic nerve. EP 33620. *B,* Posterior view of right eye that measured 28 mm anteroposteriorly, 27 mm horizontally, and 24 mm vertically. Note bulge temporally. EP 31651.

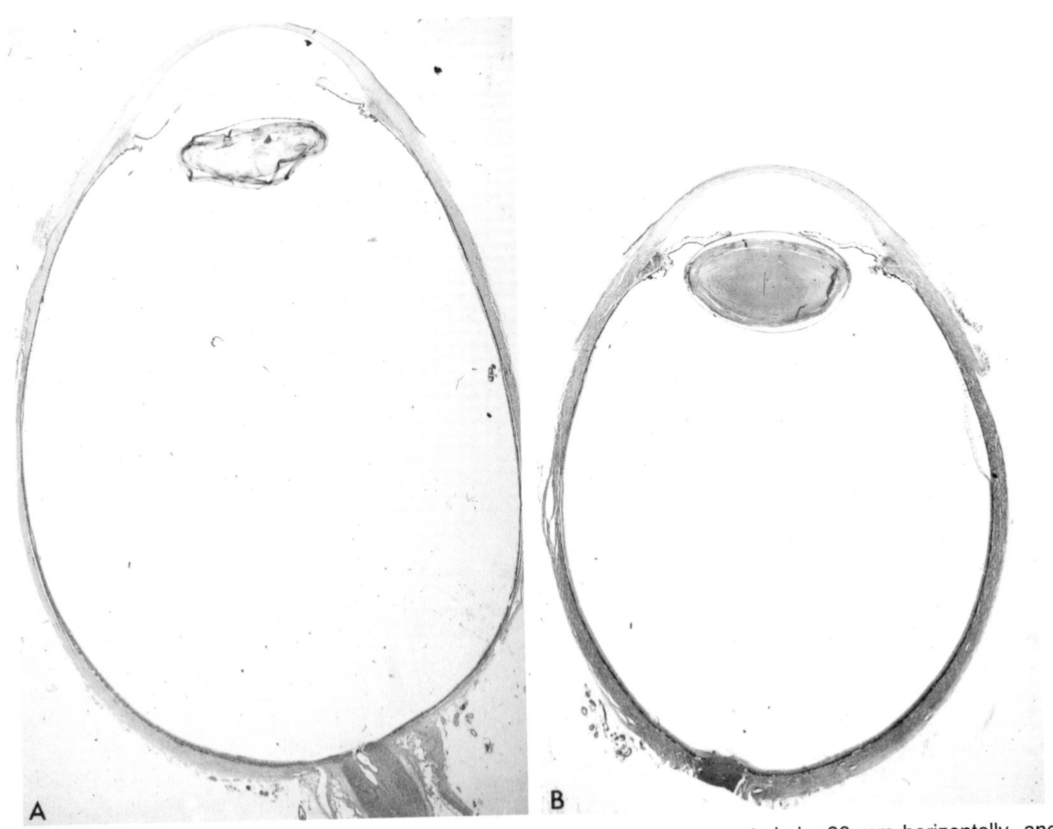

Figure 8–326. Comparison of a **myopic eye** *(A)* that measured 30 mm anteroposteriorly, 26 mm horizontally, and 25 mm vertically with an age-matched emmetropic eye *(B)* that measured 24 mm anteroposteriorly and 23 mm in horizontal and vertical places. Both, H and E. ×3.5. *A,* EP 31520. *B,* EP 39824.

pal cell in this condition appears to be retinal pigment epithelium (see more detailed discussion on page 710).

MYOPIA

Goldschmidt (1968) suggests that myopia exists in at least three different forms: simple or stationary; late; and high, pathologic or degenerative.

1. *Simple or stationary myopia* is the most frequent type. It develops during the period of body growth and is usually mild, rarely exceeding 6 to 9 diopters. Simple myopia is mainly genetically determined by a polygenic mode of inheritance.

2. *Late myopia* begins after somatic growth ceases. It is rarely severe and seems to be related to environmental conditions—excessively close visual work, for instance. These first two forms of myopia are rarely accompanied by significant pathologic changes.

3. *Pathologic or degenerative myopia* has been found to be the seventh leading cause of blindness in the United States. In this condition, myopia develops during youth and progresses throughout life, often reaching high degrees of refractive error. The process is more common in women and is associated with many ocular and systemic diseases: ocular albinism, pigmentary retinal degeneration, retrolental fibroplasia, Mar-

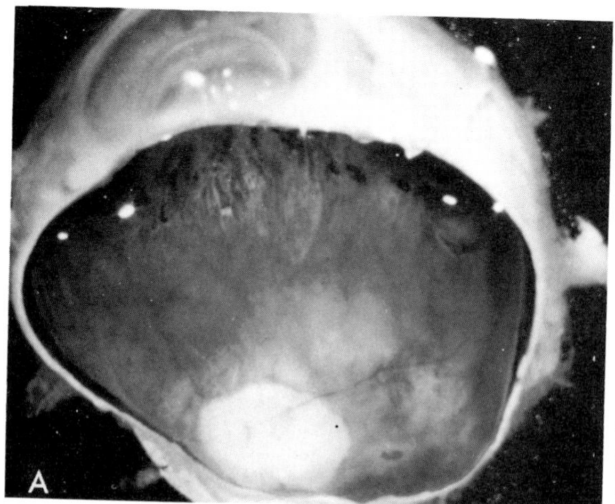

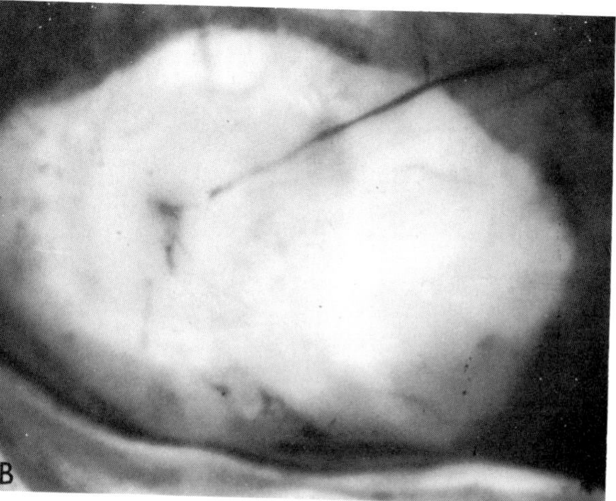

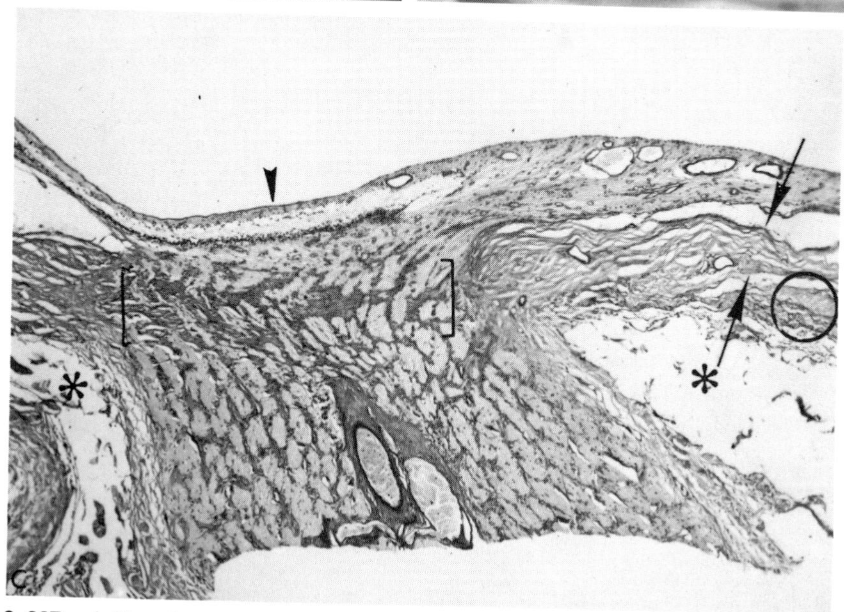

Figure 8–327. *A,* **Myopic eye,** 32 mm anteroposteriorly, 26 mm horizontally, and 25 mm vertically, with a peripapillary staphyloma. *B,* Closer view of peripapillary area, showing that most of the changes are temporal to the optic nerve head. *C,* Optic nerve head and peripapillary area, showing extension of retina (arrowhead) over the nasal two thirds of the optic disk, absence of choroid and retinal pigment epithelium in the temporal peripapillary area (arrows), lamina cribrosa (between brackets), much thinning of peripapillar sclera (between arrows), and marked enlargement of arachnoid and subdural spaces (asterisks), with lateral displacement of attachment of dura (circle). PAS, ×35. EP 50043.

fan's syndrome, Down's syndrome, and Ehlers-Danlos syndrome. Goldschmidt (1968) concludes that both heredity and environment play a role in the etiology of high myopia, with one factor more or less predominating in any particular patient.

With pathologic myopia, as the name implies, there are characteristic pathologic ocular changes. The basic feature is enlargement of the eyeball, with lengthening of the posterior segment. As seen grossly, the eye becomes elongated and egg-shaped rather than globoid (Figs. 8–325 and 8–326). Subsequently, myopic refractive errors and degenerative fundus changes develop in proportion to the magnitude of ocular axial elongation (Curtin, Karlin, 1971). Although this is generally true, there are exceptions. Zauberman and Merin (1969) studied 20 cases of myopic anisometropia greater than 5 diopters and found peripheral retinal degenerative conditions in 7 of the nearly emmetropic eyes.

Elongation of the globe in the anteroposterior (AP) dimension occurs by progressive thinning of the posterior sclera. This eventually gives rise to what is seen grossly as a posterior ectasia or staphyloma. Curtin (1977) found these defects to involve the posterior pole, macular area, peripapillary zone, nasal area, or inferior fundus (Figs. 8–327 through 8–331). Compound and complex forms were also described. Light microscopic examination of the thinned ectatic sclera (Curtin, Teng, 1958) reveals meridional collagen bundles that are thinned, with a reduction in refringency, a loss of dark longitudinal fiber striations, and fibrous bundle dissociation. Cross-sectioned equa-

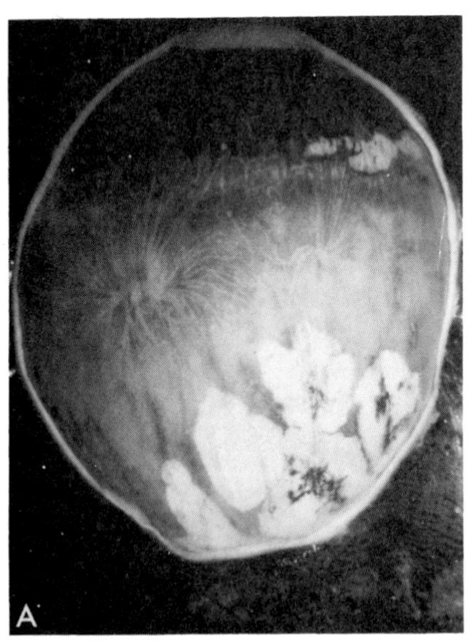

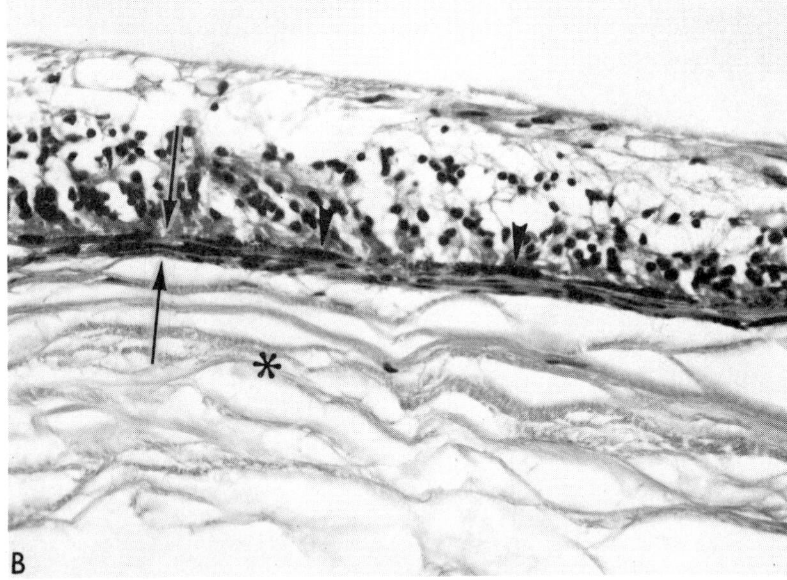

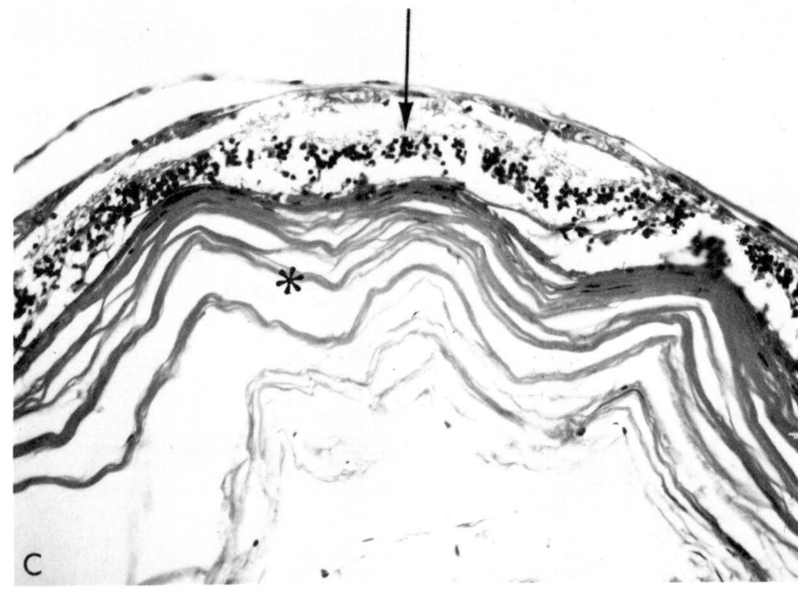

Figure 8–328. *A,* Gross appearance of superotemporal **staphyloma** with severe atrophy of retinal pigment epithelium (RPE) and choroid in an eye that measured 27 mm anteroposteriorly, 33 mm vertically, and 30 mm horizontally. *B,* Area of staphyloma located about 4 mm superotemporal to the optic disk. Thin sclera (asterisk) is artifactitiously separated. Very thin choroid (between arrows) is intact, as are RPE (arrowheads) and some photoreceptor cells. H and E, ×300. *C,* Area of most marked changes in staphyloma. Sclera (asterisk) measured about 80 microns in thickness. Choroid and RPE are absent, and inner nuclear layer (arrow) rests against sclera. H and E, ×185. EP 50781.

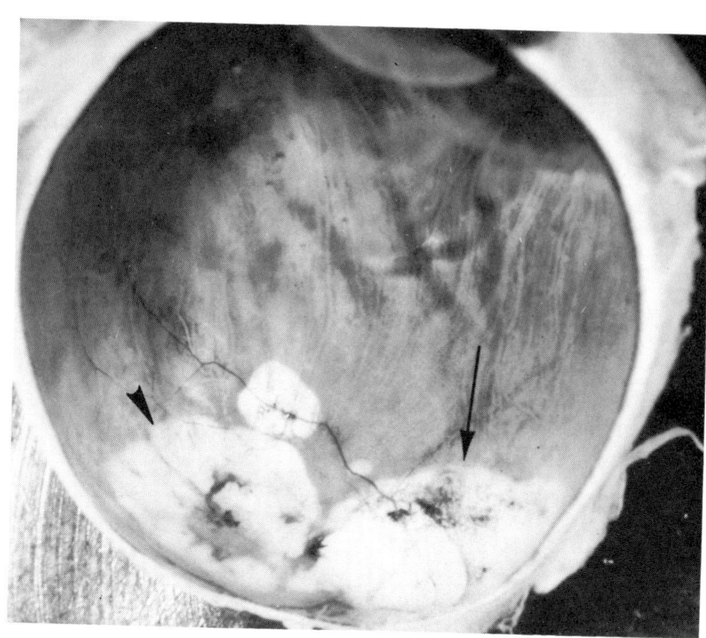

Figure 8–329. Scleral thinning with **staphyloma** and atrophy of choroid and retinal pigment epithelium in peripapillary (arrow) and posterior pole (arrowhead) areas in eye that measured 31 mm anteroposteriorly and 27 mm horizontally and vertically. EP 33581.

torial bundles show fibers that are separated, reduced in size, and splayed in the AP plane. With higher grades of myopia, the thinned sclera may even appear lamellar (like cornea) or amorphous. In the posterior sclera of five staphylomatous eyes studied with transmission electron microscopy, Curtin, Iwamoto, Renaldo, (1979) noted a predominantly lamellar arrangement of the collagen fiber bundles. The collagen fibrils within the bundles were seen to be smaller, more dispersed, and more uniform than in normal sclera. They also had a unique star-shaped pattern on cross-section. These changes were interpreted as being compatible with an abnormal proteoglycan composition of interfibrillary substance in the ectatic sclera.

Posterior *staphylomas* were observed in 19 per cent of myopic eyes with axial lengths of 26.5 mm or more (Curtin, Karlin, 1971). They are also more prevalent with increasing age. Posterior staphylomas have a guarded visual prognosis, because 19.6 per cent of these eyes in one study were legally blind. After the age of 60 years, 53.3 per cent of eyes with staphylomas were legally blind (Curtin, 1977).

With progressive elongation of the globe and ectasia of the posterior sclera, associated chorioretinal changes occur. Histologically, there is a generalized thinning of the choroid, which progresses to loss of the choriocapillaris and leads toward absence of the choroid, especially at the base of the staphyloma. With choroidal atrophy, splits may develop occasionally in Bruch's membrane. Fluorescein angiographic data from Klein and Curtin (1975) suggest that these splits heal to form fine, irregular yellow lines that often branch and criss-cross about the posterior pole. These lines, called *lacquer cracks* (Fig. 8–332), are seen in only 4.3 per cent of highly myopic eyes (axial length of 26.5 mm or more), and they affect predominantly young men (Curtin, Karlin, 1971). This predominance in men is not present in continued studies. Also, in the Klein and Curtin study of 22 eyes with lacquer cracks, all had staphylomas and temporal crescents. Significantly, seven eyes also showed choroidal hemorrhages along the course of lacquer cracks.

It might be expected that a process that produces breaks in Bruch's membrane would predispose to sub-RPE neovascular membrane formation with subsequent hemorrhage and disciform scarring. Such is the case in myopia, in which 5.2 per cent of highly myopic eyes have been observed to have a small pigmented lesion in the area centralis (Curtin, Karlin, 1971). Called a *Fuchs' spot* (Fuchs, 1901), this lesion differs from senile macular degeneration by its increased tendency to pigment deposition and its occurrence in areas of myopic chorioretinal atrophy (Levy, Pollack, Curtin, 1977). Most Fuchs' spots are associated with choroidal neovascularization that locally penetrates Bruch's membrane and extends beneath the RPE and may lead to serous and hemorrhagic RPE detachments.

Histologically, the spot appears as a fibrovascular scar containing hyperplastic RPE and basement membrane that extends into the retina (Fig. 8–333). Some Fuchs' spots have retinochoroidal vascular anastomosis. When these areas of choroidal neovascularization and retinochoroidal anastomoses are totally surrounded by hyperplastic RPE, the lesions may not stain with or leak fluorescein.

With degeneration of the choriocapillaris and

Text continued on page 921

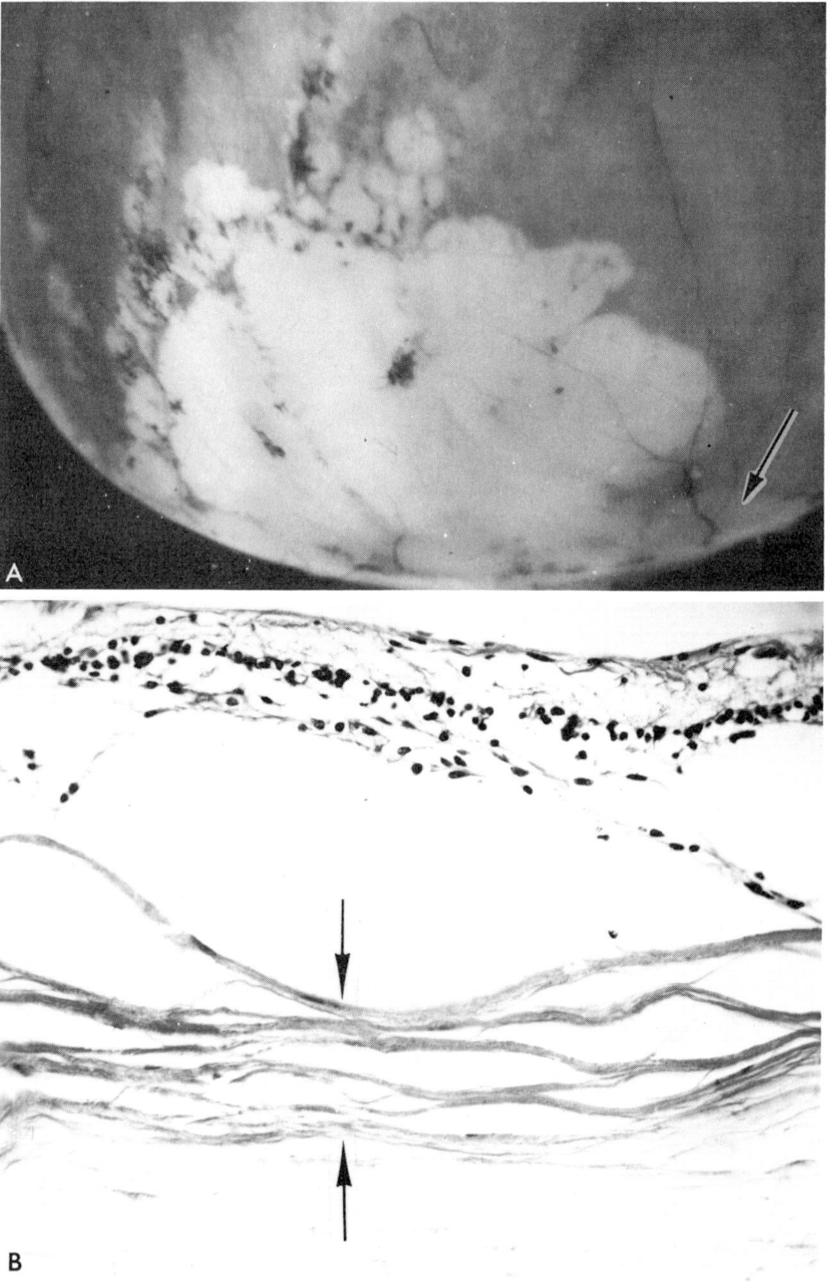

Figure 8–330. *A,* Gross appearance of **staphyloma** temporal to optic nerve head (arrow), with loss of retinal pigment epithelium (RPE) and choroid. *B,* Thinned sclera (between arrows) is less than 100 microns in thickness, and choroid and RPE are absent. H and E, ×300. EP 33096.

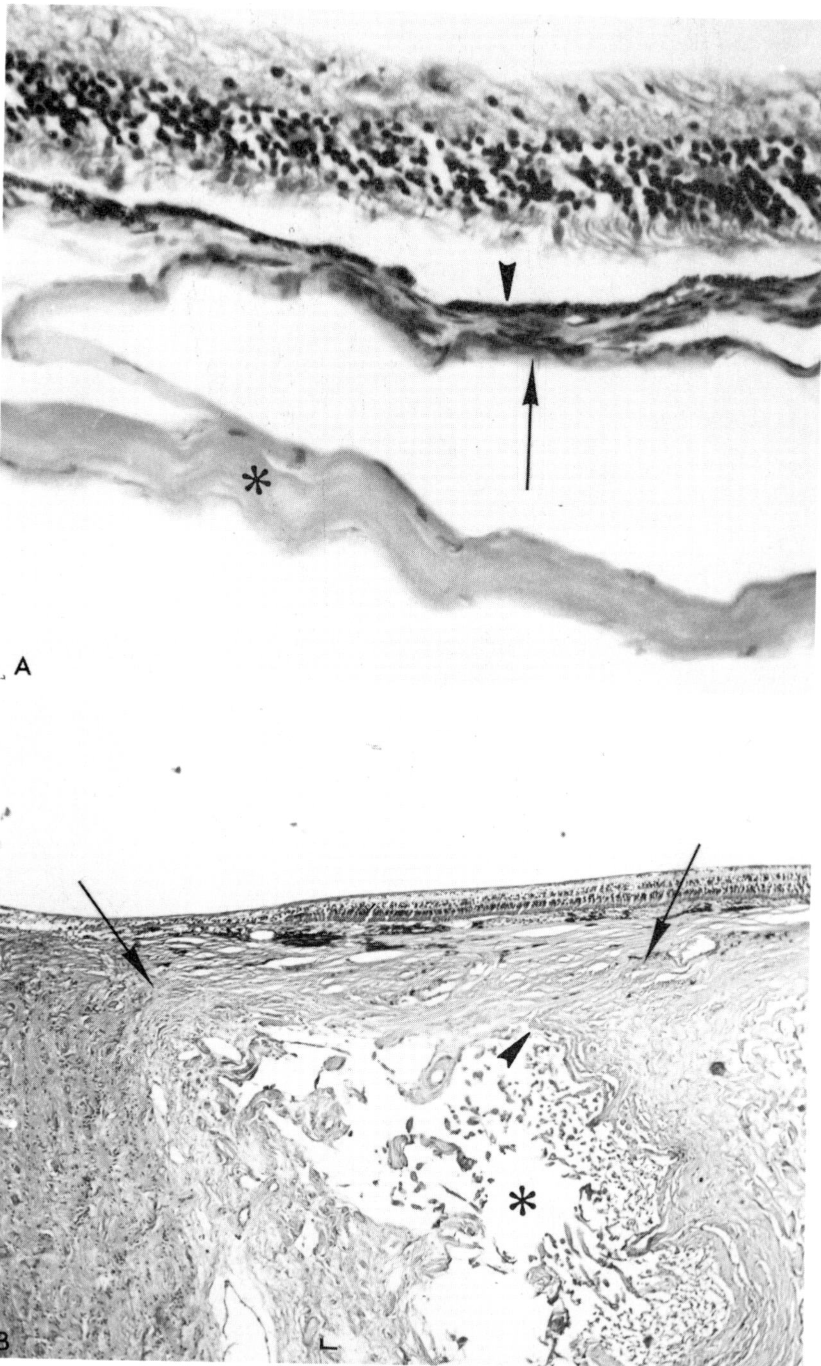

Figure 8–331. *A,* Area of temporal **staphyloma** of eye shown in Figure 8–327,*B.* Sclera (asterisk) measures about 60 microns in thickness. It is amazing that choroid (arrow) is present, but thinned. Retinal pigment epithelium (arrow) and retina are relatively intact. H and E, ×270 EP 31651. *B,* Optic nerve head and temporal peripapillary area of eye illustrated in Figure 8–328,*A* shows extreme stretching of sclera (between arrows), resulting in lateral displacement of dural attachment (arrowhead) and widening of subdural space (asterisk). H and E, ×35. EP 31520.

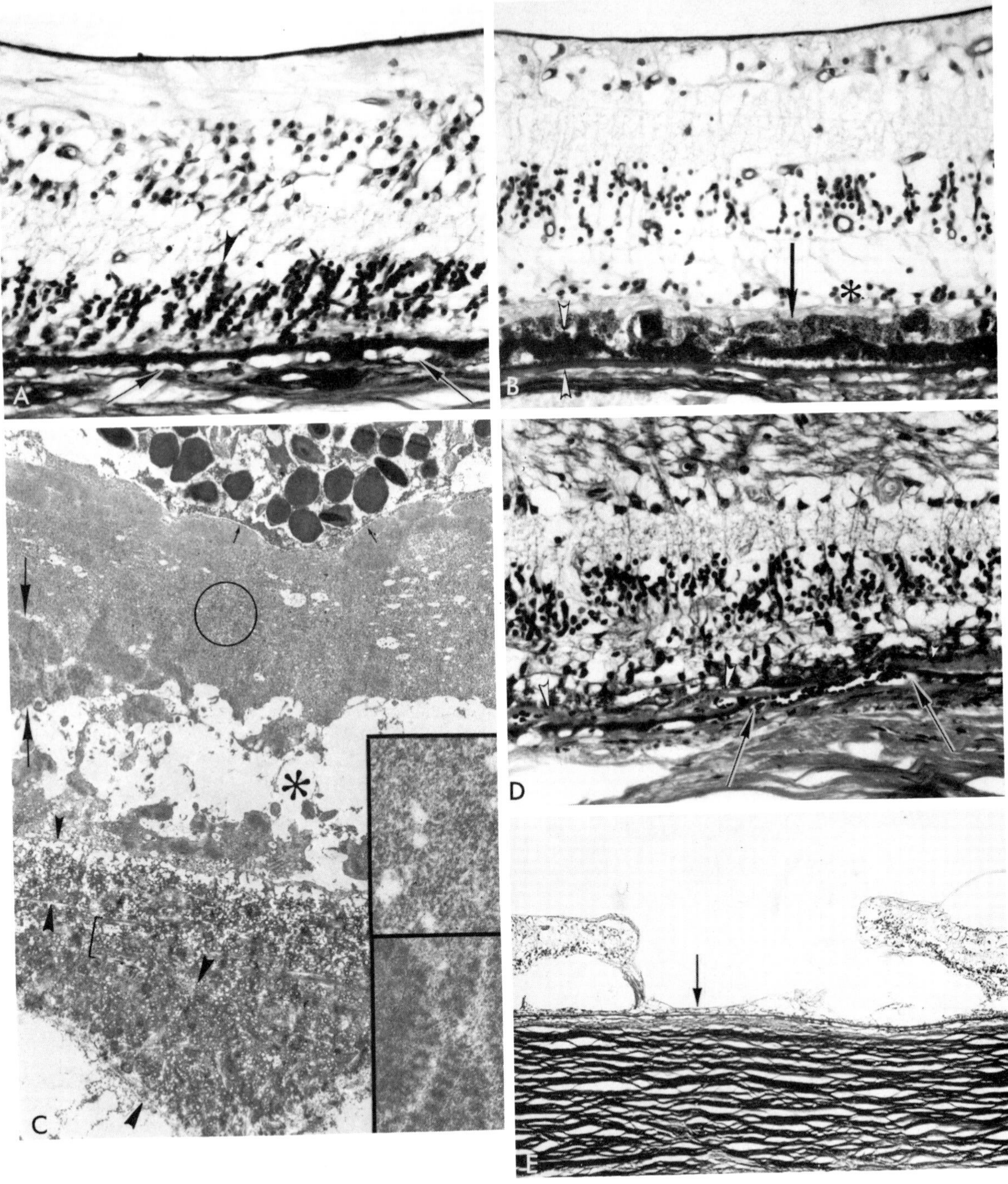

Figure 8–332 *See legend on opposite page*

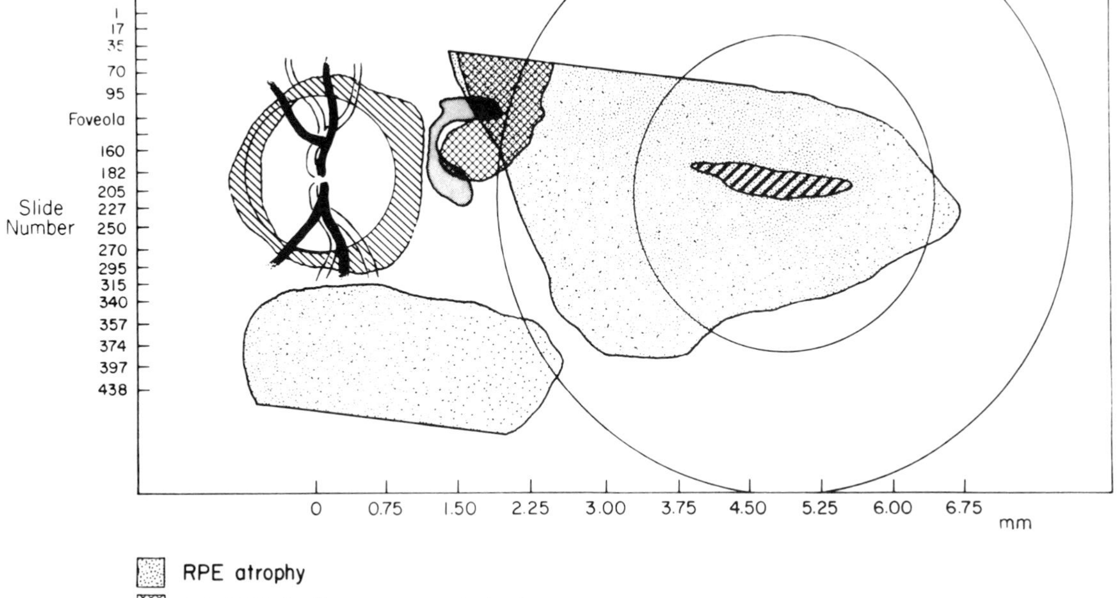

Figure 8–332. Unilateral high myopia in an eye that measured 31 mm anteroposteriorly, 27 mm horizontally, and 25 mm vertically. *A,* Diffuse areolar retinal pigment epithelium (RPE) atrophy in posterior pole. Choriocapillaris (arrows) is intact, RPE is absent, and inner nuclear layer (arrowhead) rests against a slightly thickened Bruch's membrane. Verhoeff–van Gieson, ×470. *B,* An area outside areolar atrophy shows marked thickening of the inner aspect of Bruch's membrane (between arrowheads), an intact RPE (arrow), loss of inner and outer segments of photoreceptors, and much thinning of the outer nuclear layer (asterisk).

C, Area similar to *B.* Tissue taken from paraffin and processed for electron microscopy. Basement membrane of RPE is normal (smaller arrows). Elastic layer of Bruch's membrane (bracket) and outer, and what appears to be inner, collagenous layers are thickened by small vesicles and electron-dense material (between arrowheads). There are deposition of abundant fine fibrillar-granular material (circle and lower inset) and large aggregates of wide-spaced collagen (larger arrows and upper inset). Splitting (asterisk) has occurred in the thick, new layer between the RPE and the degenerated inner collagenous zone of Bruch's membrane. ×7460; insets, ×45,200.

D, Section of linear break in Bruch's membrane ("lacquer crack") (between arrows) at which point choroidal vessels (arrowheads) extend under the RPE. Verhoeff–van Gieson, ×55. *E,* Lamellar macular hole. A thin layer of retinal tissue (arrow) extends across the posterior aspect and defect. Margins of lamellar hole are rounded, and thin preretinal membrane is present. PAS, ×90. *F,* Two-dimensional reconstruction of posterior region of eye from study of serial sections. It shows size, shape, and relation of various histopathologic features. EP 42508.

(From Green WR, Key SN III: Senile macular degeneration: A histopathologic study. Trans Am Ophthalmol Soc *75*:180–254, 1977.)

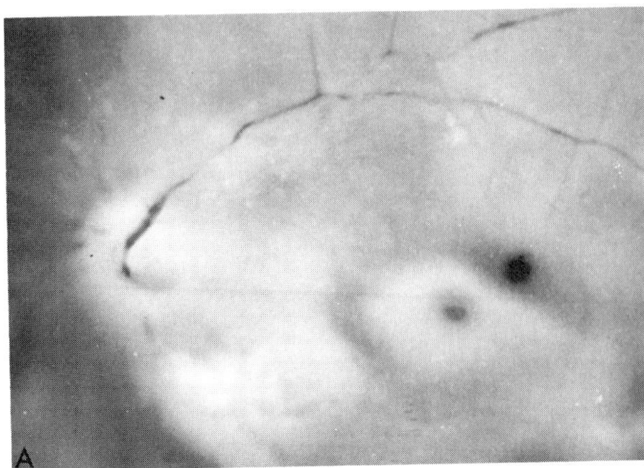

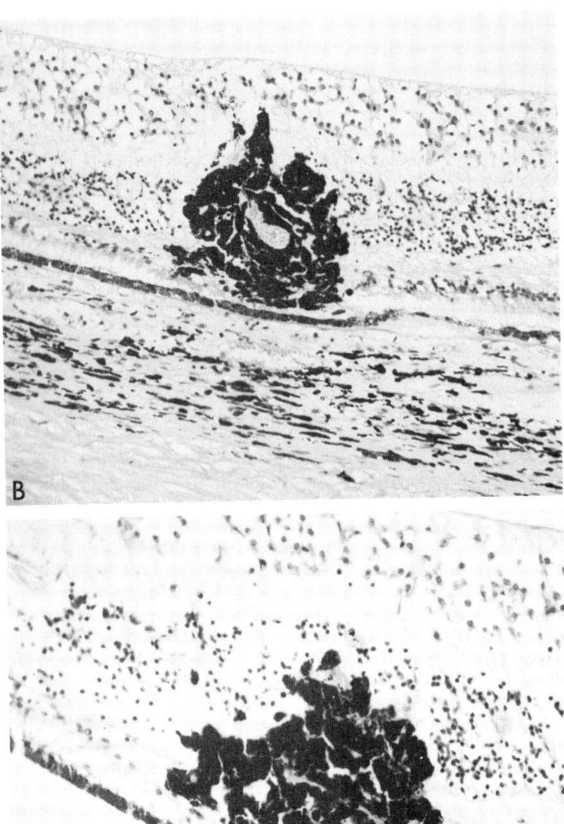

Figure 8–333. *A,* Gross appearance of a **Fuchs' spot.** EP 33092. *B,* Fuchs' spot consists of an intraretinal vascular abnormality surrounded by hyperplastic retinal pigment epithelium. PAS, ×185. EP 36664. *C,* With serial sections, retinal vascular abnormality (arrow) could be traced into choroid. PAS, ×300. EP 36665.

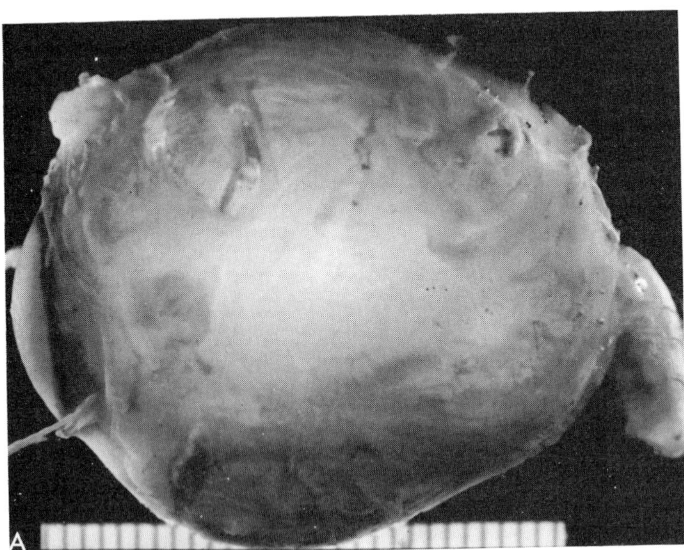

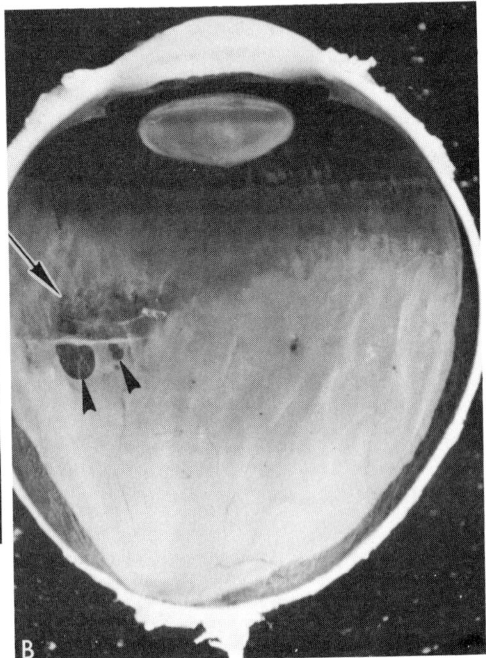

Figure 8–334. *A,* Unilateral **myopic eye** that measured 29 mm anteroposteriorly, 25 mm horizontally, and 24 mm vertically. *B,* A large area of lattice degeneration (arrows) of the retina, with holes (arrowheads) at the posterior margin, is present at the superonasal equator. EP 32238.

the remainder of the choroid, there is a subsequent degeneration of the RPE and outer retinal layers. Curtin and Karlin (1971) have found the ophthalmoscopic presence of chorioretinal atrophy to be directly related to ocular axial length and age. Furthermore, they observed such atrophy most commonly in the posterior pole in association with staphyloma (77.5 per cent) and annular-type myopic crescents (56 per cent).

Peripherally, one sees chorioretinal involvement, including white-without-pressure, pavingstone degeneration, pigmentary degeneration, and lattice degeneration. In a study of 1437 eyes, Karlin and Curtin (1976) made a positive association between the prevalence of all four of these changes and ocular axial length. Furthermore, they found white-without-pressure (an ophthalmoscopic finding) to be more prevalent in young myopic eyes, whereas pigmentary degeneration and pavingstone degeneration were more common in the aged. Lattice degeneration, which has a prevalence of 1 to 10 per cent in normal eyes, occurs with considerable variability in myopes, but can be seen in up to 20 per cent of these eyes (Fig. 8–334) (Kirker, McDonald, 1971).

The chorioretinal changes just discussed predispose the myopic retina to breaks and thus to retinal detachment. Retinal breaks usually occur in areas involved with chorioretinal lesions, but they may also arise in areas of apparently normal retina (Dumas, Schepens, 1966). A minority of these breaks will progress to rhegmatogenous retinal detachment (Hyams, Meir, Ivry, et al, 1974). In myopes who do develop retinal detachment, Menezo, Suarez-Reynolds, Frances, and Vila (1977) found the "horseshoe" type and "punched-out" round retinal tears to be the most common. This tendency of the myopic retina to progress from breaks to detachment accounts for the 34 to 79 per cent prevalence of myopia in retinal detachment patients, as opposed to the 5 to 18 per cent prevalence of myopia in the general population (Schepens, Marden, 1966). In fact, with each increment in the degree of myopia the risk of retinal detachment also increases. It has been estimated (Kaluzny, 1970) that the risk of retinal detachment for 5 diopter myopia is 15 times that for emmetropia; for 20 diopter myopia the likelihood is 110 times that of normal.

As some myopic eyes enlarge, the retinal vessels do not lengthen as much as the remainder of the retina does. This results in what is termed *stretch schisis* of the retina (Fig. 8–335). Such a mechanism results in separation of the larger retinal vessels and internal limiting membrane from the remainder of the retina in a reticular cystoid or schisis-like picture (Fig. 8–335,*D*). In other areas, only the retinal vessels are separated from the retina. This leads to a picture that may resemble retinal pits (Fig. 8–335,*F* and *G*) but is due to a different mechanism than that of retinal pits.

At the optic nerve head are classic myopic changes. Ophthalmoscopically, the optic nerve head may appear tilted toward, and flattened on, the temporal side. There is an apparent increase in the optic cup to optic disk area ratio, which varies directly with the ocular axial length (Tomlinson, Phillips, 1969). Temporal to the disk, there may be a bright white crescent of sclera that is again rimmed by a pigmented and rather vascular choroidal crescent. The pigmented crescent is caused by hypertrophy and sometimes hyperplasia of the RPE. This ophthalmoscopic picture is the myopic or temporal crescent, which, in the classic viewpoint of Schnabel (1874) results from choroid and lamina vitrea (Bruch's membrane) being pulled or pushed posteriorly into an ectasia. This in turn draws and stretches these structures away from their normal position at the optic disk. The incidence of temporal crescent varies directly with axial length, being 0 per cent in short eyes and 100 per cent in long eyes (Curtin, Karlin, 1971).

Histopathologically, in the presence of a temporal crescent, the optic nerve pursues an oblique course through the scleral canal. At the temporal side of the disk, RPE and Bruch's membrane stop some distance from the disk margin. In this way, a variable amount of choroid is left uncovered by pigment epithelium as the RPE thins on its approach to the optic nerve head. Usually the choroid itself terminates short of the disk edge and thus leaves underlying sclera and optic canal exposed. In contrast to the temporal side, nasally the RPE, Bruch's membrane, and choroid are seen to extend over the scleral lip and to cover a variable portion of the optic foramen. This histologic feature is sometimes termed supertraction or supervolution of the retina.

Vitreous changes, including degeneration, liquefaction, and opacities, are quite common in high myopia (Kirker, McDonald, 1971).

Changes in the anterior segment are few in pathologic myopia. The anterior chamber depth is often increased from enlargement of the globe. The ciliary body is usually more flattened in high myopia, and the circular and radial muscles are less conspicuous and are located slightly more posterior than in nonmyopic eyes. Peripheral iris remnants and processes are present in approximately 50 per cent of the eyes with posterior staphylomas, and these abnormalities correlate with ocular hypertension and glaucoma (Curtin, 1981).

Open-angle glaucoma is common in myopia, affecting 23.1 per cent of myopic eyes measuring above 30.5 mm in axial length (Diaz, 1966). Lastly, the frequency of cataract formation (es-

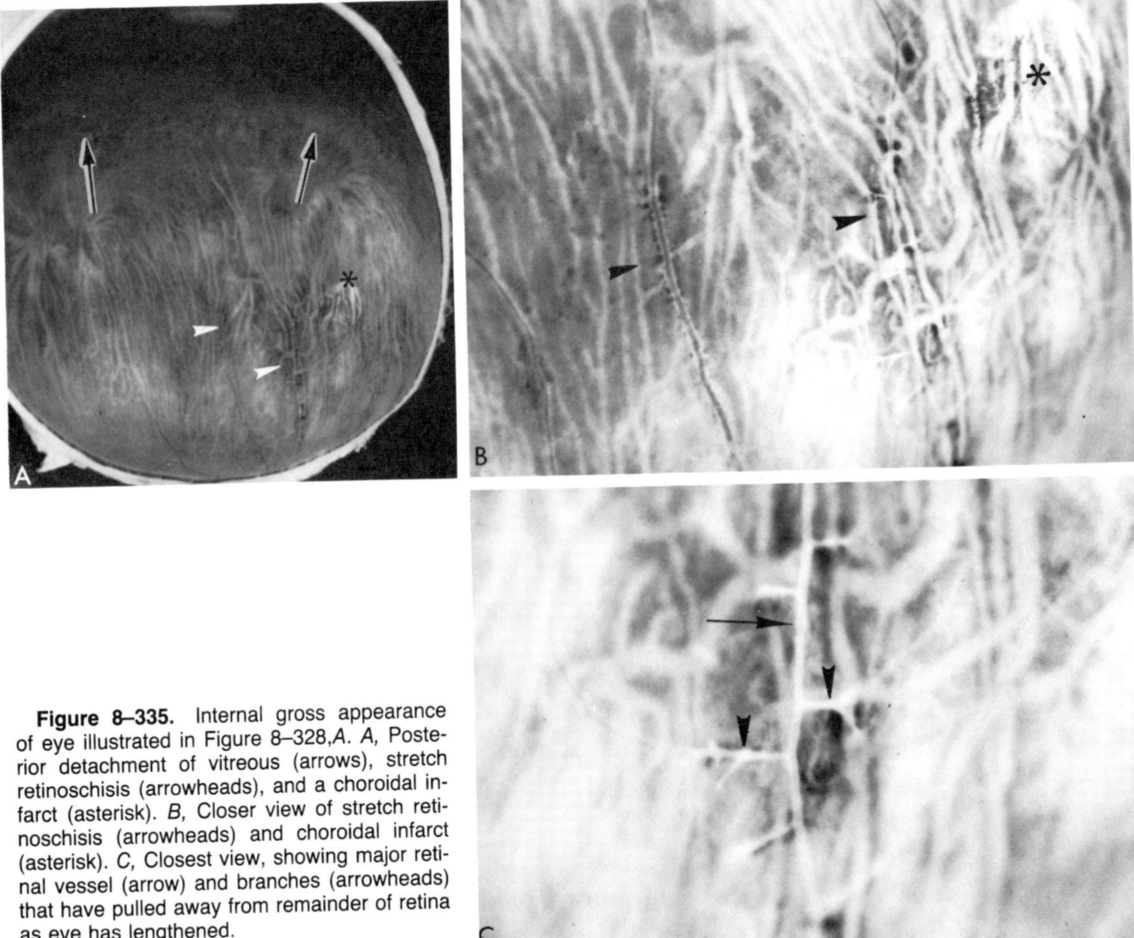

Figure 8–335. Internal gross appearance of eye illustrated in Figure 8–328,*A*. *A,* Posterior detachment of vitreous (arrows), stretch retinoschisis (arrowheads), and a choroidal infarct (asterisk). *B,* Closer view of stretch retinoschisis (arrowheads) and choroidal infarct (asterisk). *C,* Closest view, showing major retinal vessel (arrow) and branches (arrowheads) that have pulled away from remainder of retina as eye has lengthened.

Illustration continued on opposite page

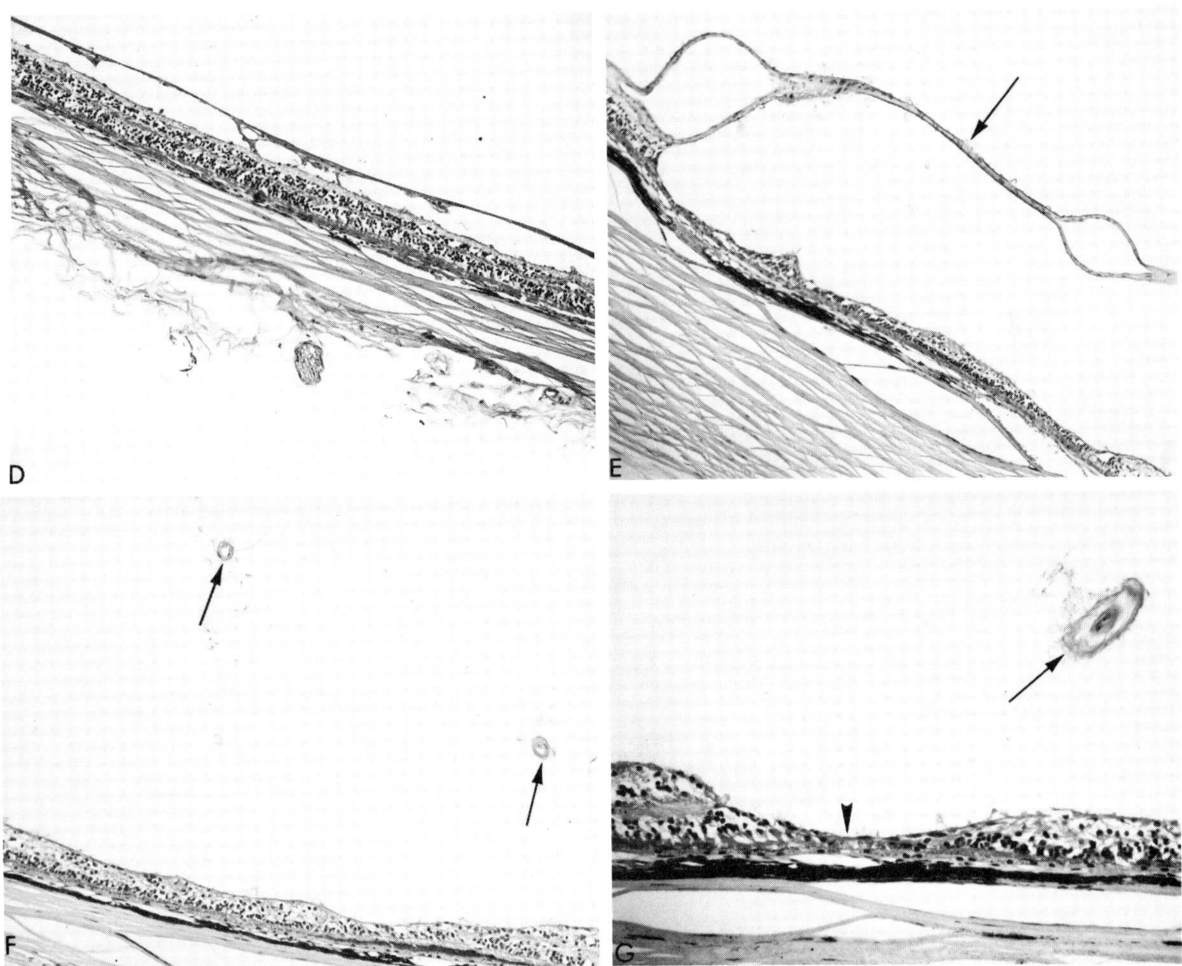

Figure 8–335. *Continued D,* Area of retinoschisis in nerve fiber layer adjacent to area where retinal vessels have detached from retina. H and E, ×100. *E,* Posterior margin of stretch retinoschisis, showing retinal vessel (arrow) separated from irregular and thinned outer layer of retina. H and E, ×120. *F,* Middle of lesion, showing retinal vessel (arrows) traversing outer vitreous cavity. H and E, ×120. *G,* Higher power view of occluded retinal vessel (arrow) in vitreous cavity and pitlike change (arrowhead) in irregular retinal layer. H and E, ×220. EP 31520.

pecially a stellate posterior subcapsular configuration), vitreous degeneration and detachment, lattice degeneration of the retina, and retinal detachment is higher in degenerative myopia than in nonmyopic eyes.

Using data from the 1971 to 1972 National Health and Nutrition Examination Survey, Sperduto, Seigel, Roberts, and Rowland (1983) found the prevalence of myopia of the right eye to be 25 per cent in persons between the ages of 12 and 54 years. Prevalence rates were significantly lower for men than for women and for blacks than for whites. These investigators noted that myopia prevalence rose with family income and educational level. Higher income and educational levels may be associated with a greater use of near vision—a factor that has been implicated in the pathogenesis of myopia.

PATHOLOGY OF THE MACULA

The term *macula* (macula lutea) has no histologic counterpart, and the term stems from the deposition of a pigment, carotenoid, in an oval pattern in the posterior pole of the retina. The presence of this pigment in the macular area varies and has been shown to be related to diet in experimental studies in monkeys (Malinow, Feeney-Burns, Peterson, et al, 1980). Those investigators found that the yellow pigmentation was absent in monkeys fed a diet that was free of xanthophyll content.

The *area centralis* and its components have definite histologic features and are defined on the basis of the number of ganglion cells, the number and ratio of rods and cones, and other criteria (see Fig. 8–11) (Hogan, Alvarado, Weddell, 1971, pages 491–498).

By convention, most ophthalmologists consider the term macula to refer to the central portion of the *area centralis,* inclusive of the parafoveal area. Some authors, however, equate the foveal area with the macula (Orth, Fine, Fagman, Quirk, 1977).

Congenital Anomalies of the Macula. These include aplasia and folds. Aplasia of the macula has been presumed on clinical grounds in regard to aniridia and persistent hyperplastic primary vitreous, but this has not been confirmed histologically. Curran and Robb (1976) observed isolated foveal hypoplasia in nine patients with varying degrees of congenital nystagmus and no other associated abnormalities. Yoshizumi, Thomas, and Hirose (1979) observed one patient with foveal hypoplasia associated with peripheral retinal rosettes and postulated the etiology to be an intercurrent infection during the late stages of embryogenesis. Macular aplasia has been confirmed histologically in X-linked ocular albinism and oculocutaneous albinism (see albinism discussion, page 609).

Horizontally oriented folds in the macular retina (Fig. 8–336) may be seen in high hypermetropia (Uemura and Morizane, 1970).

In occasional eyes there is heterotopia of the macula, with the foveomacular region being displaced either downward or temporally. It has been postulated that the heterotopia is related to fine abnormalities in the development of retinovitreal structures, leading to displacement of the fovea.

Epiretinal membranes outside the macular area may contract and lead to distortion and hetero-

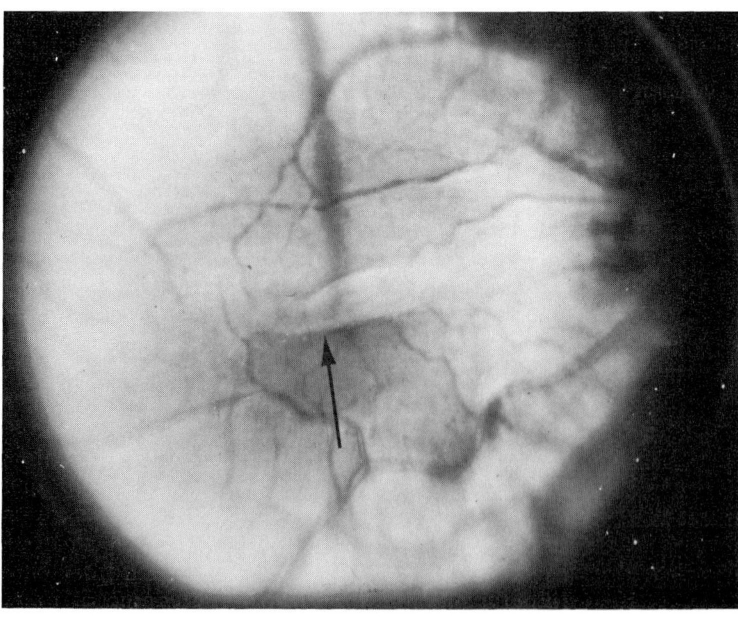

Figure 8–336. Horizontal fold in macula (arrow) in high hyperopia. (Courtesy of Dr. S.L. Fine.)

topia of the macula. Macular heterotopia has been observed with vitreoretinal traction and epiretinal membrane formation in eyes with diabetic retinopathy (Bresnick, Haight, de Venecia, 1979).

Most cases of macular heterotopia are acquired, and many are related to traction from peripheral preretinal fibrovascular or fibroinflammatory tissue proliferation, as in retrolental fibroplasia, nematode endophthalmitis, exudative vitreoretinopathy of Creswick and Schepens, persistent hyperplastic primary vitreous, and others.

Macular Dystrophies. The term *dystrophy* implies a condition that is inherited, is not necessarily evident at birth, and is unassociated with systemic diseases. In contrast, degenerations are conditions that occur as a result of aging or from a known exogenous cause.

A variety of heredomacular dystrophies without central nervous system disease have been described. Table 8–3 classifies macular dystrophies tentatively on the basis of the presumed or known site of principal involvement.

Most often the disease is restricted to the macula; it may be symmetric or asymmetric, but eventually both eyes are affected. These diseases have varying age of onset, some being of the infantile variety (Best type), some being juvenile (Stargardt type), while others appear in adolescence or early adulthood. The morphologic changes in most of these dystrophies have not been ascertained, and those that have been studied have been in eyes in the late stages, when there are few clues about their pathogenesis.

Table 8–3. CLASSIFICATION OF MACULAR DYSTROPHIES

Nerve fiber layer
- X-linked juvenile retinoschisis

Photoreceptor cell
- Cone-rod dystrophy
- Pericentral retinitis pigmentosa
- Progressive atrophic macular dystrophy

Retinal pigment epithelium (RPE)
- Vitelliform dystrophy (Best's disease)
- Fundus flavimaculatus (Stargardt's disease)
- Fundus albipunctatus
- Butterfly-shaped dystrophy
- Sjögren's reticular dystrophy (autosomal recessive)
- Macroreticular dystrophy
- Autosomal-dominant pigmentary dystrophy of RPE
  - Fundus pulverulentus
  - Reticular dystrophy of Benedikt and Werner
  - Pattern dystrophy of Marmor and Byers
- Benign concentric annular dystrophy (olivopontocerebellar degeneration)
- Patterned dystrophies of RPE (pigmentary dystrophies)*
  - Butterfly-shaped dystrophy
  - Macroreticular dystrophy
- Adult-onset foveomacular pigment epithelial dystrophy (foveomacular vitelliform dystrophy; pseudovitelliform macular degeneration)

*Watzke, Folk, Lang, 1982.

Stargardt's Disease (Stargardt's Juvenile Macular Degeneration; Juvenile Macular Degeneration). A most lucid discussion of Stargardt's disease and its relationship to fundus flavimaculatus is presented by Krill (1977), and that discussion is paraphrased here (see also Fundus flavimaculatus, page 1213). Stargardt (1909) described members of two families with a disease having these characteristics: probable autosomal recessive transmission; loss of vision prior to definite ophthalmoscopic changes; the development of an atrophic macular degeneration with yellowish flecks in the macular or posterior region; essentially normal peripheral visual fields and no night blindness throughout life; and only mild loss of color vision even with severe visual loss.

As Krill points out, Stargardt and most subsequent workers did not recognize the uniqueness of the two pedigrees in the original publication. Subsequent reports, even one by Stargardt (1913), included other conditions under the designation of the original report.

In 1963, Franceschetti described an entity identical to that in the original report by Stargardt and named the condition fundus flavimaculatus.

The various conditions that have been reported erroneously under the name of Stargardt's disease include vitelliform macular dystrophy, X-linked juvenile retinoschisis, X-linked vitreoretinal degeneration with myopia, cone degeneration, and fundus flavimaculatus.

Krill also noted that further confusion has arisen from the use of the designation of Stargardt's disease with peripheral involvement (centroperipheral tapetoretinal dystrophy). Some of these cases appear to be examples of early diffuse choriocapillaris—retinal pigment epithelial atrophy (diffuse choroidal sclerosis). Others appear to be fundus flavimaculatus with advanced atrophy that may be observed in the midperiphery as well as in the posterior pole. Krill noted that most of the literature dealing with fundus flavimaculatus has dealt only or mainly with the stage showing the typical transient flecks. When the natural course of fundus flavimaculatus is appreciated, there is no need for a special term to include "peripheral involvement."

Stargardt's disease and fundus flavimaculatus are the same disease and the term preferred by Krill is fundus flavimaculatus. The pathology of this condition has been studied in a number of eyes. The three oldest reports (Behr, 1921; Harms, 1904; Nagel, 1875) include drawings of lesions and are difficult to interpret. Most of the studies have been of patients who have been quite old, after severe changes have occurred (Klien, 1950; Vail, Schoch, 1965; Blodi, 1966). Most of these investigators described loss of RPE and the photoreceptor cell layer in the macular area. Some RPE hyperplasia was noted at the

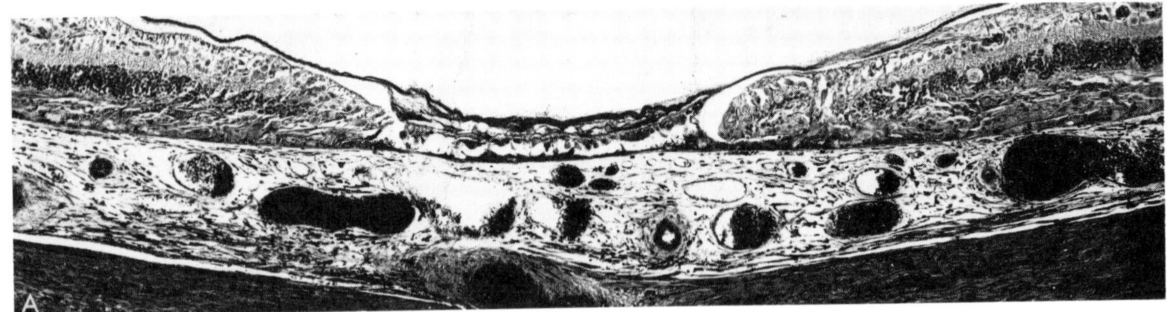

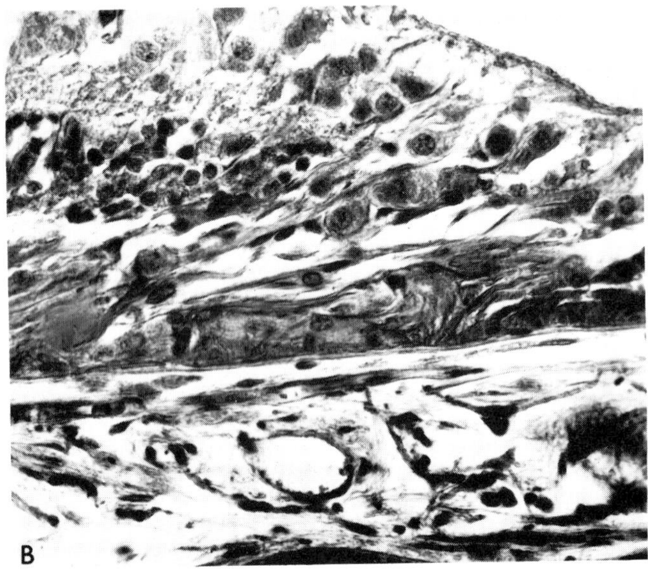

Figure 8–337. *A*, **Stargardt's disease,** showing loss of retinal pigment epithelium (RPE) and photoreceptor cells in foveal and parafoveal areas. All retinal cells are lost in foveolar area. PAS, about × 10. *B*, Higher power view showing loss of RPE and photoreceptor cells. A fibrocellular tissue is present between inner nuclear layer and Bruch's membrane. H and E, about × 40. (From Paufique L, Hervouet F: Anatomie pathologique d'un cas de maladie de Stargardt. Bull Soc France Ophtalmol *76*:108–114, 1963.)

margin in some instances. In addition, cystoid edema changes were noted in the remaining outer retinal layers, and some drusen were present.

Better specimens were studied by Brihaye-van Geertruyden (1962) and Paufique and Hervouet (1963). In these two papers the histologic findings were quite similar. There was an abrupt loss of RPE centrally at the site of the macular degeneration, with loss of rods, cones, and outer nuclear layer. The inner nuclear layers and ganglion cells were normal. The retina was fused to the choroid by noninflammatory adhesions (Fig. 8–337). Choroidal neovascularization was observed in one case.

Eagle, Lucier, Bernardino, and Yanoff (1980), in a study of the eyes of a 24 year old man with well-documented fundus flavimaculatus (see page 1213) and Stargardt's maculopathy, found marked heterogeneity in the size of the RPE cells. Some RPE cells were greatly enlarged and hypopigmented. The RPE was packed with a periodic acid–Schiff–positive material that was found to be an abnormal form of lipofuscin. A disturbance in lipopigment metabolism was postulated.

Frangieh, Green, Maumenee, et al (1982) studied the eyes of a patient that over a 40 year period evolved from displaying a flecked retina to diffuse RPE atrophy (see page 1213).

Best's Vitelliform Dystrophy. This dominant heredomacular dystrophy affects both males and females and has an early onset in life, usually by age 3 to 10 years. It is characterized initially by sharply delineated, yellowish-white lesions that may persist for considerable periods before disintegrating. Occasionally at the time of disintegration there may be hemorrhage into the retina. The only histopathologic report of this condition is that of McFarland (1955). There was an absence of RPE, photoreceptors, and outer nuclear layer of the retina. Bruch's membrane was calcified, and the choriocapillaris was absent. It is emphasized that the case reported by McFarland was in an older person, thus it is difficult to know whether the changes might be secondary to aging changes in the macula.

Andersen (1970) examined four patients with vitelliform degeneration of the macula. There was marked loss of the RPE and photoreceptor cells in a 3 disk diameter area of the macula. Bruch's membrane was thin but intact, and the choriocapillaris appeared atrophic. The RPE in the remaining posterior half of the eye seemed to be thin and hypopigmented.

Frangieh, Green, and Fine (1982) have studied an additional case by light and electron microscopy and found the following features: RPE and photoreceptor cell atrophy in the macula, accumulation of abnormal lipofuscin in residual RPE cells, deposition of abnormal filamentous structures below the RPE, apical displacement of the nuclei of the RPE, deposition of granular material in the photoreceptor area, and a break in Bruch's membrane with choroidal neovascularization (Fig. 8–338).

Weingeist, Kobrin, and Watzke (1982) have studied the light and electron microscopic features of Best's macular dystrophy of a 28 year old patient who had a "scrambled egg" lesion in the macula and some features of a "pseudohypopyon." These investigators found a generalized abnormal accumulation of lipofuscin in the retinal pigment epithelium. By light microscopy, the inner retinal layers were normal except for edema. There was irregular atrophy of the outer segments of the photoreceptors. Pigmented macrophages were present between the retina and the retinal pigment epithelium (RPE) (Fig. 8–339,*A*). The RPE was diffusely abnormal and distended with periodic-acid–Schiff–positive material, especially in the macular area. The RPE displayed marked autofluorescence, and choroidal neovascularization was observed in the macular area, which corresponded with the large yellowish deposits noted clinically. By electron microscopy, the RPE throughout showed fewer melanosomes and more lysosomes or lipofuscin granules than normal (Fig. 8–339,*B*,*C*). These investigators suggest that an abnormality in the RPE results in an abnormal accumulation of lipofuscin.

Pseudovitelliform Macular Degeneration. In recent years a number of studies have reported patients with ophthalmoscopically visible lesions similar to those of Best's vitelliform dystrophy but in whom the electro-oculograms were normal or only slightly abnormal (Birndorf, Dawson, 1973; Gass, 1974c; Fishman, Trimble, Rabb, Fishman, 1977; Kingham, Lochen, 1977; Marmor, 1979; Epstein, Rabb, 1980; Vine, Schatz, 1980; Skalka, 1981). This condition, or these conditions, have been referred to as pseudovitelliform degeneration (Fishman, et al, 1977; Sabates, Pruett, Hirose, 1982).

In a clinicopathologic study of the eyes of one patient with bilateral foveal lesions resembling vitelliform dystrophy, Gass (1974c) observed the RPE to be discontinuous and associated with photoreceptor cell degeneration (Fig. 8–340). Pigmented cells were present in the subretinal area and outer layer of the retina. Gass considered this condition to be a foveomacular dystrophy that primarily affects the RPE and is possibly related to dominantly inherited drusen.

Doyne's Colloid Degenerations. This condition was described soon after the invention of the ophthalmoscope in 1850, but the first histopathologic examination was done by Collins in 1913. Collins found large drusen and areas of absent RPE and choriocapillaris. The photoreceptors had degenerated, and the outer retina was in contact with Bruch's membrane. Farkas, Krill, Sylvester, and Archer (1971) and Wolter and Falls (1962) described similar cases. In their patients there was a hereditary pattern to the disorder, and the drusen were confluent as in Collins' case. It is interesting that these investigators found all the RPE cells in the retina to be abnormal, with enlargement and cytoplasmic changes.

A variety of colloid degeneration is known as *malattia leventinese*. Clinically, this condition greatly resembles Doyne's degeneration. It has been studied histopathologically by Forni and Babel (1962). The findings were identical to those in the reports of Collins and Farkas and associates.

Senile Macular Degeneration. The changes that occur in the macular region and elsewhere cause a variety of clinical states that are in part due to changes in the outer portion of the retina and the RPE and in part due to alterations in Bruch's membrane and possibly the choriocapillaris. Originally it was believed that the choroidal blood supply and changes in the choriocapillaris were responsible for this disease (Friedenwald, 1929; Rones, 1938; Wood, 1915), but eventually it was shown that the primary origin of the changes is in the outer retina, the RPE, and perhaps the choroid.

Senile macular degeneration is a fairly common disease. It was observed in 9 per cent of the population in the Framingham study (Kini, Leibowitz, Colton, et al, 1978) and in 33 per cent of eyes obtained post mortem from persons over the age of 65 years (Kornzweig, 1965).

Before discussing senile macular degeneration, we should consider the aging changes in the outer retina and inner choroid that can eventually lead to disease. Most of these observations have come through evaluation of eyes with the electron microscope.

Commencing at about age 20 years, the RPE shows changes that are the result of its constant activity over a period of years. Cytoplasmic changes include depigmentation with migration of pigment granules into the basal portion of the cell. There is an increased accumulation of lipofuscin granules in the cytoplasm of these cells. These granules are due in part to phagocytosis of the rod and cone outer segments and their enclosure in phagosomes (Fig. 8–341). Within the phagosomes there is gradual digestion of the disks of the outer segments, eventually producing structures known as "residual bodies."

Many of the incompletely digested disks and phagosomes are extruded into Bruch's membrane and into the area between the basal cell membrane of the RPE cell and its basement membrane. Large amounts of residual bodies can be

Text continued on page 936

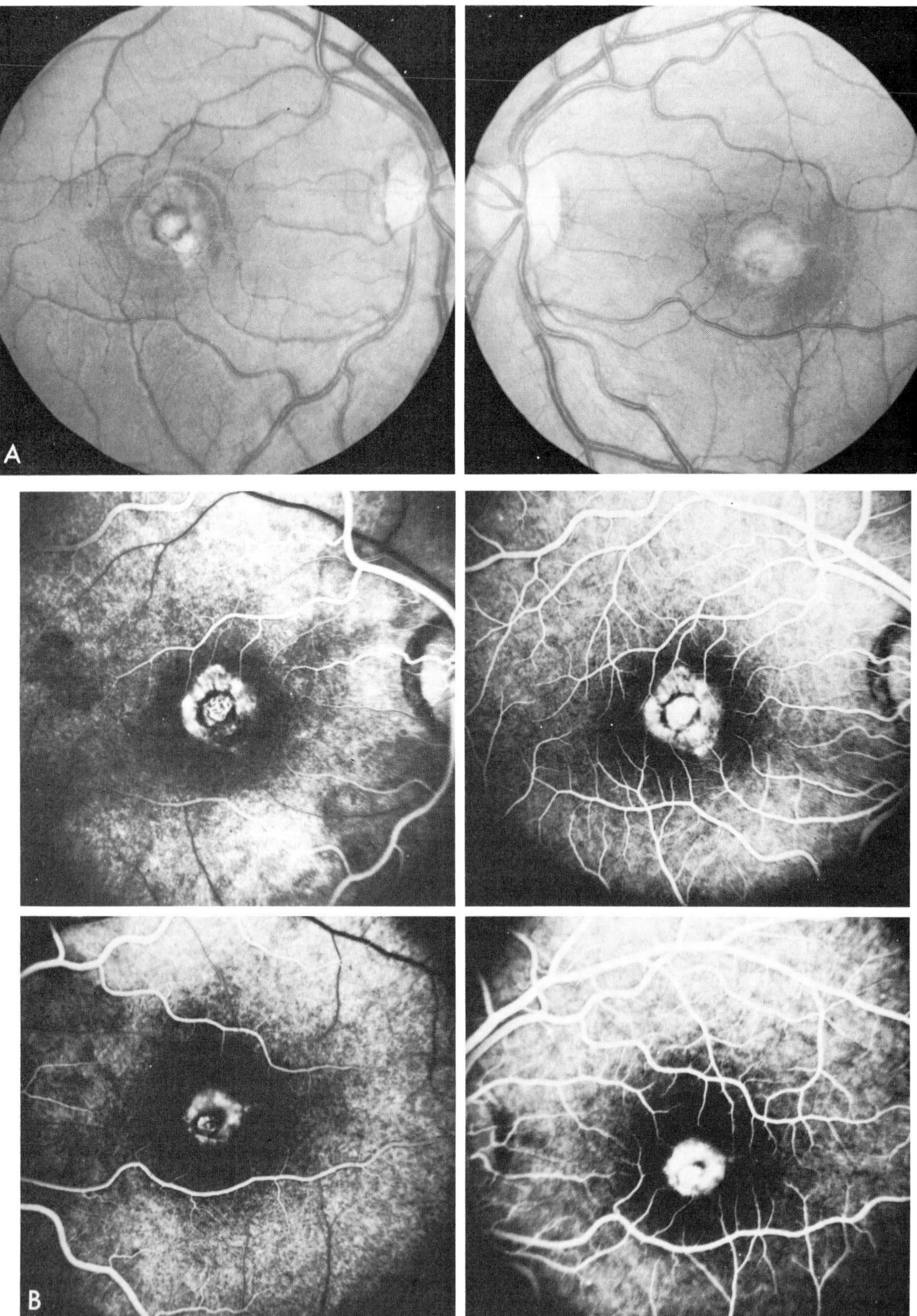

Figure 8–338. Best's macular dystrophy. Clinicopathologic study of an 80 year old woman.

A, Ophthalmoscopic appearance of macular lesions of proband at age 73 years. *B,* Fluorescein angiographic appearance of macular lesion of both eyes, showing choroidal neovascularization. Neovascular membrane fluoresces early (top left and bottom left) and stains late (top right and bottom right).

Illustration continued on opposite page

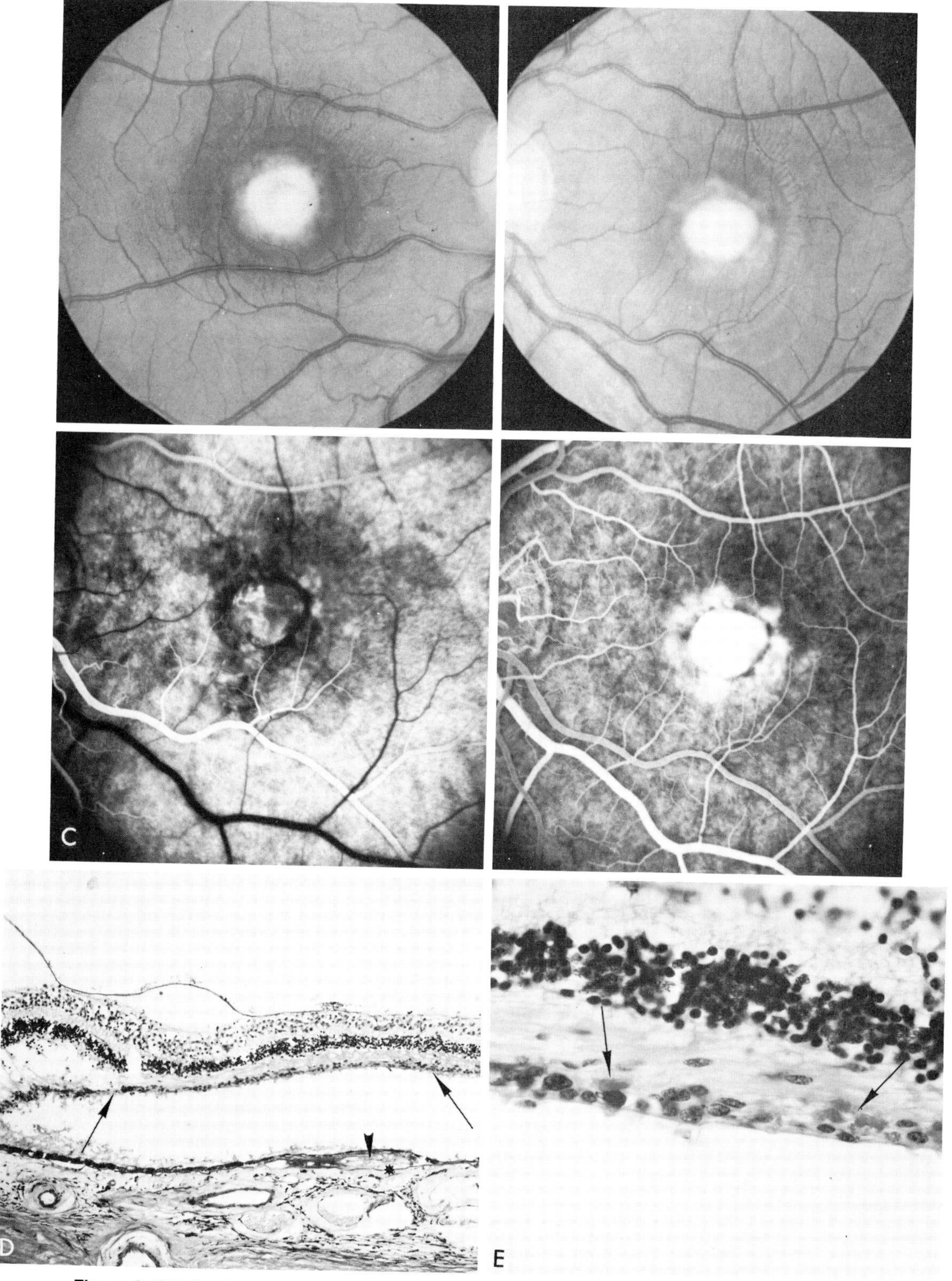

Figure 8–338 *Continued C,* Ophthalmoscopic appearance of 8 year old niece of proband. Fluorescein angiographic appearance of macular lesion of left eye showing choroidal neovascularization. Neovascular membrane fluoresces early (bottom left) and stains late (bottom right).

D, Section through macular area of left eye showing small, flat, vascularized, disciform scar (arrowhead) located between Bruch's membrane (asterisk) and attenuated retinal pigment epithelium (RPE). There is total loss of the outer segments of the photoreceptor cells and only a few stubby inner segments remain. Outer nuclear layer (between arrows) is notably attenuted. PAS, ×100. *E,* Higher-power view of macular area shows PAS-positive, diastase-resistant material (arrows) in remaining outer nuclear layer. No photoreceptors were present in this area. PAS, ×550.

Illustration continued on following page

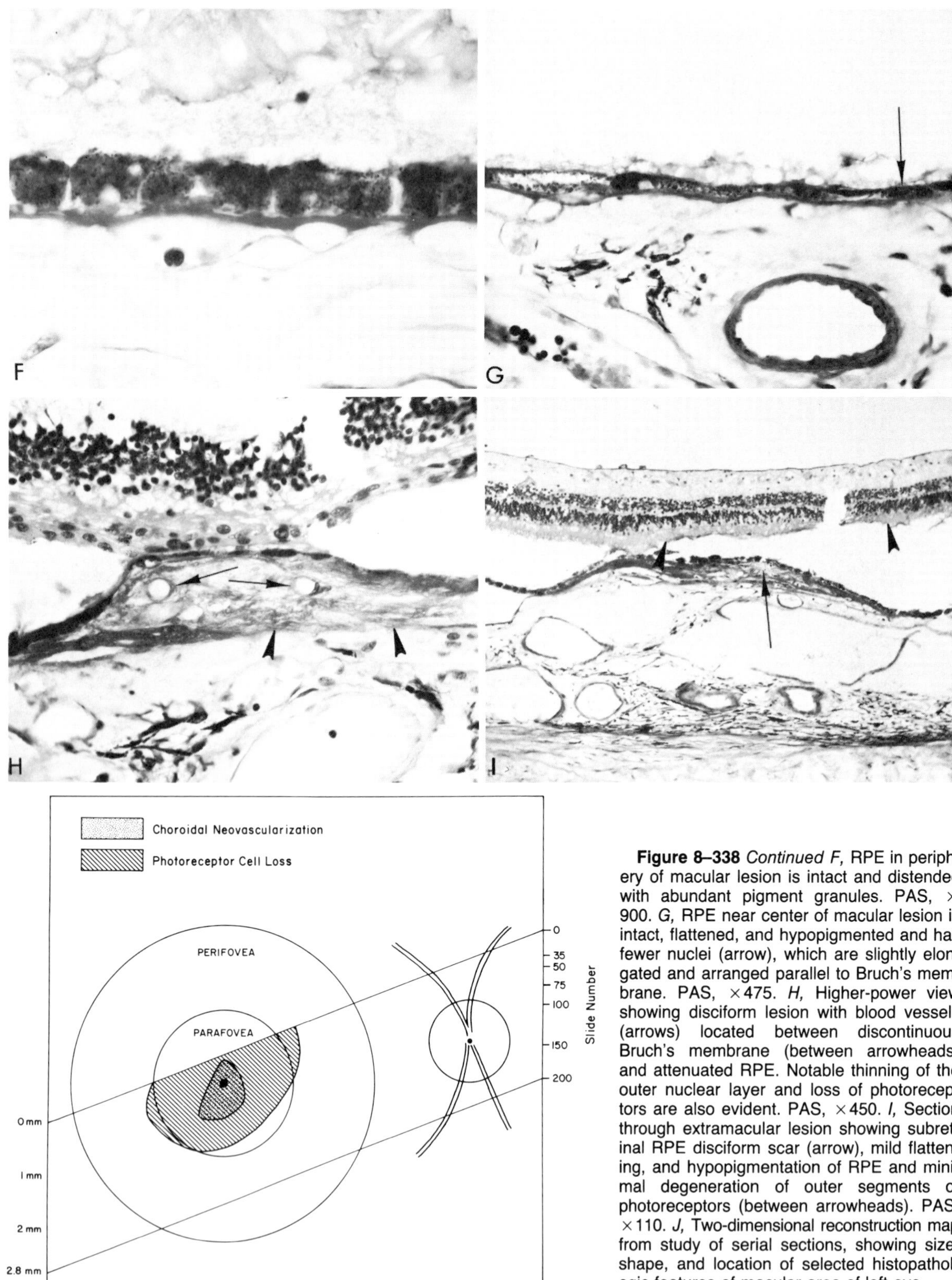

Figure 8–338 *Continued F,* RPE in periphery of macular lesion is intact and distended with abundant pigment granules. PAS, × 900. *G,* RPE near center of macular lesion is intact, flattened, and hypopigmented and has fewer nuclei (arrow), which are slightly elongated and arranged parallel to Bruch's membrane. PAS, ×475. *H,* Higher-power view showing disciform lesion with blood vessels (arrows) located between discontinuous Bruch's membrane (between arrowheads) and attenuated RPE. Notable thinning of the outer nuclear layer and loss of photoreceptors are also evident. PAS, ×450. *I,* Section through extramacular lesion showing subretinal RPE disciform scar (arrow), mild flattening, and hypopigmentation of RPE and minimal degeneration of outer segments of photoreceptors (between arrowheads). PAS, ×110. *J,* Two-dimensional reconstruction map from study of serial sections, showing size, shape, and location of selected histopathologic features of macular area of left eye.

Illustration continued on opposite page

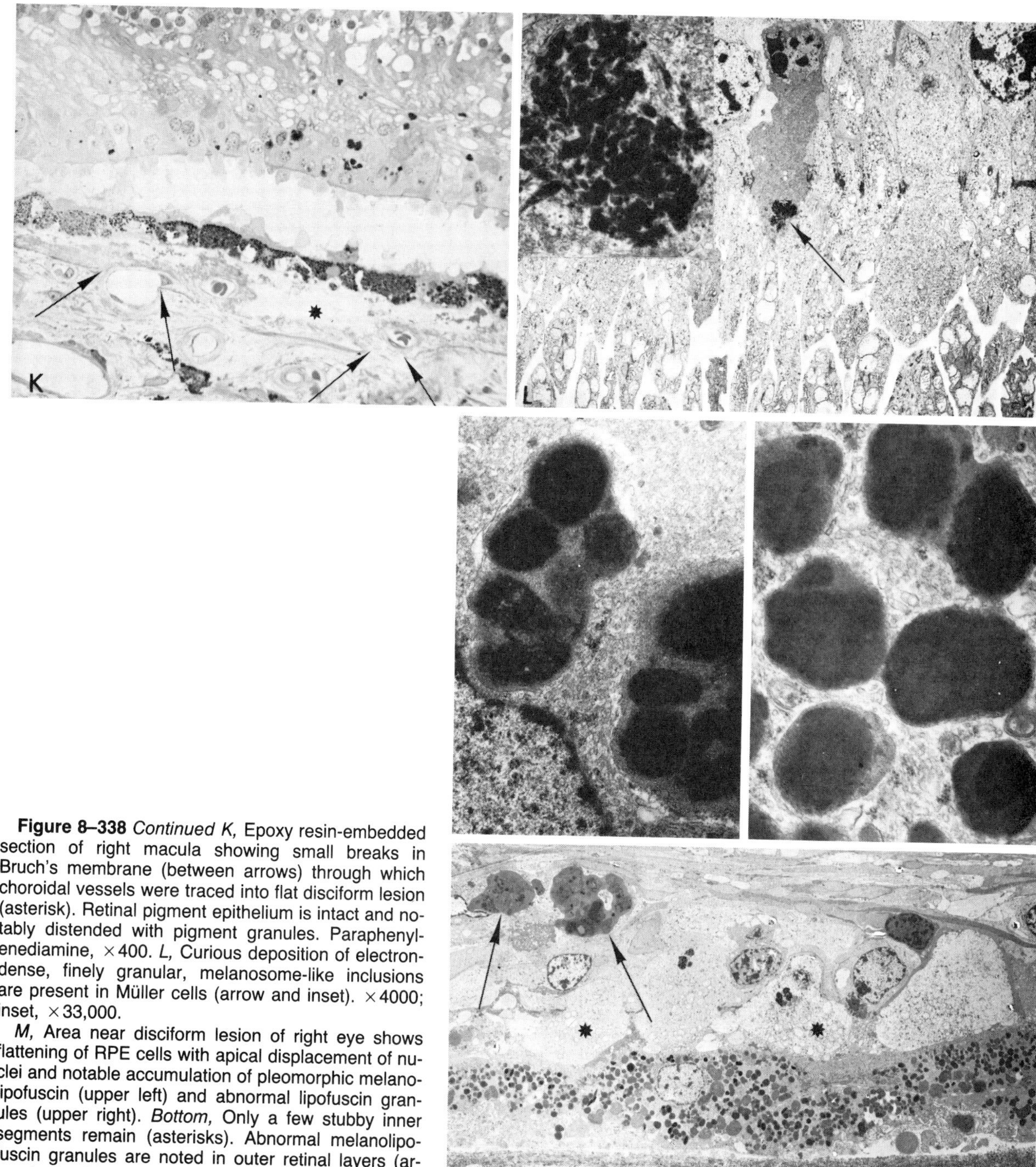

Figure 8–338 *Continued K,* Epoxy resin-embedded section of right macula showing small breaks in Bruch's membrane (between arrows) through which choroidal vessels were traced into flat disciform lesion (asterisk). Retinal pigment epithelium is intact and notably distended with pigment granules. Paraphenylenediamine, ×400. *L,* Curious deposition of electron-dense, finely granular, melanosome-like inclusions are present in Müller cells (arrow and inset). ×4000; inset, ×33,000.

M, Area near disciform lesion of right eye shows flattening of RPE cells with apical displacement of nuclei and notable accumulation of pleomorphic melanolipofuscin (upper left) and abnormal lipofuscin granules (upper right). *Bottom,* Only a few stubby inner segments remain (asterisks). Abnormal melanolipofuscin granules are noted in outer retinal layers (arrows). Bruch's membrane and choriocapillaris are intact. ×2100; insets, ×22,000. EP 51341.

(From Frangieh GT, Green WR, Fine SL: A histopathologic study of Best's macular dystrophy. Arch Ophthalmol *100*:1115–1121, 1982.)

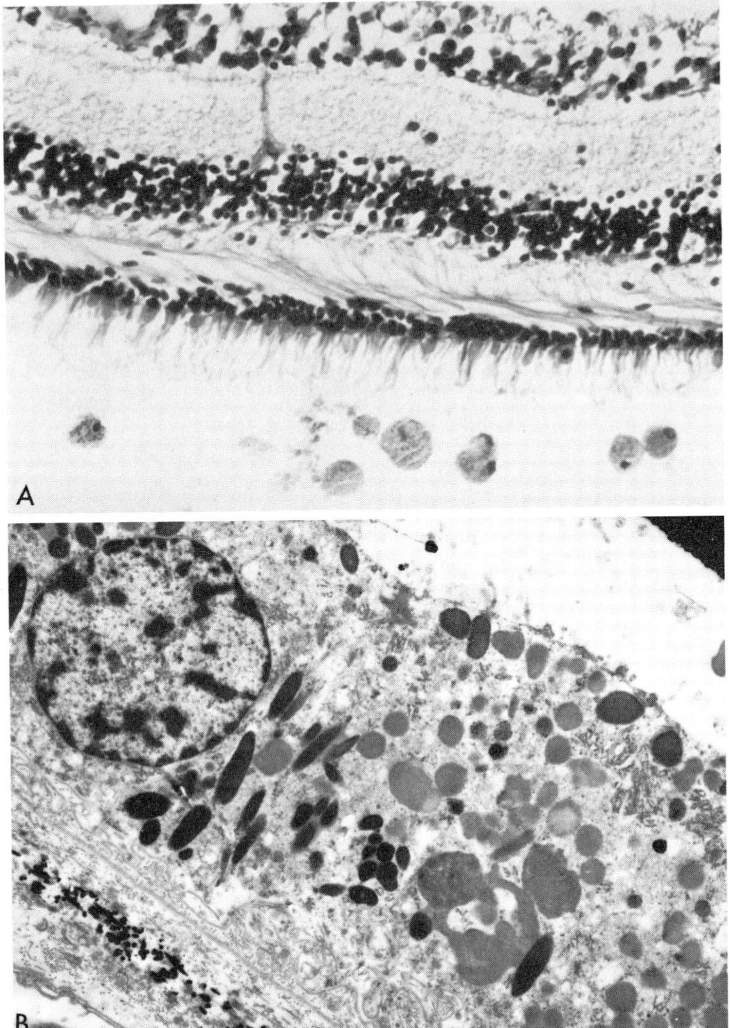

Figure 8–339. Best's macular dystrophy. *A,* Light micrograph of macula with subretinal pigment-laden macrophages. H and E, × 320. *B,* Electron micrograph of retinal pigment epithelium cells disclosing a few melanosomes and many lipofuscin granules within the cytoplasm. There is calcific degeneration of Bruch's membrane. × 7200.

Illustration continued on opposite page

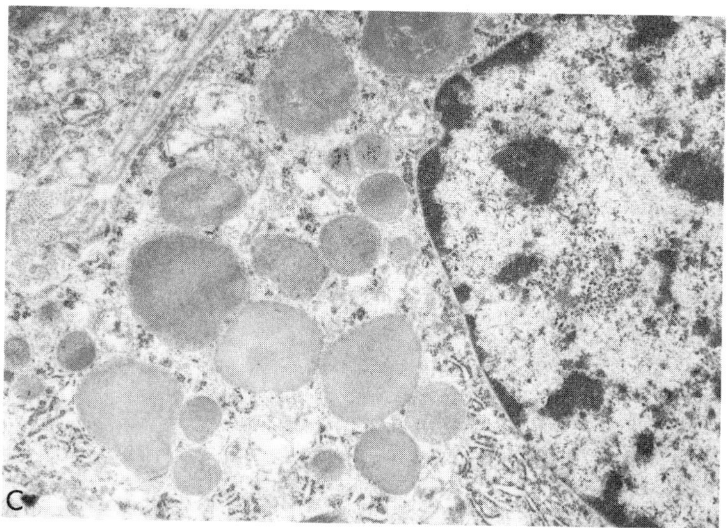

C, Electron micrograph of a retinal pigment epithelium cell showing lipofuscin granules. × 18,000. (From Weingeist TA, Kobrin JL, Watzke RC: Histopathology of Best's macular dystrophy. Arch Ophthalmol *100*:1108–1144, 1982.)

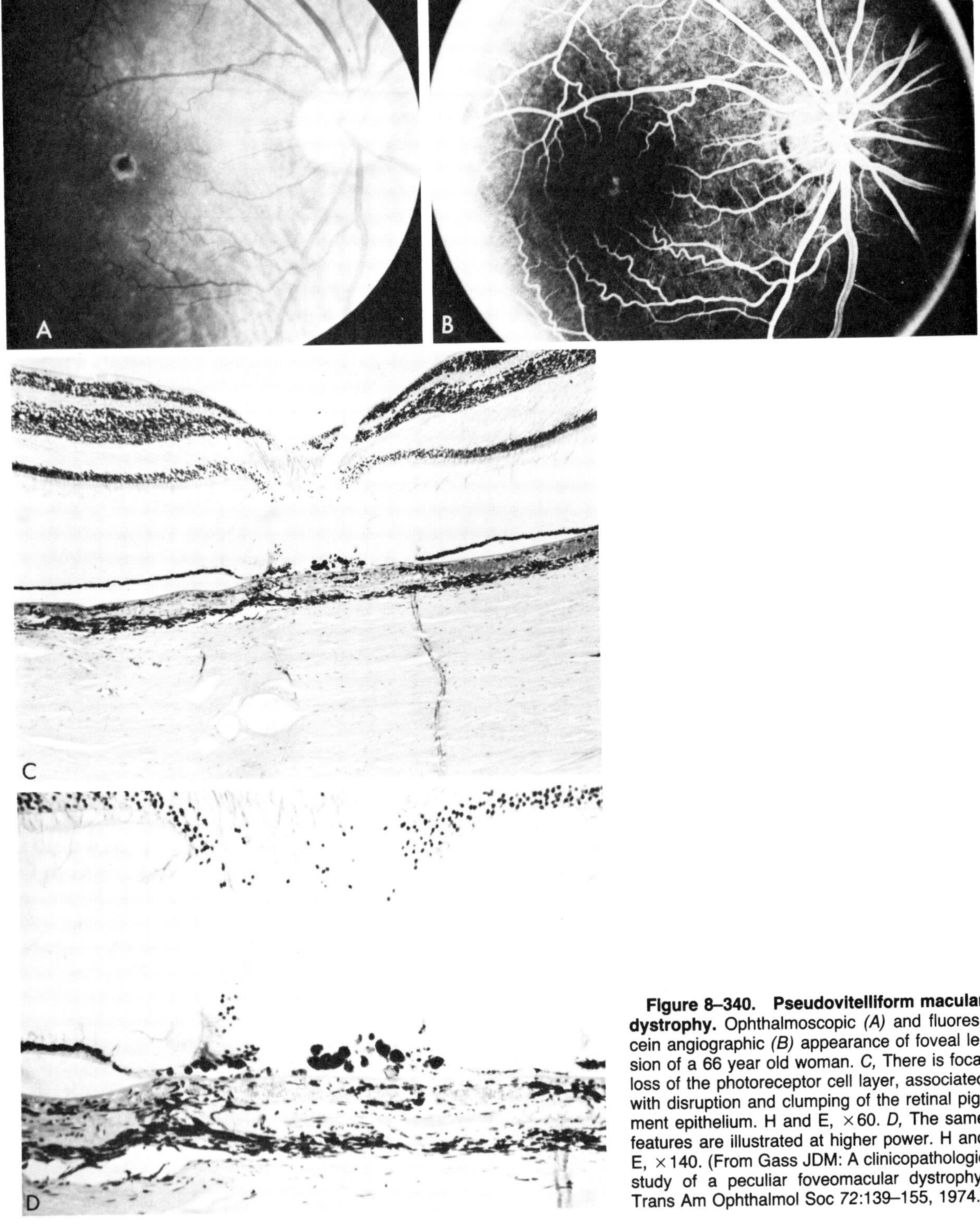

Figure 8–340. Pseudovitelliform macular dystrophy. Ophthalmoscopic *(A)* and fluorescein angiographic *(B)* appearance of foveal lesion of a 66 year old woman. *C,* There is focal loss of the photoreceptor cell layer, associated with disruption and clumping of the retinal pigment epithelium. H and E, ×60. *D,* The same features are illustrated at higher power. H and E, ×140. (From Gass JDM: A clinicopathologic study of a peculiar foveomacular dystrophy. Trans Am Ophthalmol Soc *72*:139–155, 1974.)

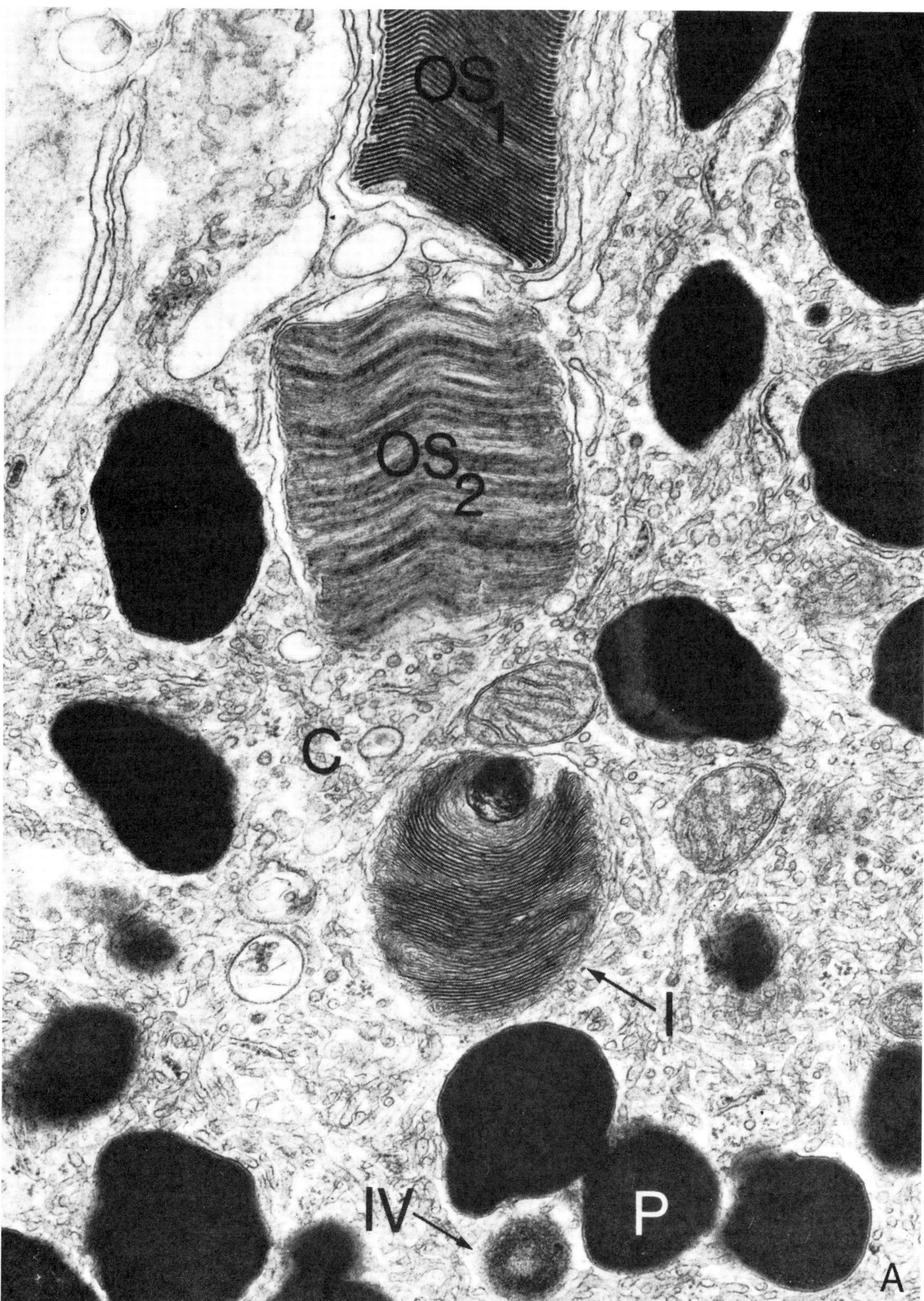

Figure 8–341. The retinal pigment epithelial cell cytoplasm is at *C* and a melanin pigment granule at *P*. An outer segment with its disk is seen at OS_1. Sequestered disks are seen at OS_2. A recently formed phagosome (*I*) contains rod disks. A phagosome in the end-stage of hydrolytic digestion is seen at *IV*. × 28,800. (From Hogan MJ, Alvarado JA, Weddell JE: Histology of the Human Eye. Philadelphia, W.B. Saunders Company, 1971, p 422.)

seen in most eyes at about age 40 to 60 years, and by age 80 years there is considerable accumulation of these structures. Other breakdown products of the cell, including mitochondria and the membranes of endoplasmic reticulum, also are enclosed in phagosomes in the cytoplasm and undergo digestion. The lipid may remain in the cytoplasm or be extruded into Bruch's membrane. Some of the extruded residual undigested material passes through Bruch's membrane into the choriocapillaris, where it is removed by the circulation.

The vacuoles in the RPE cytoplasm seen with the light microscope have been found by electron microscopy to be membrane-bound inclusions containing undigested material in the cytoplasm (Garron, 1963). The basal enfoldings of the pigment epithelial cells also may show changes characterized by an accumulation of residual bodies, lipid material, and fibrils. Some of these structures remain between the cell membrane and basement membrane, while others pass through the basement membrane into the adjacent portion of Bruch's membrane. The fibrils that form in this region are of several types. Some are sheaves of very fine fibrils without cross striations; others are collagenous and of the dimension of reticulin; still others are short clumps of banded fibers that are known as "wide-spaced collagen." The latter two types of fiber are found in the inner part of Bruch's membrane in abundance with increasing age.

Bruch's membrane shares in the changes that occur in the RPE cells during the preceding processes. With the light microscope, the membrane is seen to become somewhat more eosinophilic because of the changes in its collagen. It also becomes more PAS-positive from alterations in the amount of ground substance and basement membrane material.

Areas of basophilia were first described in Bruch's membrane by Verhoeff and Sisson (1926). The membrane becomes basophilic with hematoxylin and eosin stains in patchy areas but usually in the posterior portion of the eye and especially in the macular region. The basophilia is due to a change in pH of the collagenous fibers and deposition of calcium salts in the elastoid tissue of Bruch's membrane. Fractures may occur across the calcified membrane; if the fracture happens to occur through an adjacent choroidal capillary, bleeding may occur into the membrane and lead to a separation or splitting of Bruch's membrane (hemorrhagic detachment of RPE).

Spencer (1965) described the increased sudanophilia of Bruch's membrane with increasing age. This sudanophilia is related to accumulation of lipid substances from the RPE. Changes in the collagen occur, with an increased amount of collagen and a coating of the collagenous fibrils with an osmiophilic material, which is probably altered ground substance and calcium. The collagenous changes extend longitudinally along the inner portion of Bruch's membrane, but in older eyes they may be found also in the outer portion of the membrane. There is an associated increased amount of collagen in the region of the choriocapillaris and also in the inner capillary region, where it tends to spread capillaries farther apart. The ground substance also is altered more in older persons, accounting for the increased periodic acid–Schiff (PAS) positivity.

Drusen. Since drusen appear to be an important associated and predisposing feature of senile macular degeneration, we should consider these prior to the histopathologic features of senile macular degeneration.

Drusen (colloid bodies) are localized depositions of a hyaline-like material between the RPE and Bruch's membrane (Fig. 8–342). Drusen occur as an aging process and as a hereditary condition (dominantly inherited drusen) and may also arise secondary to various intraocular processes, such as inflammations, trauma, and chronic retinal detachment.

Drusen occurring as an aging change are consistently seen after the age of 60 years, are very frequent after the age of 45 years, and are occasionally seen in persons in the third decade.

Clinically, the typical druse is a very small, yellowish-white lesion located deep to the retina in the posterior pole and to a lesser degree in the peripapillary and peripheral areas. With fluorescein angiography, the lesion lights up early and stains late with no leakage. The extent to which these drusen are seen ophthalmoscopically, without fluorescein, depends on their size, the degree of effacement of the overlying RPE (Fig. 8–343), and the degree of surrounding RPE hypertrophy (Fig. 8–344). Drusen may become calcified (Fig. 8–345) and presumably then have a more glistening appearance.

The clinical distinction between a large druse and a small serous detachment of the RPE is arbitrary, because the ophthalmoscopic and fluorescein angiographic appearances are very similar. Some lesions that appear to be drusen may not be drusen. For example, Frank, Green, and Pollack (1973) found small serous detachments of RPE in the macular areas of a patient post mortem, who had been followed for several years for what was considered to be early senile macular degeneration with prominent drusen in the macula of both eyes.

Histopathologically, the typical druse is a rounded, dome-shaped structure lying between Bruch's membrane and the lifted-up RPE and its basement membrane. It is densely periodic acid–Schiff–positive and stains lightly positive with special staining techniques for lipid. Drusen are

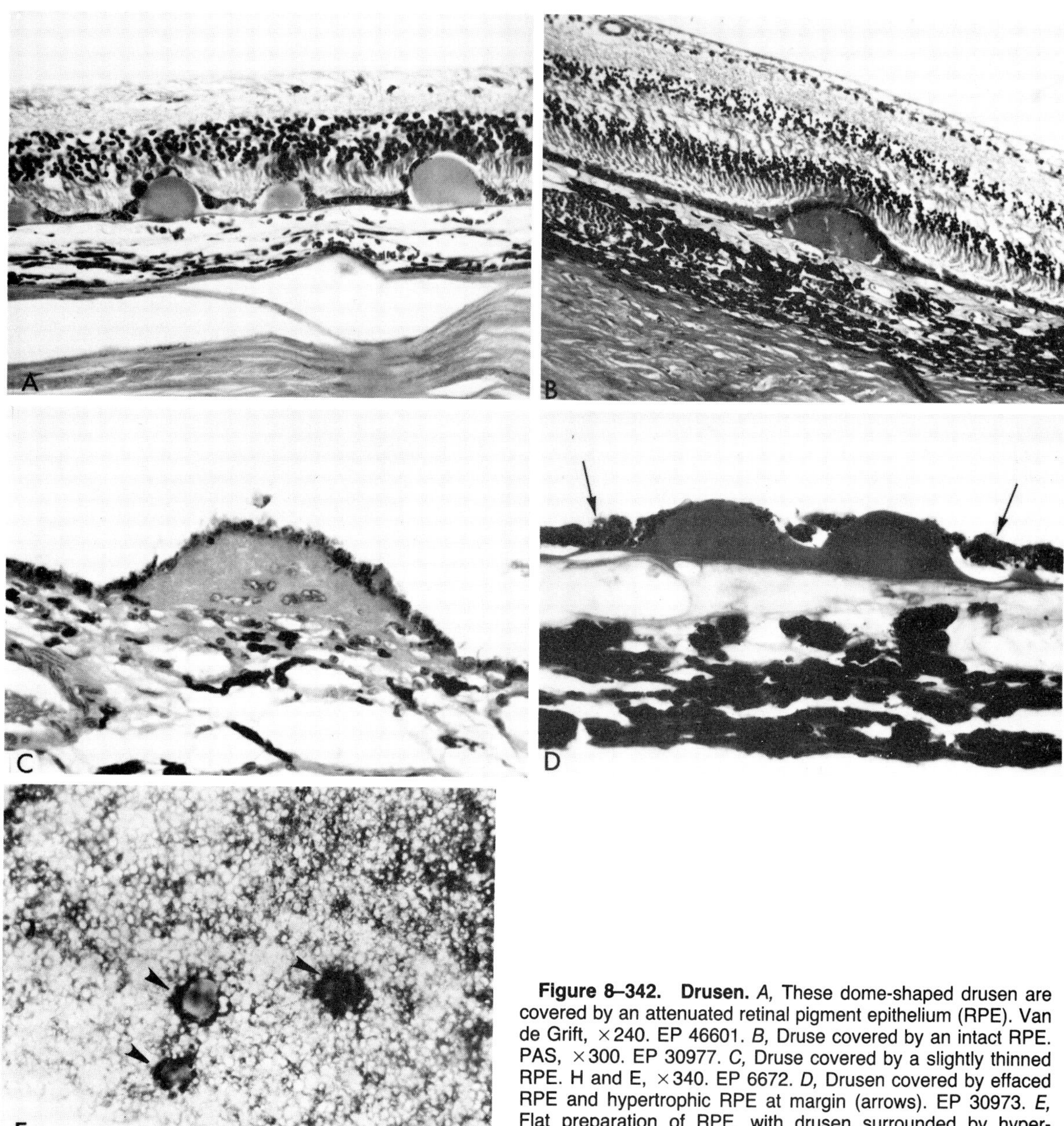

Figure 8–342. Drusen. *A,* These dome-shaped drusen are covered by an attenuated retinal pigment epithelium (RPE). Van de Grift, ×240. EP 46601. *B,* Druse covered by an intact RPE. PAS, ×300. EP 30977. *C,* Druse covered by a slightly thinned RPE. H and E, ×340. EP 6672. *D,* Drusen covered by effaced RPE and hypertrophic RPE at margin (arrows). EP 30973. *E,* Flat preparation of RPE, with drusen surrounded by hypertrophic RPE (arrowheads). H and E, ×250.

eosinophilic but may become basophilic because of the accumulation of calcium.

By electron microscopy, typical drusen are composed of various cell products, presumably derived from the RPE. These products include small-to-large clumps of lipid that is osmiophilic and not affected by the fluids used to prepare specimens. Various other structures are crystalline (probably calcium) residual bodies, granular material (Figs. 8–346 and 8–347) that is probably derived from the basement membrane, fibrils, collagen (Fig. 8–348), and a heterogeneous mixture of unidentified substances. Some drusen are more uniform in appearance and have a somewhat crystalline structure, presumably caused by insoluble lipid material that is precipitated as a mass in the inner portion of Bruch's membrane.

In clinicopathologic studies of 512 eyes from 300 patients, Sarks (1980) observed that drusen appear to change in consistency and become more fluid as senile macular degeneration develops. The softening of drusen was most evident in those eyes in which choroidal neovascularization was present.

Localized and diffuse thickening of the inner aspect of Bruch's membrane (Figs. 8–348 through 8–350) is also a commonly observed aging change, which has been clinically and histopathologically interpreted as a form of drusen. Sometimes this thickening may have a multilaminated appear-

Text continued on page 947

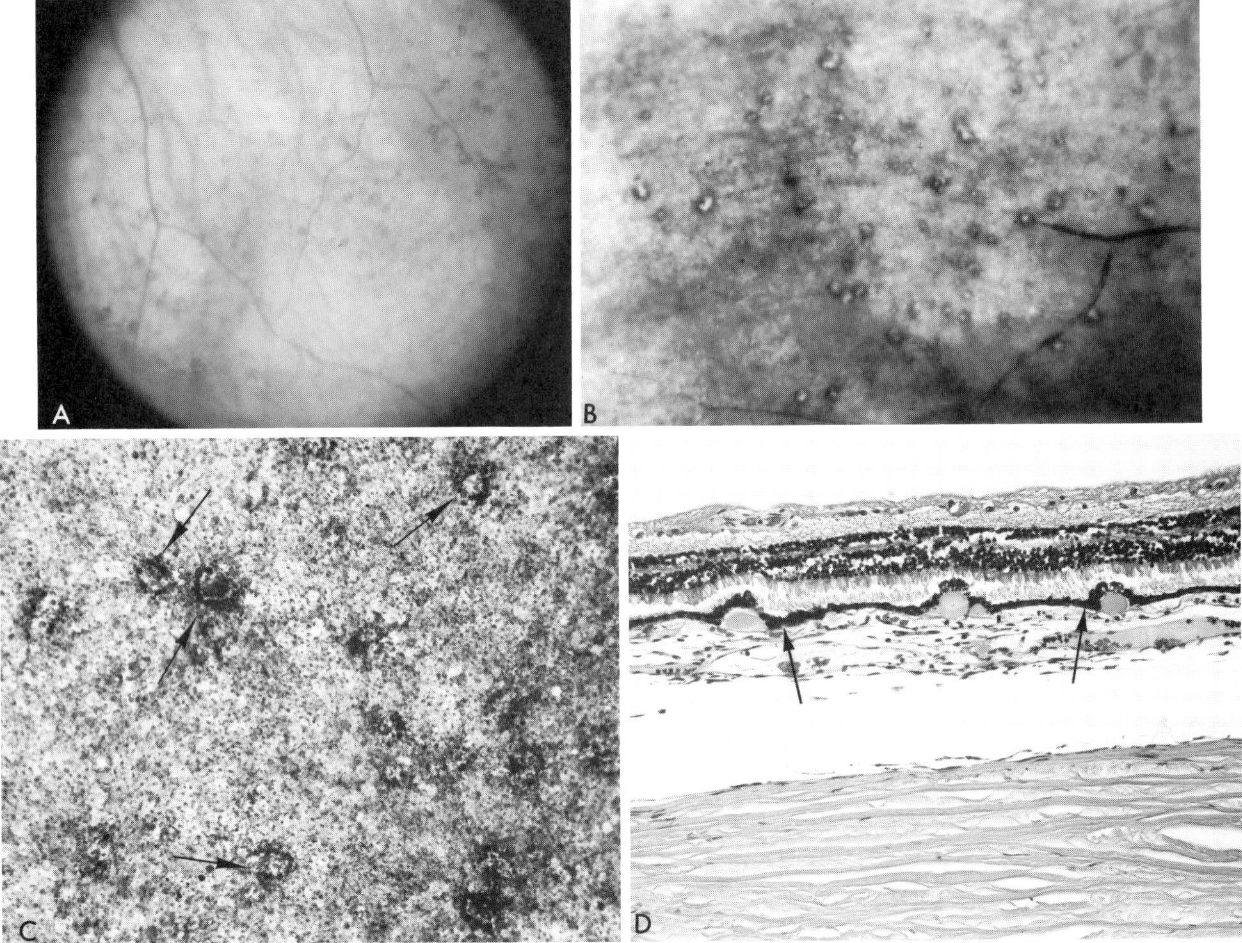

Figure 8–343. Peripheral drusen highlighted by hypertrophic retinal pigment epithelium. *A,* Ophthalmoscopic appearance. *B,* Gross view, showing a darker appearance around drusen. *C,* Flat preparation of RPE, showing drusen (arrows) surrounded by a narrow zone of RPE that is darker than elsewhere. Unstained, ×100. *D,* Drusen from same patient. RPE at margin has a darker appearance (arrows). H and E, ×190. EP 46601.

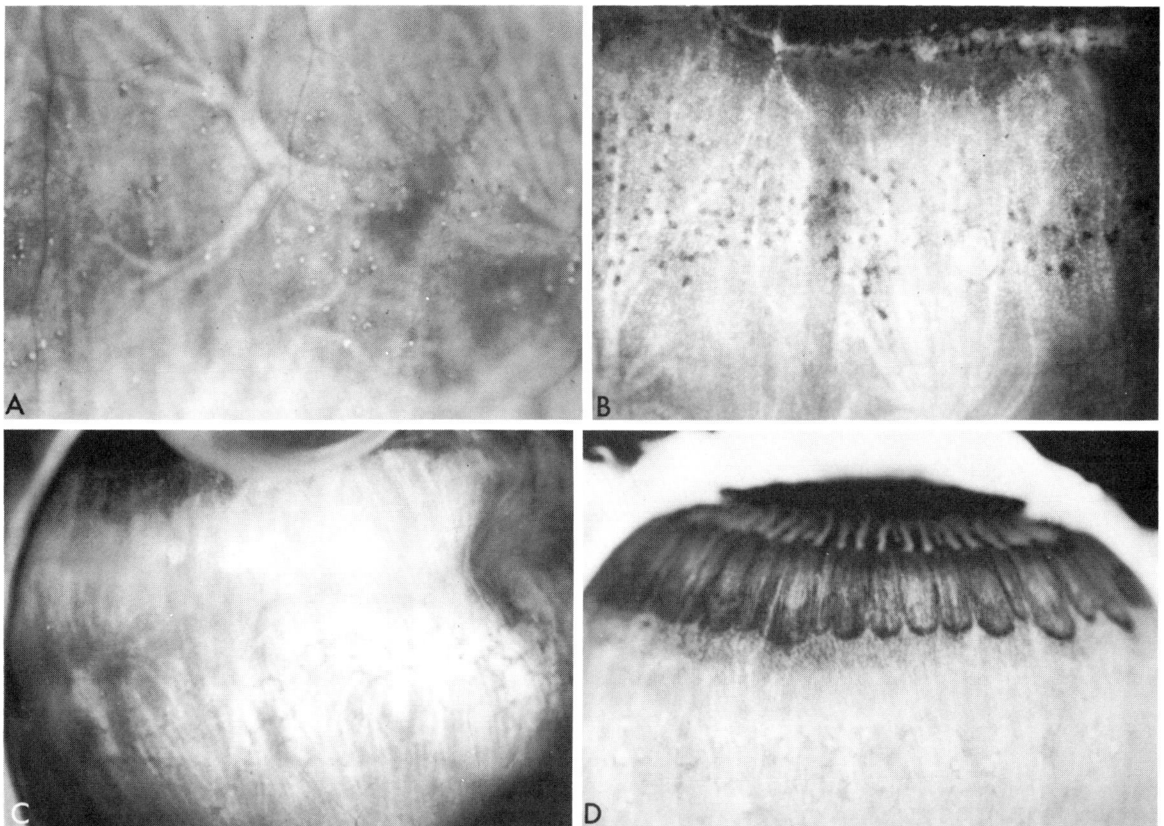

Figure 8–344. Peripheral drusen. *A,* Drusen with overlying effaced retinal pigment epithelium (RPE) and no hypertrophy. EP 30836. *B,* Drusen with hypertrophic RPE. EP 51644. *C,* Flat or confluent drusen with surrounding RPE hypertrophy, giving a reticulated appearance. EP 47146. *D,* Reticulated pattern at equator caused by RPE hypertrophy surrounding drusen. EP 31313.

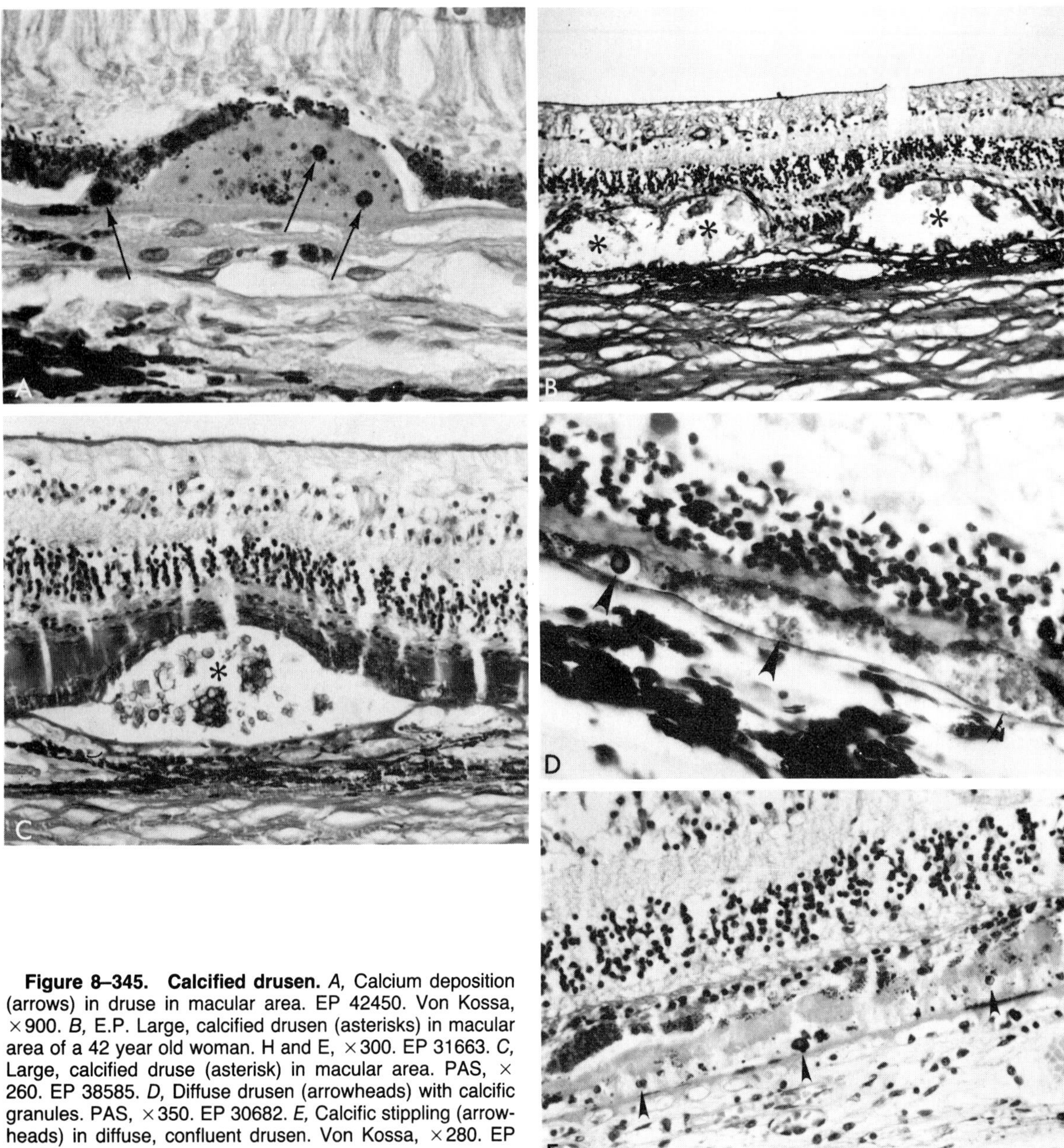

Figure 8–345. Calcified drusen. *A,* Calcium deposition (arrows) in druse in macular area. EP 42450. Von Kossa, ×900. *B,* E.P. Large, calcified drusen (asterisks) in macular area of a 42 year old woman. H and E, ×300. EP 31663. *C,* Large, calcified druse (asterisk) in macular area. PAS, × 260. EP 38585. *D,* Diffuse drusen (arrowheads) with calcific granules. PAS, ×350. EP 30682. *E,* Calcific stippling (arrowheads) in diffuse, confluent drusen. Von Kossa, ×280. EP 31489.

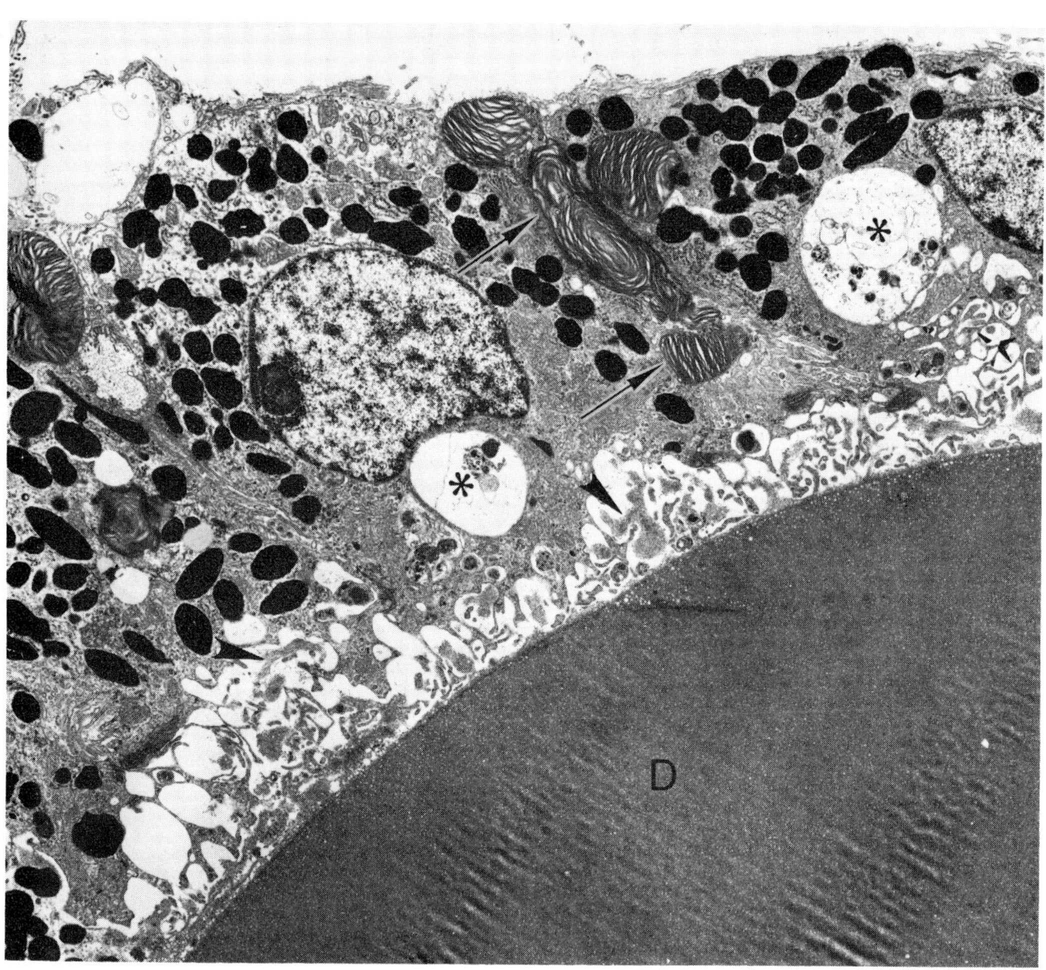

Figure 8–346. Large druse *(D)* composed of a fine granular material. Similar material (arrowheads) is also present within basal infoldings of retinal pigment epithelium (RPE). RPE contains phagocytosed outer segment disks (arrows). Large vacuoles (asterisks) are present in cytoplasm of RPE. ×6000. EP 36601.

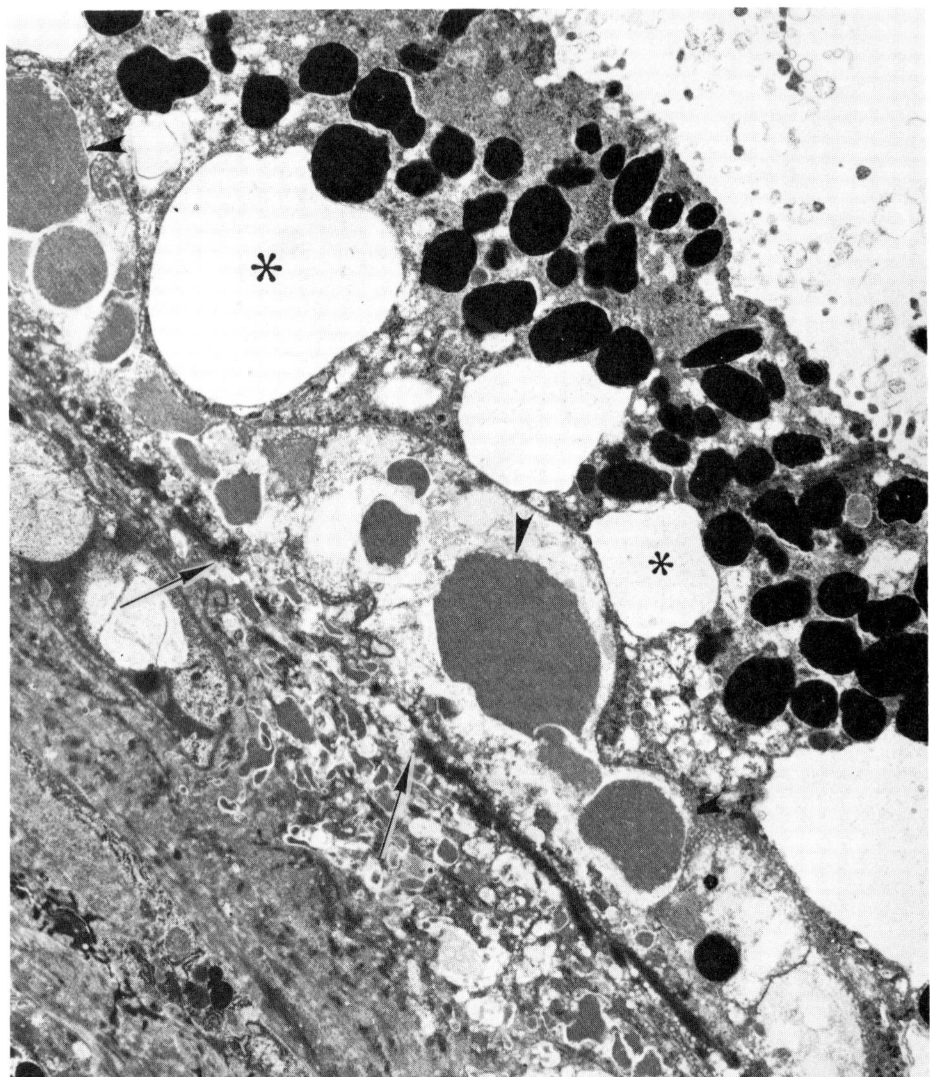

Figure 8–347. Finely granular material (arrowheads) **between retinal pigment epithelium (RPE) and Bruch's membrane.** RPE has several large cytoplasmic vacuoles (asterisks) and large pigment granules. A discontinuity is present in the elastic portion of Bruch's membrane (between arrows). ×11,000. EP 48710.

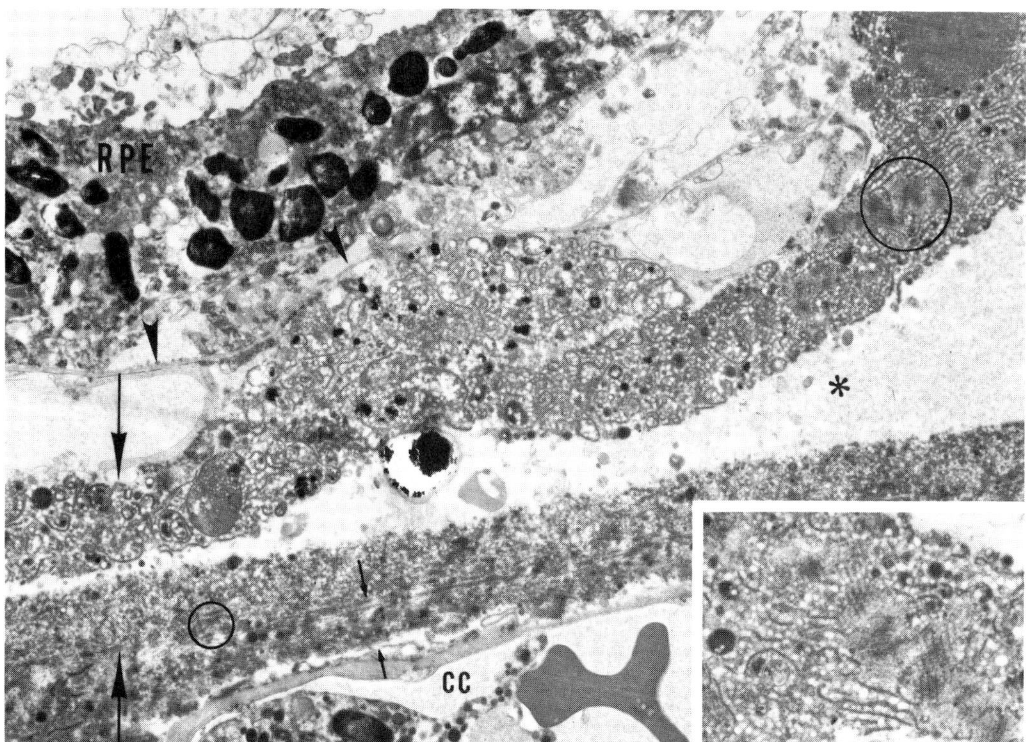

Figure 8–348. Electron microscopic appearance of **Bruch's membrane and diffuse drusen**. Retinal pigment epithelial *(RPE)* basement membrane is intact and normal (arrowheads). Inner collagenous zone of Bruch's membrane is greatly thickened (between larger arrows) by accumulation of small vesicles, electron-dense particles, fibrils, and clusters of widely spaced collagen (large circle and inset in lower right corner). Middle elastic layer of Bruch's membrane (small circle) is essentially normal. Outer collagenous zone (between smaller arrows) is mildly thickened, with accumulation of material similar to that seen in inner zone. Splitting of thickened inner collagenous zone (asterisk) has occurred, with accumulation of a finely granular material, membranous structures, and electron-dense particles. *CC,* choriocapillaris. ×3950; inset, ×6560. EP 42450.

(From Green WR, Key SN III: Senile macular degeneration: A histopathological study. Trans Am Ophthalmol Soc *75*:180–254, 1977.)

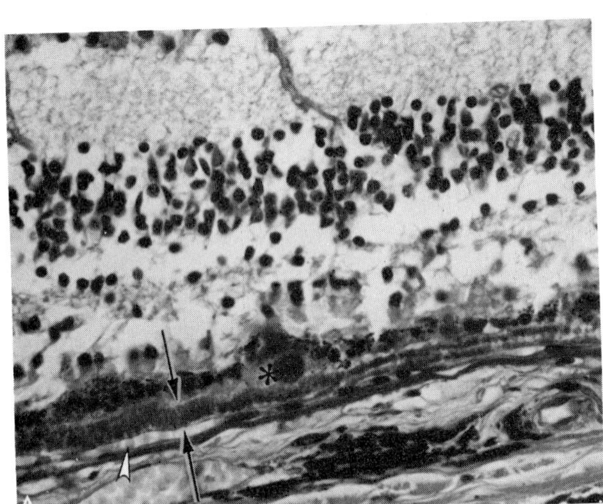

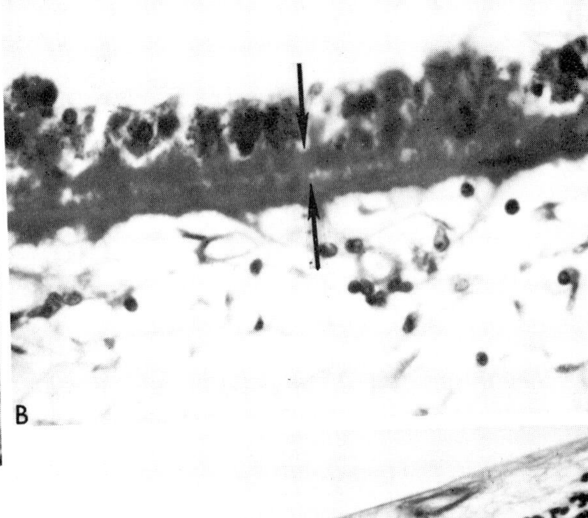

Figure 8–349. Diffuse drusen. *A,* Diffuse thickening of inner aspect of Bruch's membrane (between arrows) in macular area. Nodules (asterisk) are also present. The retinal pigment epithelium is intact but attenuated. The photoreceptor cell layer is much thinned. A small blood vessel (arrowhead) lies between the thickened inner aspect and the remainder of Bruch's membrane. PAS, ×450. EP 39707. *B,* Diffuse thickening (between arrows) of inner aspect of Bruch's membrane. PAS, ×550. EP 31489. *C,* Diffuse confluent drusen (between arrows) in periphery. PAS, ×400. EP 31041. (From Green WR, Key SN III: Senile macular degeneration: A histopathological study. Trans Am Ophthalmol Soc *75*:180–254, 1977.)

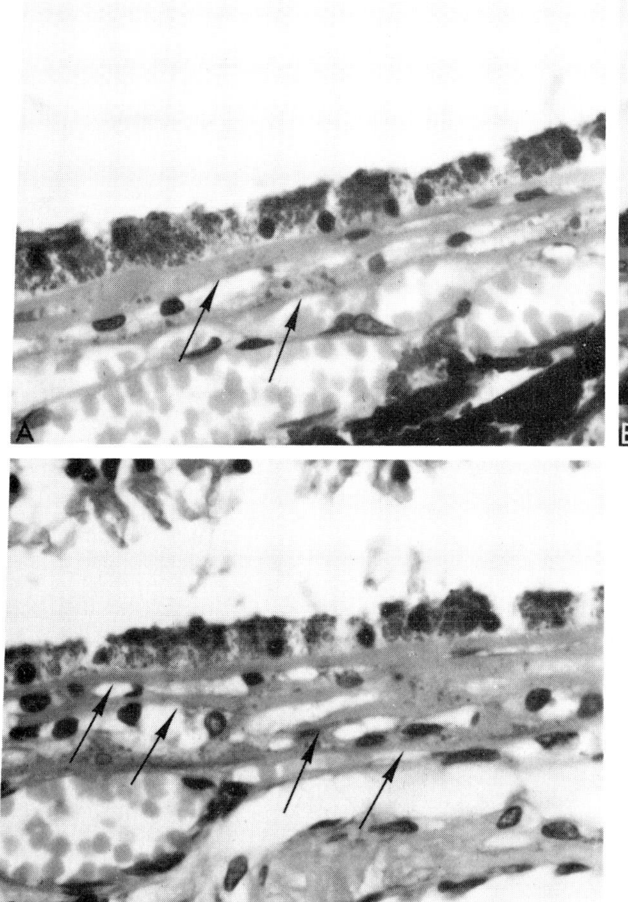

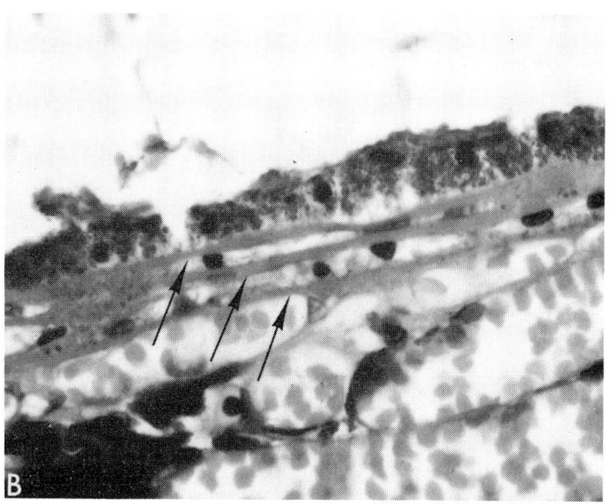

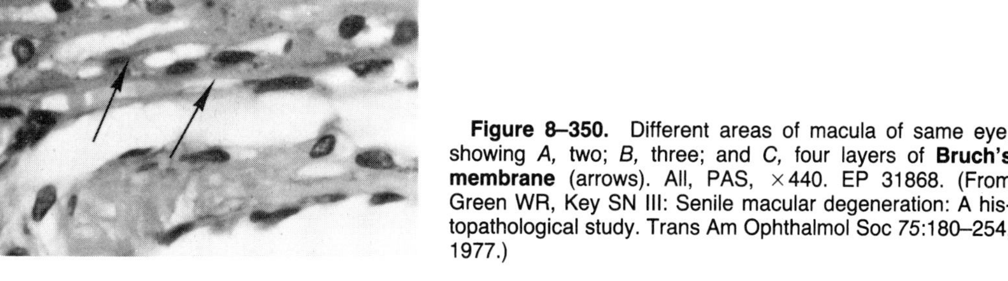

Figure 8–350. Different areas of macula of same eye, showing *A,* two; *B,* three; and *C,* four layers of **Bruch's membrane** (arrows). All, PAS, ×440. EP 31868. (From Green WR, Key SN III: Senile macular degeneration: A histopathological study. Trans Am Ophthalmol Soc *75*:180–254, 1977.)

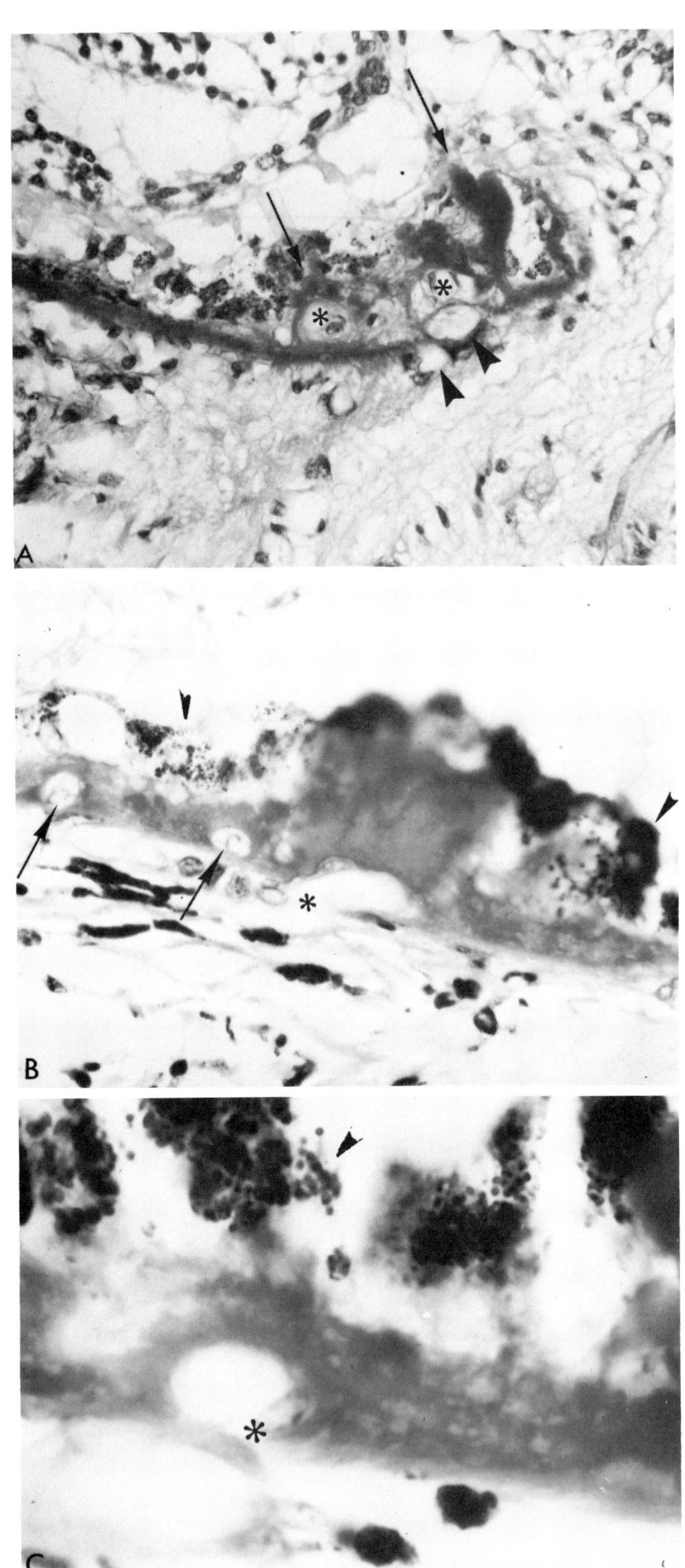

Figure 8–351. Peripapillary vascularized drusen. *A,* Vessels (asterisks) within drusen (arrows). Overlying retinal pigment epithelium (RPE) is hypertrophic, with large, spherical pigment granules. A capillary-like vessel (arrowheads) extends through a small break in Bruch's membrane. PAS, ×420. EP 45251. *B,* Vascularized (arrows) peripapillary drusen, covered by hypertrophic RPE (arrowheads). A choroidal vessel (asterisk) extends into druse through a break in Bruch's membrane. H and E, ×500. *C,* A second break in Bruch's membrane, with vessel transversing (asterisk). Large, spherical pigment granules (arrowhead) of hypertrophic RPE are more clearly shown. H and E, ×800. EP 37361. (From Green WR: Pathology of the retina, in Lancaster Course in Ophthalmic Histopathology. Frayer WC (ed): Unit 9. Philadelphia, F.A. Davis, 1981.)

ance (Fig. 8–350). Ultrastructural studies of a number of examples of this change have shown the principal constituent of the thickened material to be aggregates of widely spaced collagen or abnormal basement membrane (Green, Key, 1977; Sarks, 1973b). Sarks referred to this material as "basal laminar deposits." Mueller in 1855 also noted generalized thickening of the cuticular portion of Bruch's membrane in eyes of older persons and believed that drusen take their origin from this substance.

The diffuse thickening of the inner aspect of Bruch's membrane weakens the area and predisposes to separation of the RPE, along with the associated drusen and the inner portion of the thickened layer (Green, Key, 1977; Green, 1980a).

Another change that occurs with typical drusen or colloid bodies and more frequently with the diffuse thickening of the inner aspect of Bruch's membrane is choroidal neovascularization occurring through associated breaks in Bruch's membrane. This neovascular change can be observed in the peripapillary (Fig. 8–351), peripheral (Fig. 8–352), and macular (Fig. 8–353) areas. This change predisposes to hemorrhage and disciform scarring, especially in the macular area and to a lesser degree in the peripheral and peripapillary areas.

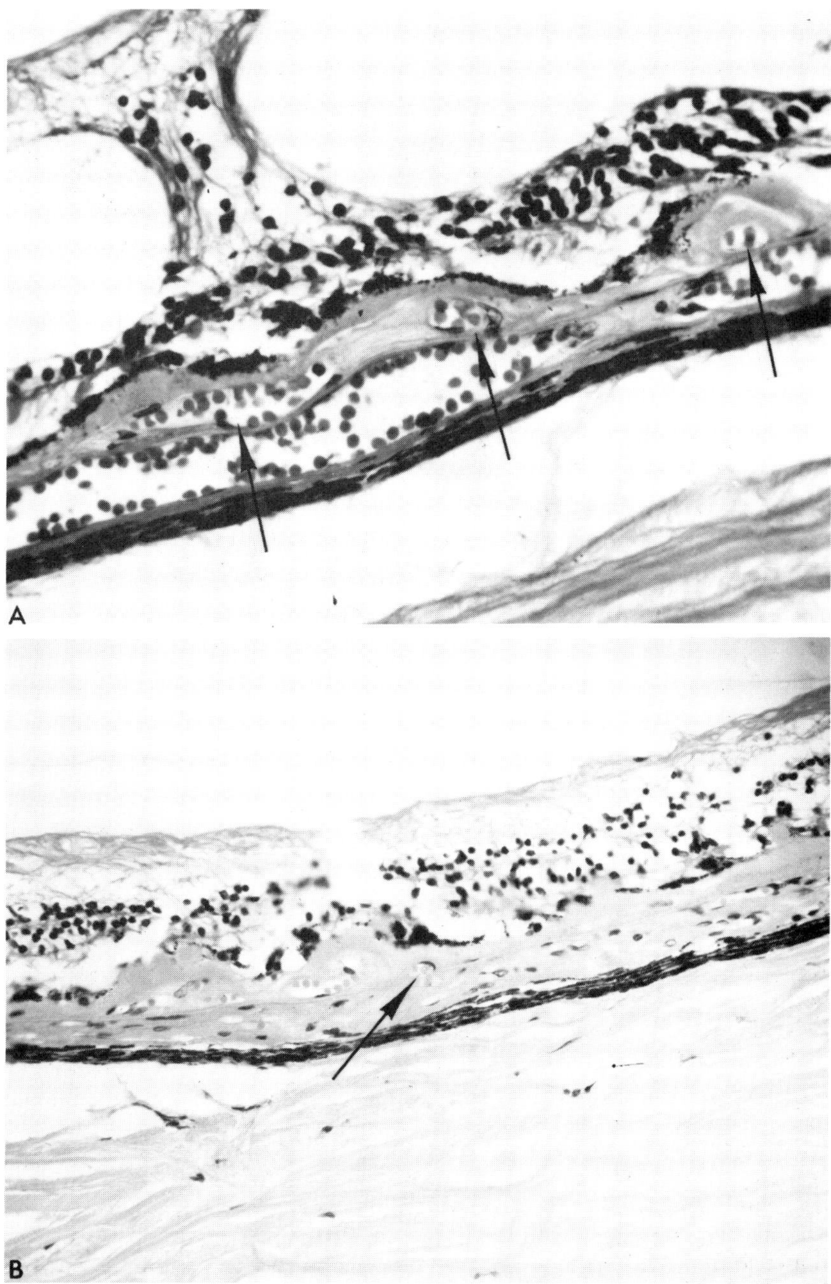

Figure 8–352. *A,* Peripheral **vascularized drusen** (arrows). H and E, ×300. *B,* A choroidal, capillary-like vessel (arrow) extends through a small break in Bruch's membrane. H and E, ×250. EP 31313.

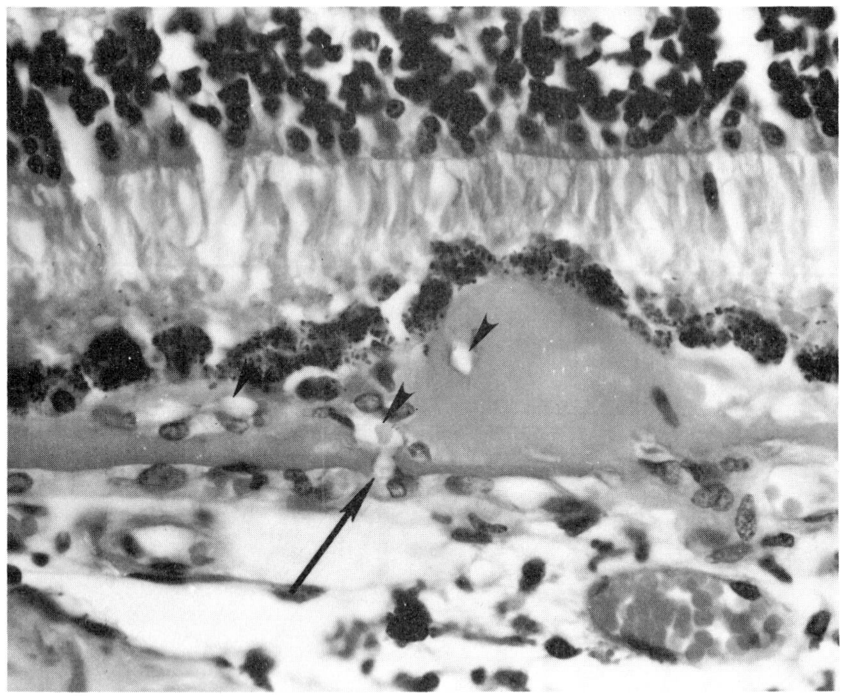

Figure 8–353. Vascularized drusen (arrowheads) in macular area. Overlying retinal pigment epithelium is hypertrophic, with large spherical granules; a choroidal, capillary-like vessel (arrow) transverses a small break in Bruch's membrane. H and E, ×450. EP 36415. (From Small ML, Green WR, Alpar JJ, Drewry RE Jr: Senile macular degeneration. A clinicopathologic correlation of two cases with neovascularization beneath the retinal pigment epithelium. Arch Ophthalmol *94*:601–607, 1976.)

It is not certain what the stimulus is for this neovascularization. It could be postulated that there may be outer retinal ischemia and that there is an attempt on the part of the choriocapillaris to overcome the ischemic state. There is progressive thickening of the intercapillary collagenous septa. The capillaries of the choriocapillaris become encased on their lateral and posterior sides by this connective tissue, which can become very dense.

Weighing against the ischemic theory is the absence of retinal neovascularization, the lack of the typical outer ischemic atrophy of the retina, and the consistent absence of occlusion of the choriocapillaris.

Burns and Feeney-Burns (1980) have studied human eyes from persons aged 1 to 92 years, with particular emphasis on the composition and temporal sequence of the formation of drusen. These investigators described the following ultrastructural features: thinning of basal lamina of RPE, deposition of material resembling cytoplasm beneath the basal lamina of the RPE (Fig. 8–354,*A*), rupture of small cytoplasmic bags with condensation and formation of "bent tubules," loss of infolding at basal surfaces of the RPE cells, loss of melanin granules in RPE cells overlying the area of drusen and increased melanin in adjacent RPE cells, migration of RPE intracellular junctional complexes from apicolateral to basolateral positions, and deposition of mineralized deposits resembling calcium salts in older drusen.

Burns and Feeney-Burns (1980) have suggested that apoptosis (Fig. 8–354,*B*), a process in which whole cell fragmentation occurs, plays a role in the development of drusen. Apoptosis is a recognized mechanism for controlled cellular deletion in tissue, involution, atrophy, remodeling, and tumor regression. The nucleus and cytoplasms condense, are partitioned, and shed as fragments that may be phagocytosed by macrophages.

Using the electron microscope, changes can be seen in the endothelial cells, with formation of tonguelike processes that extend into the collagenous tissue of Bruch's membrane. These could be the beginnings of an attempt at neovascularization (Friedman, Smith, 1965; Klien, 1964).

The pathogenesis of drusen is unknown. Some previous investigators have suggested that drusen represent an aberrant secretory activity of the RPE, while others have suggested that they represent a transformation of degenerating RPE cells. Both these theories still seem to have merit.

Rones (1938) reported that two processes were involved in the production of drusen. One was the production of material by the RPE cells and its deposition in Bruch's membrane in the case of typical senile drusen. The second involves the transformation of RPE cells into lipoidal material that is deposited under the RPE. Occasionally, individual RPE cells have been observed to undergo a form of lipoidal degeneration with the accumulation of numerous cytoplasmic lipid inclusions (Fig. 8–355). One could speculate that the adjacent RPE proliferates over this degenerating cell to encase the RPE-derived lipid-rich

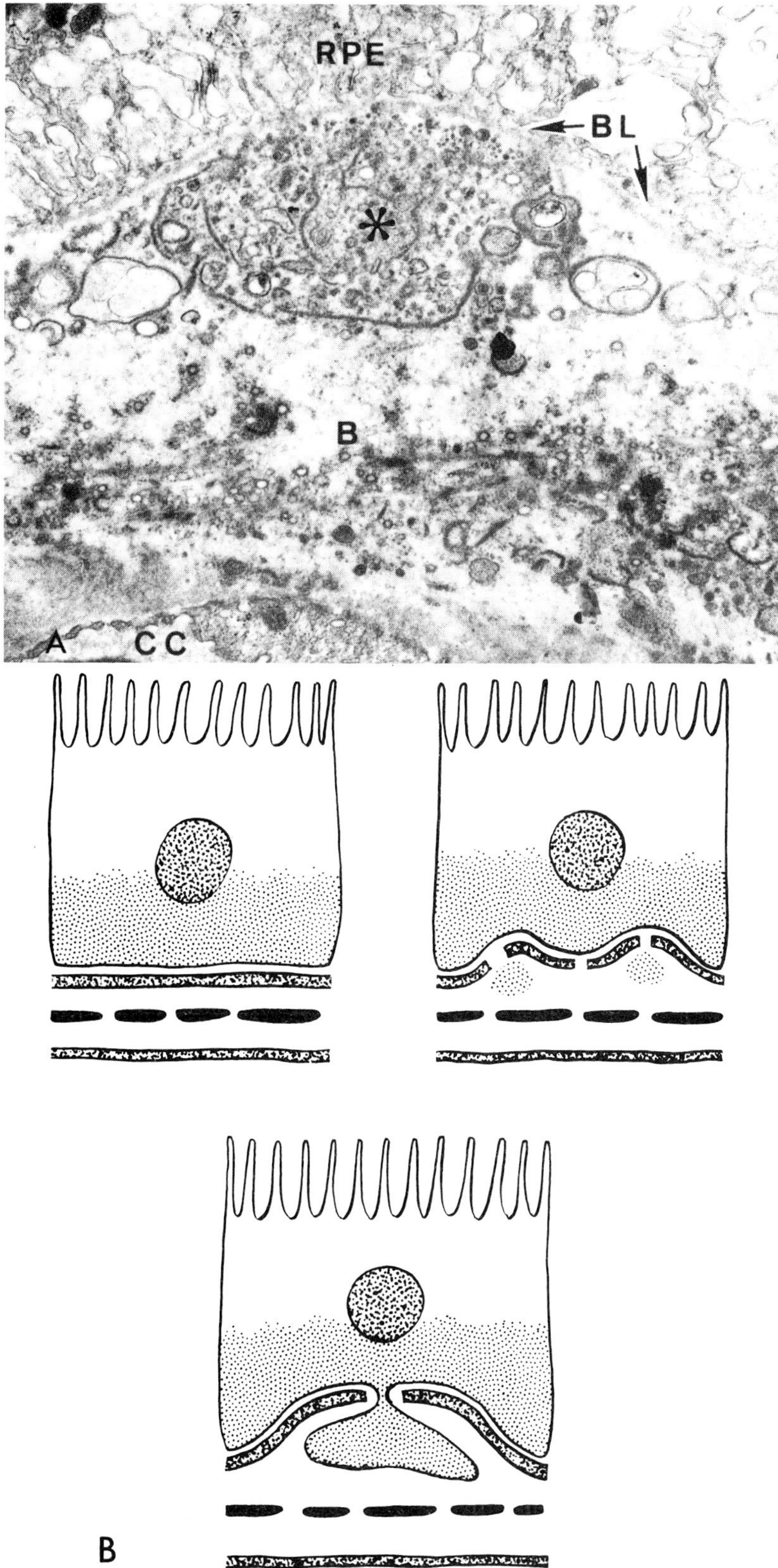

Figure 8–354. *A*, Mound of cytoplasmic debris (asterisk) between basal lamina (*BL*) of retinal pigment epithelium (*RPE*) and Bruch's membrane (*B*) in 30 year old eye. *CC*, choricocapillris. × 7000. *B*, Apoptosis of RPE. (From Burns RP, Feeney-Burns L: Clinicopathologic correlations of drusen of Bruch's membrane. Trans Am Opthalmol Soc *78*:206–225, 1980.)

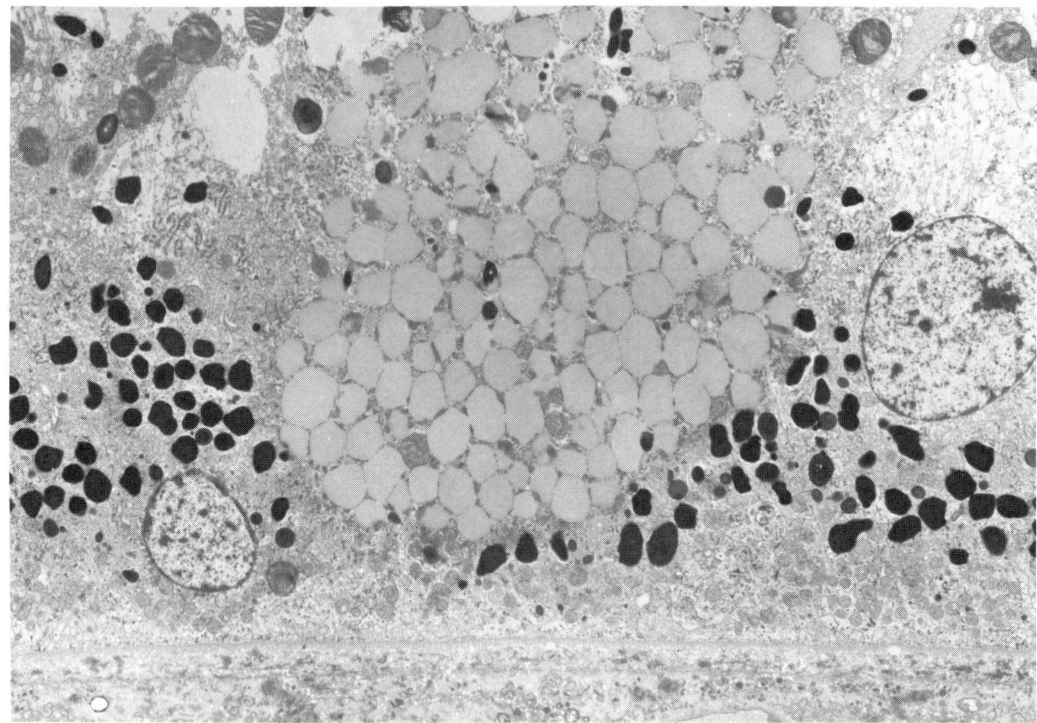

Figure 8–355. Lipid inclusions in an individual retinal pigment epithelium cell. ×3790. EP 42276. (From Green WR: Clinicopathologic studies of senile macular degeneration, *in* Nicholson DH (ed): Ocular Pathology Update. New York, Masson, 1980, p 118.)

material and form a druse. Fine (1981) has observed similar lipoidal degeneration of RPE cells in the macular area of older rhesus monkeys.

It has become increasingly evident that drusen are related to activity of the RPE and to changes in the epithelial cells, with accumulation of material in Bruch's membrane (Farkas, Krill, Sylvester, Archer, 1971; Farkas, Sylvester, Archer, Altona, 1971; Friedman, Smith, 1965; Farkas, 1971).

In the diffuse type of drusen, abnormal basement membrane production by the RPE appears to be a pathogenetic factor. In dominant hereditary drusen, the drusen have the same appearance as typical drusen. They differ only in number and size; with the electron microscope, they have the same fine structure.

Numerous investigators have indicated that senile macular degeneration is a heredodegenerative disease (Behr, 1920; Elwyn, 1955; Klien, 1950; Falls, 1949). Gass (1973b) has presented extensive evidence that drusen predispose the eye to the development of the various forms of senile macular degeneration.

Our knowledge of senile macular degeneration in the past decade or so has increased as the result of the development of fluorescein angiography and more extensive clinicopathologic correlative studies. Numerous observers have noted the clinical association of drusen with disciform degeneration of the macula (Gass, 1973b; Teeters, Bird, 1973). Recent clinical studies have disclosed that RPE atrophy (areolar atrophy) and sub-RPE neovascularization (Teeters, Bird, 1973; Sarks, 1976) also occur in association with drusen.

These studies have led to the general impression that persons with drusen in the macula are at

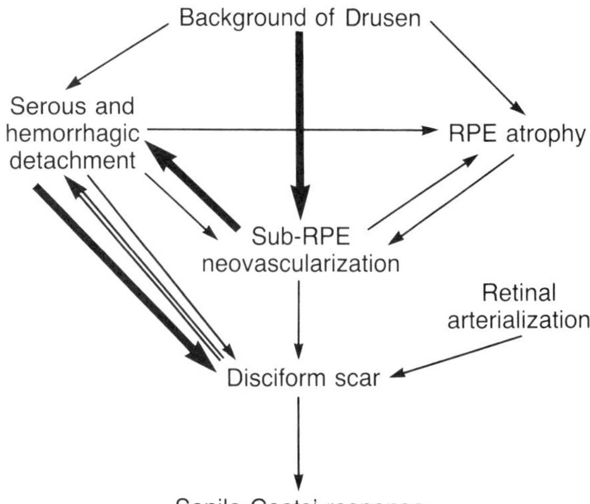

Figure 8–356. Different morphologic forms of senile macular degeneration. Larger and darker arrows indicate the more common pathways from drusen to disciform scarring. Smaller and lighter arrows indicate other pathways and associated features that may be observed. See text. (From Green WR, Key SN III: Senile macular degeneration: A histopathologic study. Trans Am Ophthalmol Soc *75*:180–254, 1977.)

a greater risk of developing senile macular degeneration (SMD). The lesions of SMD may take various morphologic forms, either singly or in various combinations. Figure 8–356 is a flow diagram of the interrelationships of the different morphologic forms of SMD. The larger and darker arrows indicate the more common pathway from drusen to disciform scarring. The smaller and lighter arrows indicate other pathways and associated features that may be observed. Older persons with drusen and diffuse thickening of the inner aspect of Bruch's membrane may develop "wet" sequelae, such as serous or hemorrhagic detachment of the retina (Fig. 8–357) or RPE (Figs. 8–358 through 8–360). Such persons may also develop RPE (areolar) atrophy (Figs. 8–361 through 8–363). Usually this occurs without associated serous or hemorrhagic detachment. Drusen also may be associated with sub-RPE neovascularization (Figs. 8–364 through 8–366).

Areolar atrophy and sub-RPE neovascularization frequently coexist (Fig. 8–367); thus the arrows go in both directions between these two cat-

Text continued on page 961

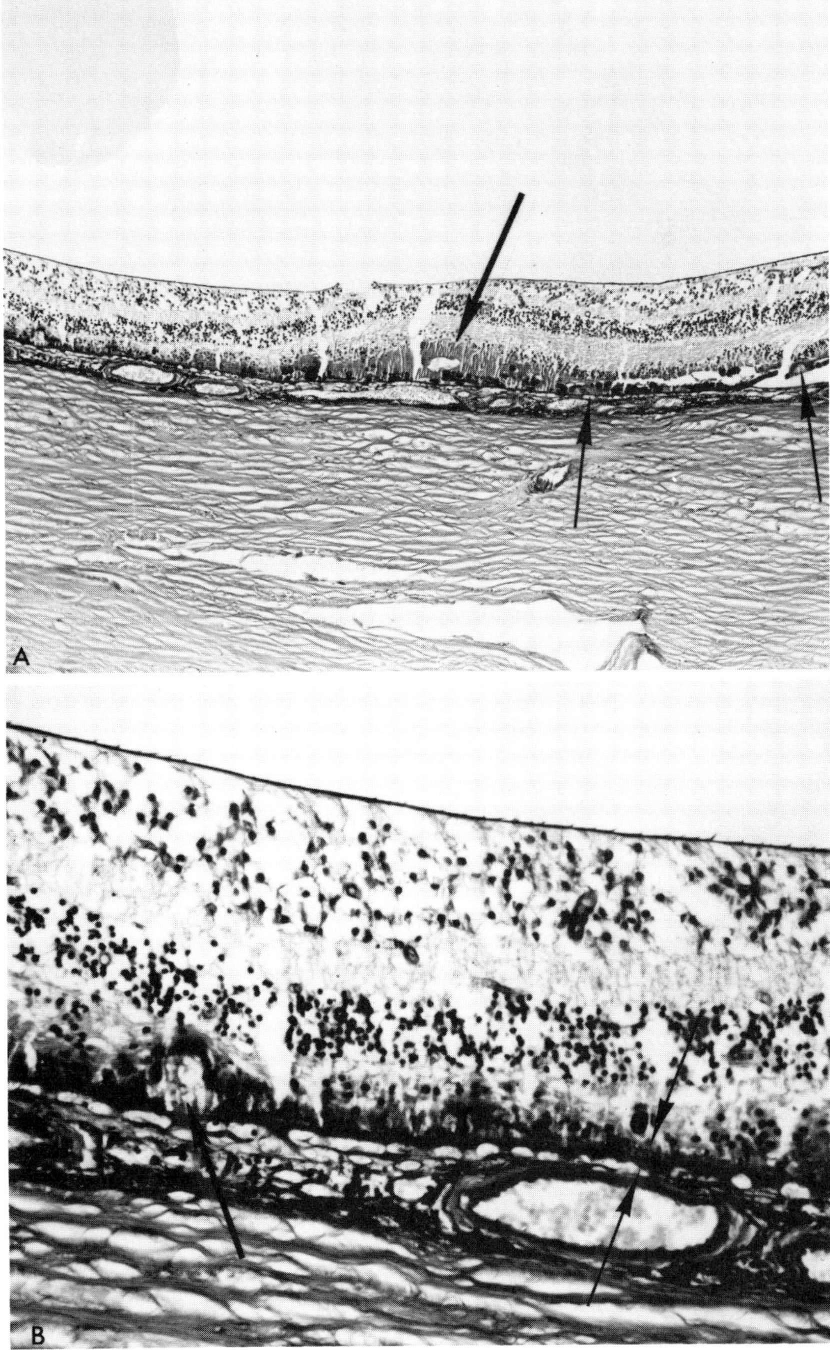

Figure 8–357. *A,* Small, serous **detachment of retina** (large arrow) associated with drusen (small arrows). PAS, ×40. *B,* Adjacent area showing drusen (large arrow), thickening of Bruch's membrane (between arrows), and atrophy of retinal pigment epithelium and photoreceptor cell layer. PAS, ×210. EP 40664. (From Green WR, Key SN III: Senile macular degeneration: A histopathological study. Trans Am Ophthalmol Soc *75*:180–254, 1977.)

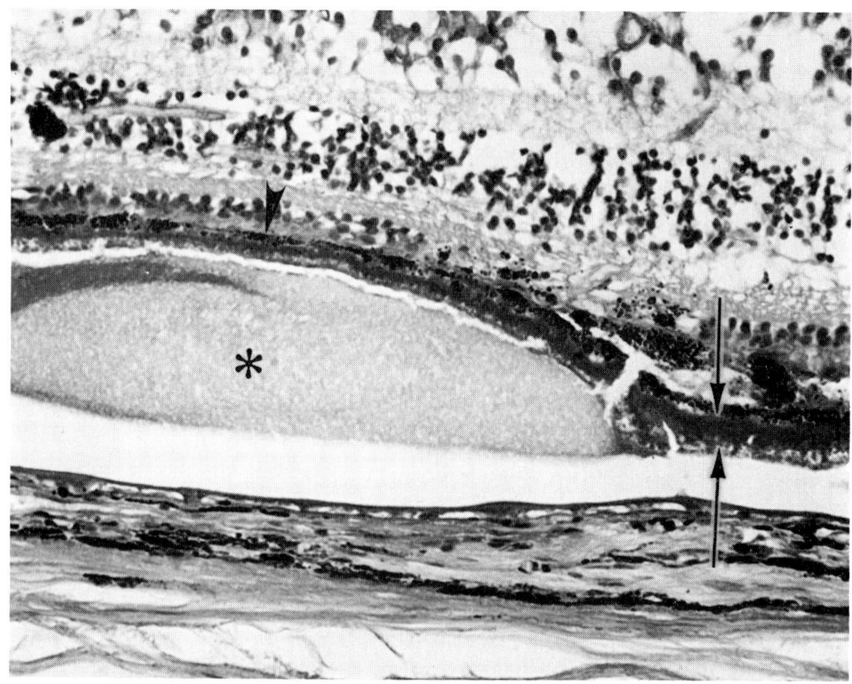

Figure 8–358. Macular area of right eye, showing much thickening of inner aspect of Bruch's membrane (between arrows) and a serous, intra-Bruch's membrane, (sub-RPE) detachment. Overlying retinal pigment epithelium (arrowhead) is intact, but attenuated. Photoreceptor cell layer is thinned. PAS, ×245. EP 38171. (From Green WR, Key SN III: Senile macular degeneration: A histopathological study. Trans Am Ophthalmol Soc 75:180–254, 1977.)

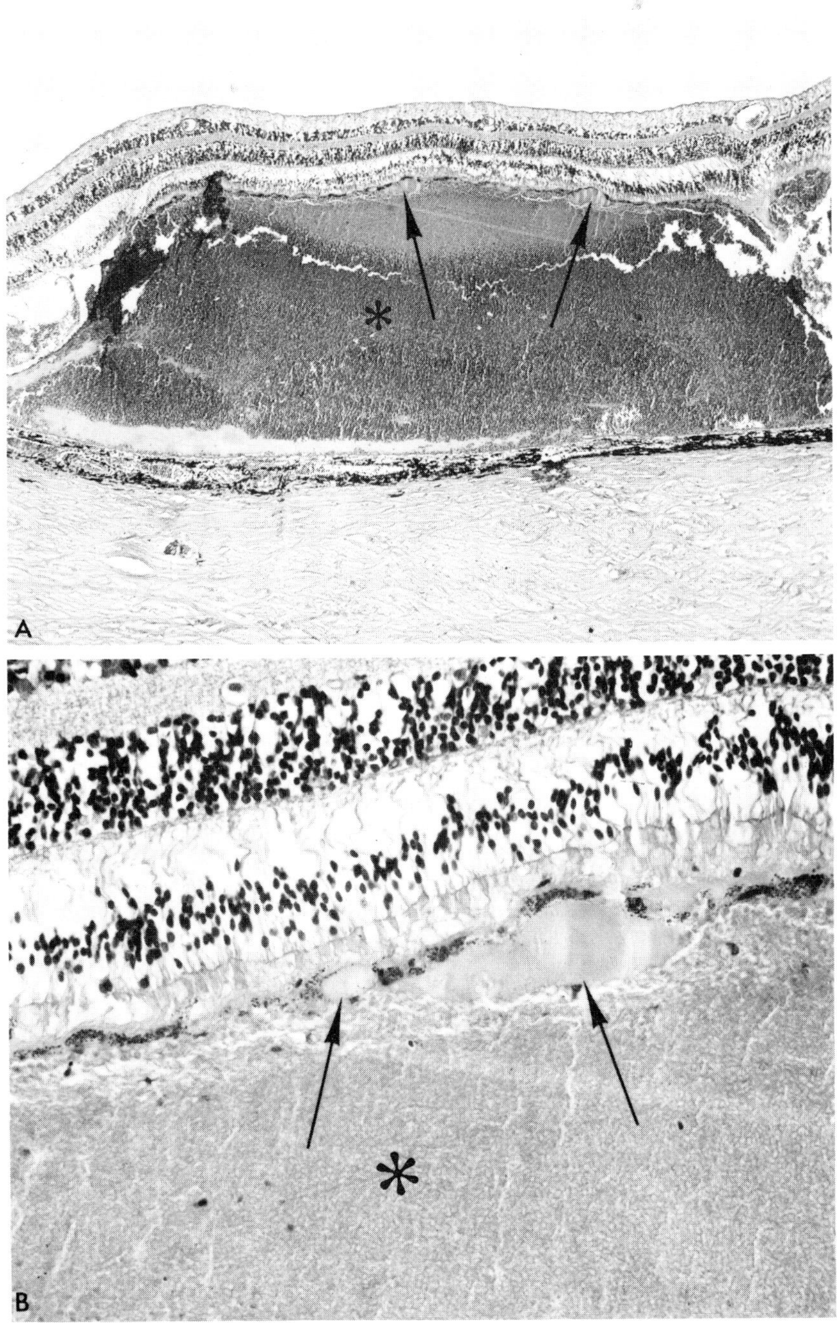

Figure 8–359. *A,* **Hemorrhagic detachment of retinal pigment epithelium (RPE)** (asterisk) in an eye that was considered to have a malignant melanoma. Drusen are detached (arrows) along with RPE. H and E, ×40. *B,* Higher power view shows drusen (arrows) and RPE detached by hemorrhage (asterisk). RPE is intact but attenuated, and the photoreceptor cell layer is generally intact. H and E, ×240. EP 27032. (From Green WR, Key SN III: Senile macular degeneration: A histopathological study. Trans Am Ophthalmol Soc *75*:180–254, 1977.)

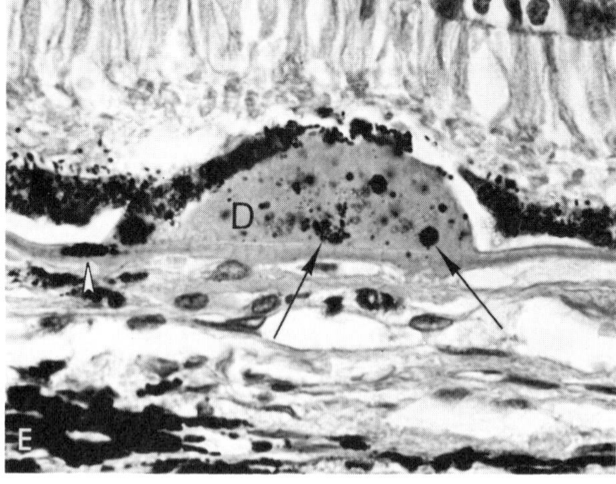

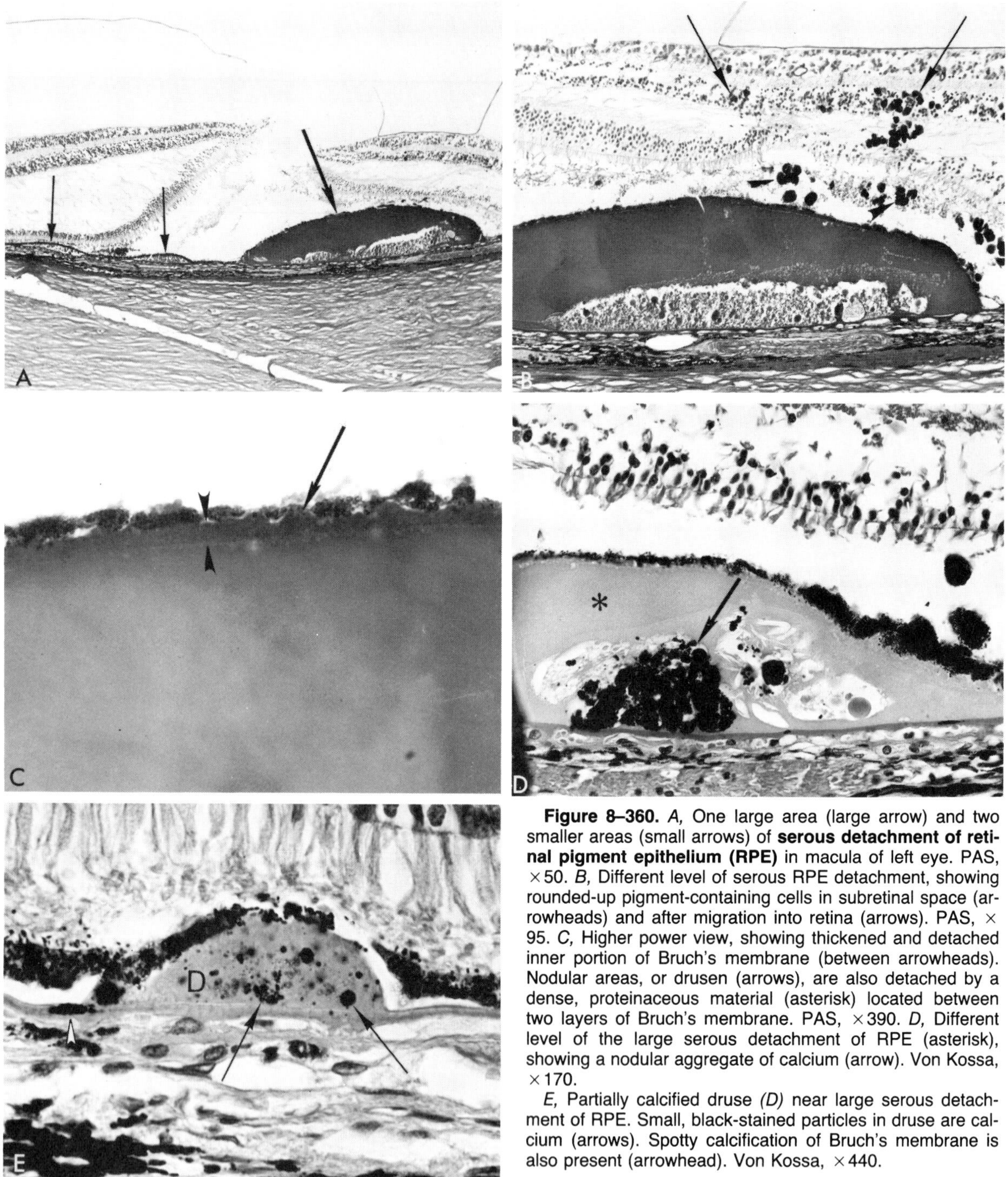

Figure 8–360. *A,* One large area (large arrow) and two smaller areas (small arrows) of **serous detachment of retinal pigment epithelium (RPE)** in macula of left eye. PAS, ×50. *B,* Different level of serous RPE detachment, showing rounded-up pigment-containing cells in subretinal space (arrowheads) and after migration into retina (arrows). PAS, × 95. *C,* Higher power view, showing thickened and detached inner portion of Bruch's membrane (between arrowheads). Nodular areas, or drusen (arrows), are also detached by a dense, proteinaceous material (asterisk) located between two layers of Bruch's membrane. PAS, ×390. *D,* Different level of the large serous detachment of RPE (asterisk), showing a nodular aggregate of calcium (arrow). Von Kossa, ×170.

E, Partially calcified druse *(D)* near large serous detachment of RPE. Small, black-stained particles in druse are calcium (arrows). Spotty calcification of Bruch's membrane is also present (arrowhead). Von Kossa, ×440.

Illustration continued on opposite page

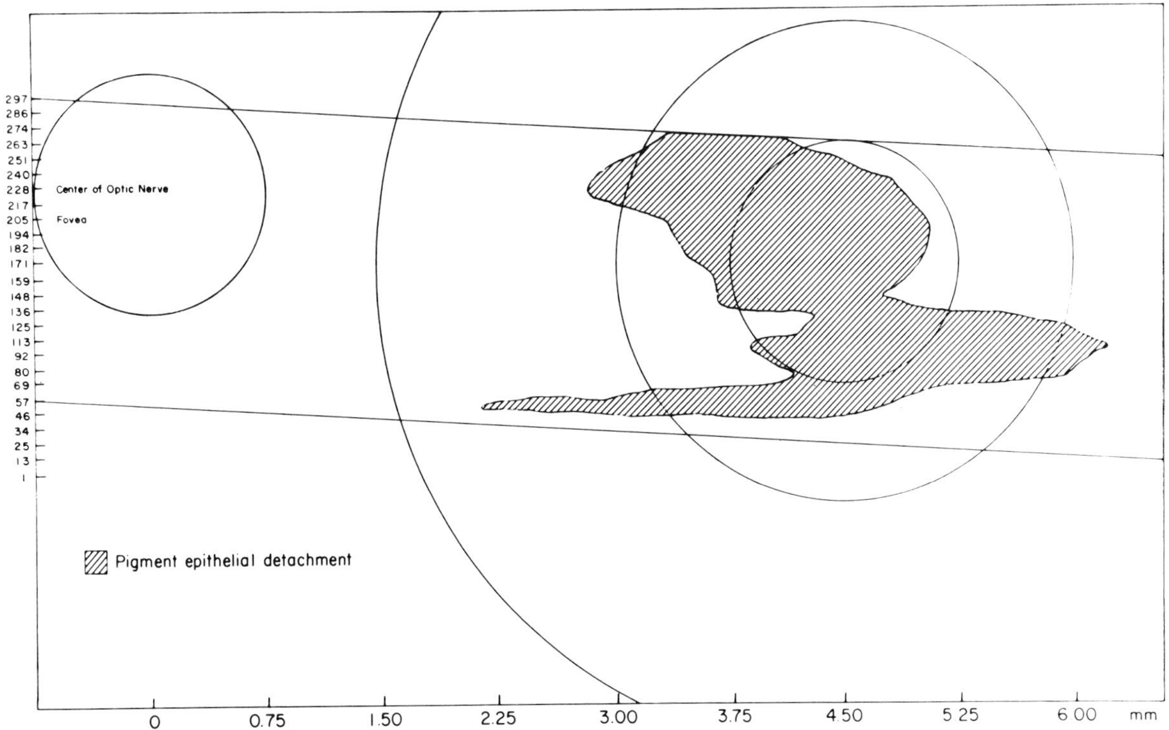

F

Figure 8–360. *Continued F,* Two-dimensional reconstruction from study of serial sections showing size and location of a large serous detachment of RPE. See Figure 8–348 for ultrastructural features of the thickened inner aspect of Bruch's membrane of this case. EP 42450. (From Green WR, Key SN III: Senile macular degeneration: A histopathological study. Trans Am Ophthalmol Soc *75*:180–254, 1977.)

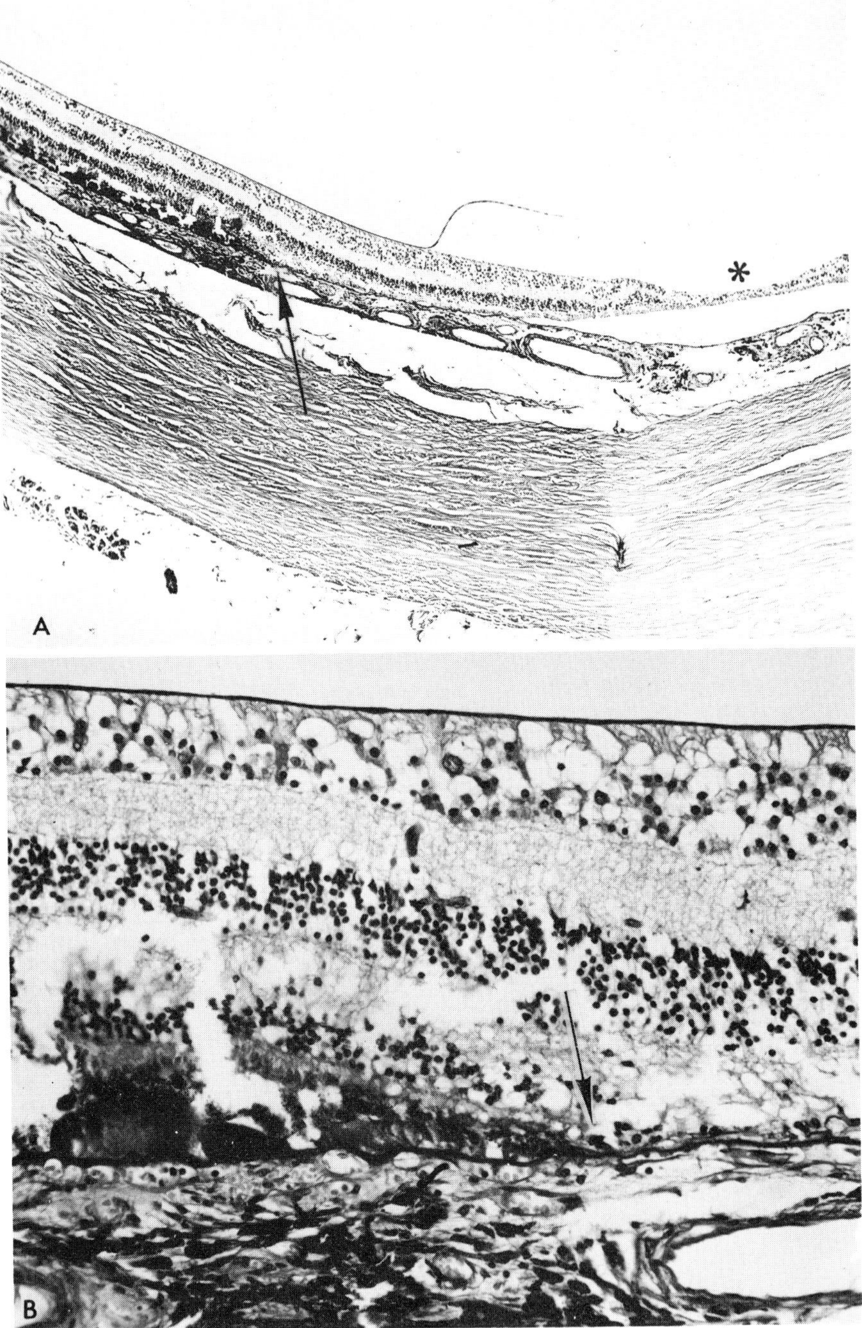

Figure 8–361. *A,* Section through foveola (asterisk) of left eye showing retinal pigment epithelium (RPE) areolar atrophy and drusen, outside area of atrophy, where RPE and retina are intact. There is total loss of photoreceptor cell layer in the area of areolar atrophy. Arrow marks junction between drusen area (to left) and areolar atrophy (to right). PAS, ×40. *B,* Higher power view of abrupt junction (arrow) between areolar and drusen areas. PAS, ×240. EP 33614. (From Green WR, Key SN III: Senile macular degeneration: A histopathological study. Trans Am Ophthalmol Soc *75*:180–254, 1977.)

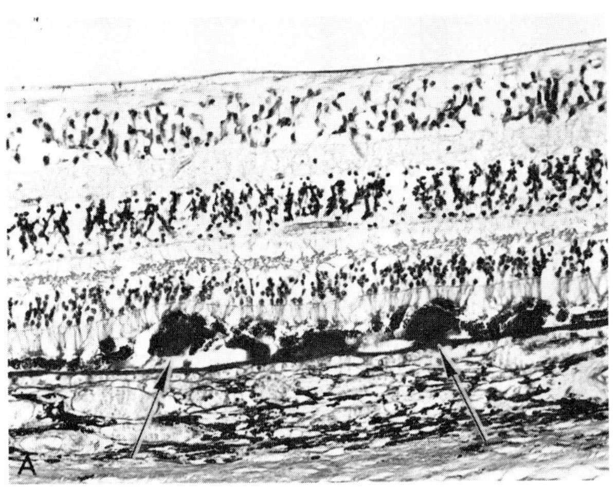

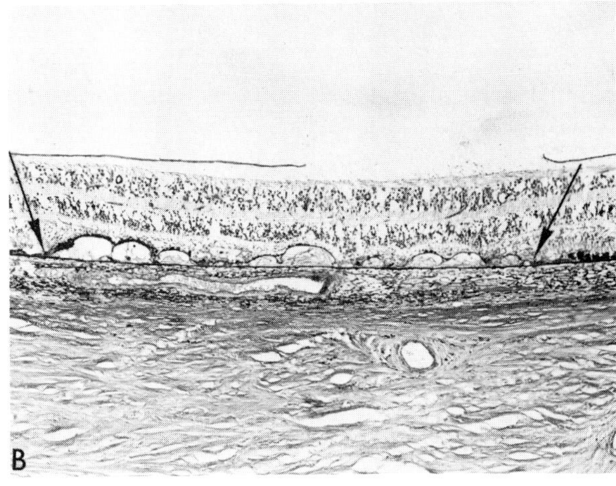

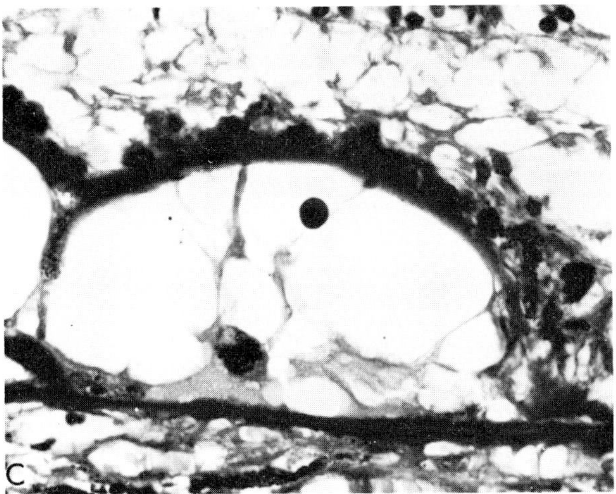

Figure 8–362. *A,* Right eye showing a **druse** (arrows) with an intact retinal pigment epithelium (RPE) and photoreceptor cell layer. PAS ×165. *B,* Druse with RPE and photoreceptor cell layer atrophy (between arrows). PAS, ×40. *C,* Higher power view of druse with separation of inner, thickened portion of Bruch's membrane. Some of drusen material appears to have been "washed out." PAS, ×465. EP 34138. (From Green WR, Key SN III: Senile macular degeneration: A histopathological study. Trans Am Ophthalmol Soc *75*:180–254, 1977.)

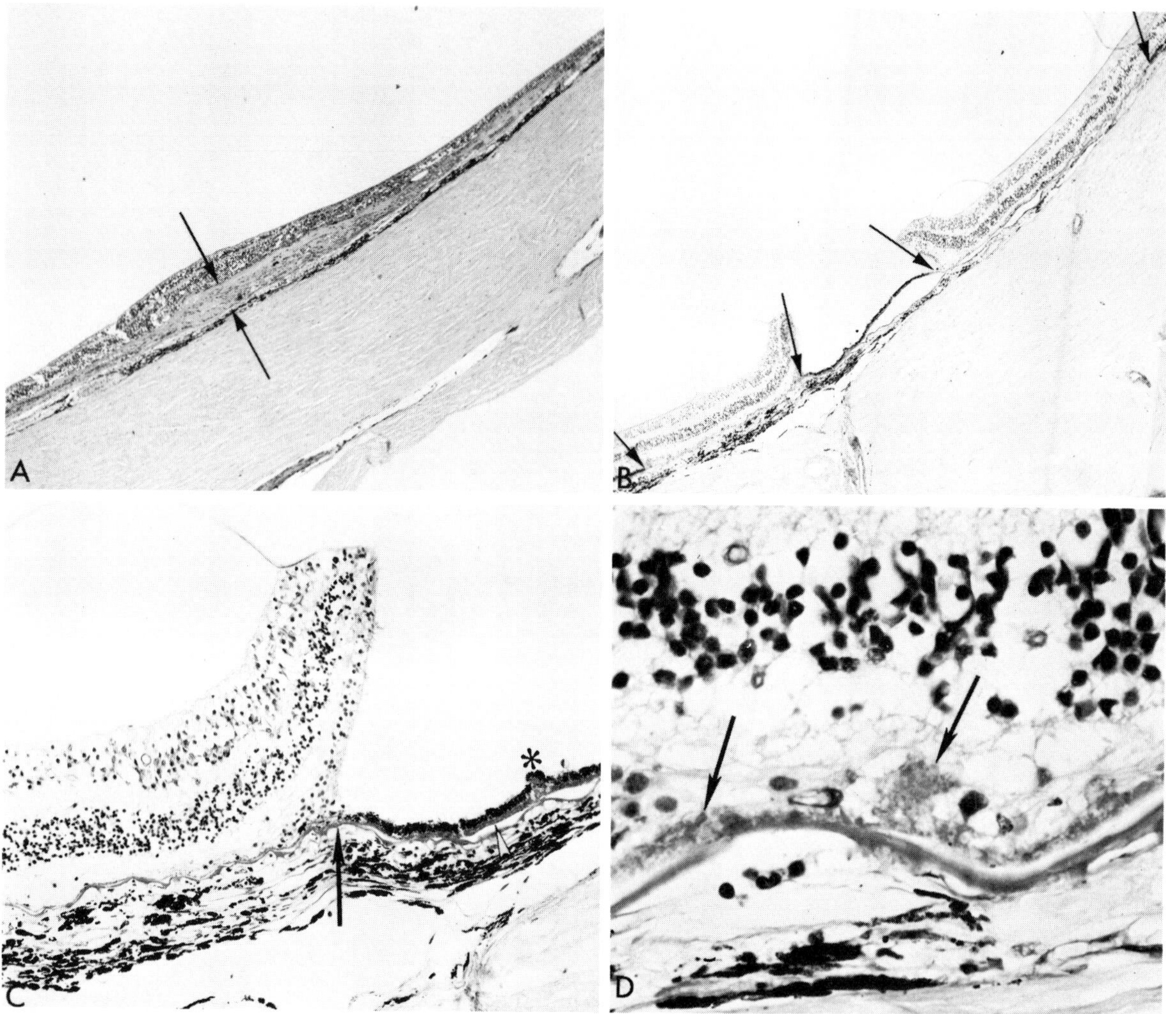

Figure 8–363. *A,* Flat, disciform lesion (between arrows) of right eye. H and E, ×19. *B,* Doughnut-shaped area of areolar atrophy of retinal pigment epithelium (RPE) and photoreceptor cell layer (between arrows). A macular hole is present in the foveola where the RPE is intact. PAS, ×19. *C,* Higher power view of junction (arrow) between areolar area (to the left) and central zone where RPE is intact and there is prominent thickening of the inner aspect of Bruch's membrane (arrowhead) and drusen (asterisk). PAS, ×100. *D,* Areolar area showing residual drusen-like material (arrows). PAS, ×385. EP 37750.

(From Green WR, Key SN III: Senile macular degeneration: A histopathological study. Trans Am Ophthalmol Soc *75*:180–254, 1977.)

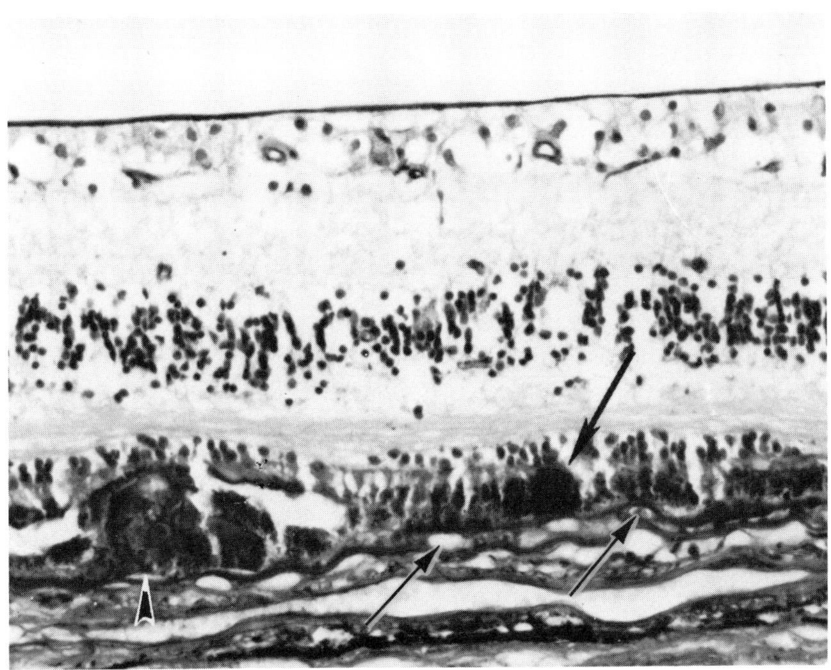

Figure 8–364. Left eye showing drusen (arrowhead) and sub-retinal pigment epithelium (intra-Bruch's membrane) neovascularization (smaller arrows). RPE is intact, but shows some clumping (larger arrow). PAS, ×280. EP 40789. (From Green WR, Key SN III: Senile macular degeneration: A histopathological study. Trans Am Ophthalmol Soc *75*:180–254, 1977.)

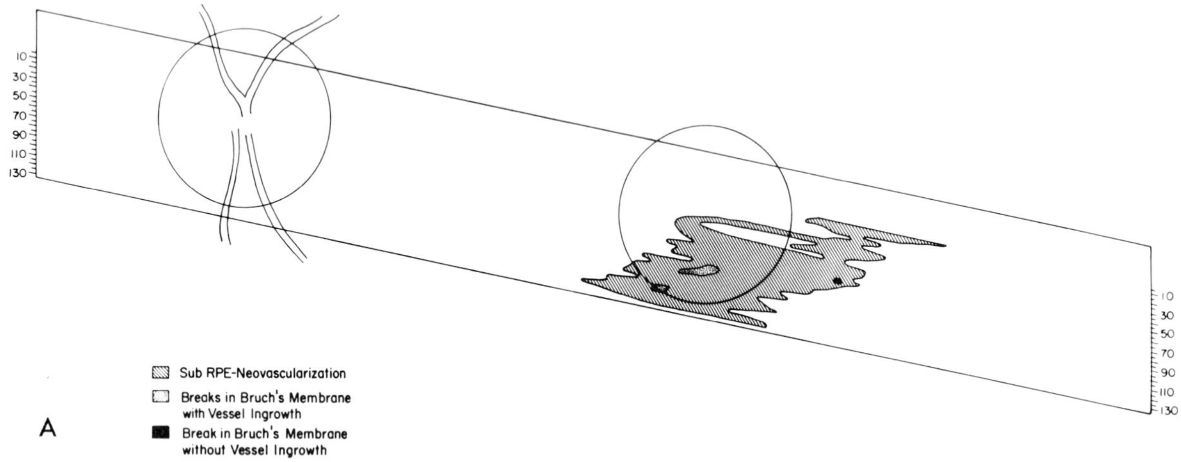

Sub RPE-Neovascularization

Breaks in Bruch's Membrane with Vessel Ingrowth

Break in Bruch's Membrane without Vessel Ingrowth

A

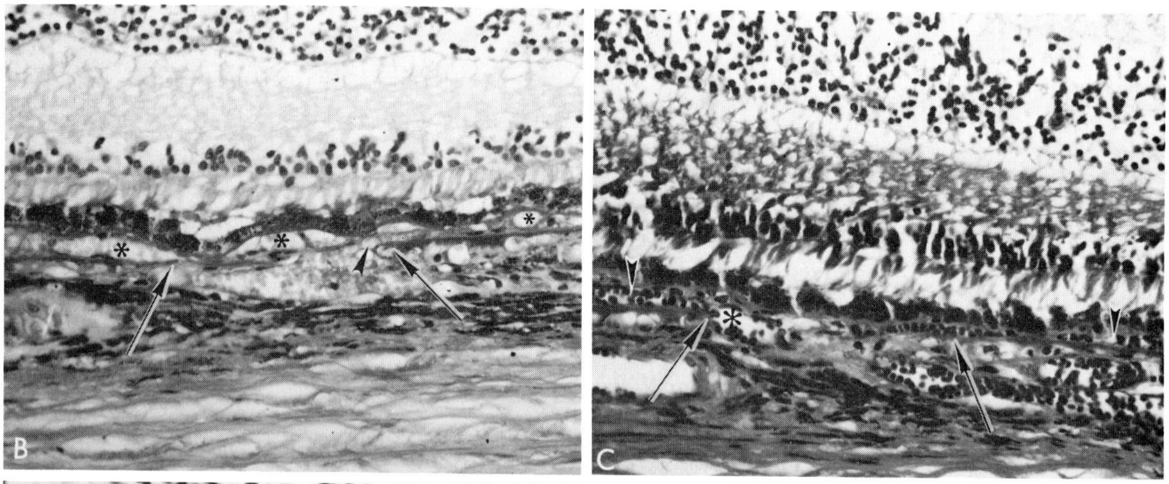

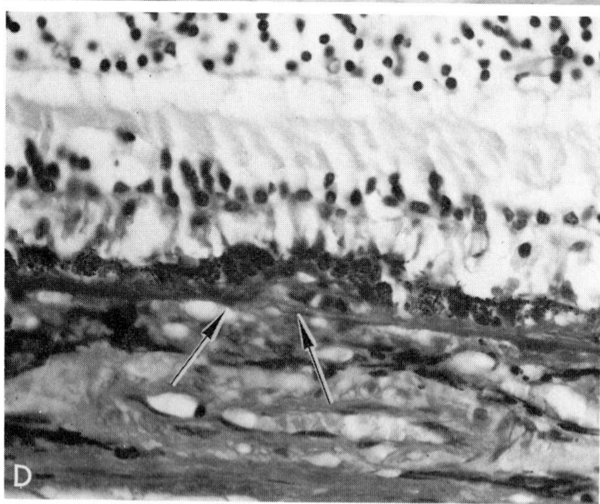

Figure 8–365. Sub-retinal pigment epithelium (RPE) neovascularization associated with drusen. *A,* Two-dimensional reconstruction from study of serial sections showing location, size, and shape of sub-RPE neovascular membrane and three discontinuities of Bruch's membrane—two of which have capillary-like choroidal vessels transversing the opening. *B,* Section through larger break in Bruch's membrane (between arrows) through which a choroidal vessel (arrowhead) traverses. New vessels (asterisks) extend under intact RPE beyond margin of breaks. PAS, × 320. *C,* A second break in Bruch's membrane (between arrows) with choroidal vessel (asterisk) extending through break and under (arrowheads) intact RPE. Van de Grift, ×320. *D,* A third and smaller break in Bruch's membrane (between arrows) has no choroidal neovascularization. PAS, ×560. EP 45027.

(From Green WR, Key SN III: Senile macular degeneration: A histopathological study. Trans Am Ophthalmol Soc *75*:180–254, 1977.)

egories. Sub-RPE neovascularization leads to serous (Fig. 8–368) and hemorrhagic (Figs. 8–369 and 8–370) detachment of the RPE or the retina, and this, in turn, may lead to disciform scarring (Figs. 8–371 through 8–380).

After the evaluation of a disciform scar, additional serous or hemorrhagic detachment of the retina or the RPE or both may occur (Figs. 8–381 through 8–384).

Retinal vascular contribution to the disciform lesion (Figs. 8–376,*B*, 8–377, 8–378, and 8–385) may occur (Green, Gass, 1971; Gold, Friedman, Wise, 1973; Green, Key, 1977). The new vasculature of some disciform lesions leaks profusely and produces marked intra- and subretinal exudation that may be rich in lipid material (Figs. 8–386 and 8–387) ("exudative senile maculopathy," "senile Coats' response").

A study of over 200 eyes with SMD, many with clinicopathologic correlation, showed prominent coexistence of the various morphologic forms of senile macular degeneration (Green, Key, 1977). A relatively high incidence of sub-RPE neovascularization from the choroid is found, which may not be appreciated clinically, even with the help of fluorescein angiography.

Sarks (1973b) and Green and Key (1977) have noted the considerable frequency of diffuse thickening of the inner aspect of Bruch's membrane in eyes of older persons with drusen. Much of this thickened material appears to be abnormal basement membrane material. This thickening appears to weaken this area and predispose to sub-RPE (or, more accurately, intra-Bruch's membrane) serous or hemorrhagic detachment and choroidal neovascularization.

Senile macular degenerations comprise a spectrum of abnormalities, commencing with advanced alterations in the pigment epithelium and Bruch's membrane with increasing age. The transition to actual *disease* is gradual. In some individuals there is a rapid course, and in others the process may require years. In some situations the changes are mild and involve only alterations in the RPE, while in others they are more dramatic and are manifested by massive hemorrhage from the new-formed vessels that have invaded Bruch's membrane. A variety of clinical and histopathologic pictures are seen, and an attempt has been made to classify the changes into groups. Such classification may be useful because in many individuals the condition may appear and remain stationary for long periods of time, while in others there is rapid progression to the various stages of senile macular degeneration.

Although choroidal vascular insufficiency has been implicated in the pathogenesis of senile macular degeneration (Klien, 1964), histopathologic studies have consistently shown the choriocapillaris to be relatively intact, and the picture of outer retinal ischemic atrophy is not present (Kornzweig, Feldstein, Schneider, 1959; Green, Key, 1977).

Classification. Senile macular degeneration can be conveniently classified as follows:

1. Areolar (geographic) retinal pigment epithelial atrophy.
2. Subretinal pigment epithelial neovascularization (choroidal neovascularization beneath the RPE).
3. Senile exudative macular degeneration.
4. Senile hemorrhagic macular degeneration.
5. Disciform macular degeneration.

All these forms in which choroidal neovascularization is present can be accompanied by lipid deposits in the macula and paramacular region and also drusen. In some patients the process is bilateral and equal. In others the eyes may show pigmentary changes in one macula and either serous or hemorrhagic changes in the fellow eye. In general, if hemorrhagic or serous changes have occurred in one eye, they usually will eventually appear in the fellow eye.

AREOLAR RETINAL PIGMENT EPITHELIAL ATROPHY. This is one of the commonest forms of senile macular degeneration. It is found in a considerable number of people beyond age 60 years and increases in prevalence so that it is present in about 15 per cent of eyes at age 80 years. Ophthalmoscopically, there is disturbance of the RPE, with areas of depigmentation in some regions and fine clumping and proliferation in others. The pattern of atrophy varies considerably. In the milder forms, vision is affected only slightly, but, as the disease progresses, vision is gradually lost. This form of disease may last 5 to 10 years without further changes occurring, or there may be a sudden, dramatic change to the serous or hemorrhagic type. As noted, it may coexist with sub-RPE neovascularization from the choroid.

Microscopically, the observed changes include alterations in the RPE cells, with depigmentation, migration, and proliferation of cells into the photoreceptor region. The most affected cells show degenerative changes in the cytoplasm and massive accumulations of lipid. In advanced stages, the RPE undergoes complete degeneration so that the photoreceptors are lost and the inner nuclear layer comes to lie adjacent to Bruch's membrane. The outer retinal structures show changes that are associated with this degenerative process, including loss of the outer nuclear layer and collapse of the outer plexiform layer. The pattern of atrophy observed in this condition is not that seen in outer retinal ischemia, for the inner nuclear layer remains intact and the choriocapillaris is relatively intact. With choroidal occlusive disease, the outer aspect of the inner nuclear layer also degenerates. If the retinal circulation is in-

Text continued on page 986

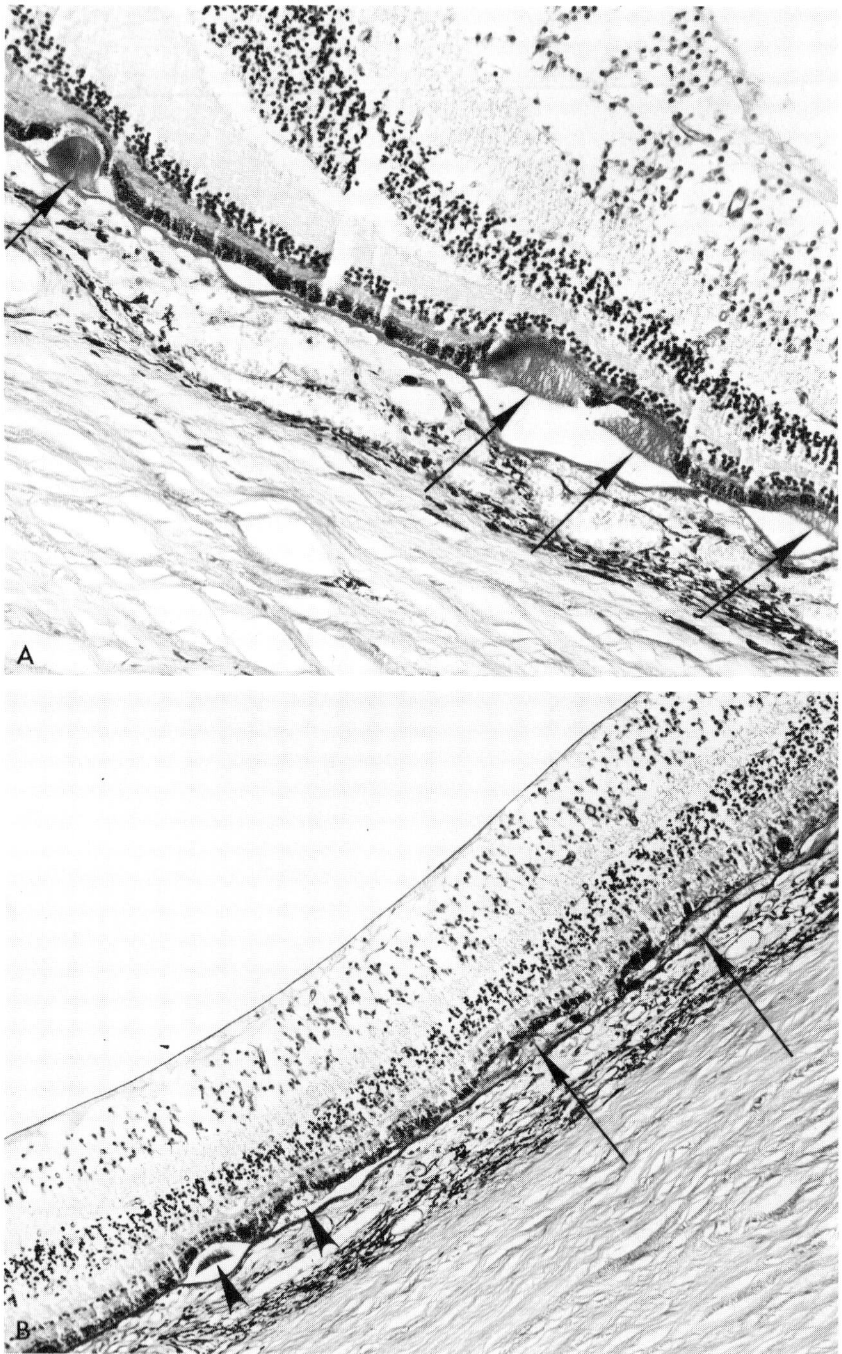

Figure 8–366. *A,* Section of left eye showing drusen (arrows). PAS, ×180. *B,* Right eye with drusen (arrowheads) and sub-retinal pigment epithelium (RPE) neovascularization (arrows). PAS, ×105.

Illustration continued on opposite page

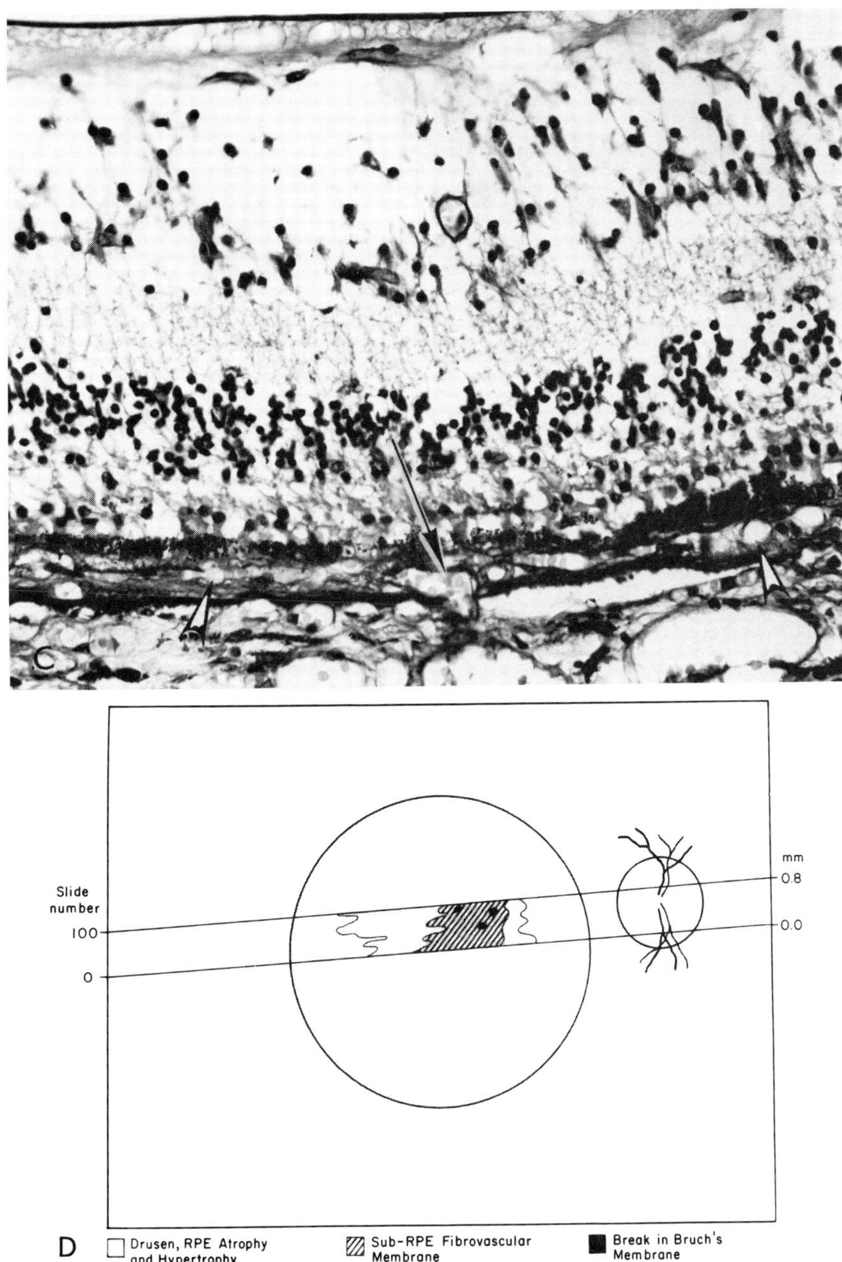

Figure 8–366 *Continued C,* One of three breaks (arrow) in Bruch's membrane through which choroidal vessels extend to form the sub-RPE vascular membrane (arrowheads). PAS, ×290. *D,* Two-dimensional reconstruction of macular lesion of right eye from study and mapping of serial sections, illustrating relative size and location of breaks in Bruch's membrane, sub-RPE neovascularization, and RPE changes. EP 40239. (From Green WR, Key SN III: Senile macular degeneration: A histopathological study. Trans Am Ophthalmol Soc *75*:180–254, 1977.)

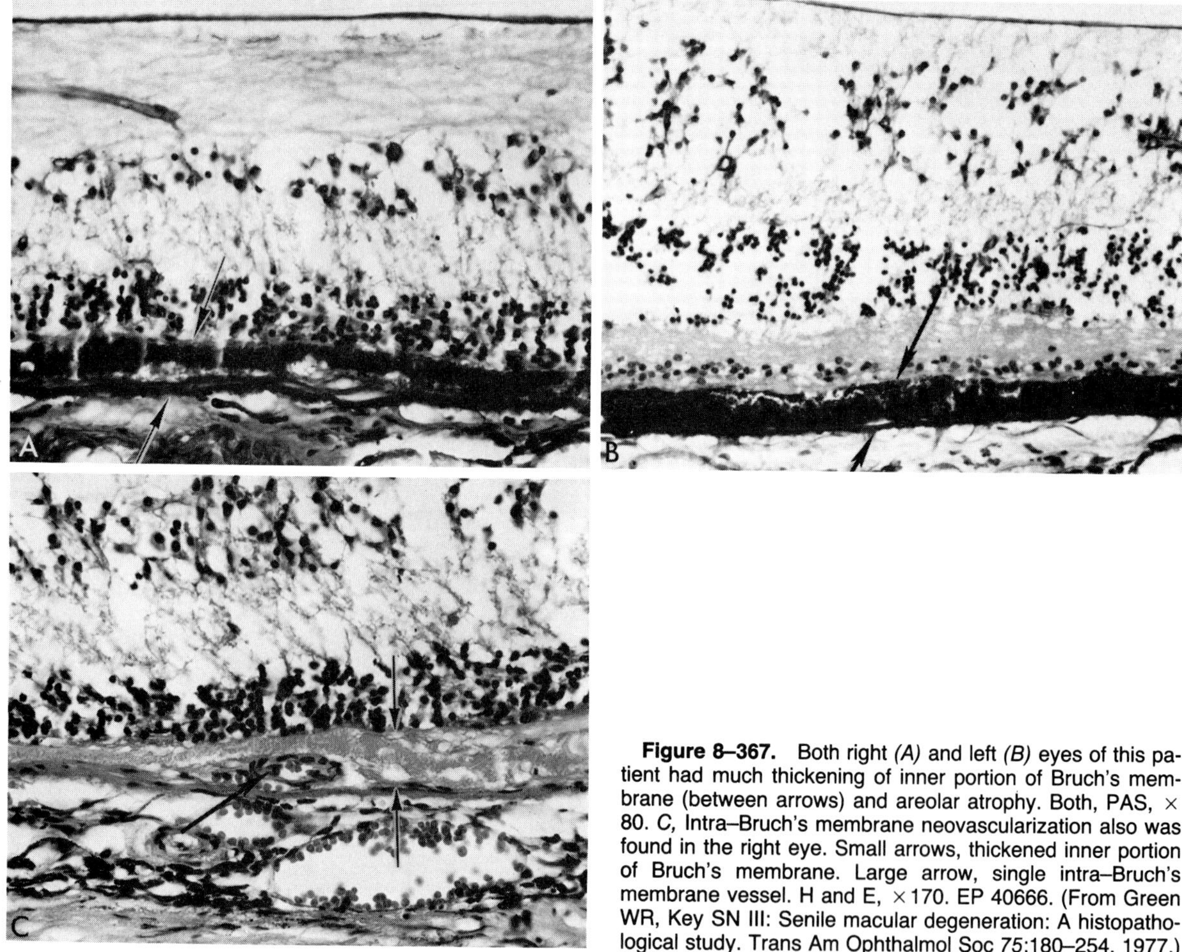

Figure 8–367. Both right *(A)* and left *(B)* eyes of this patient had much thickening of inner portion of Bruch's membrane (between arrows) and areolar atrophy. Both, PAS, × 80. *C,* Intra–Bruch's membrane neovascularization also was found in the right eye. Small arrows, thickened inner portion of Bruch's membrane. Large arrow, single intra–Bruch's membrane vessel. H and E, × 170. EP 40666. (From Green WR, Key SN III: Senile macular degeneration: A histopathological study. Trans Am Ophthalmol Soc *75*:180–254, 1977.)

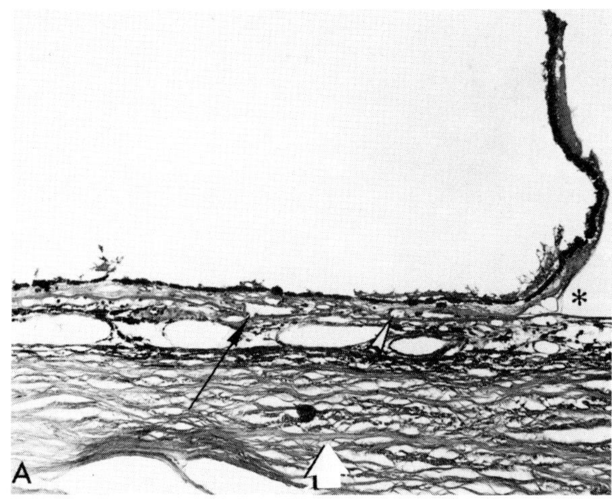

Figure 8–368. *A,* Area showing a break in Bruch's membrane with a choroidal vessel transversing (arrow) to form a sub-retinal pigment epithelium (RPE) vascular web (arrowhead). At one point (asterisk), sub-RPE neovascularization merges into a serious detachment of RPE. RPE is intact, but shows mild clumping. H and E, ×65. *B,* Higher power view of break in Bruch's membrane (between arrowheads) showing choroidal vessel through break (arrow). H and E, ×270. *C,* Inferior area of flat serous detachment (asterisk) of RPE (arrows), and cystic degeneration in outer plexiform layer of retina. H and E, ×65. *D,* Two-dimensional reconstruction map of macular area from study of serial sections, showing distribution of drusen, plus the size, shape, and location of sub-RPE neovascularization and its relation to the serous detachment of RPE and retina. EP 37432.

(From Small ML, Green WR, Alpar JJ, Dreury RE, Jr: Senile macular degeneration: A clinicopathologic correlation of two cases with neovascularization beneath the retinal pigment epithelium. Arch Ophthalmol *94*:601–607, 1976.)

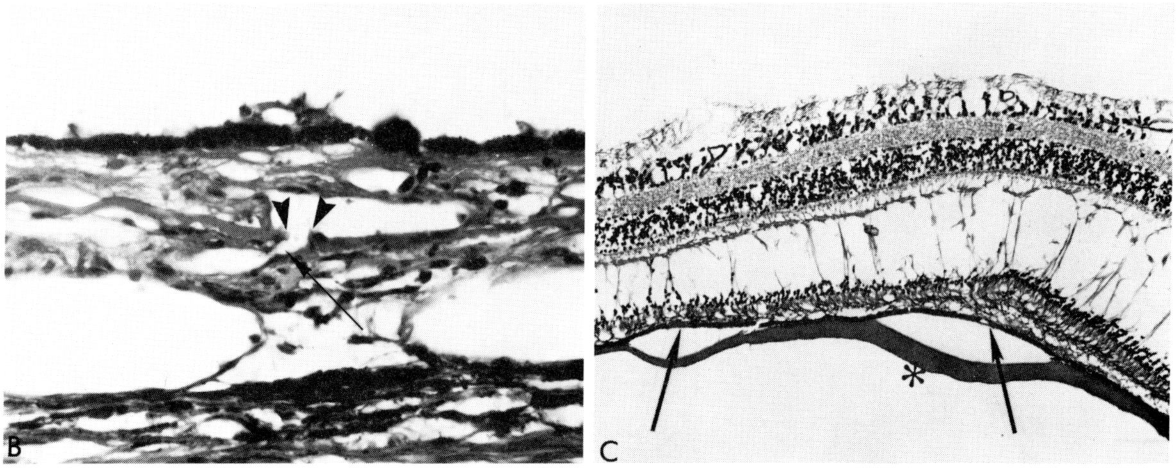

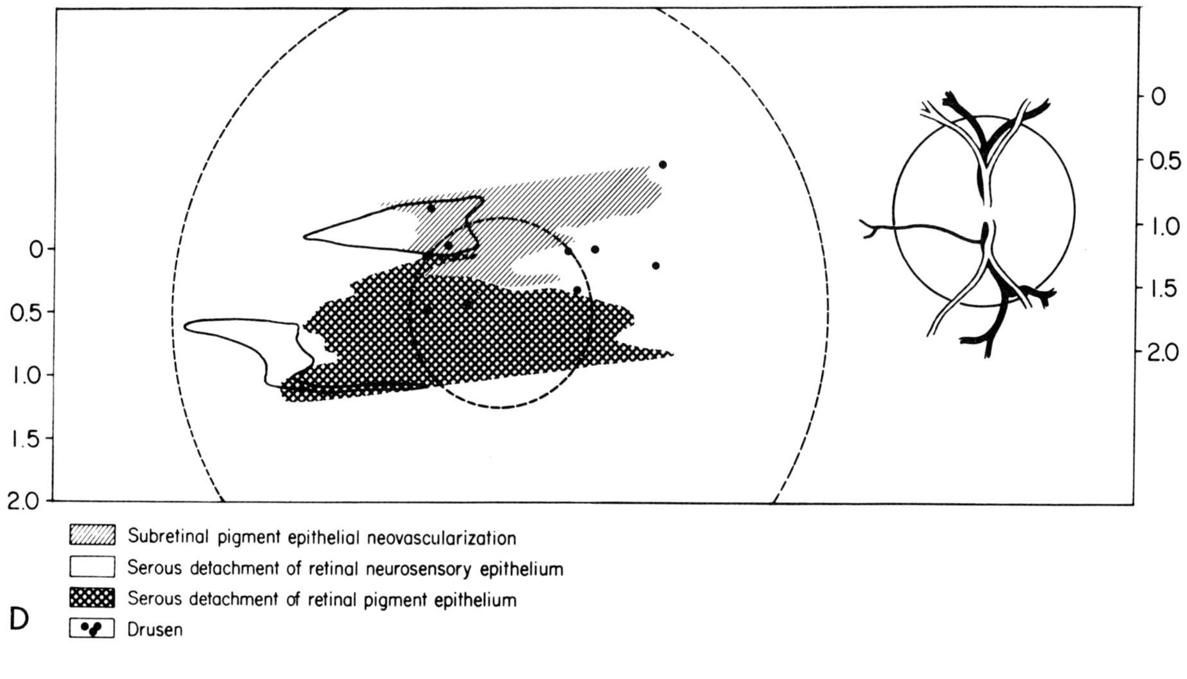

Subretinal pigment epithelial neovascularization
Serous detachment of retinal neurosensory epithelium
Serous detachment of retinal pigment epithelium
Drusen

D

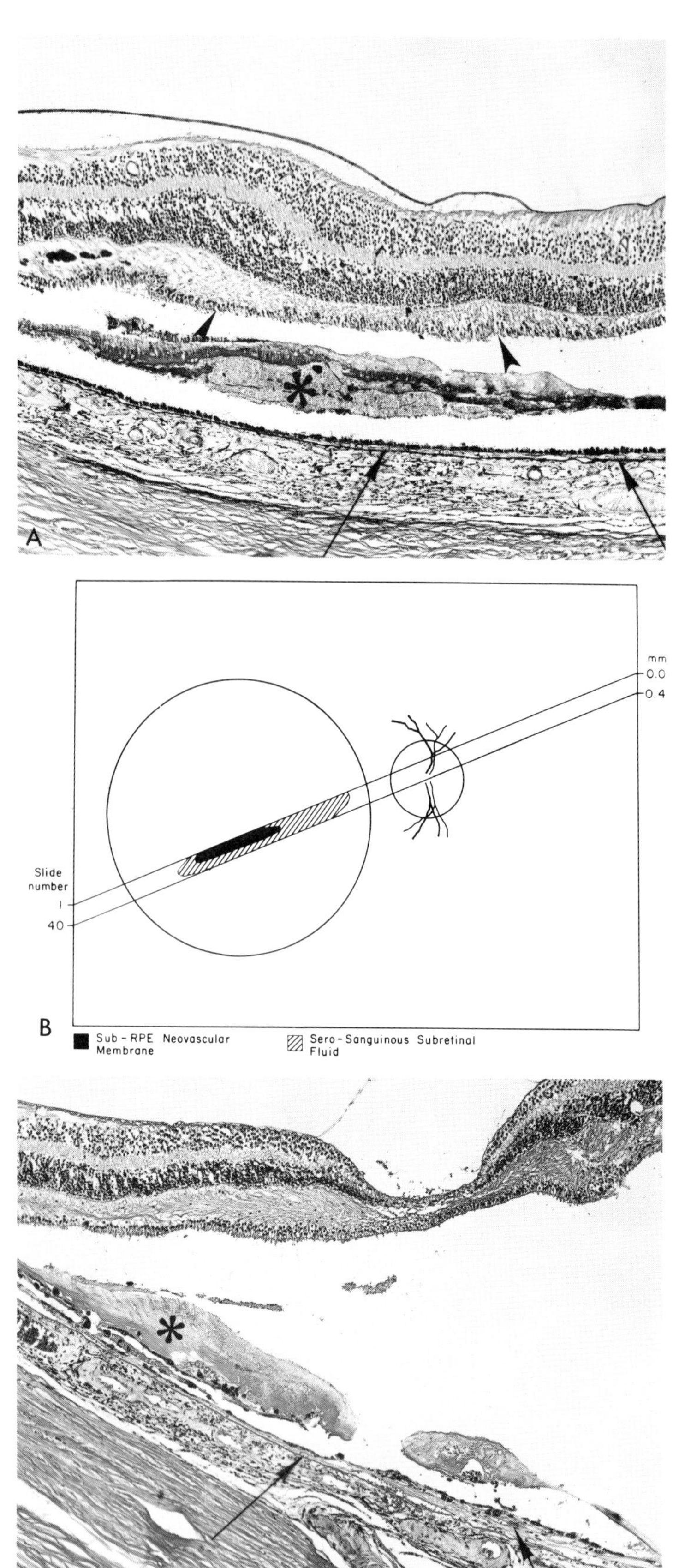

Figure 8–369. *A,* Macular area of right eye, showing extensive sub-retinal pigment epithelium (RPE) neovascularization (arrows) and a serosanguineous retinal detachment (asterisk). Some thinning of the photoreceptor cell layer is present (arrowheads). PAS, ×60. *B,* Two-dimensional reconstruction of macular lesion of right eye from study of serial sections, showing size and location of sub-RPE neovascular membrane and serosanguineous retinal detachment. *C,* Section through foveola of left eye, showing extensive sub-RPE neovascular membrane (arrows) and serosanguineous detachment of macula (asterisk). Thinning of outer nuclear layer is evident. PAS, ×60.

Illustration continued on opposite page

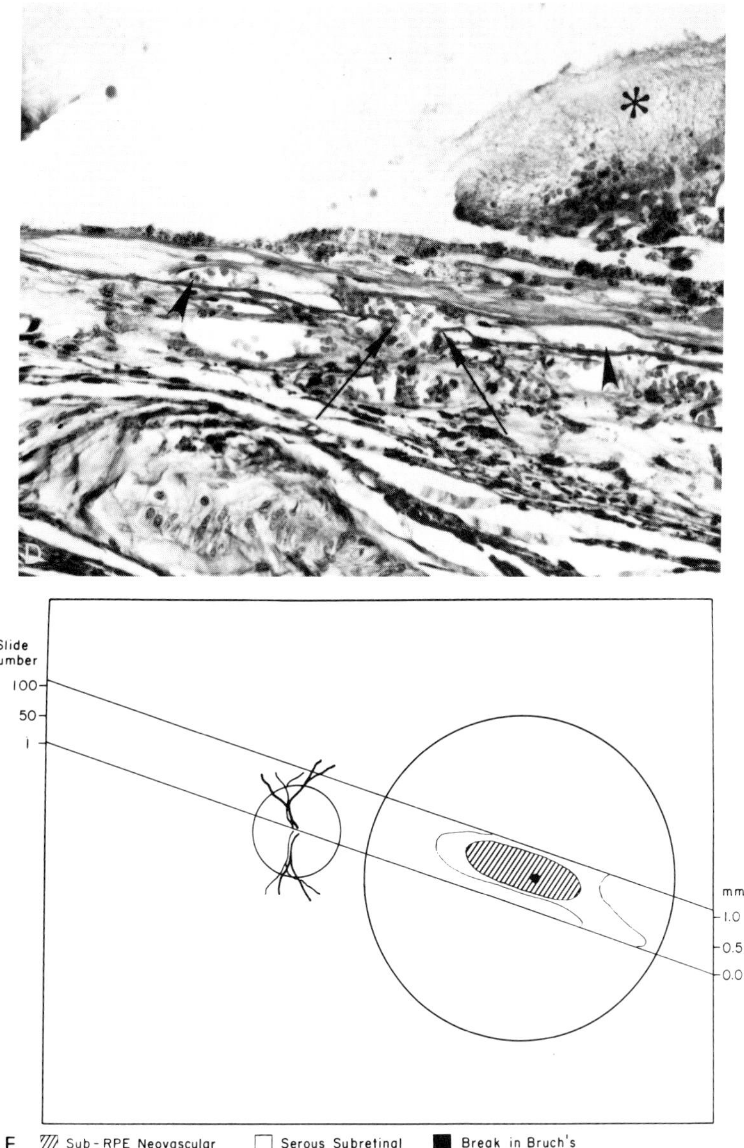

Figure 8–369 *Continued D,* Higher power view showing a single break in Bruch's membrane with traversing choroidal vessel (arrows), sub-RPE vascularization (arrowheads), and serosanguineous subretinal material (asterisk). PAS, ×240. *E,* Two-dimensional reconstruction of macular lesion of left eye, showing size and location of single break in Bruch's membrane, sub-RPE neovascularization, and serosanguineous retinal detachment. EP 38677.

(From Green WR, Key SN III: Senile macular degeneration: A histopathological study. Trans Am Ophthalmol Soc *75*:180–254, 1977.)

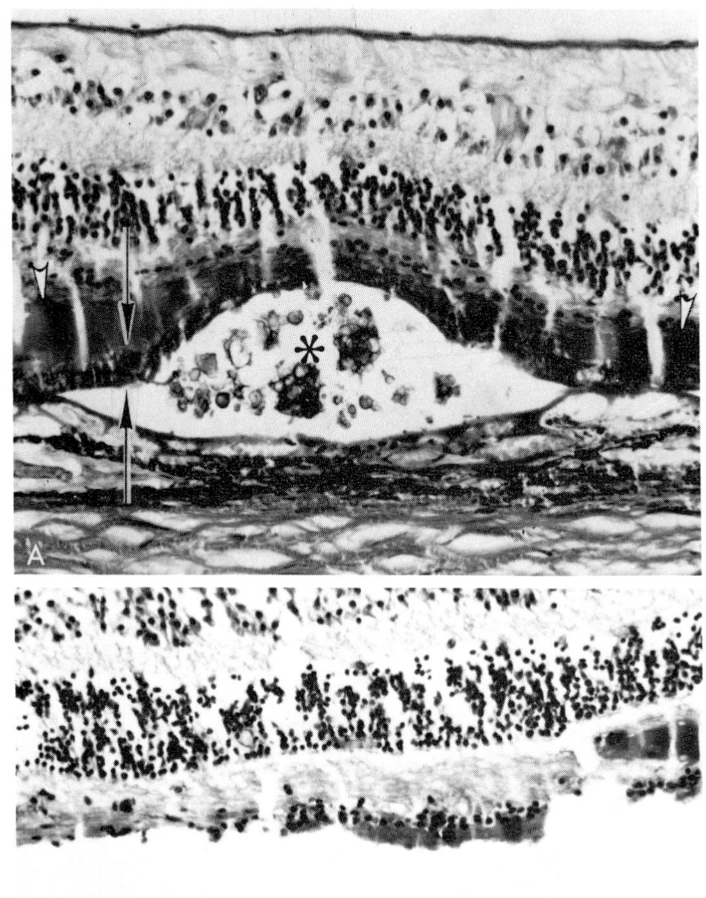

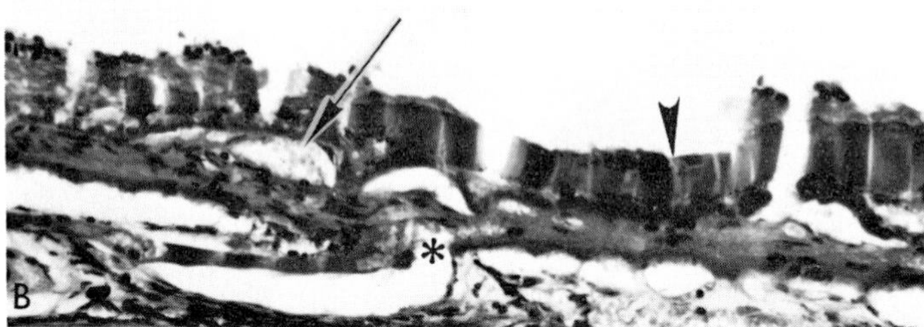

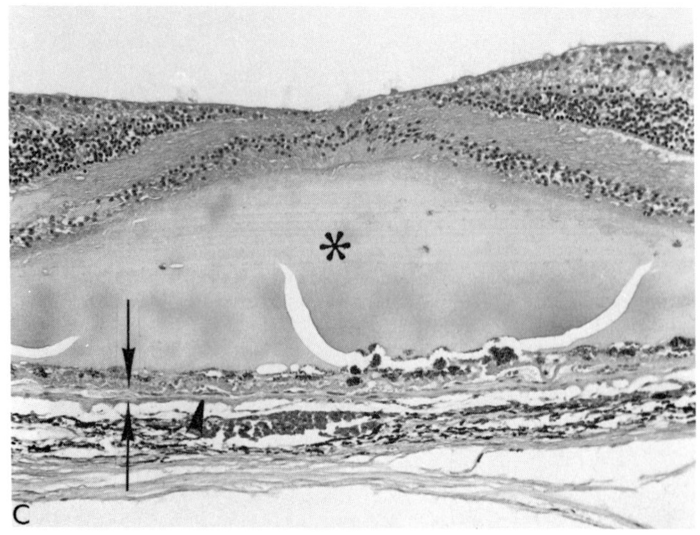

Figure 8–370. Left eye. *A,* Moderately large, partially calcified druse (asterisk) in macular area. Inner aspect of Bruch's membrane is much thickened (between arrows), and a small amount of proteinaceous material is present in subretinal space (arrowheads). PAS, ×100. *B,* Different level, showing a break in Bruch's membrane with traversing choroidal vessel (asterisk), serous fluid in subretinal space (arrowhead), and sub-RPE neovascularization (arrow). H and E, ×105. *C,* A dome-shaped, central serous retinopathy–like detachment was present in foveal area (asterisk). Inner aspect of Bruch's membrane is thickened (between arrows), and a few fine blood vessels (arrowheads) are located between two layers of Bruch's membrane. Retinal pigment epithelium is intact but shows some clumping and irregular pigmentation. H and E, ×85. EP 38585.

(From Green WR, Key SN III: Senile macular degeneration: A histopathological study. Trans Am Ophthalmol Soc *75*:180–254, 1977.)

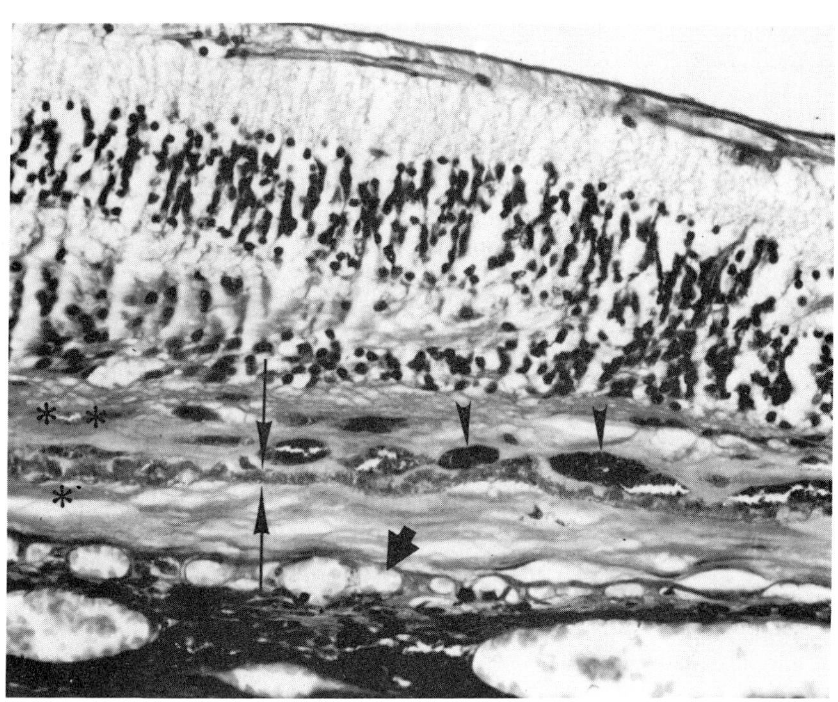

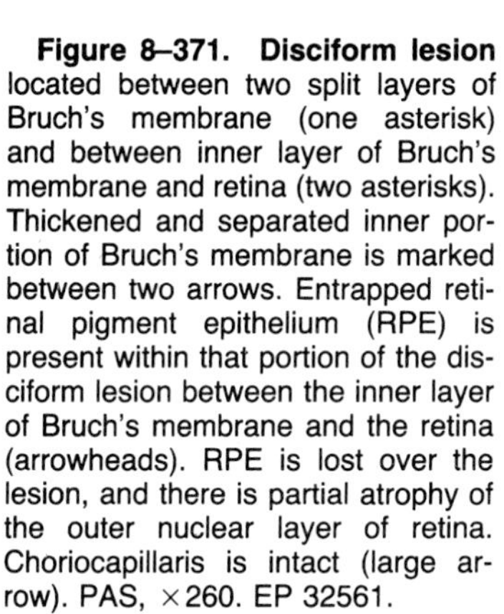

Figure 8–371. Disciform lesion located between two split layers of Bruch's membrane (one asterisk) and between inner layer of Bruch's membrane and retina (two asterisks). Thickened and separated inner portion of Bruch's membrane is marked between two arrows. Entrapped retinal pigment epithelium (RPE) is present within that portion of the disciform lesion between the inner layer of Bruch's membrane and the retina (arrowheads). RPE is lost over the lesion, and there is partial atrophy of the outer nuclear layer of retina. Choriocapillaris is intact (large arrow). PAS, ×260. EP 32561.

(From Green WR, Key SN III: Senile macular degeneration: A histopathological study. Trans Am Ophthalmol Soc *75*:180–254, 1977.)

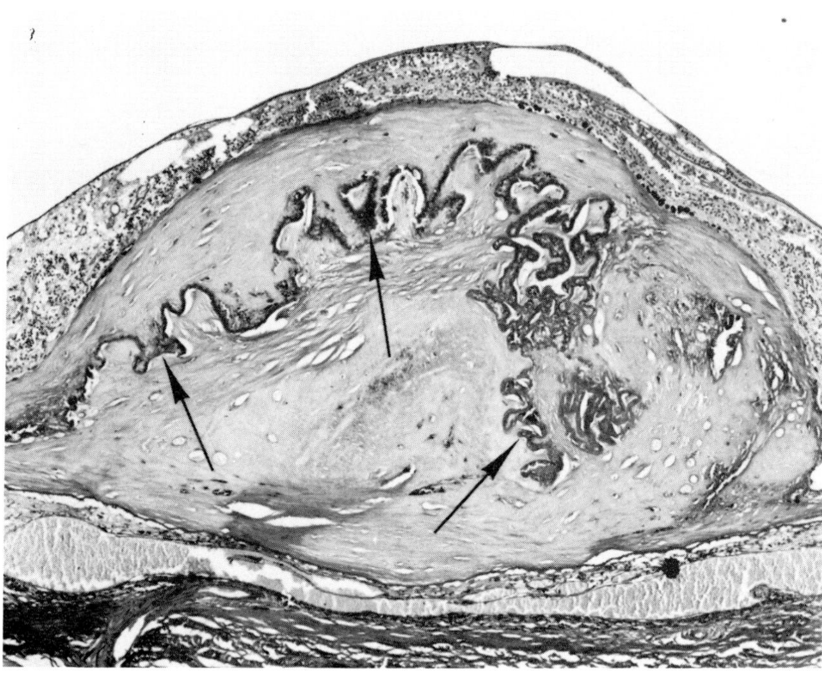

Figure 8–372. Very large **disciform lesion**, the larger portion of which is located between two layers of Bruch's membrane, and the smaller portion between the inner layer of Bruch's membrane and thin and degenerated retina. Inner layer of Bruch's membrane is much thickened and redundant (arrows). PAS, ×60. EP 33299. (From Green WR, Key SN III: Senile macular degeneration: A histopathological study. Trans Am Ophthalmol Soc *75*:180–254, 1977.)

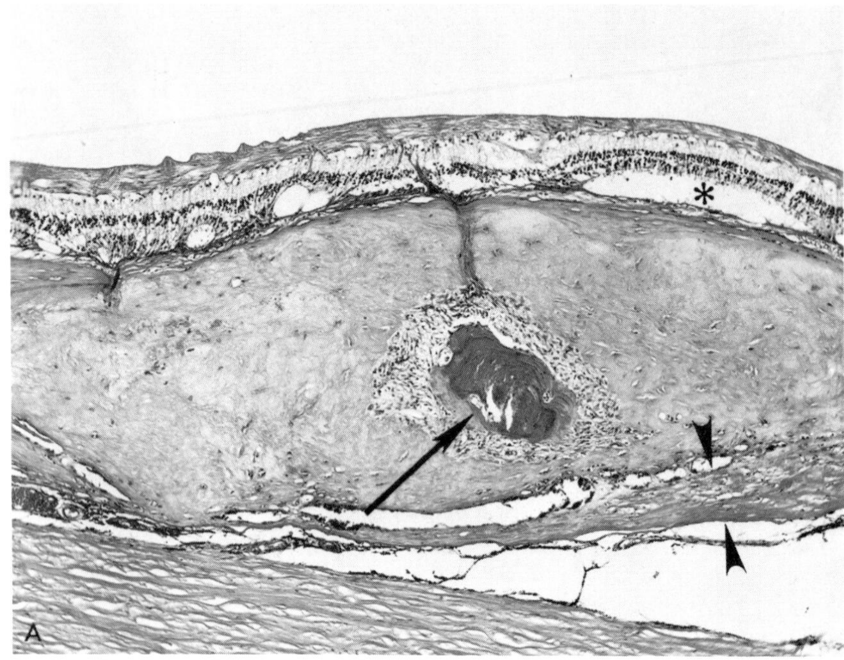

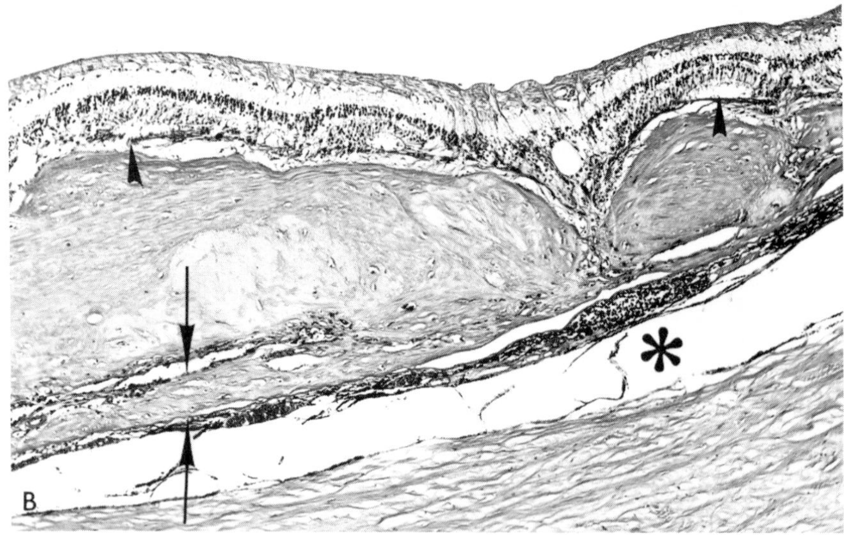

Figure 8–373. Right eye. *A*, Large, **disciform lesion** with a central area of bone formation (arrow). Only a small portion of disciform lesion is located between two split layers of Bruch's membrane (between arrowheads), and remainder is between the inner layer of Bruch's membrane and retina. It is amazing that the photoreceptor cell layer is relatively intact over some of the lesion (asterisk). H and E, ×65. *B*, Different level of disciform lesion, showing intra–Bruch's membrane component (between arrows). Prominent aggregate of lymphocytes is present in subjacent choroid (asterisk). Outer nuclear layer is intact in some areas over lesion (arrowheads). PAS, ×145. EP 40749.

(From Green WR, Key SN III: Senile macular degeneration: A histopathological study. Trans Am Ophthalmol Soc *75*:180–254, 1977.)

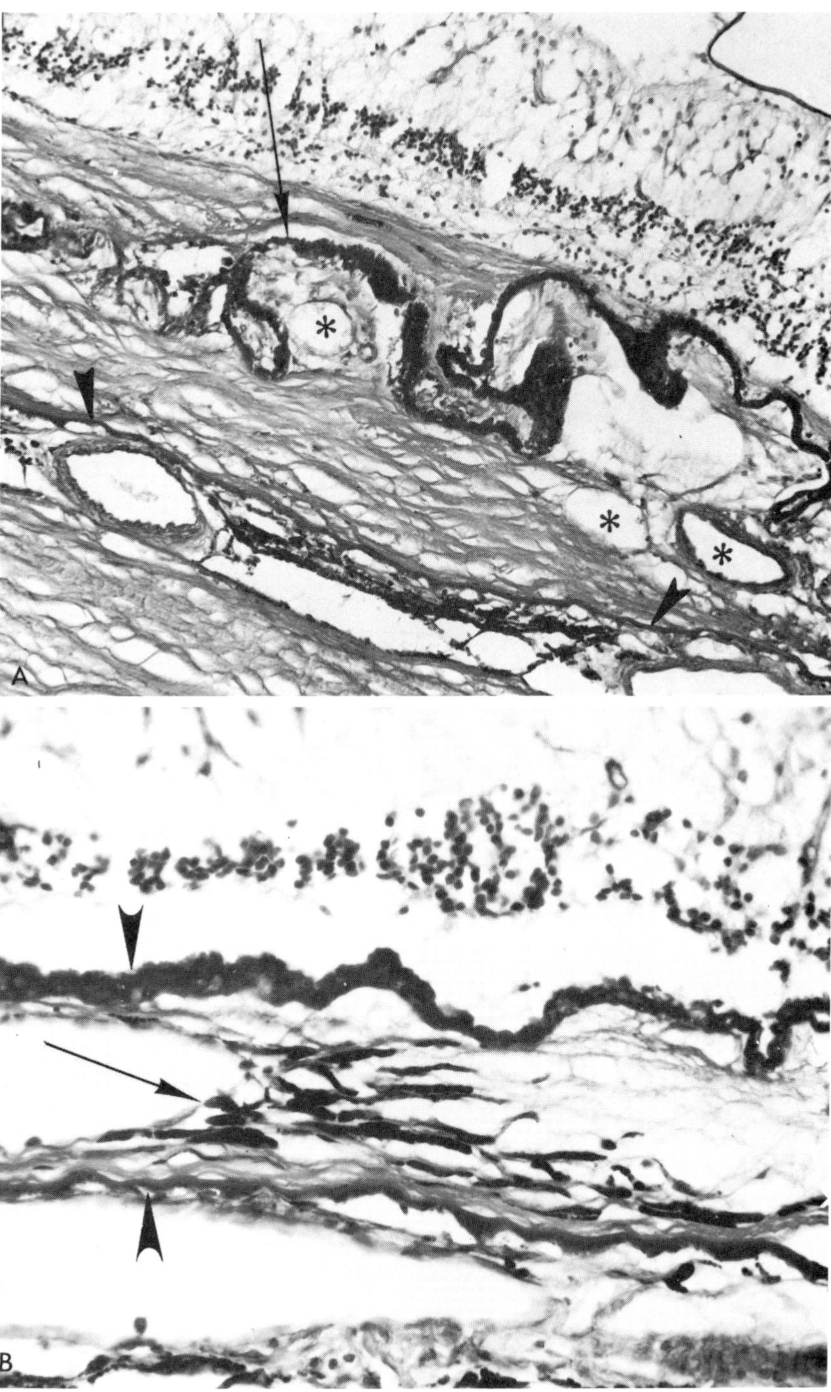

Figure 8–374. Left eye. *A,* **Disciform lesion** located between thickened and separated inner (arrow) and outer (arrowheads) layers of Bruch's membrane. A small portion is located between the inner layer of Bruch's membrane and retina. Retinal pigment epithelium and photoreceptor cell layer are absent. Choroidal neovascularization is present in intra–Bruch's membrane portion of disciform lesion (asterisks). PAS, × 145. *B,* Branching dendritic melanocytes (arrow), presumably from choroid, are located in disciform lesion between two layers of Bruch's membrane (arrowheads). PAS, ×305. EP 40749. (From Green WR, Key SN III: Senile macular degeneration: A histopathological study. Trans Am Ophthalmol Soc *75*:180–254, 1977.)

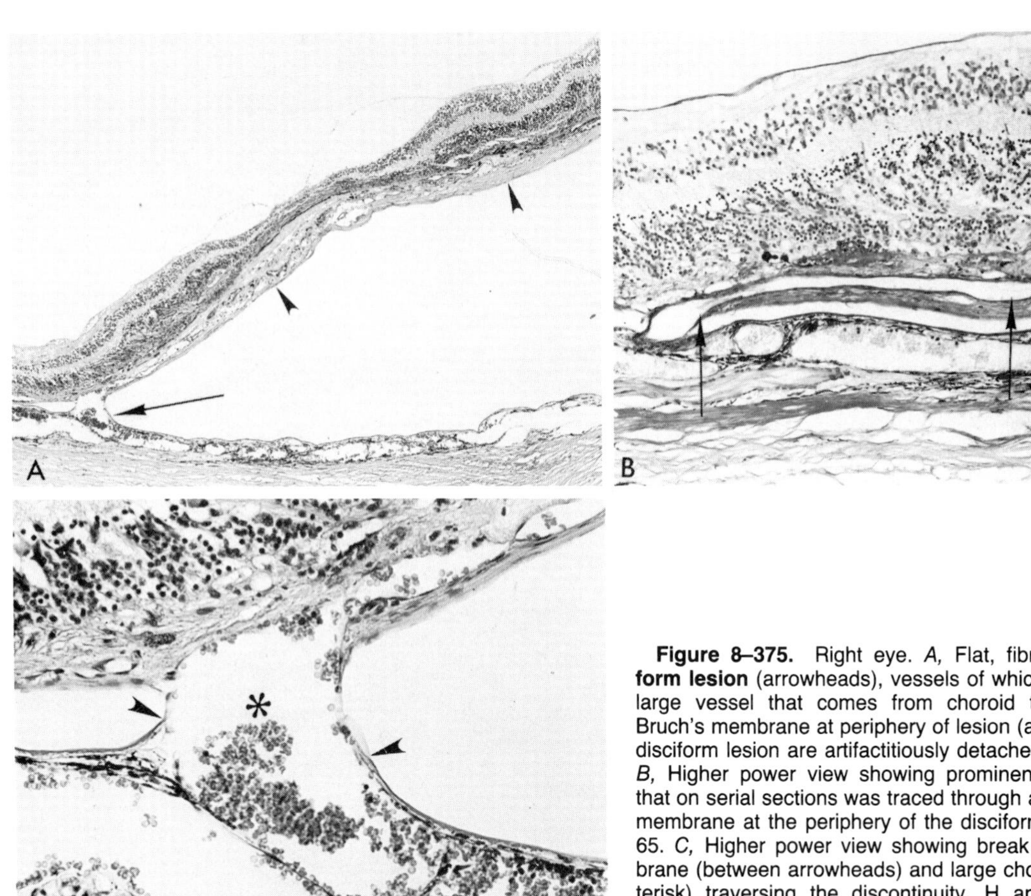

Figure 8–375. Right eye. *A,* Flat, fibrovascular, **disciform lesion** (arrowheads), vessels of which are supplied by large vessel that comes from choroid through break in Bruch's membrane at periphery of lesion (arrow). Retina and disciform lesion are artifactitiously detached. H and E, ×25. *B,* Higher power view showing prominent vessel (arrows) that on serial sections was traced through a break in Bruch's membrane at the periphery of the disciform lesion. PAS, × 65. *C,* Higher power view showing break in Bruch's membrane (between arrowheads) and large choroidal vessel (asterisk) traversing the discontinuity. H and E, ×125. EP 38421. (From Green WR, Key SN III: Senile macular degeneration: A histopathological study. Trans Am Ophthalmol Soc *75*:180–254, 1977.)

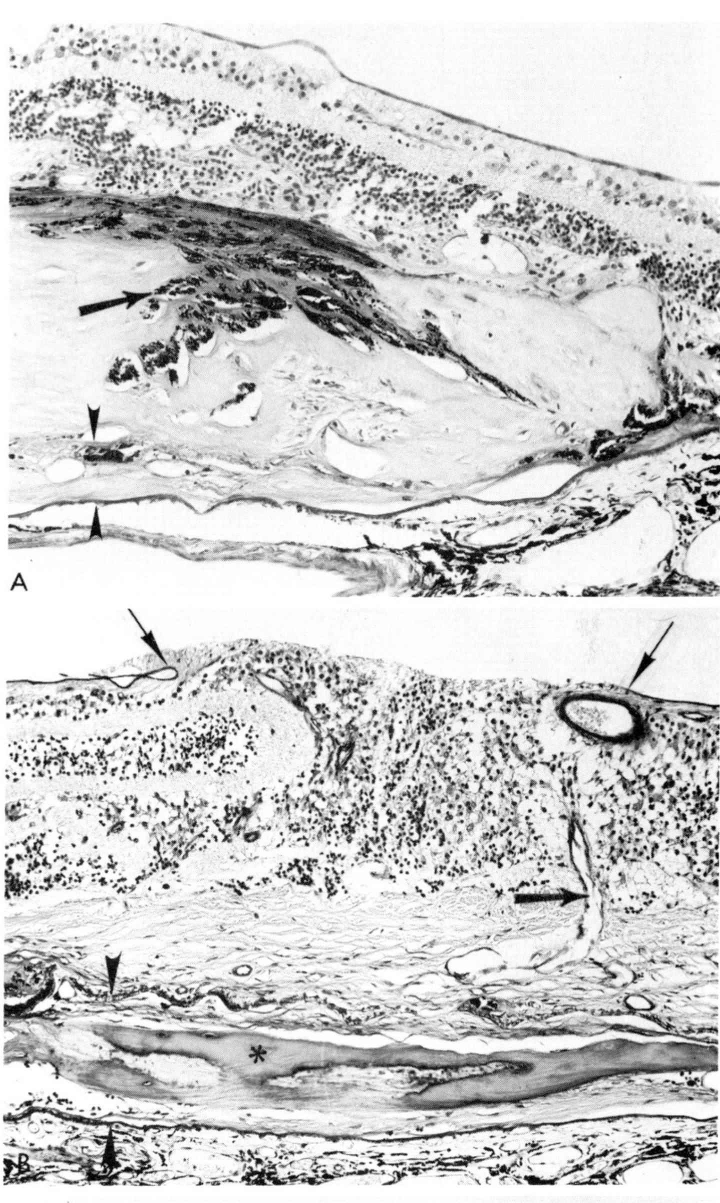

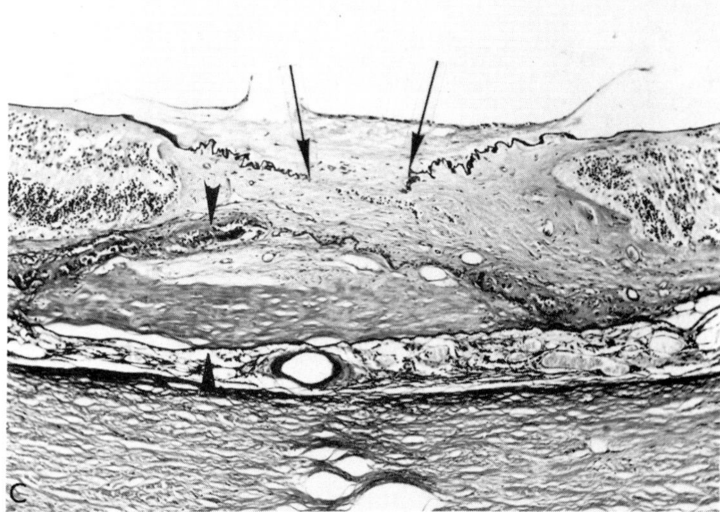

Figure 8–376. Left eye. *A,* **Disciform lesion** located between two layers of Bruch's membrane (arrowheads) and between inner layer of Bruch's membrane and retina. The latter area has a prominent area of retinal pigment epithelium hyperplasia (arrow). PAS, ×75. *B,* Different level, showing bone formation (asterisk) in that portion of the disciform lesion located between two layers of Bruch's membrane (arrowheads), retinal vascular supply to subretinal disciform lesion (large arrow), and a discontinuity in internal limiting membrane (ILM) of retina (between small arrows). PAS, ×55. *C,* A third level, showing disciform lesion between two layers of Bruch's membrane (arrowheads), internal to the inner layer of Bruch's membrane and extending through a break in the ILM (arrows) to be continuous with a fibrous nodule on the inner surface of the retina. PAS, ×30. EP 38421. (From Green WR, Key SN III: Senile macular degeneration: A histopathological study. Trans Am Ophthalmol Soc *75*:180–254, 1977.)

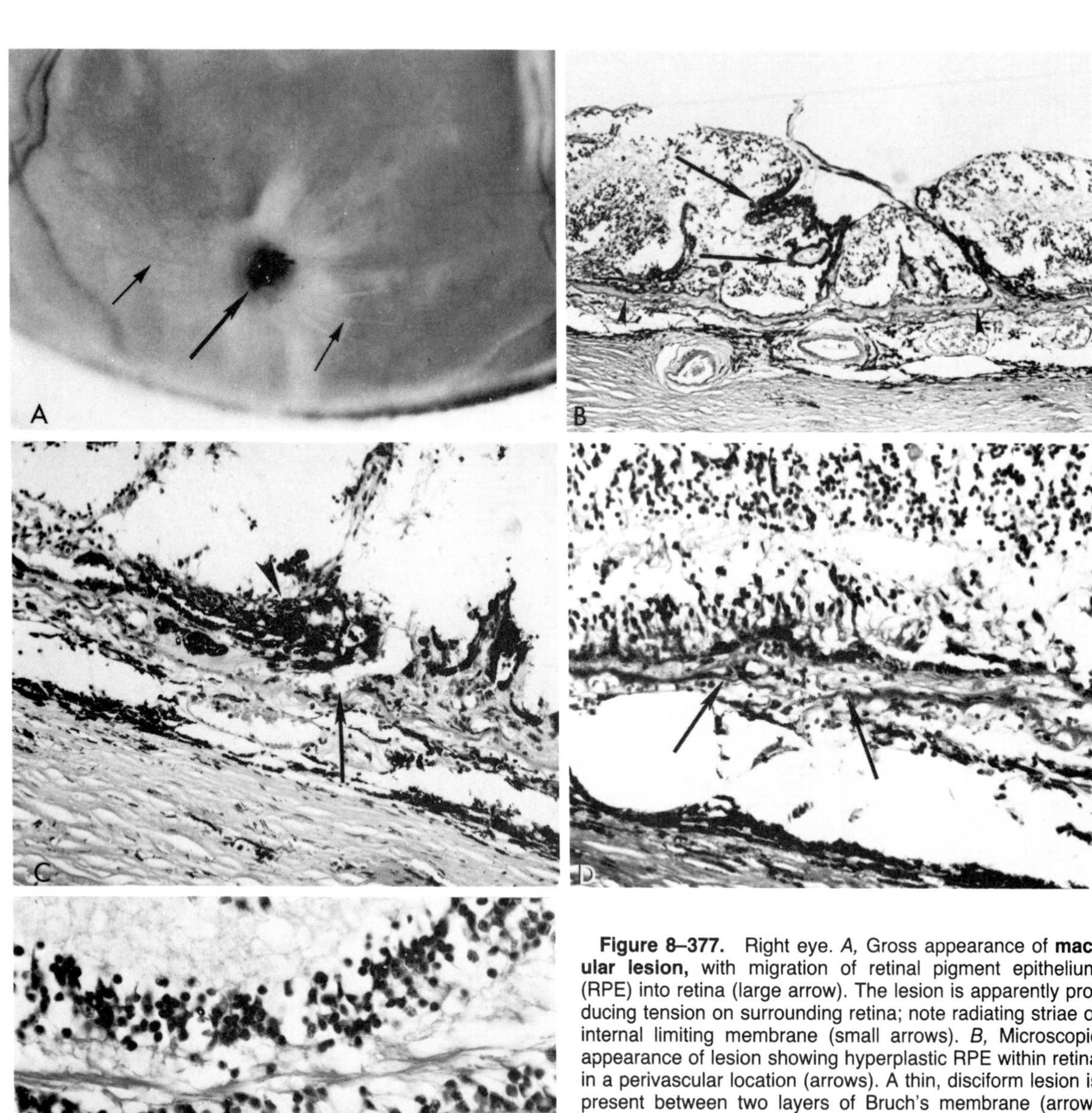

Figure 8–377. Right eye. *A,* Gross appearance of **macular lesion,** with migration of retinal pigment epithelium (RPE) into retina (large arrow). The lesion is apparently producing tension on surrounding retina; note radiating striae of internal limiting membrane (small arrows). *B,* Microscopic appearance of lesion showing hyperplastic RPE within retina in a perivascular location (arrows). A thin, disciform lesion is present between two layers of Bruch's membrane (arrowheads). Several retinal vessels extend down to the disciform lesion. *C,* Break in Bruch's membrane (arrow) through which a choroidal vessel traversed and could be traced in serial sections to anastomose with a retinal vessel. Nodule of hyperplastic RPE is present (arrowhead). H and E, ×100.

D, Sub-RPE neovascularization extends beyond central area. Additional break in Bruch's membrane (between arrows) through which a choroidal vessel extended into the sub-RPE area. Masson trichrome, ×145. *E,* Outside the neovascular area, the inner aspect of Bruch's membrane is much thickened (between arrows), and the overlying RPE and outer nuclear layer are intact. Occasional thicker, drusen-like nodules are present (arrowhead). H and E, ×475. EP 38230. (From Green WR, Key SN III: Senile macular degeneration: A histopathological study. Trans Am Ophthalmol Soc *75*:180–254, 1977.)

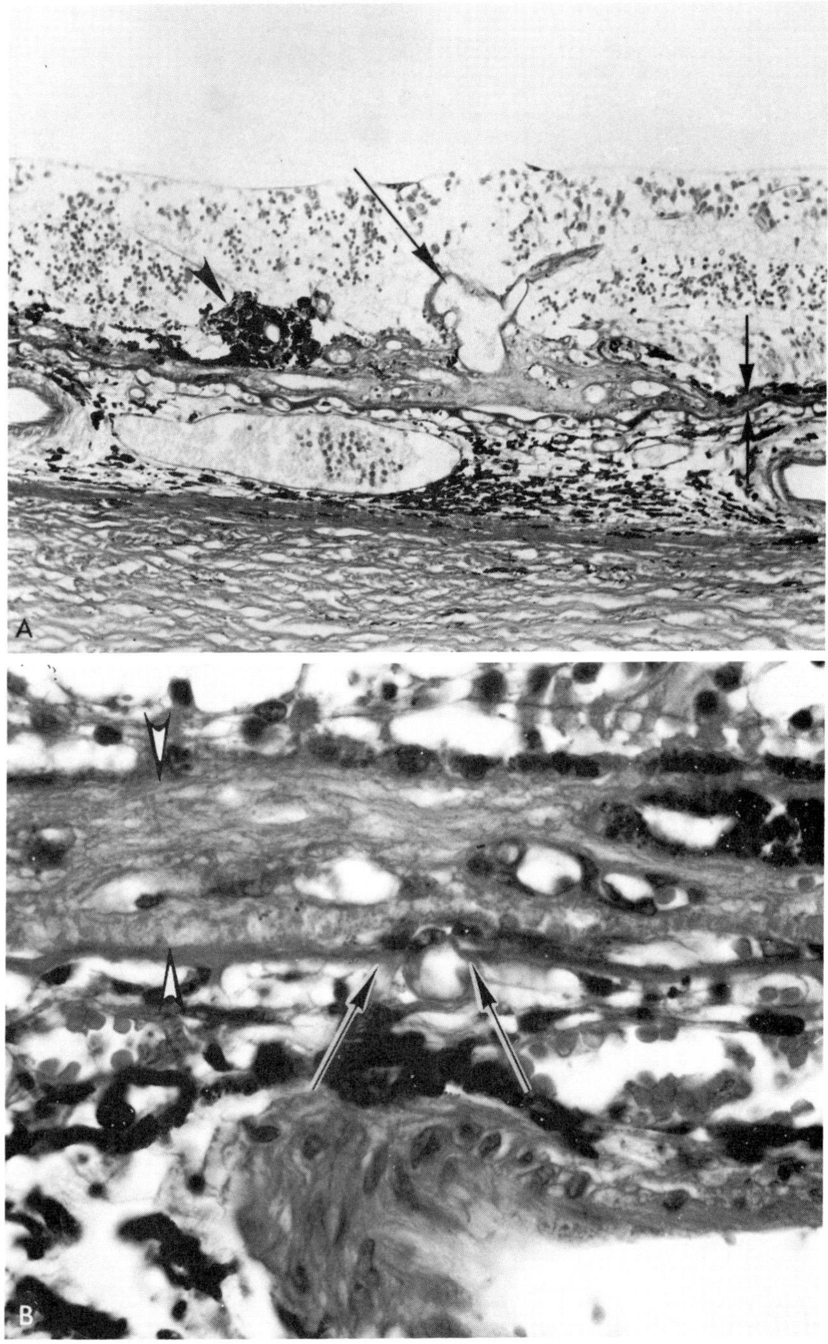

Figure 8–378. Left eye. *A,* Flat **disciform lesion** with prominent retinal vascular contribution (large arrow), nodules of hyperplastic retinal pigment epithelium (RPE) (arrowhead), and much thickening of inner aspect of Bruch's membrane (small arrows). H and E, ×475. *B,* Area of disciform lesion (arrowheads) located between Bruch's membrane and partially atrophic RPE (arrowheads). A small break in Bruch's membrane (arrows), with a choroidal vessel traversing, is present. H and E, ×600. EP 38230. (From Green WR, Key SN III: Senile macular degeneration: A histopathological study. Trans Am Ophthalmol Soc *75*:180–254, 1977.)

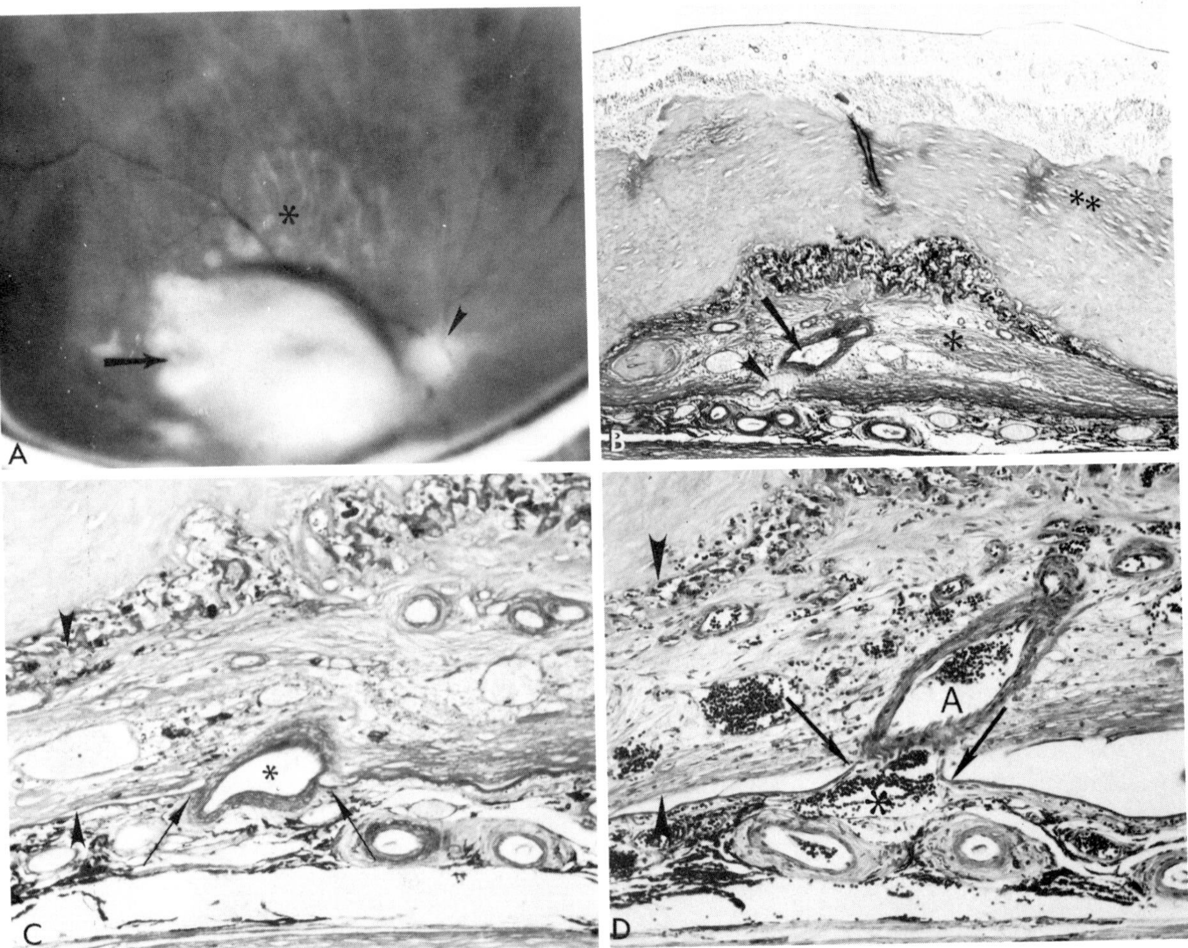

Figure 8–379. Long-standing **disciform macular scar** with choroidal vessels that have characteristics of an artery and vein. *A,* Gross appearance of disciform lesion (arrow) in macular area. Arrowhead marks optic disc. Areolar retinal pigment epithelium atrophy (asterisk) is present. *B,* Disciform macular scar with two components. One is vascularized and located between two layers of Bruch's membrane (one asterisk); the other (two asterisks) is nonvascularized and located between neurosensory retina and detached thickened inner layer of Bruch's membrane. Intra–Bruch's membrane component is highly vascularized and has a large artery (arrow) and vein (arrowhead) that were traced in serial sections and found to originate in choroid. PAS, ×60.

C, Level showing larger choroidal artery (asterisk) traversing a break in Bruch's membrane (between arrows) and extending into vascularized intra–Bruch's membrane component (between arrowheads) of disciform scar. PAS, ×145. *D,* Different level, where a choroidal vein (asterisk) extends through a break in Bruch's membrane (between arrows) and into vascularized intra–Bruch's membrane component of disciform scar (between arrowheads). *A,* artery. Van de Grift, ×150. EP 42880.

(From Green WR, Key SN III: Senile macular degeneration: A histopathological study. Trans Am Ophthalmol Soc *75*:180–254, 1977.)

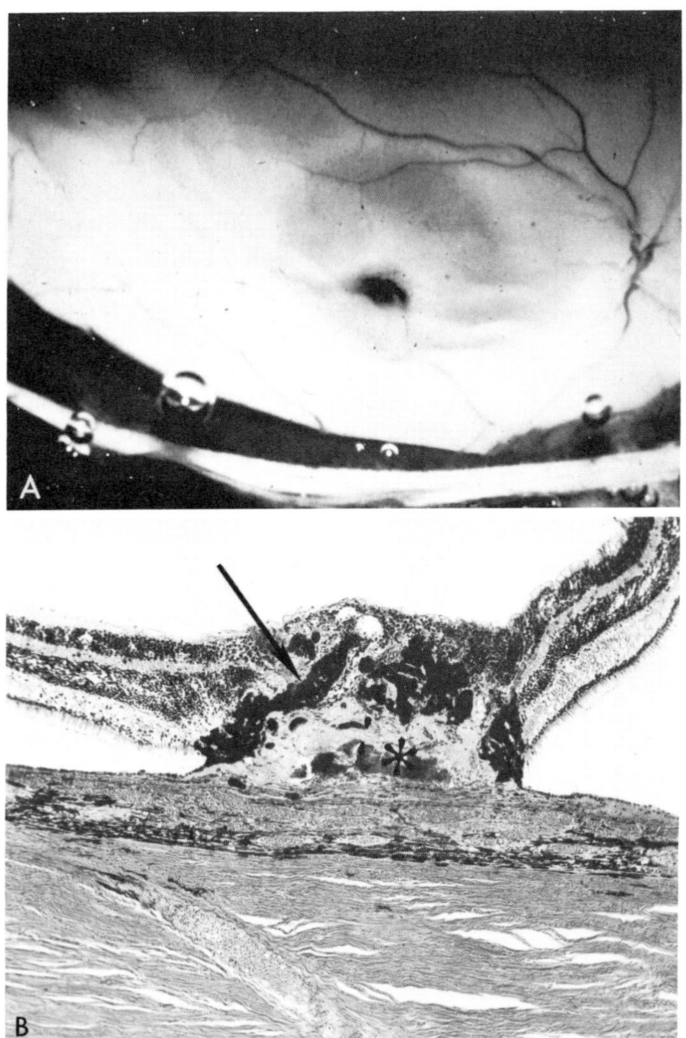

Figure 8–380. *A,* Gross appearance of a **disciform macular scar** with marked retinal pigment epithelium (RPE) hyperplasia that was confused with malignant melanoma. *B,* Section shows a vascularized and partially calcified component (asterisk) and an inner component of RPE hyperplasia (arrow). H and E, × 80. AFIP Neg. 57-14318. (From Ferry AP: Lesions mistaken for malignant melanoma of posterior uvea: A clinicopathologic analysis of 100 cases with ophthalmoscopically visible lesions. Arch Ophthalmol *72*:463–469, 1964.)

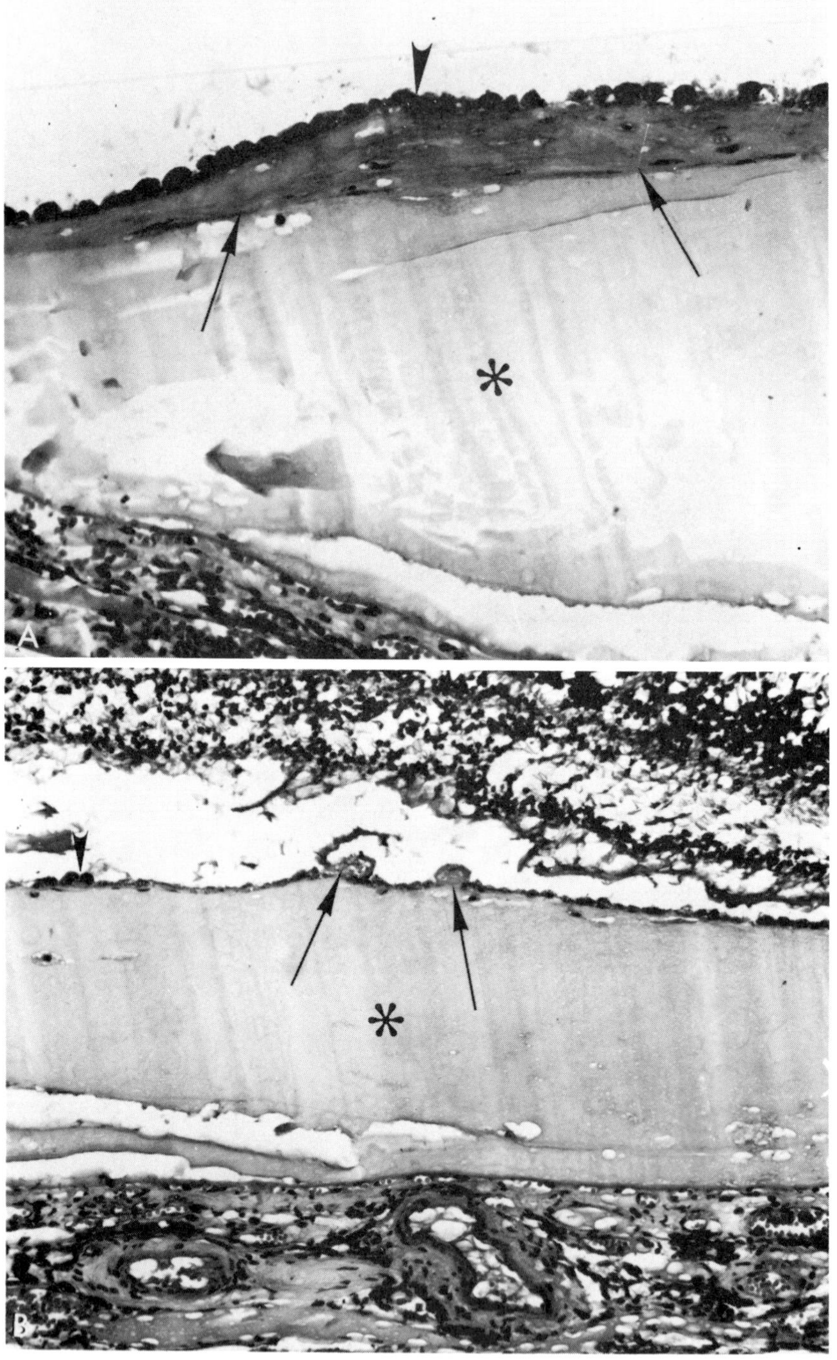

Figure 8–381. *A,* Small, flat **disciform lesion** (arrows) is detached along with retinal pigment epithelium (RPE) (arrowhead) and drusen by proteinaceous material (asterisk). H and E, ×115. *B,* Different area, showing drusen (arrows) detached along with RPE (arrowhead) by proteinaceous material (asterisk). PAS, ×75.

Illustration continued on opposite page

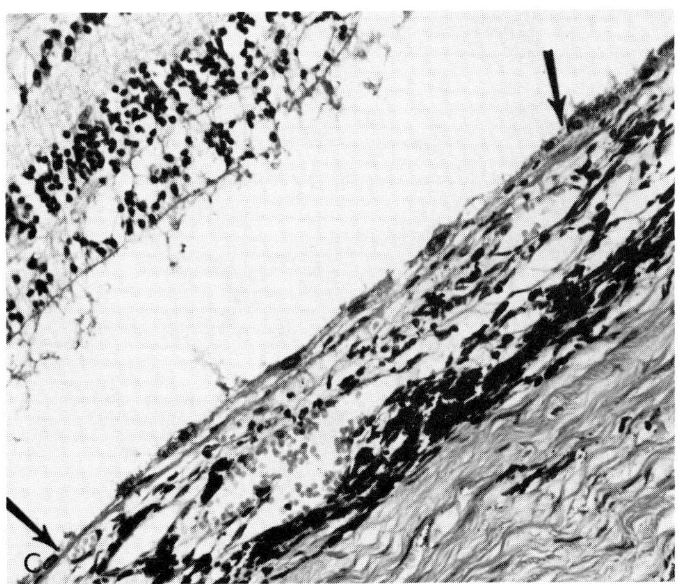

Figure 8–381. *Continued C,* Outside the area of detachment was a localized area of RPE window defect (arrows). Here epithelium is intact, but has fewer and larger nuclei than normal and has lost most or all of its pigment granules. H and E, ×120. EP 37386.

(From Green WR, Key SN III: Senile macular degeneration: A histopathological study. Trans Am Ophthalmol Soc *75*:180–254, 1977.)

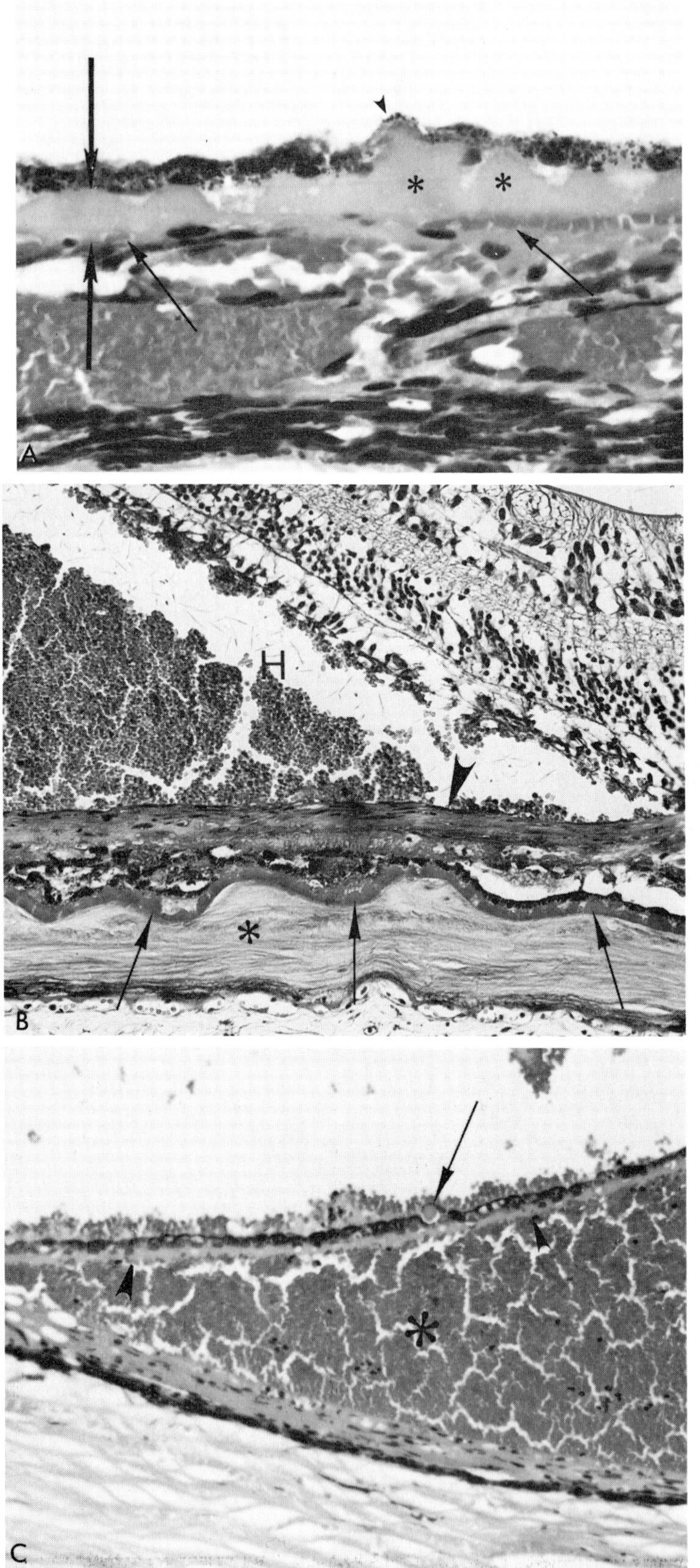

Figure 8–382. *A,* Diffuse thickening of inner aspect of Bruch's membrane (between larger arrows), with areas of nodular excrescences (asterisks) of diffuse and localized drusen. Retinal pigment epithelium (RPE) is effaced over nodular drusen (arrowhead). Choriocapillaris is intact (small arrows). H and E, ×345. *B,* Fibrous disciform lesion with a portion located between two split layers of Bruch's membrane (asterisk) and between the inner layer of Bruch's membrane and the retina (arrowhead). Hemmorrhage *(H)* is present beneath retina. There are diffuse nodular drusen (arrows) throughout the separated inner portion of Bruch's membrane. Verhoeff van Giesen, ×130. *C,* Hemorrhagic detachment (asterisk) of thickened, inner portion of Bruch's membrane (arrowheads), drusen (arrow), and RPE. H and E, ×105. EP 41158.

(From Green WR, Key SN III: Senile macular degeneration: A histopathological study. Trans Am Ophthalmol Soc *75*:180–254, 1977.)

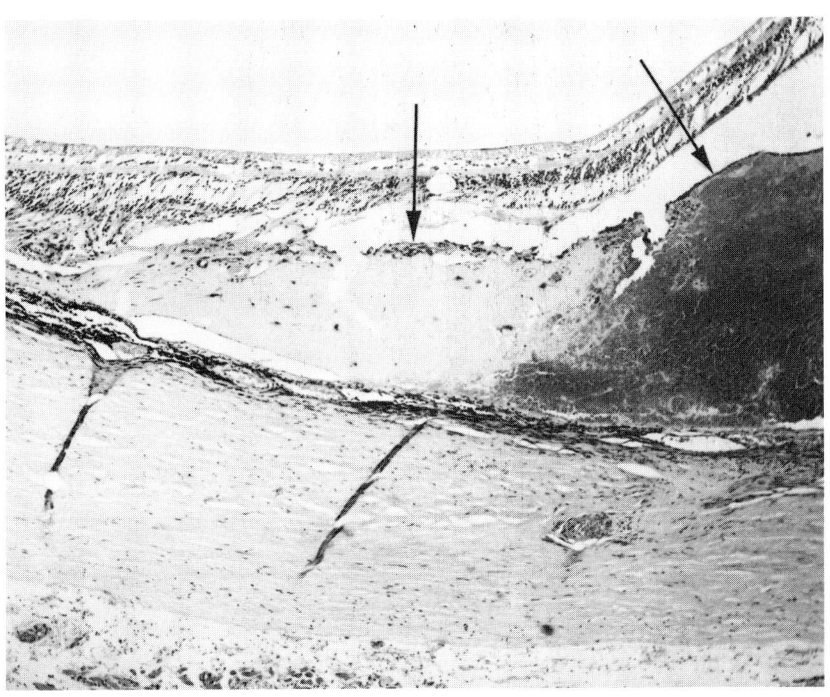

Figure 8–383. Serosanguineous detachment of retinal pigment epithelium (arrows) adjacent to a disciform macular scar. As RPE detachment increased in size, it was thought clinically to be a malignant melanoma. AFIP Acc. 1224270. (From Berkow JW, Font RL: Disciform macular degeneration with subpigment epithelial hematoma. Arch Ophthalmol *82*:51–56, 1969.)

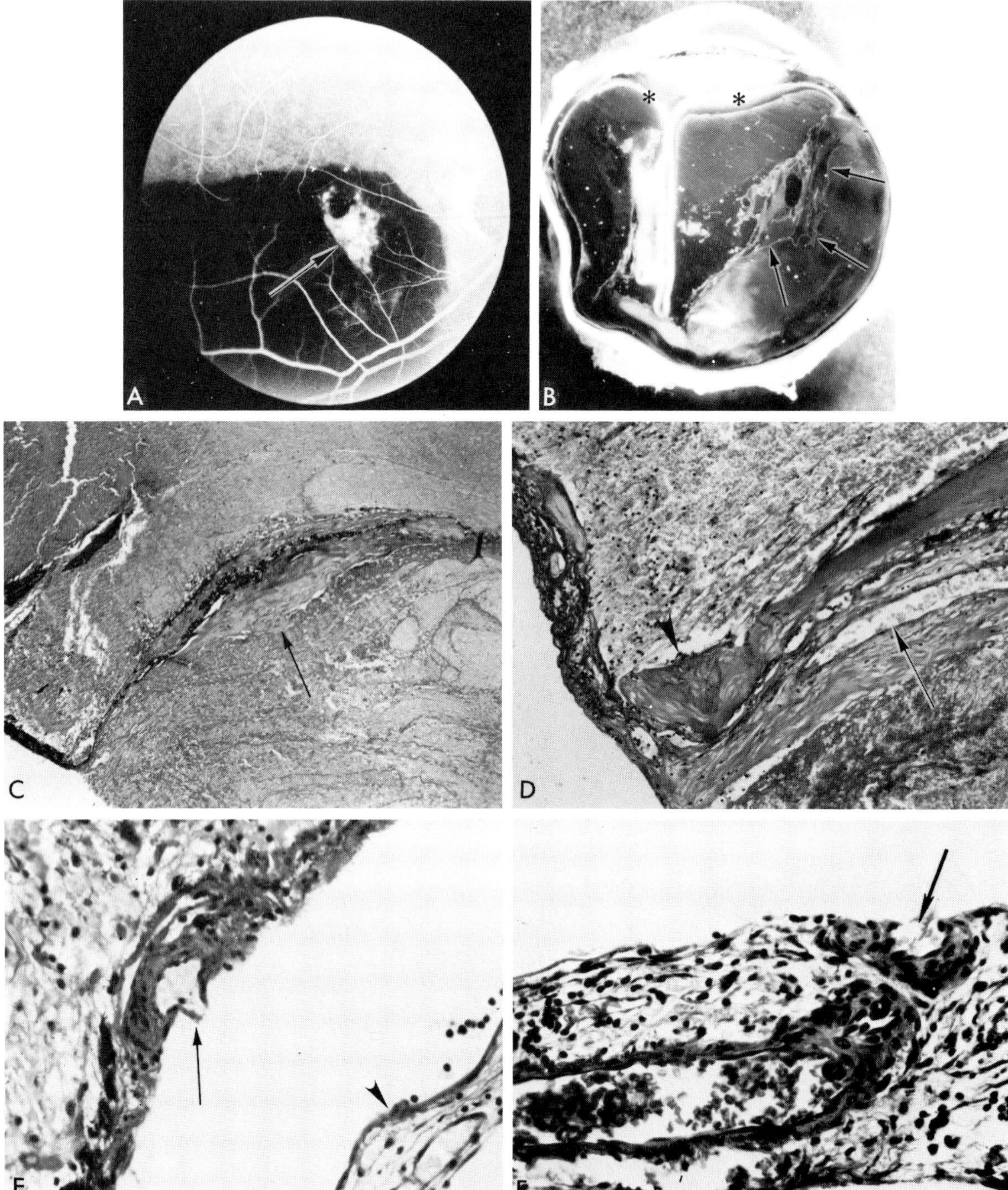

Figure 8–384. Massive **hemorrhagic detachment of disciform scar, retinal pigment epithelium (RPE) and retina** in a patient on warfarin sodium (Coumadin) therapy. *A,* Late fluorescein staining (arrow) of disciform scar (arrow) with surrounding hemorrhagic detachment of retina. Later, retina became totally detached and eye was enucleated. *B,* Gross appearance of eye with superior cap removed. Retina (asterisks) is totally detached. Vague outline of hemorrhagically detached RPE is evident (arrows). *C,* Low-power view of hemorrhagic detachment of disciform scar (arrow) and RPE. PAS, ×100.

D, Nasal margin of hemorrhagically detached disciform scar (arrowhead) with prominent artery-like vessel (arrow). Vessel was traced in serial sections and found to be disrupted at another level (see *E*). Van de Grift, ×175. *E,* Disrupted artery (arrow) at nasal margin of detached disciform scar. Bruch's membrane, arrowhead. Van de Grift, ×220. *F,* Area of choroid that corresponds to area shown in *E*. There is a discontinuity in Bruch's membrane where a choroidal artery is disrupted (arrow), the presumed site of arterial bleeding. Van de Grift, ×250.

Illustration continued on opposite page

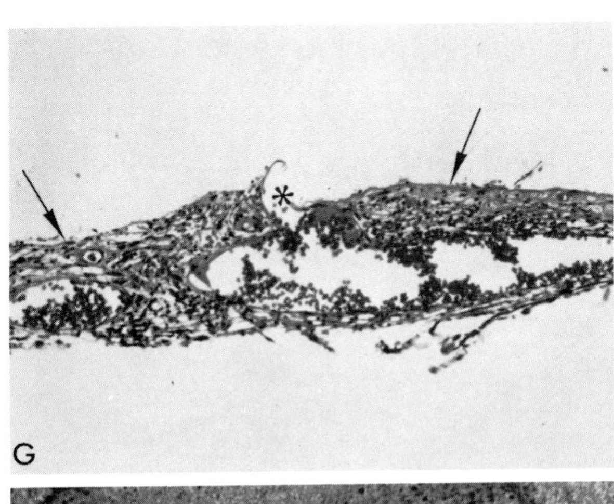

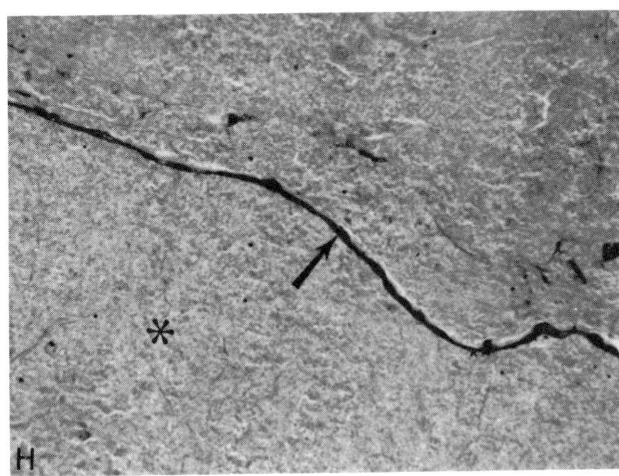

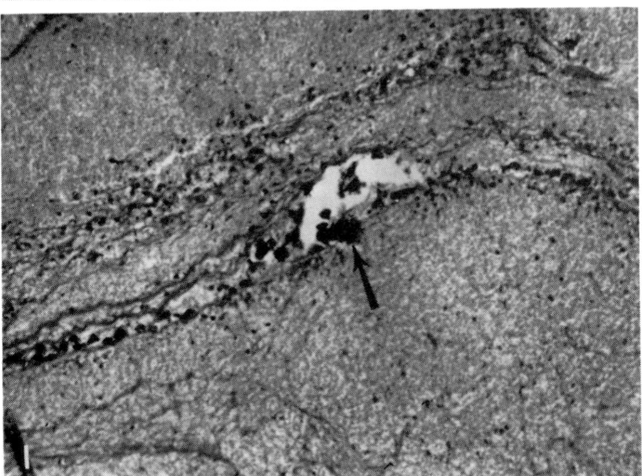

Figure 8–384. *Continued G,* A second disruption of Bruch's membrane (between arrows), with a torn choroidal vein (asterisk) traversing, is present at a different level. Van de Grift, ×220. *H,* Midperipheral area showing detached RPE (arrow). Blood is present in sub-RPE (asterisk) and subretinal spaces. Van de Grift, ×110. *I,* More posteriorly, RPE is degenerated but a tract of RPE can be noted by the presence of drusen (arrow). Van de Grift, ×130. EP 46577. (Case contributed by Dr. William H. Jarrett, II.)

(From Green WR: Clinicopathologic studies of senile macular degeneration, *in* Nicholson DH (ed): Ocular Pathology Update. New York, Masson, 1980, p 137.)

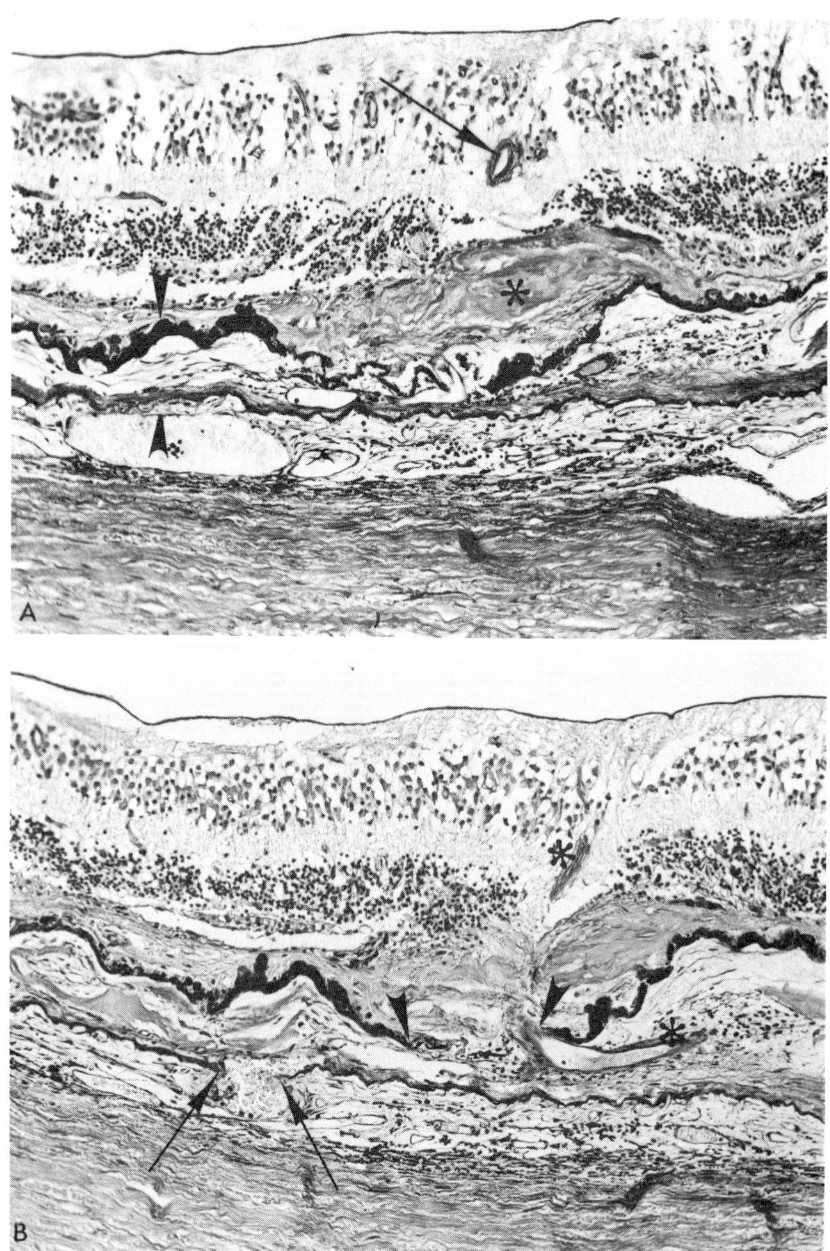

Figure 8–385. Bilateral **disciform macular degeneration** showing retinal arterialization. *A,* Right eye showing two components of disciform scar. A fibrous portion (asterisk) is located between sensory retina and detached and thickened inner portion of Bruch's membrane. A retinal artery (arrow) was traced in serial sections to extend through the inner fibrous component of scar, through a break in separated inner layer of Bruch's membrane, and into the intra–Bruch's membrane portion of scar where it anastomosed with vessels from choroid. PAS, ×115. AFIP Neg. 66-9651.

B, Different level in right eye, showing retinal artery (asterisks) dipping down and extending through break in inner layer of Bruch's membrane (between arrowheads) and into intra–Bruch's membrane component of scar, where it anastomosed with a choroidal vessel that is traversing a break in the outer layer of Bruch's membrane (between arrows). PAS, ×110. AFIP Neg. 66-9657.

AFIP Acc. 1194649. (From Green WR, Gass JDM: Senile disciform degeneration of the macula: Retinal arterialization of fibrous plaque demonstrated clinically and histopathologically. Arch Ophthalmol *86*:487–484, 1971.)

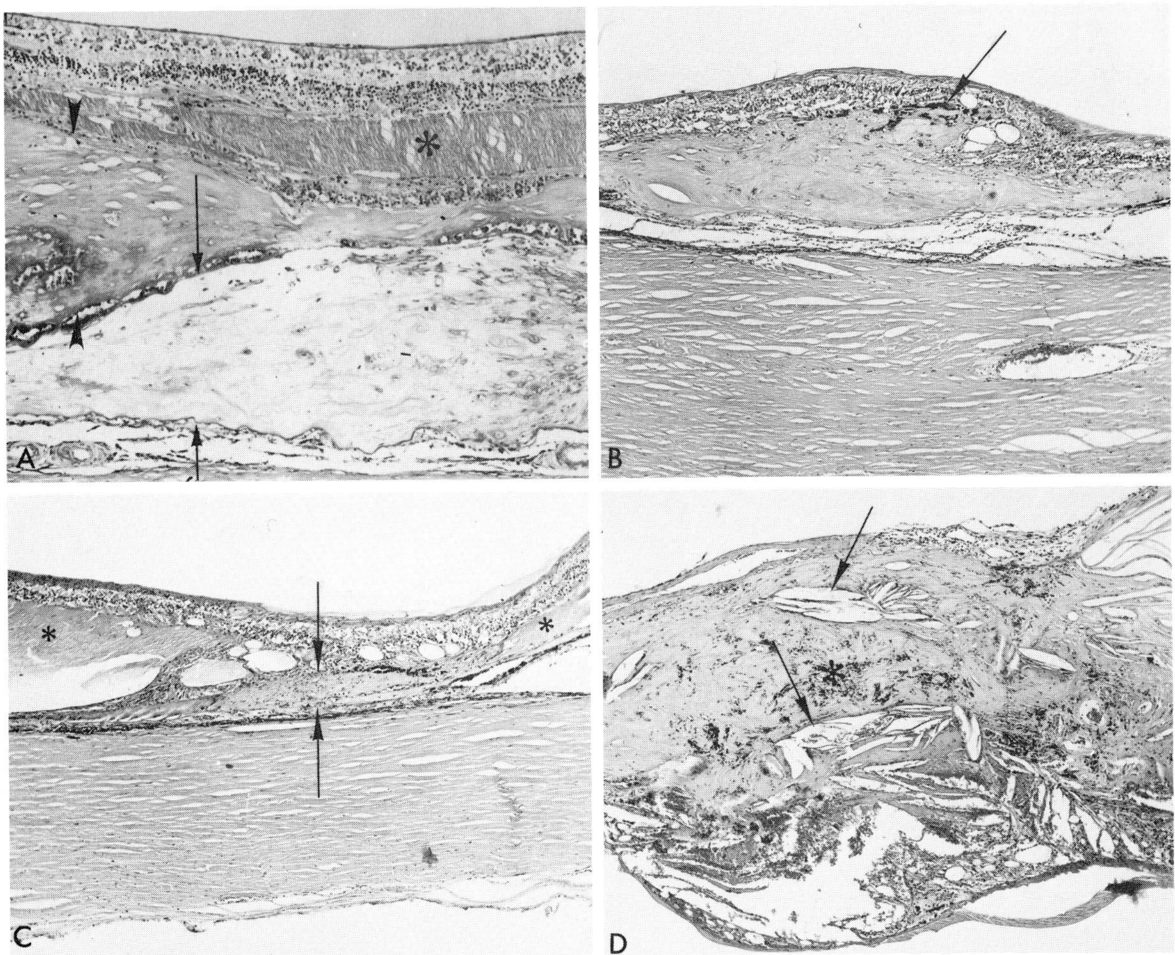

Figure 8–386. Right eye. *A,* **Disciform lesion** with components between two layers of Bruch's membrane (between arrows) and between inner layer of Bruch's membrane and retina (between arrowheads). Proteinaceous exudation is present in (asterisk) and under retina. PAS, ×40. *B,* Peripheral disciform with nodule of hyperplastic retinal pigment epithelium (arrow). H and E, ×30. *C,* Second peripheral disciform lesion (between arrows), with cystic retinal edema and subretinal exudation (asterisks). H and E, ×30. *D,* Third peripheral disciform lesion, with exudation, lipid vacuoles, cholesterol slits (arrows), and hemosiderin staining (asterisk). H and E, ×30. EP 38596.

(From Green WR, Key SN III: Senile macular degeneration: A histopathological study. Trans Am Ophthalmol Soc *75*:180–254, 1977.)

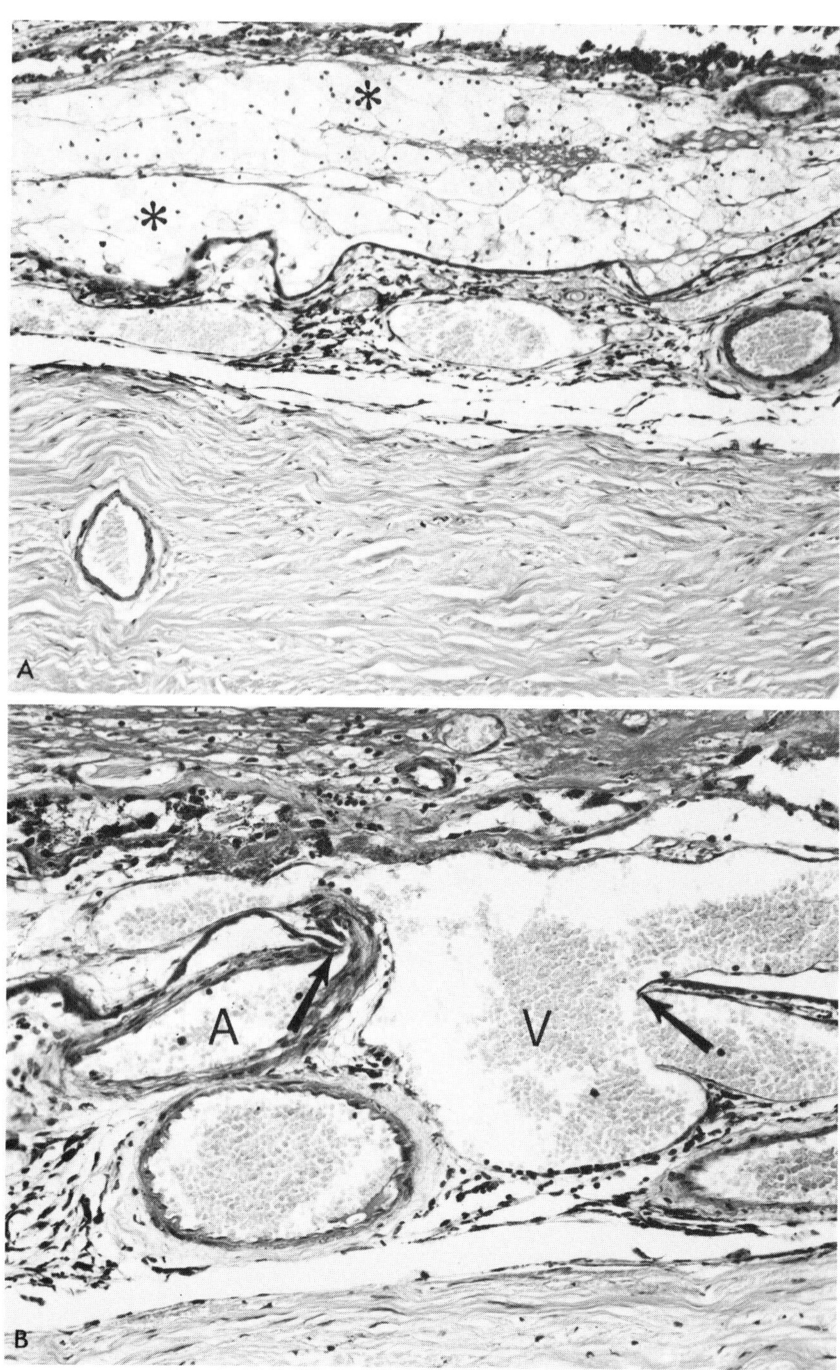

Figure 8–387. *A,* **Disciform degeneration of macula,** with accumulation of lipid-laden histiocytes (asterisks) between two layers of Bruch's membrane. PAS, ×120. *B,* Break in Bruch's membrane (between arrows) through which a choroidal artery *(A)* and vein *(V)* extend into the disciform lesion. PAS, ×220. EP 46902.

tact, no changes are seen in the inner portion of the retina. Retinal pigment epithelial window defects may precede areolar atrophy.

By electron microscopy, all the changes that have been described by light and electron microscopy as an aging process in Bruch's membrane are present, and the RPE cells show massive accumulation of lipofuscin granules and cytoplasmic alteration, with loss of organelles and displacement of the nucleus toward the periphery of the cell. The apical villi of the RPE cells are lost, and there is degeneration of the disks of the outer segments and an accumulation of debris and altered disks in the photoreceptor region. Macrophages accumulate as a result of these changes; they phagocytize pigment and debris, and either migrate into the retina or form clumps in the photoreceptor region.

Gass (1972a) studied clinically 60 patients with geographic RPE atrophy at the time of initial presentation. The disease was bilaterally symmetric in two thirds of the patients. A five-year average follow-up was obtained in this group. A large percentage of these patients had, or developed, serous detachment of the RPE and signs of choroidal neovascularization. In his group of patients with senile maculopathy, there was senile reticular degeneration at the equator with drusen in about a third of the cases. Histologically, equatorial reticular degeneration is characterized by the presence of typical drusen and diffuse confluent drusen associated with variable areas of RPE hypopigmentation, atrophy, hypertrophy, and minor hyperplasia.

Blair (1975) pointed out that the aerolar atrophy of senile macular degeneration and central areolar choroidal sclerosis differ with respect to age of onset, family history, and associated features.

The areolar atrophy may occur in areas of marked drusen formation and after previous serous detachment of the RPE (Willerson, Aaberg, 1978).

SUBRETINAL PIGMENT EPITHELIAL NEOVASCULARIZATION (SUB-RPE). Sub-RPE neovascularization is actually within Bruch's membrane, where it is located between the thickened inner aspect and the remainder of Bruch's membrane. The capillary-like vessels come from the choroid through a break in the outer aspect of Bruch's membrane. This feature of senile macular degeneration occurs more often than has been realized. This lesion was observed in 30 of 150 eyes (20 per cent) of 80 patients with senile changes in the macular region (Sarks, 1973b). In another study, sub-RPE neovascularization was observed in 46 of 176 eyes (25 per cent) from patients with senile macular degeneration (Green, Key, 1977).

Early it may occur under a relatively intact RPE and may not be appreciated clinically, even with the use of fluorescein angiography. In 17 of the 30 eyes (56.6 per cent) with choroidal neovascularization studied clinically and histopathologically by Sarks (1973b), the neovascularization had been undetected clinically. This was also true in a number of instances in the study by Green and Key (1977).

In some cases, sub-RPE neovascularization may be detected by fluorescein angiography, especially if there is depigmentation or partial or complete loss of the overlying RPE. The condition may remain rather dormant for variable periods of time. Eventually, it leads to "wet" complications, such as serous or hemorrhagic detachment of the RPE or the neurosensory retina or both. This then sets the stage for the development of three additional morphologic forms of senile macular degeneration—the exudative, hemorrhagic, and disciform types. Two reliable ophthalmologic signs of choroidal neovascularization are hemorrhage and exudates. Additional features include subretinal or subretinal pigment epithelial blood or both; intra- or subretinal exudates or both; turgid subretinal fluid; subretinal pigment epithelial ring formation; and subretinal pigment epithelial plaque or mound formation. By fluorescein angiography, the features are seen to include a vascular cartwheel or seafan configuration, with surrounding halo, one or more "hot spots" of leakage, and late staining.

The Macular Photocoagulation Study Group (1982) a multi-center group, in a randomized clinical trial found that vision could be preserved by laser photocoagulation of choroidal neovascular membranes that occurred outside the fovea. After 18 months' follow-up, 60 per cent of untreated and 25 per cent of treated eyes had severe loss of vision. These investigators recommend that patients with senile macular degeneration who are at risk for the development of choroidal neovascularization be examined periodically so that if symptomatic neovascularization develops, treatment can be considered before irreversible visual loss occurs.

It is of interest that choroidal neovascularization occurs also in the peripapillary area and the fundus periphery. Sarks observed choroidal neovascularization in the peripapillary area in 14 per cent, and in the periphery in 24.6 per cent, of 150 eyes of 80 patients studied clinically and histopathologically. Serous and hemorrhagic sequelae and disciform scarring also may occur in these extramacular sites (Mazow, Ruiz, 1973) but less commonly than in the macular area.

The finding of intra-Bruch's membrane blood vessels in the periphery in eyes of children (Spitznas, 1977) suggests that these vessels may be a normal variation in children and not neovascularization.

SENILE EXUDATIVE MACULAR DEGENERATION. In this form of senile macular degeneration, there is an accumulation of fluid under the RPE in and under the neurosensory retina. This accumulation reflects the changes that occur in Bruch's membrane and is most often a result of long-term aging changes, with decompensation of the circulation and leakage of plasma into the tissues. Implicated are severe changes in Bruch's membrane, with choroidal neovascularization. The neovascularization may not be detected clinically (Teeters, Bird, 1973). Clinically, a circumscribed area of elevation of the macular retina is seen, and in most patients the RPE can be shown to be elevated by either a clear or turbid fluid; with fluorescein angiography, vessels are often not identified. Note that small RPE detachments can be confused with drusen ophthalmoscopically and by fluorescein angiography (Frank, Green, Pollack, 1973).

Histologically, there are the usual senile changes in Bruch's membrane and the pigment epithelium, and the RPE is elevated by serous fluid that may be coagulated and granular in appearance. This elevation of the RPE may extend beyond the actual site of the most intense changes. Frequently the RPE cells are degenerated over the greatest accumulation of fluid, and there is extension of fluid through the pigment layer into the photoreceptor region. The photoreceptors and outer retina show extensive degenerative changes. Occasional macrophages may be present in the fluid in the photoreceptor region. Bruch's membrane may show basophilia. Fractures and gaps are almost always found in Bruch's membrane at the site of the accumulation of serous fluid.

Sarks (1973b) examined histologically 150 eyes from 80 patients who had been observed clinically and followed for up to 1 year. All these patients showed senile changes in the macular region. Gaps in Bruch's membrane were found in all. New vessels were found in the macular area in about 20 per cent of the eyes. This intra-Bruch's membrane choroidal neovascularization was not appreciated clinically in about 50 per cent of the eyes.

Senile hemorrhagic macular degeneration. Clinically, the hemorrhagic form of senile maculopathy is most dramatic. Often the initial clinical manifestation is a dark, moundlike sub-RPE detachment, which sometimes resembles the findings in choroidal melanoma. In some cases the hemorrhage breaks through the RPE into the retina or subretinal space or both. The hemorrhagic lesion is usually circumscribed, and, after the initial severe bleeding, it remains stationary and proceeds to the healed stage (disciform macular degeneration). Occasionally, a patient will develop recurrent bleeding into the original lesion or at its periphery.

This hemorrhagic form of senile maculopathy is simply the advanced stage of the preceding conditions. Neovascularization of Bruch's membrane and the sub-RPE region is the predecessor of the vascular accident that leads to the bleeding. The blood coagulates in the subepithelial or subretinal region, becomes organized, and forms a circumscribed scar.

In some eyes the bleeding may occur from an area not under the macula, with the peripapillary region being the most common alternate site. The temporal peripapillary region is the most common source of the hemorrhage (Reese, Jones, 1962). In such cases the bleeding elevates the retina in the peripapillary region and extends outward toward the macula. Histologically, a break is most often found in Bruch's membrane, to which vessels have proliferated widely under the epithelium; the hemorrhage results from an interruption of one or more vessels that have proliferated into this area.

Other eccentric hemorrhagic lesions can occur in various positions with respect to the macula, either inferior or superior to the macula (Mazow, Ruiz, 1973) and the periphery (Annesley, 1980). Eccentric lesions of this type usually have a somewhat better prognosis than those that occur in the foveal region, because the eccentric lesions spare the delicate macular retina.

Disciform macular degeneration. The development of fibrous disciform scars in the macular area in senile macular degeneration occurs usually, but not exclusively, as the result of the serous and hemorrhagic sequelae of sub-RPE neovascularization. Fibrous tissue, along with choroidal neovascularization, develops between the split layers of Bruch's membrane. Fibrous tissue proliferation may develop also between the separated inner layer of Bruch's membrane and the retina. The presence of hemosiderin within the disciform plaque suggests that fibrous organization of a hemorrhage plays a role in the evolution of the disciform lesion. Retinal pigment epithelium also contributes to the disciform lesion. Laminated areas of basement membrane are observed in some disciform lesions, and these suggest successive layers of RPE hyperplasia. Frank hyperplasia of RPE is a conspicuous feature of many macular disciform lesions. Some of these lesions in the past have been confused with malignant melanoma. A case of pseudomelanomas from the Armed Forces Institute of Pathology series studied by Ferry (1964) is illustrated in Figure 8–380.

Occasional infiltrates of lymphocytes may be observed in the choroid subjacent to disciform scars in senile macular degeneration (see Fig. 8–370,*B*). The significance of this infiltrate is not known.

The retina overlying the disciform scar undergoes cystic degeneration and loss of the photoreceptor cell layer. Secondary changes may occur within disciform scars and may include bone formation (Fig. 8–373,*A*), retinal arterialization (Figs. 8–376 through 8–378), and in some instances retinochoroidal anastomosis (Green, Gass, 1971) (Fig. 8–385).

Profuse serous exudation from vessels within the disciform lesion may lead to large accumulations of intra- and subretinal lipid-rich exudate (Figs. 8–386 and 8–387). The resultant fundus picture has been referred to as "senile Coats' disease," "Coats-like response," and "exudative senile maculopathy" (Schatz, Patz, 1973).

Even after rather quiescent periods of disciform macular scars, "wet" complications can occur (Figs. 8–381 through 8–384). These include serous or hemorrhagic detachment of the RPE or neurosensory retina or both. Some of these in the past have been confused with malignant melanoma (Berkow, Font, 1969; Wolter, Benz, Roth, 1965; Green, Key, 1977). Patients on anticoagulant therapy may be at greater risk of developing this complication, and the hemorrhage may be massive, with extension into the subretinal space and vitreous cavity.

Disciform Macular Degeneration in Young Persons. The nature of this condition has not been settled. It was first described by Junius as an example of juvenile exudative macular retinitis. Two apparent forms are now considered in this category; they may or may not be related, but often produce similar symptoms and findings.

One form is similar clinically to central serous retinopathy and has not been studied histopathologically. The second form is essentially the same as senile macular disciform degeneration, and it occurs in associated hemorrhage from the sub-RPE choroidal neovascularization. Vision is immediately reduced. On ophthalmoscopic examination, the vitreous is clear, and the retina is elevated by various amounts of macular hemorrhage. Recurrences of small hemorrhages are the rule, and in about 50 per cent of patients the condition becomes bilateral. Often the lesion is located eccentrically from the macula and gradually extends into the macula. Subsequently, the hemorrhage becomes organized, in much the same manner as does senile hemorrhagic maculopathy.

Microscopic examinations have been made on advanced lesions of this type, and the changes resemble those of the senile type. Early examinations have been done in a few cases, notably by Maumenee (1959), with the observation of hemorrhage under the pigment epithelium or hemorrhage that has broken through the RPE and spread beneath the retina. A disciform scar evolves in most cases and is associated with degenerative changes in the photoreceptor cell layer and loss of central vision. Histopathologic studies (Ashton, Sorsby, 1951) of eyes from two members of the family reported by Sorsby, Mason, and Gardener (1949) showed thickening of Bruch's membrane, choroidal neovascularization with breaks in Bruch's membrane, drusen, disciform scarring, and choriocapillaris atrophy.

This process apparently can occur without significant drusen, can have an inflammatory appearance, and can be transmitted as an autosomal dominant trait (Carr, Noble, Nasaduke, 1977).

Secondary Macular Degeneration with Loss of the Maculopapillary Bundle. This pattern of atrophy produces a central or centrocecal scotoma and results in loss of the foveal reflex. Conditions in which this pattern of atrophy may occur include chronic alcoholism (nutritional amblyopia) (page 1156), chloramphenicol toxicity from chronic use in patients with fibrocystic disease of the kidney (page 805), Leigh's disease (subacute necrotizing encephalomyelitis) (page 1159), and multiple sclerosis (page 1156; also Chap. 9, page 2008). The histopathologic features are essentially the same and are illustrated elsewhere.

Macular Edema (Cystoid Macular Edema). Cystoid macular edema may be associated with a wide range of intraocular inflammatory diseases (Fig. 8–388), and also retinal vascular diseases, intraocular surgery (especially cataract extraction), retinitis pigmentosa, epinephrine and nicotinic acid toxicity, radiation retinopathy, surface-wrinkling retinopathy, some choroidal lesions with submacular RPE defects, and idiopathic forms (Irvine, 1976).

Cystoid macular edema is an important cause of reduced vision after cataract extraction (Irvine-Gass syndrome), pars planitis (chronic cyclitis) (see Fig. 8–200,*C*), branch and central (see Figs. 8–72,*A*,*B* and 8–102) vein occlusion, and diabetic retinopathy. The stellate pattern of edema as shown with fluorescein angiography is attributed to the anatomic arrangement of the horizontally oriented fibers in the outer plexiform layer in the macular area. This appears to allow for more free collection of edema fluid than elsewhere in the retina. Cystoid macular edema, because of retinal vascular leakage, involves both the outer plexiform and inner macular layers (Fig. 8–389). When cystoid macular edema is related to RPE abnormalities, the edema involves the same layers but is usually more marked in the outer plexiform layer (see Figs. 8–428, 8–447, 8–456, and 8–457).

On careful ophthalmoscopic examination, using red-free light and slit lamp with contact lens, fine radiating cystoid spaces can be seen in the parafoveal area. The spaces collect fluorescein.

When the cystoid macular edema is marked and chronic, atrophy of the retinal layers may ensue. The spaces may coalesce and form a schisis cavity, which may proceed to a lamellar or complete macular hole.

Irvine-Gass Syndrome. Macular changes associated with vitreous alterations in the aphakic eye were described by S. Rodman Irvine in 1953. The features of this condition were more clearly delineated after the development of fluorescein angiography (Gass, Norton, 1966). In a prospective angiographic study, Hitchings and Chisholm (1975) found an incidence of cystoid edema in 46.7 per cent of patients examined 6 to 7 weeks after uncomplicated cataract extraction. Whether or not they received topical steroids postoperatively made no difference. In these 36 eyes, the condition resolved in 16, improved in 8, was stable in 5, and the status was unknown in 8, at 6 months. (There is a discrepancy in the authors' figures.) No predisposing factor was found. Visual acuity continued to improve, so that after 2 years, only four eyes had macular edema, and vision had improved in all of them (Hitchings, 1977). In a sim-

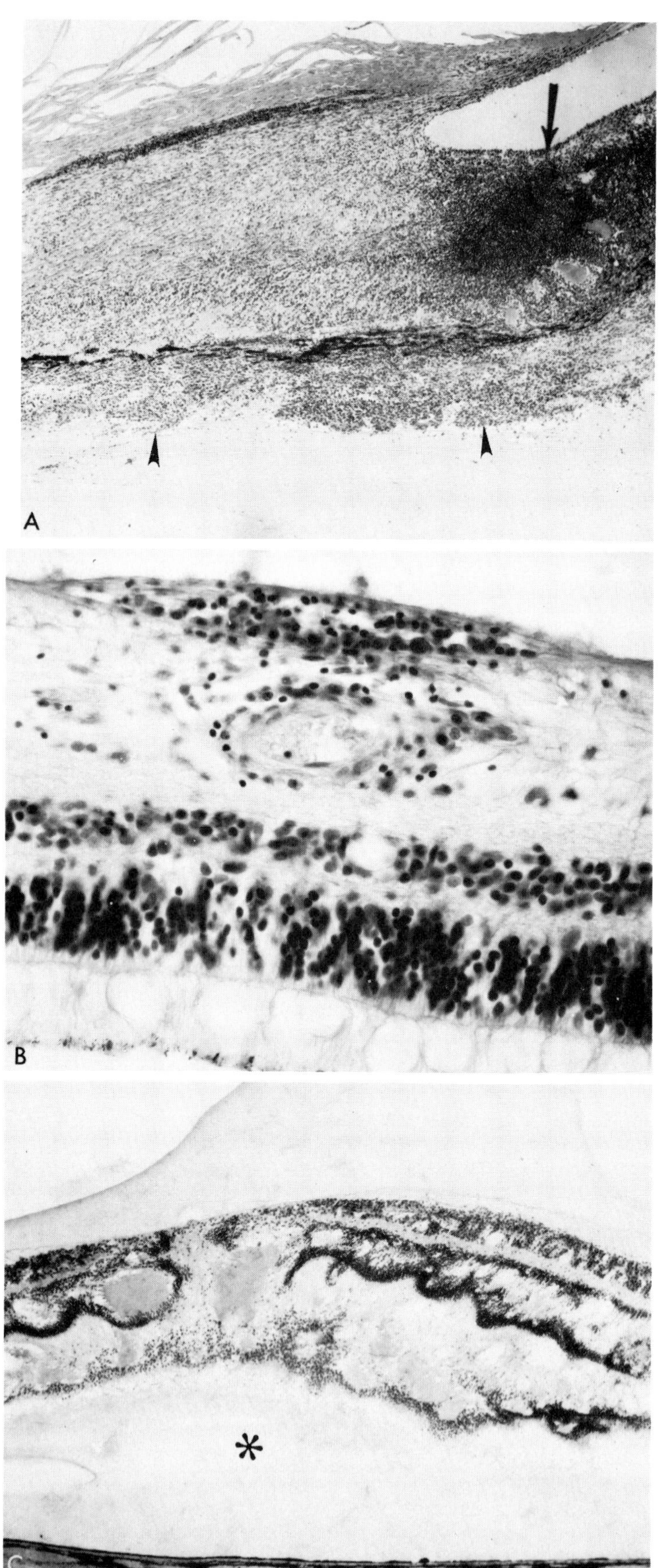

Figure 8–388. Chronic iridocyclitis with retinal phlebitis and cystoid macular edema. *A,* Base of iris and anterior portion of ciliary body are intensely infiltrated by lymphocytes (arrow). Moderately intense, diffuse infiltration by lymphocytes and plasma cells is present in the remainder of the ciliary body and along its inner surface (arrowheads). H and E, ×60. *B,* Retinal phlebitis. Lymphocytes and some plasma cells are in the wall of a retinal vein and surrounding area. H and E, ×380. *C,* Cystoid macular edema involving the outer plexiform and inner nuclear layers. A serous detachment (asterisk) of the macula is present. H and E, ×60. AFIP 578128.

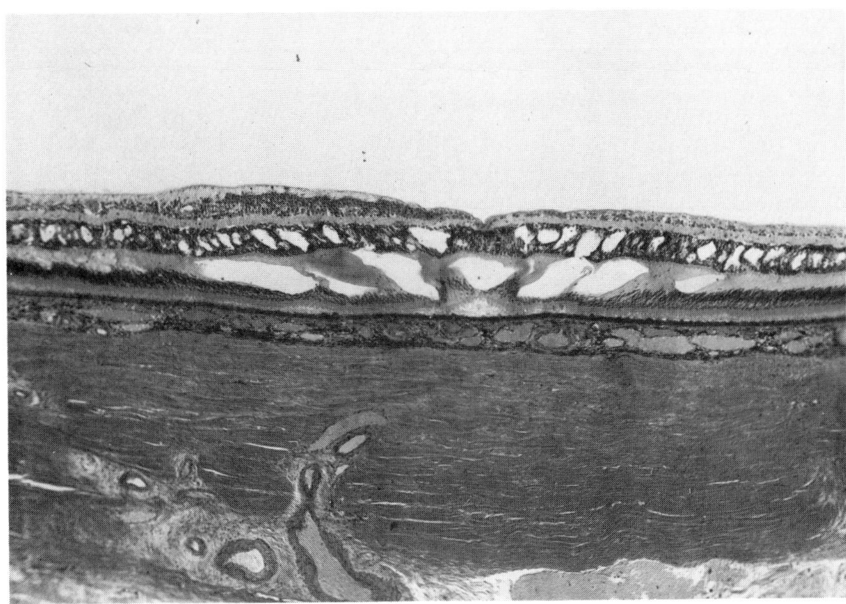

Figure 8–389. Cystoid macular edema involving inner nuclear and outer plexiform layers. H and E, ×45. AFIP 183941.

ilar prospective angiographic study, Meredith et al (1976) observed perifoveal capillary leakage in 60 per cent of 50 eyes at 2 weeks and in 17 eyes (34 per cent) at 6 weeks after cataract extraction. Cystoid macular edema has been reported to occur as late as 13 years after cataract extraction (Epstein, 1977).

The peak incidence of aphakic cystoid macular edema occurs between 3 and 6 weeks after surgery. Klein and Yannuzzi (1976) observed this condition in only 4 of 75 eyes (5 per cent) within the first week of cataract extraction.

The precise cause of retinal edema in the Irvine-Gass syndrome is not known. It is, however, more common in eyes with anterior segment complications of cataract extraction, such as iris or vitreous incarceration in the wound. These complicating factors produce mild inflammation of the ciliary body and vitreous. The state of surgical aphakia, the complicating factors, and secondary mild inflammation appear to contribute to retinal vascular instability and, consequently, the retinal edema that accumulates in the macular and peripapillary areas. In a study of eyes with this syndrome obtained post mortem, Martin, Green, and Martin (1977) found most to have some anterior segment complicating factor, such as iridovitreal synechiae, mild cyclitis and vitritis, and retinal phlebitis (Figs. 8–390 and 8–391). The evaluation of the effects of steroids on the Irvine-Gass syndrome is difficult because it often shows spontaneous remission. The possible role of light toxicity in the Irvine-Gass syndrome has been discussed elsewhere (see page 811). Indomethacin may be beneficial in the prevention and treatment of early cases (Miyake, 1978; Yannuzzi, Landan, Klein, 1980).

Macular Cysts and Holes. Macular cysts are most often the result of chronic edema with coalescence of smaller cysts into a single (Figs. 8–400, 8–401,*A*, and 8–401,*C*) or several larger cysts (Figs. 8–401,*B* and 8–402). In some instances, the thin inner layer of the cyst may rupture, producing a lamellar macular hole (Figs. 8–397,*A* and *B*; 8–398,*A* and *B*; 8–399,*A* and *B*) (Gass, 1976).

Macular holes may occur from chronic cystoid macular edema associated with inflammatory diseases (Fig. 8–394,*A*), retinal edema following trauma (Fig. 8–393,*A* through *D*), and possibly vitreous traction (Figs. 8–394,*A*, 8–396,*A*, and 8–397*A*, top) (Yoshioka, 1968). In a study of 90 macular holes, Aaberg, Blair, and Gass (1970) believed trauma to be involved in nine instances and localized vitreous traction in two. The remaining cases were idiopathic, although ametropia and systemic hypertension were possible factors.

Retinal pigment epithelial hypertrophy and hyperplasia may be seen in the area of both lamellar and complete macular holes (Figs. 8–392,*B*, 8–394,*A*, 8–395,*B* and *C*, and 8–397*A*).

Outer lamellar macular holes may be seen with breakdown of the blood ocular barrier at the RPE (Fig. 8–400, top).

Retinal glial cells may grow onto the inner surface of the retina at the margin of a lamellar or complete macular hole (Figs. 8–392,*A* and *B*, 8–393,*A* and *B*, 8–394,*A* and *B*, 8–395,*B*, 8–397,*B*, 8–398,*A* and *B*, and 8–401,*A*). Occasionally, a hole or attenuated area in an epiretinal membrane in the macular area may simulate a macular hole.

Frangieh, Green, and Engel (1981) have studied the histopathologic features of 44 eyes from

Text continued on page 1014

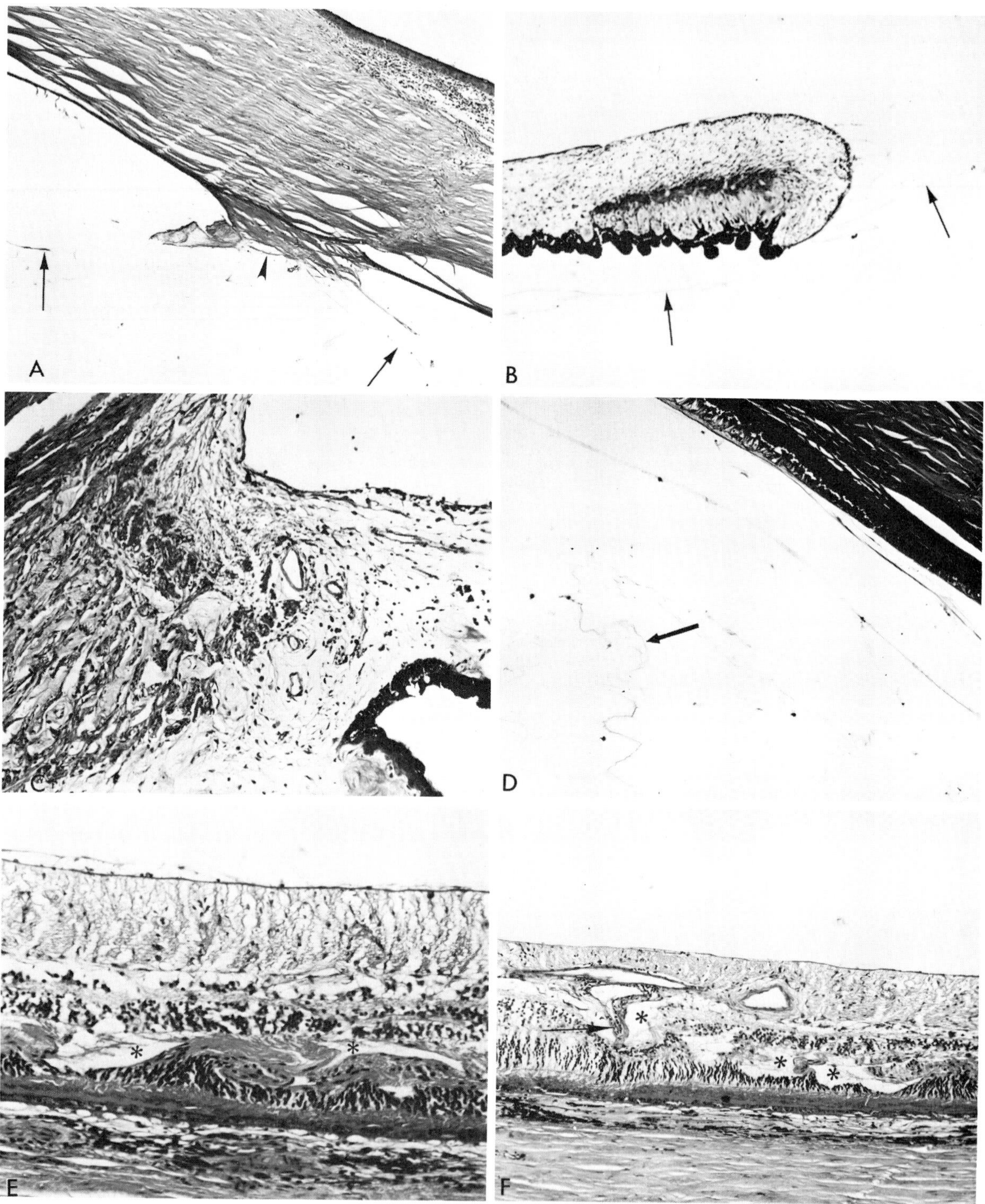

Figure 8–390. Irvine-Gass syndrome. *A,* Vitreous (arrows) incarceration in scar of cataract incision wound. A small plaque of fibrous tissue proliferation (arrowhead) is present at the inner aspect of scar. H and E, ×60. *B,* Iridovitreal synechia. A delicate strand of vitreous (arrows) is adherent to a slightly entropic iris pupillary margin. H and E, ×60. *C,* Mild cyclitis. H and E, ×160. *D,* Mild vitritis. Posterior vitreous detachment (arrow) is present. H and E, ×120. *E,* Macular edema with cystic spaces (asterisks) in outer plexiform layer. H and E, ×190. *F,* Area near posterior pole showing edema (asterisks) and phlebitis (arrow). H and E, ×110. EP 33079.

(From Martin NF, Green WR, Martin LW: Retinal phlebitis in the Irvine-Gass syndrome. Am J Ophthalmol *83*:377–386, 1977.)

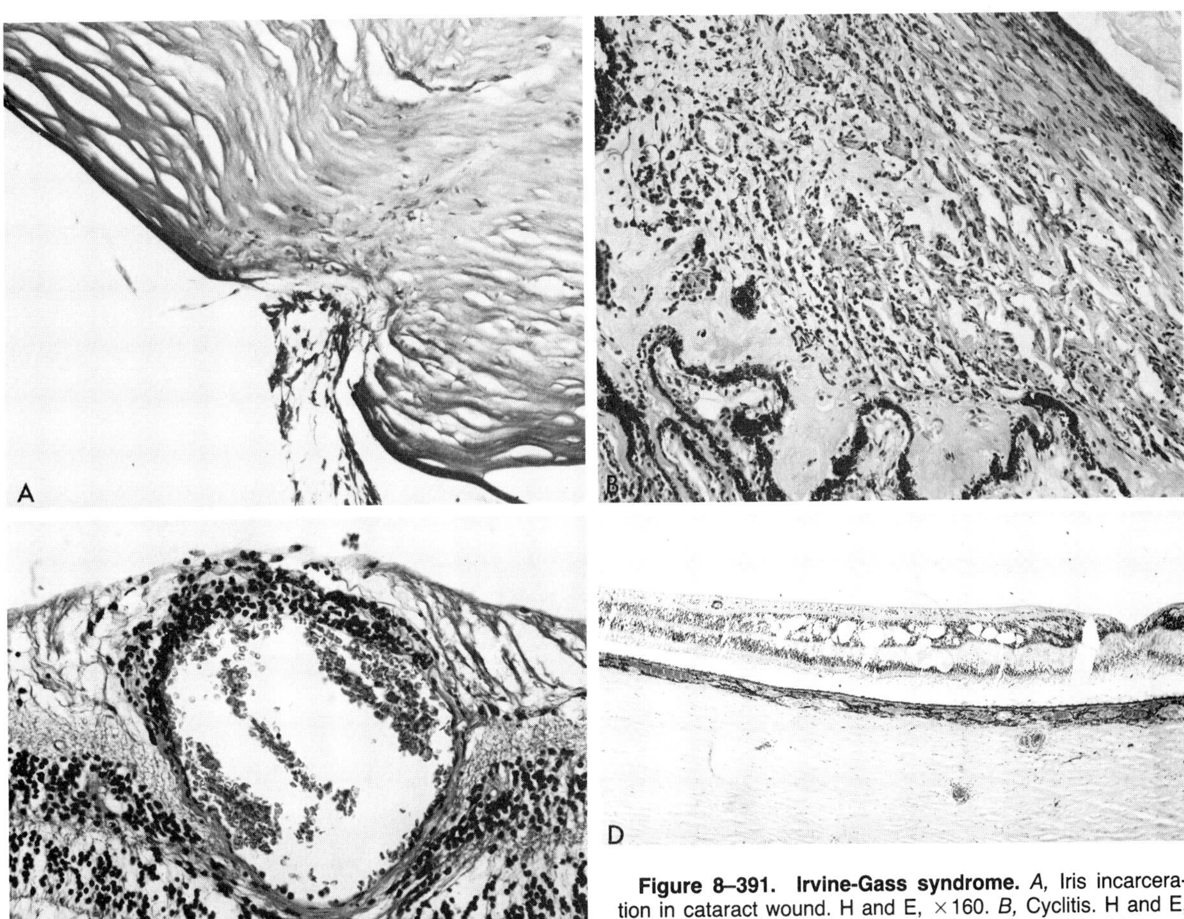

Figure 8–391. Irvine-Gass syndrome. *A,* Iris incarceration in cataract wound. H and E, ×160. *B,* Cyclitis. H and E, ×185. *C,* Retinal phlebitis. H and E, ×240. *D,* Cystoid macular edema (CME). Edema is mostly in the inner nuclear layer. H and E, ×35. AFIP 1214121.

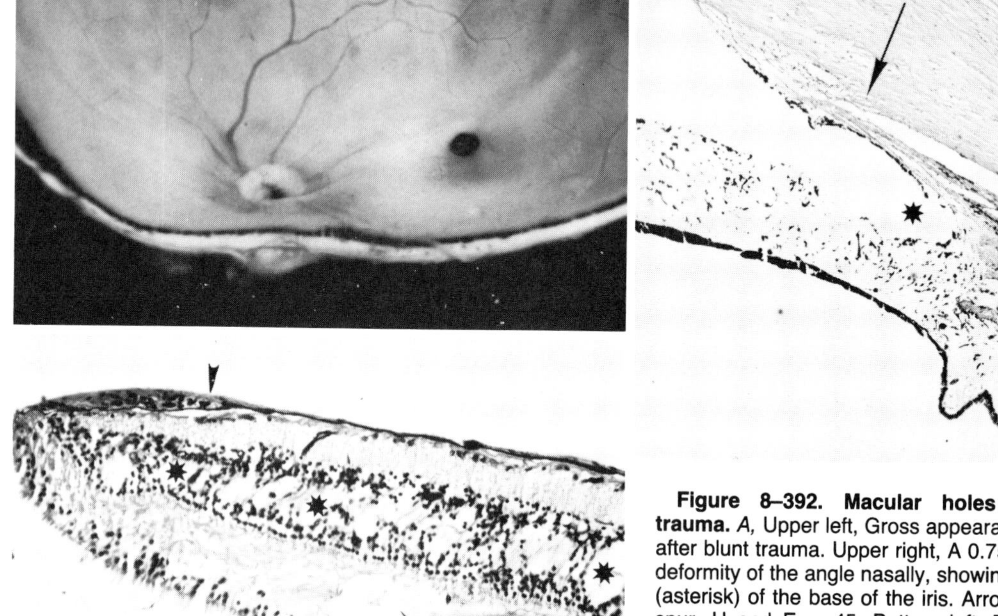

Figure 8–392. Macular holes associated with trauma. *A,* Upper left, Gross appearance of macular hole after blunt trauma. Upper right, A 0.75 mm postcontusion deformity of the angle nasally, showing retrodisplacement (asterisk) of the base of the iris. Arrow marks the scleral spur. H and E, ×45. Bottom left, Temporal margin of macular hole showing a fibroglial preretinal membrane (arrowhead) and cystic edema in the inner nuclear (asterisks) and outer plexiform (arrow) layers. PAS, ×120. EP 32803.

Illustration continued on opposite page

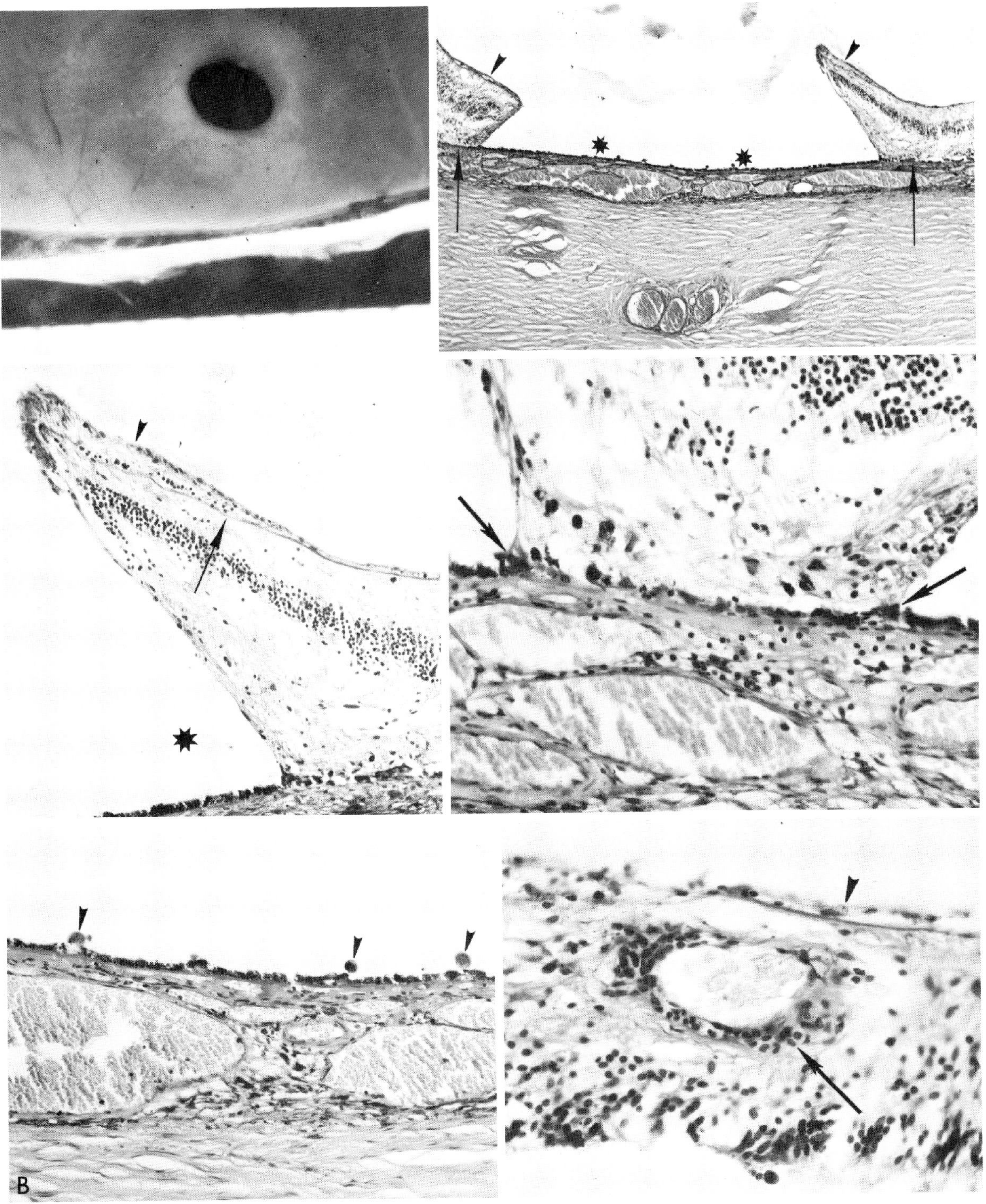

Figure 8–392 *Continued B,* Upper left, Gross appearance of macular hole following remote blunt trauma. Upper right, Low-power view of macular hole showing small area of detachment, "demarcation" chorioretinal adhesions (arrows), a fibroglial preretinal membrane on either side (arrowheads), and retinal pigment epithelium (RPE) changes in area of hole (asterisks). PAS, ×50. Middle left, Higher-power view of temporal margin of hole, showing fibroglial preretinal membrane (arrowhead) on the surface of the internal limiting membrane (arrow), a small area of retinal detachment (asterisk) and chorio-RPE-retinal adhesion. PAS, ×185. Middle right, Higher-power view of demarcation chorioretinal adhesion (between arrows), showing partial loss of RPE and adherence of retinal tissue to Bruch's membrane and residual RPE. PAS, × 300. Bottom left, Center of macular hole showing an intact RPE with areas of hypertrophy and individual pigmented cells (arrowheads) that have become dislodged internally. PAS, ×205. Bottom right, Lymphocytes in wall of retinal vein (arrow). A fibrocellular and inflammatory preretinal membrane (arrowhead) is present. PAS, ×350. EP 37860. (From Frangieh GT, Green WR, Engel HM: A histopathologic study of macular cysts and holes. Retina *1*:311–336, 1981.)

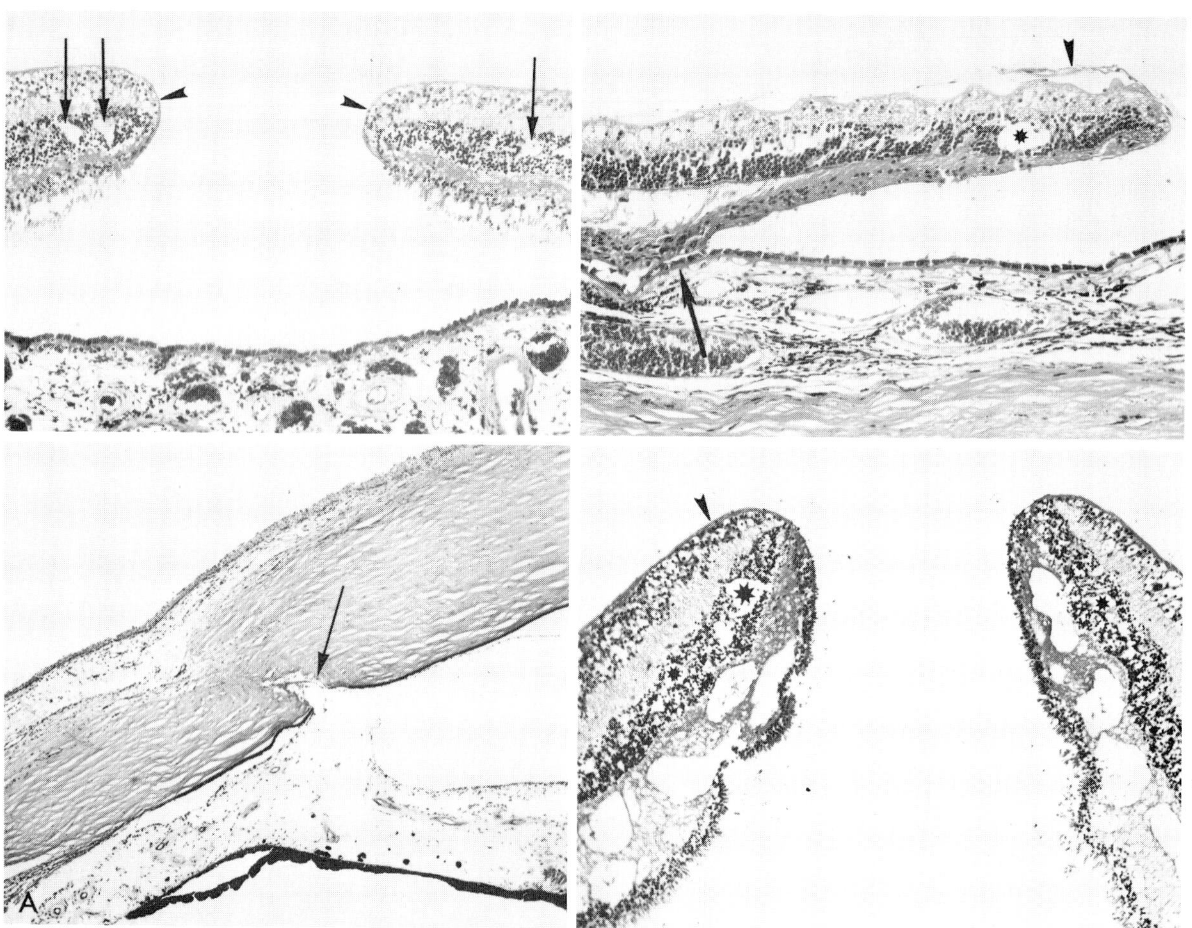

Figure 8–393. Macular holes associated with trauma. *A,* Top left, Macular hole with rounded margins (arrowheads), an intact retinal pigment epithelium (RPE), and minor cystic edema in the inner nuclear layer (arrows). H and E, ×100. EP 51635. Top right, Temporal margin of macular hole showing minor cystic edema of the inner nuclear layer (asterisk), preretinal membrane (arrowhead) with wrinkling of the internal limiting membrane, a small zone of retinal detachment, and a demarcation chorioretinal adhesion (arrow). H and E, ×110. EP 52519. Bottom left, Iris incarceration in posterior portion of scar of cataract wound (arrow). PAS, ×40. EP 51036. Bottom right, Section of macular hole showing rounded margins and cystic edema in the outer plexiform layer and to a lesser extent in the inner nuclear layer (asterisks). The preretinal membrane (arrowhead) is hardly perceptible. H and E, ×110. EP 51036.

Illustration continued on opposite page

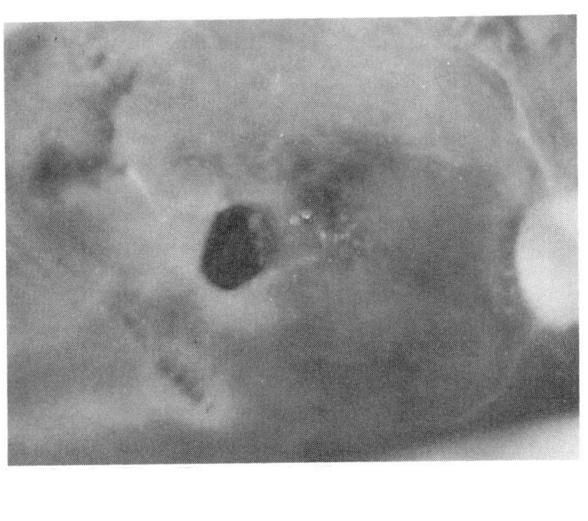

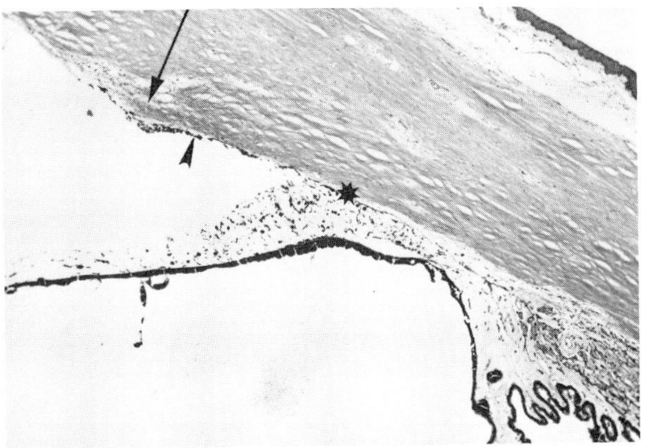

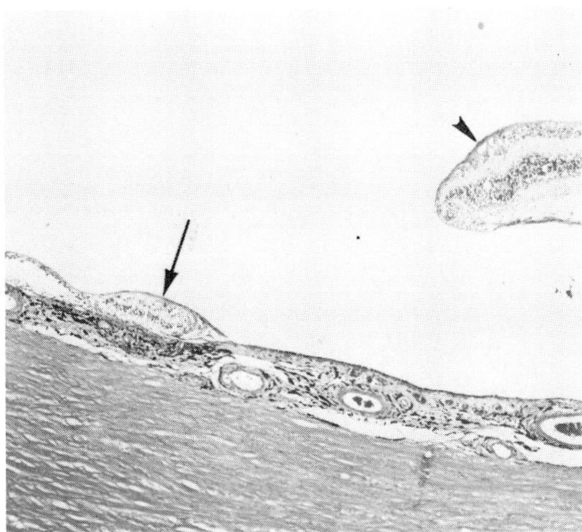

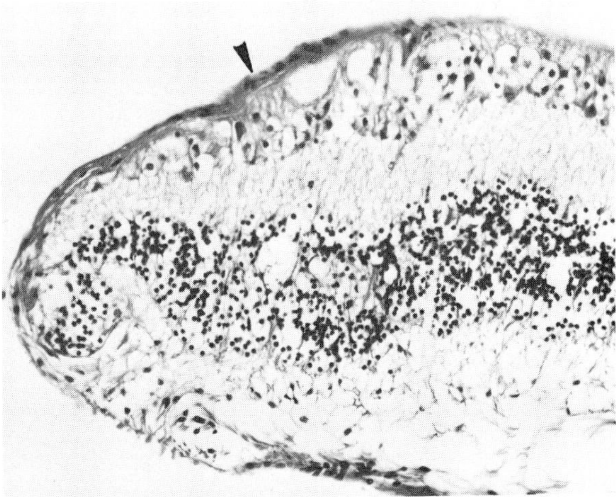

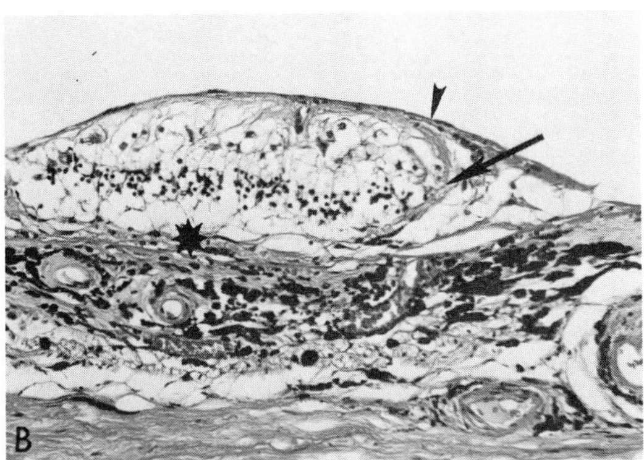

Figure 8–393 *Continued B,* Top left, Gross appearance of macular hole following trauma. Top right, Appearance of healed cyclodialysis. The ciliary body and base of iris are retrodisplaced about 2 mm from the scleral spur (arrow). The bare sclera is covered posteriorly by adherent peripheral iris (asterisk) and anteriorly by proliferation of iris melanocytes (arrowhead). H and E, ×35. Middle left, Section through macular hole showing detached temporal margin (arrowhead) and adherent nasal margin (arrow). H and E, ×35. Middle right, Higher power view of temporal margin, showing loss of the photoreceptor cell layer and a thin fibroglial preretinal membrane (arrowhead). H and E, ×195. Bottom left, Higher-power view of nasal margin of macular hole (arrow), showing marked retinal thinning, chorioretinal adhesion (asterisk), and a thin fibrocellular preretinal membrane (arrowhead). H and E, ×85. EP 48144.

Illustration continued on following page

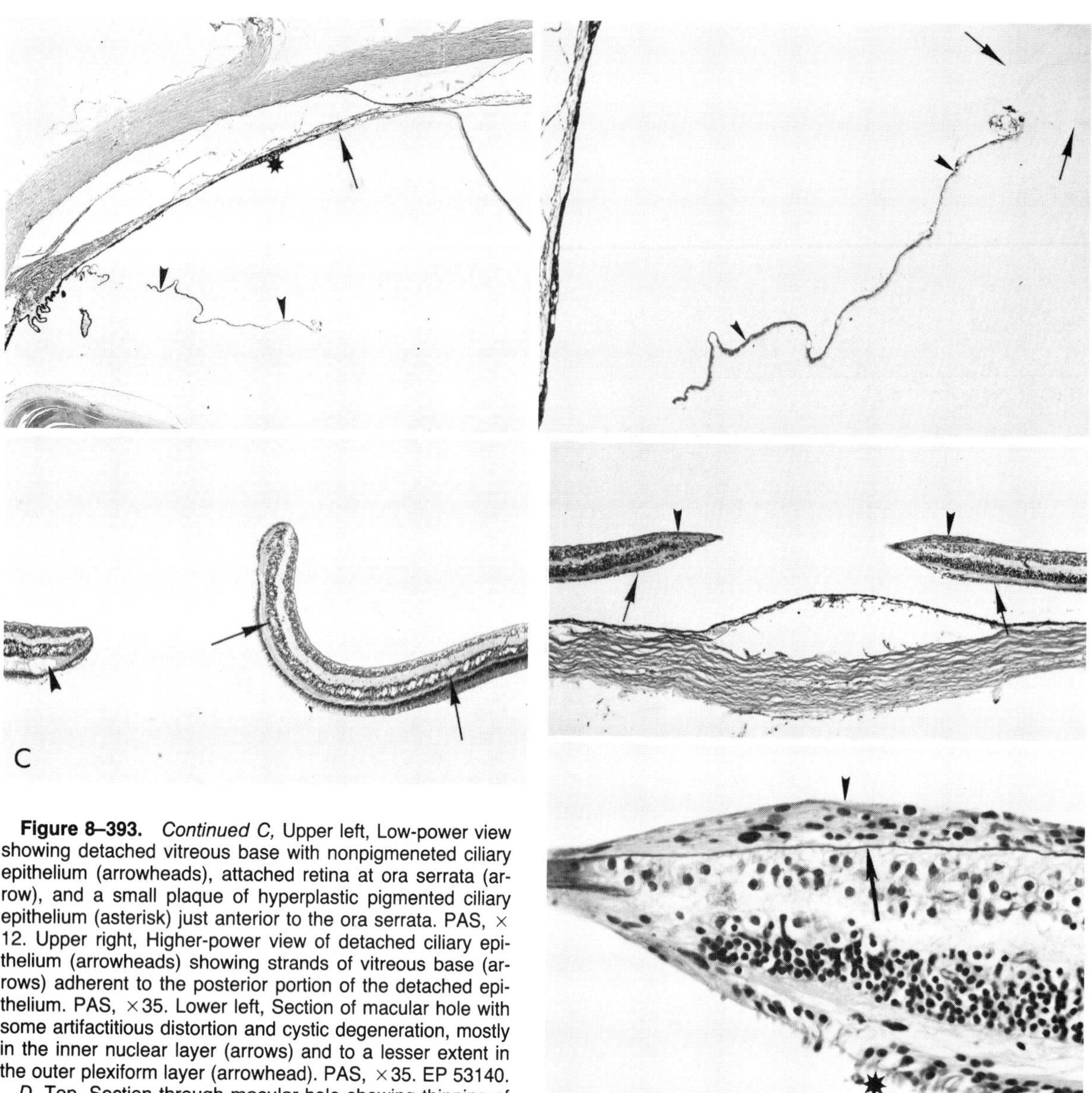

Figure 8–393. *Continued C,* Upper left, Low-power view showing detached vitreous base with nonpigmeneted ciliary epithelium (arrowheads), attached retina at ora serrata (arrow), and a small plaque of hyperplastic pigmented ciliary epithelium (asterisk) just anterior to the ora serrata. PAS, × 12. Upper right, Higher-power view of detached ciliary epithelium (arrowheads) showing strands of vitreous base (arrows) adherent to the posterior portion of the detached epithelium. PAS, ×35. Lower left, Section of macular hole with some artifactitious distortion and cystic degeneration, mostly in the inner nuclear layer (arrows) and to a lesser extent in the outer plexiform layer (arrowhead). PAS, ×35. EP 53140. *D,* Top, Section through macular hole showing thinning of photoreceptor cell layer (arrows) in the area of detachment and a relatively thick fibroglial preretinal membrane (arrowheads). PAS, ×60. Bottom, Higher-power view showing fibroglial membrane (arrowhead) on the inner surface of the internal limiting membrane (arrow) and thinning of the photoreceptor cell layer (asterisk) in the area of retinal detachment. PAS, ×300. EP 50043. (From Frangieh GT, Green WR, Engel HM: A histopathologic study of macular cysts and holes. Retina *1*:311–336, 1981.)

Figure 8–394. Macular holes associated with trauma. *A,* Top left, Area of limbal cataract wound and iridencleisis with an associated intense inflammatory reaction. H and E, ×35. Top right, Higher-power view showing iris in the episcleral area with an intense granulomatous inflammatory cell infiltration. Some epithelioid and giant cells display pigment phagocytosis. H and E, ×250. Middle left, Slightly thickened choroid with a granulomatous inflammatory cell infiltration. H and E, ×510. Middle right, Section of macular hole showing detached vitreous (arrowheads) with adherent operculum (asterisk), cystoid edema in outer plexiform and inner nuclear layers, a small area of surrounding detachment, demarcation chorioretinal adhesions on both sides (large arrows), and occasional pigmented cells (small arrows) internal to intact retinal pigment epithelium. H and E, ×55. Bottom left, Higher-power view showing a thin hypocellular preretinal membrane (arrrowhead), marked cystic edema, and demarcation adhesion (arrow). H and E, ×140. EP 5314. B, Appearance of macular hole with a rounded margin superiorly (asterisk). A fibroglial tissue (arrow) extends from the retina at the inferior margin, across the hole, and onto the inner surface of the retina at the superior margin (arrowhead). PAS, ×75. EP 49987. (From Frangieh GT, Green WR, Engel HM: A histopathologic study of macular cysts and holes. Retina *1*:311–336, 1981.)

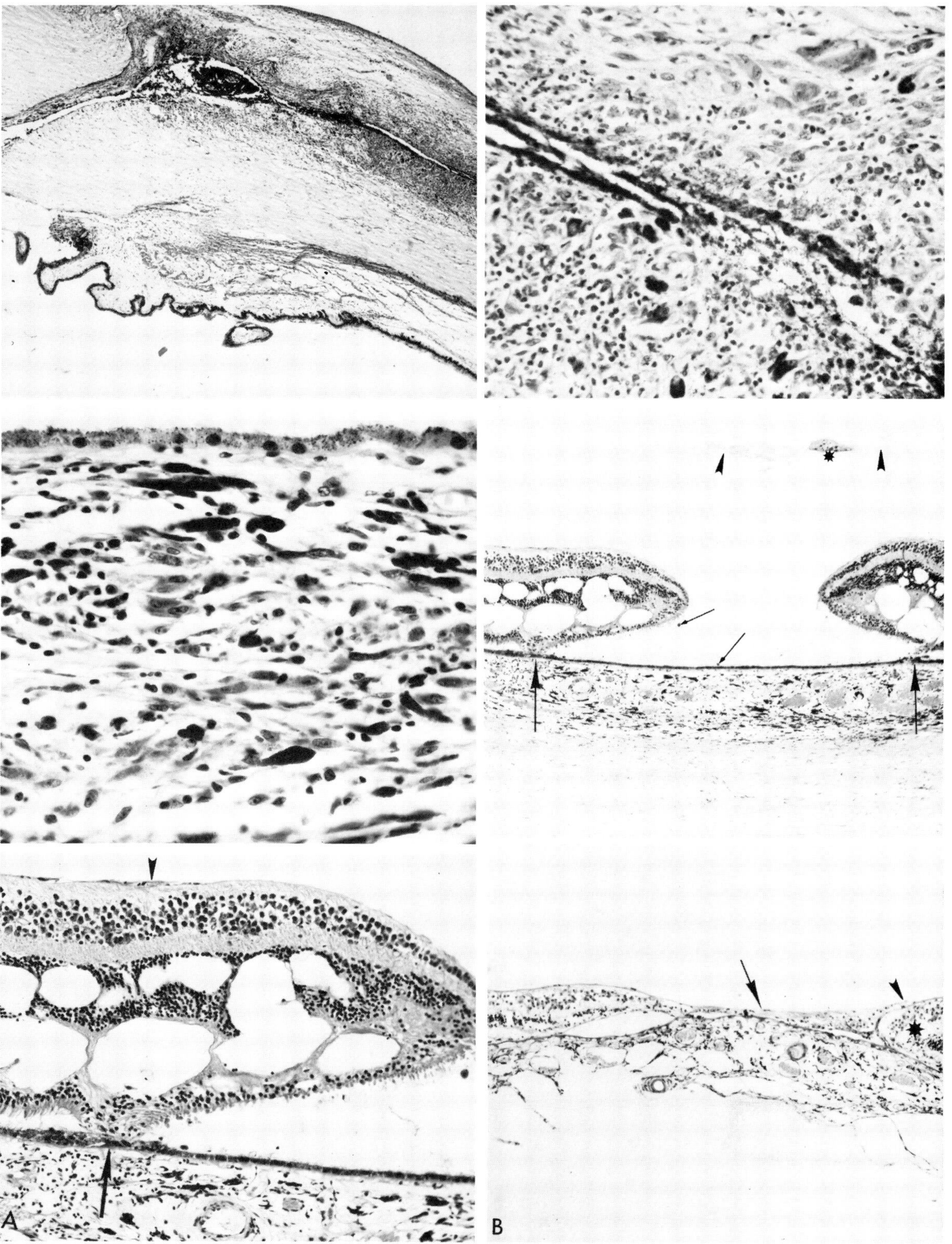

Figure 8–394 *See legend on opposite page*

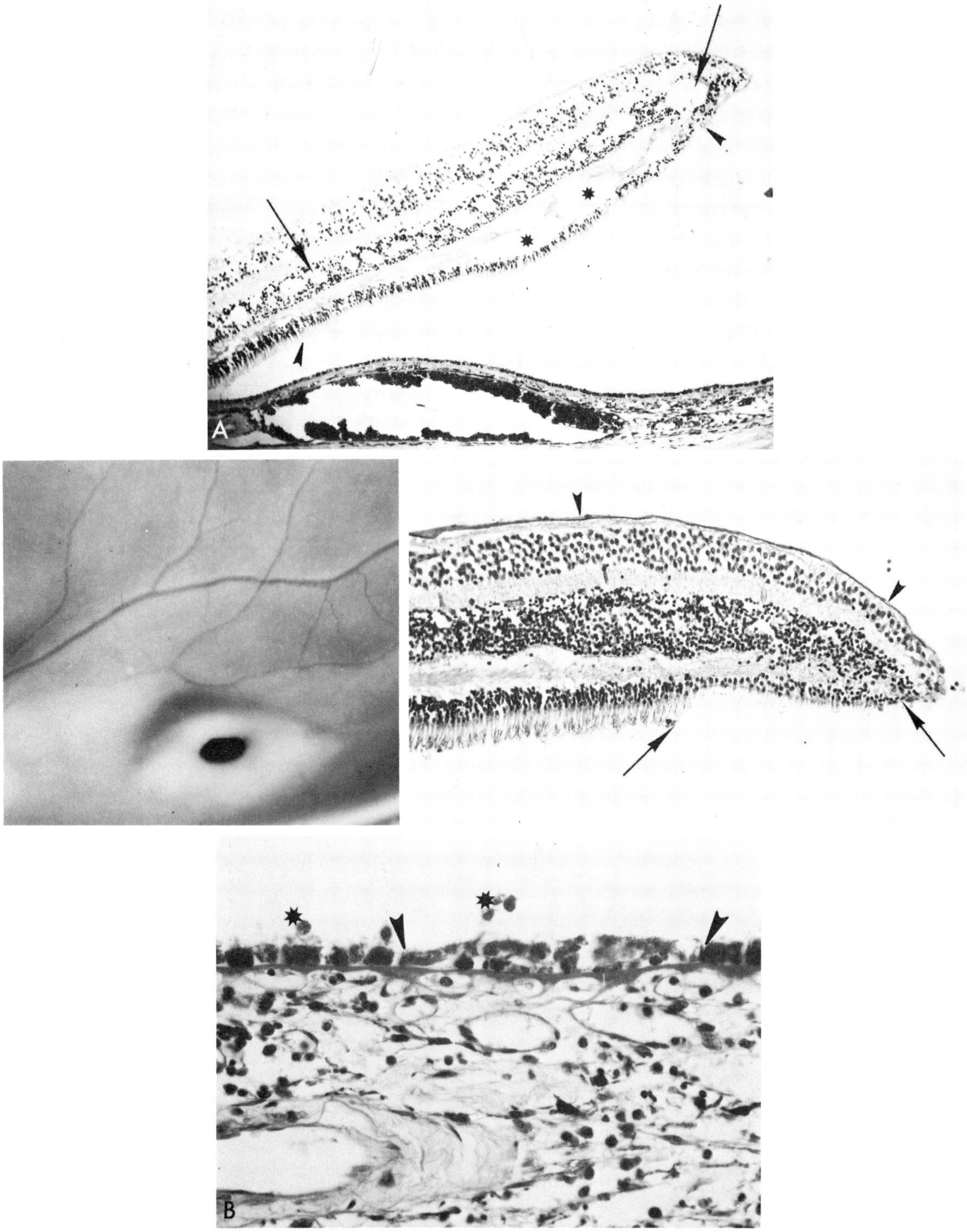

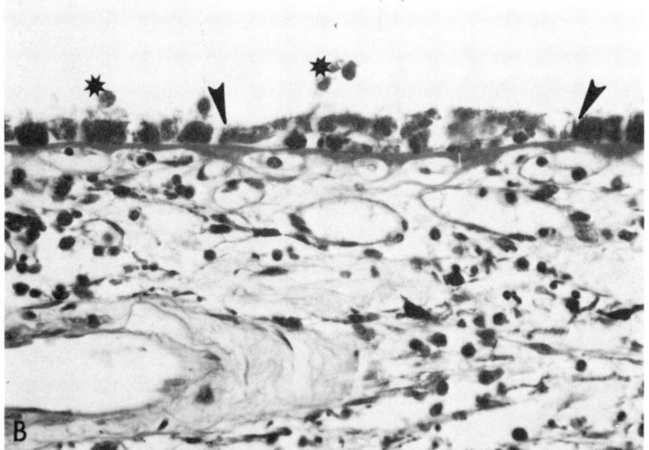

Figure 8–395. Macular holes unassociated with trauma. *A,* One margin of a macular hole, showing cystic edema in the inner nuclear layer (arrows) and to a lesser extent the outer plexiform layer (asterisks). Thinning of the photoreceptor cell layer (between arrowheads) marks an area of detachment, although no demarcation adhesion is present. H and E, ×100. EP 43245.

B, Top left, Gross appearance of macular hole of right eye. Top right, Margin of hole, showing a thin, delicate, hypocellular preretinal membrane (arrowheads) and a narrow zone of partial photoreceptor cell atrophy (between arrows). PAS, ×185. Bottom left, Area of macular hole showing minor hyperplasia and irregularity of retinal pigment membrane (RPE) (between arrowheads) and separated, pigment-containing cells (asterisks). PAS, ×400. EP 50156.

Illustration continued on opposite page

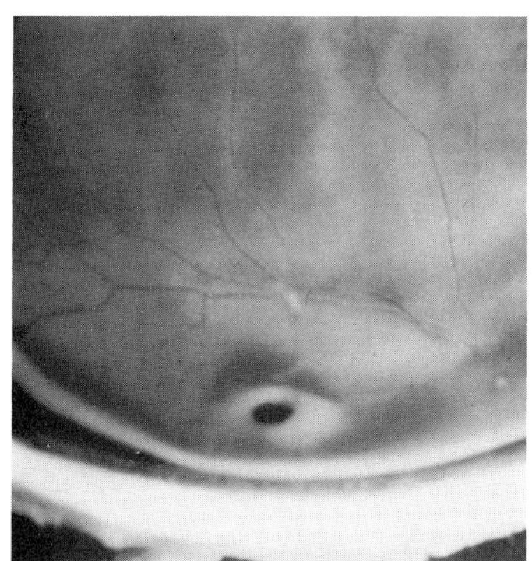

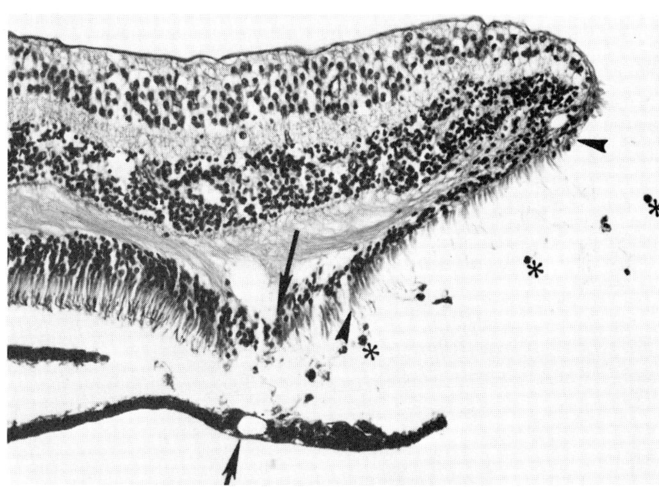

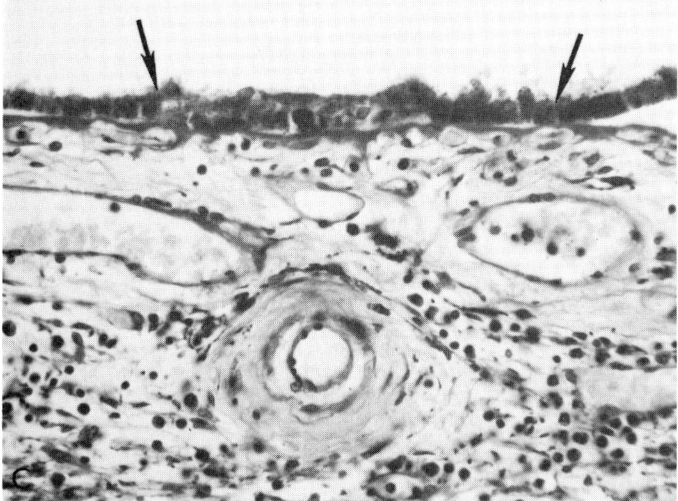

Figure 8–395 *Continued C,* Top left, Gross appearance of macular hole in left eye. Top right, Margin of hole showing artifactitiously separated point of demarcation with retinal-RPE adhesion (between arrows), an area of retinal detachment with partial loss of photoreceptor cell layer (between arrowheads), and separated, pigment-containing cells internal to the RPE (asterisks). PAS, ×210. Bottom left, Minor RPE alteration (between arrows) in area of macular hole. Subjacent choroid contains leukemic cell infiltration. PAS, × 330. EP 51056.

(From Frangieh GT, Green WR, Engel HM: A histopathologic study of macular cysts and holes. Retina *1*:311–336, 1981.)

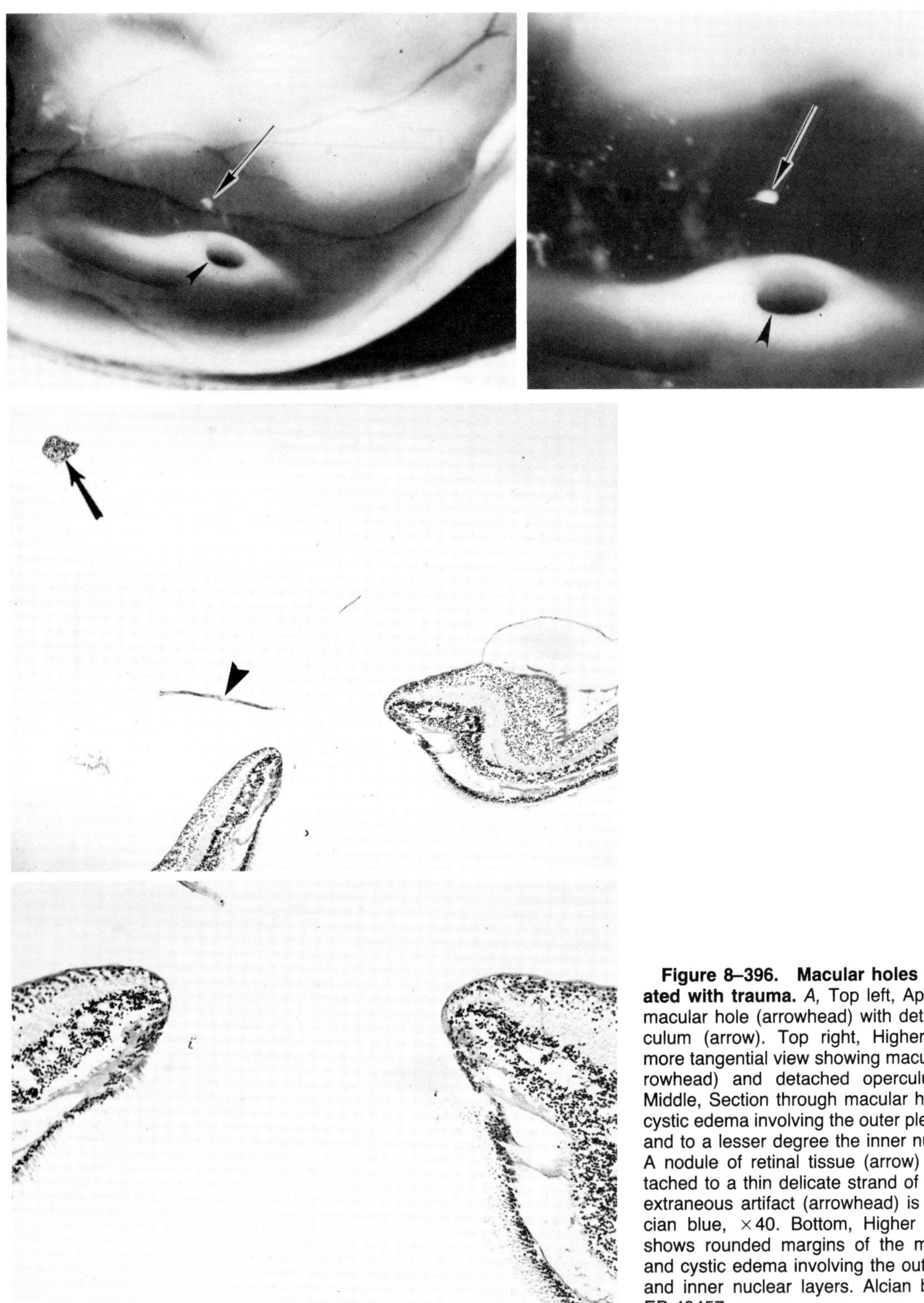

Figure 8–396. Macular holes not associated with trauma. *A,* Top left, Appearance of macular hole (arrowhead) with detached operculum (arrow). Top right, Higher-power and more tangential view showing macular hole (arrowhead) and detached operculum (arrow). Middle, Section through macular hole showing cystic edema involving the outer plexiform layer and to a lesser degree the inner nuclear layer. A nodule of retinal tissue (arrow) remains attached to a thin delicate strand of vitreous. An extraneous artifact (arrowhead) is present. Alcian blue, ×40. Bottom, Higher power view shows rounded margins of the macular hole and cystic edema involving the outer plexiform and inner nuclear layers. Alcian blue, ×105. EP 48457.

Illustration continued on opposite page

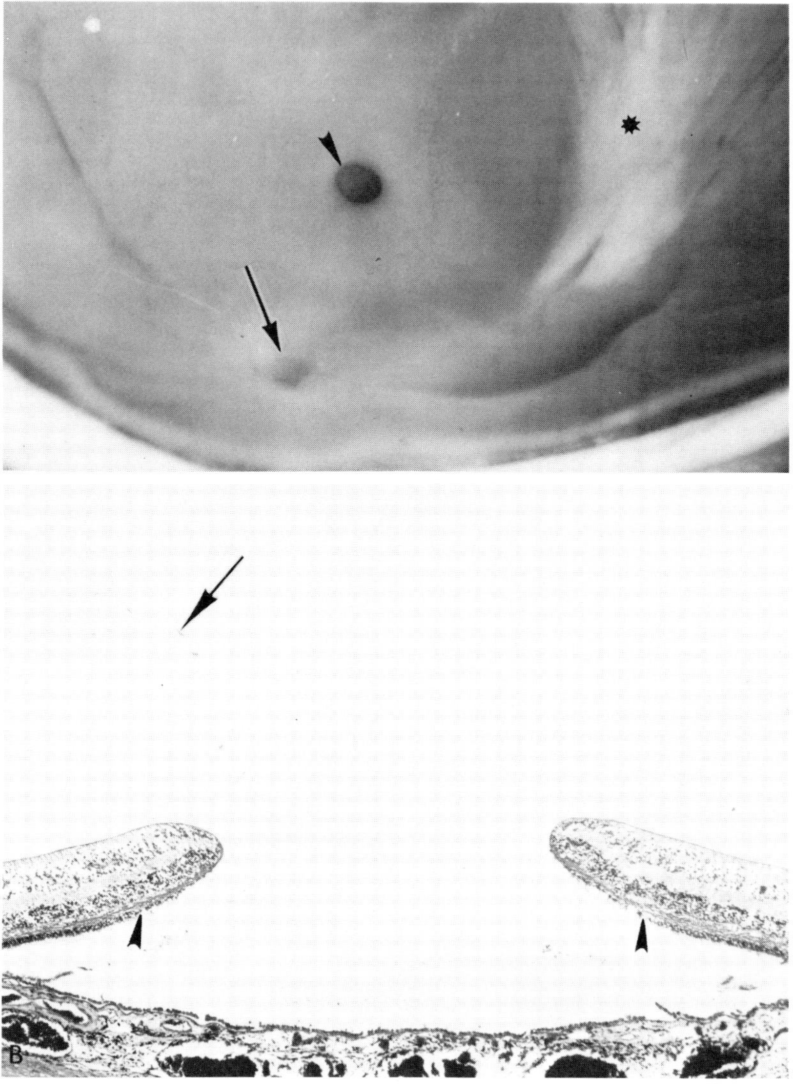

Figure 8–396 *Continued B,* Top, Gross appearance showing disk (arrow), macular hole (arrowhead), and myelinated nerve fibers (asterisk). Bottom, Section through hole showing a delicate strand of vitreous (arrow), which extends down to the area of the macular hole but is not connected to retina. A surrounding area of retinal detachment is evidenced by partial photoreceptor cell degeneration (arrowheads). H and E, ×45. EP 49373.

(From Frangieh GT, Green WR, Engel HM: A histopathologic study of macular cysts and holes. Retina *1*:311–336, 1981.)

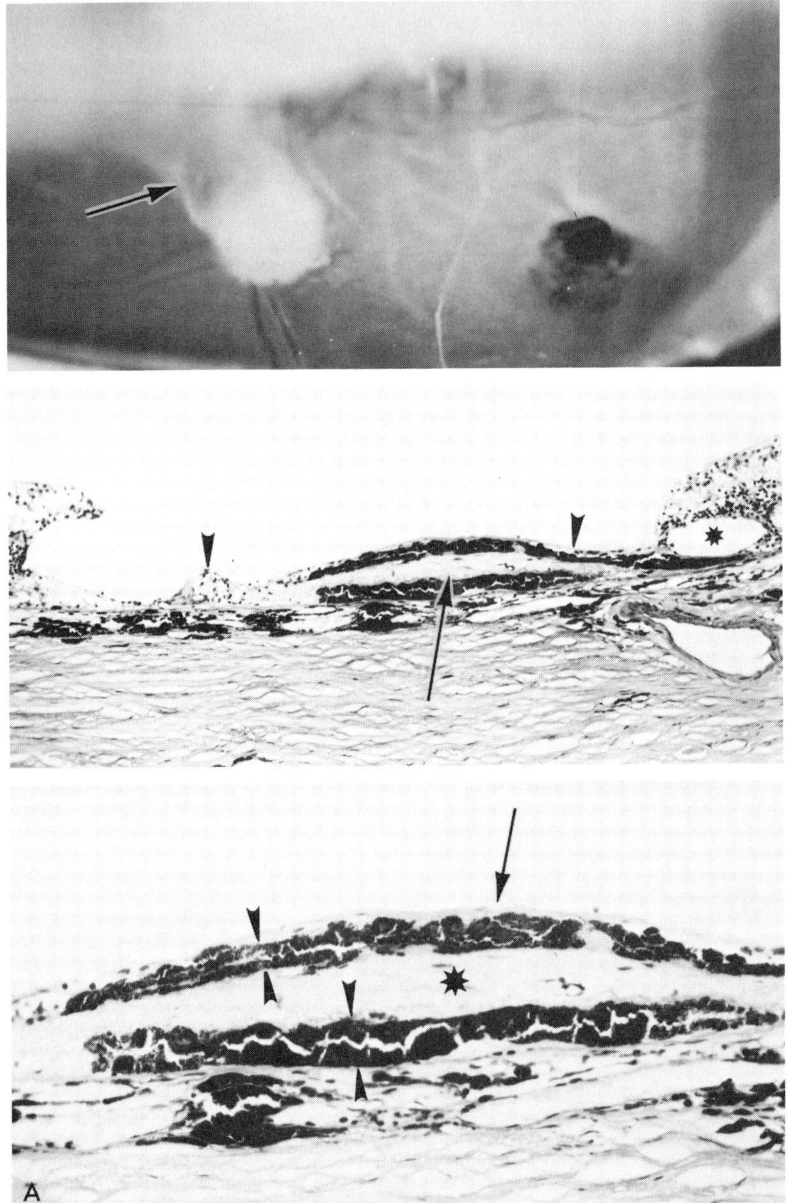

Figure 8–397. Lamellar macular holes associated with trauma. *A,* Top, Gross appearance of macular hole with pigmentation. Vitreous is detached except at the optic nerve head (arrow). Middle, Section through lamellar macular hole showing a thin layer of retinal tissue (arrowheads) lining a small disciform scar (arrow). Cystic edema in outer plexiform layer (asterisk) is present. Retinal pigment epithelium (RPE) areolar atrophy is also noted. PAS, ×100. Bottom, Higher power view of disciform scar shows it to be composed of a layer of fibrous tissue (asterisk) located between two layers of hyperplastic RPE arranged in a double-layered configuration (between arrowheads). A thin layer of retinal tissue (arrow) lies internal to the disciform scar. PAS, ×200. EP 30981.

Illustration continued on opposite page

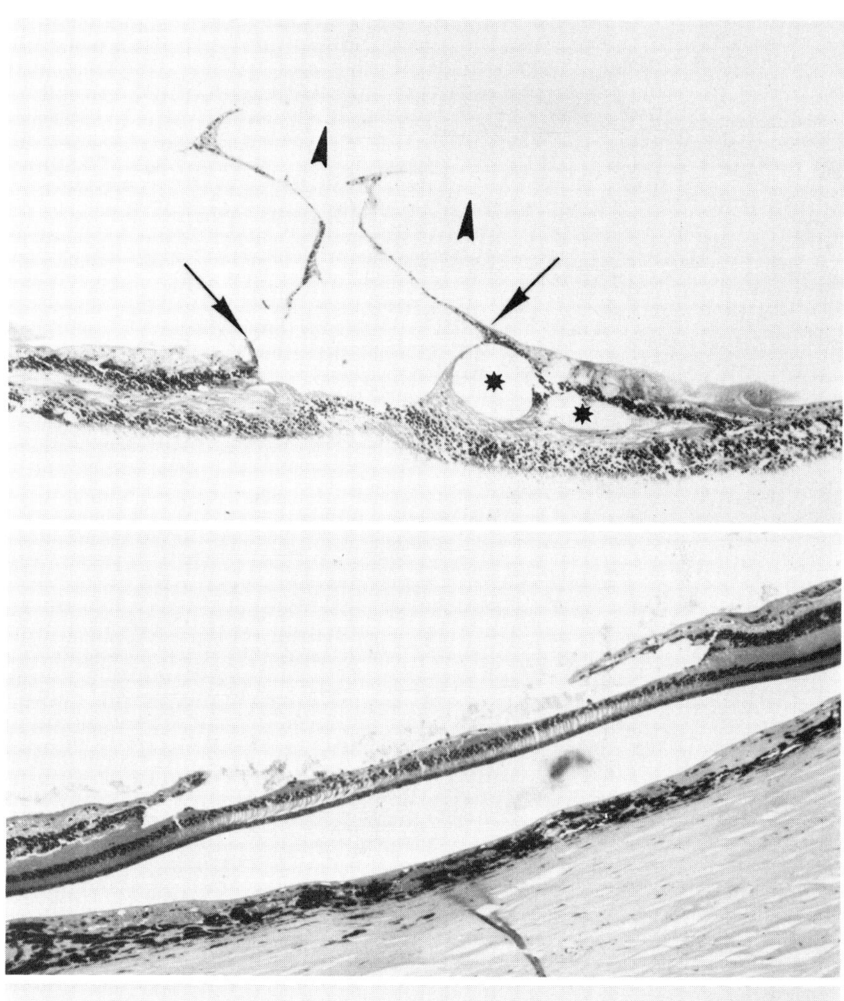

Figure 8–397 *Continued B,* Top, Section of macular shows an inner lamellar macular hole (between arrows), with strands of vitreous (arrowheads) attached to margins of the hole. Cystic spaces (asterisks) are present. H and E, ×65. EP 44228. Middle, Section through lamellar macular hole. RPE and photoreceptor cells are intact. There is extreme glaucomatous atrophy, with loss of nerve fiber and ganglion cell layers. H and E, ×75. EP 51852. Bottom, Section through a lamellar macular hole (asterisk). A fibroglial preretinal membrane (arrowheads) is present on either side. PAS, ×115. EP 48459.

(From Frangieh GT, Green WR, Engel HM: A histopathologic study of macular cysts and holes. Retina *1*:311–336, 1981.)

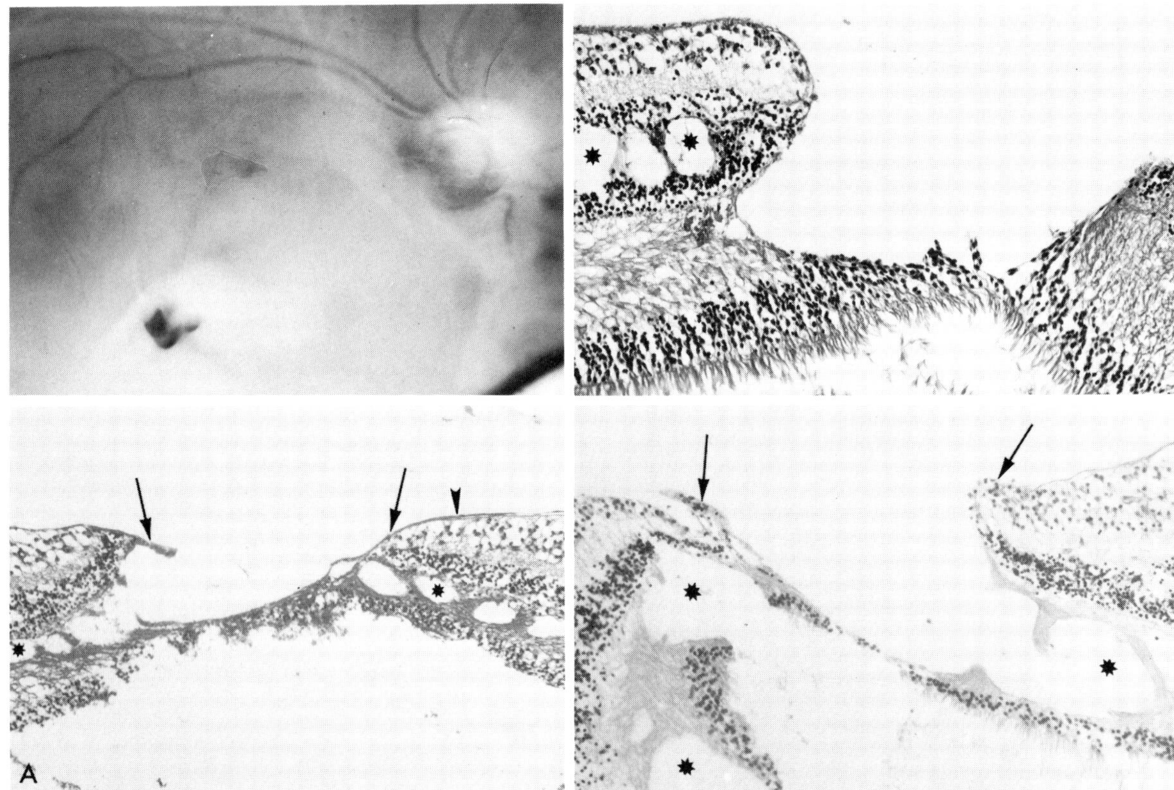

Figure 8–398. Lamellar macular holes unassociated with trauma. *A,* Upper left, Gross appearance of irregular lamellar macular hole. Upper right, Section through lamellar macular hole showing cystic edema (asterisk) involving the inner nuclear layer. H and E, ×185. EP 48036. Bottom left, Lamellar macular hole (between arrows) associated with a thin, preretinal membrane (arrowhead) and cystic edema involving the outer plexiform layer. H and E, ×100. EP 49373. Bottom right, Lamellar macular hole (between arrows) associated with cysts (asterisks) in the outer plexiform layer, associated with a small serous detachment of the retinal pigment epithelium (RPE). PAS, ×140. EP 46139.

Illustration continued on opposite page

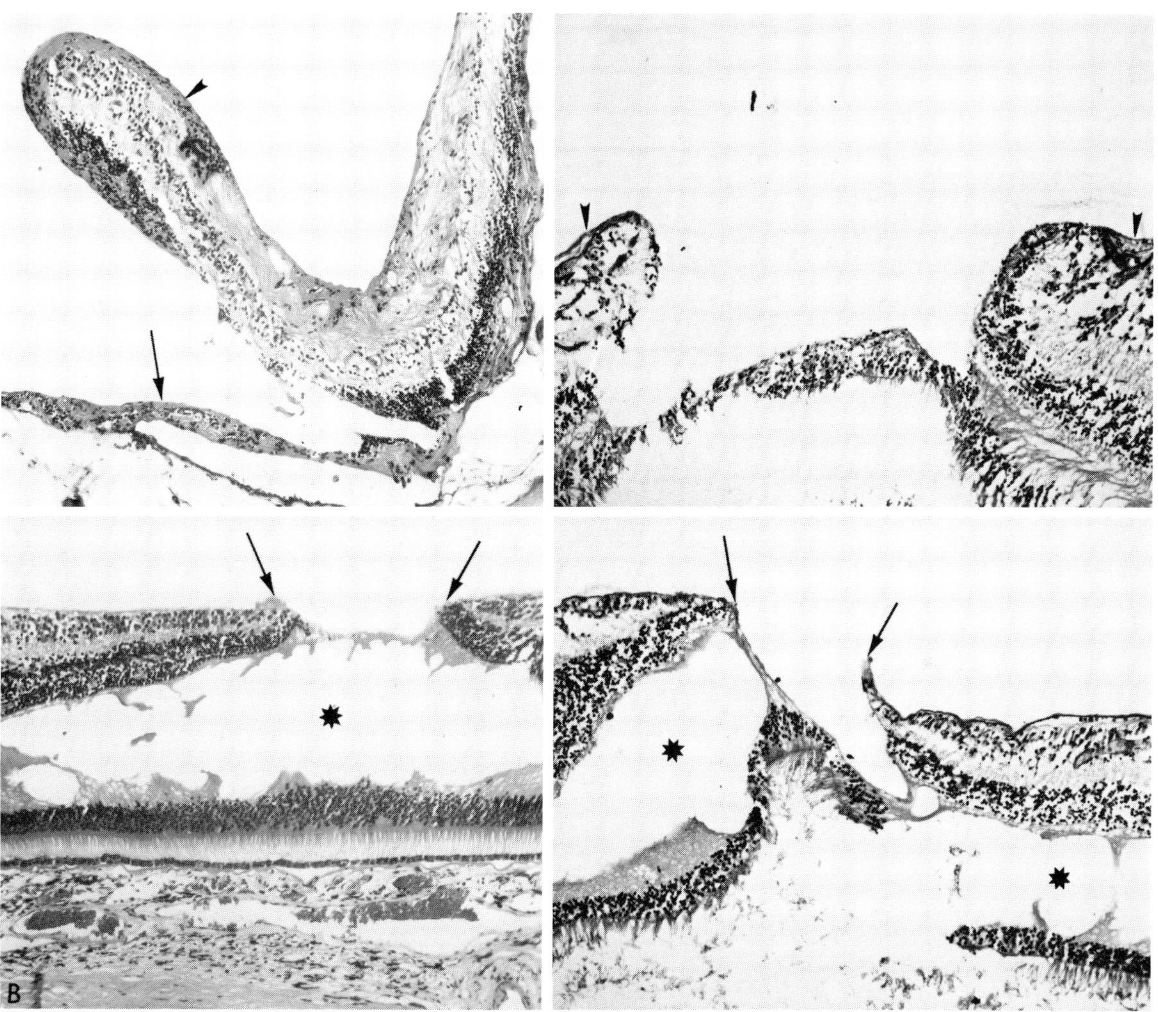

Figure 8–398 *Continued* B, Top left, Section through lamellar macular hole showing a thicker inner layer (arrowhead) and a thin gliotic outer layer (arrow). H and E, ×90. EP 50043. Top right, Lamellar macular hole with associated preretinal membrane (arrowheads). PAS, ×100. 40568. Lower left, Area showing a small inner lamellar macular hole (between arrows) and a large area of cystic edema–retinoschisis (asterisk). RPE is intact. H and E, ×100. EP 52986. Lower right, Small lamellar macular hole (between arrows) associated with extensive cystoid edema (asteriks) involving the outer plexiform layer. PAS, ×120. EP 49746.

(From Frangieh GT, Green WR, Engel HM: A histopathologic study of macular cysts and holes. Retina *1*:311–336, 1981.)

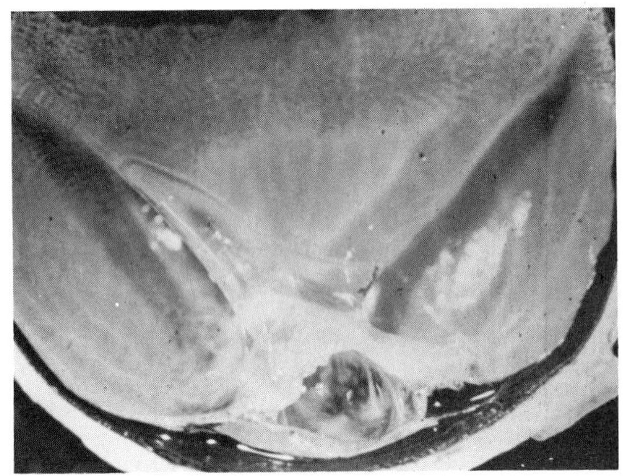

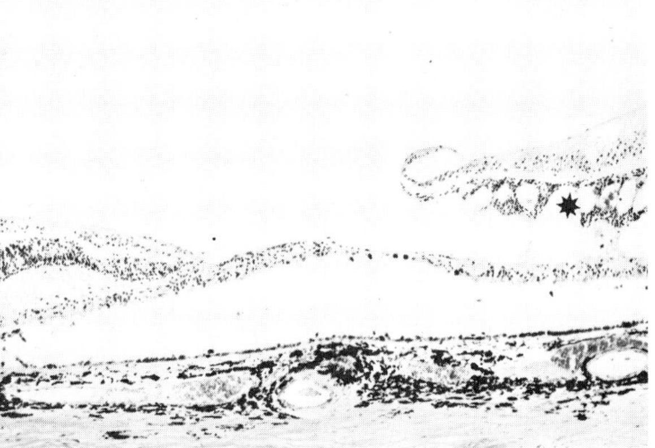

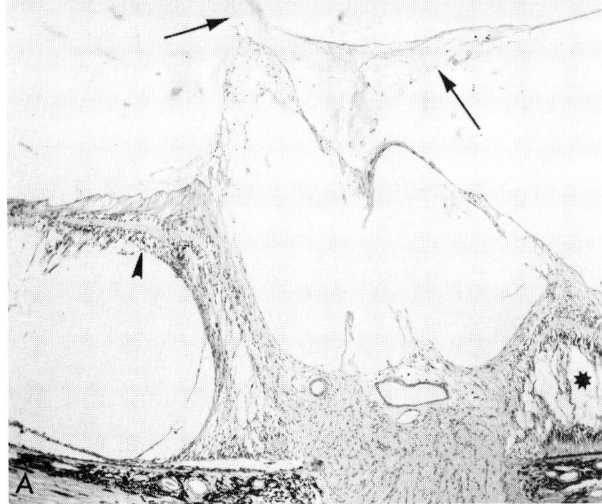

Figure 8–399. Lamellar macular holes unassociated with trauma. *A,* Top left, Gross appearance of partial posterior vitreous detachment and traction effects on retina. Top right, Macular area with lamellar hole and cystic edema involving the inner nuclear (asterisk) and outer plexiform layers. The underlying retinal pigment epithelium (RPE) is irregular and shows areas of hypo- and hyperpigmentation. H and E, ×65. Lower left, Neovascular tissue (arrows) at optic nerve head inducing tractional cystic degeneration (asterisk) and tractional retinal detachment (arrowhead). PAS, ×30. EP 37625.

Illustration continued on opposite page

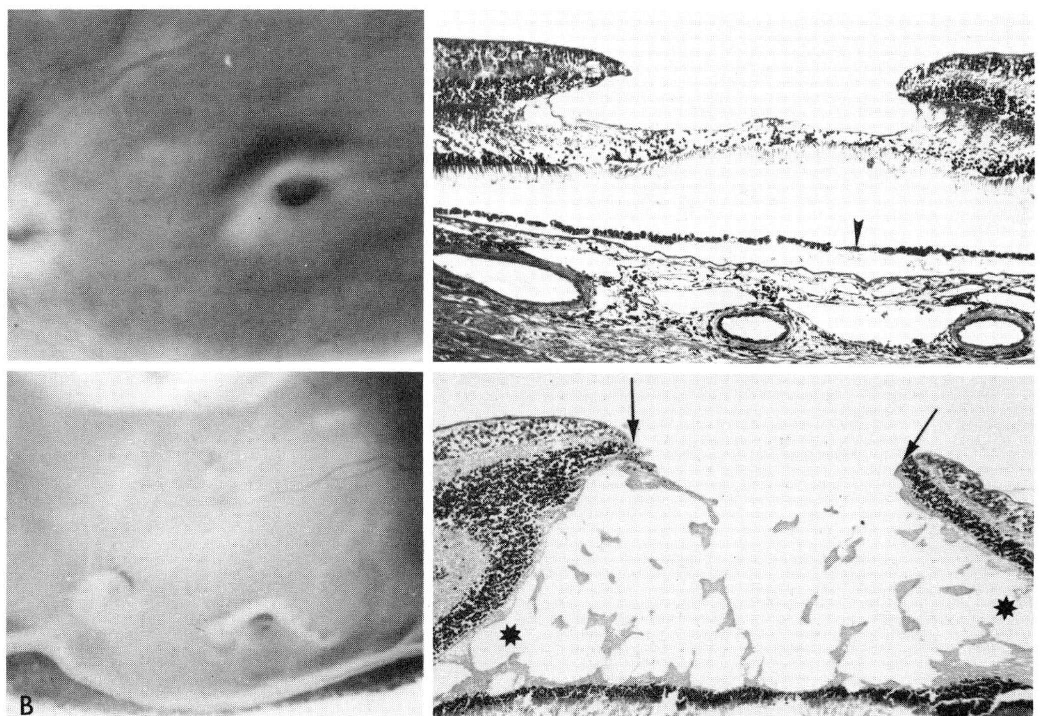

Figure 8–399 *Continued B,* Top left, Gross appearance of lamellar macular hole. Top right, Lamellar macular hole. Intact retina consists of partially degenerated photoreceptor cell layer. RPE is artifactitiously detached. It shows areas of hypopigmentation (arrowhead). H and E, ×100. EP 50046. Bottom left, Gross appearance of lamellar macular hole. Bottom right, Microscopic appearance of lamellar macular hole (between arrows) continuous with extensive cystic degeneration (asterisks) in outer plexiform layer. PAS, × 90. EP 47170.

(From Frangieh GT, Green WR, Engel HM: A histopathologic study of macular cysts and holes. Retina *1*:311–336, 1981.)

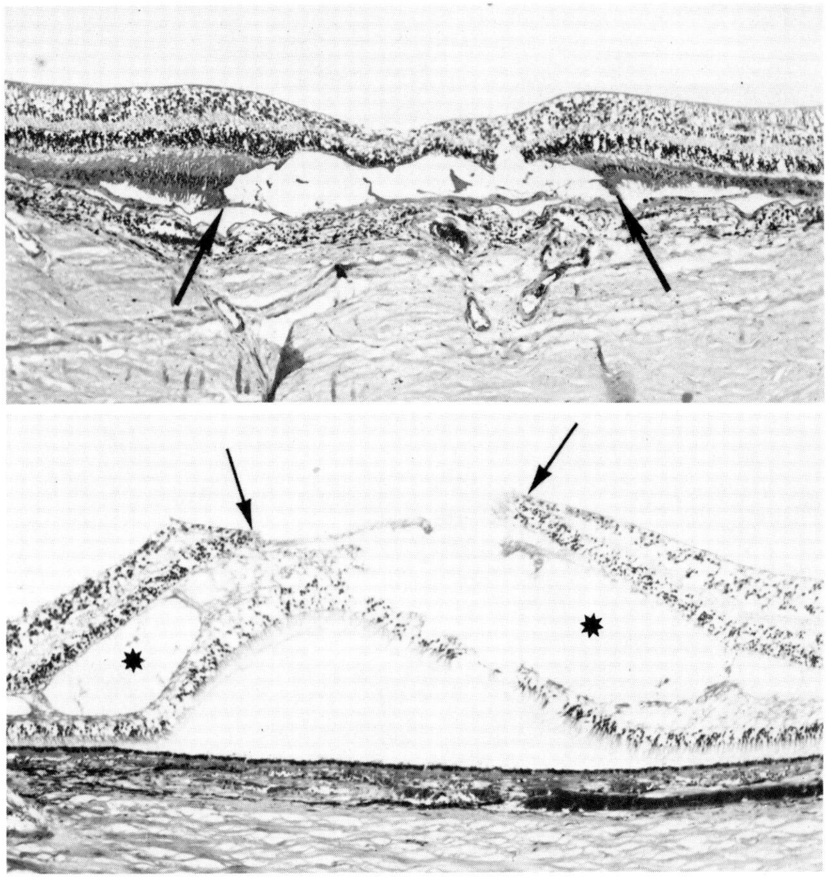

Figure 8–400. Macular cysts associated with trauma. Top, Area near center of macula showing loss of photoreceptor cell and outer plexiform layers (between arrows) associated with retinal pigment epithelium (RPE) atrophy. H and E, ×50. EP 52775. Bottom, Inner lamellar defect (between arrows) associated with marked cystoid changes in outer plexiform layer (asterisk). RPE is intact. H and E, ×75. EP 43245. (From Frangieh GT, Green WR, Engel HM: A histopathologic study of macular cysts and holes. Retina *1*:311–336, 1981.)

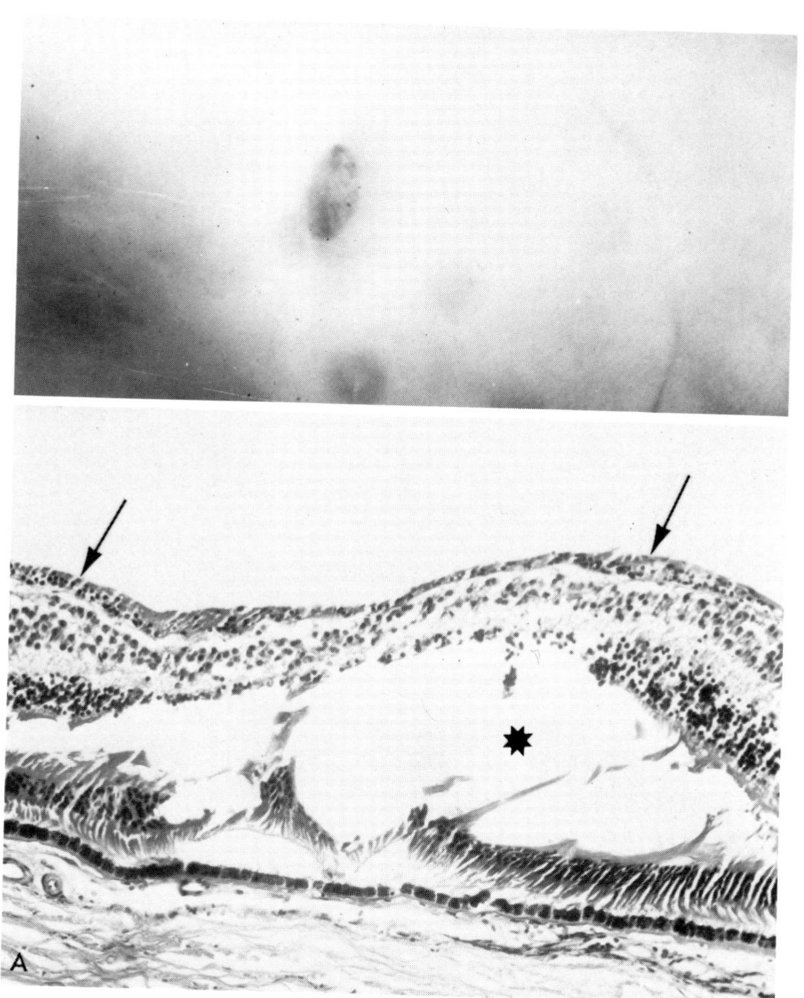

Figure 8–401. Macular cysts unassociated with trauma. *A*, Top, Gross appearance of macular lesion that was macroscopically thought to be a hole but was found histopathologically to be a cyst. Bottom, Cyst (asterisk) in outer plexiform layer associated with extensive fibrocellular preretinal membrane (arrows) and intact retinal pigment epithelium. H and E, ×145. EP 46885.

Illustration continued on following page

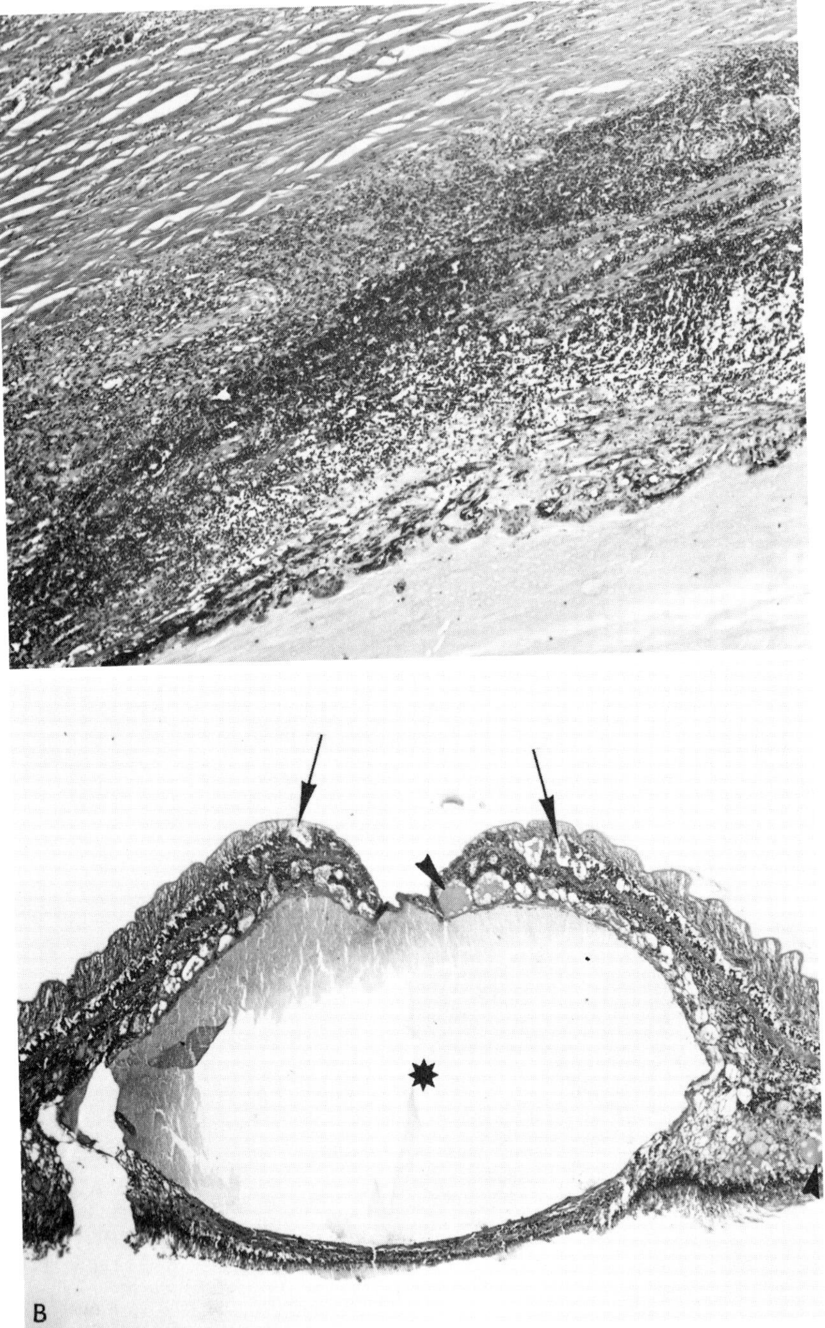

Figure 8–401 *Continued B,* Top, Ciliary body with intense lymphocytic infiltration. H and E, ×55. Bottom, Section through center of macula showing large cyst filled with a proteinaceous material (asterisk) Small cysts are present in outer plexiform (arrowheads) and ganglion cell (arrows) layers. H and E, ×40. EP 43854.

Illustration continued on opposite page

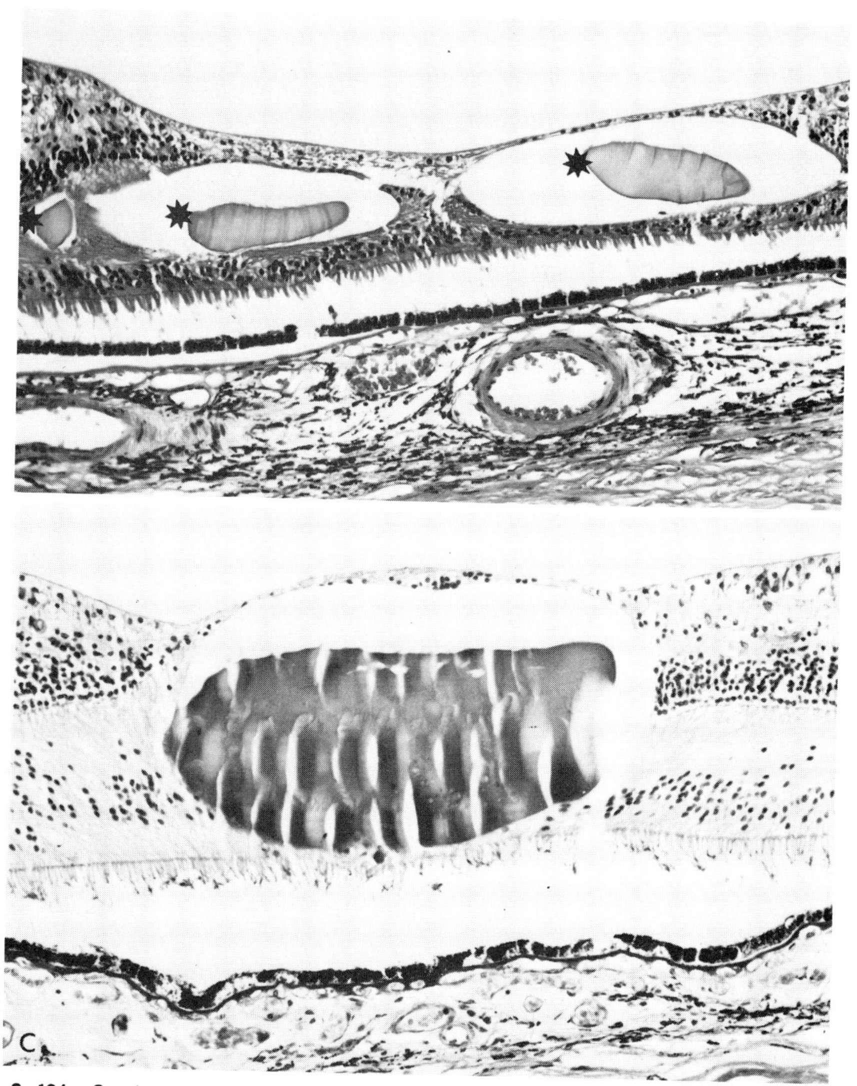

Figure 8–401 *Continued C,* Top, Two large and one small macular cysts (asterisks) filled with proteinaceous material. H and E, ×140. EP 50247. Bottom, Cyst is filled with a dense proteinaceous material and is limited anteriorly and posteriorly by thin retinal layers. PAS, ×160. EP 48820.
(From Frangieh GT, Green WR, Engel HM: A histopathologic study of macular cysts and holes. Retina *1*:311–336, 1981.)

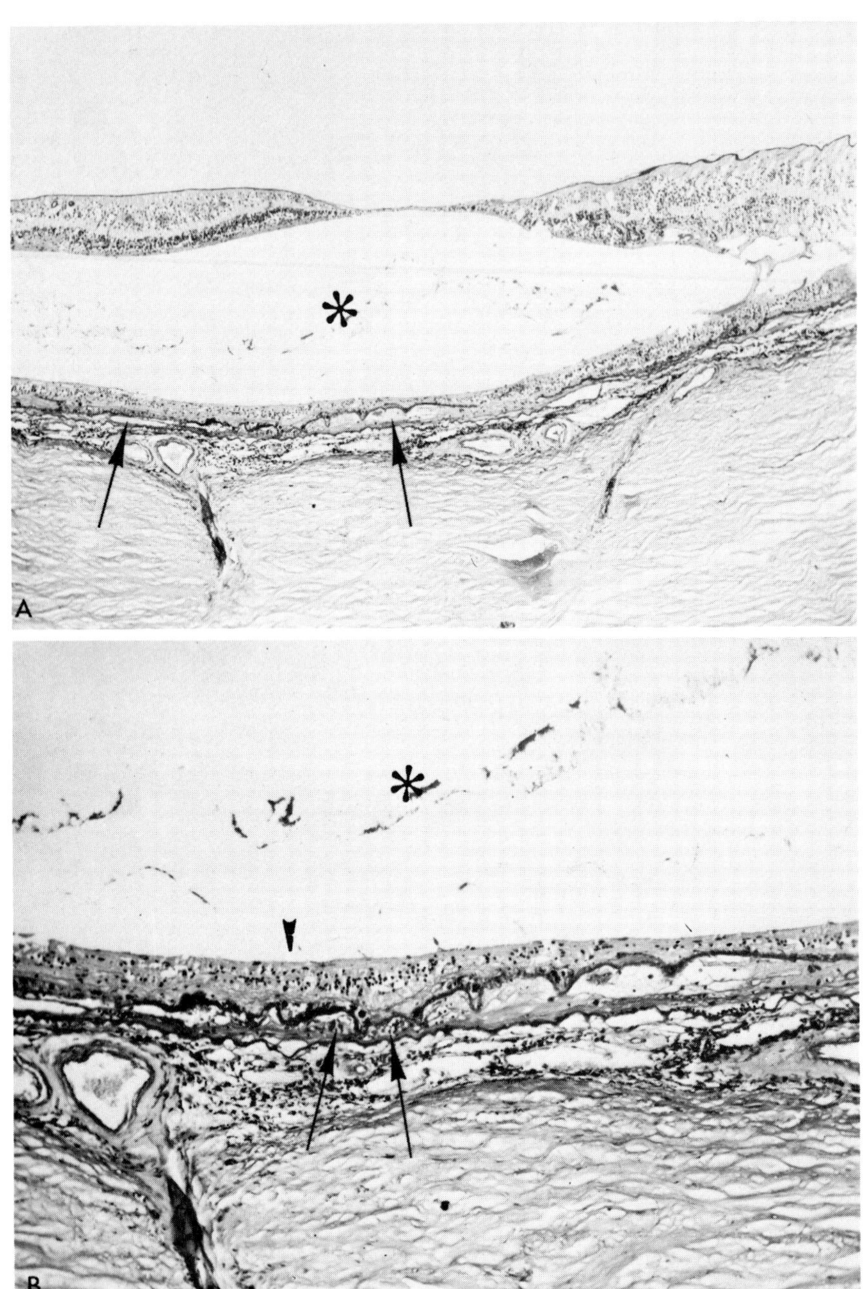

Figure 8–402. *A,* Large macular **cyst-schisis** (asterisk) with areolar retinal pigment epithelium (RPE) atrophy and intra–Bruch's membrane vascularization (arrows). PAS, ×35. *B,* Higher power view shows cystic cavity (asterisk), outer layer of retina (arrowhead), loss of RPE and photoreceptor cell layers, and intra–Bruch's membrane neovascularization (arrows). PAS, ×90. EP 44443. (From Frangieh GT, Green WR, Engel HM: A histopathologic study of macular cysts and holes. Retina *1*:311–336, 1981.)

39 patients with either lamellar macular holes (17 eyes), full-thickness macular holes (18 eyes), or macular cysts (9 eyes). These cases were classified into macular holes with trauma (Figs. 8–392 through 8–394); macular holes unassociated with trauma (Figs. 8–395 and 8–396); lamellar macular holes associated with trauma (Figs. 8–397 through 8–399); lamellar macular holes unassociated with trauma (Fig. 8–399); macular cysts associated with trauma (Fig. 8–400); and macular cysts unassociated with trauma (Figs. 8–401 and 8–402). Lamellar and full-thickness holes were frequently found in eyes of patients with a history of trauma or ocular surgery. Diabetes mellitus was the most common condition associated with macular cysts (Figs. 8–398,*B*, top left and right; 8–399,*A*, and 8–401,*C*, bottom). Six lamellar holes, eight full-thickness holes, and one macular cyst developed on an idiopathic basis. Residual cystoid macular edema was the most prevalent accompanying pathologic feature. Cystoid macular edema also was noted in the opposite eye in seven cases of lamellar and full-thickness holes. A preretinal glial membrane, thought to be a secondary change, was found at or near the edges of the lamellar or full-thickness holes or over the macular cyst in the majority of cases. Wrinkling of the ILM was present in five cases. Vitreous traction, with or

without an operculum, was infrequently associated with these entities.

In a clinical study of 52 patients (39 women and 13 men; mean age: 65 years) with idiopathic macular cysts and holes, McDonnell, Fine, and Hillis (1982) noted the following features: 17 patients had bilateral involvement, half of the cysts progressed to holes, no holes developed in fellow eyes without cysts on the initial examination, posterior vitreous detachment was present in all eyes with holes and was intact in all eyes with cysts, posterior detachment of the vitreous developed in those eyes with cysts that developed holes, and 31 of the 39 women had undergone hysterectomy, had taken estrogens, or both.

Serous Detachment of Retinal Pigment Epithelium. This lesion of unknown cause affects an area of 0.5 to 2 disc diameters in size and persists for 2 to 3 months. It then subsides, leaving normal vision in more than 50 per cent of the patients. It affects young adults and may be unassociated with drusen or other features of senile

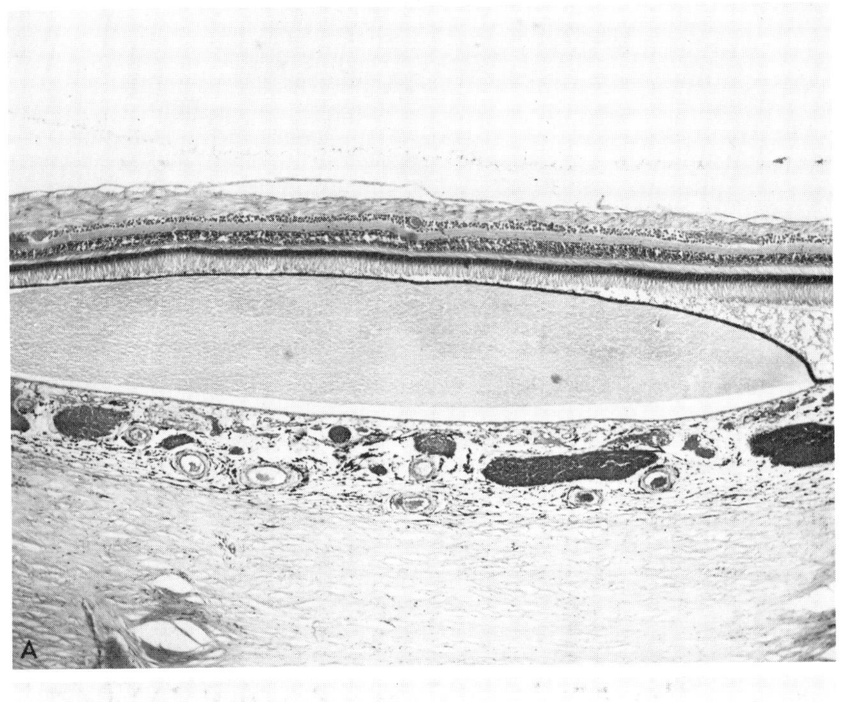

Figure 8–403. Serous detachment of retinal pigment epithelium (RPE) in a 46 year old woman with a 3 week history of reduced vision attributed to a **malignant melanoma** in the macular area. *A,* Flat, dome-shaped detachment of RPE by finely fibrillar and granular material. The overlying macular area shows preservation of photoreceptors and outer nuclear layer. H and E, ×35. *B,* Higher power view shows a thin membrane (basement membrane of RPE) (arrows) along with detached RPE. Outer segments are slightly degenerated, and rare macrophages (asterisk) are present in the vicinity of the outer segments of photoreceptors. EP 5397. (From Maumenee AE; case presented at the Ophthalmic Pathology Club, Washington, DC, April, 1948.)

macular degeneration. Serous detachment of the RPE can occur in the context of senile macular degeneration (see page 987).

This detachment most often is unilateral and affects men four times more frequently than women. If the serous elevation persists for a long period (for instance, over 6 months), secondary macular degeneration often occurs. The ophthalmoscopic appearance is typical, with a moundlike elevation. Fluorescein angiography shows that the lesion lights up early and stains late. Microscopically, there is an accumulation of serous fluid between Bruch's membrane and the RPE and its basement membrane (Maumenee, 1959—Fig. 8–403; Zimmerman, 1969—Fig. 8–404). The case studied by Zimmerman showed detachment of some drusen, along with RPE, and some accumulation of serous material under the neurosensory retina (Fig. 8–404). The choroid appeared normal, and there was no inflammation. Except in prolonged cases, the retinal receptors are normal, and the retina itself shows no evidence of edema or degeneration.

The cause of this serous outpouring of fluid is not known. In some cases there may be associated hemorrhage, which suggests that choroidal neovascularization may be a factor in such eyes.

Hemorrhagic Detachment of RPE (Hematoma of RPE). This lesion apparently can occur in middle age and is unassociated with features of senile macular degeneration (Fig. 8–405) (Reese and Jones, 1961, 1962; Tredici and Fenton, 1964).

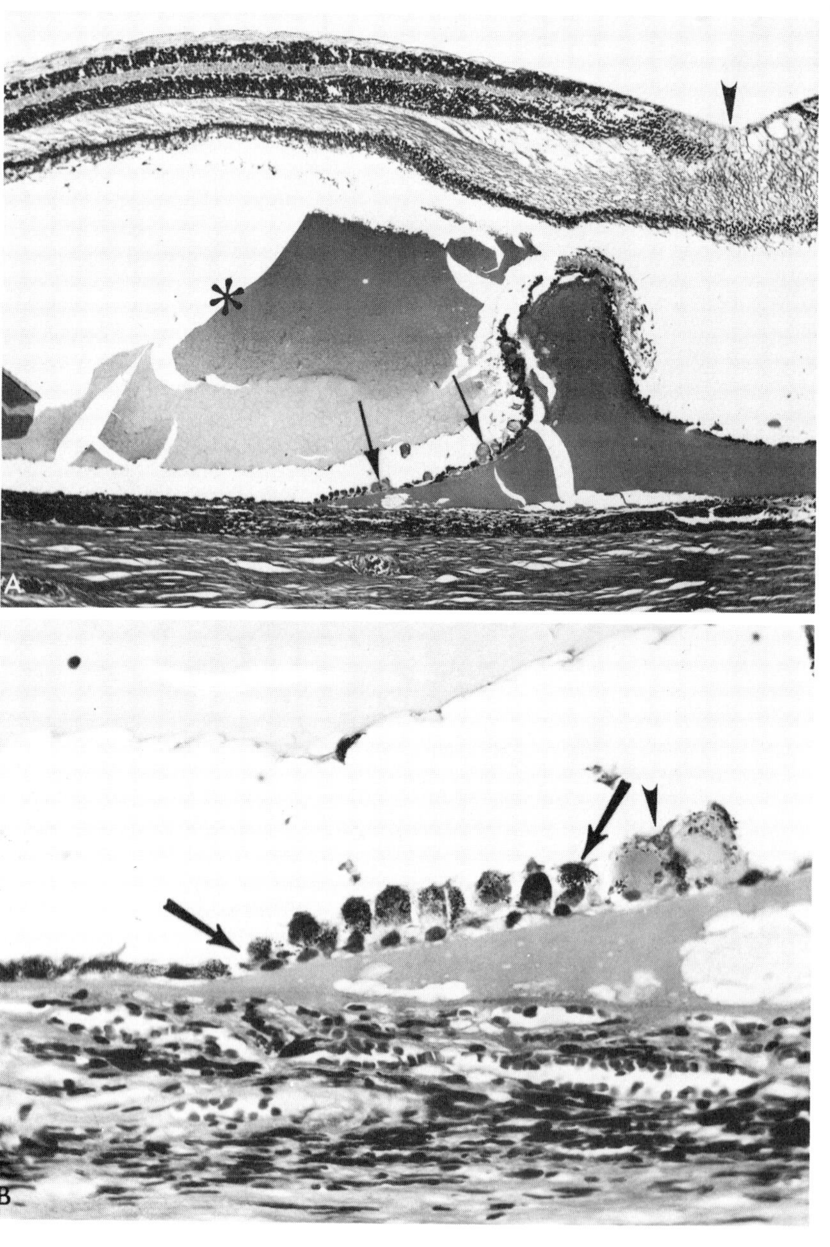

Figure 8–404. Combined serous detachment of retinal pigment epithelium (RPE) and neurosensory retina in macula. *A,* Section near foveola (arrowhead), showing proteinaceous material under retina (asterisk) and RPE. Drusen (arrows) are also detached along with the RPE. Outer segments of photoreceptor cells are degenerated. H and E, ×50. AFIP Neg. 69-3992. *B,* Higher power view at margin of serous RPE detachment shows Bruch's membrane, hypertrophic RPE (between arrows) and detached drusen (arrowhead). H and E, ×305. AFIP Neg. 69-3994. AFIP 1306261. (From Zimmerman LE; case presented at Verhoeff Society, Washington, DC, April, 1969.)

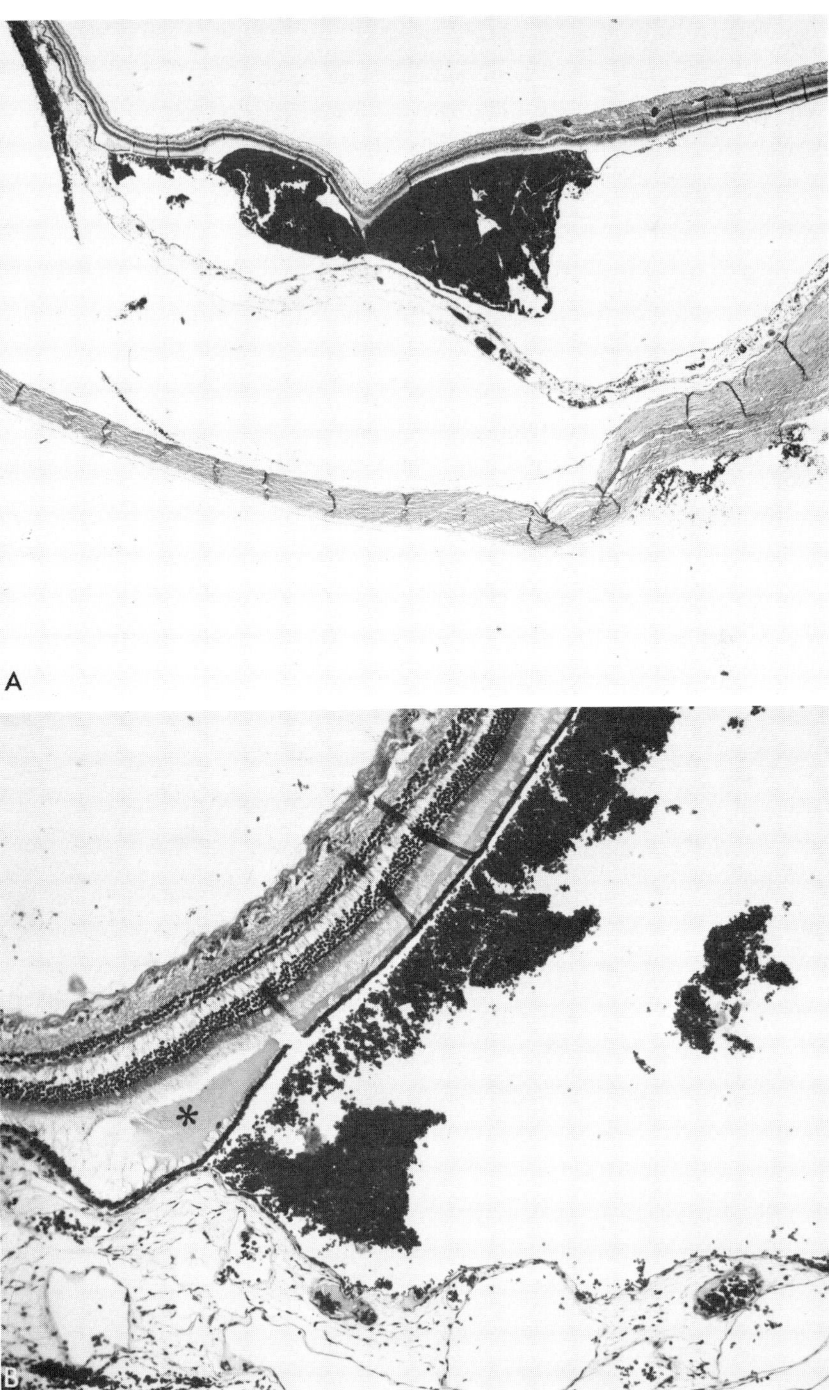

Figure 8–405. Hemorrhagic detachment of retinal pigment epithelium. (RPE) *A,* Two mounds of RPE detached by blood. H and E, ×13. *B,* Higher power view of margin of lesions. A small serous detachment of the retina is present (asterisk). H and E, ×100. (Courtesy of Dr. M.J. Reeh. Case presented at Verhoeff Society, Washington, DC, April, 1969.)

Most of these lesions are probably due to sub-RPE neovascularization. Reese and Jones (1962) felt that the hemorrhage had its origin from subretinal pigment neovascularization in the peripapillary area in the 34 eyes they studied. Serial sections or evaluation of stepped sections is necessary to rule out associated choroidal neovascularization.

Central Serous Chorioretinopathy (Central Serous Retinopathy). This is a serous detachment of the macular retina associated with a RPE defect that characteristically affects healthy young adults between 20 and 40 years of age. Men are affected more commonly than women, and often a history of emotional stress accompanies the onset of the visual complaint. Metamorphopsia, positive scotoma, micropsia, and blurring of vision are the most common complaints. These patients have a delayed retinal recovery time after exposure to bright light. Visual acuity is often only moderately decreased and may be improved to near normal with a small hyperopic correction.

The lesion usually disappears spontaneously within 3 to 4 months. A slight degree of metamorphopsia, a decrease in brightness, and an alteration in color vision may persist for many months and may be permanent. Visual acuity tends to return to normal.

Fluorescein angiography typically shows a small defect or area of detachment of the RPE, which may leak in a "smokestack" configuration into the area of subretinal serous exudation. Late fluorescein phases may outline lightly the entire area of serous retinal detachment. The area of RPE detachment may be quite large in some cases. After resolution of the macular detachment, the angiographic findings may return to normal or show a mottled pattern of hyperfluorescence early, with no late staining. This pattern is presumably due to partial loss of pigment from the RPE cell (RPE window defect).

Histopathologic studies have demonstrated a serous detachment of the macular retina (Klien, 1961; Fry and Spaeth, 1955; Ikui, 1969), but the RPE detachment or defect has escaped morphologic study.

The efficacy of laser photocoagulation for treating the RPE detachment and leakage site, when it is located outside the foveal area, has not been clearly established. Robertson and Ilstrup (1983) observed that direct laser photocoagulation of the retinal pigment epithelial area of leakage shortened the duration of central serous chorioretinopathy by about 2 months. These investigators further noted that there were no recurrences within an 18 month period in the treated group, whereas a recurrence of 34 per cent was observed in the sham or indirect photocoagulation group of patients.

A condition quite similar to that observed in humans has been produced experimentally in the monkey by repeated injections of epinephrine (Yoshioka, Katsume, Akune, 1981, 1982). Ultrastructural studies of this model have shown degeneration of a localized area of retinal pigment epithelial cells associated with damaged endothelial cells of the subjacent choriocapillaris. The region of these endothelial cell defects was covered with plateletfibrin clots (Yoshioka, Katsume, 1982).

Macy and Baerveldt (1983) have observed the association of serous detachment of the macular retina with a pin-point area of RPE defect with extracapsular cataract extraction and placement of a posterior chamber intraocular lens.

Serous Detachment of Macular Retina Associated with a Pit of Optic Nerve Head. Congenital pits or small colobomas of the optic nerve head are an important congenital abnormality to recognize, because of the occasional associated serous detachment of the macular retina—often with a central serous appearance. The serous detachment may wax or wane and undergo spontaneous resolutions, making the effects of therapy difficult to evaluate. Kranenburg (1960) outlined the clinical features, as gleaned from the literature and a report of 24 additional cases. The condition is also important because the macular detachment has been confused with malignant melanoma (Ferry, 1963).

In a clinical study of 75 eyes with a congenital pit of the optic nerve head, Brown, Shields, and Goldberg (1980) found a retinal detachment in 52 per cent of all eyes and a 63 per cent incidence of retinal detachment in those eyes with a temporally located pit.

Histopathologic studies (Ferry, 1963) have shown a defect in the lamina cribrosa that, in part, is filled with fibroglial tissue. One of Ferry's specimens (Case 7) showed only a loose fibrillar tissue separating the pit and the subretinal space (Fig. 8–406). In patients with long-standing macular detachment, partial degeneration of the photoreceptor cells and cystic degeneration of the macula were observed.

The mechanism of the macular detachment is not agreed upon and has been attributed to various types of mechanical, vascular, and radiational strain and fever (Kranenburg, 1960; Ferry, 1963); traction on the macula (Zimmerman, cited by Ferry, 1963); access of fluid from the vitreous via the pit to the subretinal space (Sugar, 1964); and access of cerebrospinal fluid to the subretinal space (Gass, 1969).

Brown, Shields, Patty, and Goldberg (1979) have studied a similar condition in dogs and found a small retinal break at the edge of the optic disc and pit. They believe that the fluid under the macula is derived from the vitreous cavity.

Photocoagulation at the edge of the disc has given variable results (Jack, 1969; Gass, 1969; Brockhurst, 1975; Theodossiadis, 1977).

Bull's Eye Macular Lesions. This is an interesting categorization of a doughnut-shaped or bull's eye configuration in the macular area that may be seen in a variety of unrelated conditions, including congenital cone dystrophy, fucosidosis, chloroquine toxicity, ceroid lipoproteinosis, benign concentric annular bull's eye macular dystrophy (Deutman, 1974), olivopontocerebellar degeneration (Duinkerke-Eerola, Cruysberg, Deutman, 1980), some cases of the areolar form of senile macular degeneration, the Sjögren-Larsson syndrome, retinal degeneration with acanthocytosis (Hallervorden-Spatz syndrome), some cases of retinitis pigmentosa, crystallin retinopathy due to presumed canthaxanthine toxicity, Sea-blue histiocytic disease (ophthalmoplegic dystonic lipidosis), and others. Most of these conditions are discussed elsewhere in this chapter.

Macular Lesions in the Presumed Ocular Histoplasmosis Syndrome. These disciform lesions (Key, Green, Maumenee, 1977; Meredith, Green, Key, et al, 1977; Makley, Craig, Long, 1977;

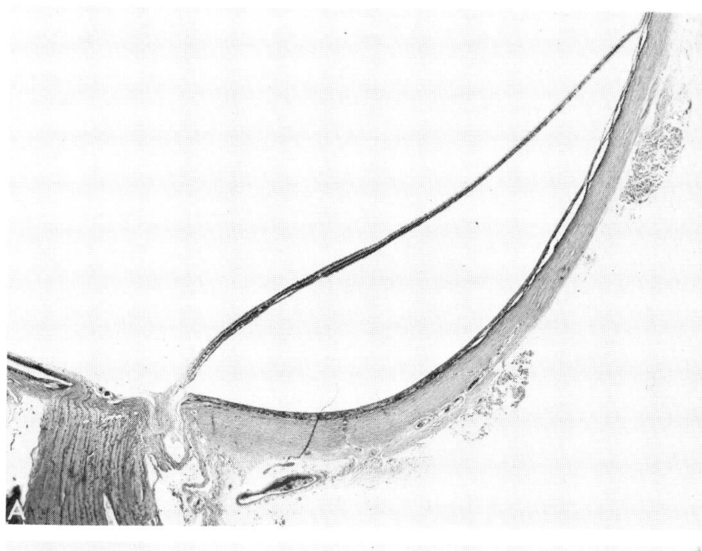

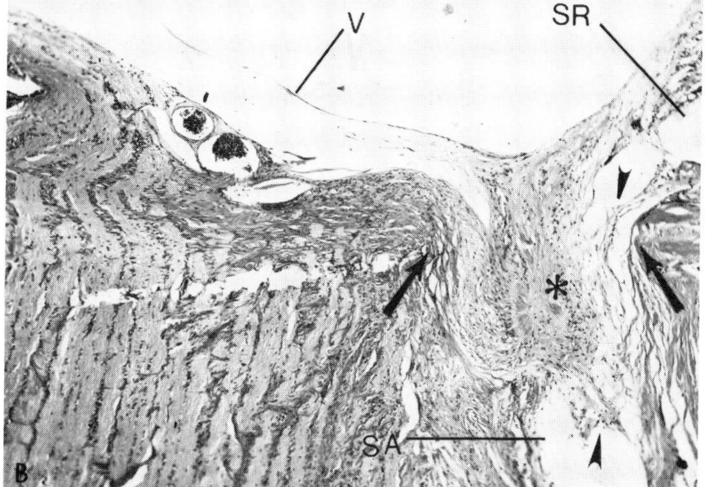

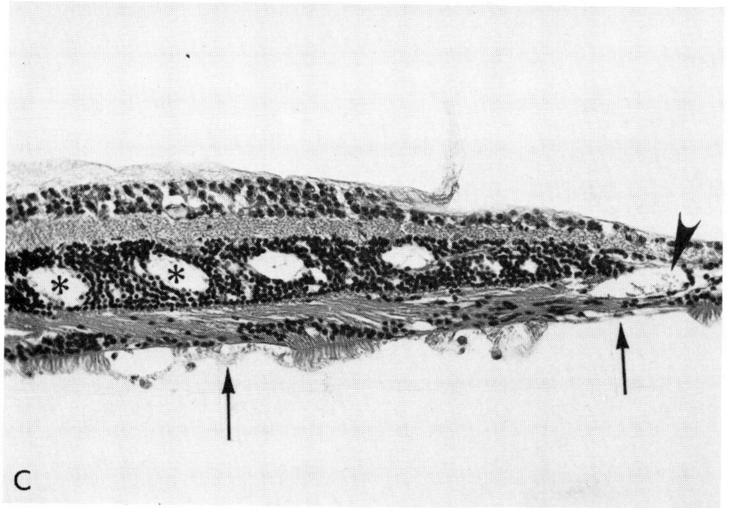

Figure 8–406. Pit of optic nerve head with **detachment of retina** in a 29 year old woman thought clinically to have a malignant melanoma. *A,* Low-power view showing a defect at the temporal margin of the optic nerve head. A fibrocellular tissue partially fills the defect. The retina is detached temporally, from the nerve head to near the equator. H and E, ×8. AFIP Neg. 62-2328. *B,* Higher power view of the optic nerve head shows a lamina cribrosa defect (between arrows) filled in by fibroglial tissue (asterisk). Only a loose fibrocellular tissue separates subretinal *(SR)* and subarachnoid *(SA)* spaces at the most temporal margin of the defect. A delicate fibrocellular strand of vitreous *(V)* is attached to fibroglial tissue that fills the defect. H and E, ×50. AFIP Neg. 62-2327. *C,* Detached macular area showing cysts in outer plexiform (arrowhead) and inner nuclear layers (asterisks). Outer segments of photoreceptors are lost throughout, and there is irregular loss of inner segments and partial loss of outer nuclear layer (arrows). H and E, ×165. AFIP Neg. 62-6585. AFIP Acc. 1010495. (From Ferry AP: Macular detachment associated with congenital pit of optic nerve head. Arch Ophthalmol *70*:346–357, 1963.)

Sheffer, Green, Fine, Kincaid, 1980) are quite similar to those seen in senile macular degeneration but usually without the association of drusen. The active lesions develop at the site of an old healed chorioretinal scar. Within such scars there is a chorioretinal adhesion with minor fibrous and RPE proliferation associated with a discontinuity in Bruch's membrane. Five, ten, or fifteen years after the initial infection, the lesion changes because of an unknown stimulus. Choroidal vessels extend through a break in Bruch's membrane and give rise to a serous or hemorrhagic detachment of the RPE. This has been mistakenly categorized as an "active" lesion and has been equated with inflammation by some observers. Irvine, Spencer, Hogan, et al (1976) reported a case that showed an unusually prominent degree of choroidal inflammation, in which the fluorescein antibody technique was interpreted as showing immunohistopathologic staining for *Histoplasma* antigens, but no organisms were identified.

None of the other cases studied histopathologically have had any appreciable inflammatory cell component, except for early cases with a large granuloma in the choroid beneath the macular area (Fig. 8–407).

Multifocal choroidal granulomas with histoplasmic organisms present have been observed in an immunologically deficient patient (Klintworth, Hollingsworth, Lusman, Bradford, 1973). The organism has been observed in the eye in other atypical cases (Hoefnagels, Pijpers, 1967; Craig, Suie, 1974).

The sub-RPE hemorrhage stimulates fibrous tissue proliferation which in part is derived from the RPE (Sheffer, Green, Fine, Kincaid, 1980). The end stage is a disciform lesion that is, as

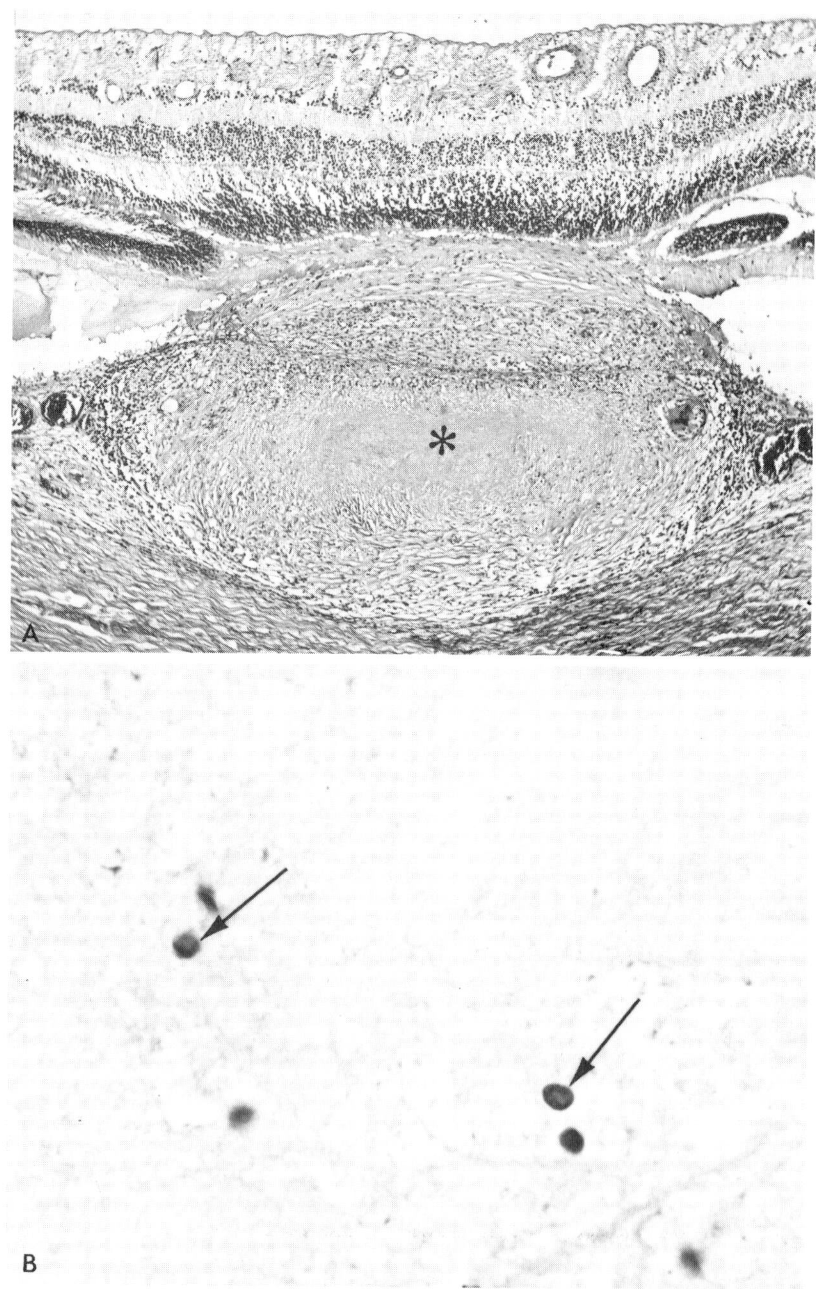

Figure 8–407. Macular lesion in right eye of a 21 year old man considered to have a malignant melanoma. Dr. Stephen J. Ryan examined the left eye years later and found typical features of the ocular histoplasmosis syndrome, including peripapillary lesions, a peripheral punched-out lesion, and one chorioretinal scar near the macula. *A,* Granuloma with central necrosis (asterisk) in submacular choroid. H and E, ×50. AFIP Neg. 66-2819. *B,* Organisms (arrows) consistent with *Histoplasma capsulatum* within granuloma. Gomori–methenamine silver, × 1260. AFIP Neg. 66-2814. AFIP 1180173. (Case originally studied by Drs. G. Naumann and L.E. Zimmerman.)

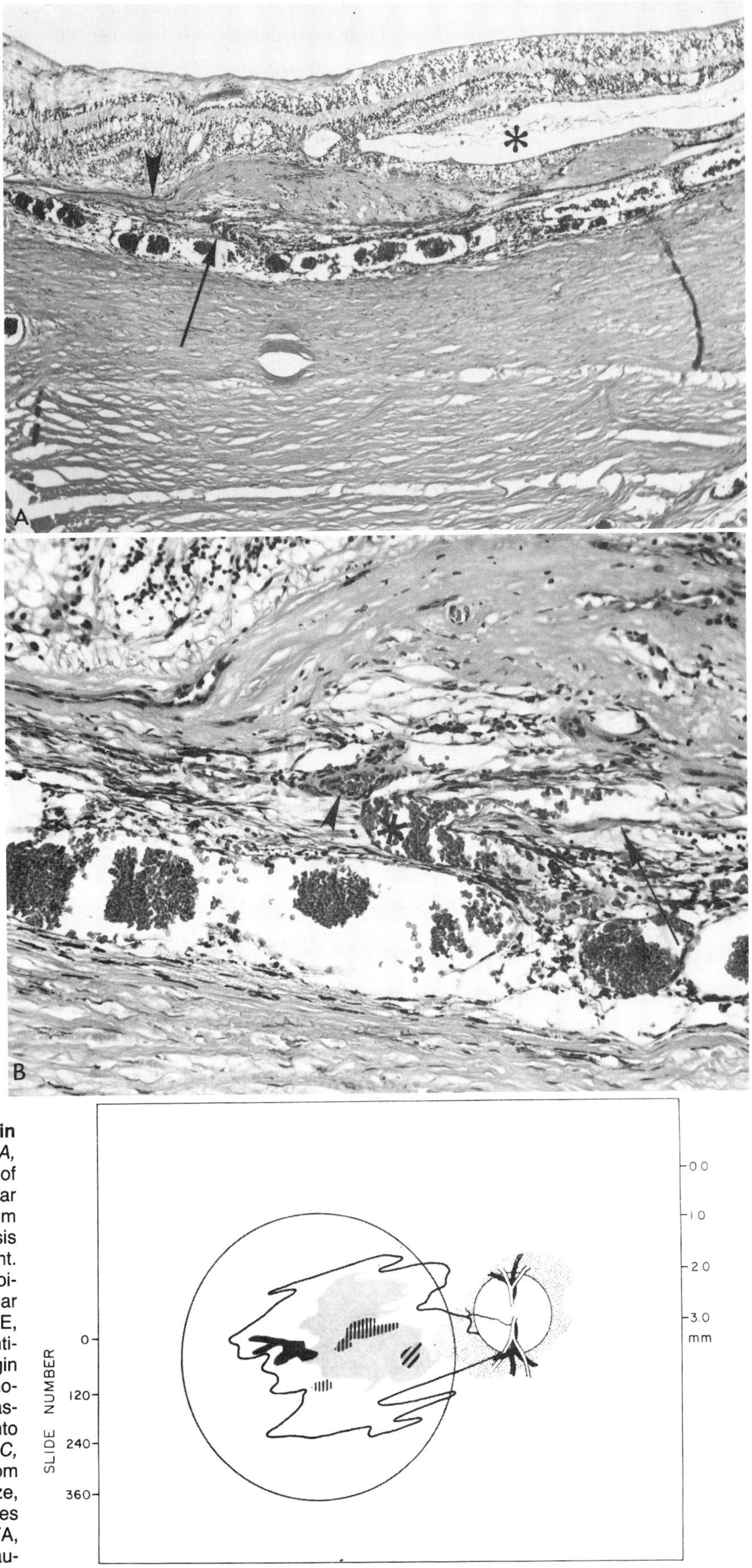

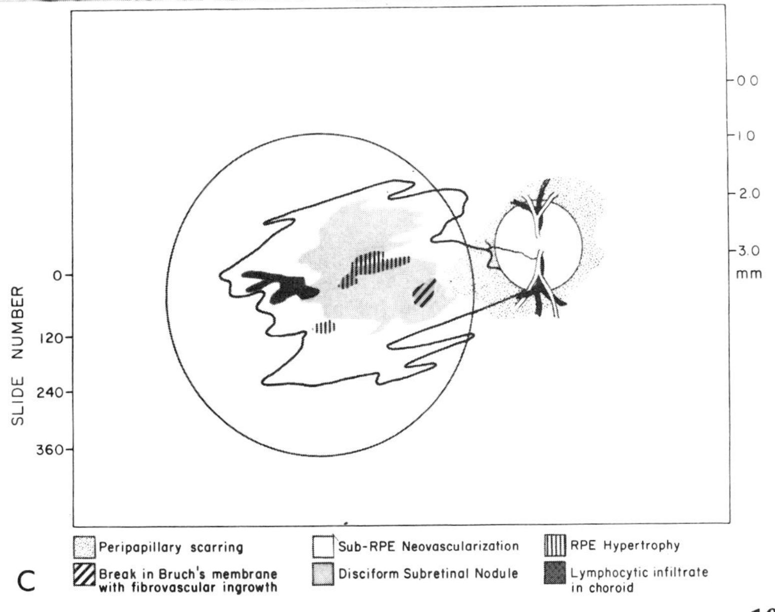

Figure 8–408. Macular lesion in ocular histoplasmosis syndrome. *A,* Disciform scar beneath macular retina of right eye. A small nasal portion of scar is covered by retinal pigment epithelium (arrowhead). Cystic edema and schisis (asterisk) of overlying retina are present. Break in Bruch's membrane with choroidal neovascularization is present near nasal margin of lesion (arrow). H and E, ×40. *B,* Higher-power view of discontinuity of Bruch's membrane. One margin of break is marked by an arrow. A choroidal artery (arrowhead) and vein (asterisk) extend through the break and into a disciform lesion. H and E, ×190. *C,* Two-dimensional reconstruction from study of serial sections showing size, shape and relations of various features of lesion. EP 38239. (From Meredith TA, Green WR, Key SN III, Dolin GS, Maumenee AE: Ocular histoplasmosis: Clinicopathologic correlation of three cases. Surv Ophthalmol *22*:189–205, 1977.)

mentioned, very similar to that seen in senile macular degeneration (Figs. 8–408 through 8–411).

The scars in the midperiphery (see Fig. 8–278) and peripapillary areas (Fig. 8–412) also have discontinuities of Bruch's membrane, but they rarely lead to choroidal neovascularization and disciform lesions.

The pathogenesis of late-onset macular lesions in ocular histoplasmosis remains in dispute. The various possibilities include active infective choroiditis, immunologic mechanisms, and vascular instability at the posterior pole. The various features for and against these possible pathogenetic mechanisms are reviewed by Thomas and Green (1981).

A close representation of the human disease has now been produced in experimental animals (Wong, 1972; Smith, Macy, Parrett, Irvine, 1978), and additional studies may help to delineate more clearly the pathogenesis of the late-onset macular lesions.

Macular Disciform Lesions Associated with Angioid Streaks (Dreyer, Green, 1978). These are

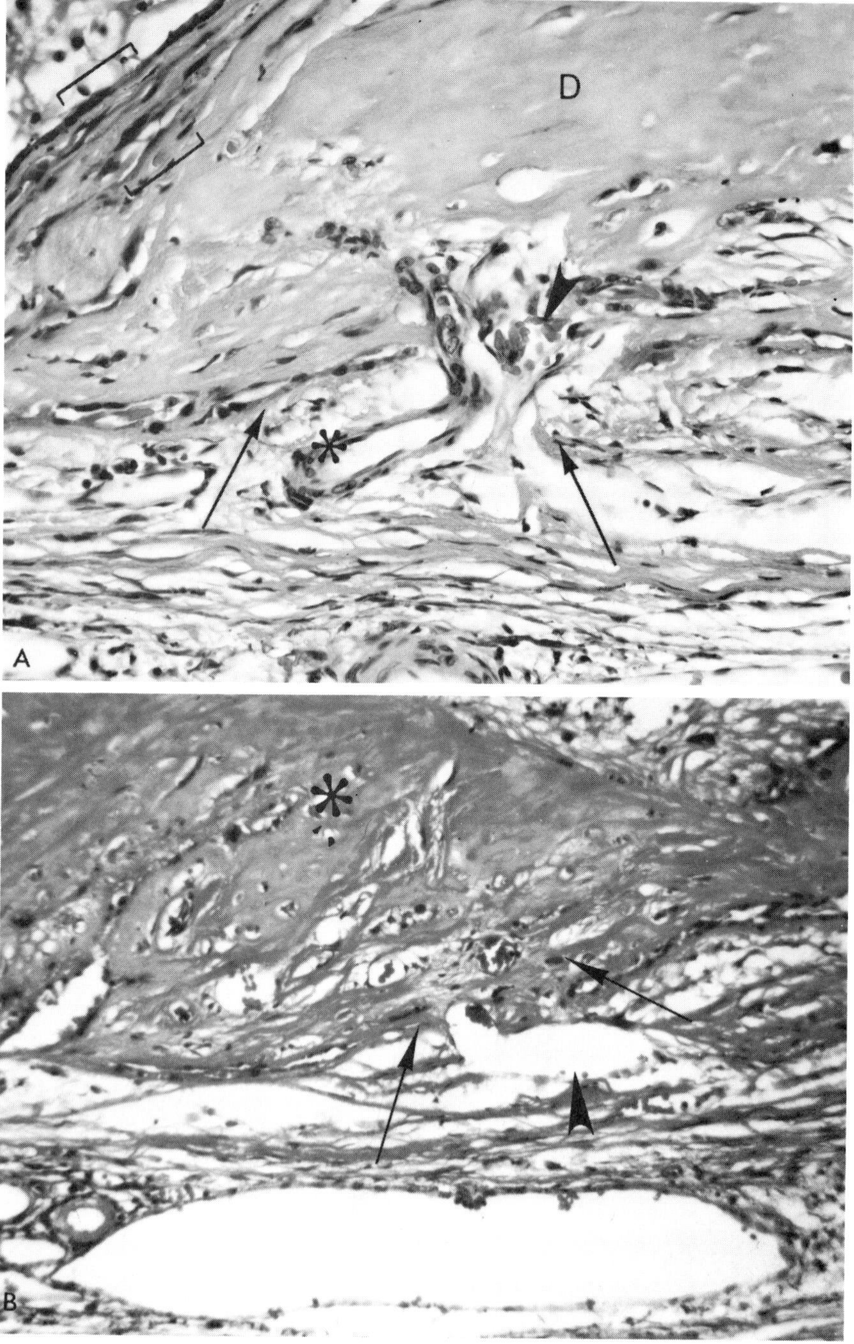

Figure 8–409. Xenon photocoagulation of **macular lesion of left eye** in ocular histoplasmosis syndrome. *A,* Disciform scar *(D)* with break in Bruch's membrane (between arrows) through which a choroidal artery (asterisk) and vein (arrowhead) extend into scar. Laminated hyperplastic retinal pigment epithelium (brackets) is present in anterior portion of scar. H and E, ×270. *B,* Different level of disciform scar (asterisk) and break in Bruch's membrane (between arrows), showing an additional choroidal vessel (arrowhead) extending into scar. H and E, ×270.

Illustration continued on opposite page

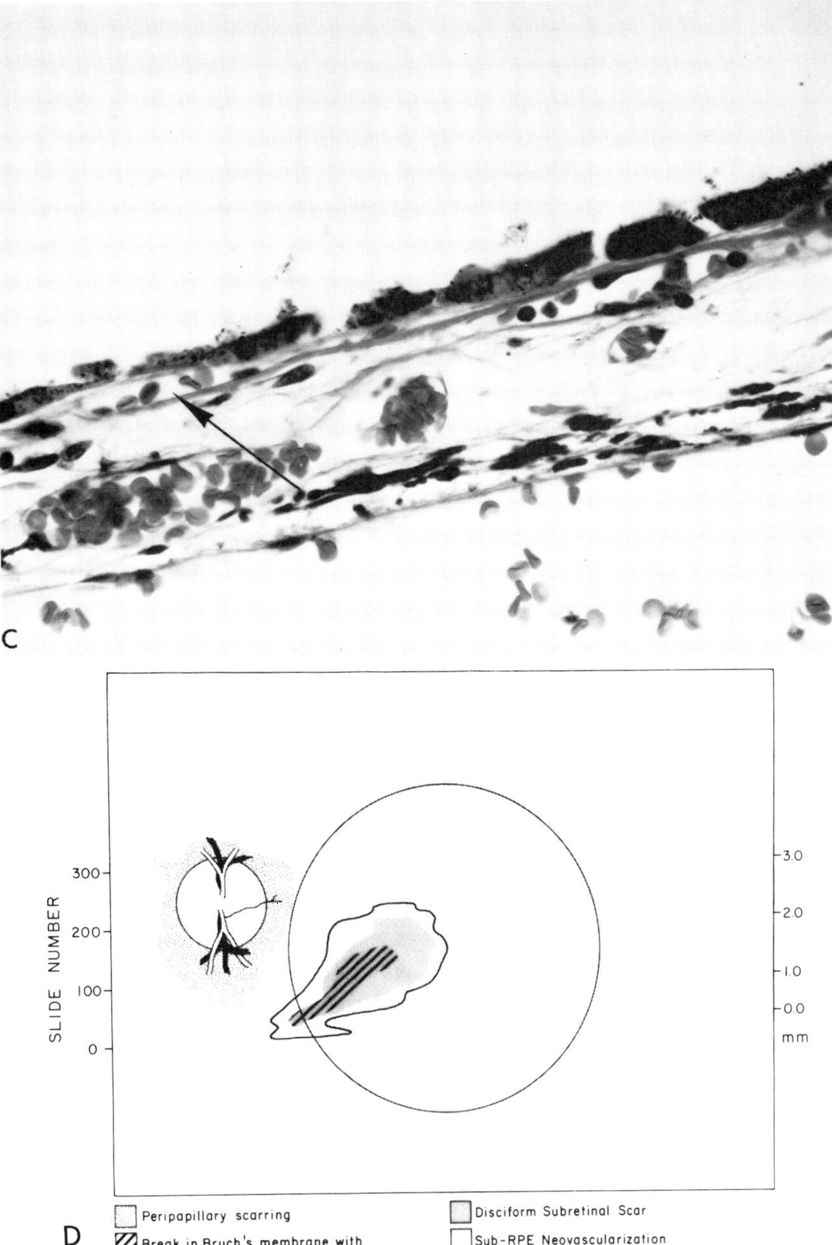

Figure 8–409 *Continued C,* Sub-RPE neovascularization (arrow) extends beyond margin of disciform scar. PAS, ×490. *D,* Two-dimensional reconstruction from study of serial sections shows size, shape, and relations of various histopathologic features. EP 38239. (From Meredith TA, Green WR, Key SN III, Dolin GS, Maumenee AE: Ocular histoplasmosis: Clinicopathologic correlation of three cases. Surv Ophthalmol *22*:189–205, 1977.)

quite similar to those seen in senile macular degeneration and the presumed ocular histoplasmosis syndrome. As the streak extends into the macular area, choroidal neovascularization ensues, leading then to serous or hemorrhagic detachment of the RPE and stimulation of fibrous tissue proliferation with a resultant disciform scar (Fig. 8–413).

Pathology of Angioid Streaks. Histopathologic studies (Boeck, 1938; Hagedoorn, 1939; Verhoeff, 1948; Paton, 1962, 1972; Gass, Clarkson, 1973; Dreyer, Green, 1978) generally have concluded that angioid streaks are breaks in a thickened and calcified Bruch's membrane. In a histopathologic study of 32 eyes from 21 patients, Dreyer and Green (1978) noted what was interpreted as the evolution of the histopathologic changes. Early, the primary change is a discontinuity in the elastic layer of Bruch's membrane, and this may be associated with thickening of the basement membrane of the RPE and loss of pigment granules in the RPE (Figs. 8–414 and 8–415). Intermediate streaks are due to full-thickness breaks in Bruch's membrane and are associated with disruption of the choriocapillaris and atrophy of the RPE and photoreceptor cells (Figs. 8–416 and 8–417). Later, there is choroidal neovascularization with fibrovascular tissue extending through the break (Fig. 8–418). This fibrovascular tissue may replace or extend under

Text continued on page 1032

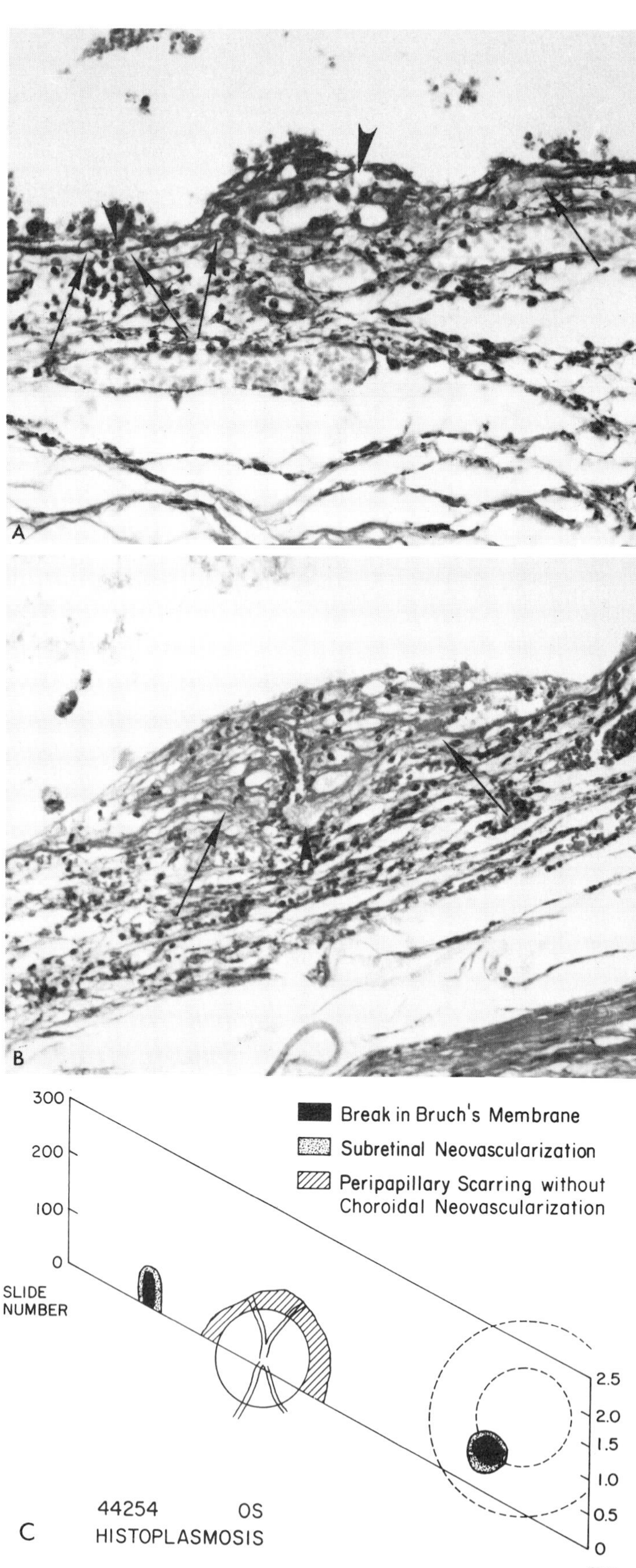

Figure 8–410. Choroidal neovascularization in untreated chorioretinal scars in macular area and adjacent to optic disc superonasally in ocular histoplasmosis syndrome. *A,* A lesion just superonasal to the disk has two breaks in Bruch's membrane (between arrows) with early choroidal neovascularization (arrowheads). The larger of the two lesions is slightly elevated in a moundlike configuration. PAS, ×300. *B,* Macular lesion is slightly larger, is mound-shaped, and has lamination suggestive of former retinal pigment epithelium (RPE) hyperplasia. Presumably the RPE has undergone degeneration and left only newly formed basement membrane, which appears laminated. There is a break in Bruch's membrane (between arrows) through which a choroidal vessel (arrowhead) can be traced into a disciform scar. Van de Grift, ×225. *C,* Two-dimensional reconstruction from study of serial sections showing features and locations of two lesions. EP 44254.

(From Sheffer A, Green WR, Fine SL, Kincaid M: Presumed ocular histoplasmosis syndrome: A clinicopathologic correlation of a treated case. Arch Ophthalmol *98*:335–345, 1980.)

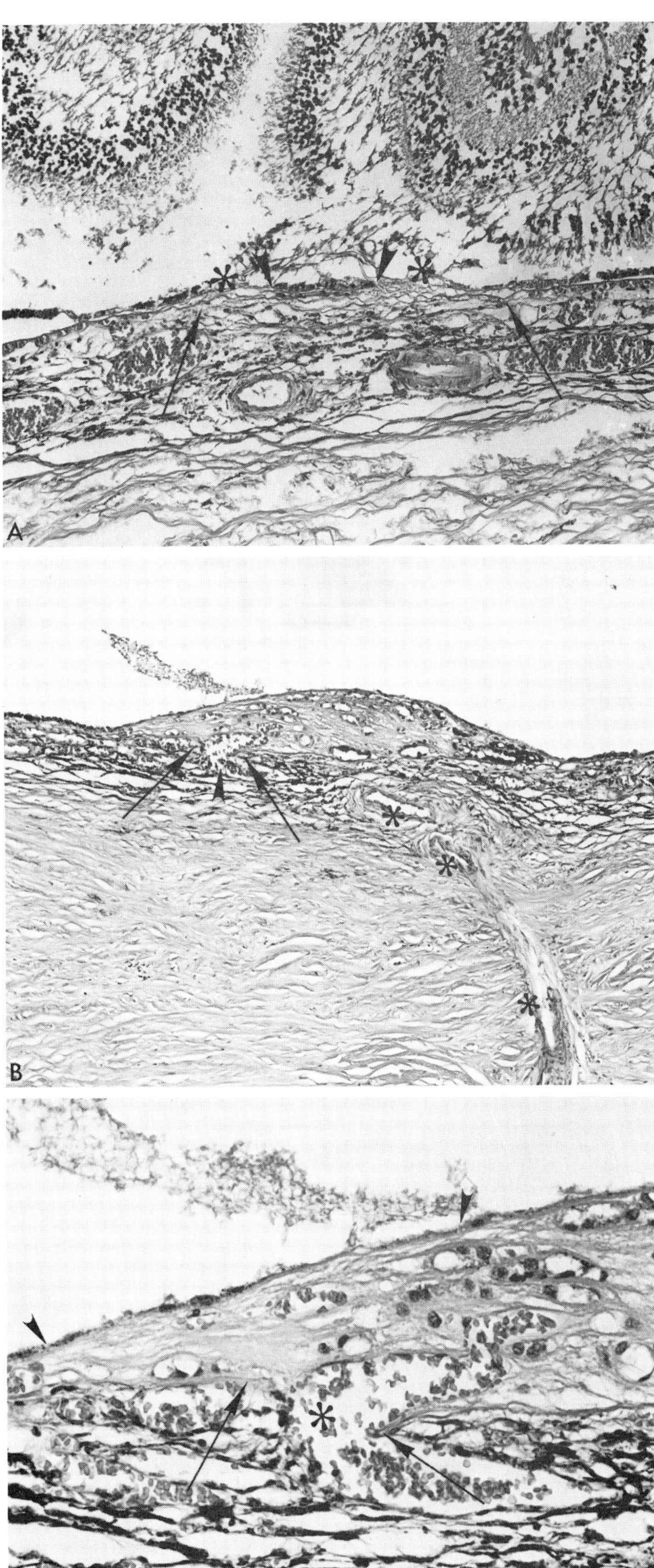

Figure 8–411. Macular lesions of ocular histoplasmosis syndrome. *A,* Chorioretinal scar in temporal aspect of macular area of right eye. Bruch's membrane is discontinuous (between arrows). The retinal pigment epithelium (RPE) is discontinuous in two areas (asterisks) but remains intact centrally (between arrowheads). Photoreceptor cells are lost in the central area of the lesion, and retina is adherent to a thin fibrillar scar in the area of discontinuous Bruch's membrane. No neovascularization is present. PAS, ×125.

B, Section through central portion of lesion located superiorly in macular area of left eye. A fibrovascular disciform lesion with an admixture of hyperplastic RPE is located between intact but attenuated and partially depigmented RPE and Bruch's membrane. A choroidal vessel (arrowhead) traverses a break in Bruch's membrane (between arrows). A prominent short ciliary artery (asterisks) enters choroid subjacent to this disciform lesion. H and E, ×75. *C,* Higher power view of macular lesion of left eye showing an intact but attenuated and partially depigmented RPE (arrowheads) over the lesion and a choroidal vessel (asterisk) extending through a break in Bruch's membrane (between arrows). H and E, ×265.

EP 41434. (From Meridith TA, Green WR, Key SN III, Dolin GS, Maumenee AE: Ocular histoplasmosis: Clinicopathologic correlation of three cases. Surv Ophthalmol *22*:189–205, 1977.)

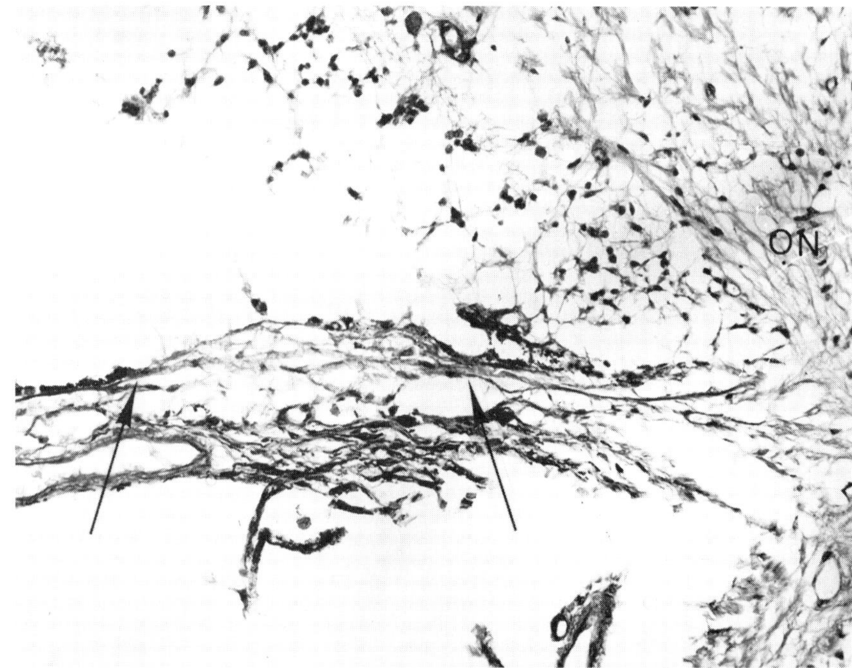

Figure 8–412. Peripapillary area in left eye showing a thin scar in area of discontinuous Bruch's membrane (between arrows). There is partial loss of retinal pigment epithelium, loss of photoreceptor cell layer, and adhesion of retina to scar. Optic nerve head (ON) is to right. PAS, ×185. EP 41434.

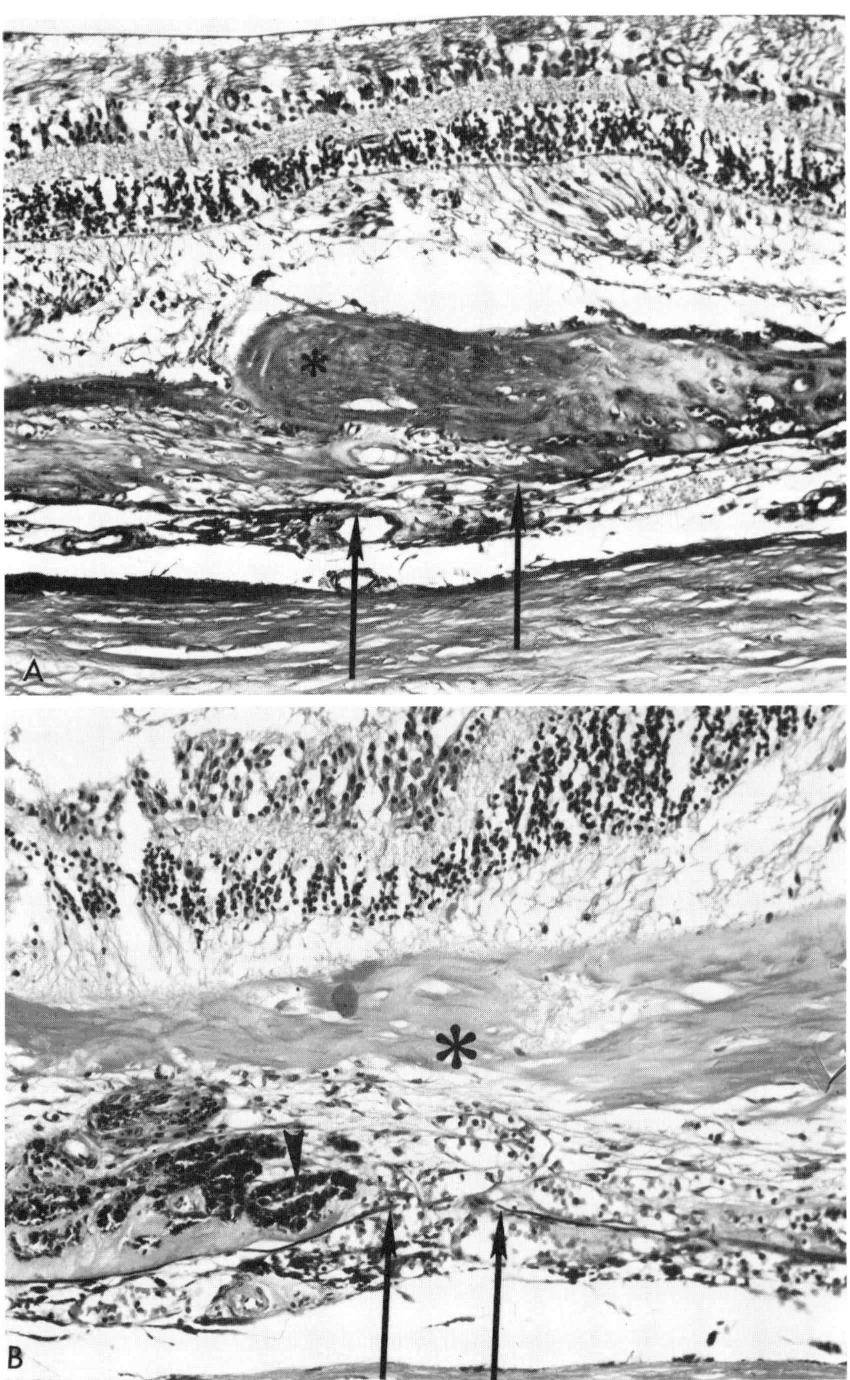

Figure 8–413. Angioid streaks in a patient with pseudoxanthoma elasticum. *A,* Histologic section through macula of right eye. Arrows delimit edges of angioid streak. Fibrovascular disciform scar (asterisk) is located between Bruch's membrane and residual retinal pigment epithelium (RPE). RPE is discontinuous over this lesion, with prominent photoreceptor loss. H and E, ×130. *B,* Histologic section through macula of left eye. Arrows delimit edges of angioid streak. Tubular configuration of hypertrophic and hyperplastic RPE (arrowhead) is present in the midst of dense fibrous scar (asterisk). H and E, ×155.

Illustration continued on following page

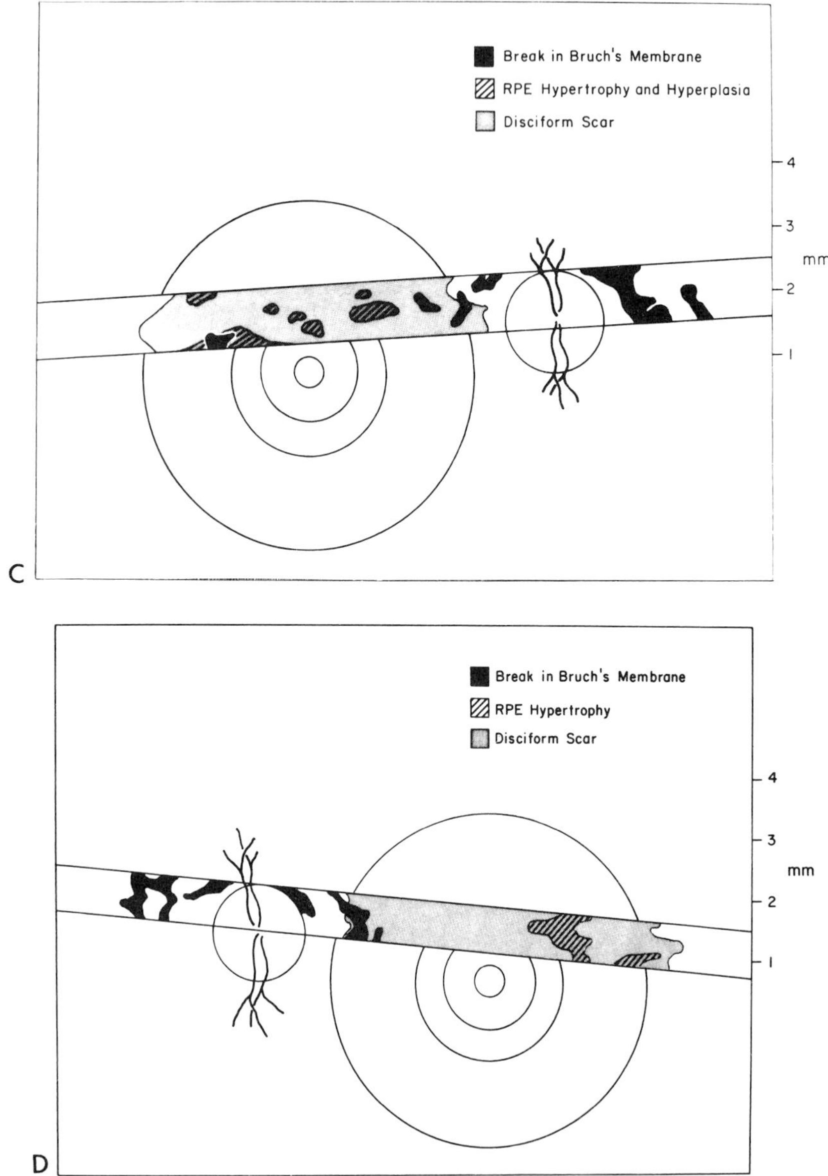

Figure 8–413 *Continued* Two-dimensional reconstruction of *C,* right and *D,* left peripapillary area of patient with bilateral disciform scars and pseudoxanthoma elasticum. In both eyes, an angioid streak in the macular area is visible. Fibrovascular membranes grew through these streaks and apparently bled, giving rise to the large disciform lesions now present. Angioid streaks are also present nasally. EP 32503. (From Dreyer R, Green WR: Pathology of angioid streaks. Trans Pa Acad Ophthalmol Otolaryngol *31*:158–167, 1978.)

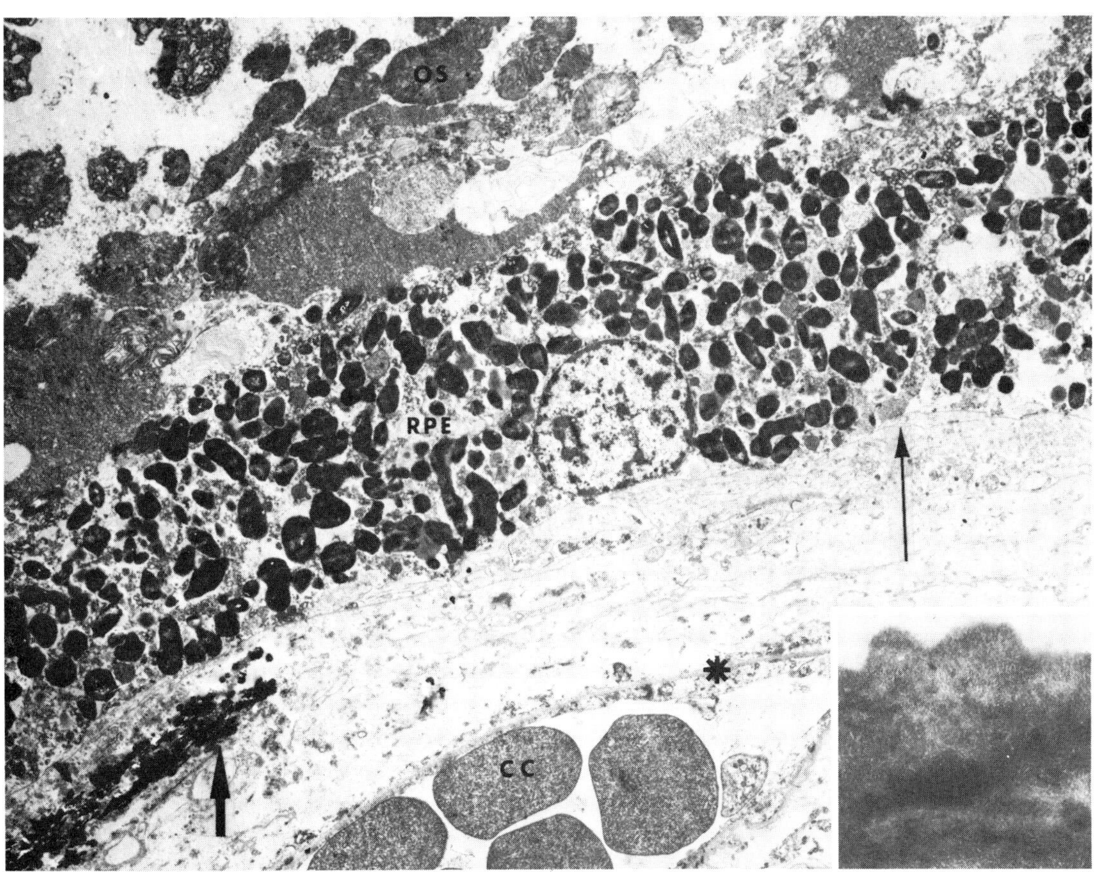

Figure 8–414. Electron micrograph of **angioid streak** from a patient with pseudoxanthoma elasticum. Calcium deposits are present in elastic layers of Bruch's membrane (large arrow). Outer segments *(OS)* are visible. The retinal pigment epithelium *(RPE)* and its basement membrane (thin arrow) and basement membrane of choriocapillaris *(CC)* (asterisk) are intact. ×4000. Inset reveals fine, granular nature of calcium deposits. ×70,000. EP 41049. (From Dreyer R, Green WR: Pathology of angioid streaks. Trans Pa Acad Ophthalmol Otolaryngol *31*:158–167, 1978.)

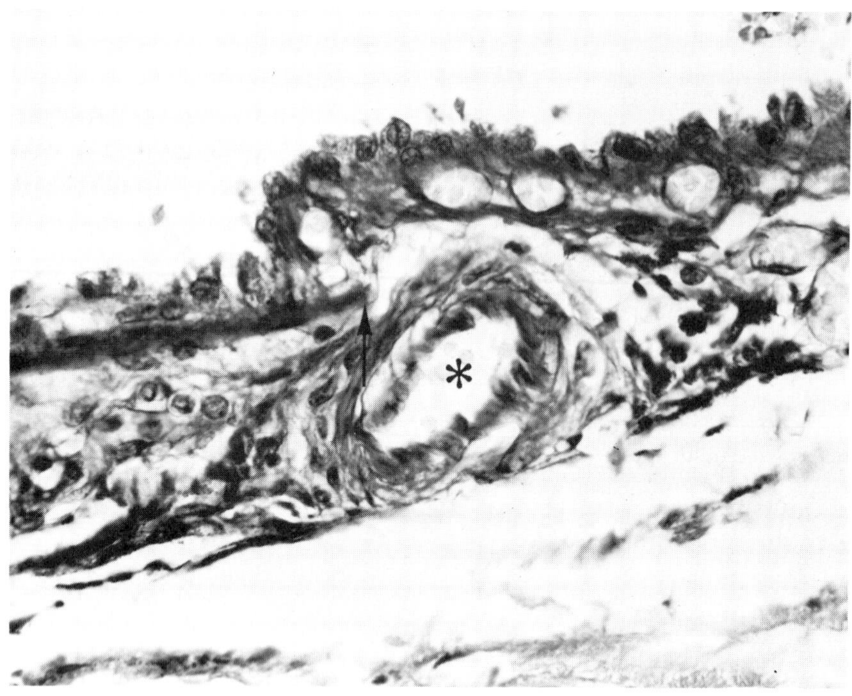

Figure 8–415. One edge of an **angioid streak** is visible (arrow). Retinal pigment epithelium (RPE) is intact but has lost its pigment granules. Choriocapillaris remains intact. A large choroidal artery (asterisk) is near angioid streak and area of depigmented RPE (window defect). PAS reaction, × 500. EP 30240. (From Dreyer R, Green WR: Pathology of angioid streaks. Trans Pa Acad Ophthalmol Otolaryngol *31*:158–167, 1978.)

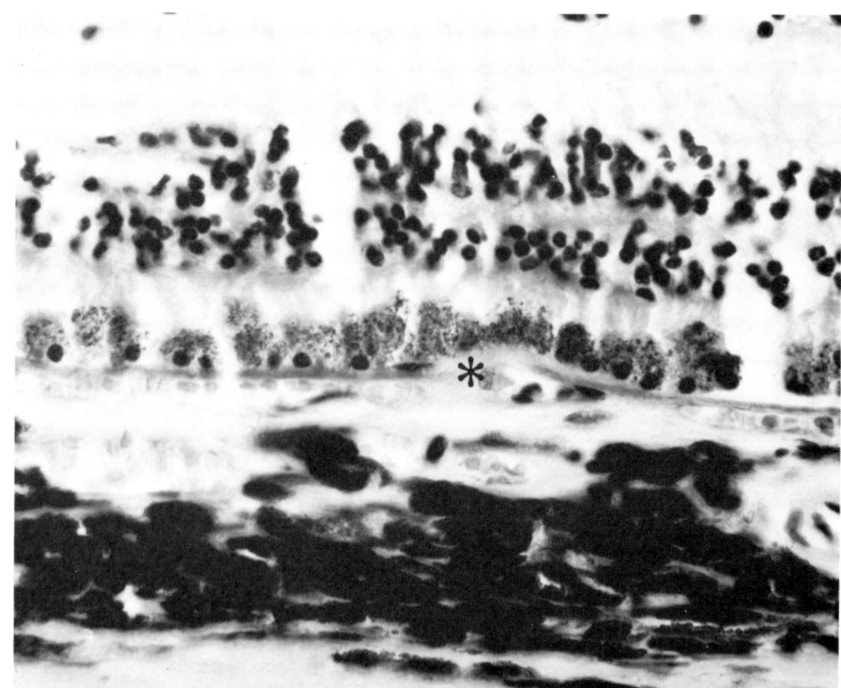

Figure 8–416. A small mound of fibrovascular tissue is interposed between the edges of an **angioid streak** (asterisk). Retina and retinal pigment epithelium are normal. H and E, × 500. EP 30240. (From Dreyer R, Green WR: Pathology of angioid streaks. Trans Pa Acad Ophthalmol Otolaryngol *31*:158–167, 1978.)

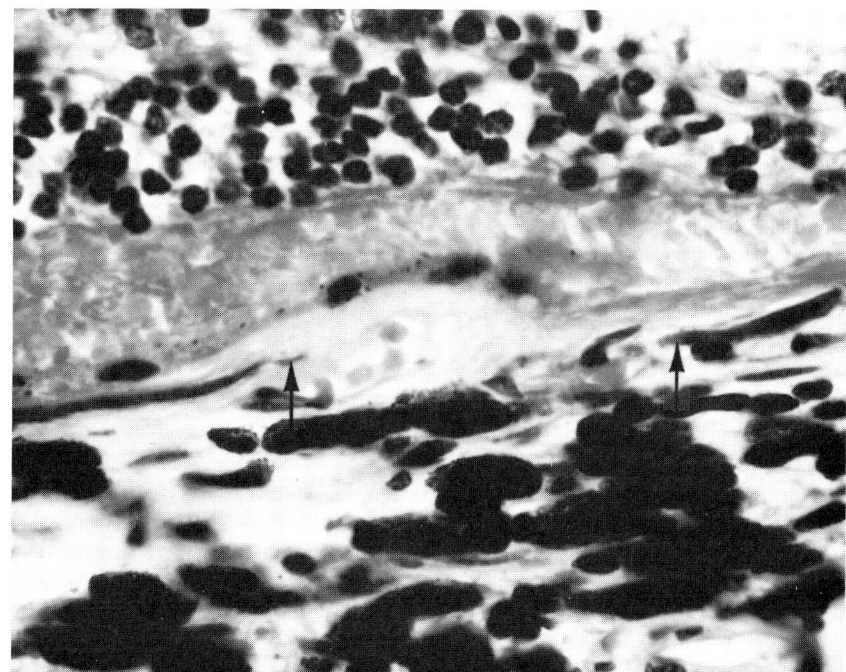

Figure 8–417. Arrows delimit **angioid streak**. Fibrovascular tissue has grown over both ends of a break in Bruch's membrane for a short distance. A vascular channel from choroid is present in this ingrowth. There is partial atrophy and near-total loss of pigment granules of retinal pigment epithelium on both sides of the streak. H and E, ×775. EP 30312. (From Dreyer R, Green WR: Pathology of angioid streaks. Trans Pa Acad Ophthalmol Otolaryngol *31*:158–167, 1978.)

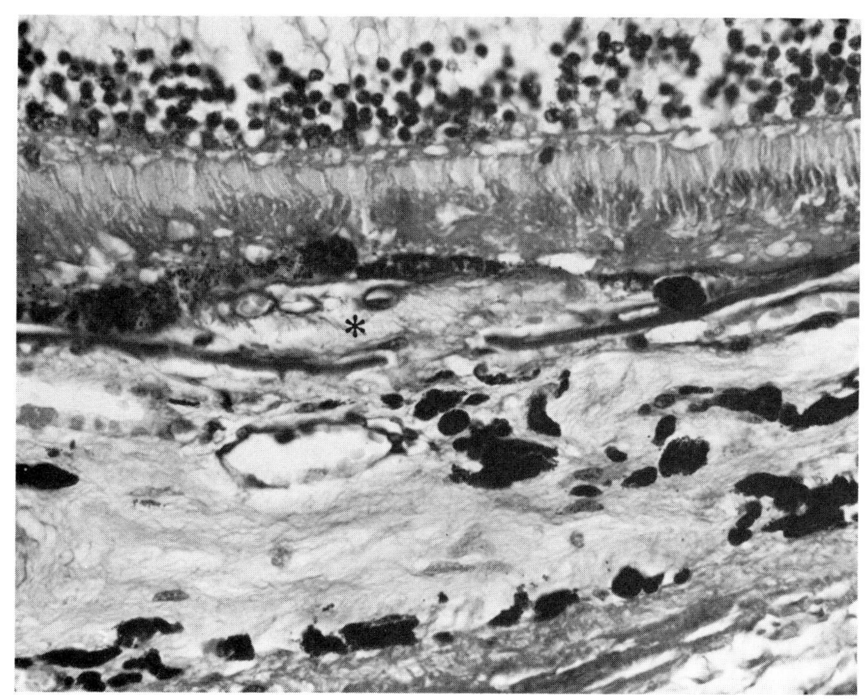

Figure 8–418. Fibrovascular tissue from choroid (asterisk) extends between retinal pigment epithelium (RPE) and Bruch's membrane to either side of the streak. There is RPE hypertrophy. PAS reaction, ×370. EP 40149. (From Dreyer R, Green WR: Pathology of angioid streaks. Trans Pa Acad Ophthalmol Otolaryngol *31*:158–167, 1978.)

the surrounding RPE. Secondary hypertrophy and hyperplasia of the RPE may occur. Serous (Fig. 8–419) or hemorrhagic detachment (Fig. 8–420) of the retina, the RPE, or both may occur.

The halo at the margin of the streaks may be due to RPE atrophy or to fibrovascular tissue from the choroid.

Diseases with which angioid streaks are associated and with which there appears to be a pathogenetic relationship include pseudoxanthoma elasticum, Paget's disease, and Ehlers-Danlos syndrome. Condon and Serjeant (1976) have observed angioid streaks in 22 per cent of patients over 40 years of age with homozygous sickle cell disease. In a study of a large series of patients with angioid streaks, Clarkson (1976) found that approximately 50 per cent of the patients had no associated systemic disorder.

Scleropachynsis Maculopathy. Conn, Green, and De La Cruz (1981) have observed the occurrence of a bilateral and symmetric macular lesion characterized by a linear area of mottling of the RPE, extending from the optic disc margin through the macular area. This area was slightly elevated. Histopathologic studies disclosed marked reduction in the thickness of the choroid, with collapse of the otherwise normal choroidal vessels; RPE hypo- and hyperpigmentation; and marked thickening of the inner two thirds of the sclera, with accumulation of mucopolysaccharide and large collagen fibrils measuring up to 3500 angstroms in diameter (Fig. 8–421).

Acute Macular Neuroretinopathy. This condition affects young adults with a sudden decrease of visual acuity or paracentral scotomas (Bos, Deutman, 1975). Examination disclosed subtle, reddish-brown dots in a wedge-shaped configuration that pointed toward the foveola, located superficially in the retina nasal to the fovea. The etiology is unknown, but the use of oral contraceptives (Bos, Deutman, 1975; Rush, 1977) and preceding viral illness (Rush, 1977) have been noted. The condition also has been described in male patients (Bos, Deutman, 1975; Priluck, Buettner, Robertson, 1978). No histopathologic studies have been conducted. Little or no improvement in vision has been noted.

Foveolar Splinter and Macular Wisps. Daily (1970b, 1973) has observed a splinter of retinal tissue protruding from the foveal pit and wisps of white tissue from the macular surface. Traction of the detaching posterior hyaloid membrane on the retina was thought to be the cause of these splinters and wisps. Patients may complain of slight distortion of vision, and visual acuity may be slightly affected. Similar lesions were found in association with retinitis pigmentosa, juvenile macular degeneration, foveomacular retinitis, after absorption of a small "prefoveal" hemorrhage, old healed chorioretinitis, and after direct and indirect concussion and whiplash injury (Daily, 1973). No histopathologic correlative studies have been conducted.

Whiplash Maculopathy. Small (50 to 100 microns) pits or depressions with whitish borders have been observed in the foveas of patients with a history of flexion-extension head and neck trauma (Kelley, Hoover, George, 1978; Grey,

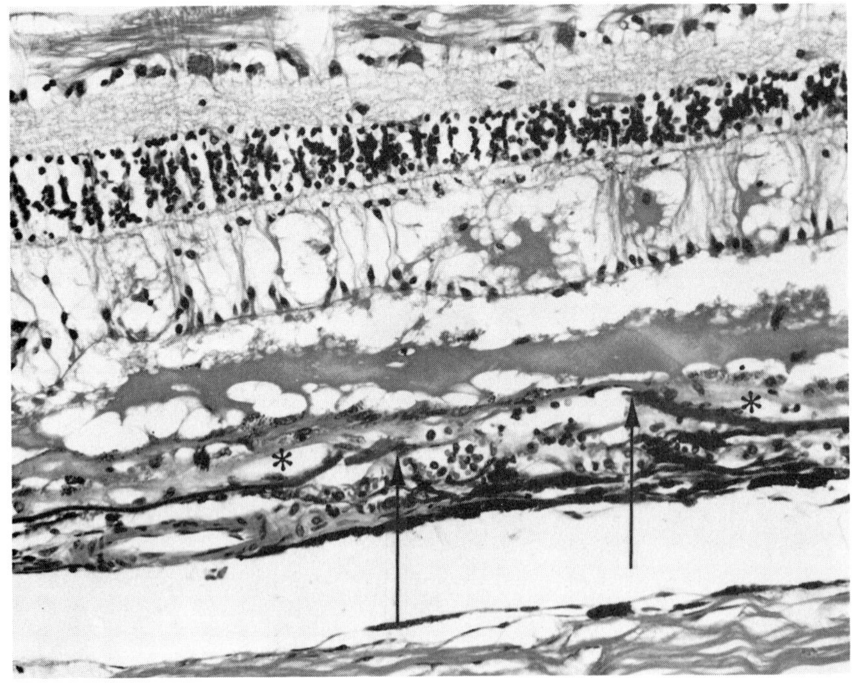

Figure 8–419. Histologic section nasal to optic disc in left eye of a patient with pseudoxanthoma elasticum. A **streak** (between arrows) was not visible ophthalmoscopically. Neovascular tissue (asterisks) extends through and to either side of a break in Bruch's membrane. A flat serous detachment of retina is present. Overlying retinal pigment epithelium remains intact, but there are fewer nuclei than normal and near-total loss of pigment granules. Cystic degeneration of retina and partial photoreceptor loss are present. H and E, ×205. EP 32503. (From Dreyer R, Green WR: Pathology of angioid streaks. Trans Pa Acad Ophthalmol Otolaryngol *31*:158–167, 1978.)

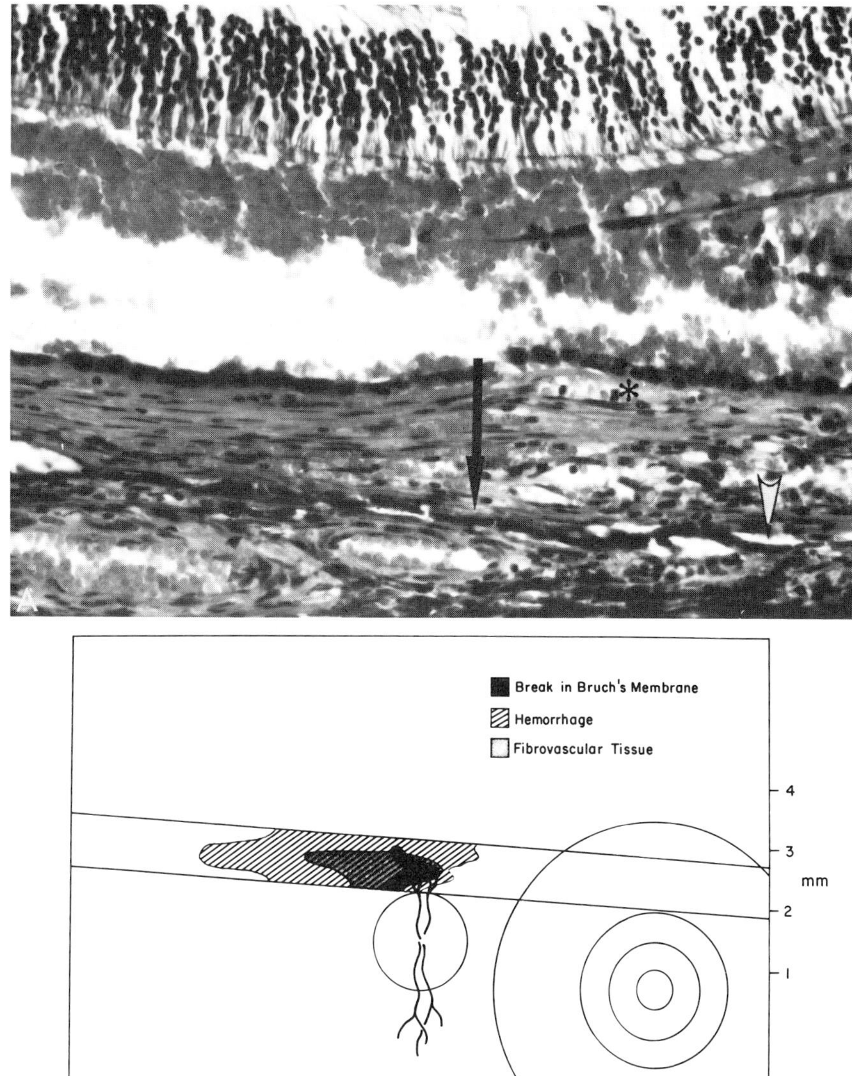

Figure 8–420. *A,* Histologic section of area adjacent to an **angioid streak,** showing fibrovascular tissue (asterisk) between retinal pigment epithelium (RPE) and Bruch's membrane (arrow), margin of streak (arrowhead), and massive hemorrhage. H and E, ×225. *B,* Two-dimensional reconstruction of superonasal hemorrhage present in *A,* showing angioid streak, sub-RPE fibrovascular tissue proliferation, and area of hemorrhage. EP 18402. (From Dreyer R, Green WR: Pathology of angioid streaks. Trans Pa Acad Ophthalmol Otolaryngol *31*:158–167, 1978.)

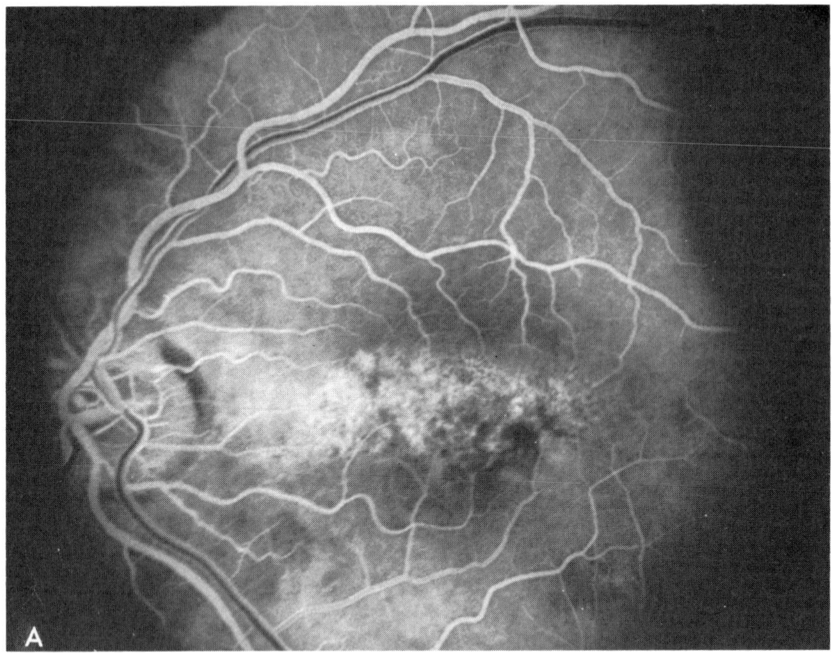

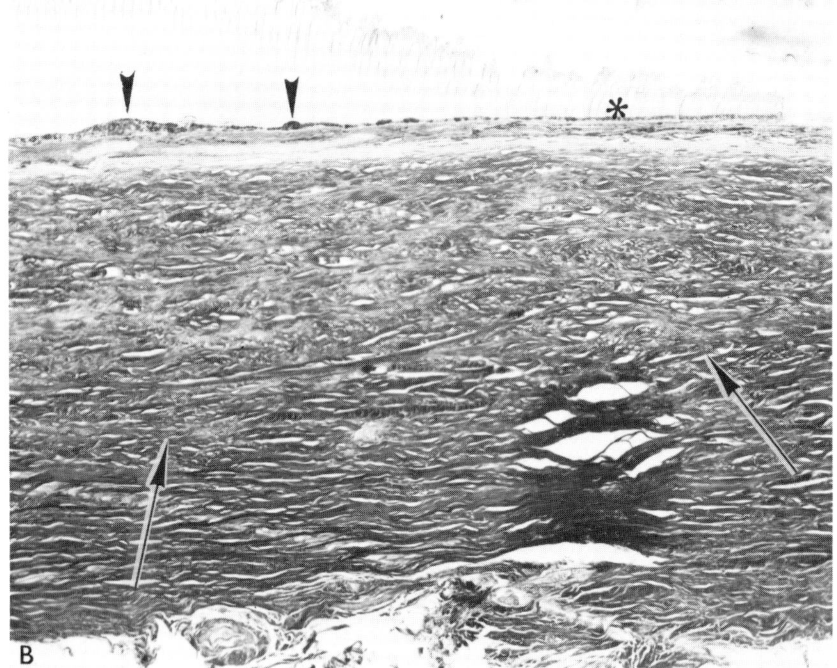

Figure 8–421. Scleropachynsis maculopathy. *A,* Linear pattern of fluorescein staining of retinal pigment epithelium (RPE). *B,* Sclera is thickened, and there is deposition of mucopolysaccharide (arrows). Choroid is compressed, and RPE shows areas of hypo- (asterisk) and hyperpigmentation (arrowheads). Alcian blue, × 60. EP 46583. (From Conn H, Green WR, de la Cruz Z, Hillis A: Scleropachynsis maculopathy. Arch Ophthalmol *100*:793–799, 1982.)

1978). Visual disturbance is mild and transient. No pathologic studies have been conducted.

Nicotinic Acid Maculopathy. See page 805.

SYSTEMIC DISEASES WITH RETINAL INVOLVEMENT

Vascular

Arteriosclerosis and Hypertension. Arteriosclerosis is a general term to designate all the diffuse arterial diseases characterized by thickening of the arterial wall. Mild thickening of the arteriolar wall in the retina of clearly nonhypertensive persons is referred to as involutional sclerosis and is identical to the changes with aging in small arteries elsewhere in the body. Arteriosclerosis is an inevitable accompaniment of systemic hypertension, and they are considered together here.

The process of involutional arteriosclerosis is accelerated by systemic hypertension. With mild hypertension, in which there is a moderate elevation in the diastolic pressure, the arterioles de-

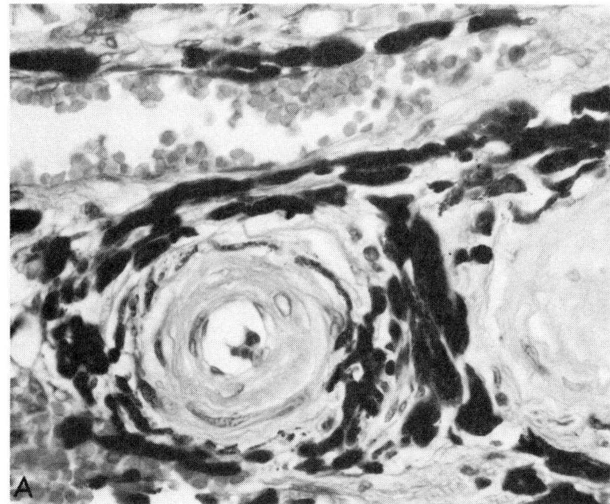

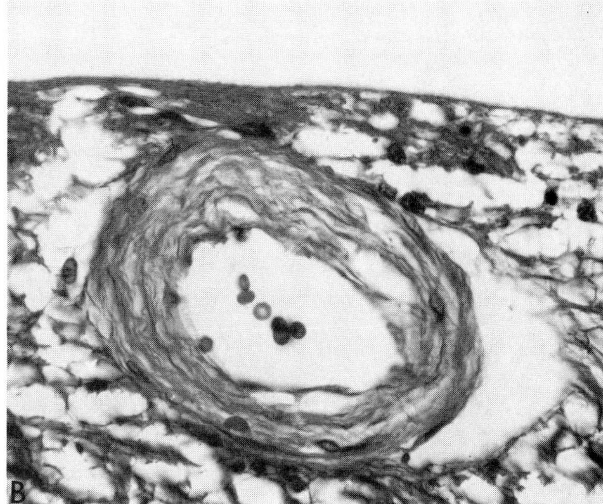

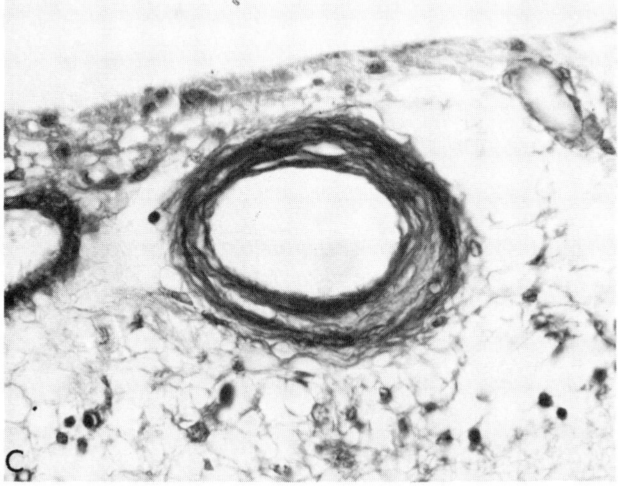

Figure 8–422. Arteriosclerosis with "onionskin" appearance. *A,* Choroidal artery. H and E, ×625. *B,* Retinal artery. H and E, ×575. *C,* Retinal artery. PAS, ×650. EP 38861.

velop further thickening of their walls as a result of intimal hyalinization, medial hypertrophy, and endothelial hyperplasia. This category of changes is referred to as arteriosclerosis, or arteriolar sclerosis, and the arterioles often have an "onion-skin" appearance in cross section (Fig. 8–422) (Harry, Ashton, 1963). This condition is also referred to as endarteritis fibrosa. Kimura (1970a) found the earliest change to be a thickening of the tissue between the endothelium and internal elastic layer. The collagen content between the muscle cells increases, the number of muscle cells decreases, and basement membrane increases in the more advanced lesions. Endothelium and muscle cells accumulate lipid inclusions in more advanced lesions. In severe sclerosis, lipid particles are also observed extracellularly in the intima. No atheromatous plaques are observed (Kimura, 1965a and b, 1966, 1967a and b, 1970a and b). Atheromatous disease may be seen at the optic nerve head (see Figs. 8–97 and 8–98) and occasionally in the peripapillary retinal arteries (Brownstein, Font, Alper, 1973).

Atheromatous disease of the ciliary (Fig. 8–423) and choroidal arteries may affect the retina and retinal pigment epithelium (RPE). When the process is sufficient to produce occlusion alone or with thrombosis, outer retinal ischemic atrophy of the affected area of the retina occurs.

Grading of retinal arteriosclerosis is based on the size of the arteriolar light reflex and the character of the arteriovenous crossings (Scheie, 1953).

Attenuation of Arteries. Arteries may show generalized or localized attenuation that can be seen clinically. General attenuation may result from diffuse vasospasm in acute hypertension or occur as a gradual process secondary to such retinal diseases as retinitis pigmentosa. Focal narrowings of the retinal arteries have been considered to be due to spasm of local areas of the wall. The histologic counterpart of focal narrowings has not been identified, but it is assumed that several possibilities can exist to produce this picture. One is that edema accumulates in and around the vessel wall, which produces narrowing of the blood column. With subsidence of the edema, the blood column resumes its normal pat-

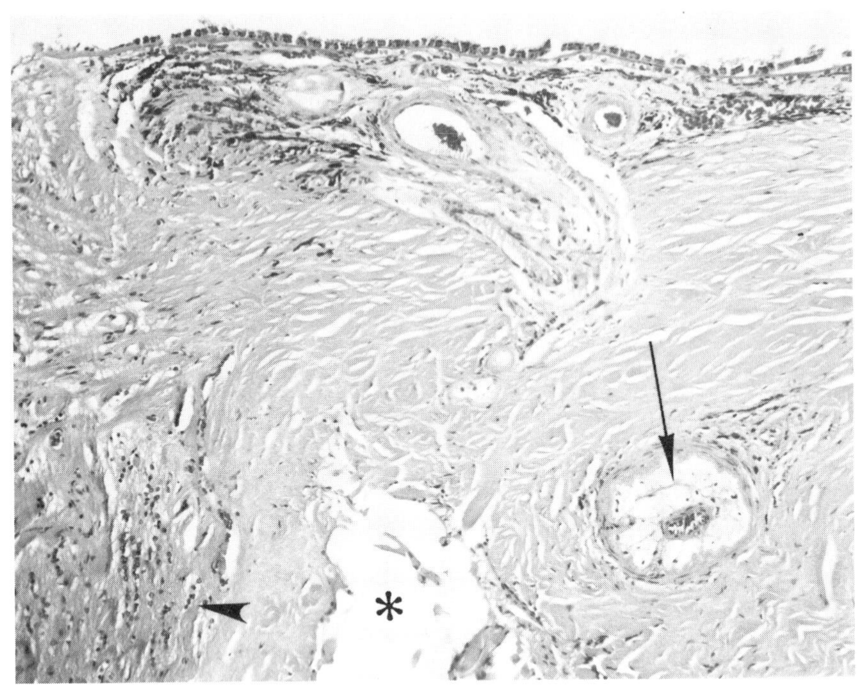

Figure 8–423. Atherosclerosis of short ciliary artery within peripapillary sclera. Vessel lumen is much narrowed by subintimal accumulation of lipid-laden histiocytes (arrow). Optic nerve, arrowhead; subarachnoid space, asterisk. H and E, ×105. EP 39922.

tern—or, if scarring and fibrosis occur in the wall, permanent localized narrowing results. Another possibility is that the local narrowing may be due primarily to spasm and not to edema, in which case it can disappear fairly rapidly or remain fixed because of fibrosis of the wall after a short period.

The earliest ophthalmologic sign of arteriosclerosis is a change in the arteriolar light reflex. The normal retina and its blood vessel walls are not visible with the ophthalmoscope, but the blood column is. The normal light reflex of the ophthalmoscope forms a bright stripe along the center of the blood column. This is produced by reflection of light from the interface between the column of blood and the vessel wall. Arteriosclerosis alters the density of the vessel wall, and therefore the reflection of light, so that the central reflex is less bright and more diffused.

The next early change is the development of a copper wire artery, in which the central light reflex becomes even more diffused and the arteriole color changes to a reddish-brown. The intensity of the ophthalmoscope light also may be a factor in this observation. Microscopically, this is brought about by an increasing sclerosis or hyalinization of the vessel wall, so that the reflection of light from the blood column is altered. The arterioles show hyalinization of the media, thickening of their walls, and luminal narrowing. The preceding changes may exist for years before other lesions develop, or the hypertension suddenly may become severe and progressive, producing rapid vascular and retinal changes.

In the slower cases, advanced sclerosis gradually becomes evident, with vascular crossing changes. One of the earliest of these is "nicking." Normally, at arteriolar-venous crossings, the adventitia forms a common sheath for the arteriole and venule, and the walls of these two vessels are intimately united, with the arteriole usually crossing internal to the vein (see Fig. 8–118).

From light and electron microscopic studies, Kimura (1967a and b, 1970a and b) concluded that pathologic vascular crossing changes were caused by proliferation of the perivascular glial cells. Ikui (1963) found that the basement membranes of the arteriole and venule are adherent, that collagen fibers are common to the walls of both vessels, and that the wall of the arteriole is thinner at the crossing point. In hypertension, there is thickening of the basement membrane and media of the arteriole. These changes were thought to impinge upon the vein and cause the crossing phenomenon. Ikui was unable to confirm the presence of an increase in glial tissue around the arteriole-venule crossing in hypertension.

Mimatsu (1963) reported that the arteriole-venule crossing phenomenon was caused by sclerotic thickening of the wall of the venule and not by compression by the arteriole. Seitz (1964) found that artery and vein had a common wall and adventitia at the point of crossing. Seitz (1961) attributes the pathologic arteriole-venule crossing phenomenon to vascular sclerosis and perivascular glial cell proliferation and not to changes in the lumen of the vein.

Arteriosclerosis, therefore, is also associated with phlebosclerosis at the crossings. Normally at the crossing the artery can be seen to cross the vein, and the blood column in both vessels can be seen quite distinctly. Increasing sclerosis interferes with visualization of the vein at the crossing. If the sclerotic process extends along the wall of the vein beyond the crossing, it interferes with visualization of the blood column here also. In addition, the vein is compressed and its lumen is narrowed.

As a result of this reduction in caliber, the vein becomes dilated distal to the crossing then tapers and seems to lose its blood column at some distance before it crosses under the arteriole. After passing under the arteriole it does not reappear visibly for a short distance; when it does, it again is tapered and reduced in caliber.

All this change, then, is produced by extension of the sclerotic process from the arteriole into the wall of the vein and from that area on beyond the crossing. A certain amount of outward displacement of the vein by the arteriole may assist in production of the phenomenon. Constant twisting movements of these vessels, caused by their normal pulsation, may lead to stress on the walls and predispose to such crossing changes in hypertension.

A second important sclerotic crossing change is deflection of the veins. This may be produced in much the same fashion as the tortuosity of the radial arteries in Monckeberg's sclerosis. Ordinarily, the radial arteries become tortuous because they elongate as they become sclerotic. The retinal arterioles may either elongate or shorten with sclerosis. The common sheath at arteriolar-venous crossings causes the vein to be deflected from its course by the change in length of the artery. Normally, the vein passes under the arteriole at a rather acute angle. If it is deflected, it crosses at a more obtuse angle. The combination of "nicking" and deflection of the veins is important for the diagnosis of arteriosclerosis.

Long-standing hypertension leads to severe arteriosclerosis, with marked thickening and hyalinization of the arterioles and reduction in caliber of the lumen. This change may interfere completely with visualization of the blood column, so that the vessels appear as "silver-wire" vessels.

In malignant or accelerated hypertension, the arterioles become thickened, as in arteriolar sclerosis. In addition, necrosis and fibrinoid deposition in the vessel wall occurs (Fig. 8–424). This process more commonly involves choroidal arteries than retinal arteries. Retinal edema (Fig. 8–425) occurs as the result of damage to retinal vessel endothelium, but retinal edema and detachment also may be attributed to breakdown of the blood ocular barrier at the level of the RPE. In malignant hypertension and severe renal hypertension, the edema fluid within the retina may have a fibrinous appearance (Fig. 8–426).

Fibrinous necrosis in the walls of arteries and papilledema (Figs. 8–427 and 8–428) are the histopathologic features that distinguish malignant hypertension. Additional features and conditions associated with and attributed to hypertension include microinfarctions in the retina (Fig.8–427,*E,F*) and optic nerve head (Fig. 8–427,*A,B*), retroretinal membranes of RPE origin (Figs. 8–427,*D* and 428,*D*), arterial macroaneurysms (see page 707), and branch retinal vein occlusion (see page 705).

Atherosclerosis per se seems not to occur in the retinal arteries but may be seen in the central retinal artery in the optic nerve and optic nerve head and in the larger choroidal arterioles. Retinal hemorrhages and nerve fiber microinfarctions (cotton-wool spots) are seen in arteriosclerosis and more commonly when there is associated hypertension. Cotton-wool spots are associated with closure of capillaries in the same area and often with microaneurysms in the bordering zone (see Fig. 8–68) (Ashton, 1959; Ashton, Harry, 1963).

In studies of experimental hypertension, Garner and Ashton (1970) and Ashton (1972) have shown endothelial damage as the source of plasma leakage.

From analysis of experimental studies of hypertension in the monkey, Garner, Ashton, Tripathi, and others (1975) proposed the following sequence of changes:

1. The arterioles constrict as the pressure rises, most likely as a result of vascular autoregulation. This may lead to occlusion of the precapillary arterioles and is associated with necrosis of vascular smooth muscle.
2. Dilatation then occurs, with insudation of plasma into the unsupported wall through a damaged endothelium. This stage probably corresponds to the autoregulatory break point and is evidenced clinically by focal leakage of fluorescein.
3. Progressive plasma insudation into the vessel wall, with further muscle necrosis, results in secondary occlusion and the typical picture of advanced fibrinoid necrosis.

In a clinicopathologic study of eyes from 30 patients who died of essential or renal hypertension, Marquardt (1969) found hyaline thickening of the artery walls and lipid deposition. These changes were more marked in renal hypertension, and the changes of the choroidal vessels were more severe than those in the retina and more closely paralleled the changes elsewhere in the body.

In a discussion of the pathophysiology of the effects of systemic hypertension on the posterior segment of the eye, Tso and Jampol (1982) broke

Text continued on page 1042

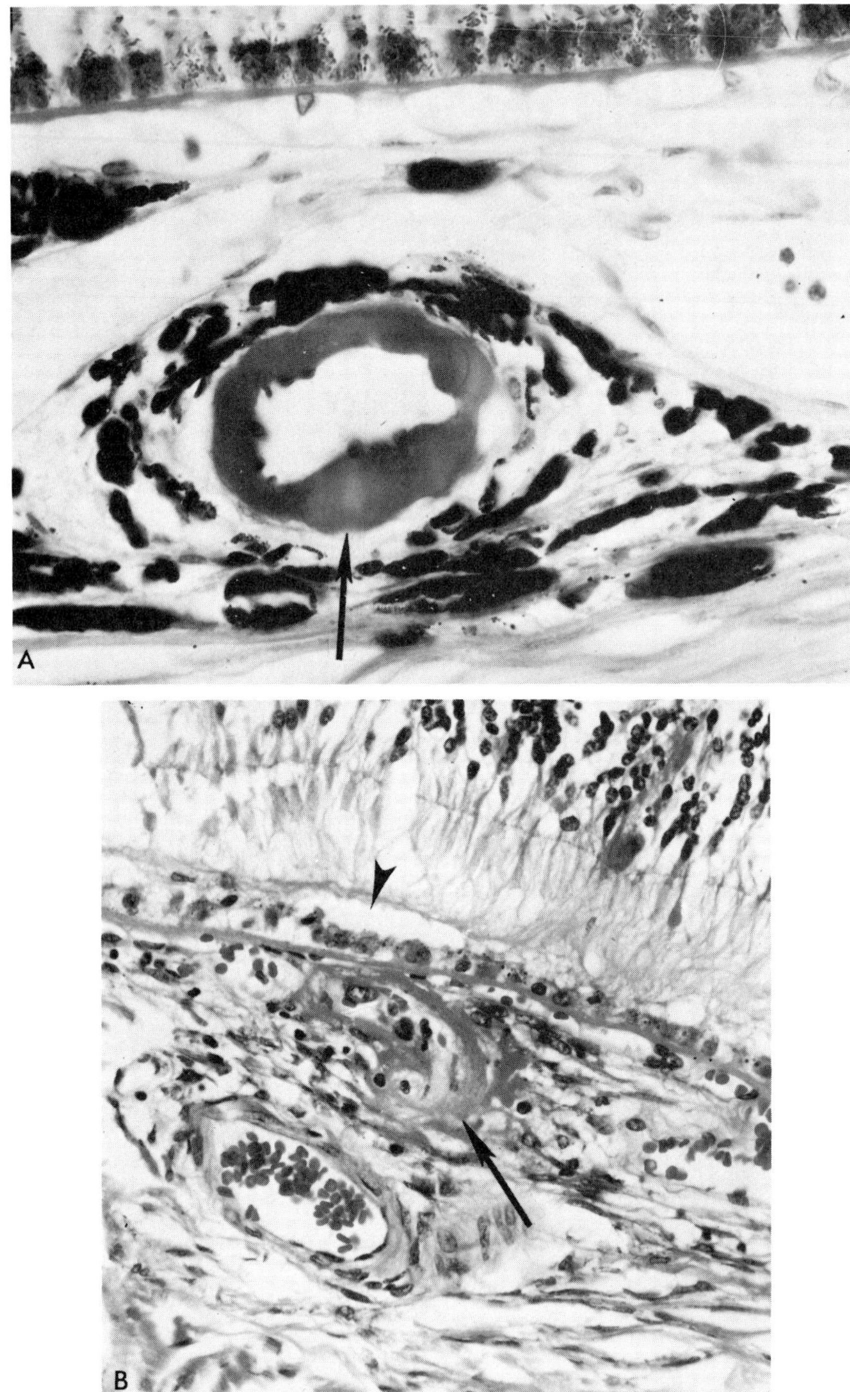

Figure 8–424. Fibrinoid deposition in wall of choroidal arteries in malignant hypertension. *A,* Wall of artery is thickened by a homogeneous material (arrow). Endothelium remains intact. PAS, ×375. EP 38841. *B,* Thrombosed choroidal artery with fibrinous necrosis (arrow). Adjacent retinal pigment epithelium is disrupted (arrowhead). H and E, ×165. EP 33307.

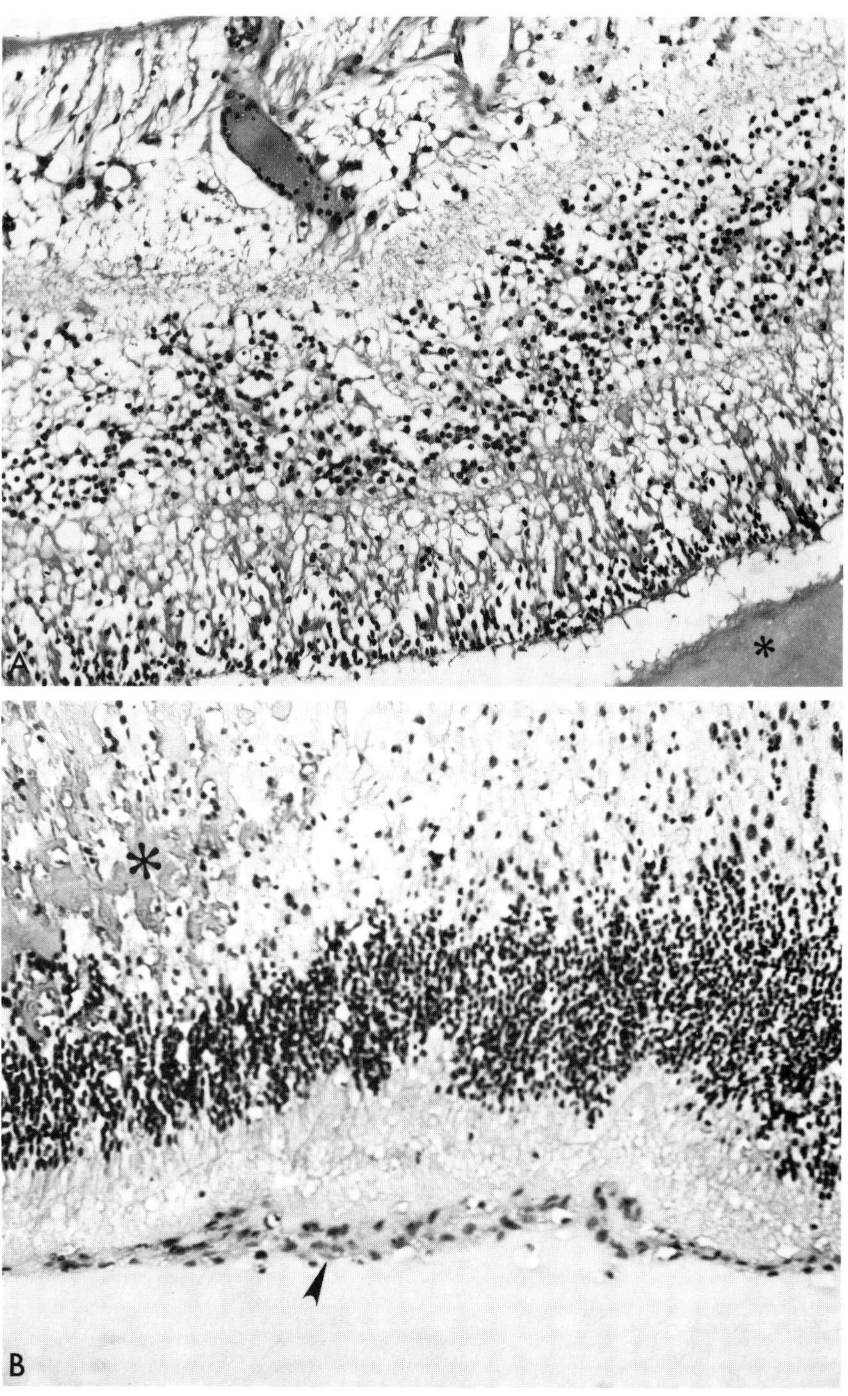

Figure 8–425. Retinal edema in malignant hypertension. *A,* Retina is diffusely thickened, with extreme microcystic formation. A proteinaceous material (asterisk) is present in the subretinal space. H and E, ×190. *B,* Another area showing accumulation of denser proteinaceous material in retina (asterisk) and a retroretinal membrane of retinal pigment epithelium origin (arrowhead). H and E, ×185. (From Frayer W; case presented at Verhoeff Society, Washington, DC, April, 1977.)

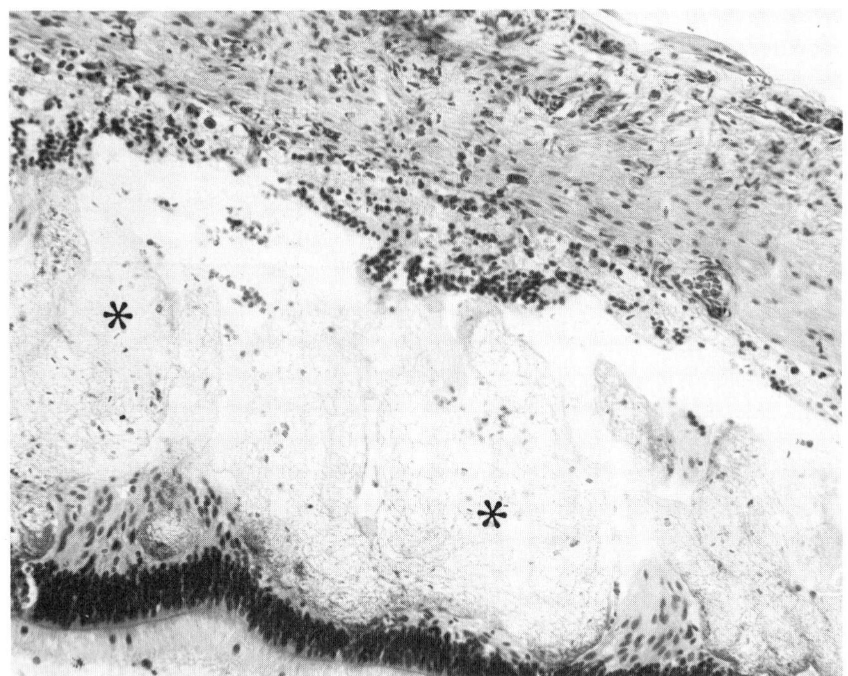

Figure 8–426. Cystic retinal edema (asterisks) with a fibrinous component in malignant hypertension. H and E, ×190. (From Heath P; case presented at Ophthalmic Pathology Club, Washington, DC, April, 1954.)

Figure 8–427. Changes in eye of a 26 year old man who died **of malignant hypertension.** *A,* Papilledema, showing partial obliteration of optic cup, thickening of peripapillary retina (between arrowheads), and peripapillary crowding of retina (arrows). Retina adjacent to nerve head has been pushed away for about 0.5 mm on both sides, and a microinfarction is present in the temporal prelaminar area of the optic nerve head (asterisk). H and E, ×30.

B, Higher power view of area of "ischemic papillitis." Disruption of nerve fibers is seen in area of infarction (arrowheads), and cytoid body formation is just anterior to lamina cribrosa (asterisks). The temporal margin of the optic disk is marked by an arrow at the termination of Bruch's membrane. H and E, ×200. *C,* Thickening of retina by edema. Some cystic spaces have a fibrinous character (asterisks). Some retinal vessels show much endothelial-cell proliferation (arrows). A thin layer of proteinaceous material is present in subretinal space (arrowhead). H and E, ×185.

D, Different area showing detached retina with total loss of outer segments of photoreceptors, near-total loss of inner segments, retinal edema, and a pigmented retroretinal membrane (arrow) of retinal pigment epithelium origin. External limiting membrane, arrowheads. H and E, ×310. *E,* Two areas of microinfarction (arrows) with much thickening of nerve fiber layer, with prominent cytoid bodies. Masson trichrome, ×185. *F,* Higher power view shows pseudonucleus from obstructed axoplasmic material in cytoid bodies. Masson trichrome, ×500. EP 4036.

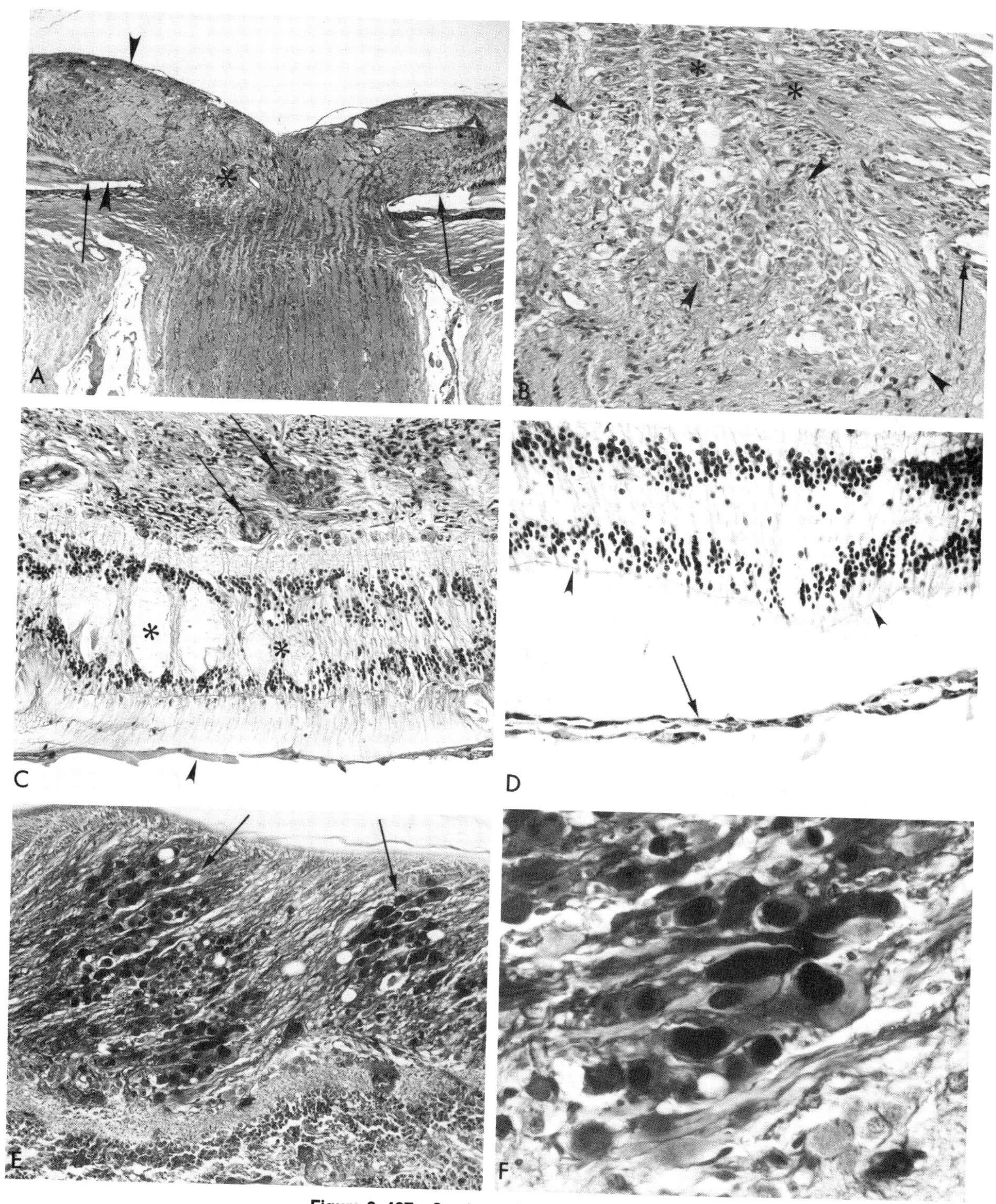

Figure 8–427 *See legend on opposite page*

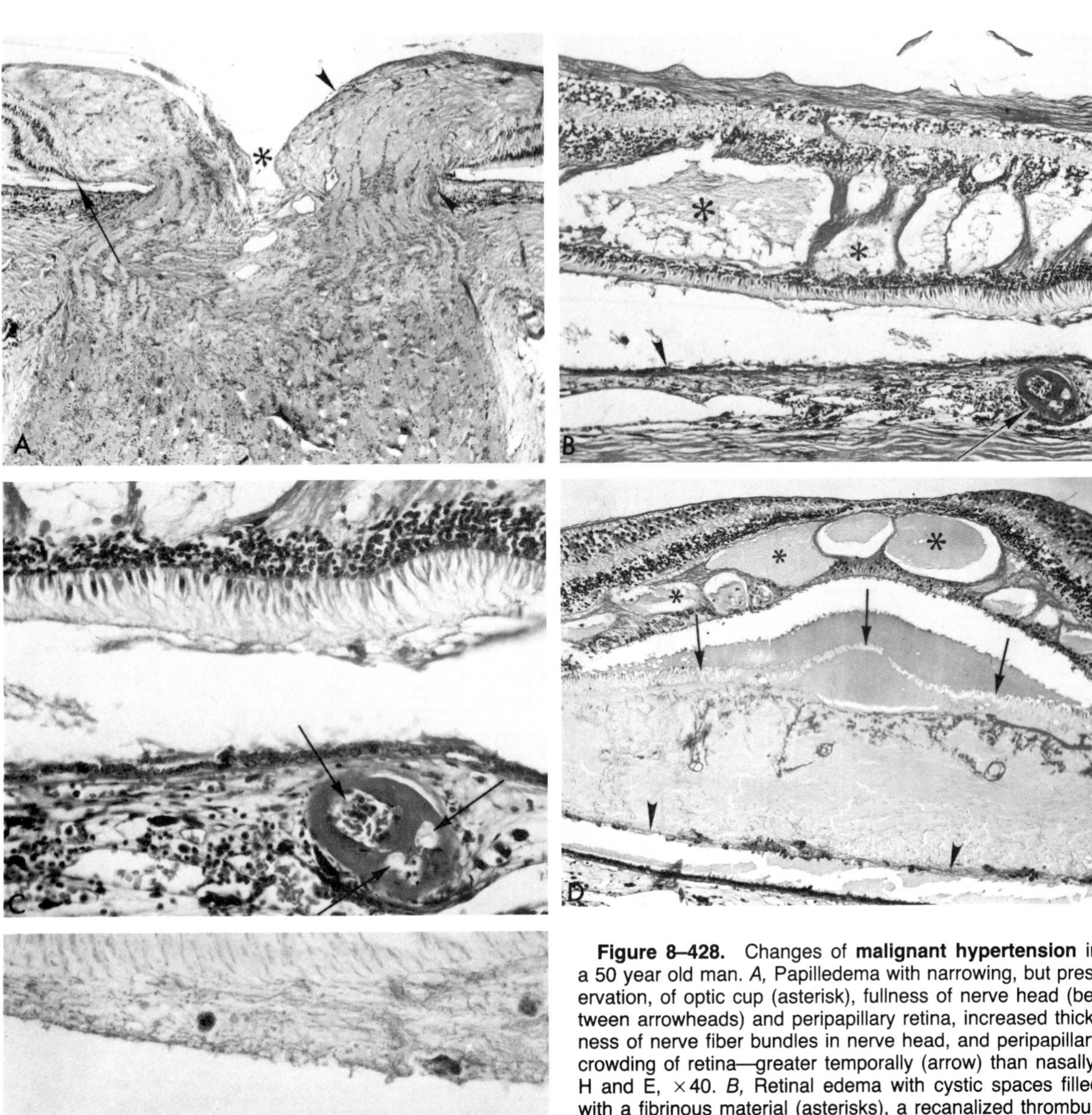

Figure 8–428. Changes of **malignant hypertension** in a 50 year old man. *A,* Papilledema with narrowing, but preservation, of optic cup (asterisk), fullness of nerve head (between arrowheads) and peripapillary retina, increased thickness of nerve fiber bundles in nerve head, and peripapillary crowding of retina—greater temporally (arrow) than nasally. H and E, ×40. *B,* Retinal edema with cystic spaces filled with a fibrinous material (asterisks), a recanalized thrombus in a choroidal artery with fibrinoid necrosis (arrow), and partially degenerated retinal pigment epithelium (RPE) (arrowhead). H and E, ×110.

C, Higher power view showing channels of recanalization (arrows) in a choroidal artery, with fibrinous material in wall. H and E, ×320. *D,* Section of macula showing cystic edema in outer plexiform layer (asterisks), a proteinaceous material with cellular elements, fibrin, and separated photoreceptors (arrows). A fibrocellular membrane with fluid on both sides extends across the subretinal space (arrowheads) in the area of macular detachment. H and E, ×100.

E, One of several areas of occlusion of choriocapillaris with fibrinoid material (between arrows). Suprajacent RPE is cystic and partially degenerated (between arrowheads). H and E, ×450. EP 4859.

down the effects into hypertensive choroidopathy, retinopathy and optic disk edema. In hypertensive choroidopathy, focal occlusion of choriocapillaris leads to necrosis and atrophy of the RPE with outer ischemic atrophy (Elschnig spots). The phases of hypertensive retinopathy include vasoconstrictive, exudative, sclerotic, and complications of arteriosclerosis. The latter include intimal thickening (endarteritis fibrosis), hyalinization of muscle cells, macroaneurysms, microaneurysms, central retinal artery and vein occlusions, epiretinal membrane formation, and vascular remodeling. Hypertensive optic disk edema is influenced by the blood supply and extracellular tissue fluid pressure of the optic nerve head. Experimental studies of hypertension in baboons showed there was an accumulation of axoplasmic material in swollen axons anterior to the lamina scleralis (Tso and Jampol, 1982).

Choroidal vascular insufficiency is thought to be the basis of the secondary retinal detachment observed in *toxemia of pregnancy* (Fastenberg, Fetkenhour, Choromokos, Shoch, 1980). Mabie and Ober (1980) presented evidence that the retinal detachment seen in toxemia was secondary to choroidal and RPE damage. Oliver and Uchenik (1980) observed that the choroidal and RPE effects of toxemia with exudative retinal detachment may occur without signs of hypertensive retinopathy.

Occlusive changes in the central and tributary arteriolar and venous channels of the eye are frequent in the sclerosis of long-standing hypertension. Branch retinal vein occlusions occur at crossings because the sclerotic process seems to compress and deflect to the vein. The upper temporal vein possibly is more often affected, because it has more crossings with branches of the central retinal artery. Central retinal vein occlusions are fairly common. Branch arteriole and central artery occlusions are less common in arteriosclerosis, probably because of the stronger construction of these vessels, lack of compression by other vessels, and their more direct course.

Long-standing hypertension with retinal vas-

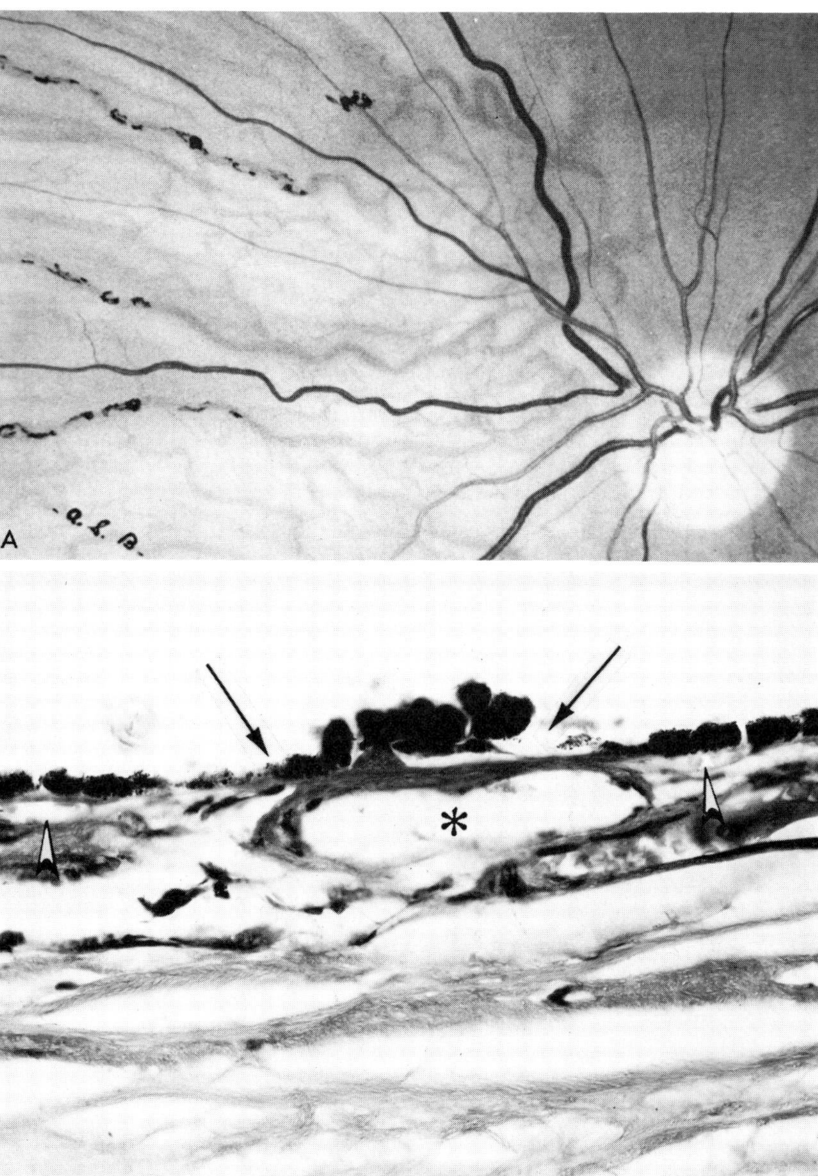

Figure 8–429. *A,* **Siegrist streaks** consist of hyperpigmentation over arteriosclerotic choroidal arteries in systemic hypertension. *B,* Hyperpigmentation is due to retinal pigment epithelium (RPE) hypertrophy and minor hyperplasia (between arrows). The sclerotic choroidal artery (asterisk) has apparently obliterated choriocapillaris in the area, and this caused the RPE changes. Choriocapillaris (arrowheads) is intact at either side of streak. PAS, ×500. EP 48087. (From Scholz RO: Epivascular choroidal pigment streaks; Their pathology and possible prognostic significance. Bull Johns Hopkins Hosp. 77:345–376, 1945.)

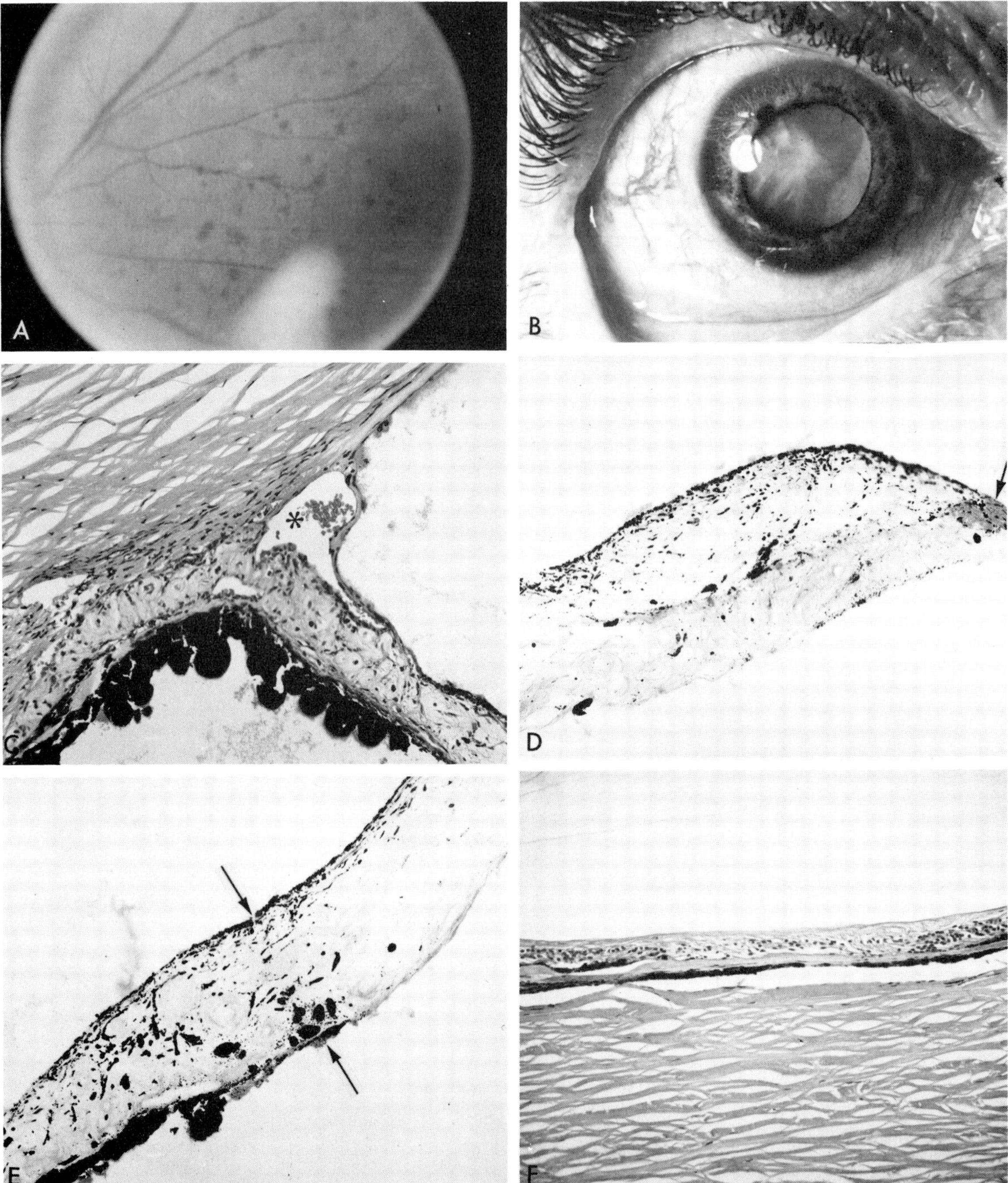

Figure 8–430. Hypotensive retinopathy in a 69 year old man, with occlusion of both internal carotids and left vertebral artery. *A,* Ophthalmoscopic appearance of retinal vascular dilatation and peripheral punctate hemorrhages. *B,* Patient developed episcleral vascular dilatation, iris atrophy, and cataract. *C,* Neovascularization of iris at anterior chamber angle. Vessels (asterisk) cross false angle at a point of peripheral anterior synechia. H and E, ×180.

D, Pupillary margin of iris, showing necrosis and loss of pigment epithelium and almost the entire sphincter muscle. Only a small portion of sphincter muscle remains (arrow). H and E, ×170. *E,* Junction (between arrows) between intact iris (left) and necrotic iris (right). H and E, ×175. *F,* Outer retinal ischemic atrophy in area of cobblestone degeneration, with loss of retinal pigment epithelium (RPE) and outer macula. The remains of the inner macular layer rest against Bruch's membrane. H and E, ×185.

Illustration continued on opposite page

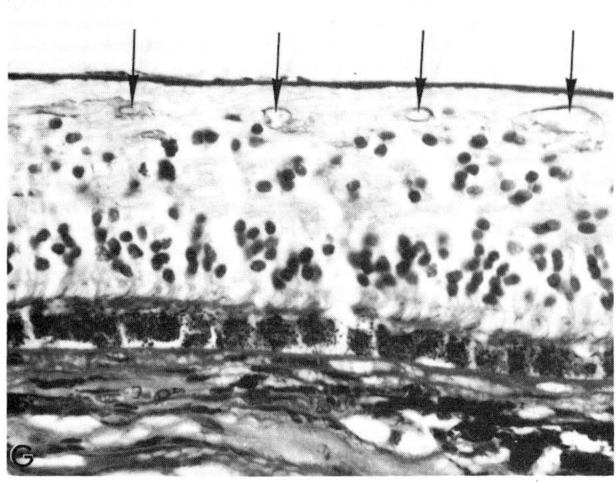

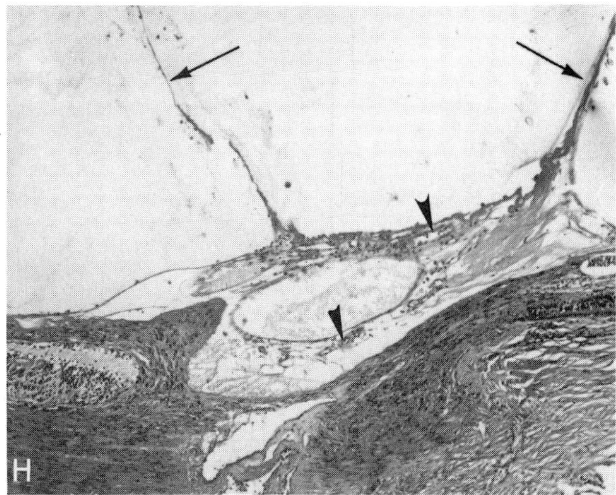

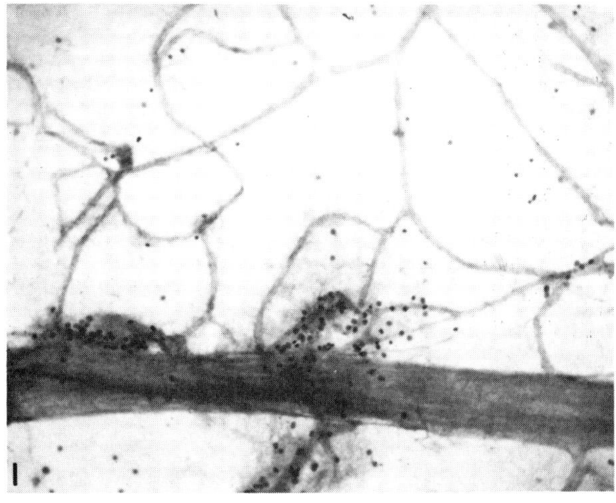

Figure 8–430 *Continued G,* Parafoveal area of macula, showing inner ischemic atrophy with loss of all inner layers down to and including the inner portion of the inner nuclear layer. Choriocapillaris, RPE, outer nuclear and outer plexiform layers, and outer portion of inner nuclear layer remain intact. Retinal capillaries (arrows) are acellular. *H,* Disk neovascularization (arrowheads). Strands of vitreous (arrows) are attached to neovascular tissue. H and E, ×165. *I,* Trypsin digestion of retina, showing total acellularity. Hematoxylin, PAS, ×185.

EP 31062. (From Michelson PE, Knox DL, Green WR: Ischemic ocular inflammation: A clinicopathologic case report. Arch Ophthalmol *86*:274–280, 1971.)

cular sclerosis can lead to gradual atrophy of the retina, with reduction in the number and size of cells and also their function. Edema and hemorrhages are not characteristic of the retinopathies related to arteriolar sclerosis, except in the case of vascular accident and accelerated hypertension.

Sheathing of the vessels can be due to severe arteriosclerotic changes along the side of the vessel wall. If the sheathing encircles the wall, it produces a silver-wire vessel, but if the sheathing is more visible along the lateral walls, the walls appear to be sheathed laterally. The microscopic counterpart is also hyalinization and sclerosis of the vessel wall, with narrowing of its lumen. Sheathing also may be due to accumulation of debris, cells, and plasma in the perivascular space, as a result of edema in various types of retinopathy. This type of sheathing is more common around veins and is transient, subsiding as soon as the process causing it disappears.

Retinal Capillaries. Ikui, Tominaga, Inomata, et al (1968) have described senescent capillary changes that included thickening of the basement membrane surrounding the pericytes and that of the endothelium in some areas, vacuoles with probable lipid droplets in the new basement membrane, and formation of reticular fibrils in the basement membrane. The term "senile retinal capillarosclerosis" is useful (Ikui and associates, 1968) to indicate these changes. Kuwabara and Cogan (1965), utilizing the trypsin digestion technique, have observed peripheral capillary acellularity as a frequent aging change. In benign hypertension there is loss of pericytes and considerable thickening of the basement membrane of the capillaries.

An uncommon change seen in chronic hypertension is *Siegrist streaks*. These are linear areas of hyperpigmentation that occur over choroidal arteries. Histopathologic studies have shown the streaks to be localized hyperplasia of the RPE overlying a markedly sclerotic choroidal artery, with compression and attenuation of the choriocapillaris (Scholz, 1945) (Fig. 8–429).

Ocular Changes Associated with Massive Blood Loss. Retinal hemorrhages and edema, disk edema, blindness, and optic atrophy may accompany large losses of blood (Pears, Pickering, 1960; Zanen, Meunier, 1961). The hemorrhages and edema are believed to be caused by ischemia. Optic atrophy and blindness are attributed to ischemic optic neuropathy in these cases.

Hypotensive Retinopathy (Retinopathy of Carotid Artery Occlusive Disease). Hypotensive retinopathy is a slowly progressive, occlusive vascular disease of the whole eye. Hypotensive retinopathy (venous stasis retinopathy—Kearns, Hollenhorst, 1963; ocular ischemic inflammation syndrome—Knox, 1965, 1969; Michelson, Knox, Green, 1971) occurs in association with partial or complete occlusion of the internal carotid artery. It is characterized by dilatation of retinal arteries and, especially, retinal veins, and blot hemorrhages in the midperiphery and periphery of the retina (Hedges, 1963) (Fig. 8–430,*A*). In some instances of hypotensive retinopathy, partial ischemic necrosis of the iris, and possibly of the ciliary body, may ensue, and signs of inflammation may be prominent (Fig. 8–430,*B*). The entire eye eventually may develop ischemic changes in both the inner (retinal) and outer (choroidal) circulations.

Histopathologic studies (Michelson, Knox, Green, 1971) have shown rubeosis iridis (Fig. 8–430,*C*), partial necrosis of iris (Fig. 8–430,*D,E*), partial atrophy of the ciliary body, cataract, extensive retinal cobblestone degeneration (outer retinal ischemic atrophy) (see Figs. 8–271 and 8–430,*F*), inner ischemic atrophy of the retina, and disk neovascularization (Fig. 8–430,*H*). The retina disintegrated almost totally when exposed to trypsin digestion. A few remaining areas showed total loss of endothelium and pericytes (Fig. 8–430,*I*). The fellow eye in that same case was studied by trypsin digestion and showed loss of pericytes and the presence of capillary microaneurysms in the periphery only (Fig. 8–43,*A* and *C*). Of interest was the finding of a normal ratio of endothelial cells to pericytes posteriorly (Fig. 8–31,*B*), a reduction of pericytes in the midperiphery, and near-total loss of pericytes with normal endothelium in the periphery (Fig. 8–431,*C*). This eye had been symptomatic, with several episodes of amaurosis fugax prior to the patient's death.

Serial sections through the optic nerve were available for restudy (Dr. W. R. Green) in the case reported by Michelson, Knox, and Green (1971). The central retinal artery and vein in the optic nerve head and the laminar and retrolaminar portions were patent without evidence of thrombosis in both eyes.

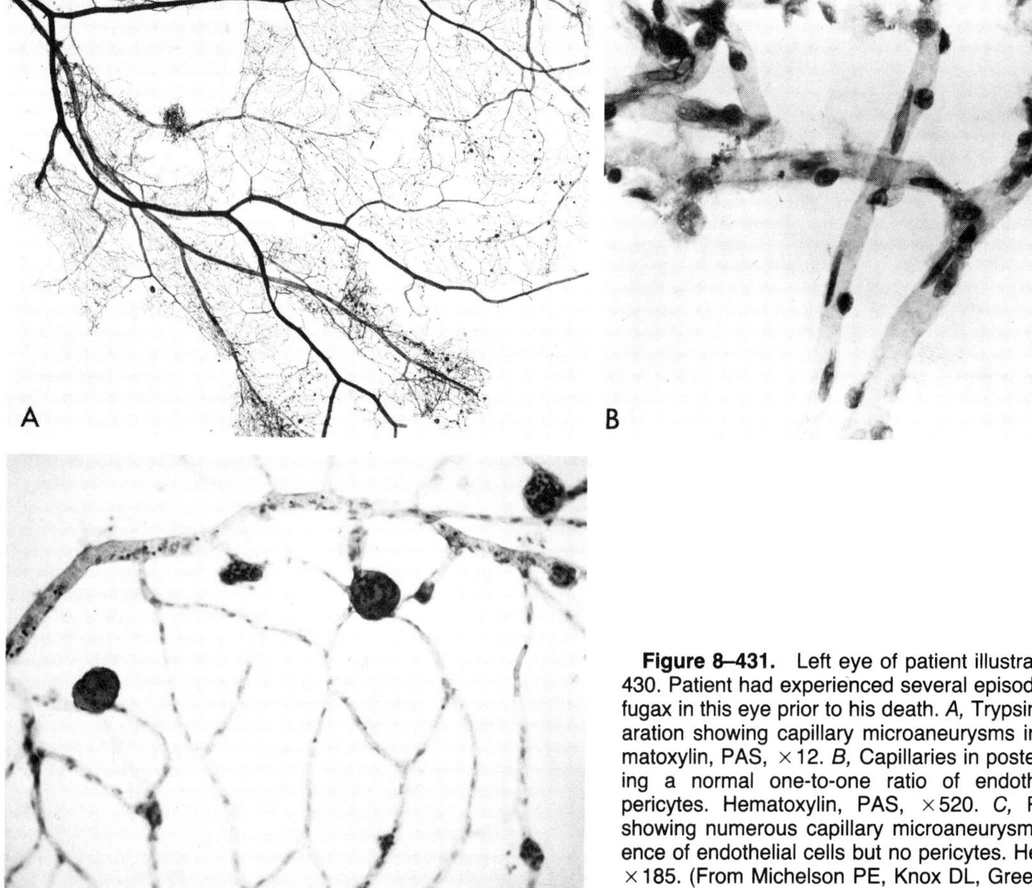

Figure 8–431. Left eye of patient illustrated in Figure 8–430. Patient had experienced several episodes of amaurosis fugax in this eye prior to his death. *A,* Trypsin digestion preparation showing capillary microaneurysms in periphery. Hematoxylin, PAS, ×12. *B,* Capillaries in posterior area, showing a normal one-to-one ratio of endothelial cells and pericytes. Hematoxylin, PAS, ×520. *C,* Peripheral area, showing numerous capillary microaneurysms and the presence of endothelial cells but no pericytes. Hematoxylin, PAS ×185. (From Michelson PE, Knox DL, Green WR: Ischemic ocular inflammation: A clinicopathologic case report. Arch Ophthalmol *88*:274–280, 1971.)

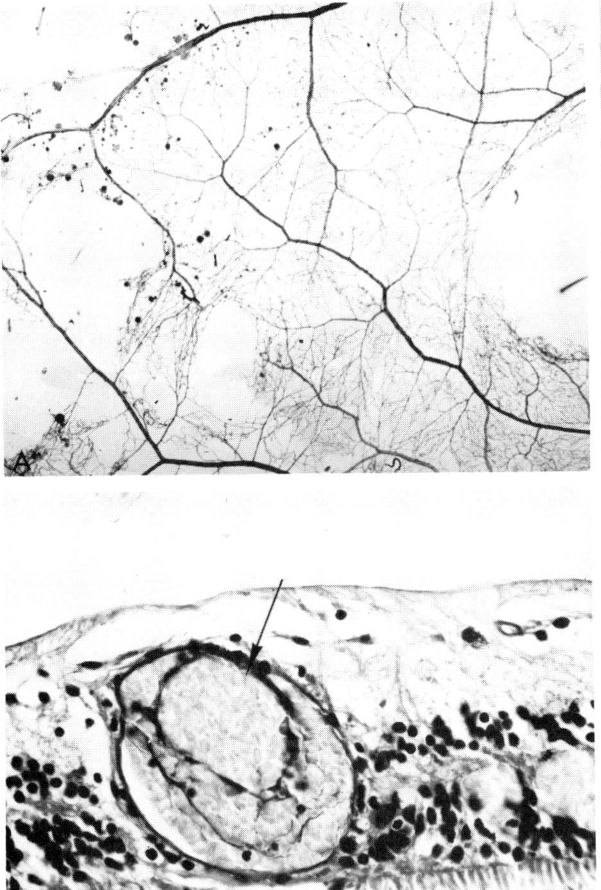
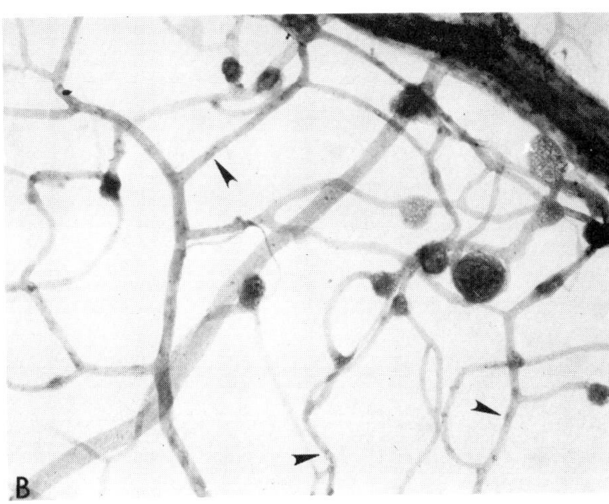

Figure 8–432. Hypotensive retinopathy. *A,* Trypsin digestion preparation of retina showing capillary microaneurysms in peripheral retina. Hematoxylin, PAS, ×40. *B,* Higher power view showing capillary microaneurysms, total loss of pericytes, and relative preservation of endothelium (arrowheads). Hematoxylin, PAS, ×100. *C,* The finding of large peripheral capillary microaneurysms in routine sections (arrow) first suggested the diagnosis of hypotensive retinopathy. PAS, ×525. EP 44444.

Hypotensive retinopathy associated with occlusion of the internal carotid was diagnosed post mortem by a study of the eyes of a 78 year old man (Fig. 8–432). An additional case of hypotensive retinopathy shows inner retinal ischemic atrophy posteriorly (Fig. 8–433,*A*) and both inner and outer ischemic atrophy in the periphery (Fig. 8–433,*B*).

Resolution of hypotensive retinopathy (venous stasis retinopathy) has been observed after carotid artery bypass surgery (Kearns, Young, Piepgras, 1980).

Pulseless Disease (Takayasu's Disease; Takayasu-Ohnishi's Disease). Takayasu's disease is a generalized disease with a predilection for the aorta and its branches (Strachan, 1964) and frequent central nervous system signs and symptoms (Riehl, 1965). The disease is considered to be an autoimmune process (Riehl, Brown, 1965; Nakao, Ikeda, Kimata, et al, 1967), and steroid therapy has been found helpful (Fraga, Mintz, Valle, Flores-Izquierdo, 1972; Spencer, Tolentino, Doyle, 1980).

It is of interest that in his original patient, Takayasu (1908) observed a wreathlike vascular anastomosis around the optic nerve head. In a discussion of this case, Ohnishi and Kagoshima (1908) reported the absence of the pulse in two cases with similar ocular findings.

A clinical and histopathologic picture similar to that described previously in carotid artery occlusion also may be seen in pulseless disease (Dowling, Smith, 1960; Font, Naumann, 1969; Pinkham, 1955).

The case reported by Font and Naumann (1969) is of interest because it showed that some blood was getting through the retinal circulation, for there was preservation of some ganglion cells only around the retinal arterioles in the peripapillary retina (Fig. 8–434,*A*). It is also interesting that there was preservation of the pericytes and loss of retinal vascular endothelium (Fig. 8–434,*B*), in contrast to the changes described in carotid occlusive disease.

Aortic Arch Syndrome. This categorization implies insufficient blood flow from the aortic arch (Hedges, 1964), and it can be caused by Takayasu's disease, arteritis of unknown etiology, syphilitic aortitis with or without aneurysm, and atherosclerosis with or without thrombosis.

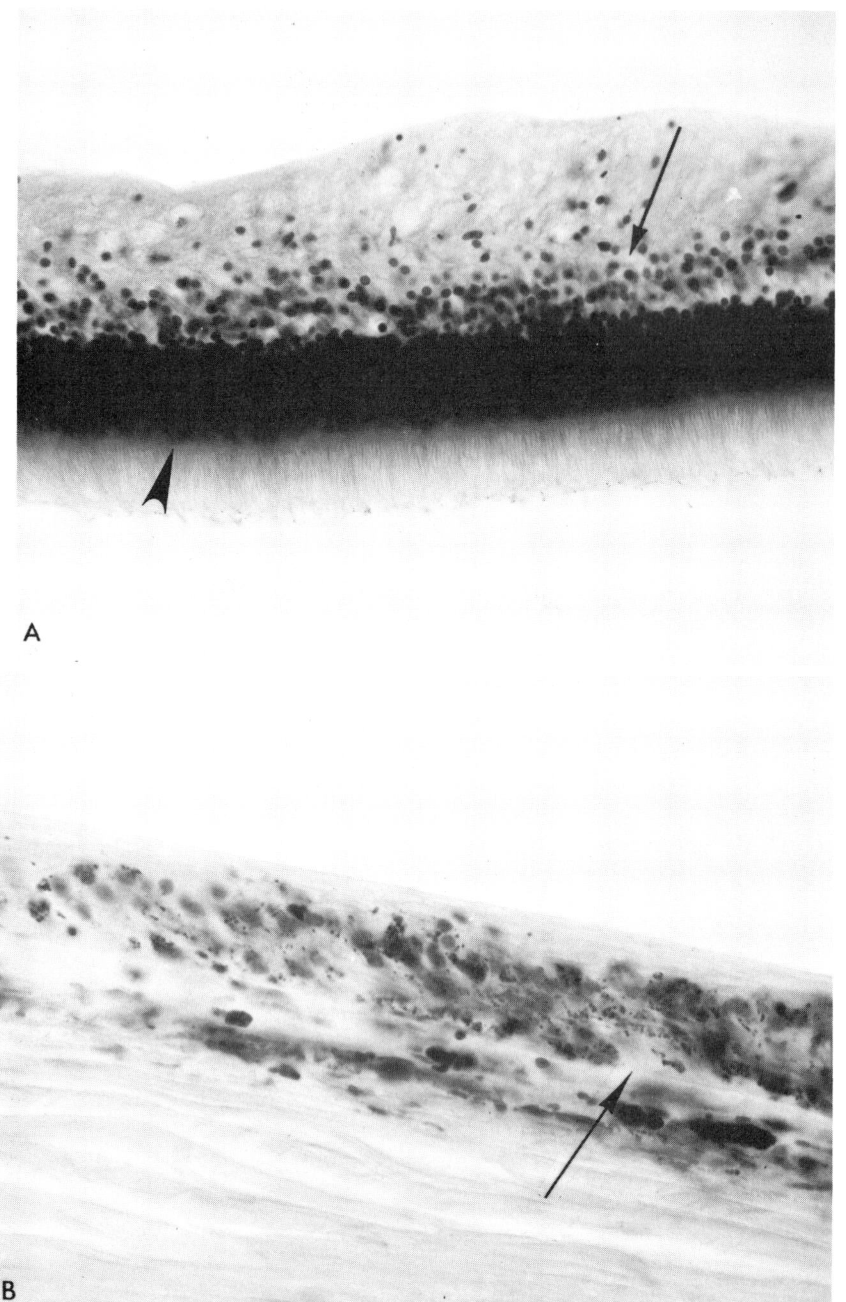

Figure 8–433. Hypotensive retinopathy. *A,* Posterior retina showing loss of inner retinal layers down to and including the inner portion of the inner nuclear layer. Retinal pigment epithelium (RPE) (out of field), photoreceptors, outer nuclear (arrowhead) and outer portion of inner nuclear layer (arrow) are preserved. H and E, ×350. *B,* Peripheral area showing a fibroglial strand of retina containing some pigment. RPE is absent. Choroid is thinned, and Bruch's membrane (arrow) is intact. H and E, ×400. EP 50925.

Metabolic Diseases

Diabetic Retinopathy. Diabetic retinopathy has become one of the most serious and important blinding diseases, in part because of the longer life span of diabetics. Diabetic retinopathy occurs in 1.5 to 2 per cent of all diabetics, and eventually the retinal changes affect 50 per cent of patients. Diabetic retinopathy was present in 2 per cent of all persons between 52 and 64 years of age in the Framingham Eye Study of a general population (Kini, Leibowitz, Colton, et al, 1978). Retinal involvement is greater with duration of the diabetes; it is rare in diabetes of less than 3 years' duration, and it occurs in about 10 per cent of diabetic patients who have had the disease 11 to 15 years, and in 70 per cent of cases lasting beyond 20 years.

The process can be described as a capillary microangiopathy (see Fig. 8–82) with microinfarctions (see Fig. 8–68), exudates (see Fig. 8–71), edema, and neovascularization (Fig. 8–83). Vitreous hemorrhage and traction and retinal detachment can cause severe loss of vision.

Diabetic retinopathy can be classified into two main types: nonproliferative and proliferative. The nonproliferative form (also called "background'' retinopathy) is characterized by intraretinal changes.

In the early 1970s, it was recognized that some background changes heralded the imminent onset of proliferative retinopathy. This was termed preproliferative retinopathy to imply the more advanced process. Early, or simple, background retinopathy includes microaneurysms, dot-and-blot hemorrhages, and hard exudates. Preproliferative retinopathy includes venous beading, cotton-wool spots, and intraretinal microvascular abnormalities (IRMA) (Murphy, Patz, in press).

Clinically, one of the earliest signs of simple background retinopathy is dilatation of the veins. Microaneurysms are found in the posterior fundus, especially on the temporal side between the superior and inferior temporal vessels. These aneurysms are located more often on the venous side of the circulation. They are of capillary origin and vary enormously in number, but only a small portion of them are seen with the ophthalmoscope. Their full extent is revealed on fluorescein angiography. As few as ten microaneurysms or up to several hundred in more advanced cases may be seen. Usually they are around 25 to 100 microns in size. They increase in number with the duration of the diabetes, especially in the area centralis. They are of two types, saccular and fu-

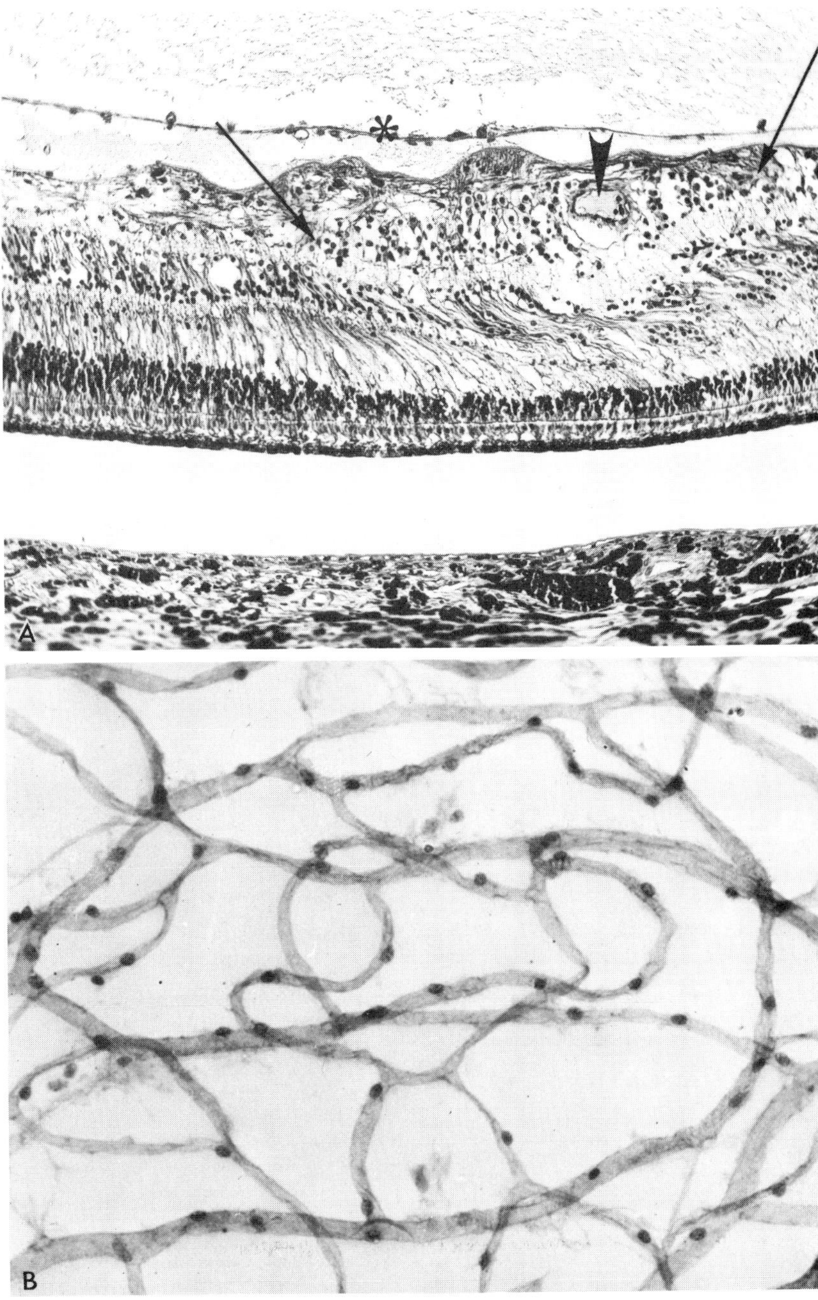

Figure 8–434. *A,* Peripapillary retina showing preservation of ganglion cells (between arrows) around a major retinal artery (arrowhead). Hypocellular epiretinal membrane (asterisk) is present. H and E, × 115. AFIP Neg. 69-468. *B,* Trypsin digestion preparation showing loss of capillary endothelium and preservation of pericytes. H and E, ×165. AFIP Neg. 69-3368. AFIP 1170584. (From Font RL, Naumann G: Ocular histopathology in pulseless disease. Arch Ophthalmol *82*:784–788, 1969.)

siform, and in the initial periods may be associated with small intraretinal exudates. They may be quiescent for years or may gradually fade as hyalinization and occlusion occur.

The hemorrhages that are seen in diabetic retinopathy arise mostly in the deeper capillary plexuses and therefore are round in shape. These hemorrhages lie in the inner plexiform, inner nuclear, and outer plexiform layers. They are small to large in size, and with increasing time they may become extensive, eventually becoming massive when hemorrhages occur from leakage of blood into the vitreous.

Diabetic exudates are a result of leakage of plasma into the retina. They tend to form in clusters, are sharply defined, and are somewhat waxen in color. Frequently they form a circinate pattern around groups of microaneurysms.

Microinfarctions of the nerve fiber layers with cotton-wool patches are also seen in the retina in the preproliferative form of diabetic retinopathy. The veins show fusiform changes and eventually develop a sausage-like appearance in the more advanced stage, described clinically as venous beading. Intraretinal microvascular abnormalities is a clinical term that includes shunt vessels, dilated capillaries, and intraretinal neovascularization (Davis, Myers, Engerman, et al, 1969) (Fig. 8–435).

Other changes can be superimposed on the diabetic retinopathy, because of the development of hypertension and arteriosclerotic changes. All the findings of hypertensive retinopathy may be present along with the diabetic changes.

Vitreous traction may lead to the production of venous loops (Fig. 8–436) (Hersh, Green, 1981). These loops consist of a telangiectatic retinal vein that is pulled into the vitreous through a discontinuity in Bruch's membrane. Venous loops may be a source of vitreous hemorrhage in background and proliferative diabetic retinopathy.

Proliferative retinopathy occurs in about 10 per cent of cases and is superimposed on the nonproliferative form. In proliferative retinopathy there

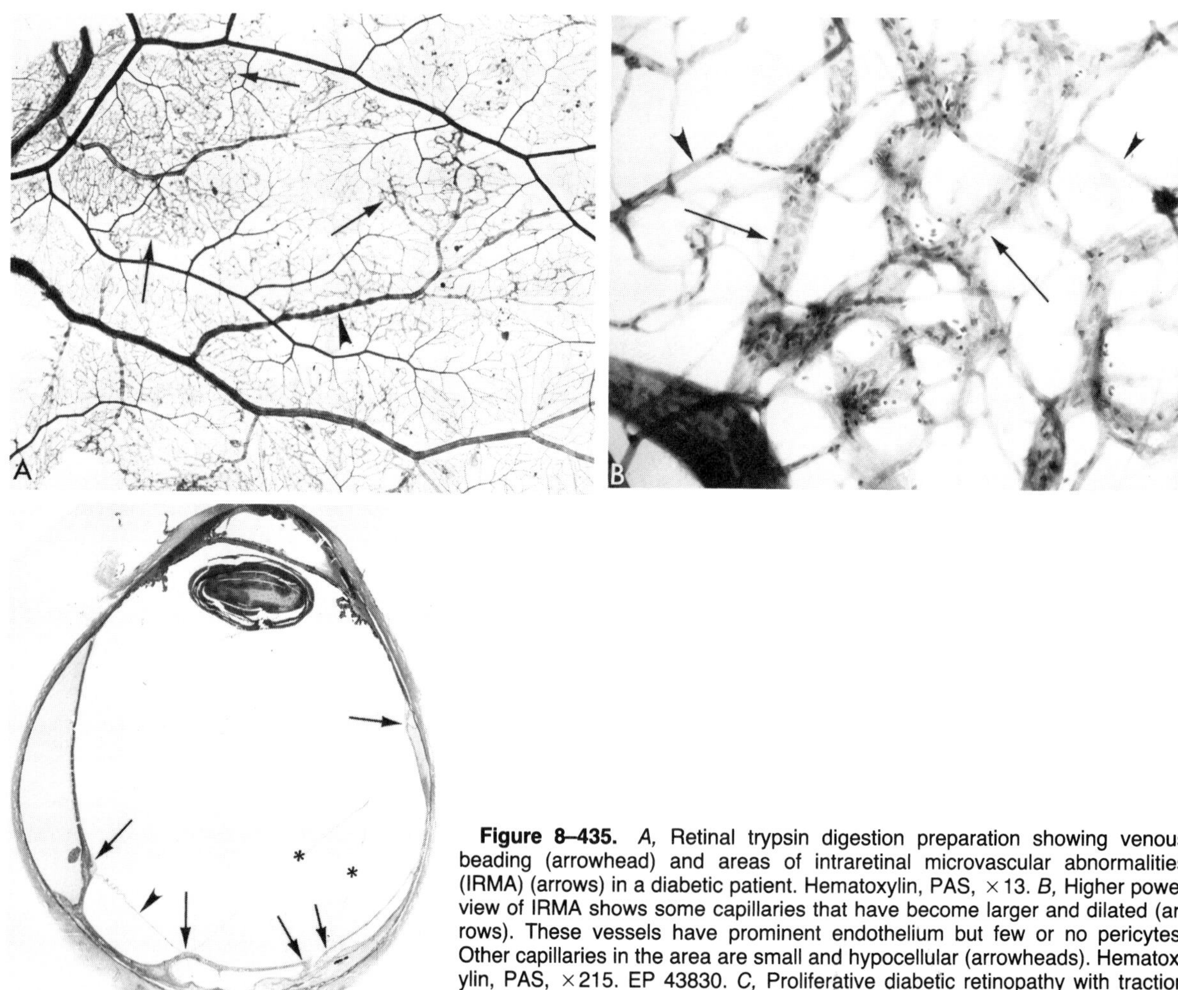

Figure 8–435. *A,* Retinal trypsin digestion preparation showing venous beading (arrowhead) and areas of intraretinal microvascular abnormalities (IRMA) (arrows) in a diabetic patient. Hematoxylin, PAS, ×13. *B,* Higher power view of IRMA shows some capillaries that have become larger and dilated (arrows). These vessels have prominent endothelium but few or no pericytes. Other capillaries in the area are small and hypocellular (arrowheads). Hematoxylin, PAS, ×215. EP 43830. *C,* Proliferative diabetic retinopathy with traction retinal detachment. There are anteroposterior (asterisks) and tangential (arrowhead) tractional bands. Retina is tented-up at each point (arrows) of attachment of these tractional vitreous membranes. H and E, ×45. EP 52444.

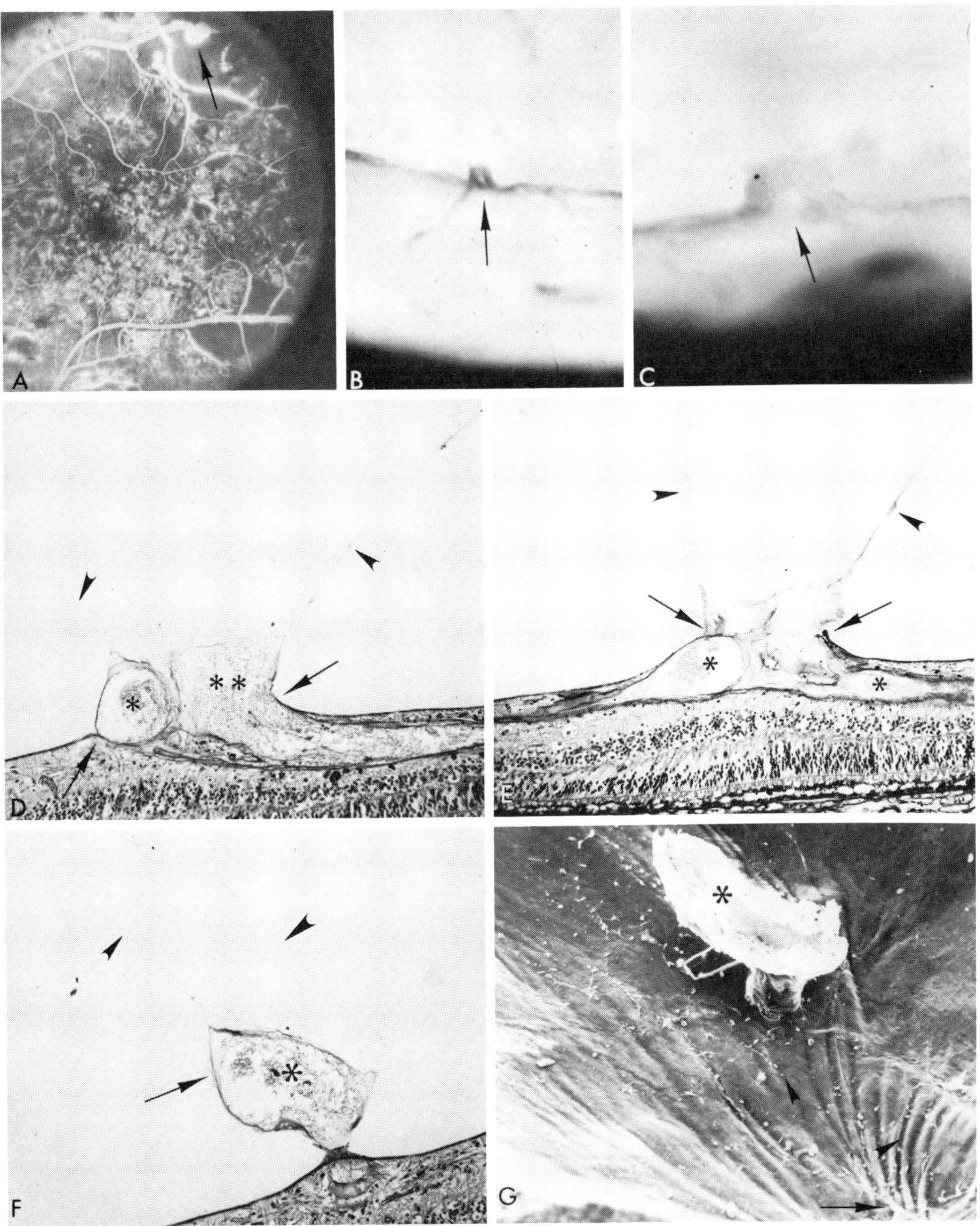

Figure 8–436. Tractional venous loops in diabetic retinopathy. *A,* Fluorescein angiographic appearance of venous loop of superotemporal vein (arrow). The wall of the loop shows staining with dye. The surrounding capillary bed is nonperfused. *B,* Gross appearance of venous loop (arrow) in left eye. *C,* Gross appearance of venous loop of right eye. The loop passes out and back into the retina. *D,* Section through the venous loop and parallel to the axis of the vein shows the anterior (asterisk) and posterior (double asterisk) components of the loop as it extends through a discontinuity in the internal limiting membrane (between arrows) of left eye. The wall of the loop is thin and tented at the points of attachment of thin delicate vitreous strands (arrowheads) anteriorly and posteriorly. PAS, ×100.

E, Different level of venous loop in left eye shows discontinuity of the internal limiting membrane (between arrows), continuity of loop with retinal vein (asterisks), and strands of vitreous (arrowheads) adherent to loop. PAS, ×100. *F,* Different level shows the attenuated wall (arrow) of the venous loop (asterisk), with strands of vitreous (arrowheads) attached. PAS, ×100. *G,* Scanning electron microscopy shows mushroom-shaped venous loop (asterisk) passing through the internal limiting membrane. Ridges in the membrane (arrowheads) are related to a localized preretinal membrane (arrow). ×60. EP 48650.

(From Hersh PS, Green WR, Thomas JV: Tractional venous loops in diabetic retinopathy. Am J Ophthalmol *92*:661–671, 1981.)

are intraretinal neovascularization and extension into the vitreous cavity in the region of the disk (NVD) and elsewhere in the retina (NVE). Intraretinal vessels form a congeries of small channels that lie in the nerve fiber and inner plexiform layers. In the papillary region, the vessels arise from the capillaries in the nerve fiber layer and proliferate as naked channels in the earliest stages. Later, fibrosis and gliosis occur around these vessels. Eventually there is bleeding from the vessels, producing recurring vitreous hemorrhages. Scarring and shrinkage tend to occur around these proliferating channels and may lead to wrinkling of the retina, to macular heterotopia (Bresnick, Haight, de Venecia, 1979), and to localized or extensive traction detachments of the retina.

Wallow, Greaser, and Stevens (1981), utilizing myosin subfragment-1 found cells in the vitreous, in a case of proliferative diabetic retinopathy with traction retinal detachment, to have abundant bundles of contractile protein actin. These investigators suggest that this feature may explain the contraction phenomenon and that the contraction might be blocked pharmacologically.

The tractional forces of such proliferative vitreous membranes may be directed anterior-posterior and tangentially (Fig. 8–435,*C*).

The histologic changes in diabetic retinopathy have been studied both in experimental animals and in human eyes. The pathogenesis of the lesions is debated, with some believing that endothelial damage leads to changes in permeability of the vessel walls and others believing that the primary change is in the basement membrane system of the retinal arterioles and capillaries. Similar changes are seen in the capillaries of the renal glomeruli, vessels that have a structure similar to those in the retina.

In experimental clinicopathologic studies of the blood ocular barriers in streptozocin (streptozotocin) diabetes, T'so, Cunha-Vaz, Shih, and Jones (1980) found that changes in the RPE were the principal site of leakage of fluorescein and horseradish peroxidase.

Some (Davis, Myers, Engerman, et al, 1969) think that diabetic retinopathy is best considered as the result of a gradually increasing ischemia, due presumably to a progressive narrowing or obliteration of capillaries and terminal arterioles.

There is general agreement that the characteristic capillary microaneurysms of diabetic retinopathy occur adjacent to acellular capillaries. Some investigators (Cogan, Kuwabara, 1963) favor the "shunt theory" to explain the sequence of changes. The shunt theory suggests that the initial change is a loss of the capillary pericytes (intramural pericytes), which leads to dilatation of capillaries, preemption of blood flow, then secondary atrophy and obliteration of the adjacent capillary bed. Others (Ashton, 1963; Levene, Horton, Gorn, 1966; Davis, Myers, Engerman, et al, 1969) believe that the capillary obliteration occurs first and is followed by dilatation of adjacent vascular channels that then accommodate a greater blood flow. The formation of capillary microaneurysms adjacent to localized acellular capillary zones is thought by some (Wise, 1956; Davis, Myers, Engerman, et al, 1969) to be abortive attempts at neovascularization.

There appears to be a selective loss of intramural pericytes in retinal capillaries in diabetes (Kuwabara, Cogan, 1963; Toussaint, Dustin, 1963; Yanoff, 1966; Speiser, Gittelsohn, Patz, 1968; Addison, Garner, Ashton, 1970). This loss is believed to weaken the capillary wall and predispose to the development of microaneurysms.

Kinoshita (1974) has demonstrated the accumulation of sorbitol in cataracts of diabetic patients. Aldose reductase mediates the conversion of glucose to sorbitol. The sorbitol accumulation and consequent osmotic effects are thought to lead to the diabetic cataract. A similar process is thought to occur in Schwann cells of the peripheral nervous system (Gabbay, Merola, Field, 1966) and the retinal mural cells (Buzney, Frank, Varma, et al, 1977). The accumulation of sorbitol is then the possible mechanism by which diabetic patients develop retinal microangiopathy, peripheral neuropathy, and cataract.

Capillary microaneurysms are weakened areas that can lead to hemorrhages and edema, the residue of which are "hard waxy" exudates (see Fig. 8–71). Adjacent to areas of ghost capillaries, the blood vessels lose their pericytes or endothelium, and saccular aneurysms form. Cellular shunt vessels are found at the periphery of these avascular areas. Early, they are very thin, and red blood cells can pass through their walls by diapedesis, but later the walls become thickened and laminated and are periodic acid–Schiff–positive. There is an increased number of nuclei within the walls of these aneurysms, and in the late stages they can undergo thrombosis. Hemorrhages are found mainly in the outer plexiform layer and are like those described in hypertensive retinopathy.

Serum leaks into the surrounding retina from the microaneurysms and neovascular tissue. The water content of the edema fluid is taken up by the blood vessels, and this leaves a lipid-rich residue that usually accumulates in the outer plexiform layer. Such exudate residues have discrete margins and may be distributed in a circinate or stellate pattern around the leaky vascular lesions. These exudates often collect in the outer plexiform layer of the parafoveal region because the anatomic configuration here allows for more distensibility of the retina and accumulation of edema and exudate residues. This lipid-rich material is mainly extracellular and is composed of polyunsaturated fats. Sometimes lipid-laden histiocytes are present within the exudate residues.

From these changes of simple background retinopathy the eye may progress to the preproliferative stage. With increasing duration of the disease, the larger vessels show changes like those previously described in arteriosclerosis from hypertension. The terminal arterioles usually show hyaline thickening and corkscrew coiling, with narrowing of their lumina. The venous changes are characterized by formation of loops and varicosities. Electron microscopy shows thickening of the basement membrane of the endothelium and the pericytes. There is separation of the layers of the capillary wall by debris and lipid material, and eventually there is loss of both endothelium and pericytes, leading to the formation of ghost capillaries that are functionless, with only the basement membrane remaining.

Gradually increasing ischemia then appears to be the initiator of the process. The most direct ophthalmoscopic sign of this ischemia is the presence of microinfarction, as evidenced by cotton-wool exudates.

Neovascularization with extension of vessels along the inner retinal surface sets the stage for development of blinding complications of diabetic retinopathy. These new blood vessels are thin walled and may have an endothelium that has fenestrations. This allows for profuse leakage of serum and often results in vitreous hemorrhage. The neovascular tissue is accompanied by fibroglial tissue. This fibrovascular and fibroglial tissue, and also contraction of the vitreous, leads to traction on the retina, with production of cystic degeneration, schisis, and retinal detachment with or without a retinal break.

Clinical pathology correlative studies of specific features in diabetic retinopathy include microaneurysm (de Venecia, Davis, Engerman, 1976; Bresnick, Davis, Myers, et al, 1977); venous loops (Hersh, Green, Thomas, 1981); and photocoagulation burns (Wallow, Davis, 1979). Other studies have utilized the trypsin digestion technique (Cogan, Toussaint, Kuwabara, 1961) to correlate retinal circulatory disturbances seen by fluorescein angiography with morphologic alterations (Kohner, Henkind, 1970; Bresnick, Engerman, Davis, et al, 1976).

Kincaid, Green, Fine, et al (1983) conducted clinicopathologic studies of the eyes of more than 50 patients with diabetic retinopathy, of whom 20 had been treated by panretinal scatter photocoagulation. Six patients were enrolled in the Diabetic Retinopathy study. Of those six patients, four had equal or better vision in the treated eye at their last visit. Two had worse vision, which was attributed mostly to cystoid macular edema. All but one patient had prominent visual field loss in the treated eye.

The Diabetic Retinopathy Study (DRS), begun in 1971 by the National Eye Institute, showed photocoagulation is of benefit in preserving vision in eyes with proliferative retinopathy (Diabetic Retinopathy Study Research Group, 1976, 1978). In the design of this study, the ocular findings were standardized (1979, 1981a, 1981b), and treatment was limited to one eye chosen at random.

Additional randomized clinical studies are currently underway to evaluate treatment of early diabetic retinopathy and the possible benefits of vitreous surgery.

Collagen Vascular Diseases

Retinal involvement in the collagen vascular diseases consists primarily of localized ischemia with the production of microinfarctions.

The intensity of cotton-wool exudates varies with the different diseases in this group. If systemic hypertension is present, there is a greater tendency for microinfarcts to occur.

Retinal hemorrhages and edema generally reflect the intensity of the disease and also may be related to the concomitant presence of hypertension.

Choroidal vascular involvement also may be observed, with the production of ciliochoroidal effusion and scondary serous retinal detachment. Choroidal changes can be observed in any of the diseases of this group but are more likely to occur in polyarteritis nodosa, Wegener's granulomatosis, and allergic angiitis.

Keratoconjunctivitis can occur in each of the disease categories but is more likely to be a problem clinically in rheumatoid arthritis and lupus erythematosus. Peripheral corneal degeneration and ulceration is a feature seen in the entire group, but, again, it is likely to be more severe in cases of rheumatoid arthritis, polyarteritis nodosa, and Wegener's granulomatosis.

The changes are mostly in blood vessels, the ground substance, and collagenous components of the affected area. The vessels and collagenous tissue show fibrinoid necrosis, with mucoid swelling of the ground substance. It is believed that most of the connective tissue diseases show variations and the cornea, sclera, uveal tract, optic nerve, and retina are affected in a variety of ways. The retina ordinarily is involved through its vascular system. The central vessels or their branches are the sites of the hypersensitivity reaction, and the tissue changes are secondary to the vascular disease. Those connective tissue dis-

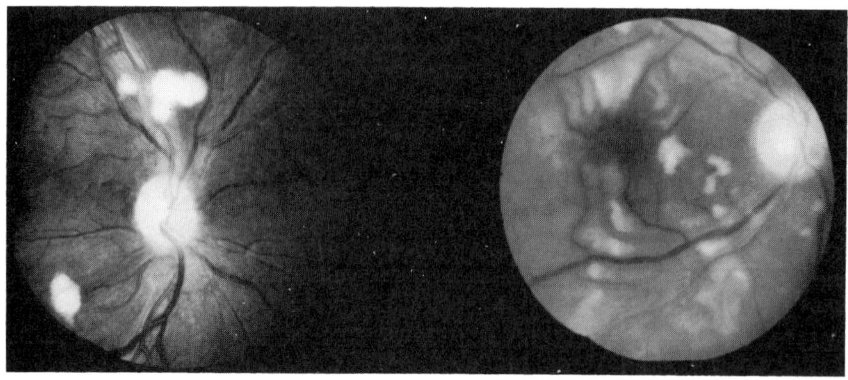

Figure 8–437. Microinfarctions in nerve fiber layer of lupus erythematosus in two patients without hypertension.

eases that induce systemic hypertension eventually produce the retinal changes of hypertension.

Systemic Lupus Erythematosus (SLE). SLE is a chronic inflammatory disease of unknown origin that may affect many different organs. The remarkably diverse clinical manifestations include fever, an erythematous rash, polyarthralgia and arthritis, polyserositis (especially pleurisy and pericarditis), anemia, thrombocytopenia, and renal, neurologic, and cardiac abnormalities (Dubois, 1966; Primer on Rheumatic Diseases, 1973).

Pathologically, there is collagenous degeneration in the walls of the blood vessels, with secondary endothelial proliferation and thrombosis. The retinal findings are mainly secondary to the vascular changes (Maumenee, 1940; Brihaye-Van Geertruyden, Danis, Toussaint, 1954; Clifton, Greer, 1955). Microinfarctions of the nerve fiber layer in the posterior pole are the main ocular finding in lupus erythematosus (Fig. 8–437). Studies of the retina from a patient with SLE and retinal microinfarctions disclosed many areas of discrete, fibrinoid necrosis of retinal arterioles that bordered on grossly observed cotton-wool spots (Yanoff, 1977, 1979). These cotton-wool patches are like those described under vascular diseases of the retina. Hemorrhage may occur as a result of the vascular damage and necrosis. There may be papilledema.

Perivasculitis has been described in the peripheral vessels (Böke, Bäumer, 1965). Extensive retinal vascular occlusion (Coppeto, Lessell, 1977) and central retinal artery occlusion (Gold, Feiner, Henkind, 1977) have been reported.

Focal RPE leakage with secondary localized retinal detachment was presumed to be caused by a vasculitis of choroidal vessels in a patient in whom choroidal mononuclear cell infiltration and deposition of immunoglobulin was demonstrated in choroidal vessels (Diddie, Ernest, 1977).

Polyarteritis Nodosa (Periarteritis Nodosa; Necrotizing Angiitis). This condition more commonly affects men in the age range of 20 to 40 years. Multiple inflammatory nodules occur in the arteriole walls, which undergo necrosis and then thrombosis. A variety of visceral, muscular, joint, cerebral, and ocular lesions develop in this disease, which is characterized by fever, malaise, weight loss, anemia, myalgias, subcutaneous nodules, skin rash, and joint pains. Ocular changes occur in about 10 to 20 per cent of patients. The retina is less commonly involved in the primary disease, but severe retinal changes follow hypertension. Central retinal artery occlusions or branch occlusions also have been described.

Clinically, the retina may show cotton-wool patches, hemorrhages, and exudate. Microscopically, there may be changes in the walls of the main arteries or arterioles, with necrosis. Inflammatory changes soon appear, and then either aneurysmal dilatations or ruptures of the vessels may form, and granulation tissue, composed mainly of chronic inflammatory cells with some macrophages and occasional giant cells, develops. The final healing stages follow, with formation of scar tissue. Exudative retinal detachment associated with scleritis has been reported (Kielar, 1976). Newman, Hoyt, and Spencer (1974) described an interesting patient with macular-sparing monocular blackouts caused by a vasculitis involving the short ciliary arteries, confirmed post mortem (Fig. 8–438). The insufficiency was not of a sufficient degree to produce outer retinal ischemic atrophy.

Wegener's Granulomatosis. Wegener's granulomatosis is characterized by necrotizing granulomatous lesions of the upper and lower respiratory tract, together wih a necrotizing glomerulonephritis and widespread disseminated vasculitis. Additionally, disseminated visceral necrotizing granulomata are present. The cause of Wegener's granulomatosis remains obscure; however, the pathologic features of granuloma formation, vasculitis, and glomerulonephritis are consistent with experimental models of hypersensitivity. The dramatic remissions with cytotoxic therapy, as well as the detection of immune complexes in renal biopsies, also support the concept of an immunologically mediated cause (Wolff, Fauci, Horn, Dale, 1974). The incidence of ocular

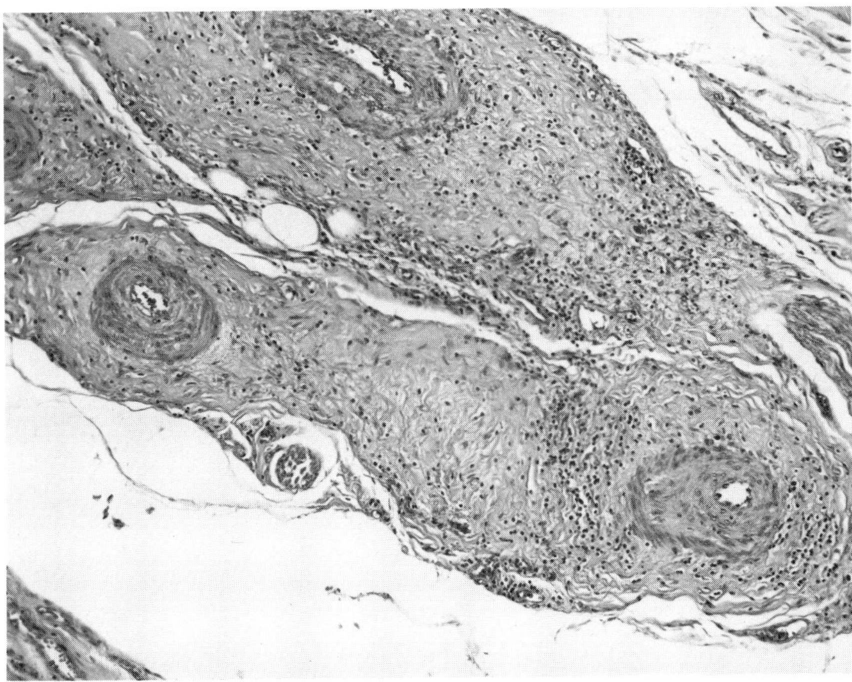

Figure 8–438. Ciliary arteries, showing marked thickening of wall, with intimal hyperplasia and extreme fibrosis of adventitia. Moderate lymphocytic infiltration of adventitia is present, and lumen of vessels is greatly narrowed. H and E, ×110. (From Newman NM, Hoyt WF, Spencer WH: Macula-sparing nonvascular blackouts: Clinical and pathologic investigations of intermittent choroidal vascular insufficiency in a case of periarteritis nodosa. Arch Ophthalmol *91*:367–370, 1974.)

involvement was about 42 per cent in two series with a total number of 141 patients (Straatsma, 1957; Cutler, Blatt, 1956).

In Straatsma's review of 44 reported cases, 19 (43 per cent) had ocular findings. In six cases, spread of granulomas from upper respiratory tract foci resulted in orbital involvement; these were classified as contiguous. Orbital signs included exophthalmos, exposure keratitis, chemosis, motility problems, retinal venous congestion, and papilledema. In 14 patients, focal ocular involvement was present in which the lesions were distinct from those of the respiratory tract. Focal signs, which are the result of focal vasculitis or granulomas, included cotton-wool exudates, narrowed retinal arterioles, uveitis, and conjunctivitis. The most common focal involvement was corneoscleral inflammation. Three patients had nonspecific episcleritis and scleritis; two other patients had paralimbal infiltrates with subsequent furrow formation.

Marginal ulceration is a common ocular manifestation and is often the first sign of Wegener's granulomatosis (Brady, Israel, Lewin, 1965; Tyner, 1960; Ferry, Leopold, 1970; Borley, Miller, 1961; Austin, Green, Sallyer, et al, 1978). The corneal involvement usually begins as paralimbal infiltrates, which lead to epithelial and stromal necrosis with subsequent furrow-like ulceration. The process may extend concentrically to form a ring ulcer or may progress centrally. There is often an overhanging leading edge, similar to a Mooren's ulcer. The base of the furrow may have a moderate degree of inflammatory cell infiltration and superficial vascularization. Eventually, perforation may result; the process is often bilateral. Scleral inflammation is invariably present, ranging from redness and induration to a localized necrotic slough.

Austin, Green, Sallyer, et al (1978) showed the peripheral corneal ulceration to be associated with an occlusive vasculitis involving the anterior ciliary arteries. Ciliochoroidal effusion (Fogle, Green, 1976) and outer retinal ischemic changes (see Fig. 8–96) also may be observed.

Dermatomyositis. The retinal changes of dermatomyositis are rather rare and consist mainly of cotton-wool patches and hemorrhages. The microscopic changes are similar to those described in the other connective tissue diseases.

Scleroderma. This condition is more common in women, and especially after infectious diseases. The skin is affected, especially that of the face, neck, and hands. The onset occurs with nonpitting edema and secondary fibrosis. The retina is not commonly affected, and the inflammatory lesions in scleroderma are not distinctive. Edema, exudates (Fig. 8–439), and hemorrhages have been described. The eyes have been examined microscopically in a number of patients with scleroderma, and no specific changes have been described except those possibly owing to hypertension (Ashton, Coomes, Garner, Oliver, 1968; Manschot, 1965). Retinal detachment has been described by Manschot (1965).

Farkas, Sylvester, and Archer (1972), in a clinicopathologic correlative study, observed the primary changes in the vasculature of the choroid. These consisted of diffuse basement membrane thickening and endothelial swelling and necrosis.

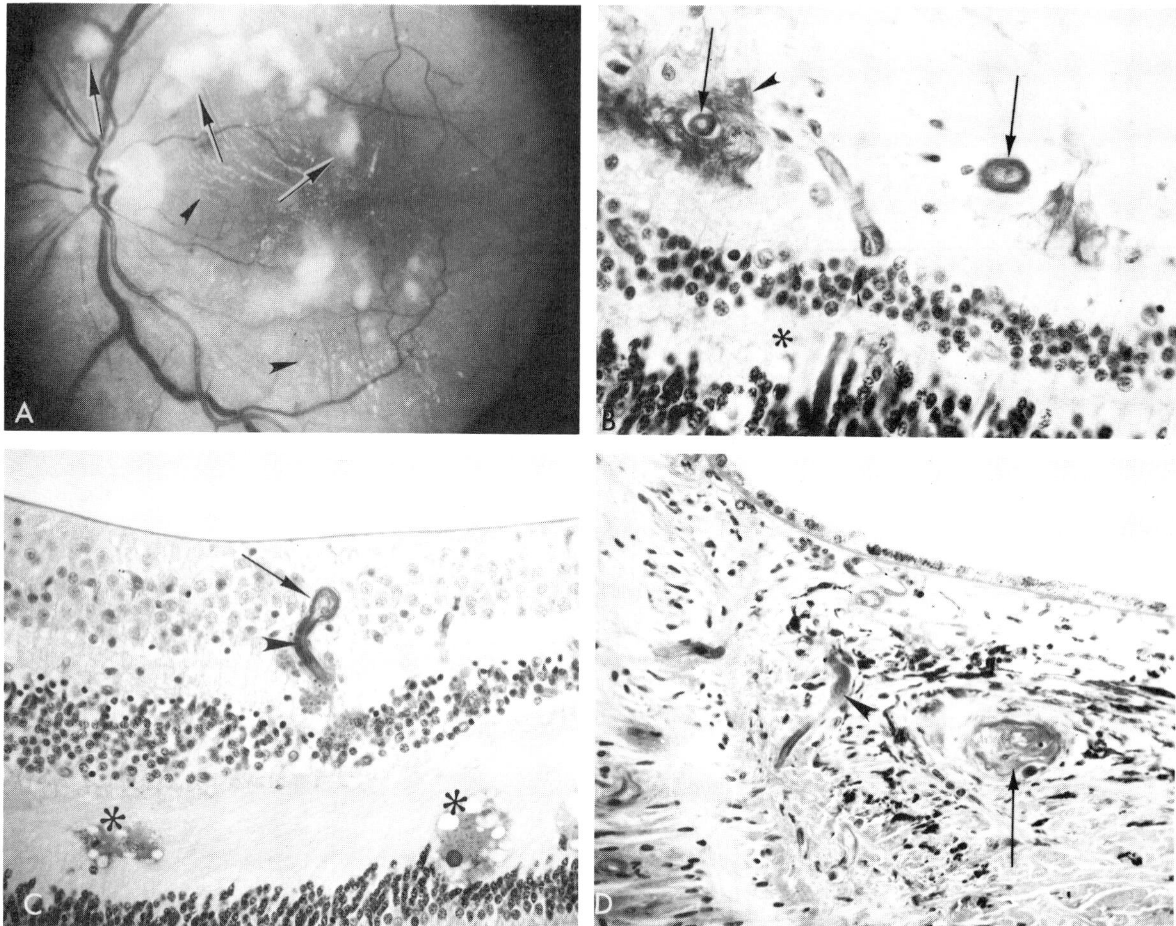

Figure 8–439. Ocular changes in scleroderma. *A,* Ophthalmoscopic appearance of "cotton-wool" exudates (arrows) and deep retinal exudates (arrowheads). *B,* Thick-walled and occluded retinal capillaries (arrows). One is surrounded by a fibrinous material (arrowhead). Deep exudates (asterisk) are present in outer plexiform and outer nuclear layers. *C,* Parafoveal area, showing a precapillary arteriole with thickened wall with fibrinoid material (arrow) that is continuous with an occluded capillary that also has a thickened wall with fibrinoid material (arrowhead). Exudate residues are present in the outer plexiform layer (asterisks). *D,* Peripapillary choroidal artery (arrow) and small vessel (arrowhead) showing occlusion and fibrinous deposition. PAS, ×315. (Courtesy of Dr. J.D.M. Gass; case presented at Association of Ophthalmic Alumni of Armed Forces Institute of Pathology, Washington, DC, June, 1969.)

They observed a weakly acidic mucopolysaccharide and lipid in and adjacent to vascular endothelial cells.

Blood Diseases

Anemia. Anemias, as in vitamin B_{12} and folic acid deficiency, iron deficiency and hemolytic states, leukemia, and polythemia, may present a similar fundus picture. All may produce edema of the optic nerve head, retinal hemorrhages, and exudates.

In a clinical study of 67 patients with anemia of diverse causes, Rubenstein, Yanoff, and Albert (1968) found that the frequency of retinal hemorrhages depended partly on the coexistence of anemia and thrombocytopenia. With anemia alone, 10 per cent of patients had retinal hemorrhages. If both anemia and thrombocytopenia were present, 40 per cent had hemorrhages. When both conditions were severe (hemoglobin less than 3 grams per dl and platelet count less than 50,000 per ml), 70 per cent had retinal hemorrhages. With thrombocytopenia alone, no patient had retinal hemorrhages.

Polycythemia. There are two forms of polycythemia, the primary and the secondary.

The *primary form* is referred to as polycythemia vera, polycythemia rubra, Vaquez-Osler disease, erythemia, or idiopathic polycythemia. It is a disease of unknown cause, characterized by a striking absolute increase in the number of erythrocytes in total blood volume and by signs of increased bone marrow activity, usually coming on in middle life (35 to 36 years). Approximately one third of the patients complain of neurologic symptoms (headaches, tinnitus, vertigo, blurring of vision, loss of consciousness, convul-

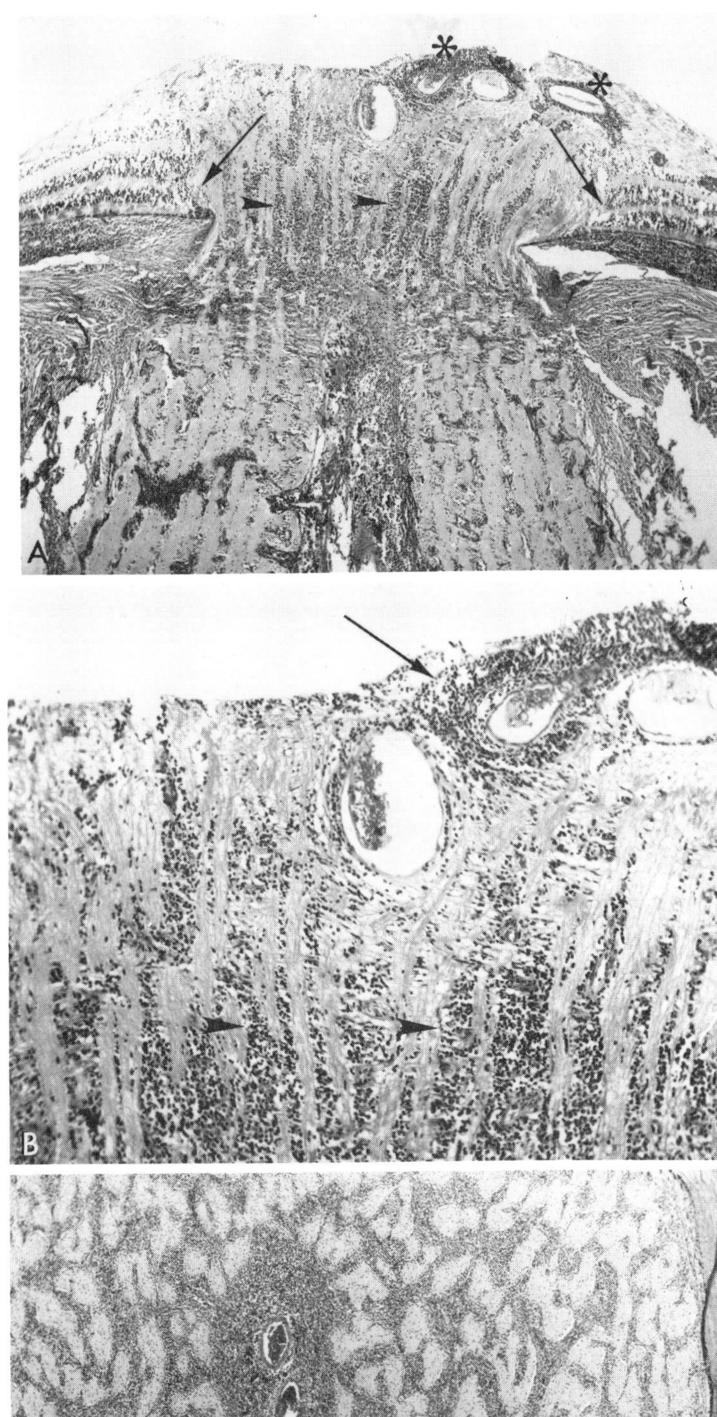

Figure 8–440. Acute leukemia. *A,* Papilledema, with fullness of optic nerve head, peripapillary crowding of retina (arrows), and sheathing of retinal veins by tumor cells (asterisks); also, leukemic infiltration of astrocytic columns of optic nerve head (arrowheads) and fibrovascular pial septae of optic nerve and around central retinal vessels in optic nerve. H and E, ×35. *B,* Higher power view of optic nerve head showing leukemic cells around a branch of central retinal vein (arrow) and within astrocytic columns (arrowhead). H and E, ×100. *C,* Cross-section of optic nerve showing marked leukemic infiltration of fibrovascular pial septae and surrounding central retinal vessels. H and E, ×65. EP 32542.

(*A* and *C* from Kincaid MC, Green WR: Ocular and orbital involvement in leukemia. Surv Ophthalmol *27*:211–232, 1983.)

sive seizures, and so on). Other complaints are dyspnea and weakness. The face and distal extremities are cyanotic—the degree of cyanosis depends on the amount of reduced hemoglobin present (which is due to slowing of blood flow as a result of increased blood viscosity). Venous thrombosis, varicosities, and phlebitis often occur. Hypertension is found in 42 per cent of patients, hepatomegaly in 50 per cent and splenomegaly in 90 per cent. Thrombosis often results in peptic ulcer, portal hypertension or esophageal varices. Sometimes the disease terminates in leukemia or anemia.

The *secondary form* is a compensatory phenomenon caused by conditions in which a subnormal amount of oxygen is taken up by the blood and delivered to the tissues. Some of these conditions are congenital heart disease, stenosis of pulmonary artery, emphysema, Ayerza's disease, methemoglobinemia, subtentorial brain tumors, and high altitude (temporary).

The general manifestations of the secondary form are similar to those of the primary form, except that cyanosis is sometimes more intense in the secondary form. No age group is affected preferentially by the secondary form.

The changes in polycythemia, whether primary or secondary, are due to hyperviscosity of the blood. These appear when the red cell count is at least 6 million. The fundus is cyanotic, the veins are engorged with severe stasis, retinal hemorrhages and optic nerve head swelling appear, and central retinal artery and vein occlusion have been reported.

Leukemia. Leukemias are of two types, myelogenous and lymphocytic. Monocytic leukemia is a type of myelogenous. Leukemias are named for their cell type (e.g., monocytic, myelocytic, myelomonocytic, granulocytic, and so on). Any bone marrow cell type can give rise to a leukemia. The most severe manifestations are seen in patients with acute leukemia that has a rapid onset and course. Retinal venous dilation and segmentation occur. Sheathing of vessels due to perivascular infiltration (Fig. 8–440), occlusion of vessels, and localized nodular infiltration by leukemic cells also may develop (Figs. 8–441 and 8–442). The vessels also may become yellower because of the increase of leukemic cells and decrease of erythrocytes.

Retinal hemorrhages (Tashiro, 1966) are caused by the vascular occlusions and by concomitant anemia and thrombocytopenia (Fig. 8–443). Some investigators (Culler, 1951; Mahneke, Videbock, 1964; Robb, Ervin, Sallan, 1978) find no really good correlation between platelet count, hemoglobin level, white blood count, and hemorrhages. The hemorrhages are most frequent in the posterior pole. They may involve all layers of the retina and may break into the vitreous cavity. Some hemorrhages contain a white component owing to the presence of leukemic cells (Fig. 8–444,*A*). Cotton-wool patches are common in the acute forms of leukemia. Occlusions of blood vessels can occur, producing localized infarctions of the retina. Branch and retinal arteries have been observed (Newman, Smith, Gay, 1972).

The retinal tissues are diffusely infiltrated with immature leukocytes; there is a tendency for local accumulation of these cells at various levels, producing small or large nodular masses (Kuwabara, Aiello, 1964). The retinal blood vessels are packed with immature white cells (Fig. 8–444,*B*), and there may be evidence of closure of the smaller capillaries by massive accumulations of cells. Perivascular accumulation of immature cells is common around the veins and some larger arterial channels. In the later stages, there is glial cell hyperplasia and neuronal degeneration of the retinal tissues.

The change in the color of the fundus can be explained on the basis of an increased number of white blood cells and a reduction of erythrocytes.

Infiltrates in the choroid may induce drusen formation and diffuse focal RPE changes ("Milky Way" pattern of fluorescein leakage) (Clayman, Flynn, Koch, Israel, 1972; Kincaid, Green, Kelley, 1979) (Figs. 8–445 through 447) and detachments of the RPE (Fig. 8–448) and retina (Burns, Blodi, Williamson, 1965). Peripheral retinal microaneurysms (Duke, Wilkinson, Sigelman, 1968; Jampol, Goldberg, Busse, 1975) and localized neovascularization (Morse, McCready, 1971; Frank, Ryan, 1972) also may be observed. The peripheral neovascularization reported by these investigators occurred in two patients, and both had chronic myelogenous leukemia with white blood counts of 340,000 and 250,000, respectively.

In their pathologic study of the eyes of patients who died of leukemia and related disorders, Allen and Straatsma (1961) noted ocular involvement in 50 per cent. The frequency of eye involvement was higher in acute than in chronic leukemia. In addition to hemorrhages, exudates, and nerve fiber layer infarctions, direct leukemic infiltration was noted in the following tissues, in descending order of frequency: choroid, sclera, conjunctiva, retina, optic nerve (especially the meninges), optic nerve head, ciliary body, iris, and vitreous. This study did not include the orbit, which also may be infiltrated with leukemic cells.

In a study of 1976 consecutive cases of eyes obtained post mortem from 1976 to 1980, Kincaid and Green (1983) found that 116 (5.9 per cent) were from patients with leukemia. Of these, 72 were acute, 27 chronic, and 17 unspecified. Fifty-five of the 72 patients with acute leukemia and 19 of the 27 patients with chronic leukemia had ocular involvement. The choroid was the most frequently involved tissue.

Text continued on page 1064

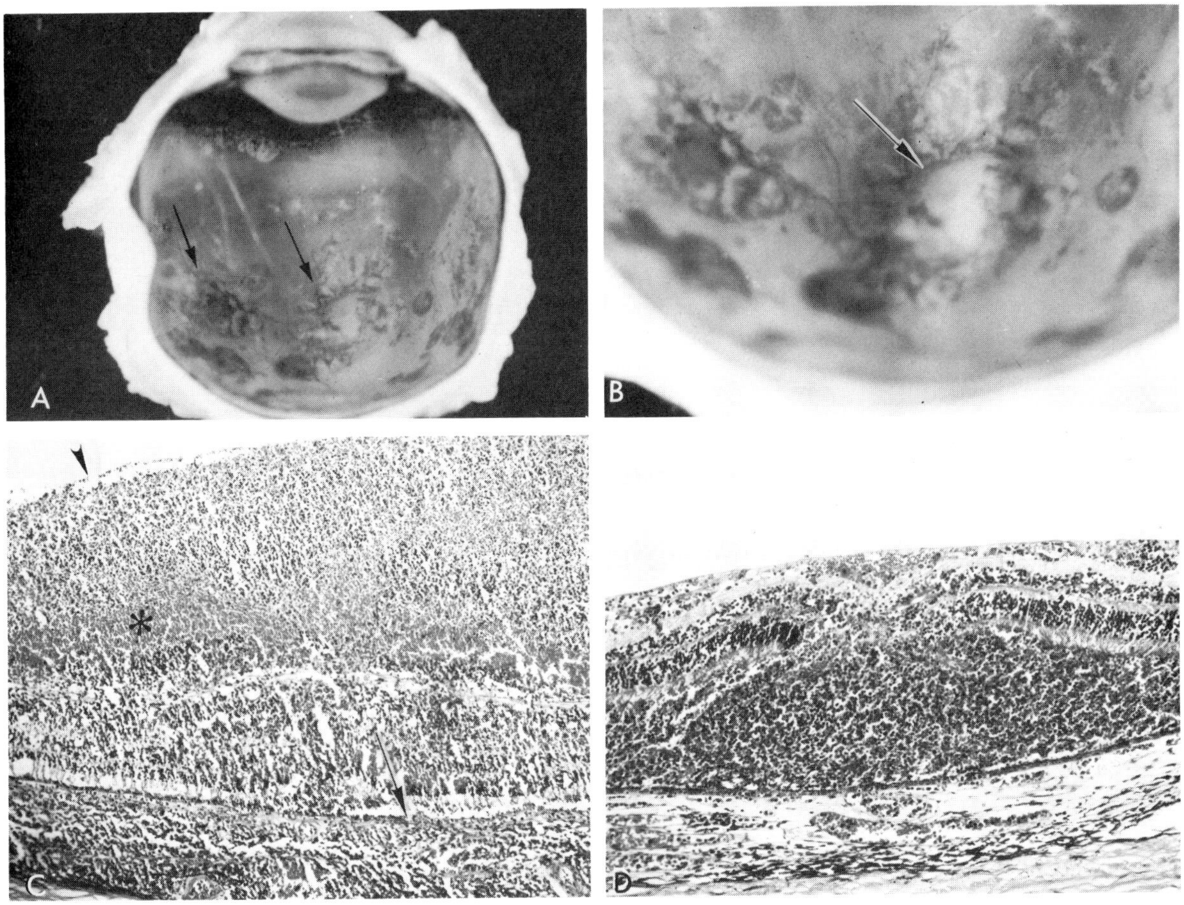

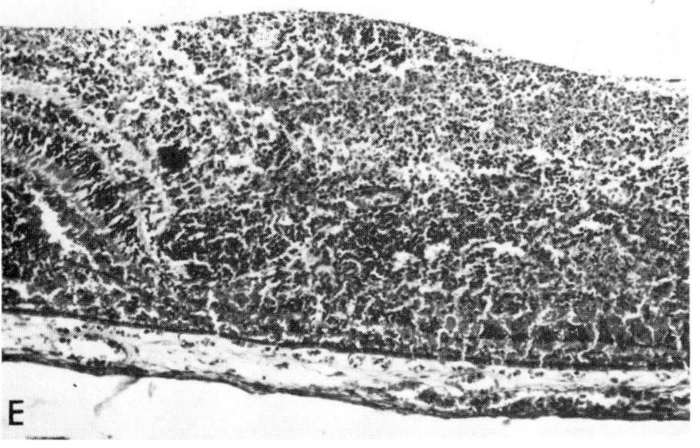

Figure 8–441. Acute leukemia. *A,* Gross appearance of tumor infiltrates (arrows) in retina. Variable amounts of hemorrhage are associated. *B,* Closer view showing one large tumor nodule (arrow) in retina. *C,* Section through nodule shows a large infiltrate under the internal limiting membrane (arrowhead), hemorrhage (asterisk), and diffuse tumor infiltrate of the remainder of the retina and choroid. Retinal pigment epithelium (RPE) is discontinuous (arrow). H and E, ×100. *D,* Retinal leukemic infiltrate that extends into subretinal space. Subjacent RPE is intact, and stroma of choroid is free of tumor. Choroidal vessels contain leukemic cells. H and E, ×130. *E,* Leukemic nodule almost totally replaces retina. H and E, × 130. EP 31209.

(*A* from Kincaid MC, Green WR: Ocular and orbital involvement in leukemia. Surv Ophthalmol *27*:211–232, 1983.)

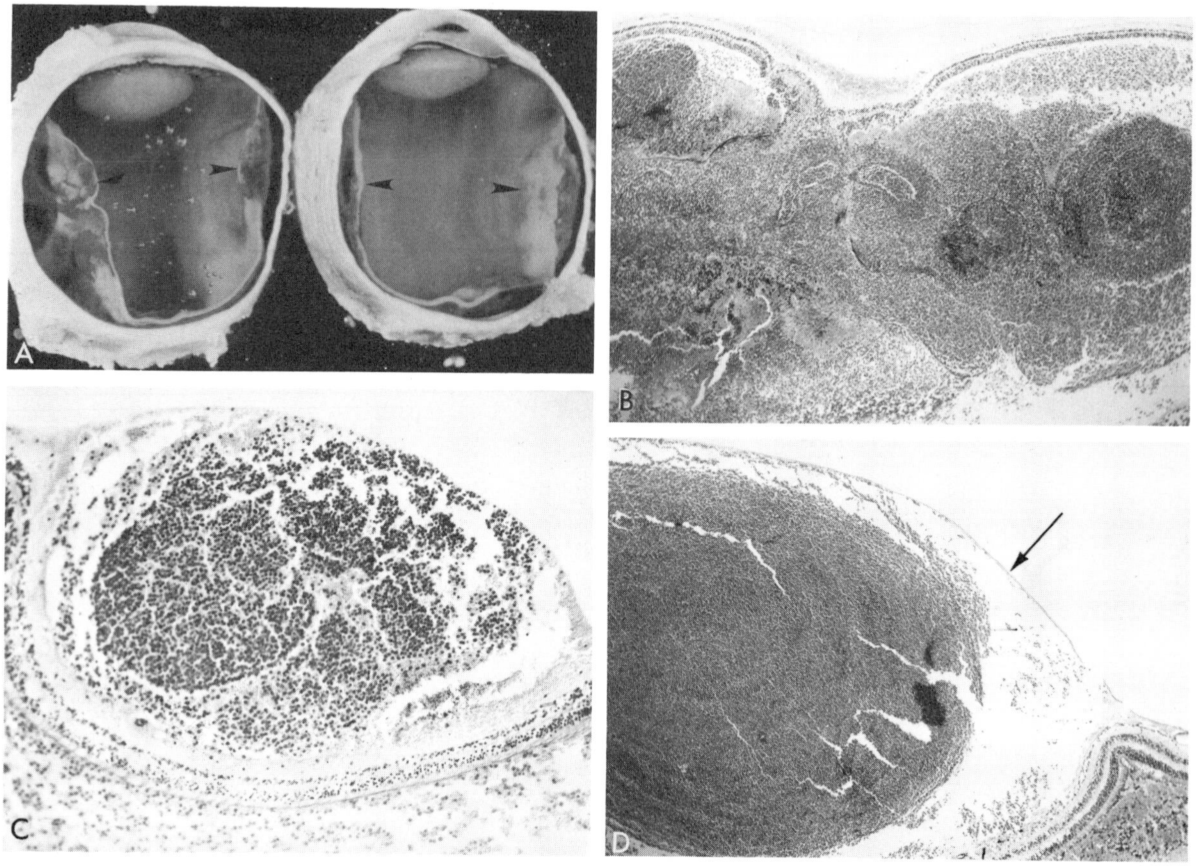

Figure 8–442. Acute leukemia. *A,* Gross appearance of massive leukemic infiltrates in retina (arrowheads). *B,* Large leukemic nodule in subretinal space. PAS, ×30. *C,* Small sub–internal limiting membrane (ILM) leukemic nodule. PAS, ×100. *D,* Large leukemic nodule between ILM (arrow) and remainder of retina. PAS, ×30. EP 30259.

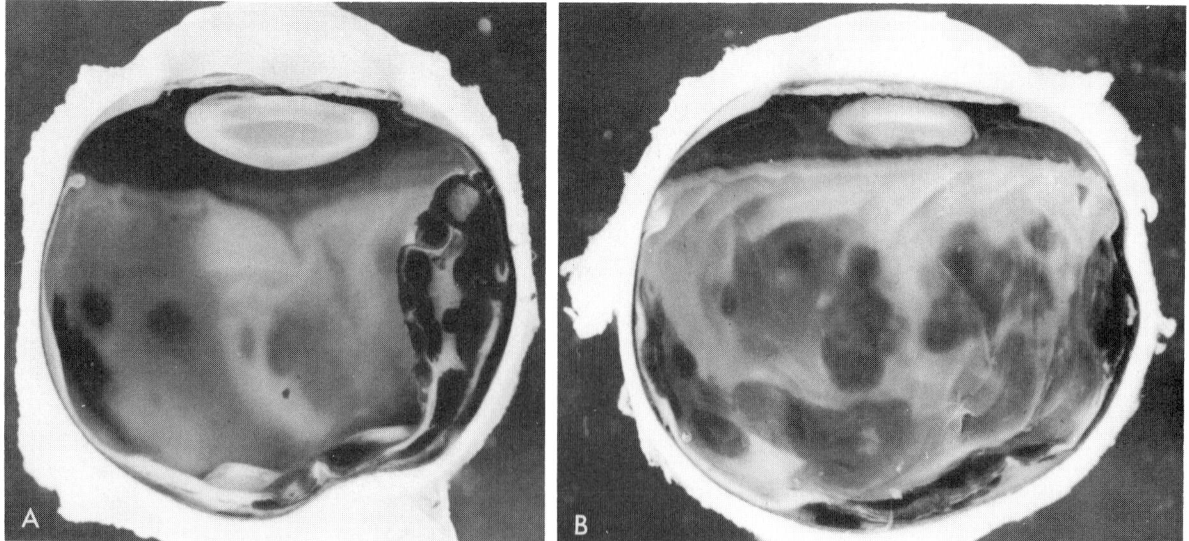

Figure 8–443. Acute leukemia with extensive retinal hemorrhage *(A* and *B)* in a child with anemia and thrombocytopenia. Leukemic infiltration was also present but was minimal. EP 32096.

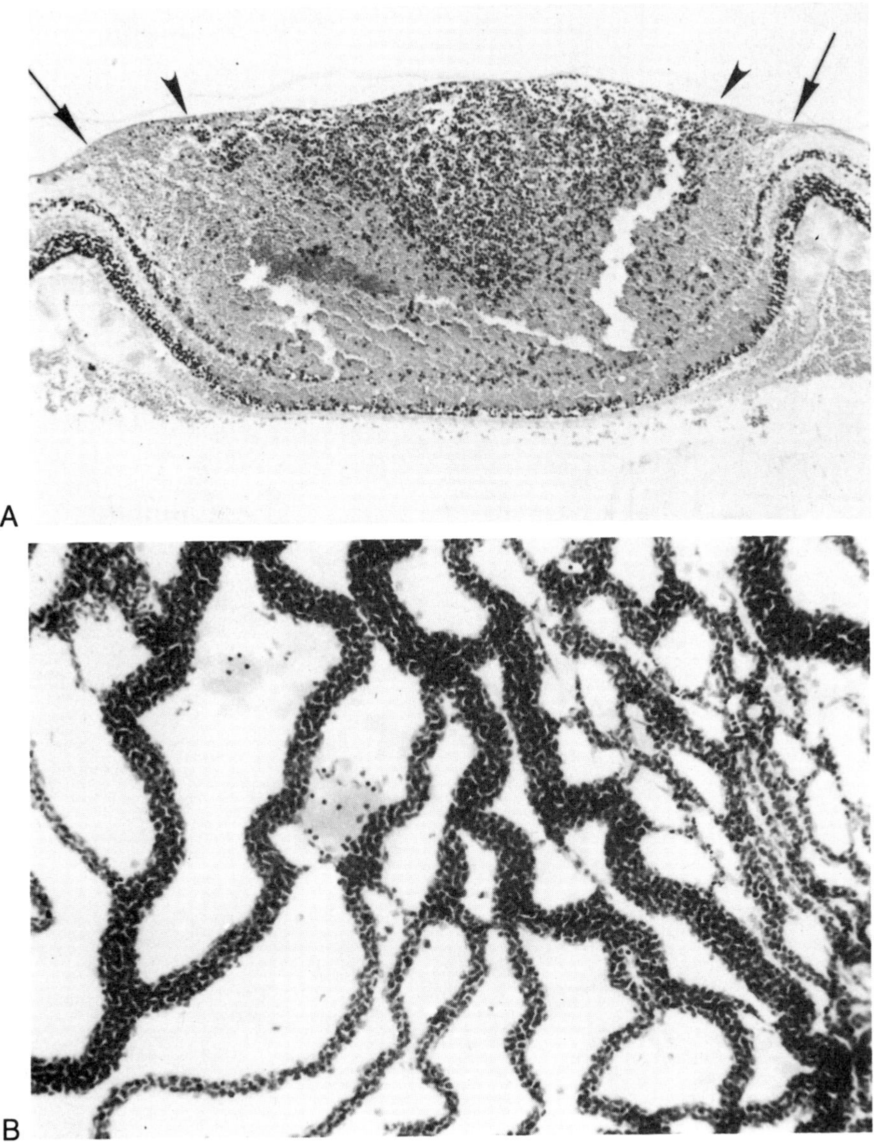

Figure 8–444. *A,* **Leukemic Roth spot.** Retinal hemorrhage (between arrows) with central area of leukemic cells (between arrowheads). H and E, ×100. *B,* Retinal trypsin digestion preparation, showing retinal vessels greatly distorted by leukemic cells. (Courtesy of Dr. W.H. Spencer; case presented at Verhoeff Society, Washington, DC, April, 1965.)

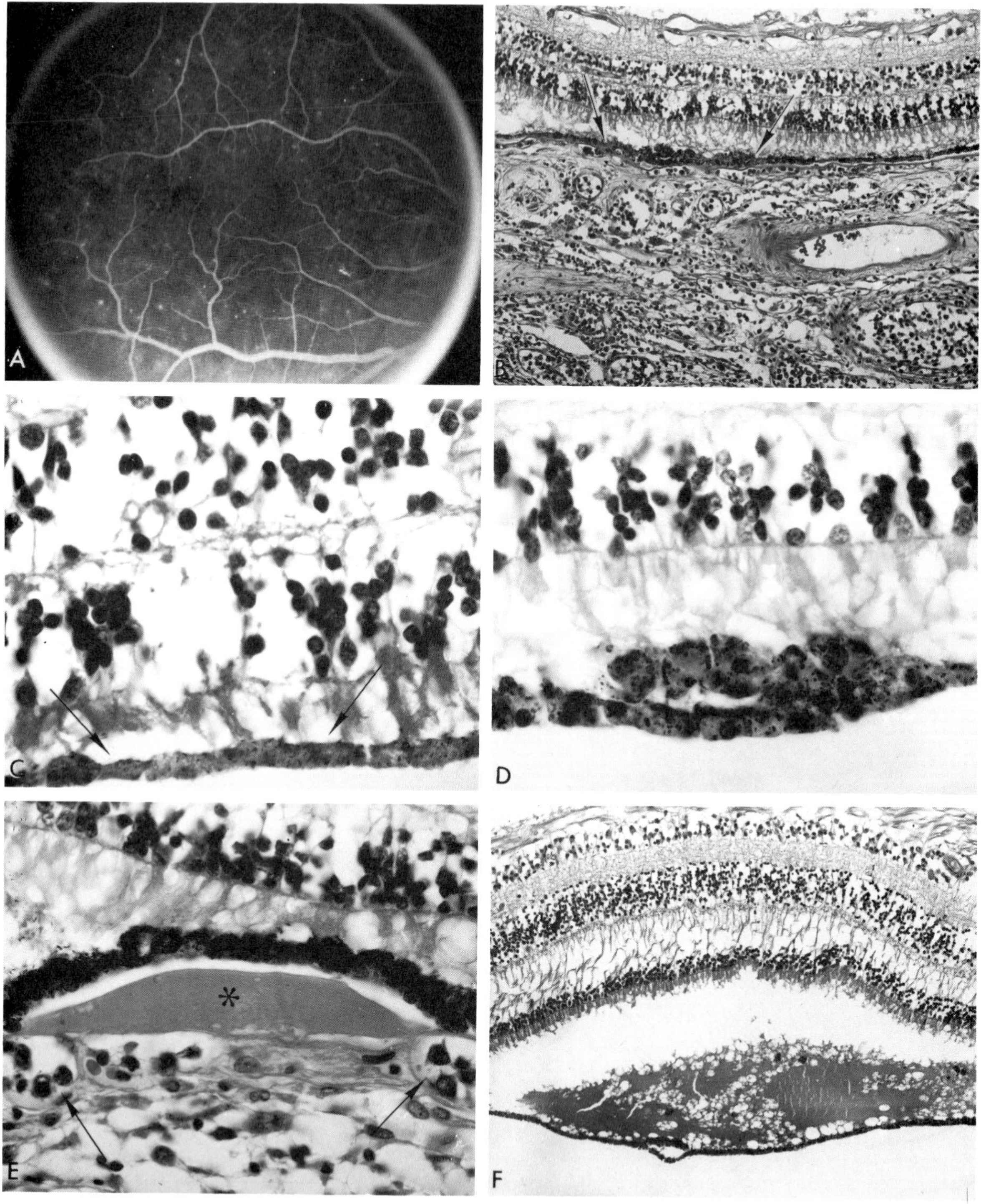

Figure 8–445. A 71 year old woman had a history of recent weight loss and bilateral decreased visual acuity, bilateral serous detachment, and mental depression. Despite extensive evaluation, cause of her weight loss and ocular process remained uncertain until her death, when post-mortem examination revealed **leukemic infiltrates** of many organs, including choroid. *A,* Fluorescein angiograms showed a myriad of retinal pigment epithelium (RPE) leakage points. *B,* Thickening of choroid by infiltration of tumor cells, mainly located within vascular spaces. Minor RPE hyperplasia is present (between arrows). H and E, ×160.

C, Area of RPE with reduced number of melanin granules (between arrows). H and E, ×875. *D,* Small area of hyperplasia of RPE. H and E, ×850. *E,* Small serous detachment (asterisk) of RPE. Tumor cells (arrows) are present in choriocapillaris. H and E, ×650. *F,* Serous detachment of retina in macular area. H and E, ×140. EP 43271.

(From Kincaid MC, Green WR, Kelley JS: Acute ocular leukemia. Am J Ophthalmol *87*:698–702, 1979.)

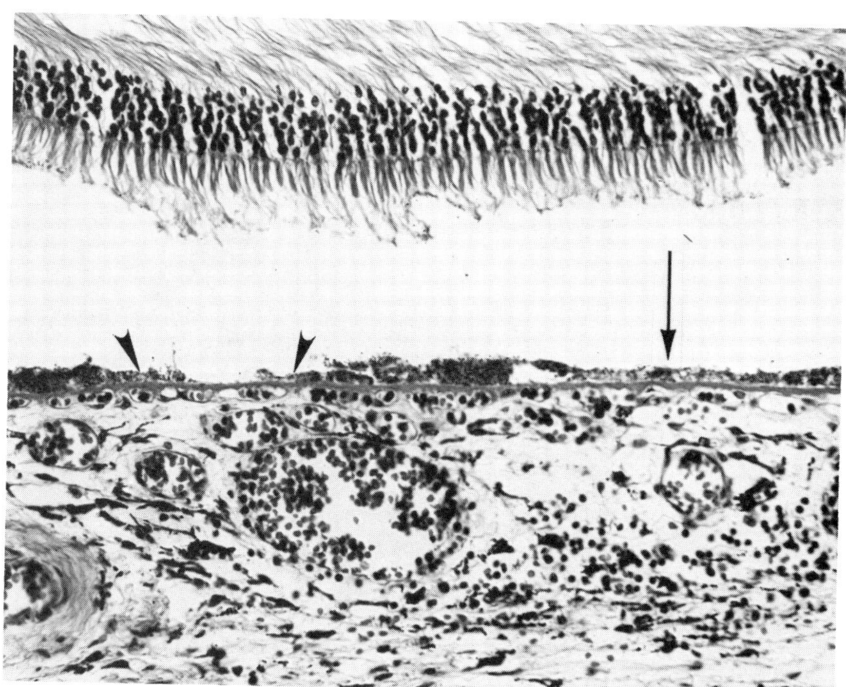

Figure 8–446. Retinal pigment epithelium defect (between arrowheads) and depigmentation (arrow) associated with choroidal infiltration by **leukemic cells**. H and E, × 215. EP 44108. (From Kincaid MC, Green WR: Ocular and orbital involvement in leukemia. Surv Ophthalmol *27*:211–232, 1983.)

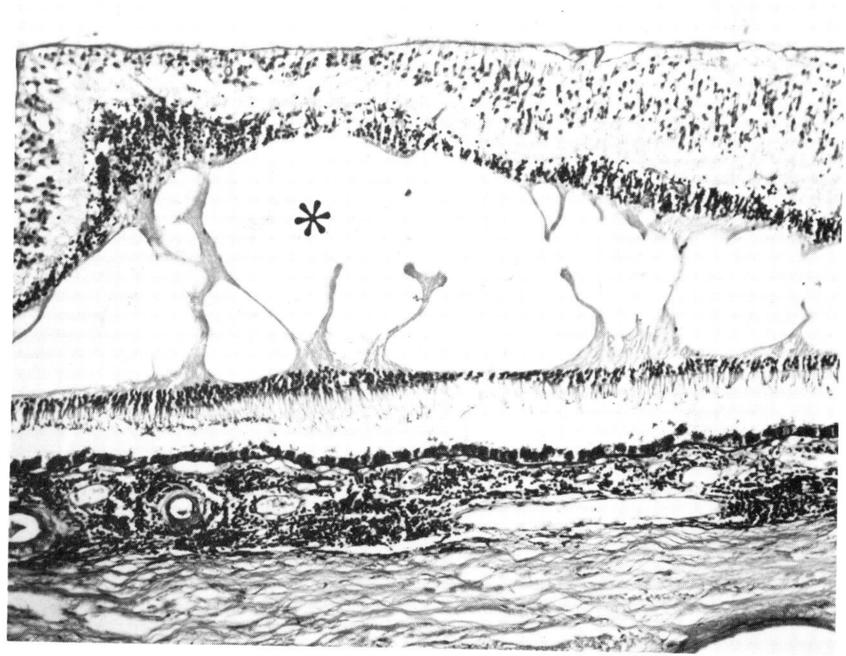

Figure 8–447. Cystoid macular edema (asterisk) with retinal pigment epithelium irregularities associated with a **leukemic infiltration** in choroid. PAS, ×105. EP 50048. (From Kincaid MC, Green WR: Ocular and orbital involvement in leukemia. Surv Ophthalmol *27*:211–232, 1983.)

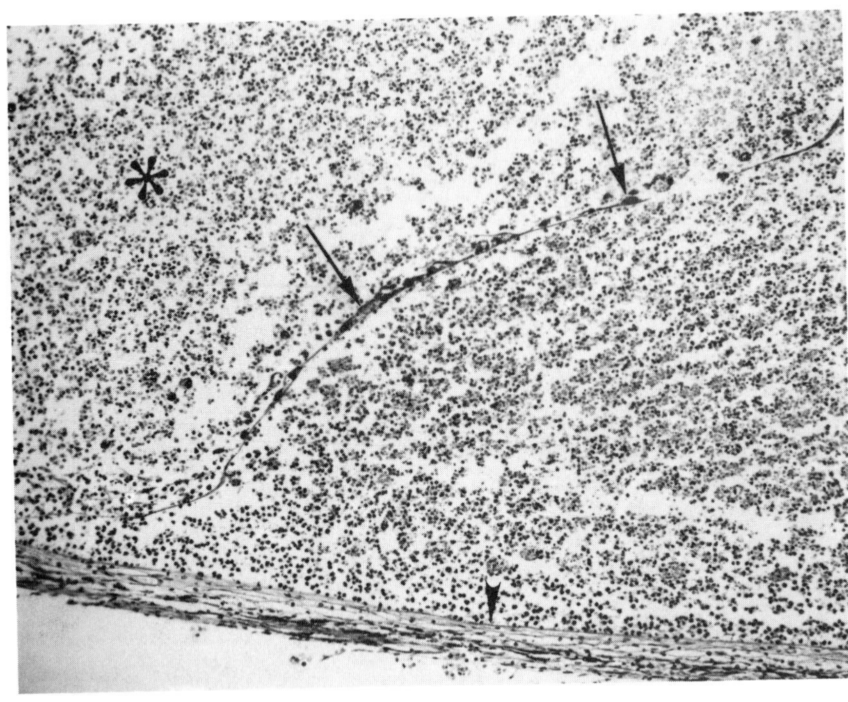

Figure 8–448. Leukemic detachment of retinal pigment epithelium (RPE) (arrows). In some areas, only basement membrane of RPE remains. Tumor is also present in subretinal space (asterisk). Bruch's membrane, arrowhead. PAS, ×110.

Retinal and optic nerve atrophy may occur from toxicity of chemotherapeutic agents (Sanderson, Kuwabara, Cogan, 1976; Green, 1975).

The case reported by de Juan, Green, Rice, and Erozan (1982) presented a particular problem. A 3 year old boy developed acute lymphocytic leukemia, with presumed ocular involvement by tumor and hemorrhages. He was successfully treated with chemotherapy and was in remission. Disk neovascularization and vitreous haze persisted. Because leukemic involvement of the vitreous could not be excluded clinically, a pars plana vitrectomy was performed, which disclosed neoplastic cells consistent with lymphocytic leukemia (Fig. 8–449).

Figure 8–449. Hyperchromatic cell with scanty cytoplasm and irregular nuclear membrane. Millipore filter, modified Papanicolaou, ×1950. EP 51001. (From De Juan E, Green WR, Rice TA, Erozan YS: Optic disc neovascularization associated with ocular involvement in acute lymphocytic leukemia. Retina 2:61–64, 1982.)

All the ophthalmoscopic signs of leukemia may be explained on the basis of one or more of the following: increased viscosity from increased numbers of leukemic cells or associated hyperproteinemia, hemorrhagic diathesis with reduction of platelets and alteration in the proteins involved in clotting, and infiltration of ocular tissues by leukemic cells.

Reticulum Cell Sarcoma (RCS). This neoplastic disease of the reticuloendothelial system varies considerably in the initial site and intensity of involvement. Rappaport (1966) prefers the term histiocytic lymphoma to reticulum cell sarcoma in designating this neoplasm. Others (Jones, Fuks, Bull, et al, 1973), using an immunologic approach, present evidence that this tumor consists of immunoblastic B cells and, to a lesser extent, immunoblastic T cells. An increase in the number of reports of ocular involvement of this disorder has been noted in the following reviews of the subject: Vogel, Font, Zimmerman, Levine (1968), Barr, Green, Payne, et al (1975), and Kim, Zakov, Albert, et al (1979).

Generally, uveal tract involvement is associated with systemic RCS, and retinal involvement with RCS of the brain. Rarely, only the eye may be involved (Barr and associates, 1975; Klingele, Hogan, 1975; Sullivan, Dallow, 1977), and, in one instance with central nervous system involvement, tumor was located only in the vitreous (Minckler, Font, Zimmerman, 1975). The disease affects adults of middle and older ages and often presents initially with signs of uveitis, with cells and flare in the anterior chamber and vitreous cells and debris (Figs. 8–450 through 8–453). Extensive infiltration of the retina and optic nerve head may lead to coagulative necrosis (Fig. 8–454). Tumor detachments of the RPE, when present, are characteristic (Figs. 8–450 and 8–451).

Because of the frequency of glaucoma, uveitis (especially bilateral uveitis), and neurologic signs, Kim, Zakov, Albert, et al (1979) have coined the mnemonic, the GUN syndrome.

When the diagnosis is suspected, the patient should be worked up systemically. In some cases the diagnosis may be established by bone marrow, lymph node, brain, or soft tissue biopsy. Often, however, there may be no evidence of systemic involvement and the diagnosis can be established by study of cells removed from the vitreous by aspiration or pars plana vitrectomy (Fig. 8–455) (Michels, Knox, Erozan, Green, 1975; Klingele, Hogan, 1975; Parver, Font, 1979). Some investigators recommend the use of the Millipore filter and staining by a modified Papanicolaou technique (Engel, De La Cruz, Jimenez-Abalahin, et al, 1982).

Once the diagnosis is established, radiation therapy is probably the treatment of choice (Margolis, Fraser, Lichter, Char, 1980). Cytotoxic agents may be of some help in controlling the diseases (Sullivan, Dallow, 1977).

Disseminated Intravascular Coagulopathy (DIC) This condition is due to a widespread tendency for formation of thrombi in small blood vessels in the course of many systemic diseases, such as abruptio placentae, leukemia, carcinoma, after renal transplantation, and after extensive tissue damage such as with burns. It also may be observed in systemic infections (particularly those due to gram-negative organisms), acute antigen-antibody reactions, drug reactions, and hypertension.

Ophthalmologic manifestations of DIC include reduction of vision from involvement of the submacular choroid or from serous retinal detachment. In some instances, an unusual streaked chorioretinopathy has been observed (Cogan, 1975). Fluorescein angiography shows multiple leaks into the subretinal space.

Histopathologically (Cogan, 1975), there is thrombotic occlusion of the choriocapillaris and adjacent choroidal arterioles and venules in the submacular and peripapillary areas, with necrosis of the RPE and serous retinal detachment (Figs. 8–456 and 8–457). In early cases, the vascular occlusions have a finely granular appearance, suggestive of platelet thrombi. In older lesions, the thrombi have a more hyaline or fibrillar appearance and may show endothelial proliferation and recanalization. Choroidal hemorrhage also may be observed.

Idiopathic Thrombotic Thrombocytopenia. This condition is considered to be the idiopathic form of disseminated intravascular coagulopathy and consists of the triad of hemolytic anemia, thrombocytopenia, and fluctuating neurologic signs. These patients may show lesions similar to those described above for DIC (Figs. 8–458 and 8–459).

Hemoglobinopathies. The sickling disorders, in which mutant hemoglobins S and C are inherited as alleles of normal hemoglobin A, are the hemoglobinopathies of interest to ophthalmologists. Sickle trait (Hb AS) affects 3 per cent of American blacks; 0.4 per cent have sickle cell disease (Hb SS), and 0.2 per cent have hemoglobin SC disease. Thalassemia and persistent fetal hemoglobin rarely cause retinopathy.

Sickle Cell Retinopathy. The sickle cell defect is transmitted as an autosomal dominant trait and results in hemoglobin that has a single substitution of an amino acid–glutamic acid for valine. This trait has been propagated in part because of the resistance of erythrocytes with sickle-type hemoglobin to the malaria parasite. Sickling of red cells containing abnormal hemoglobin occurs under conditions of decreased oxygen tension. This is seen more often in those organs with more sluggish circulation—such as the spleen, intestinal tract, lungs, joints, and bones. Under situations that may induce anoxia, sickling also can occur in other organs. Sickle cell hemoglobin is relatively insoluble in the reduced state, and then the molecule is elongated and rod-shaped. The molecules accumulate in parallel rows within the red cell and produce a change in its shape. The stiffened cells become trapped in capillaries and cause occlusions, with resulting ischemia of the affected tissues.

Ocular complications are most severe and frequent in sickle cell disease and are caused by vascular occlusion. The exact mechanism for the vascular occlusions is uncertain but appears to involve sickling, hemolysis, and stasis. The vessels that may be affected include iris, central artery and vein, macular capillaries, and, most often, the midperipheral retinal vessels.

Nonproliferative sickle retinopathy includes retinal hemorrhages, salmon patches, iridescent fundus deposits, and spiculated or stellate pigmented fundus lesions—the "black sunburst" sign. These changes have been observed in sickle cell disease, SS disease, sickle trait, sickle thalassemia (Hb S Thal), and hemoglobin C trait (Hb AC). Romayananda, Goldberg, and Green (1973) described the histopathologic correlation of these observations. They postulated that the peculiar pink-orange color of salmon patches is due to partially broken-down blood in deep retinal and subretinal hemorrhages. They showed that iridescent spots are old resorbed hemorrhages with hemosiderin deposition under limiting membrane of the retina (see Fig. 8–81). Black sunburst lesions were demonstrated to be resorbed subretinal

Text continued on page 1075

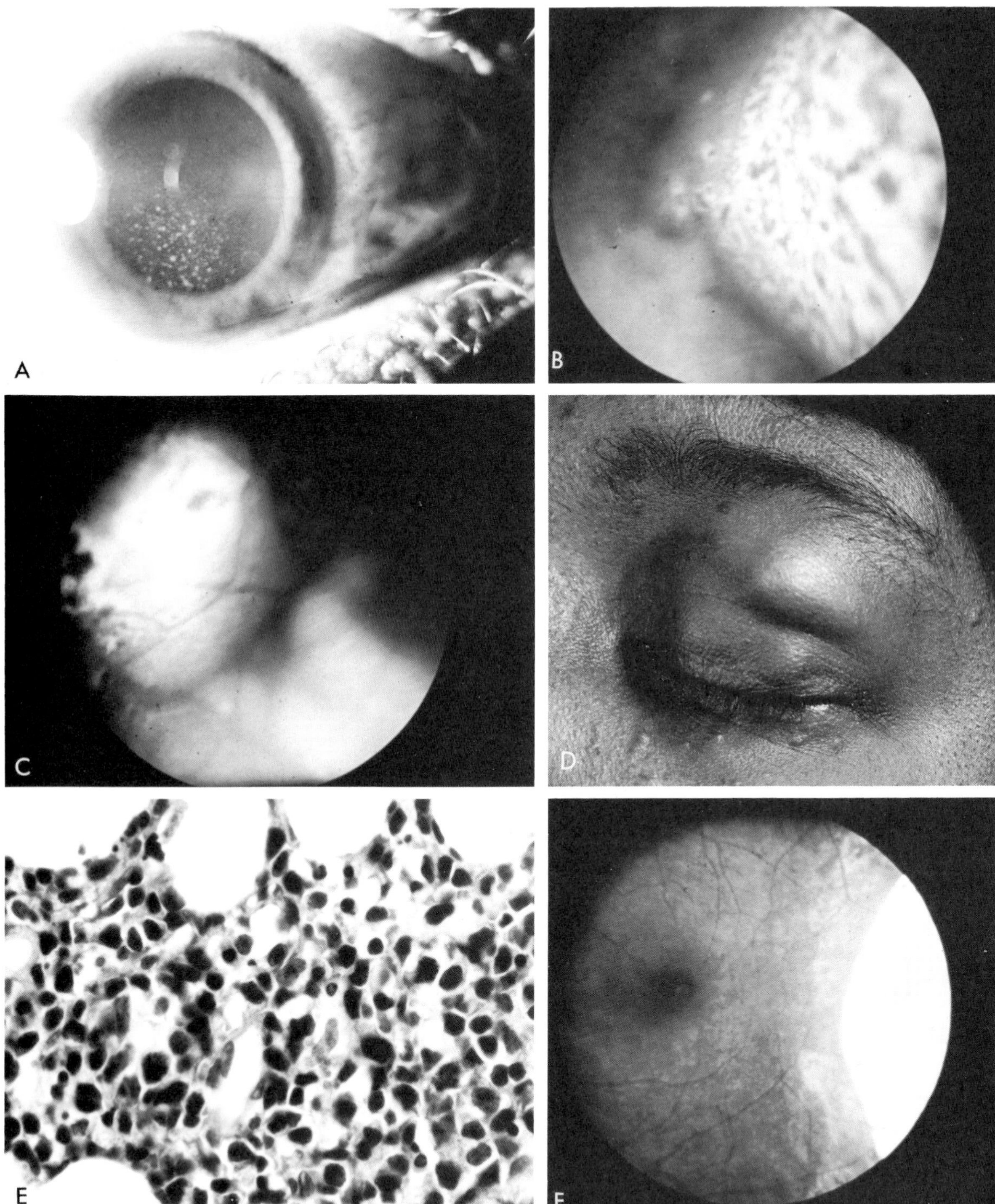

Figure 8–450. Ocular reticulum cell sarcoma in a 46 year old woman who was found postmortem to have tumor in all organs except the brain. *A,* External appearance of left eye 4 months after onset of symptoms, showing numerous large keratic precipitates. *B,* Large, partially pigmented sub-retinal pigment epithelium (RPE) mass temporal to macula of left eye, which appeared 4 months after initial symptoms. *C,* Appearance of sub-RPE mass in superior fundus of right eye 6 months after onset of symptoms. *D,* Nodule on left upper lid that appeared 6 months after onset of symptoms. *E,* Appearance of tumor excised from left upper lid. There is much hyperchromatism and moderate pleomorphism. H and E, ×900. *F,* Sub-RPE lesion of left eye 8 months after it appeared, now much smaller after irradiation.

Illustration continued on opposite page

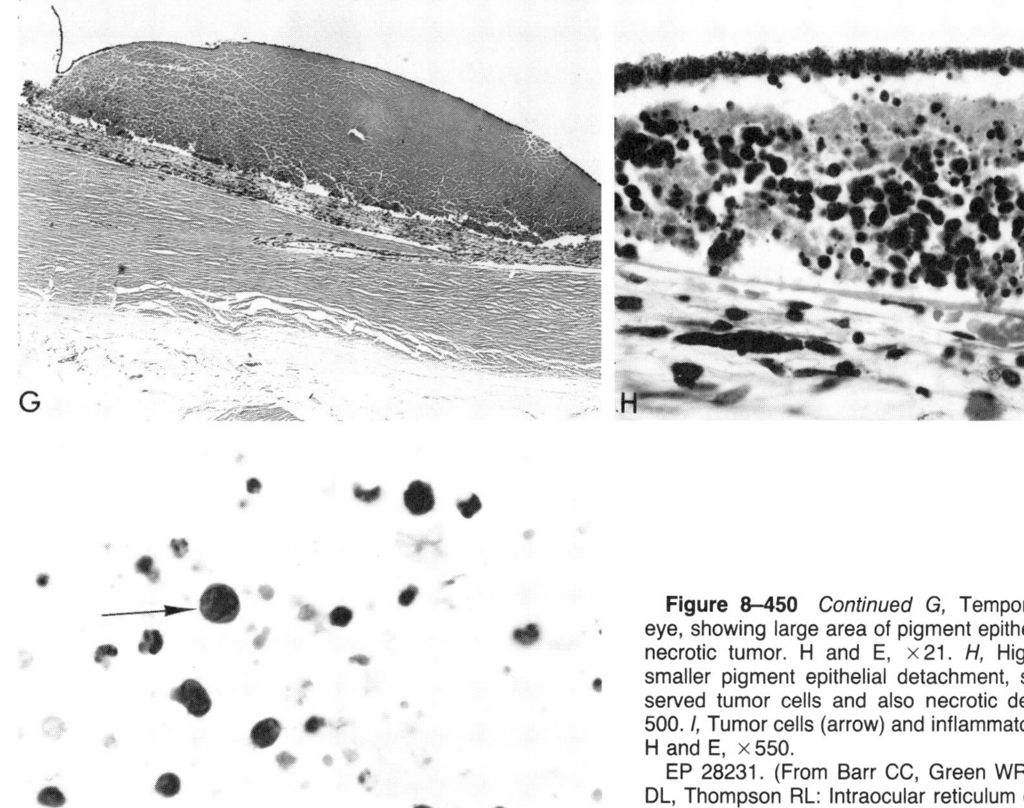

Figure 8–450 *Continued G,* Temporal portion of right eye, showing large area of pigment epithelial detachment by necrotic tumor. H and E, ×21. *H,* High magnification of smaller pigment epithelial detachment, showing more preserved tumor cells and also necrotic debris. H and E, × 500. *I,* Tumor cells (arrow) and inflammatory cells in vitreous. H and E, ×550.

EP 28231. (From Barr CC, Green WR, Payne JW, Knox DL, Thompson RL: Intraocular reticulum cell sarcoma: Clinicopathologic study of four cases and review of literature. Surv Ophthalmol *19*:224–239, 1975.)

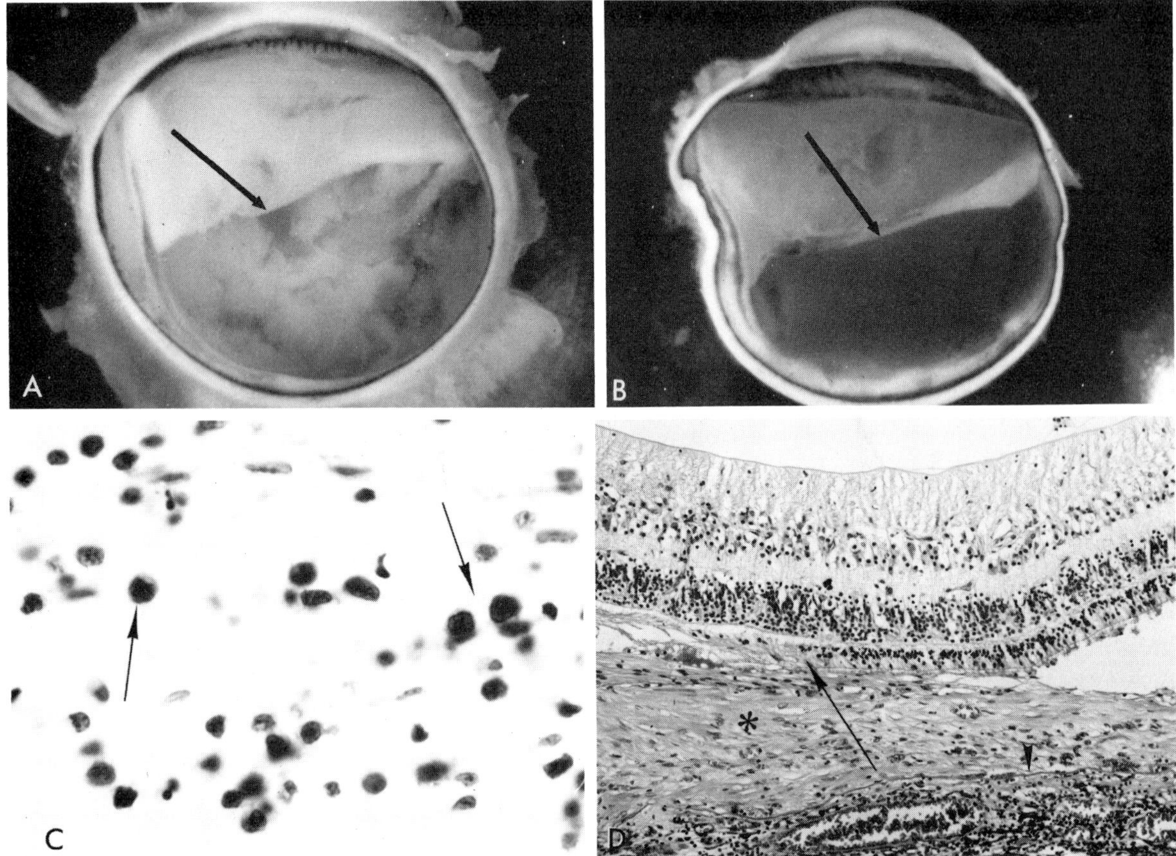

Figure 8–451. Ocular and central nervous system reticulum cell sarcoma in a 57 year old woman. *A,* Gross appearance of right eye showing detachment (arrow) and cloudiness of vitreous, with thickening of retina and choroid posteriorly. *B,* Gross appearance of left eye showing clouded detached vitreous (arrow) and thickened choroid and retina. *C,* Vitreous of right eye shows typical tumor cells with scanty cytoplasm and finger-like nuclear projections (arrows). H and E, ×1000.

D, Retina near optic disk of right eye was detached by a fibrovascular disciform membrane (asterisk) containing some chronic inflammatory cells. Photoreceptors and outer nuclear layer are partially atrophic over this membrane and in some areas (arrow) are severely degenerated. Bruch's membrane, arrowhead. H and E, ×135.

Illustration continued on opposite page

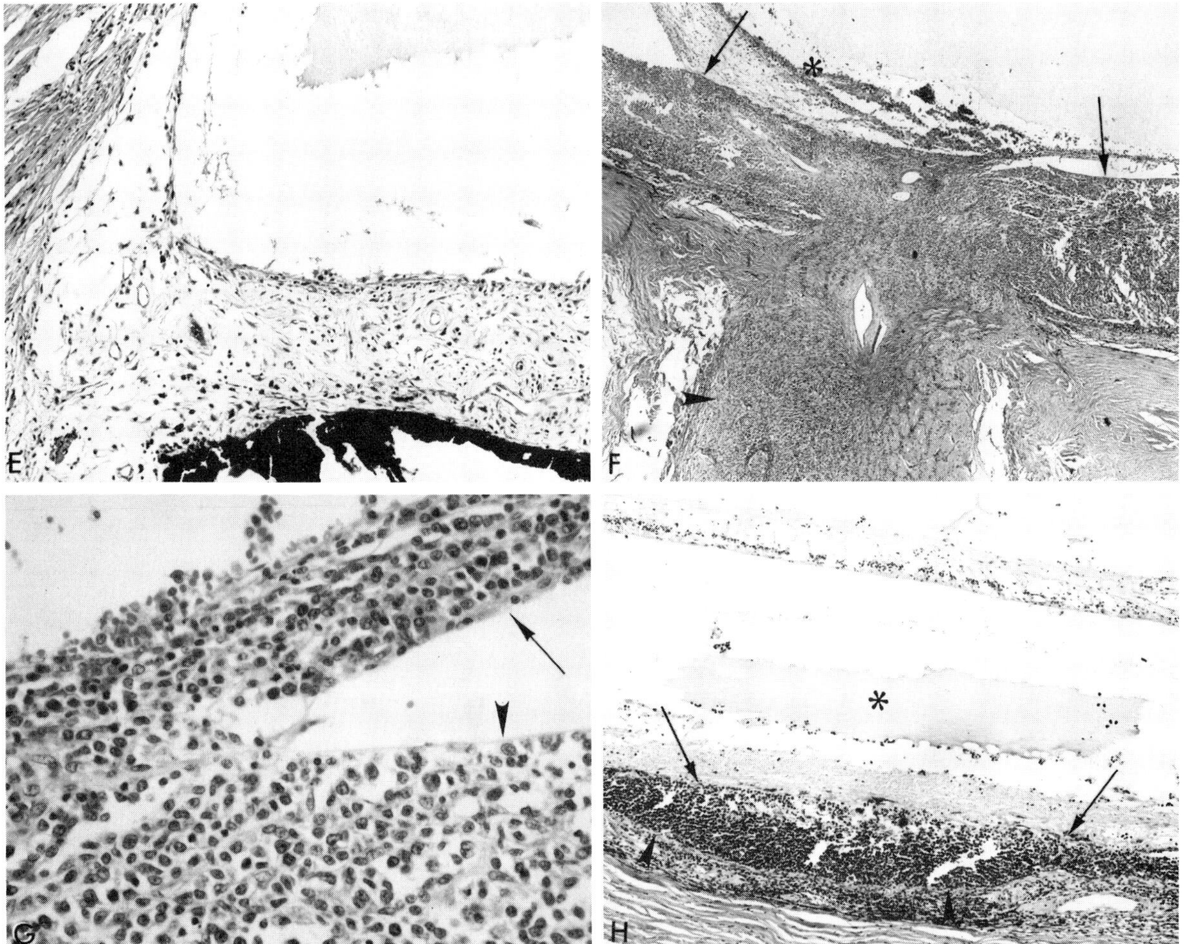

Figure 8–451 *Continued E,* Temporal angle of left eye showing peripheral anterior synechiae, chronic inflammatory cells in iris and ciliary body, and proteinaceous material in anterior chamber. H and E, ×130.

F, Optic nerve head of left eye is almost completely replaced by tumor, with extension into optic nerve (arrowhead), peripapillary retina (arrows), and vitreous (asterisk). H and E, ×21. *G,* Area of peripapillary retina of left eye showing marked tumor infiltration with extension into vitreous (arrow). Internal limiting membrane, arrowhead. H and E, ×350.

H, Midperiphery of left eye showing extensive inflammatory cellular infiltration in choroid and tumor detachment of partly atrophic retinal pigment epithelium (arrows). Retina is detached by serosanguineous material containing clumps of tumor cells and inflammatory cells (asterisk). Tumor and inflammatory cells are also present in adjacent vitreous. Bruch's membrane, arrowheads. H and E, ×50.

EP 33026. (From Barr CC, Green WR, Payne JW, Knox DL, Thompson RL: Intraocular reticulum-cell sarcoma: Clinicopathologic study of four cases and review of literature. Surv Ophthalmol *19*:224–239, 1975.)

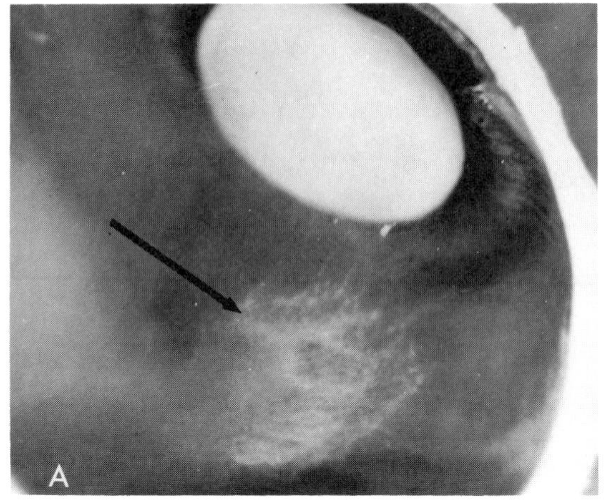

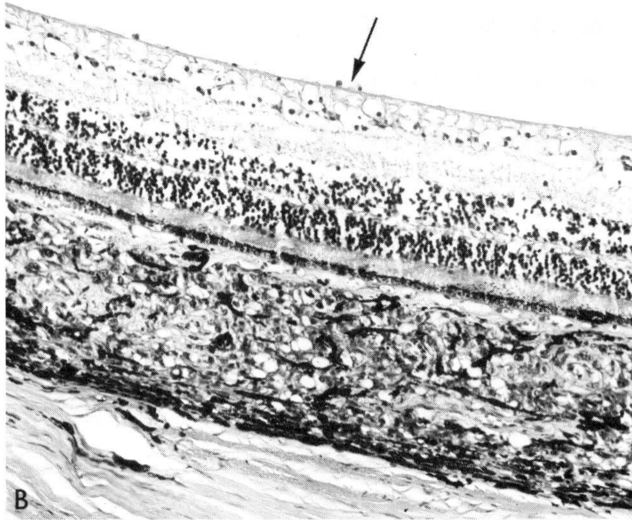

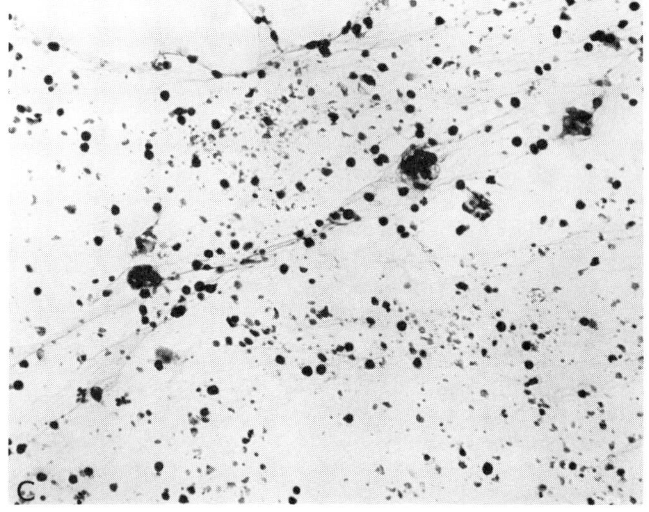

Figure 8–452. Bilateral vitreous and choroidal reticulum cell sarcoma in a 65 year old man with disseminated disease found post mortem. *A,* Gross appearance of right eye showing vitreous with dense tumor infiltrate (arrow). *B,* Area near posterior pole of right eye shows much tumor infiltration in choroid and occasional tumor cells in vitreous (arrow). H and E, × 170. *C,* Area of vitreous opacity of right eye showing individual as well as clumps of tumor cells and mononuclear inflammatory cells. H and E, ×260. EP 37421. (From Barr CC, Green WR, Payne JW, Knox DL, Thompson RL: Intraocular reticulum-cell sarcoma: Clinicopathologic study of four cases and review of literature. Surv Ophthalmol *19*:224–239, 1975.)

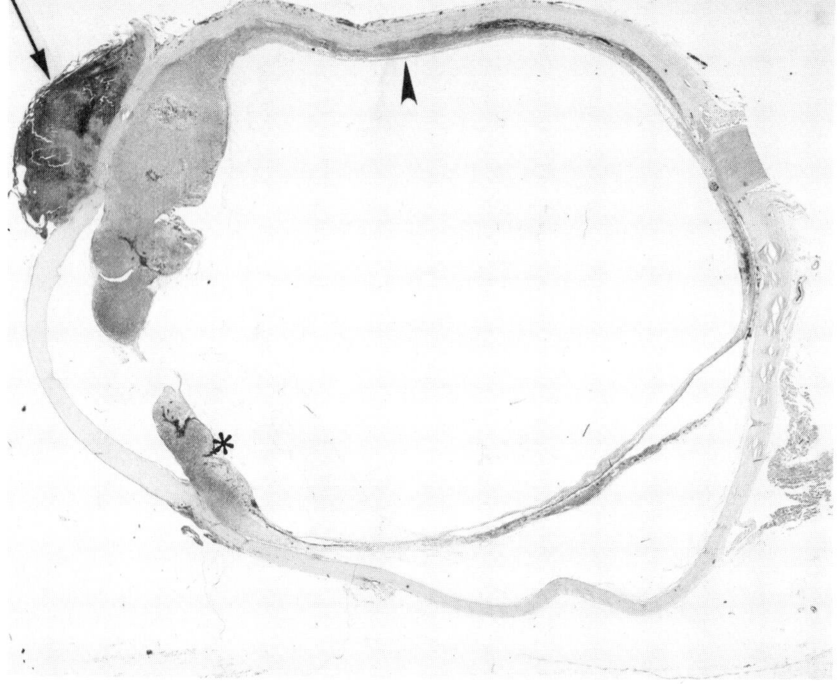

Figure 8–453. Uveal and vitreous reticulum cell sarcoma in a 57 year old woman who initially had signs of ocular inflammation and 3 years later was proved to have central nervous system reticulum cell sarcoma. Section through pupil and optic nerve, showing epibulbar (arrow), iris, and ciliary body involvement, superonasally. There is also diffuse infiltration of superonasal choroid (arrowhead) and iris and ciliary body inferotemporally (asterisk). H and E, ×45. EP 43447. (From Raju VK, Green WR: Reticulum-cell sarcoma of the uvea. Ann Ophthalmol *14*:555–560, 1982.)

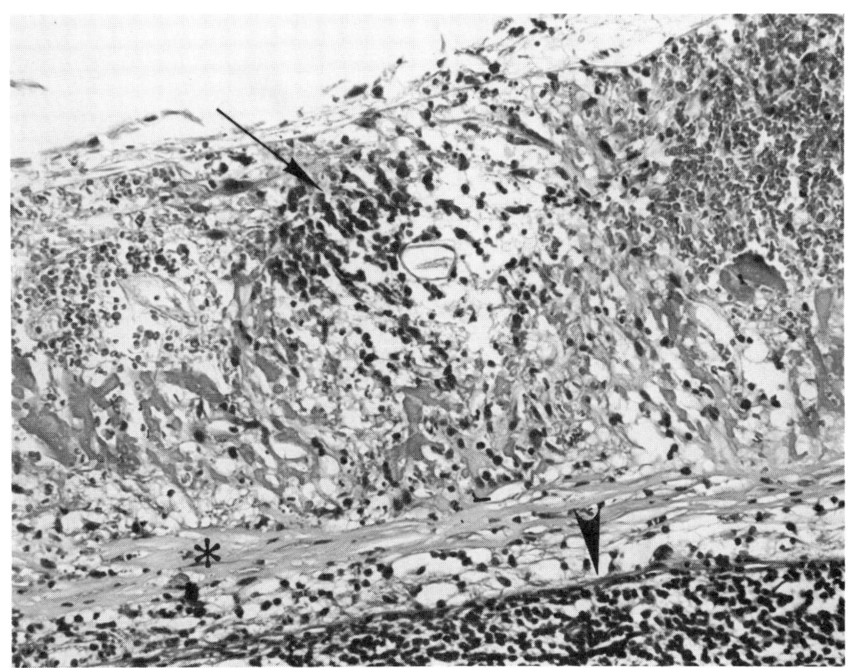

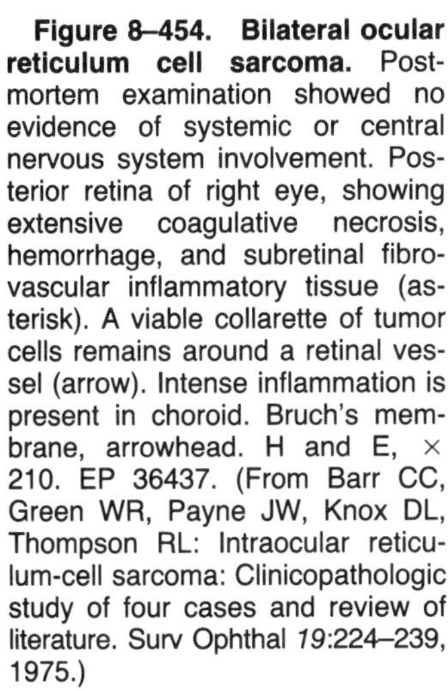

Figure 8–454. Bilateral ocular reticulum cell sarcoma. Postmortem examination showed no evidence of systemic or central nervous system involvement. Posterior retina of right eye, showing extensive coagulative necrosis, hemorrhage, and subretinal fibrovascular inflammatory tissue (asterisk). A viable collarette of tumor cells remains around a retinal vessel (arrow). Intense inflammation is present in choroid. Bruch's membrane, arrowhead. H and E, × 210. EP 36437. (From Barr CC, Green WR, Payne JW, Knox DL, Thompson RL: Intraocular reticulum-cell sarcoma: Clinicopathologic study of four cases and review of literature. Surv Ophthal *19*:224–239, 1975.)

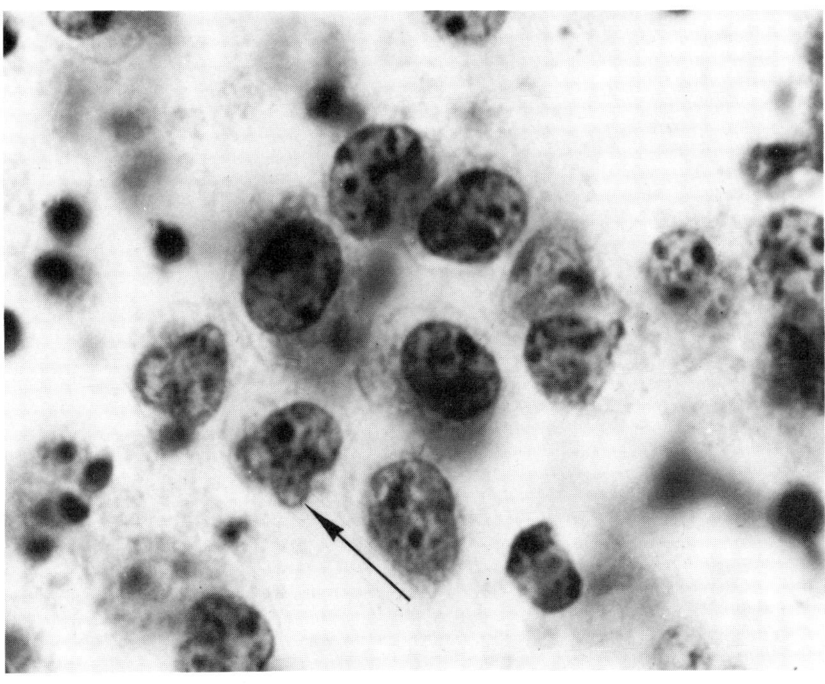

Figure 8–455. Reticulum cell sarcoma in a 61 year old man diagnosed by studies of vitreous obtained by pars plana vitrectomy. Cells are rather large, with scanty cytoplasm. Nuclei are round, oval, or bean-shaped, with one or more prominent nucleoli. Occasional nuclei show lobulation and some finger-like protrusions (arrow). Millipore filter, modified Papanicolaou stain, ×1500. EP 38606. (From Michels RG, Knox DL, Erozan YS, Green WR: Intraocular reticulum cell sarcoma: Diagnosis by pars plana vitrectomy. Arch Ophthalmol *93*:1331–1335, 1975.)

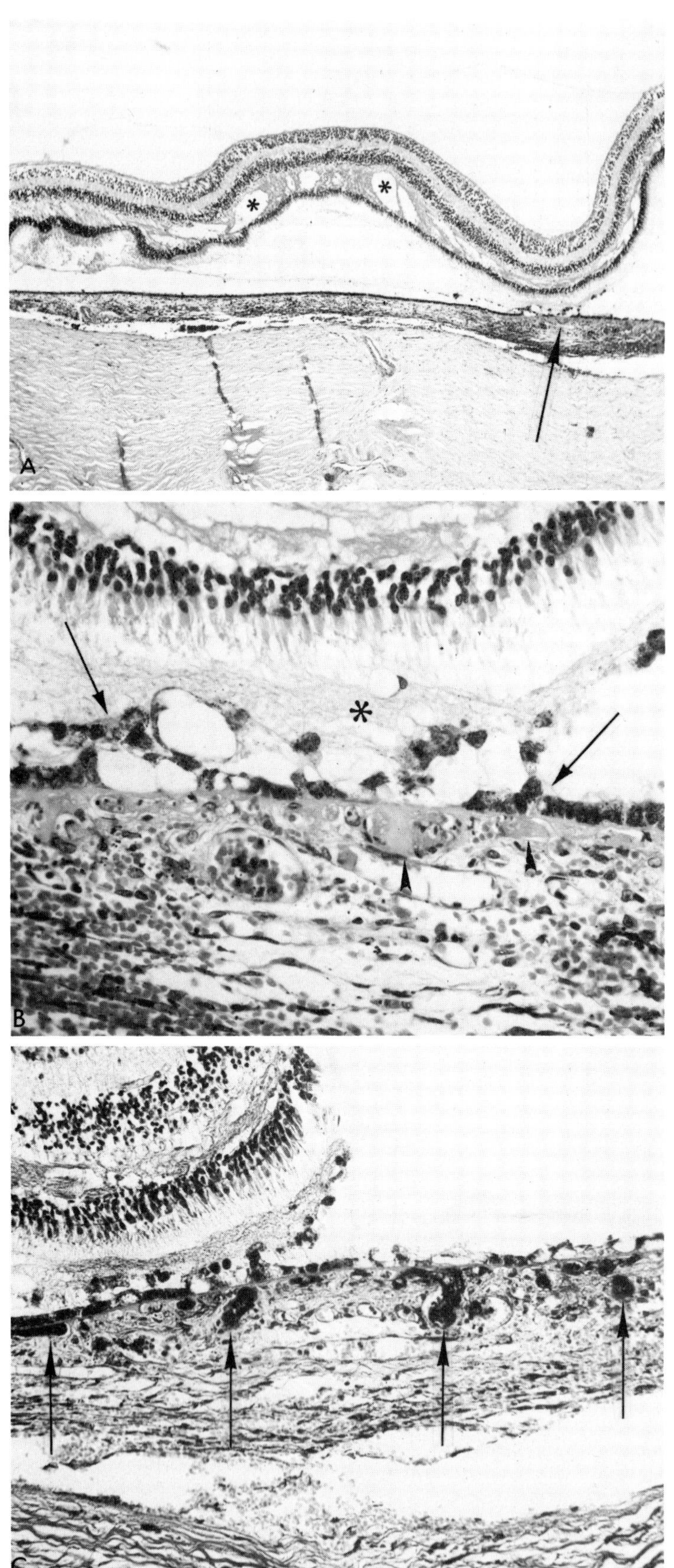

Figure 8–456. Disseminated intravascular coagulopathy in a 68 year old woman with acute renal failure and sepsis. *A,* Cystoid macular edema (asterisks) associated with area of occlusion of choriocapillaris and disruption of retinal pigment epithelium (RPE) (arrow). H and E, ×4. *B,* Higher power view shows occlusion of choriocapillaris by a homogeneous eosinophilic material (arrowheads). RPE is disrupted (between arrows), and a lightly staining material (asterisk) is present in the subretinal space. H and E, ×320. *C,* Special staining showed the fibrinous character of the occluding material (arrows). Degenerated RPE is evident. Phosphotungstic acid; hematoxylin, ×215. EP 43193.

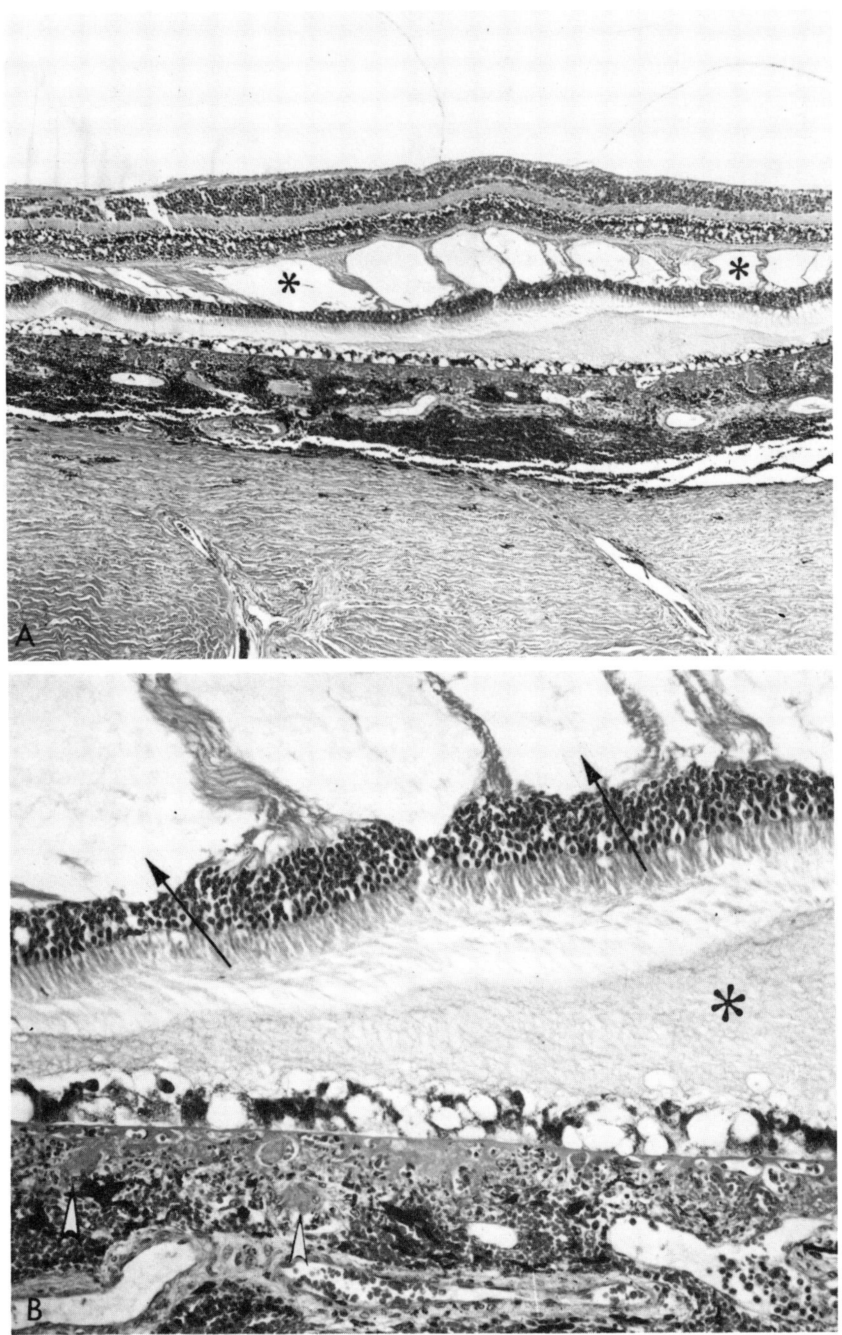

Figure 8–457. Disseminated intravascular coagulopathy in a 23 year old woman whose death was caused by sepsis and drug reaction after cesarean section. *A,* Extensive cystoid macular edema (CME) (asterisks) resulting from breakdown of the blood-ocular barrier at the level of the retinal pigment epithelium (RPE) from occlusion of the choriocapillaris. RPE has a vacuolated appearance. Flat macular detachment is present. H and E, ×40. *B,* Higher power view shows occlusion of choriocapillaris by eosinophilic material. An occasional larger choroidal vessel (arrowheads) is occluded. RPE is vacuolated and apparently disrupted, a proteinaceous material (asterisk) is present in subretinal space, and CME (arrows) is present. H and E, ×210. (Courtesy of Dr. H.K. Leathers; case presented at Association of Ophthalmic Alumni of Armed Forces Institute of Pathology, Washington, DC, June, 1973.)

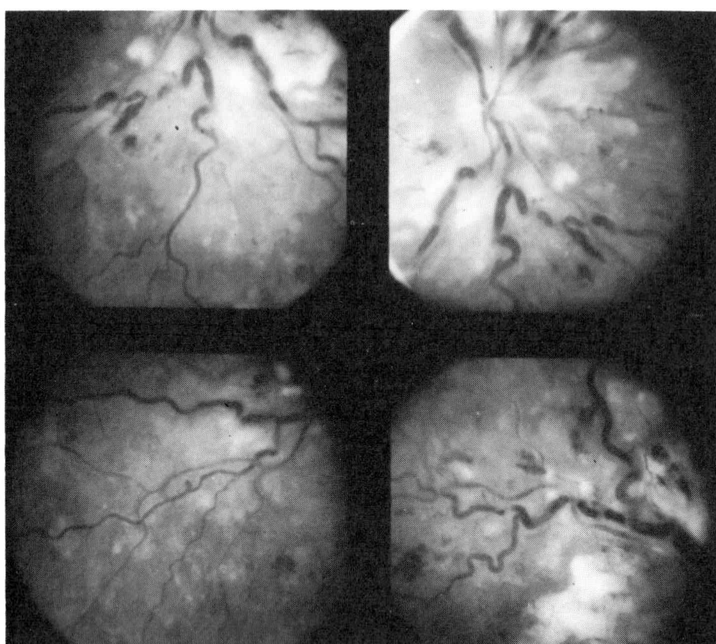

Figure 8–458. Ophthalmoscopic appearance of retinal microinfarctions, edema, hemorrhages, vascular dilatation and tortuosity, and lesions at the level of the retinal pigment epithelium in patient with **idiopathic thrombotic thrombocytopenia.**

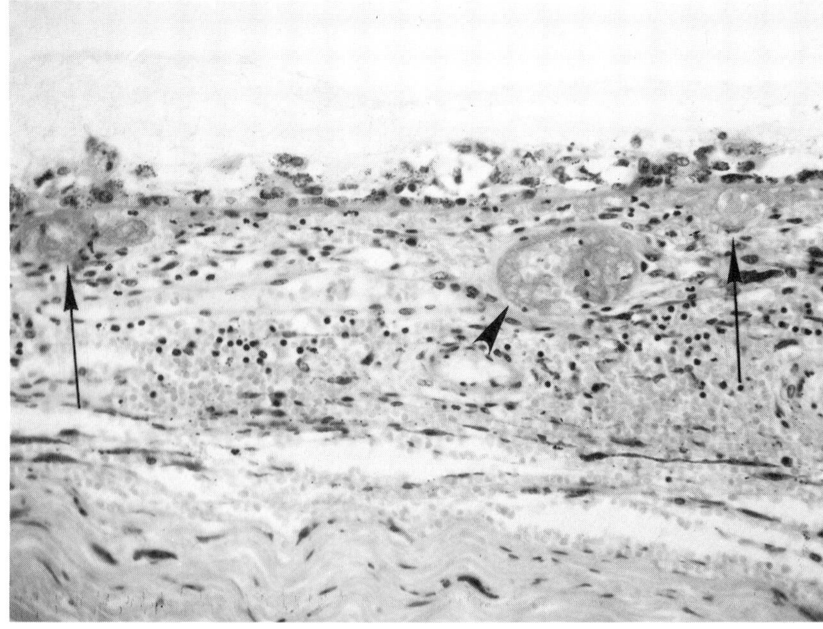

Figure 8–459. Fibrinous occlusion of choriocapillaris (arrows) and larger choroidal vessel (arrowhead) in patient with **idiopathic thrombotic thrombocytopenia**. Retinal pigment epithelium is irregular and vacuolated and shows minor hyperplasia. H and E, ×290. (Courtesy of Dr. Rene Berry; case presented at Verhoeff Society, Washington, DC, April 1970.)

hemorrhages, with secondary RPE hypertrophy, hyperplasia, and migration into the retina in a perivascular location, and hemosiderin deposition (Figs. 8–460 through 8–462). Arteriolar obstruction of the third and fourth branches of the central retinal artery occurs (Fig. 8–463). At the junction of the perfused and nonperfused retina, several changes occur, including arteriovenous looping and bending (Fig. 8–464) and localized areas of neovascularization (sea fans) (Fig. 8–465). Figure 8–466 is a flow diagram of the proposed sequence of events that occur in sickle cell retinopathy.

Goldberg (1971) classified proliferative sickle retinopathy into the following pathogenetic sequence: Stage I, peripheral arteriolar occlusions; Stage II, peripheral arteriolar-venular anastomoses; Stage III, neovascular and fibrous proliferation; Stage IV, vitreous hemorrhage; and Stage V, retinal detachment.

Proliferative sickle retinopathy also occurs, although with much less frequency, in SS disease, hemoglobin C trait, and sickle cell thalassemia.

Loss of capillaries, with macular and perimacular vascular remodeling, also may be observed (Fig. 8–467) (Knapp, 1972; Ryan, 1974; Stevens, Busse, Lee, et al, 1974; Asdourian, Nagpal, Busse, et al, 1976). Vision is variably affected and may be severely impaired by inner ischemic retinal atrophy.

Angioid streaks have been reported clinically in up to 6 per cent of cases of SS disease (Paton, 1972). They have also been reported in sickle trait (Gerde, 1974). The pathogenesis of this association is unknown, and its causal relationship is questioned by some.

Dysproteinemias. Dysproteinemias are sometimes primary, in association with macroglobulinemia or cryoglobulinemia caused by a diffuse disturbance in the reticuloendothelial system. They can be secondary to such diseases as multiple myeloma, Hodgkin's disease, and collagen vascular diseases.

The ocular fundus shows venous engorgement, retinal hemorrhages, exudates, and even venous occlusions. The frequency of ocular involvement is reported to be 30 to 50 per cent in macroglobulinemia, and less in the other disorders (Duke-Elder, 1967).

Characteristically, there are elevated or abnor-

Text continued on page 1082

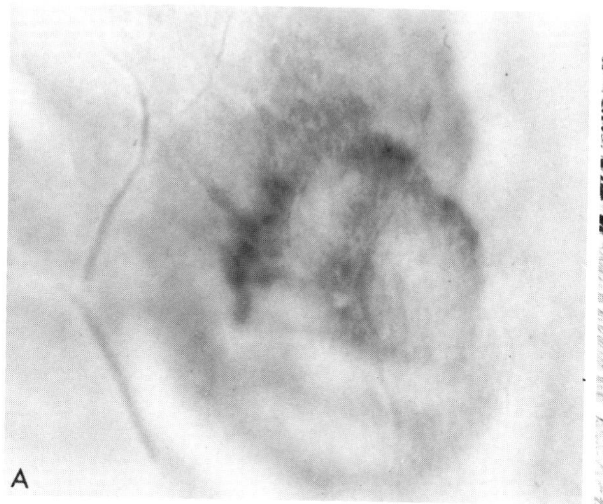

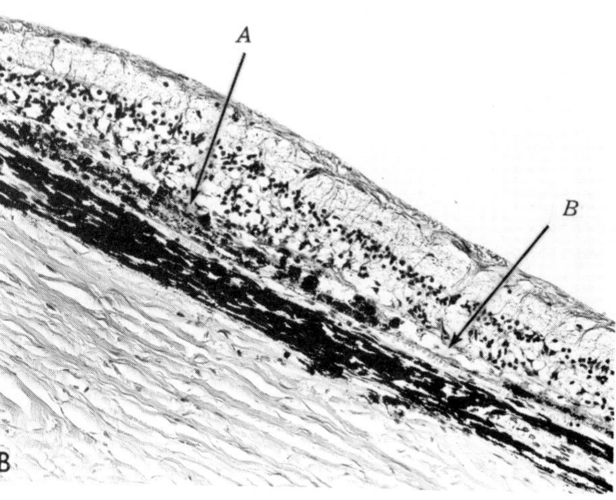

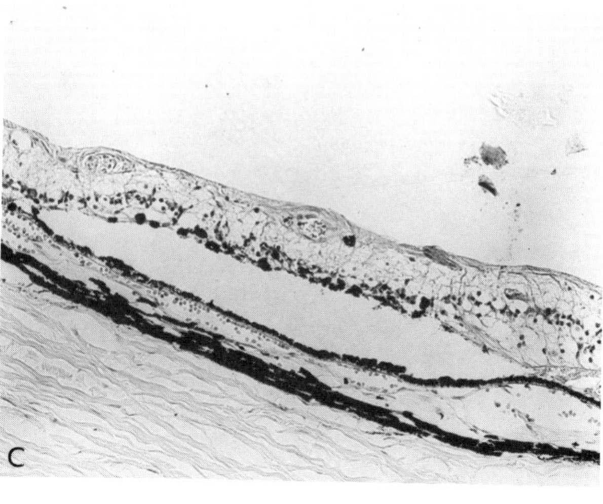

Figure 8–460. Black "sunburst" sign in **sickle cell retinopathy.** *A,* Gross: close-up view of partially pigmented lesion at inferotemporal quadrant in midperiphery (early black sunburst). *B,* Microscopic section at margin of lesion. Proliferation of retinal pigment epithelium (RPE) *(arrow A).* Area of focal loss of RPE *(arrow B).* H and E, ×112. *C,* Deeper section of lesion. Note thinning of retina, with loss of outer retinal layers and migration of RPE into partially degenerated retina. Occasional pigmented macrophages are present in and beneath the retina. Diffuse iron deposition is present throughout lesion. Prussian blue, ×112. EP 30493. (From Romayananda N, Goldberg MF, Green WR: Histopathology of sickle cell retinopathy. Trans Am Acad Ophthalmol Otolaryngol 77:652-676, 1973.)

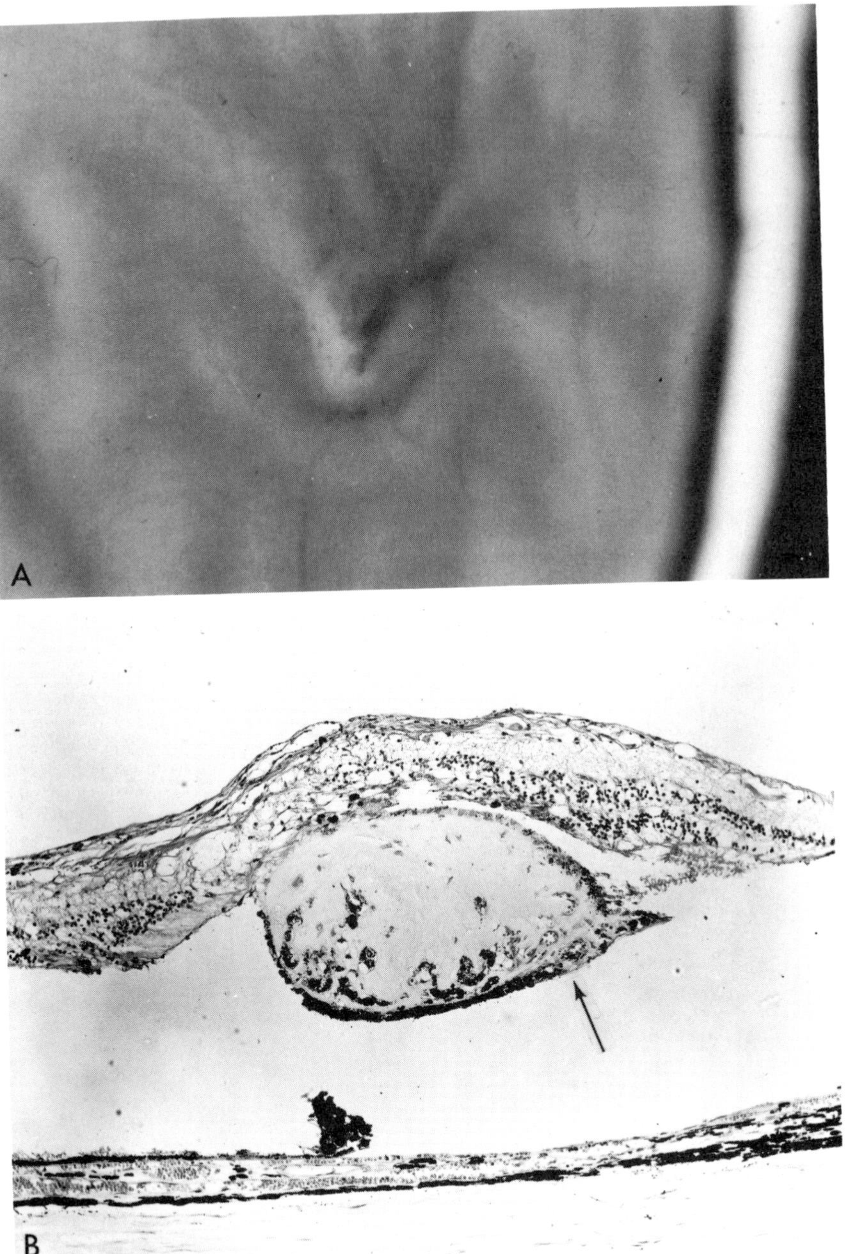

Figure 8–461. Sickle cell retinopathy. *A,* Gross: an elevated and partially pigmented area (early black sunburst). *B,* Microscopic section through lesion. Large hyaline nodule between retina and choroid. Proliferation of retinal pigment epithelium; some fibroblasts and capillaries (arrow) are present within the nodule. Partial loss of outer layers of overlying retina is seen. H and E, ×80. EP 30493. (From Romayananda N, Goldberg MF, Green WR: Histopathology of sickle cell retinopathy. Trans Am Acad Ophthalmol Otolaryngol 77:652-676, 1973.)

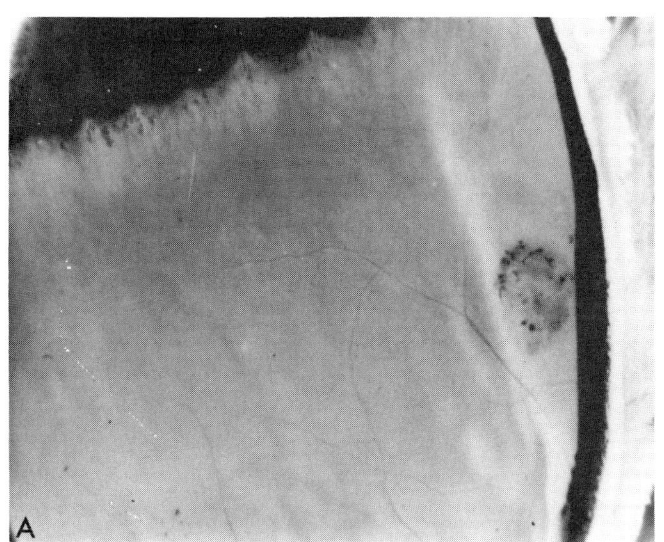

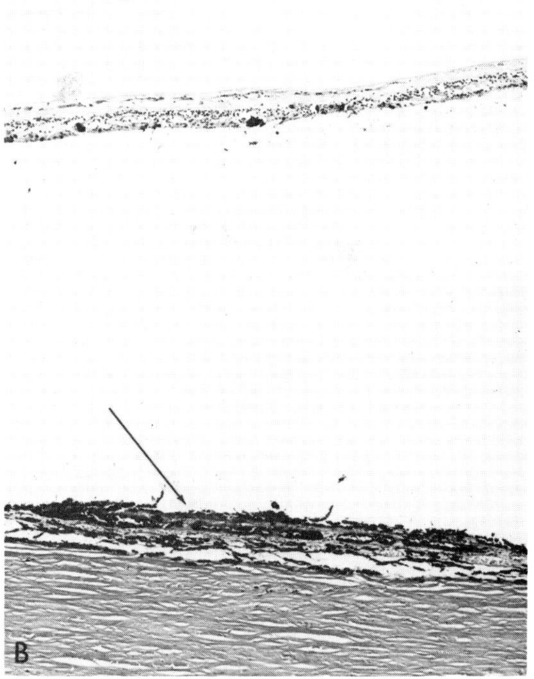

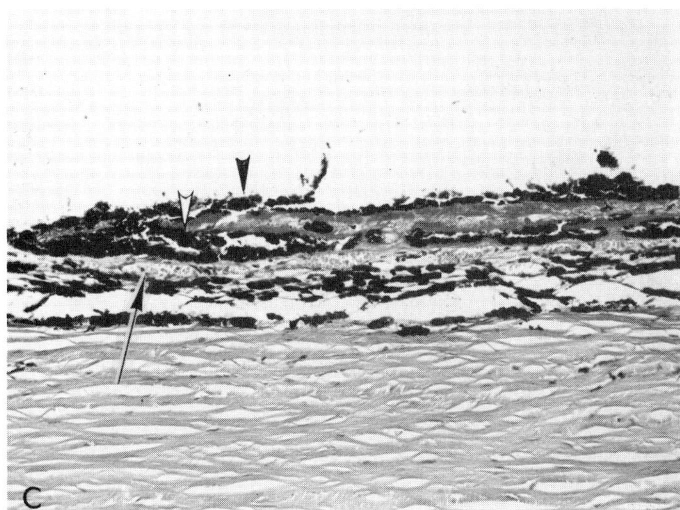

Figure 8–462. Sickle cell retinopathy. *A,* Oval retinal lesion characterized by retinal pigment epithelium (RPE) hyperplasia and migration into retina in perivascular location, giving lesion a spiculate appearance. *B,* Retina (artifactitiously detached) shows loss of outer nuclear layer and hyperplastic RPE. Coresponding area below (arrow) shows laminated hyperplastic RPE. PAS, ×50. *C,* Higher power view of hyperplastic RPE arranged in laminated pattern (arrowheads). Choriocapillaris (arrow) is normal. Special staining of an adjacent section showed hemosiderin deposits in area of hyperplastic RPE and overlying retina. H and E, ×135. EP 33444. (From Romayananda N, Goldberg MF, Green WR: histopathology of sickle cell retinopathy. Trans Am Acad Ophthalmol Otolaryngol 77:652-676, 1973.)

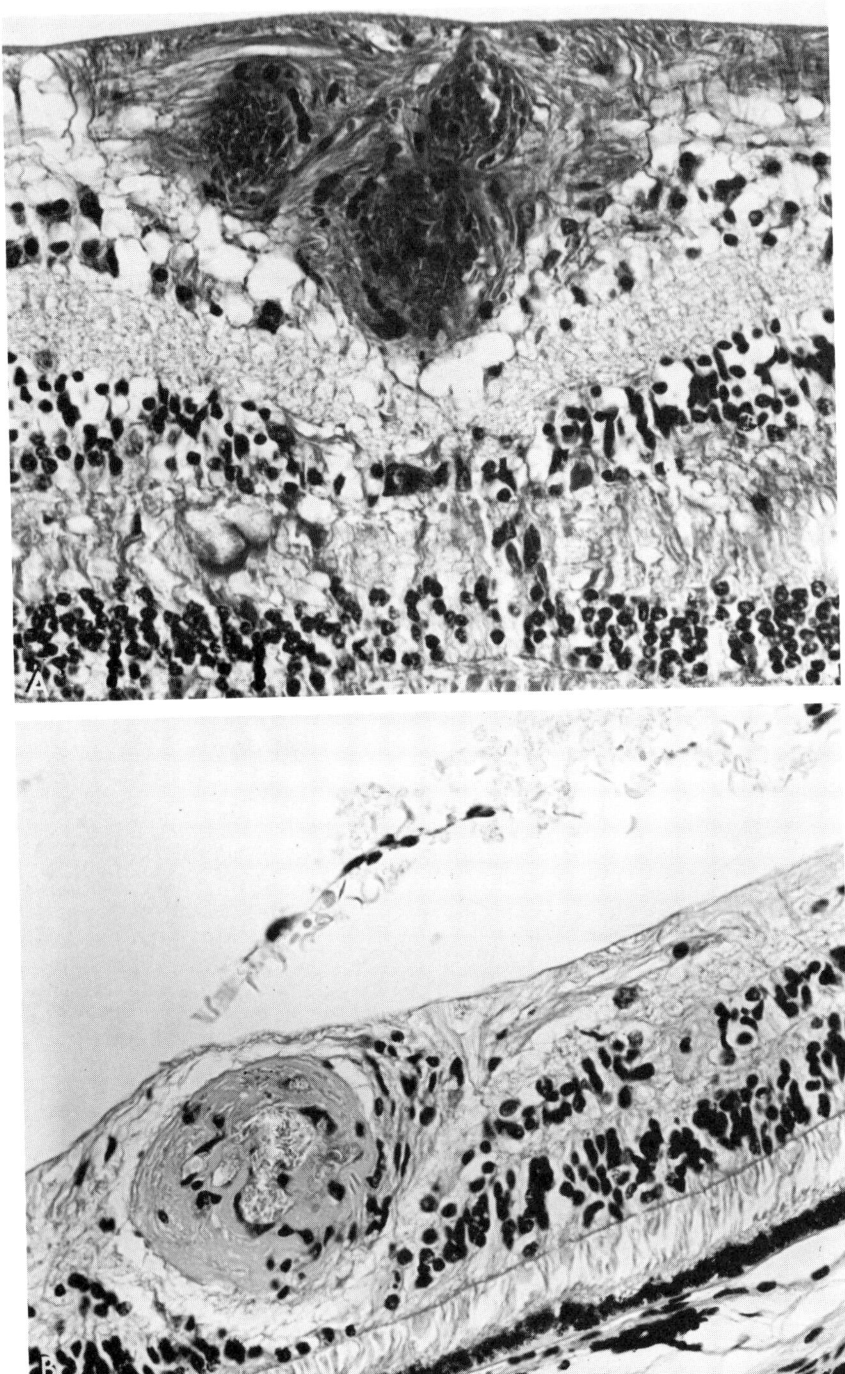

Figure 8–463. *A,* Retina shows focal **arteriolar obstruction** by compact sickled erythrocytes. H and E, ×254. *B,* Arteriolar obstruction. Recanalized thrombus. H and E, ×195. EP 30356. (From Romayananda N, Goldberg MF, Green WR: Histopathology of sickle cell retinopathy. Trans Am Acad Ophthalmol Otolaryngol *77*:652-676, 1973.)

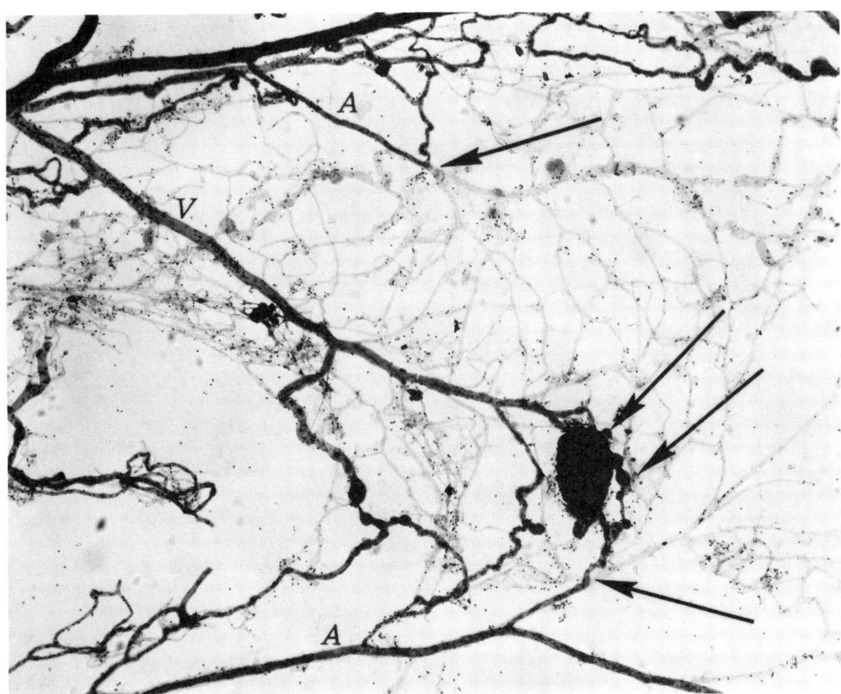

Figure 8–464. Sickle cell retinopathy. Retina, trypsin digestion preparation. Abrupt arteriolar obstruction (single arrows) with distal ischemic atrophy. Arteriolar-venular loop with beading is present (double arrows). *A,* arteriole; *V,* venule. PAS, H and E, ×29. EP 30356. (From Romayananda N, Goldberg MF, Green WR: Histopathology of sickle cell retinopathy. Trans Am Acad Ophthalmol Otolaryngol 77:652-676, 1973.)

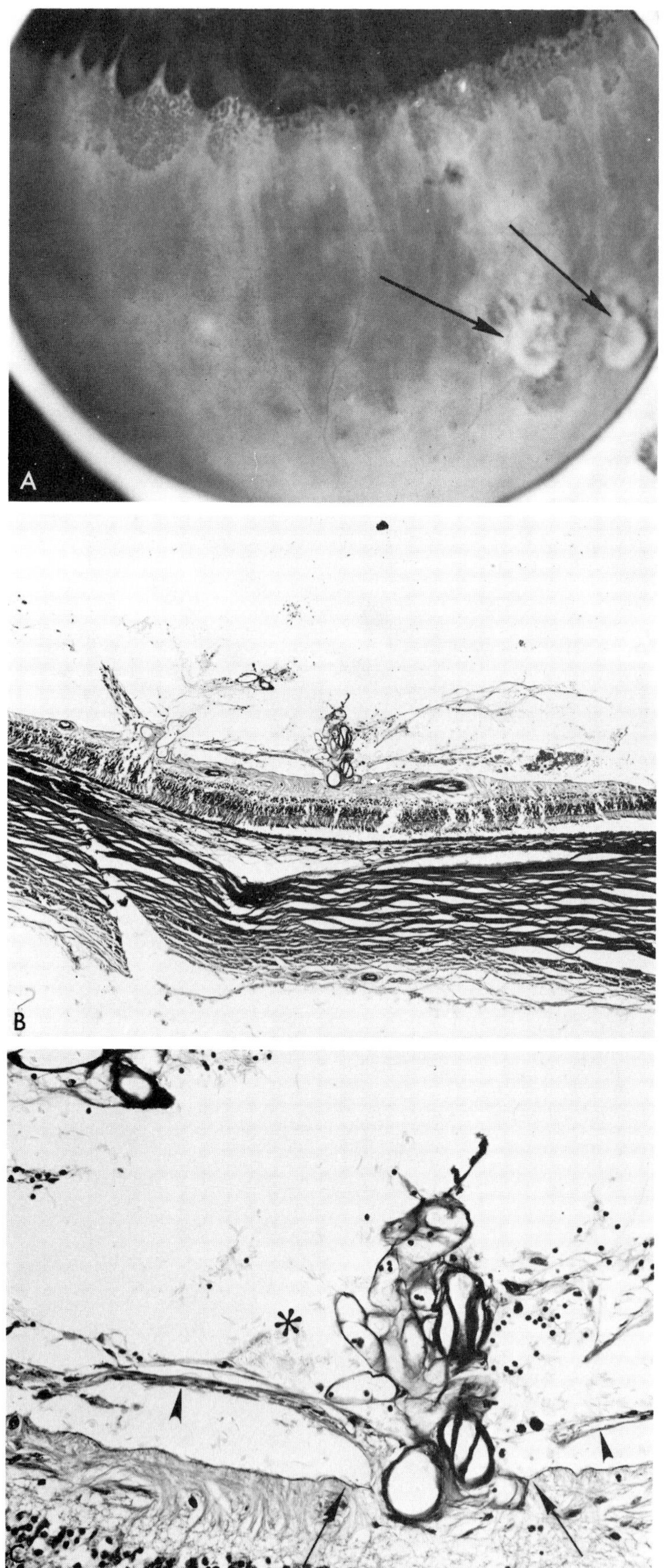

Figure 8–465. Sickle cell retinopathy. *A,* Gross appearance of two "sea-fans" with surrounding hemorrhage. *B,* Section of one of sea-fans shows two areas where vessels extend into the vitreous from the retina. H and E, ×38. *C,* Higher power view showing discontinuity of retinal internal limiting membrane (between arrows) through which vessels extend into vitreous. Fibroglial membranes (arrowheads), a few lymphocytes, and numerous sickled erythrocytes are present in vicinity of sea-fan. PAS, ×210. EP 30356. (From Romayananda N, Goldberg MF, Green WR: Histopathology of sickle cell retinopathy. Trans Am Acad Ophthalmol Otolaryngol *77*:652–676, 1973.)

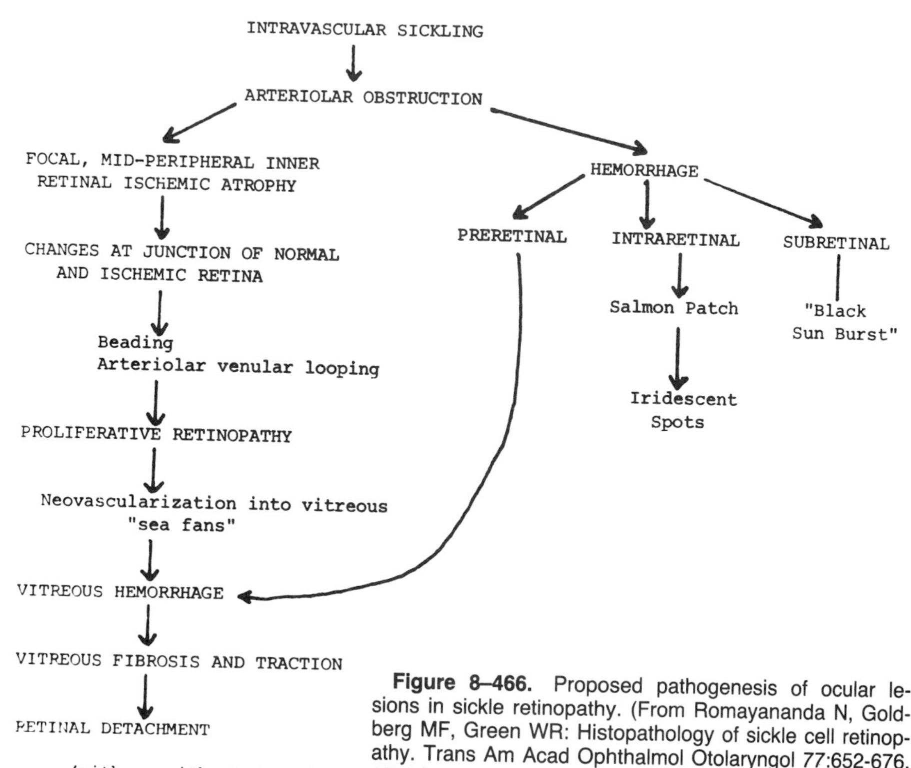

Figure 8–466. Proposed pathogenesis of ocular lesions in sickle retinopathy. (From Romayananda N, Goldberg MF, Green WR: Histopathology of sickle cell retinopathy. Trans Am Acad Ophthalmol Otolaryngol *77*:652-676, 1973.)

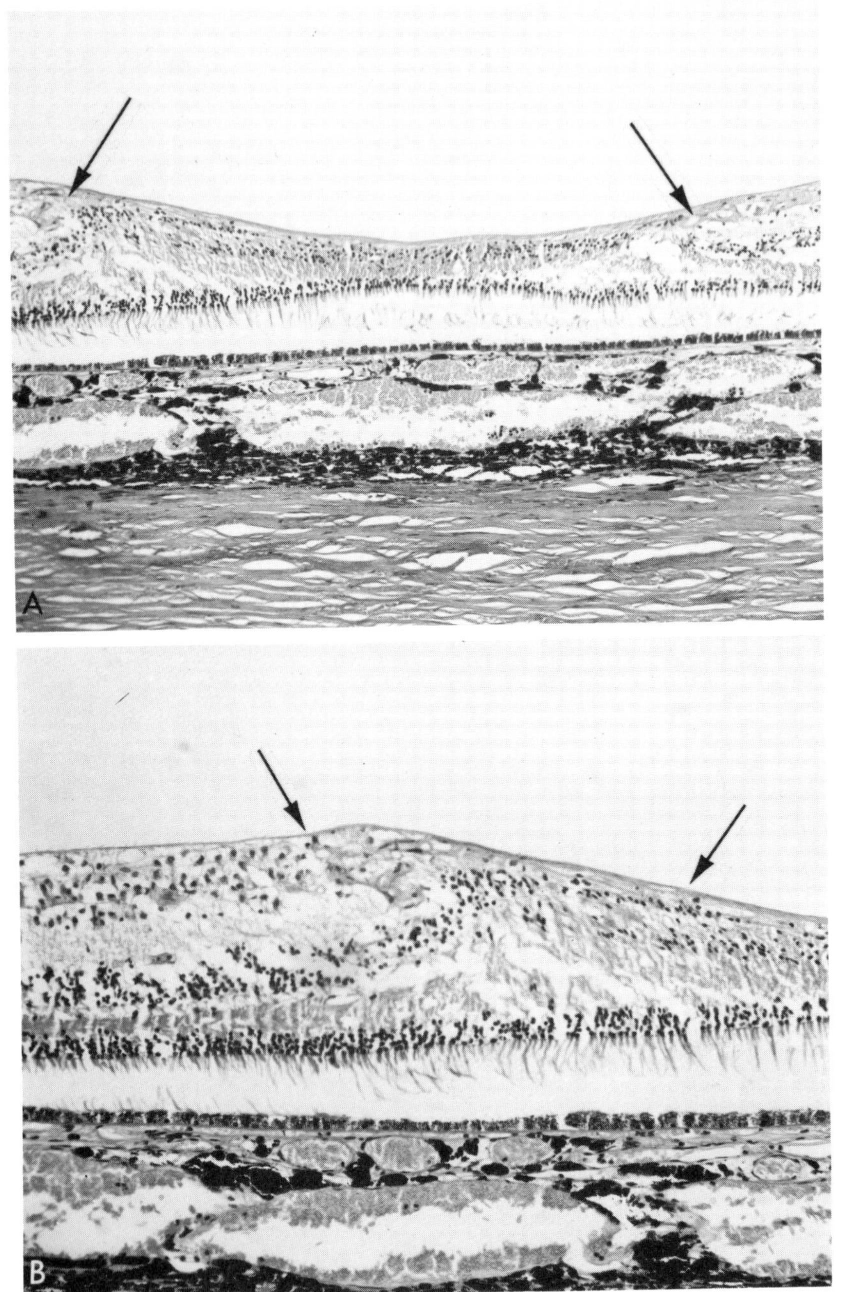

Figure 8–467. Macular vascular "remodeling" in **sickle cell retinopathy**. *A,* Section through foveola shows loss of ganglion cell layer in foveal area (arrows). H and E, × 100. *B,* Parafoveal area and clivus of macular area. Ganglion cells normally begin to associate about midway in clivus and build up to 5 to 7 layers in parafoveal area. Ganglion cells are totally absent in clivus and inner portion of parafoveal area (between arrows). H and E, ×200. EP 30356.

mal high-molecular-weight globulins in the blood, which induce increased viscosity. The increased viscosity leads to reduction in blood flow in the retina and secondary ischemia (Carr, Henkind, 1963). Clinically, in the very early stages the main changes are in the veins, which are dilated and somewhat tortuous. As the process progresses they begin to show segmentation and sausage-like dilations and constrictions. Later there are intraretinal hemorrhage (Fig. 8–468), exudation, and cotton-wool patches, and finally there may be occlusion of tributary veins or even the central retinal vein. Clearing of the retinopathy may be observed following plasmapheresis (Fig. 8–468), but vision can be permanently reduced (Thomas, Olk, Markman, et al, 1983).

Histopathologic studies (Spalter, 1959; Timm, 1960; Ackerman, 1962; Carr, Henkind, 1963; Ashton, Kok, Foulds, 1963) have shown venous dilatation, retinal hemorrhages and exudates, microthrombi in smaller retinal vessels, and serous detachment of the macula.

Ashton, Kok, and Foulds (1963) studied flat preparations of the retina from individuals with dysproteinemia. They found characteristic changes, consisting of many microaneurysms distributed in the peripheral portion of the retina (Fig. 8–469). The affected vessels in the retinal

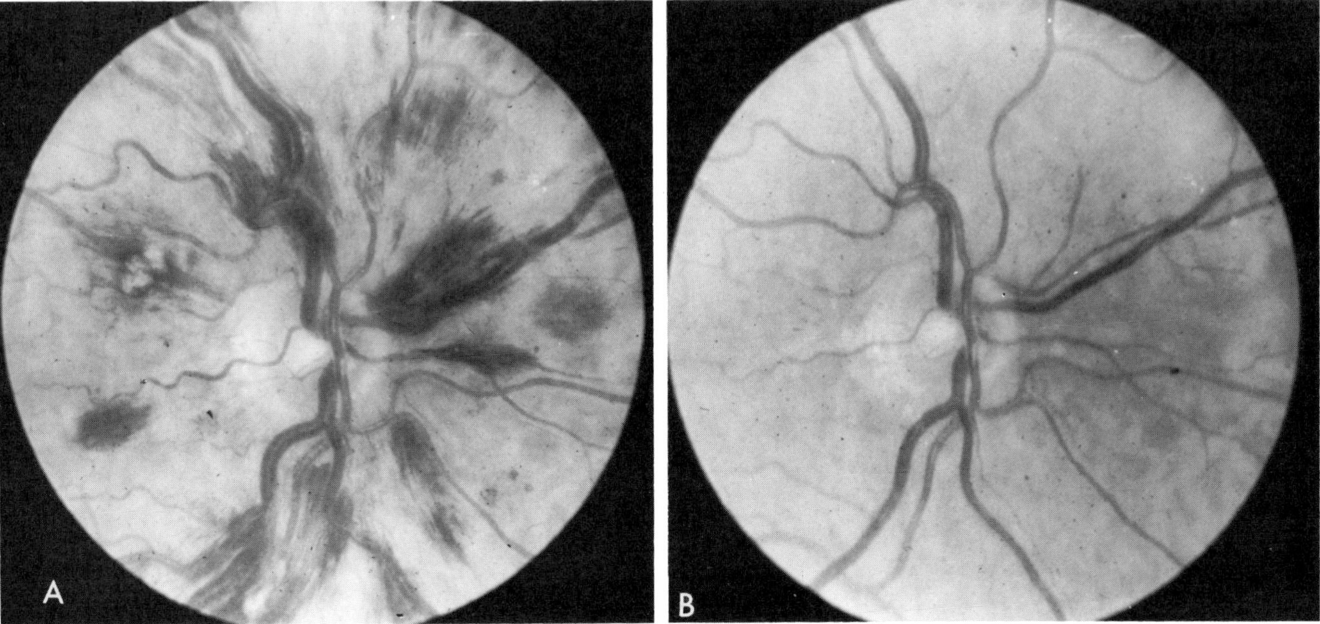

Figure 8–468. Waldenström's macroglobulinemia, *A,* before and *B,* after plasmapheresis. Before therapy, much vascular dilatation and tortuosity, flame-shaped hemorrhages, and cotton-wool patches are evident. (Courtesy of Dr. Joseph Olk.)

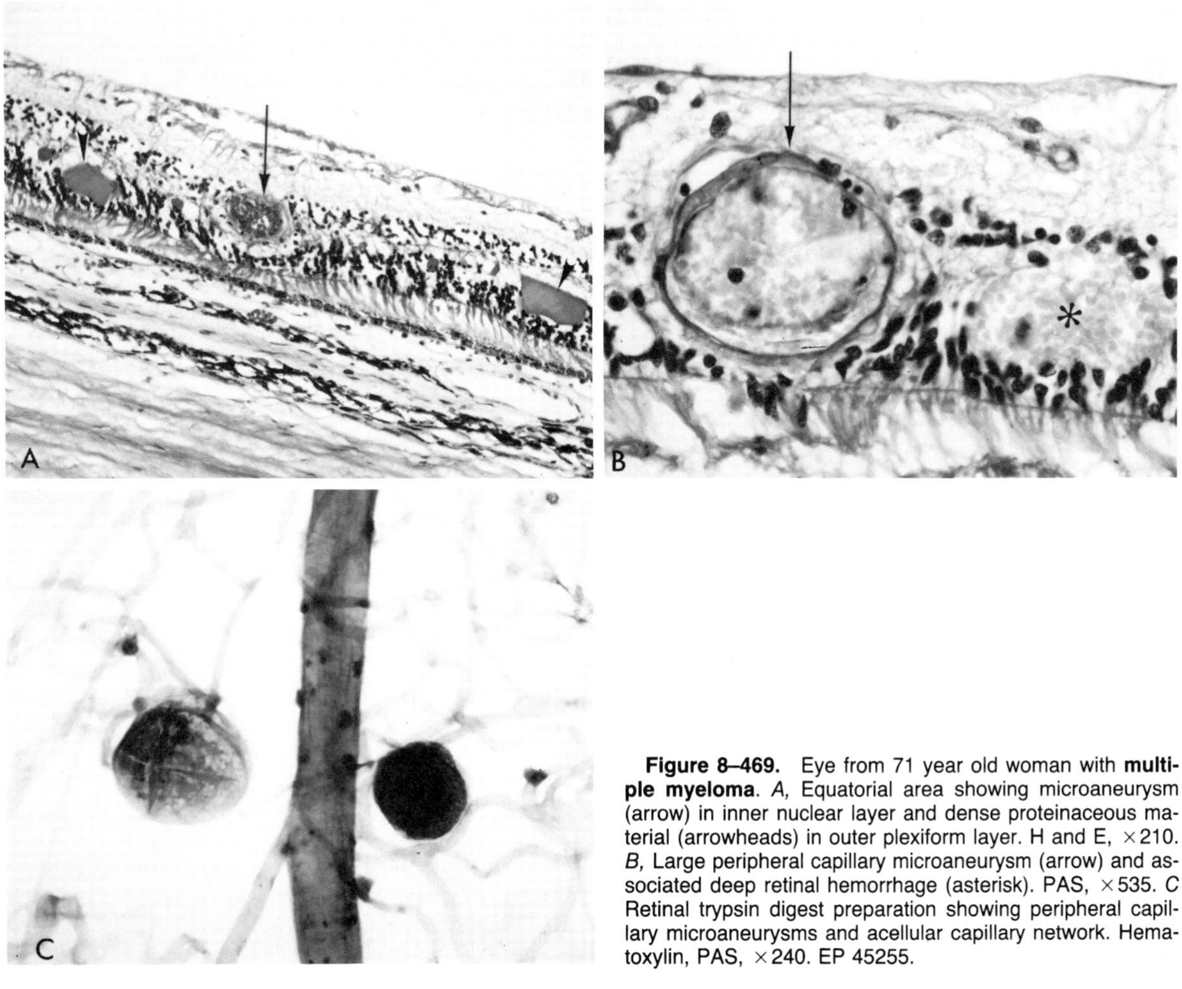

Figure 8–469. Eye from 71 year old woman with **multiple myeloma**. *A,* Equatorial area showing microaneurysm (arrow) in inner nuclear layer and dense proteinaceous material (arrowheads) in outer plexiform layer. H and E, ×210. *B,* Large peripheral capillary microaneurysm (arrow) and associated deep retinal hemorrhage (asterisk). PAS, ×535. *C* Retinal trypsin digest preparation showing peripheral capillary microaneurysms and acellular capillary network. Hematoxylin, PAS, ×240. EP 45255.

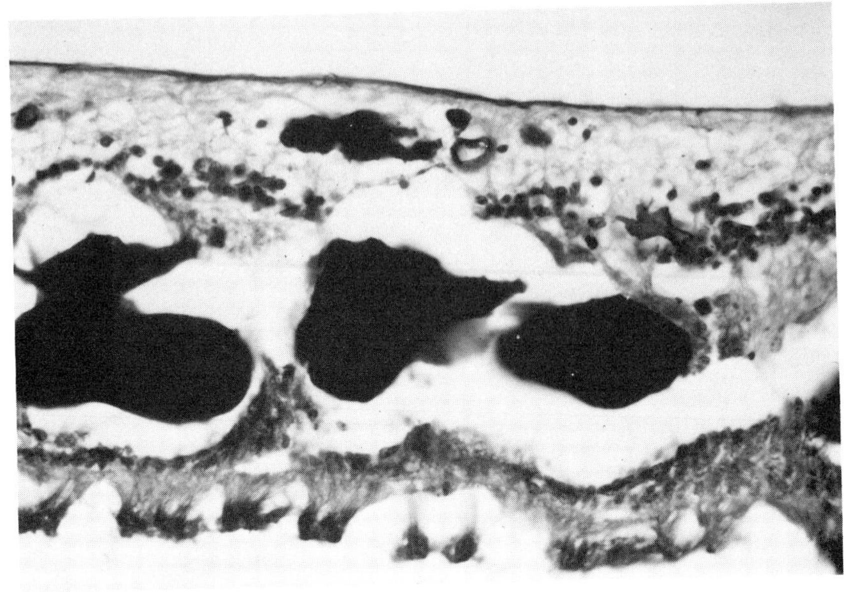

Figure 8–470. Midperiphery of retina with dense proteinaceous deposits in patient with **Waldenström's macroglobulinemia.** (From Friedman AH, Marchevsky A, Odel JG, Gerber MA, Thung SN: Immunofluorescent studies of eye in Waldenström's macroglobulinemia. Arch Ophthalmol *98*:743-746, 1980.)

periphery showed a loss of endothelial cells and pericytes; at the equator there were some microaneurysms that contained an increased number of endothelial cells, as if the endothelium had migrated from the periphery toward the intermediate portions of the retina. Such changes also may suggest an attempt at neovascularization. These changes are presumably caused by vascular stasis and secondary hypoxic damage to retinal vessels. Similar findings by trypsin digestion were observed by Toussaint (1966).

Friedman, Marchevsky, and others (1980), in a study of eyes obtained post mortem from a patient with Waldenström's macroglobulinemia (K light chain), found IgM deposits by an immunofluorescent technique in cystic spaces in the outer plexiform layer and inner layers of the retina (Fig. 8–470) and around the photoreceptors. In addition, retinal hemorrhages and capillary microaneurysms were observed.

Cysts of the ciliary epithelium occur in multiple myeloma (Johnson, Storey, 1970) and in other hypergammaglobulinemias (Johnson, 1970). These cysts contain the elevated or abnormal serum protein (see Figs. 8–247 and 8–248). Ciliochoroidal effusions sometimes occur with hyperproteinemic states (Fogle, Green, 1976) (see Fig. 8–247,*B*). It is presumed that the material in the effusion, like that in the pars plana cysts, is the same as the increased serum protein. Additional findings (Lewis, Falls, Troyer, 1975) include conjunctival vascular sludging, deposits in the cornea, plasma cell infiltrates in the orbit, and copper deposition in the cornea.

Genetic/Metabolic Diseases

Mucopolysaccharidoses. The genetic mucopolysaccharidoses are a group of inborn errors of mucopolysaccharide metabolism that result in at least six well-defined clinical syndromes. All are transmitted as autosomal recessive traits, except type II (Hunter) which is sex-linked recessive. The main ophthalmologic changes include progressive corneal clouding, retinal pigmentary degeneration, and optic atrophy. In each syndrome there are specific defects of catabolic lysosomal exoenzymes that are necessary for degradation of dermatan sulfate and heparin sulfate. The differential features of the systemic mucopolysaccharidoses are listed in Table 8–4. Dwarfism, gargoylism, and coarse facies occur to a variable degree in patients with this group of diseases. External features are present to some degree in all types. Dwarfism is a feature in types I, II, IV, and VI, and gargoylism is seen in types I, II, and VI. Coarse facies is a feature of types I-S and III.

Corneal clouding is observed clinically in types I-H, I-S, IV, and VI-A (Topping, Kenyon, Goldberg, Maumenee, 1971) and is variable in type III. Corneal involvement is not observed clinically in type II (Hunter), some cases of type III (San Filippo), or type VI-B (Maroteaux-Lamy, mild phenotype) (Quigley, Kenyon, 1974), but increased amounts of mucopolysaccharide (MPS) can be observed by light and electron microscopy.

Retinal pigmentary degeneration in the mucopolysaccharidoses has the same clinical and histopathologic features as in retinitis pigmentosa and is seen in MPS types I-H, I-S, II-A, II-B, III, and IV. There are hypertrophy, hyperplasia, and migration of RPE into the midperipheral retina in a perivascular location, which gives a spiculate appearance.

Retinal ganglion cells may have a distended appearance from deposition of complex lipid and acid mucopolysaccharides. The lipid is evident electron microscopically by the presence of

Table 8–4. DIFFERENTIAL FEATURES OF THE SYSTEMIC MUCOPOLYSACCHARIDOSES

		Systemic Features		Ocular Features			Urinary AMP Excess			
MPS Type	**Genetics**	***Skeletal Dysplasia***	***Mental Retardation***	***Corneal Clouding***	***Retinal Pigmentary Degeneration***	***Optic Atrophy***	***Heparan Sulfate***	***Dermatan Sulfate***	***Keratan Sulfate***	**Deficient Enzyme**
I-H: Hurler	AR } allelic	+ + +	+ + +	+ + +	R	R	+ +	+ + +	—	α-L-Iduronidase
I-S: Scheie (formerly MPS V)	AR } allelic	+	±	+ + +	R	R	+ +	+ + +	—	α-L-Iduronidase (partial)
II: Hunter A: Severe phenotype	XR } allelic	+ + +	+ + +	—	R	R	+ +	+ +	—	Sulfoiduronate sulfatase
B: Mild phenotype	XR } allelic	+ +	±	+*	R	R	+ +	+ +	—	Sulfoiduronate sulfatase
III: Sanfilippo A: Sulfatase-deficient	AR } allelic	±	+ + +	—	R	R	+ + +	—	—	Heparan sulfatase
B: Glucosaminidase-deficient	AR } allelic	±	+ + +	—	R	R	+ + +	—	—	*N*-Acetyl-α-D glucosaminidase
IV: Morquio	AR	+ + +	±	+ +	NR	R	—	—	+ + +	?
V: Vacant, now MPS I-S										
VI: Maroteaux-Lamy A: Severe phenotype	AR } nonallelic	+ + +	—	+ +	NR	R	—	+ + +	—	?
B: Mild phenotype	AR } nonallelic	+	—	+ +	NR	NR	—	+ + +	—	?

*Positive by slit lamp biomicroscopy in some older patients.

AR, autosomal recessive; XR, X-linked recessive; R, reported; NR, not reported; —, absent/not elevated; ±, variable; +, mild; + +, moderate; + + +, marked.

After Kenyon KR: Ocular ultrastructure of inherited metabolic disease, *in* Goldberg MF (ed): Genetic and Metabolic Eye Diseases. Boston, Little Brown, 1974, p 141.

membranous lamellar inclusions, and the mucopolysaccharides by fibrillogranular inclusions.

Optic atrophy and commensurate retinal atrophy have been observed in all MPS types except VI-B.

There are marked thinning of the outer nuclear layer and loss of the outer segments of the photoreceptor cells. The RPE contains excessive acid mucopolysaccharides and lipofuscin. This material may be demonstrated histochemically, and it appears as fibrogranular inclusions by electron microscopy. It is postulated that the abnormal accumulations in the RPE may lead to the photoreceptor cell degeneration by interfering with the biochemical interplay between RPE and photoreceptor cells.

There is also deposition of MPS in the iris pigment epithelium, nonpigmented ciliary epithelium, and endothelium of the trabecular meshwork. Thickening of the sclera by accumulation of MPS has been observed histopathologically in MPS types I-H, II-A, III-A, III-B, and VI-A.

Neufeld and Cantz (1971) have found that the enzyme defect in cells grown in tissue culture from patients with the various forms of MPS can be corrected when the abnormal cells are grown with cells from normal individuals or with cells from a patient with a different form of MPS. There is also preliminary evidence that serum from normal patients can effect a partial correction in vivo (Maumenee, 1973). Such research efforts may lead to the isolation of specific corrective factors that can be used in the treatment of patients with these conditions.

Electron microscopic study of conjunctival biopsies may be helpful in the initial evaluation of a patient suspected of having one of the systemic mucopolysaccharidoses (Fig. 8–471) (Kenyon, Quigley, Hussels, Wyllie, 1972).

Systemic Mucopolysaccharidosis I-H (MPS I-H; Hurler's Disease) (Hurler, 1919). The light microscopic features of the entire eye of patients with MPS I-H have been reported by Newell and Koistinen (1955) and by Chan, Green, Maumenee, and Sack (1983).

Since the late 1960s, various ocular tissue specimens obtained from patients with the Hurler syndrome have been studied by the newer methods of histochemistry and electron microscopy. Generally, single membrane-limited cytoplasmic vacuoles, with predominantly fibrillogranular or occasionally membranous lamellae, were found in the conjunctiva (Van Hoof, Hers, 1964; Kenyon, Quigley, Hussels, Wyllie, 1972), cornea (Pouliquen, Faure, Bisson, et al, 1967; Rosen, Haust, Yamashita, et al, 1968; Matsuda, Satake, Katsumata, 1970; Reim, Rohen, Dittrick, 1971), sclera (Spellacy, Kennerley-Bankes, Crow, et al, 1980), trabecular meshwork (D'Epinay, Reme, 1978), and iris (Spellacy, Kennerley-Bankes, Crow, et al, 1980).

Chan, Green, Maumenee, and Sack (1983) re-

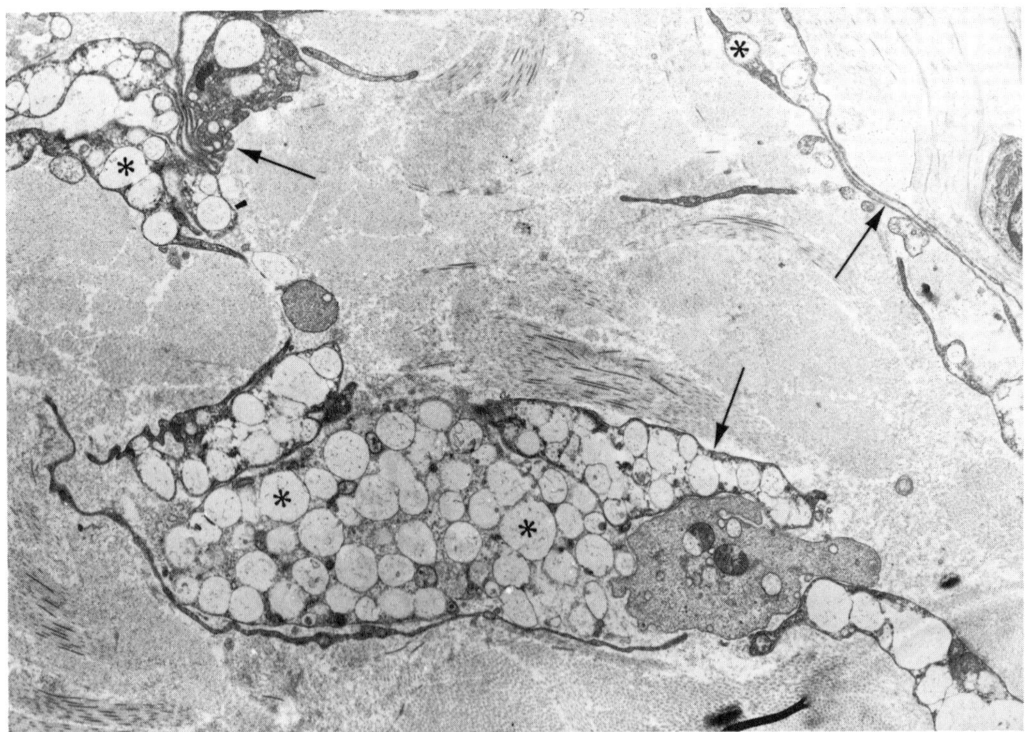

Figure 8–471. Conjunctival biopsy showing fibrocytes (arrows) with distended, membrane-bound inclusions containing fibrillogranular material (asterisks) in a patient with **Hurler's disease (MPS I-H)**. ×7500. EP 41186.

ported the results of light and electron microscopic study on eyes in two cases of MPS I-H. They observed numerous fine fibrillogranular inclusions in conjunctival fibrocytes, vascular endothelium, and pericytes (Fig. 8–472,*A*); corneal epithelium, keratocytes (Fig. 8–472,*B*), and endothelium (Fig. 8–472,*C*); endothelium of trabecular meshwork (Fig. 8–472,*D*); uveal melanocytes and fibrocytes (Fig. 8–472,*E*); iris pigment epithelium (Fig. 8–472,*F*); ciliary epithelium (Fig. 8–472,*G*); smooth muscle cells of ciliary body; pericytes (Fig. 8–472,*H*); lens epithelium (Fig. 8–472,*I*); retinal pigment epithelium (Fig. 8–472,*J*); ganglion cells; and sclerocytes (Fig. 8–472,*K*). Some multimembranous inclusions were noted in Schwann cells, keratocytes, trabecular endothelium (Fig. 8–472,*D*), uveal fibrocytes and melanocytes (Fig. 8–472,*E*), iris pigment epithelium (Fig. 8–472,*F*), retinal ganglion cells (Fig. 8–472,*L*), sclerocytes (Fig. 8–472,*K*), optic nerve astrocytes (Fig. 8–472,*M*), and vascular pericytes (Fig. 8–472,*A* and *H*). Extracellular fibrillogranular material was present in the corneal stroma, Descemet's membrane, and scleral stroma. The extensive involvement of the ocular tissues in those two cases indicates that the Hurler syndrome is the most severe form of the systemic mucopolysaccharidoses.

Chan, Green, Maumenee, and Sack (1983) also found inclusion of melanin pigment granules in storage vacuoles containing fibrillogranular and membranous material in the iris pigment epithelium, ciliary epithelium, and RPE. Many such melanin granules appeared to be undergoing degradation, with replacement by a fine fibrillogranular substance. This change suggests that a process of autophagocytosis of melanin pigment has taken place, resulting in relative depigmentation of the pigmented epithelia. This observation was also noted in cases of Sanfilippo disease, MPS III-A (Lavery, Green, Jabs, et al, 1983) and MPS III-B (Del Monte, Maumenee, Green, Kenyon, 1983).

Systemic Mucopolysaccharidosis I-S (MPS I-S; Scheie syndrome) (Scheie, Hambrick, Barness, 1962). This condition is a mild variant of MPS I-H. Although the whole eye has not been studied, the following tissues have been studied: cornea and conjunctiva (Scheie, Hambrick, Barness, 1962); conjunctiva (Rasteiro, 1977); skin and conjunctiva (Quigley, Goldberg, 1971); and limbal tissue (Quigley, Maumenee, Stark, 1975).

Systemic Mucopolysaccharidosis II (MPS II; Hunter Syndrome) (Hunter, 1917). Histopathologic and histochemical studies of the eyes of patients with MPS II have been reported by Goldberg and Duke (1967). Electron microscopic studies have been conducted by Topping, Kenyon, Goldberg and Maumenee (1971) and Danis and Toussaint (1971).

Systemic Mucopolysaccharidosis III-A (MPS III-A; Sanfilippo syndrome) (Sanfilippo. Podosin, Langer, Good, 1963). Light microscopic studies of the eyes from patients with MPS III-A have been reported by Jensen (1971) and by Vogel, Müller, and Witting (1974).

Del Monte, Maumenee, Green, and Kenyon (1983) examined by light and electron microscope the eyes of a 19 year old Caucasian female with MPS III-A who had poor vision (questionable light perception), flat electroretinogram, and fundus changes similar to those of classic retinitis pigmentosa (Fig. 8–473,*A*). (A similar microscopic appearance is seen in MPS VI-A [Fig. 8–473,*B*].) Phase-contrast and electron microscopy showed extensive intracellular accumulation of fibrillogranular (acid mucopolysaccharide, AMPS) and membranous lamellar (complex lipid) vacuoles in cornea, trabecular meshwork (Fig. 8–473,*C*), iris, lens, ciliary body (Fig. 8–473,*D*), and sclera (Fig. 8–473,*E*). Retinal ganglion cells (Fig. 8–473,*F*), RPE (Fig. 8–473,*G* and *H*), and optic nerve glia (Fig. 8–473,*I*) were similarly involved. Retinal pigment epithelial hyperplasia and hypopigmentation, intraretinal RPE migration (Fig. 8–473,*J*), vascular attenuation, and marked photoreceptor loss (Fig. 8–473,*K*) were prominent and closely resembled those occurring in inherited retinitis pigmentosa. The patient's blindness was attributed to photoreceptor cell loss, since the ganglion cells and optic nerve appeared intact. Although the etiology of photoreceptor loss is unclear, the massive storage of AMP and lipofuscin within the RPE might disturb its essential metabolic functions and lead to photoreceptor degeneration.

Systemic Mucopolysaccharidosis III-B (MPS III-B). Light microscopic and electron microscopic studies have been conducted by Lavery, Green, Luckenbach, et al (1983). Widespread partial degeneration of the photoreceptor cells was observed (Fig. 8–474,*A* and *B*). External migration of cone nuclei in the posterior pole was observed (Fig. 8–474,*A*). No migration of RPE into the retina was observed. The RPE was hypopigmented and markedly distended by vacuoles (Fig. 8–474,*C*). Cytoplasmic, single membrane-bound vacuoles containing the major storage product, acid mucopolysaccharide, were found in virtually every ocular tissue. Some of these are illustrated as follows: keratocytes (Fig. 8–474,*D*), endothelium of trabecular meshwork (Fig. 8–474,*E*); fibrocytes in the iris (Fig. 8–474,*F*); iris pigment epithelium (Fig. 8–474,*G*); cell bodies of the iris dilator muscle cells (Fig. 8–474,*H*); lens epithelium and lens fibers (Fig. 8–474,*I*); pigmented and nonpigmented ciliary epithelium (Fig. 8–474,*J*); fibrocytes and vascular endothelium and pericytes of the ciliary body (Fig. 8–474,*J*); retinal ganglion cells (Fig. 8–474,*K*); retinal pigment ep-

Text continued on page 1114

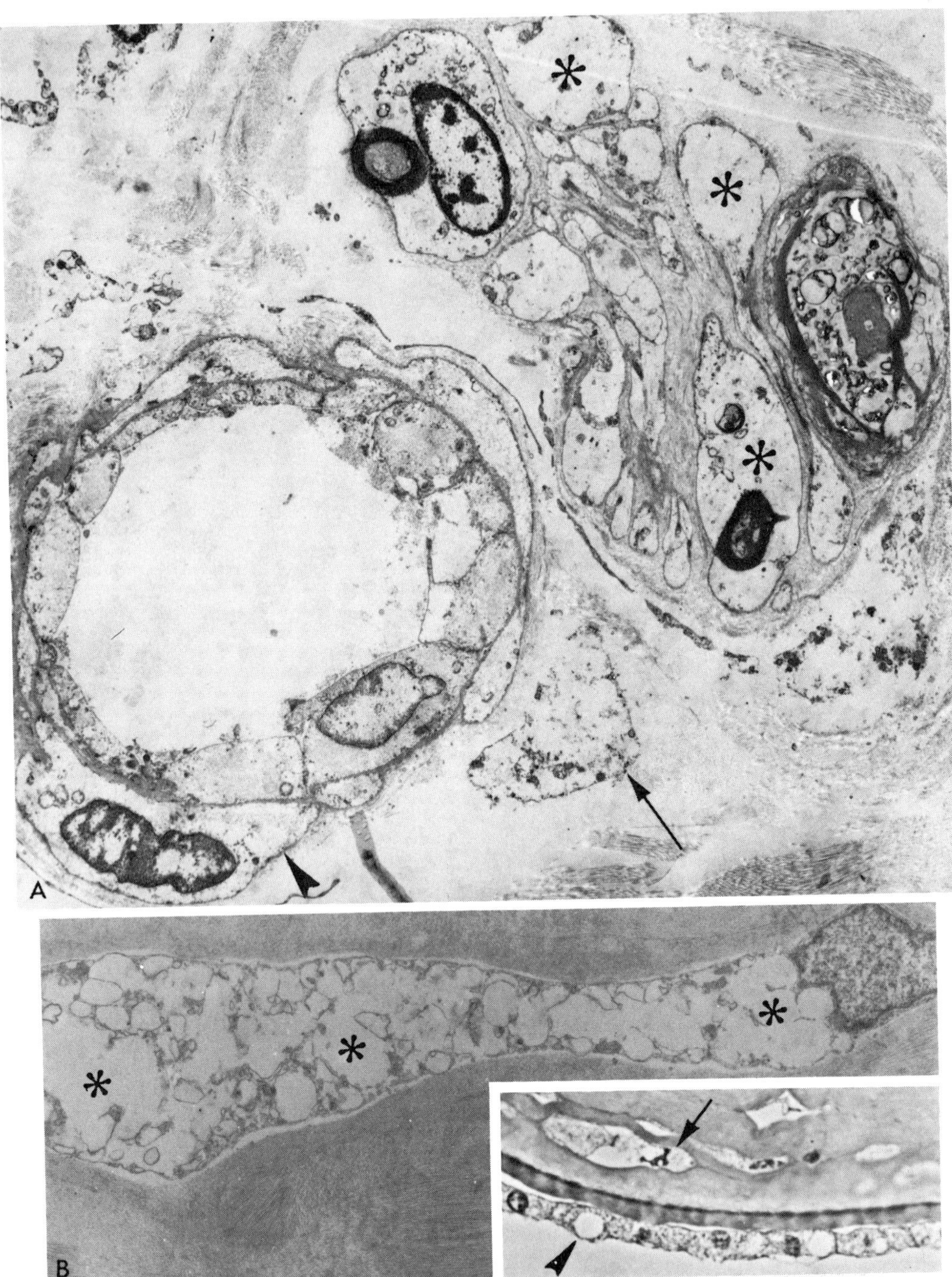

Figure 8–472. Systemic mucopolysaccharidosis IH (MPS-IH). *A,* Conjunctiva with numerous inclusions containing fibrillogranular material in fibrocytes (arrow), vascular endothelium and pericytes (arrowhead), and Schwann cells of a peripheral nerve (asterisks). ×3,800. *B,* Inset: Keratocytes (arrow) and corneal endothelium (arrowhead) are distended by vacuoles. Paraphenylenediamine, ×480. Main figure: electron microscopy reveals that distended fibrocytes contain large inclusions (asterisks) containing the fibrillogranular material. ×8,300.

Illustration continued on opposite page

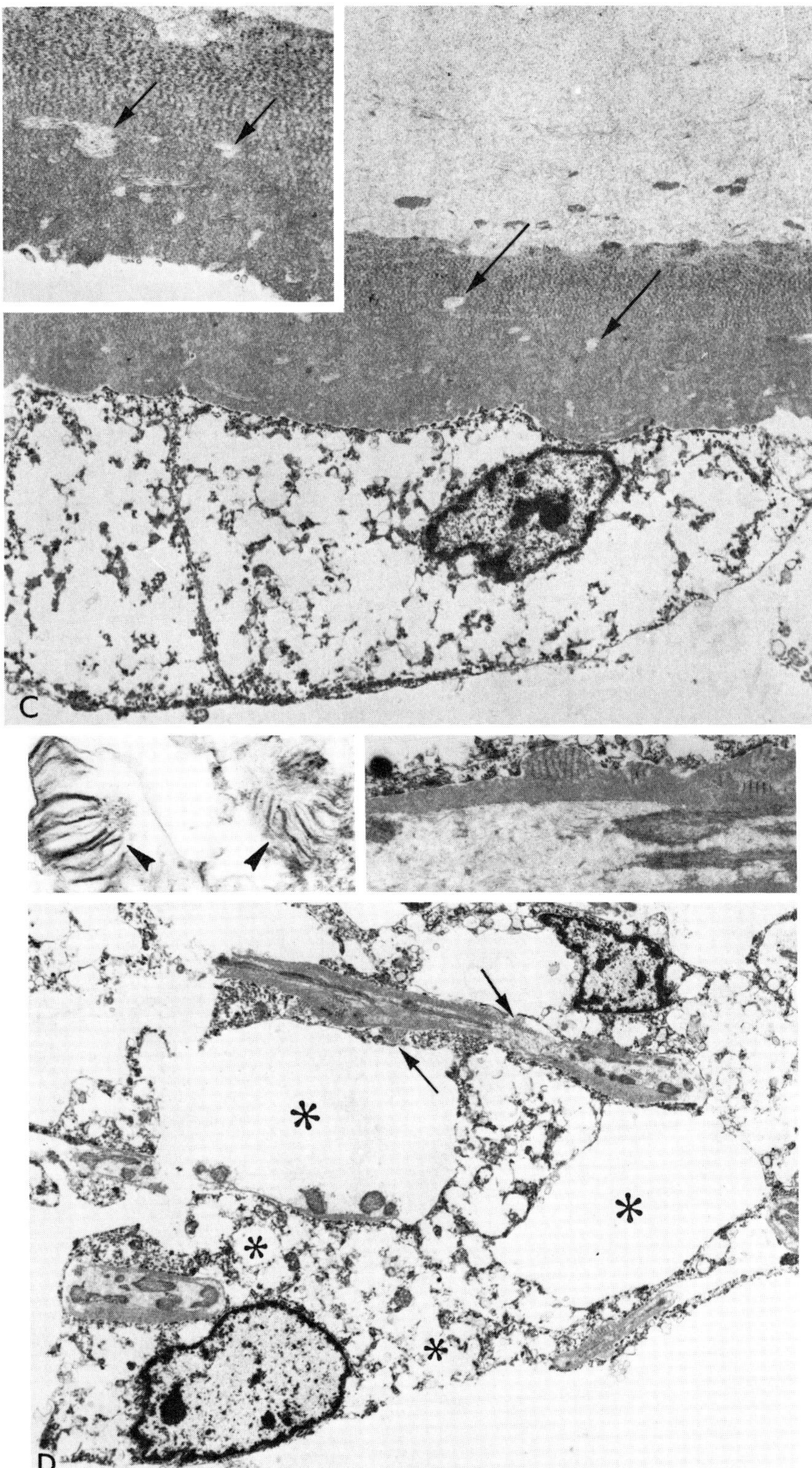

Figure 8–472. *Continued C,* The posterior portion of Descemet's membrane contains small deposits of fibrillogranular material (arrows and inset). Endothelium is markedly distended by numerous inclusions containing fibrillogranular material. ×7000; inset, ×10,250. *D,* Endothelial cells of the trabecular meshwork are considerably distended by vacuoles (asterisks) containing fibrillogranular material and some multimembranous material (arrowheads, upper left inset). The basement membrane is thickened and nodular and contains large collagen fibrills that have a periodicity of 1000 angstroms (arrows and upper right inset). ×5500; insets: upper left, ×40,000; upper right, ×11,250.

Illustration continued on following page

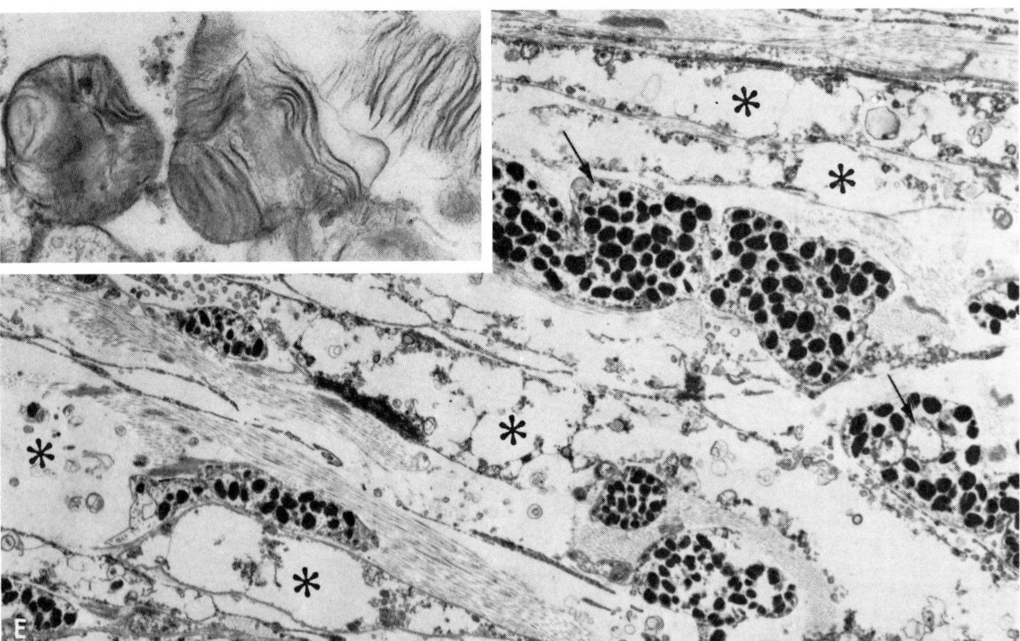

Figure 8–472 *Continued E,* Choroidal fibrocytes contain mostly fibrillogranular inclusions (asterisks) and a few membranous inclusions (inset). Melanocytes contain only a few fibrillogranular inclusions (arrows). ×5300; inset, ×33,300.

Illustration continued on opposite page

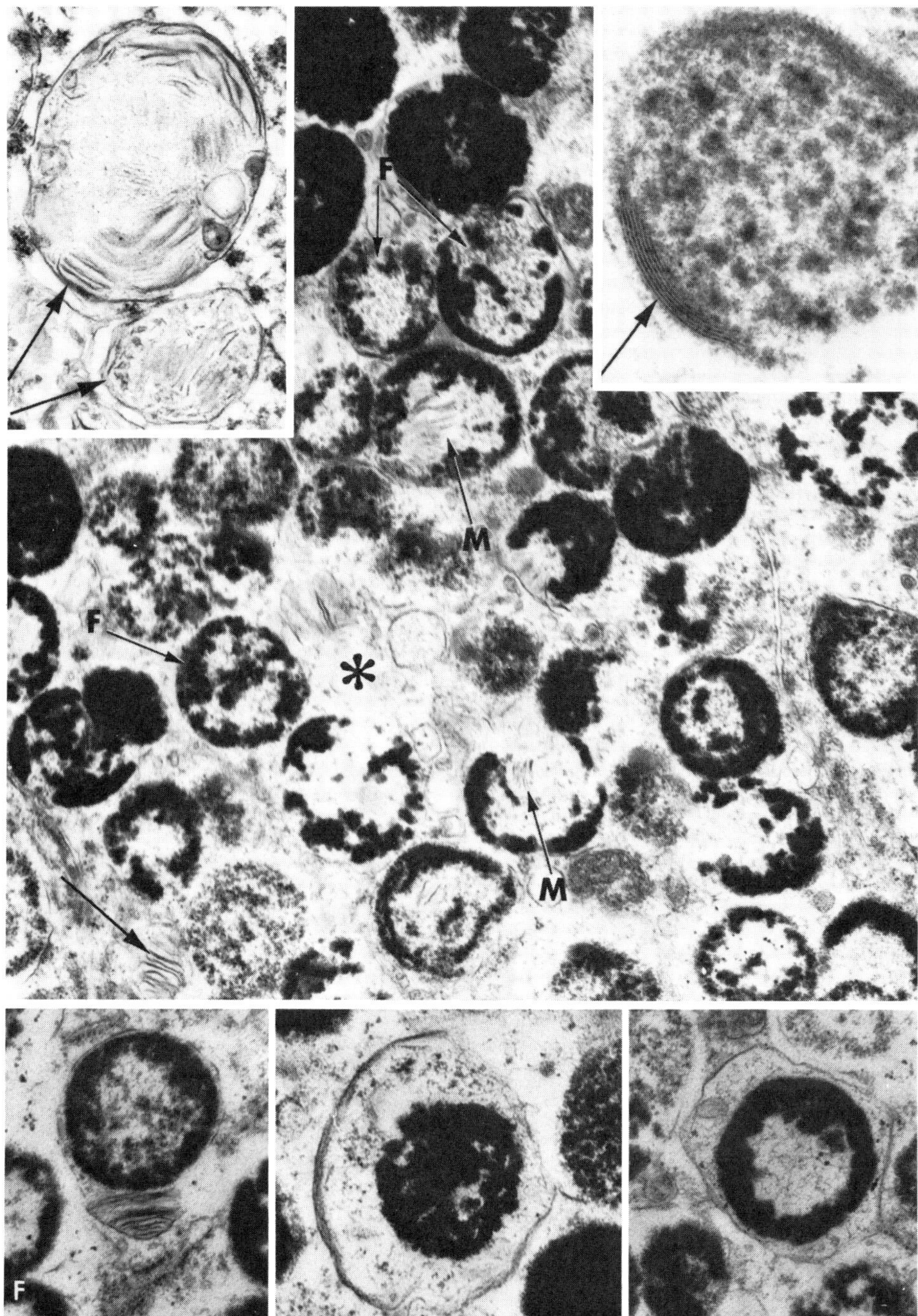

Figure 8–472 *Continued F,* Inclusions in iris pigment epithelium contain fibrillogranular material (asterisk) and occasional multimembranous material (arrows and upper left inset). Melanin pigment granules in various stages of degradation contain both fibrillogranular (F) and membranous materials (M and upper right inset). Some partially degenerated melanin granules are present within membrane-bound inclusions that contain fibrillogranular material (lower middle and right insets) or fibrillogranular and membranous material (lower left inset). Main figure, ×22,000; insets: upper left, ×29,200; upper right, ×62,500; lower left, ×31,900; lower middle, ×29,400; lower right, ×31,700.

Illustration continued on following page

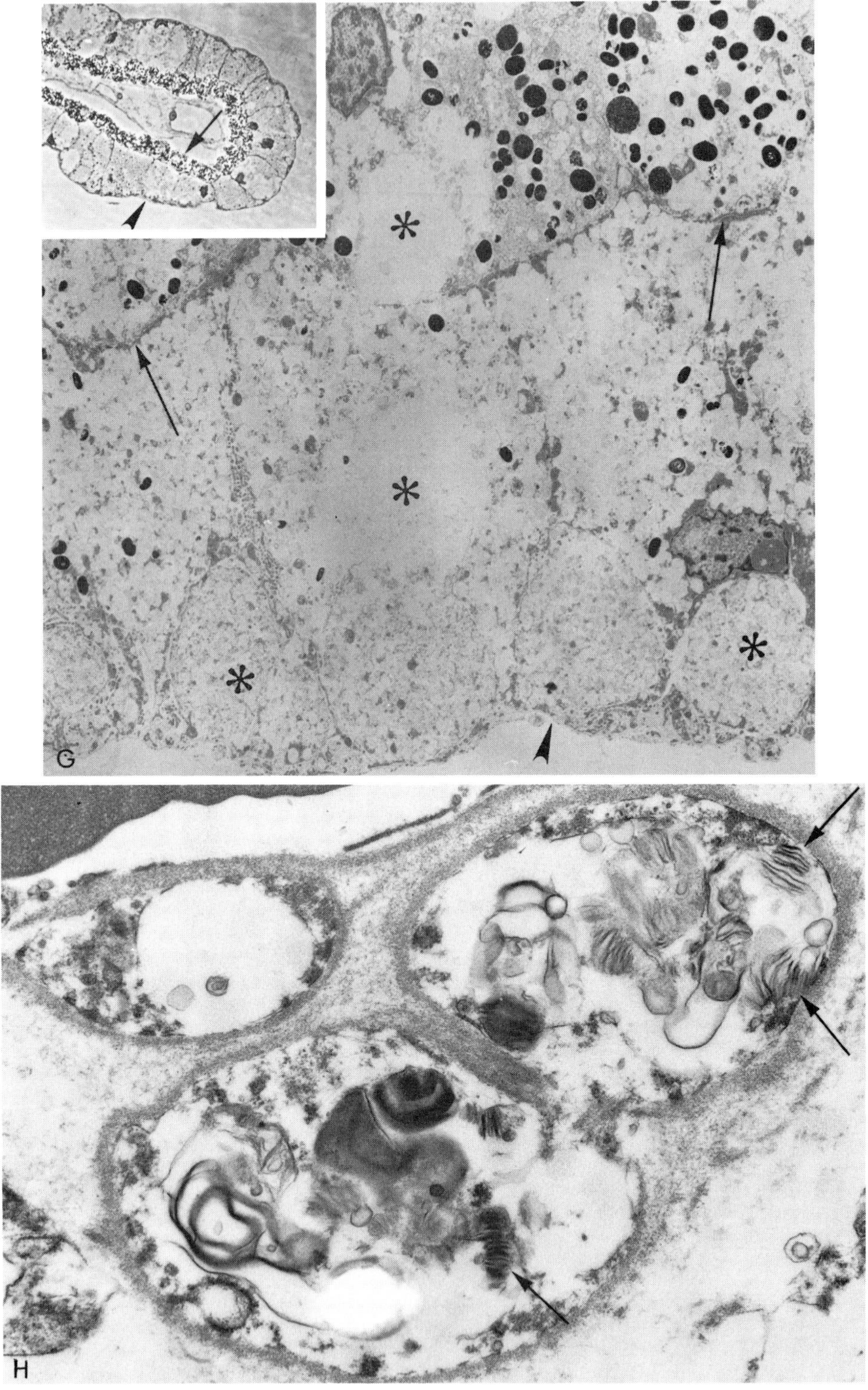

Figure 8–472 *Continued G,* The nonpigmented (arrowhead) and to a lesser degree, the pigmented (arrows) ciliary epithelia are distended by vacuoles, which are large inclusions that contain fibrillogranular material (asterisks). Main figure, ×3700; inset, paraphenylenediamine, ×480. *H,* Pericyte of vessel in optic nerve contains many multimembranous inclusions (arrows). ×26,000.

Illustration continued on opposite page

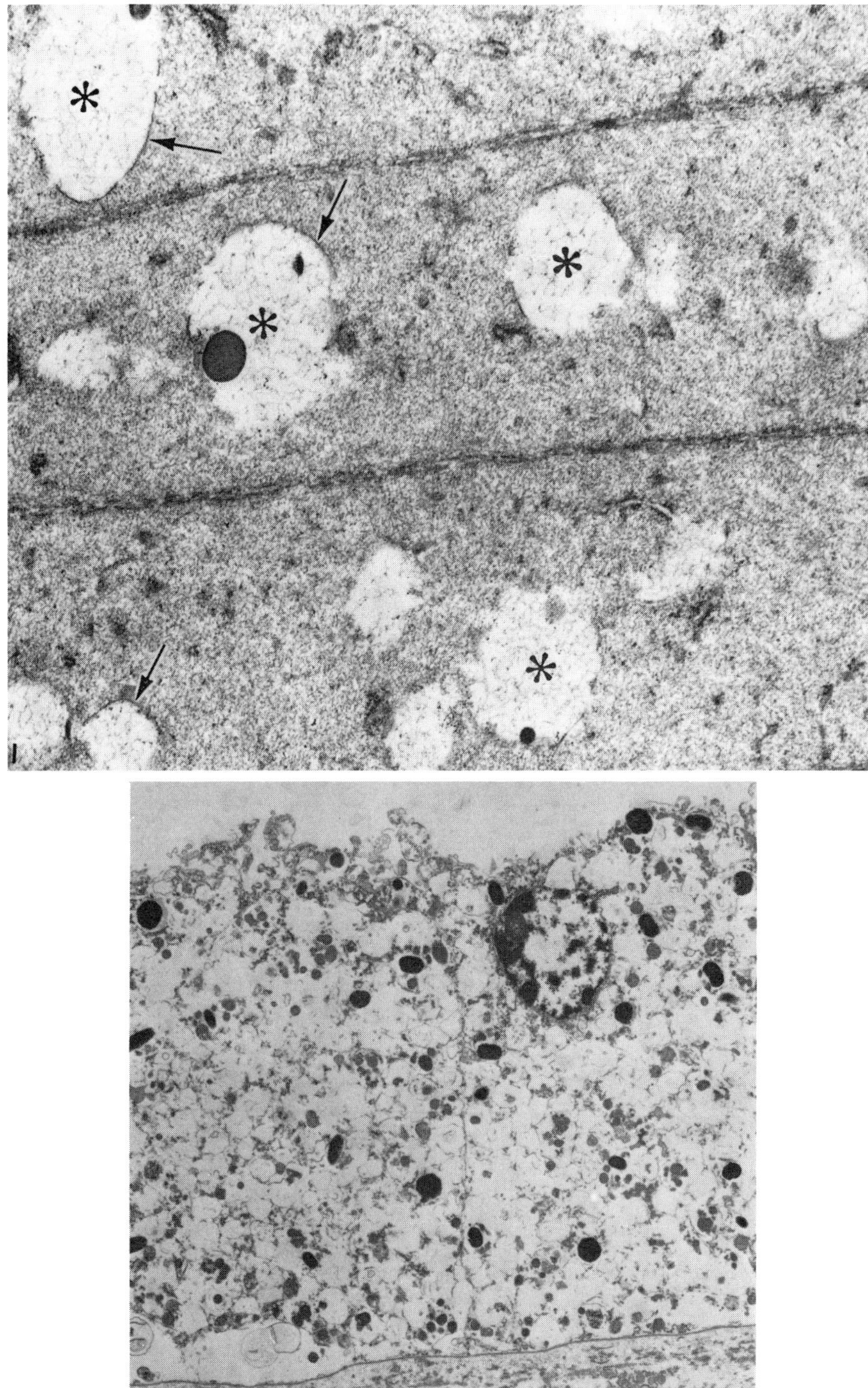

Figure 8–472 *Continued I,* Membrane-bound inclusions (arrows) with fibrillogranular material (asterisks) are present in equatorial lens cortical fibers. ×28,000. *J,* Retinal pigment epithelium is hypopigmented and greatly distended by inclusions containing fibrillogranular material. ×5500.

Illustration continued on following page

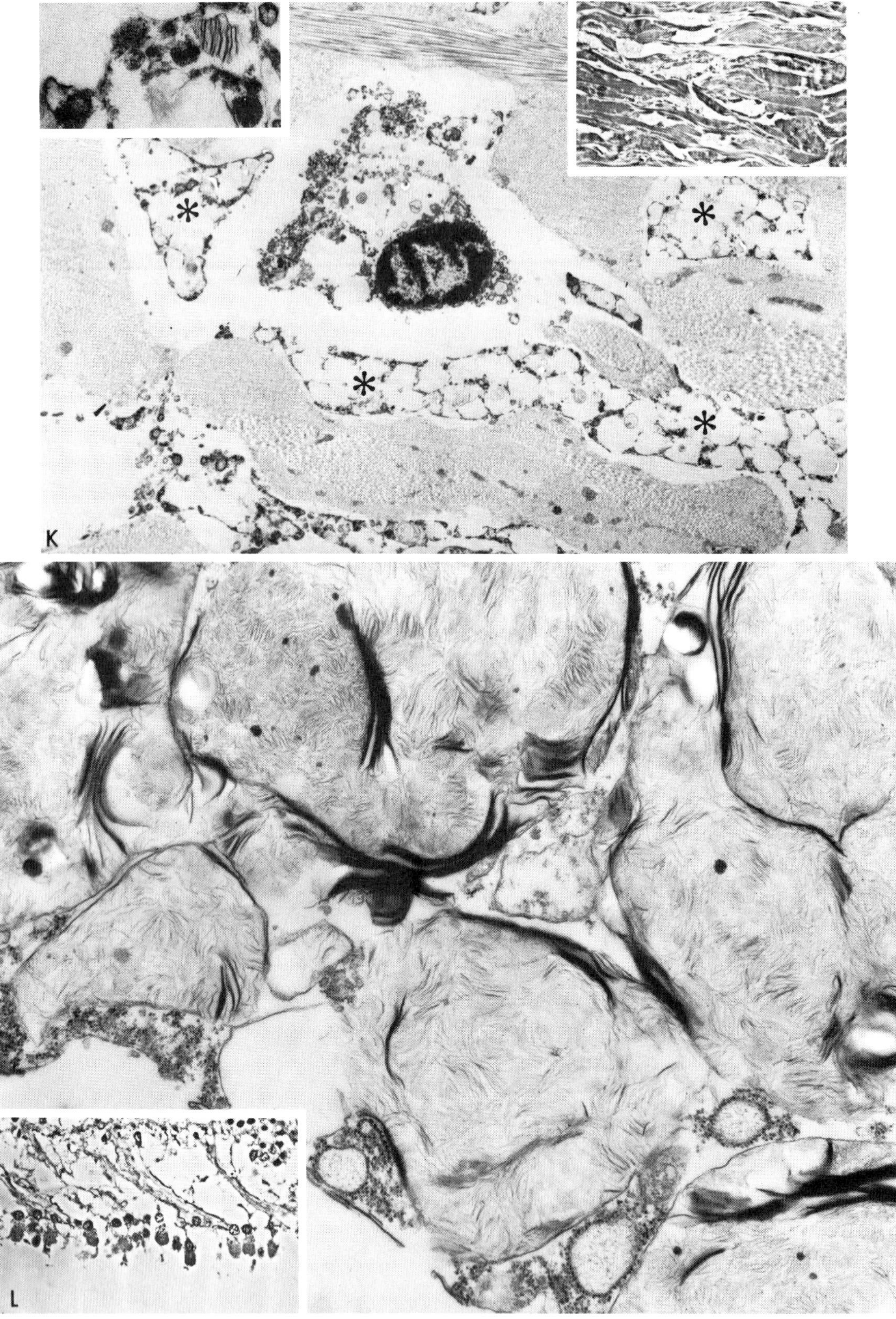

Figure 8–472 *Continued K,* Scleral fibrocytes are markedly distended by vacuoles (upper right inset), which by electron microscopy are seen to be inclusions containing fibrillogranular material (asterisks) and little multimembranous material (upper left inset). ×5300; insets: upper left, ×23,000; upper right, paraphenylenediamine, ×480. *L,* Retinal ganglion cell is quite distended by inclusions containing large aggregates of multimembranous material. ×26,000. Macular retina (inset) shows much atrophy of the photoreceptor cell layer, with only one layer of nucleus in the outer nuclear layer and total loss of outer segments; the few remaining inner segments are short and stubby. Paraphenylenediamine; phase contrast, ×480.

Illustration continued on opposite page

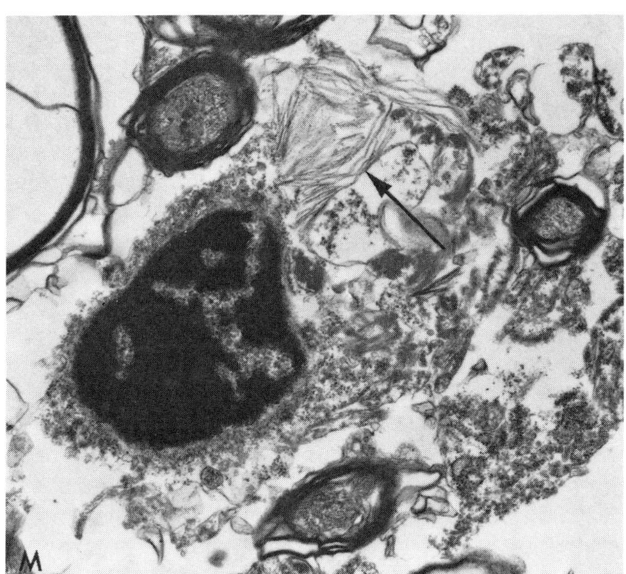

Figure 8–472 *Continued M,* Astrocyte of optic nerve contains multimembranous material (arrow). ×14,000.

(From Chan CC, Green WR, Maumenee IH, Sack GH Jr: Ocular ultrastructural studies of two cases of the Hurler syndrome (systemic mucopolysaccharidosis I-H). Ophthalmic Paediatr Genet *2*:3–19, 1983.)

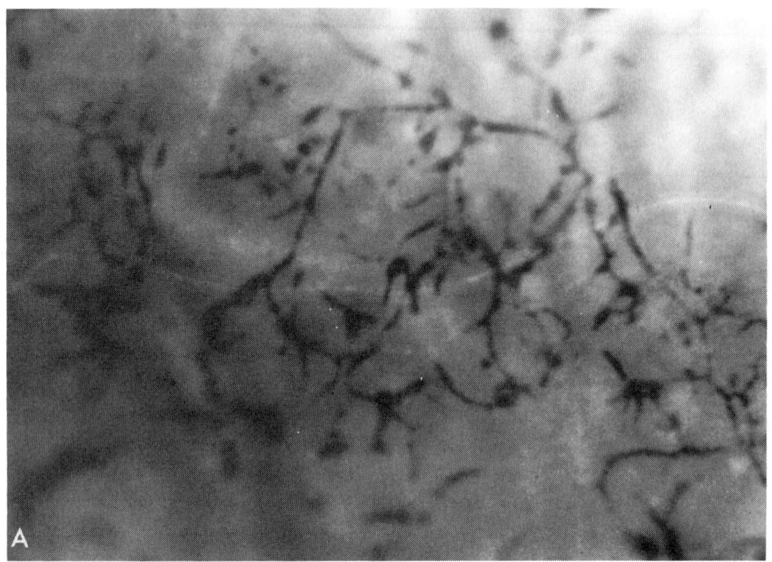

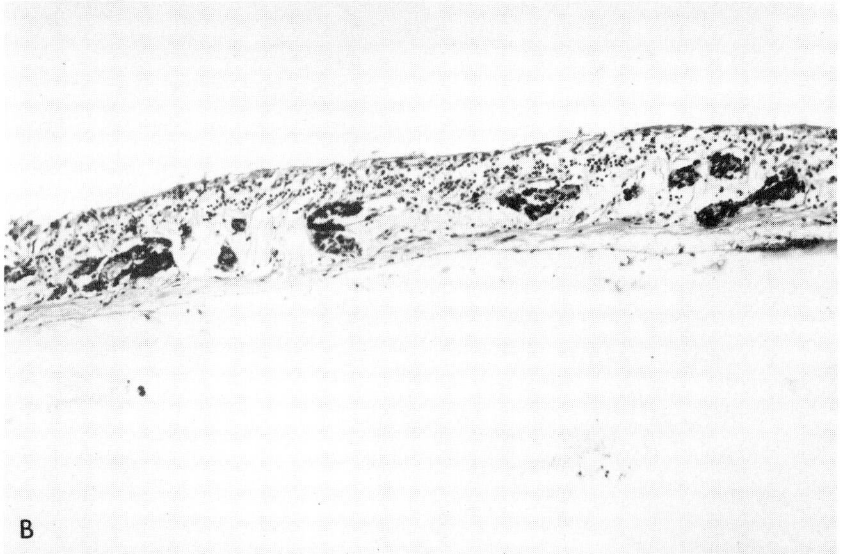

Figure 8–473. Sanfilippo syndrome (mucopolysaccharidosis III-A). *A,* Retinitis pigmentosa–like appearance due to hyperplasia of retinal pigment epithelium (RPE), with migration into retina in perivascular location. *B,* Microscopic appearance of equatorial area showing photoreceptor cell loss and RPE hyperplasia, with migration into retina in perivascular location, in eye from patient with MPS VI-A. EP 26277.

Illustration continued on opposite page

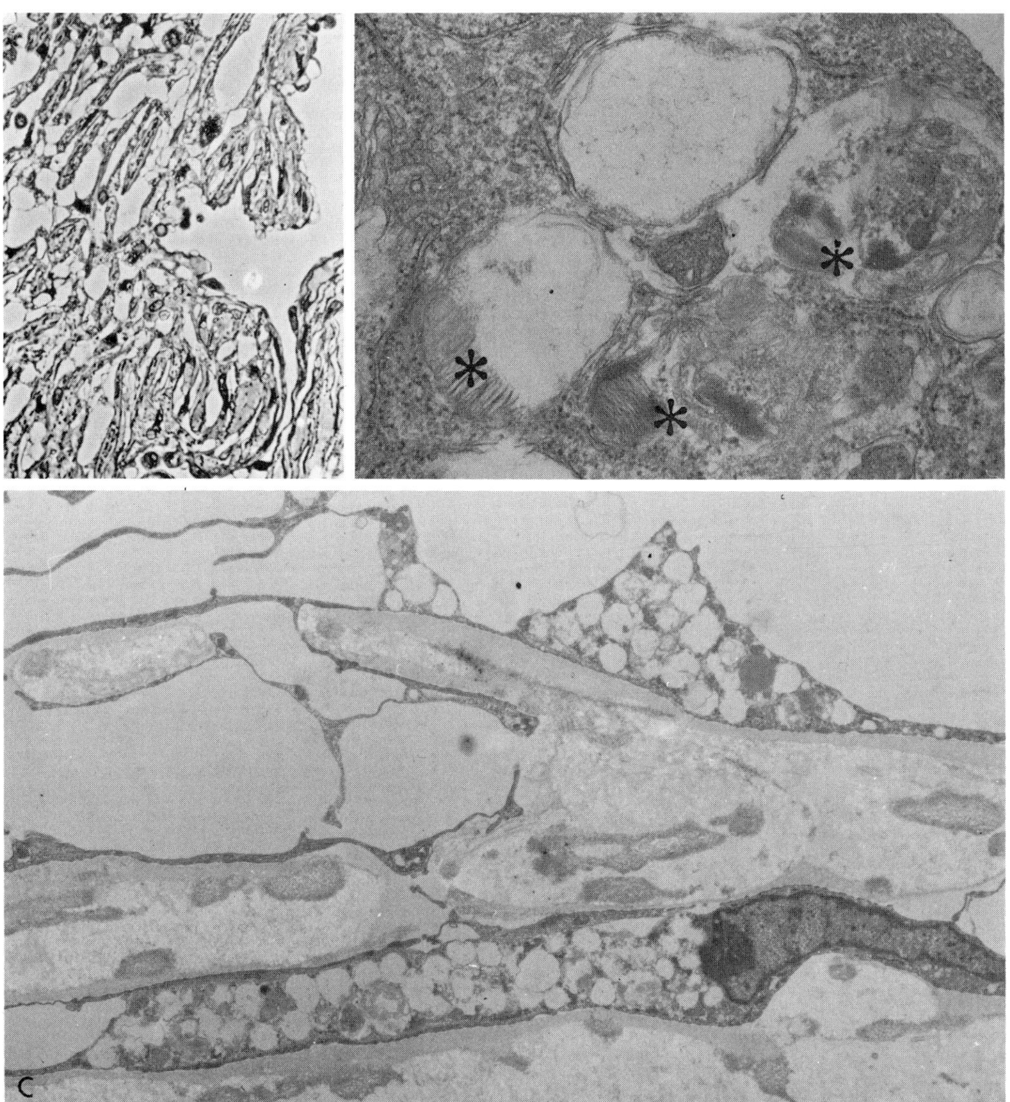

Figure 8–473 *Continued C,* Trabecular meshwork. Top left, Phase contrast photomicrograph shows angle structures to be normal except for vacuolation of trabecular endothelial cells. Paraphenylenediamine, ×250. Bottom, Survey transmission electron micrograph resolves that the trabecular endothelial cells are filled with intraplasmic vacuoles. No extracellular abnormalities are evident. ×6000. Top right, Higher magnification transmission electron micrograph reveals membrane-limited intracytoplasmic vacuoles containing sparse granular substance plus substantial amounts of membranous lamellar lipid material (asterisks). ×45,000.

Illustration continued on following page

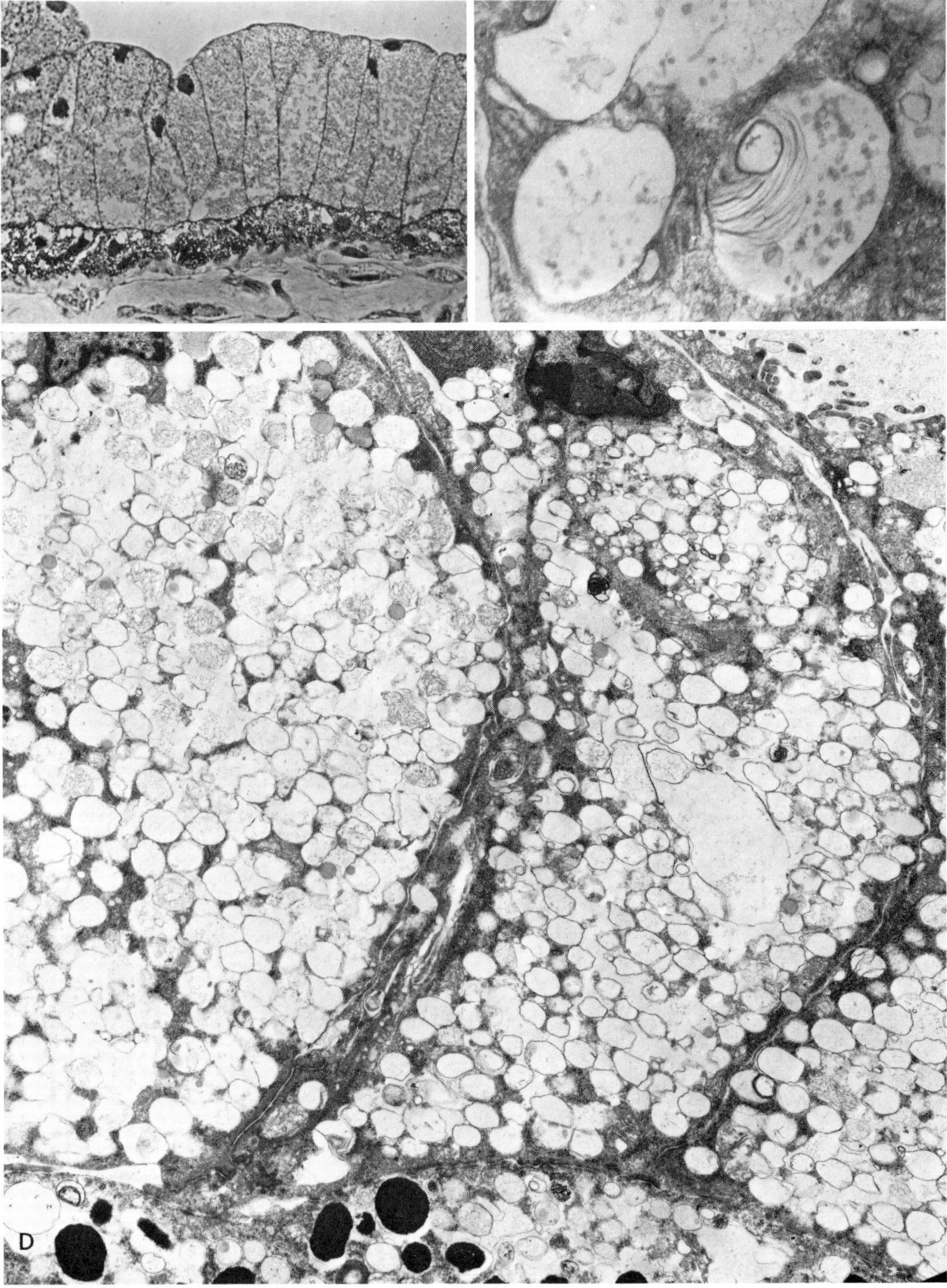

Figure 8–473 *Continued D,* Ciliary body. Top left, Phase contrast photomicrograph reveals enormous distension of nonpigmented ciliary epithelium by foamy cytoplasmic material, in comparison with pigmented ciliary epithelium that shows no evidence of accumulated material. Paraphenylenediamine, ×400. Bottom, Survey transmission electron micrograph of corresponding area shows nonpigmented ciliary epithelium to be enormously distended with single, membrane-limited vacuoles having predominantly fine granular content. Note that the pigmented ciliary epithelium at the bottom also shows a mild accumulation of ultrastructurally similar material. ×7000. Top right, Higher magnification transmission electron micrograph of nonpigmented ciliary epithelium resolves limiting membranes of cytoplasmic inclusions as well as contents ranging from fine granular material to membranous material. ×50,000.

Illustration continued on opposite page

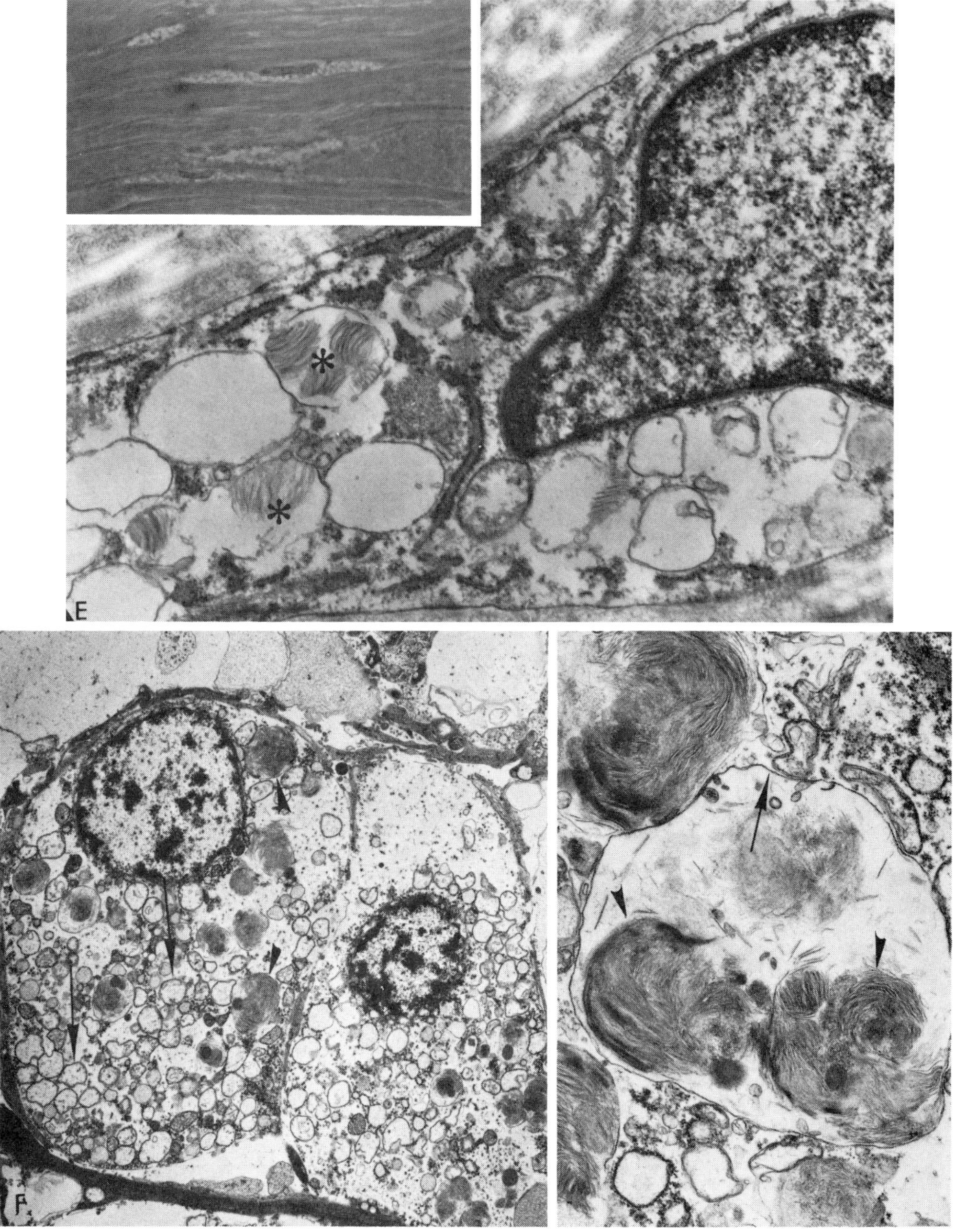

Figure 8–473 *Continued E,* Sclera. Inset, Phase contrast photomicrograph shows sclerocytes with foamy cytoplasm. Extracellular collagen appears unremarkable. Paraphenylenediamine, ×500. Main figure shows transmission electron micrograph of scleral fibrocyte with numerous membrane-limited vacuoles having sparse granular material or membranous lamellae (asterisks) within. Other cytoplasmic components appear unremarkable. ×28,000. *F,* Left, Distended ganglion cell with fibrillogranular (arrows) and multilaminated membranous (arrowheads) membrane-bound inclusion. ×6000. Right, Higher power view of membranous inclusions (arrowheads) that are membrane bound (arrow). ×17,500.

Illustration continued on opposite page

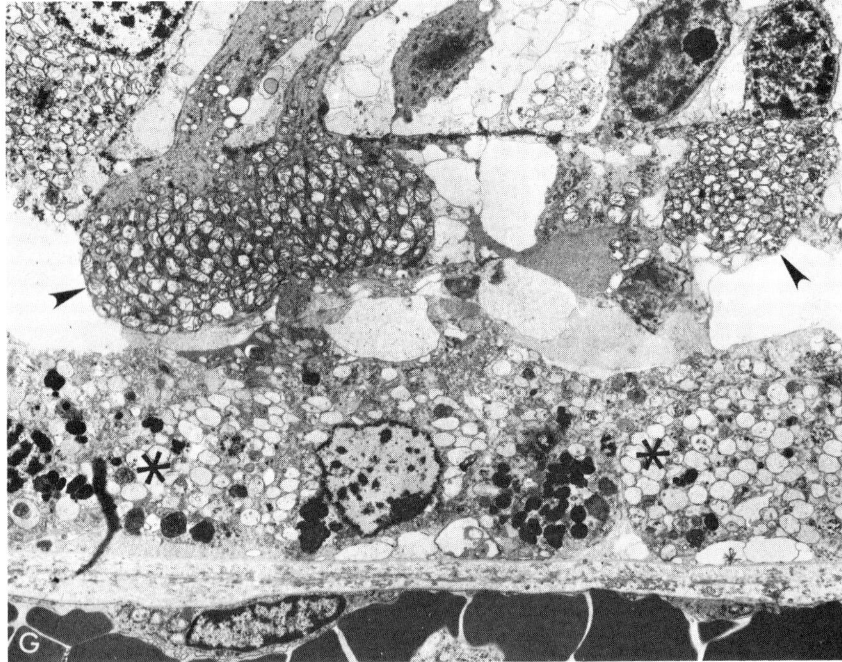

Figure 8–473 *Continued G,* The retinal pigment epithelium is distended by numerous inclusions of fibrillogranular material (asterisks). Outer segments of photoreceptors are absent, and only a few stubby inner segments remain (arrowheads). The outer nuclear layer is greatly reduced. Choriocapillaris and Bruch's membrane are normal. ×4000. *H,* Retinal pigment epithelium and choroid. Inset, Fluorescence microscopy shows marked autofluorescence in RPE cells corresponding to lipofuscin accumulation. ×400. Main figure shows, by transmission electron microscopy, RPE cells greatly distended by innumerable fibrillogranular inclusions, with scattered melanosomes; large, lipofuscin-containing residual bodies (asterisks) are also evident. Bruch's membrane and the choriocapillaris appear unremarkable. ×12,000.

I, Optic nerve. Top left, Phase contrast photomicrograph of optic nerve in cross-section shows maintenance of nerve fiber bundles with extensively vacuolated glial cells (asterisks). Paraphenylenediamine, × 500. Top right, Markedly thickened optic nerve sheath also reveals severely vacuolated connective tissue cells (asterisks). Paraphenylenediamine, ×500. Bottom, By transmission electron microscopy, glial cell vacuolization is predominantly the result of membranous lamellar material within membrane-limited inclusions. ×20,000.

Illustration continued on opposite page

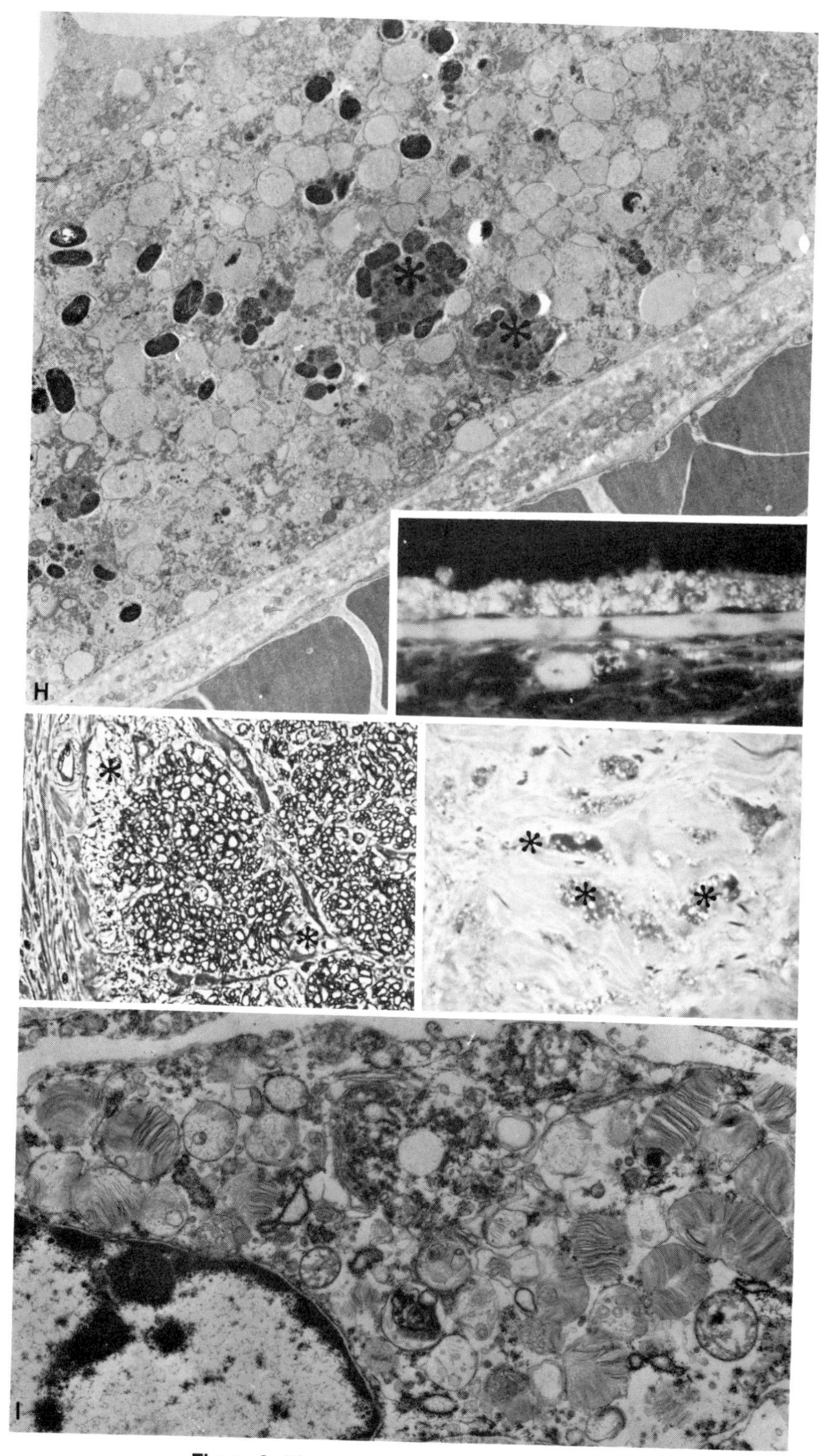

Figure 8–473 *See legend on opposite page*

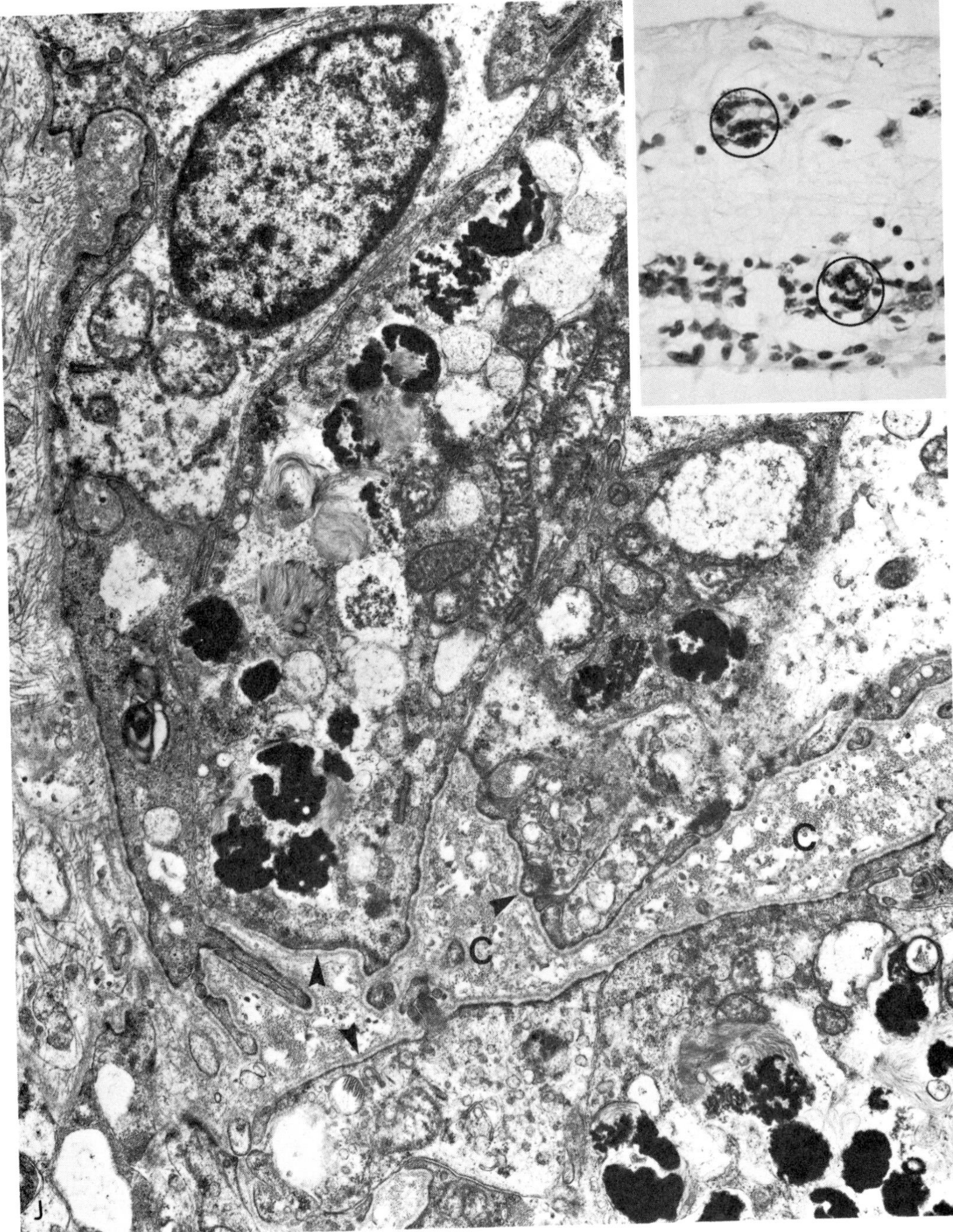

Figure 8–473 *Continued J,* Peripheral retina. Inset, Light microscopy shows migratory pigment epithelial cells in perivascular configurations (circled) and virtual absence of photoreceptors. H and E, ×200. Main figure shows transmission electron micrograph of corresponding area, which demonstrates the pigment epithelial origin of intraretinal pigmented cells as confirmed by their extracellular elaborations of basement membrane material (arrowheads) and collagen fibrils *(C.)* Numerous membranous lamellar vacuoles as well as melanosomes are apparent intracellularly. ×12,000.

Illustration continued on opposite page

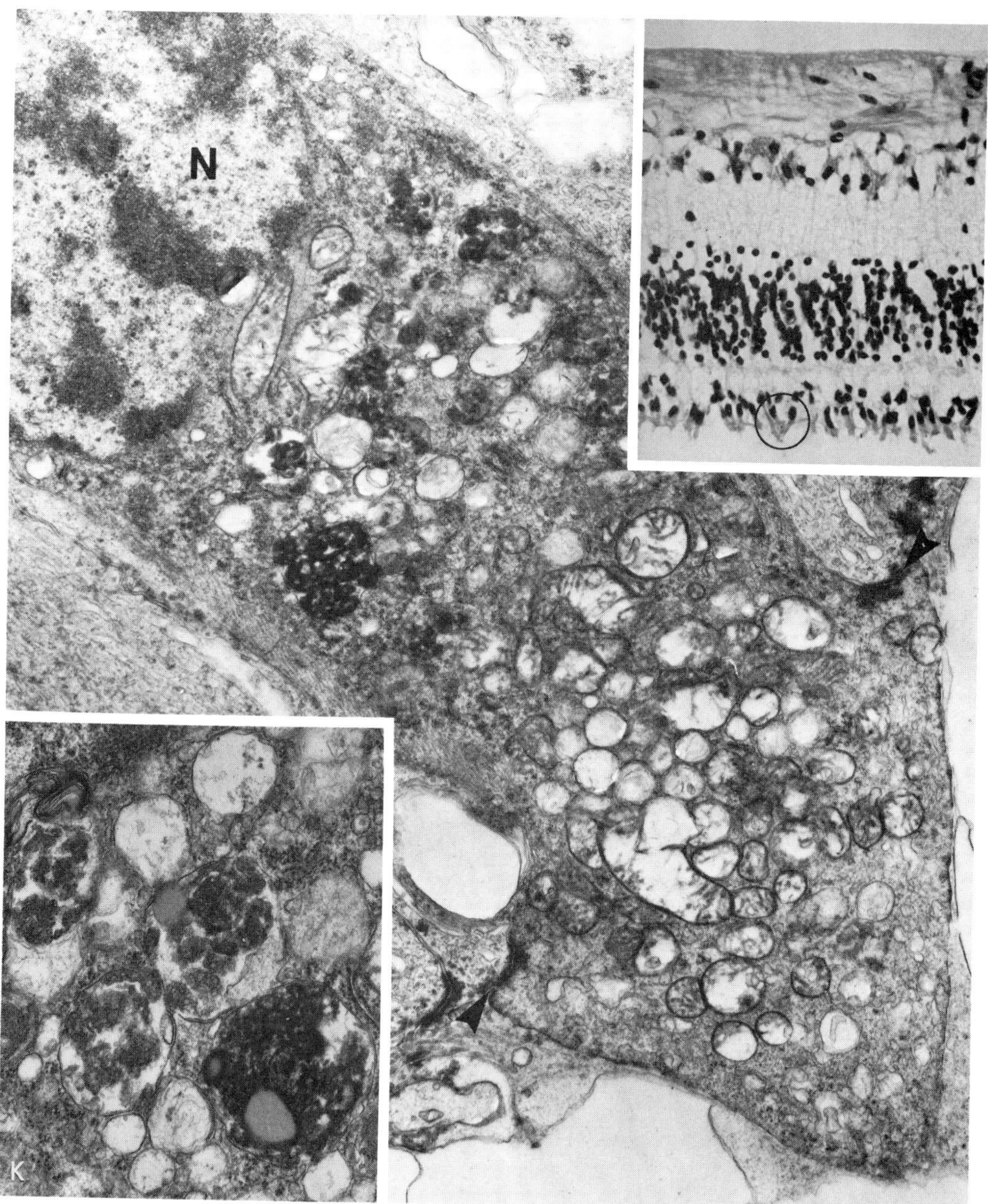

Figure 8–473 *Continued K,* Posterior retina. Top right, Survey light photomicrograph of posterior retina illustrates vacuolization of ganglion cells and thinning of outer nuclear layer with photoreceptor elements (circled) nearly devoid of outer segments. PAS, ×200. Main figure, transmission electron micrograph shows a single photoreceptor cell to have a normal nucleus (N), a myoid portion containing electron-dense bodies, and numerous mitrochondria within the shortened inner segments. No outer segment material is evident. The outer limiting membrane is designated by arrowheads. ×12,000. Bottom left, Higher magnification of photoreceptor cell residual bodies reveals their pleomorphic content of globular and membranous lamellar lipids in addition to fine granular material within limiting membranes. ×28,000.

A and *C* through *K,* EP 38028. (From Del Monte MA, Maumenee IH, Green WR, Kenyon KR: Histopathology of the Sanfilippo syndrome (mucopolysaccharidosis type IIIA). Arch Ophthalmol *101*:1255–1262, 1983.)

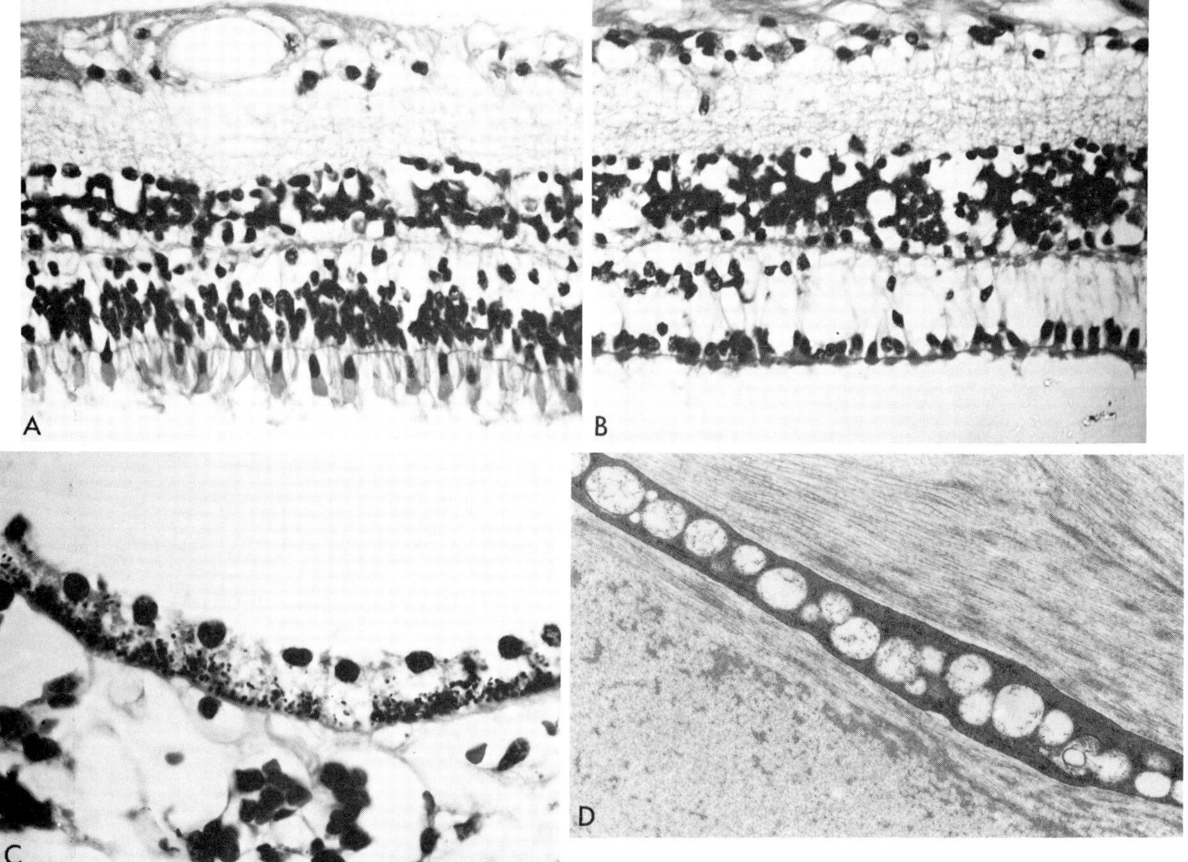

Figure 8–474. Sanfilippo syndrome (mucopolysaccharidosis III–B). *A*, Temporal midperipheral retina, showing mild thinning of the outer nuclear layer, moderate loss of inner segments, prominent loss of outer segments, and migration of cone nuclei into the inner segment zone. H and E, ×460. *B*, Posterior nasal retina, showing much thinning of the outer nuclear layer, total loss of outer segments, and severe loss of inner segments of photorecepter cells. H and E, ×460.

C, Hypopigmented retinal pigment epithalium (RPE) in temporal midperiphery. The remaining pigment granules are located at the base of the cells, and nuclei are displaced toward the apex of the cells. ×900. *D*, Keratocytes contain cytoplasmic inclusions that measure up to 0.5 micron in diameter and contain fibrillogranular material. ×19,200.

Illustration continued on opposite page

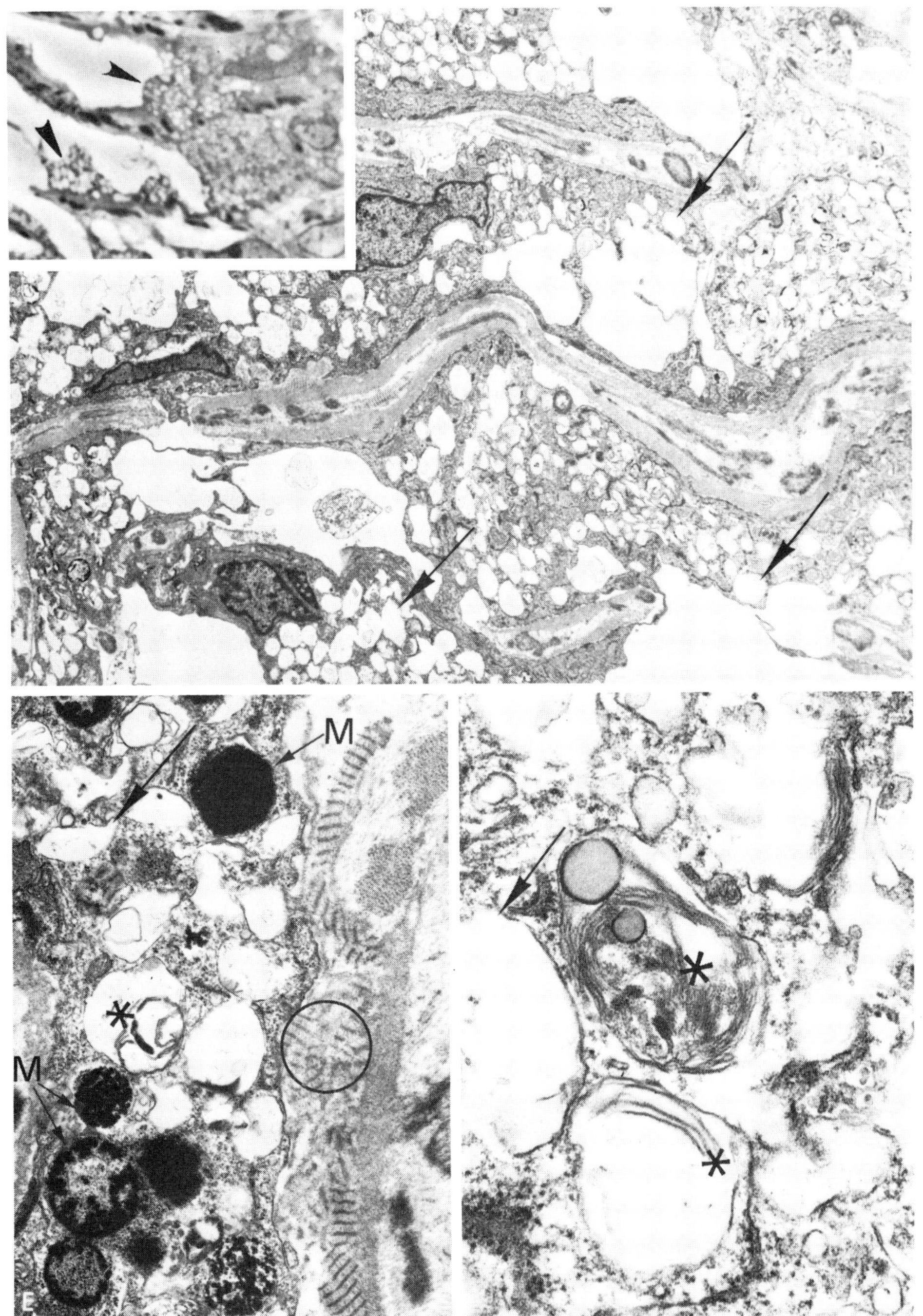

Figure 8–474 *Continued E*, Endothelium of trabecular meshwork is distended by vacuoles (arrowheads, upper left inset), which, by electron microscopy, are seen to be membrane-bound inclusions that contain fibrillogranular material (arrows) and occasional membranous material (asterisks) (main figure and lower insets). Some endothelial cells contain melanin granules (*M*) in various states of degradation (lower left). Abundant wide-spaced collagen (circle) is present between endothelial cells and basement membrane (lower left). ×4500; upper inset, phase-contrast, paraphenylenediamine, ×1250; lower left, ×13,500; lower right, ×39,000.

Illustration continued on following page

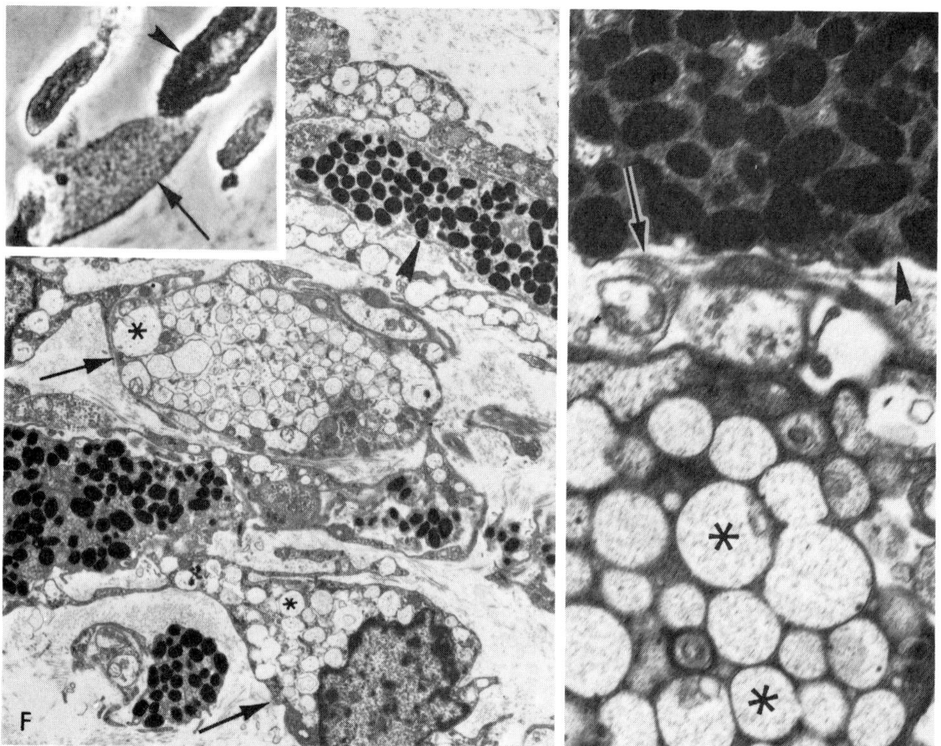

Figure 8–474 *Continued F*, Iris stroma. Fibrocytes (arrows) are distended by vacuoles (upper left, inset) which, by electron microscopy, are seen to be membrane-bound inclusions (asterisks) that contain fibrillogranular material. Melanocytes (arrowheads) are normal and do not have inclusions. Left main figure, ×4500; right figure, ×18,800; upper left inset, paraphenylenediamine, ×1200.

Illustration continued on opposite page

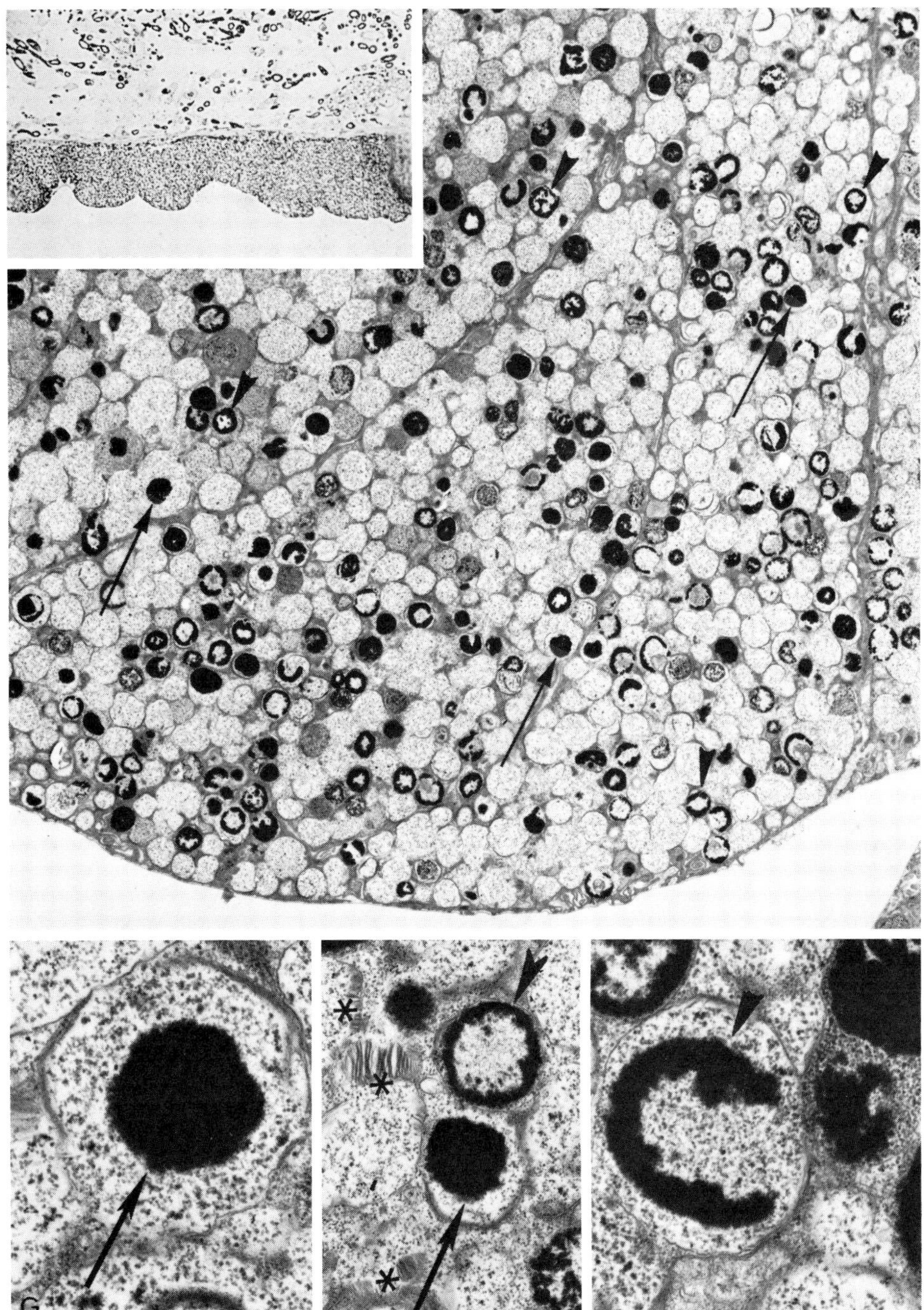

Figure 8–474 *Continued G*, Iris pigment epithelium is greatly distended by vacuoles (upper inset) which, by electron microscopy, are seen to be membrane-bound inclusions containing fibrillogranular material, with intact and also partially degraded melanin granules. Rarely, stacks of membranous inclusions are observed at higher power (asterisks, lower middle). The melanin granules within storage vacuoles have various appearances. These granules may be relatively intact and located centrally (arrows and lower left and middle figures), have a central area of fibrillogranular material (arrowheads, middle and right lower figures), or show various patterns of greater degrees of destruction. ×4350; upper left inset, paraphenylenediamine, ×1250; lower left, ×27,600; lower middle, ×16,000; lower right, ×25,600.

Illustration continued on following page

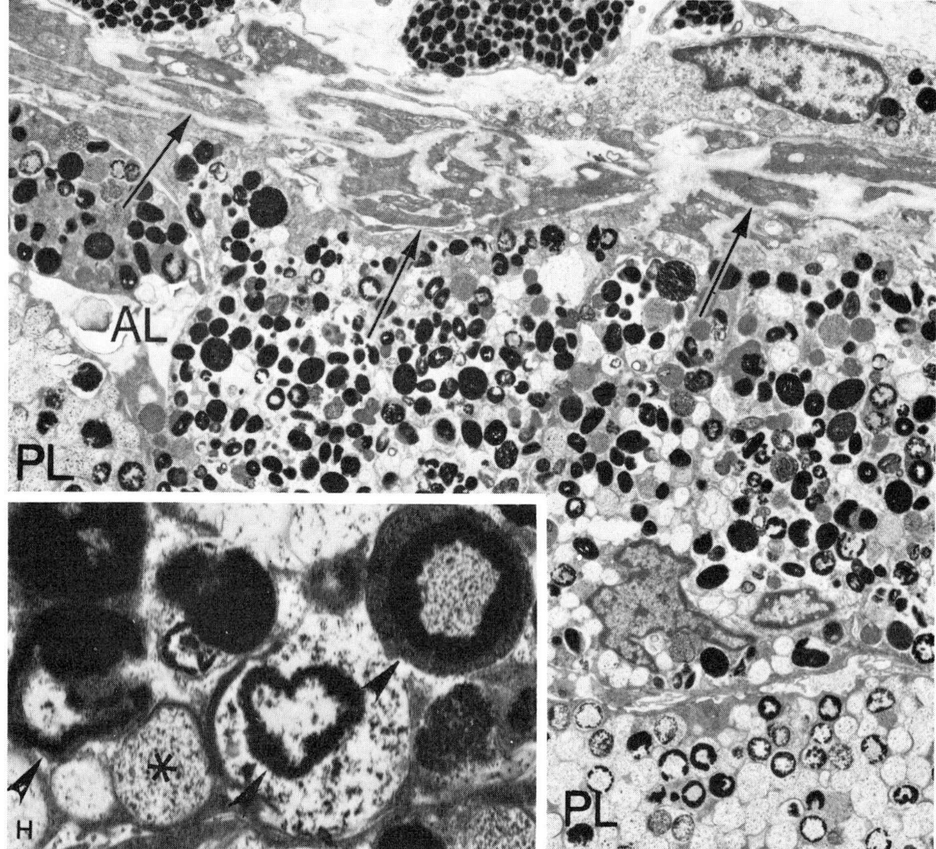

Figure 8–474 *Continued H*, Anterior epithelial layer (*AL*) of iris (dilator muscle). The cell body is distorted by membrane-bound inclusions containing fibrillogranular material (asterisk) and melanin pigment granules in various stages of degradation (arrowheads) (main figure and inset). The smooth muscle processes of these cells (arrows) are free of inclusions. The anterior epithelial layer (*AL*) has more pigment granules and fewer fibrillogranular inclusions than the does posterior epithelial layer (*PL*). ×4500; inset, ×18,800.

Illustration continued on opposite page

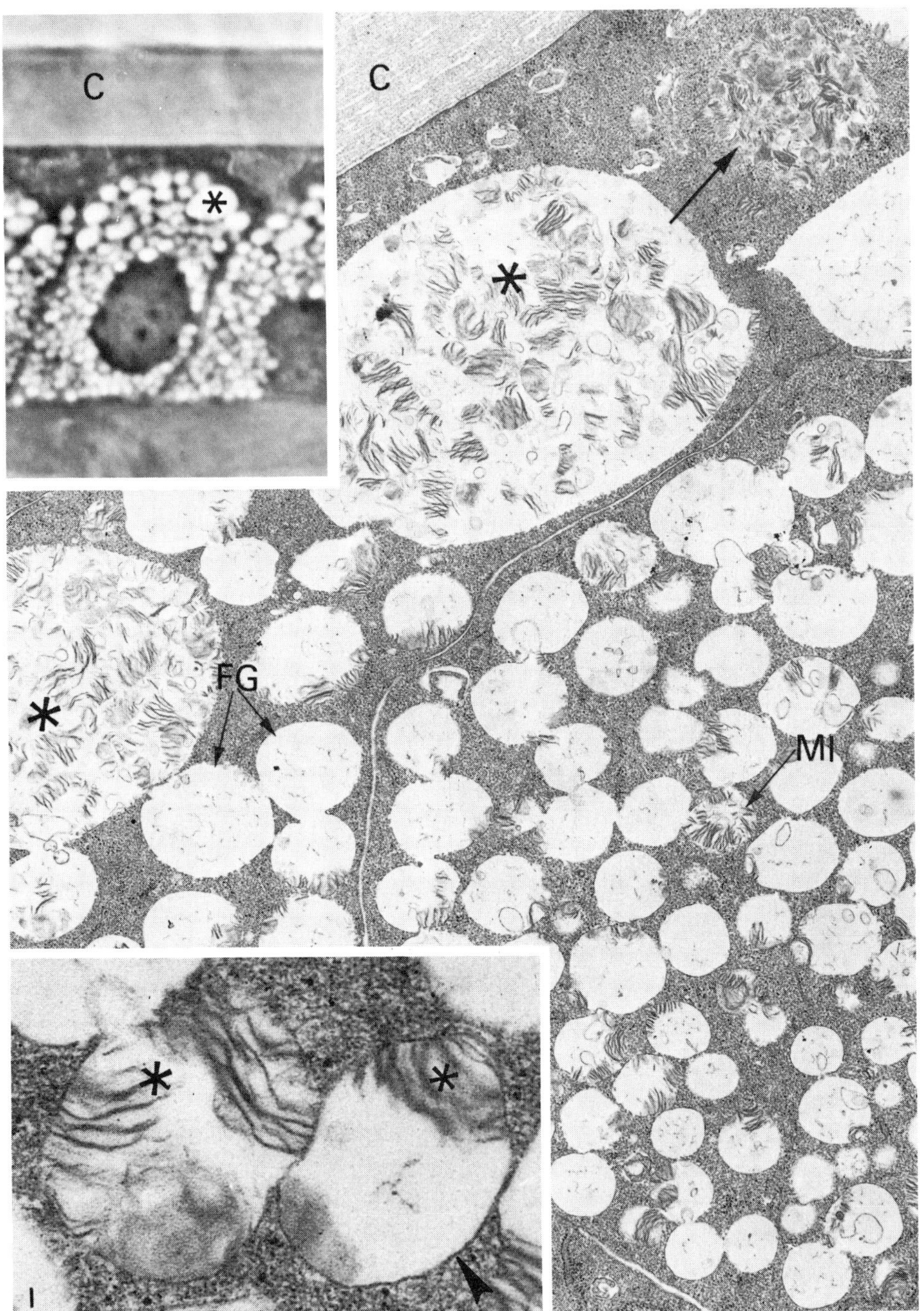

Figure 8–474 *I*, Equatorial area of lens, showing capsule (*C*) and epithelium. The epithelium is quite distended by vacuoles (upper inset), which, by electron microscopy, are seen to be membrane-bound inclusions that contain fibrillogranular material and many membranous inclusions arranged in stacks, usually perpendicular to the limiting membrane (arrowhead). Some inclusions contain only fibrillogranular material (*FG*); most contain both types of inclusion material, and some have a predominance of membranous material (*MI*). Occasional larger vacuoles (asterisks) lack a surrounding membrane, appear to be the result of the coalescence of smaller inclusions, and contain both types of inclusion material. Rarely, large vacuoles (arrow) contain only membranous material. ×13,000; upper inset, paraphenylenediamine, ×1800; lower inset, × 53,800.

Illustration continued on following page

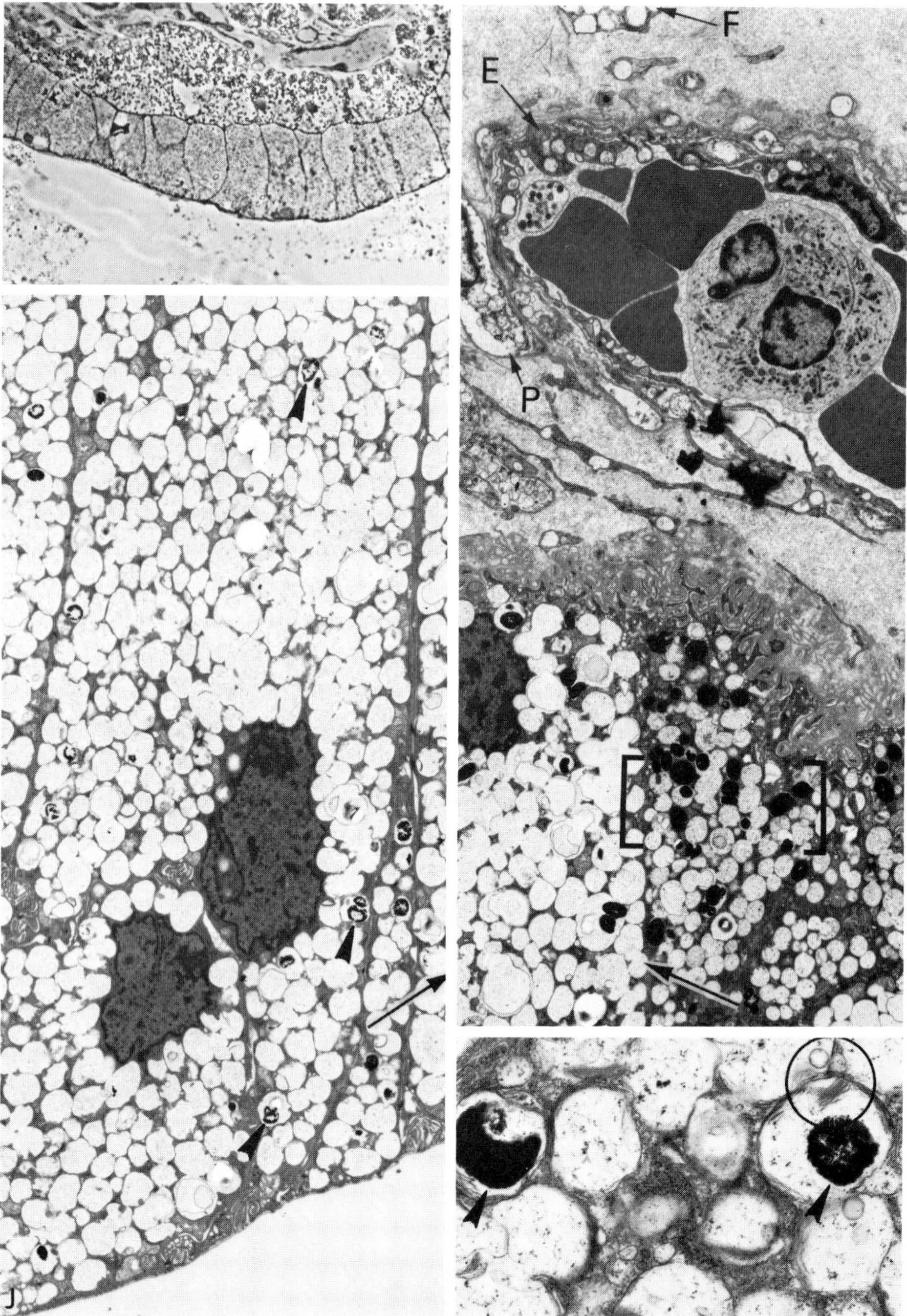

Figure 8–474 *Continued J*, Nonpigmented (left) and pigmented (right) ciliary epithelia. Both are greatly distended by vacuoles (upper left, inset) which, by electron microscopy, are shown to consist mainly of fibrillogranular material. Occasional melanin pigment granules (arrowheads) in various stages of degradation are present within the inclusions in the nonpigmented epithelium. This feature is increased in the pigmented epithelium (right and lower inset). Some of the cells (between arrows) in the pigmented layer are greatly depigmented and contain inclusions with lightly staining fibrillogranular material. An adjacent cell (between brackets) contains more melanin pigment granules, some of which are in various stages of degradation within inclusions (arrowhead, lower inset) and have smaller inclusions with a more densely staining fibrillogranular material. Only rarely is membranous material present in the inclusions of either layer (pigmented layer, circle, lower inset). Fibrillogranular inclusions are also present in vascular endothelium (*E*), pericytes (*P*), and fibrocytes (*F*) in the vascular layer of the ciliary body. Both main figures, ×4180; upper left, paraphenylenediamine, ×1250; lower inset, ×20,400.

Illustration continued on opposite page

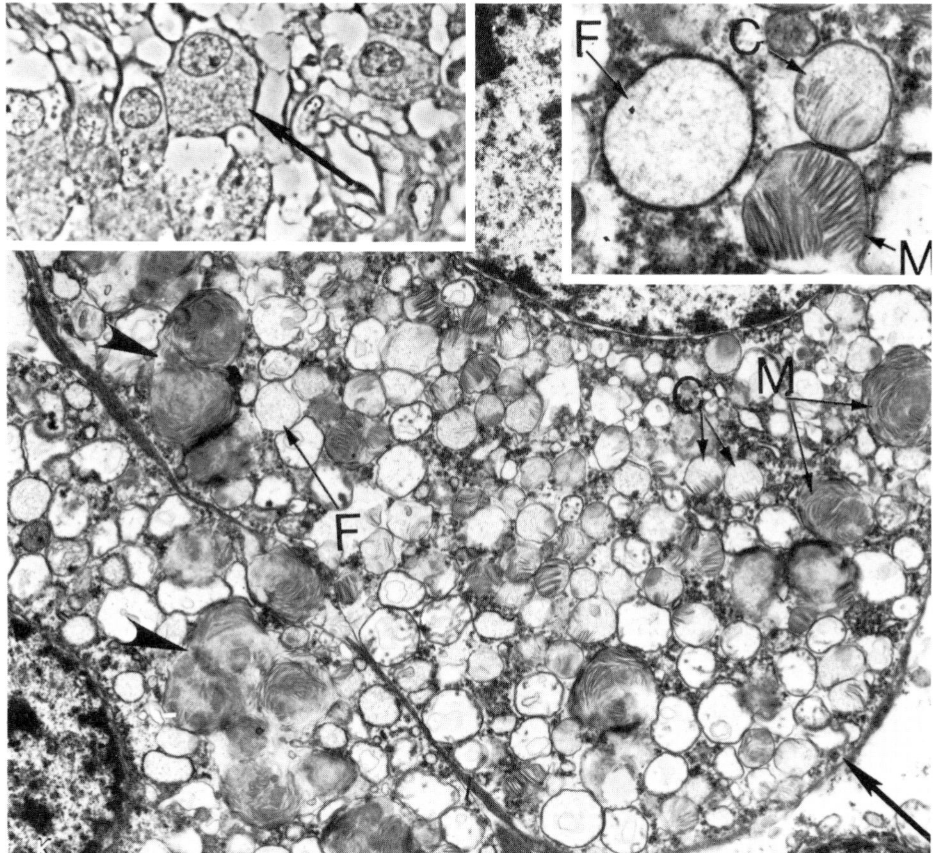

Figure 8–474 *Continued K*, Retinal ganglion cells are distended by granular material and vacuoles (arrow, upper left inset) which, by electron microscopy, are shown to be inclusions, some of which have only fibrillogranular material (*F*); but most of them have a combination of fibrillogranular and membranous material (*C*), and many of them have only membranous material (*M*). All three of these types of inclusions are shown in the main figure and at higher power in the upper right inset. Occasional large aggregates of apparently confluent membranous inclusions (arrowheads) are present. ×10,400; upper left, paraphenylenediamine, ×1250; upper right, ×27,400.

Illustration continued on following page

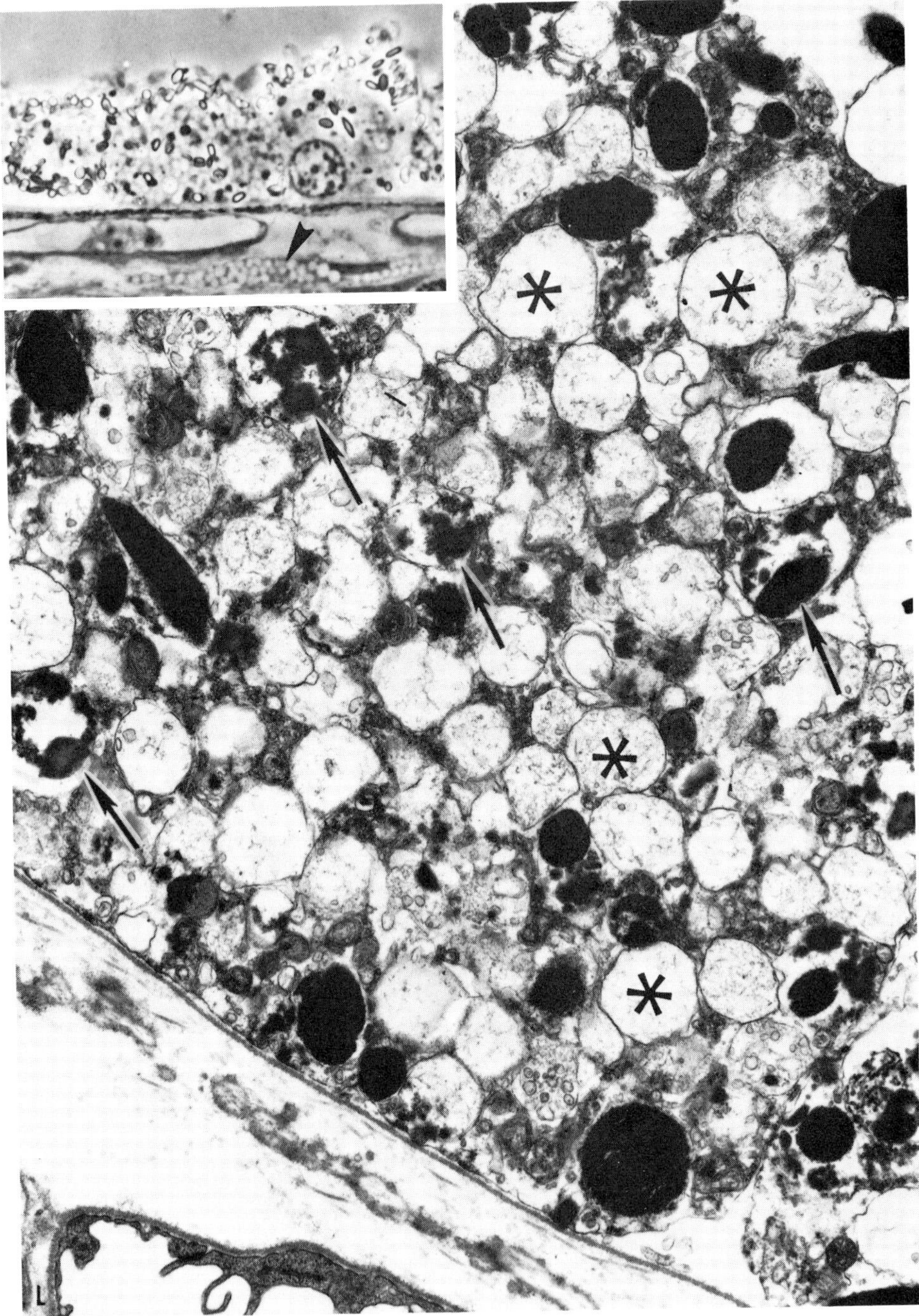

Figure 8–474 *Continued L,* The RPE is partially depigmented and is distended by vacuoles (inset) which, by electron microscopy, are seen to be membrane-bound inclusions containing fibrillogranular material (asterisks). Many inclusions contain melanin pigment (arrows) in various stages of degradation. A fibrocyte in the choroid (arrowhead, inset) is distended by vacuoles. ×13,500; inset, paraphenylenediamine, ×1250.

Illustration continued on opposite page

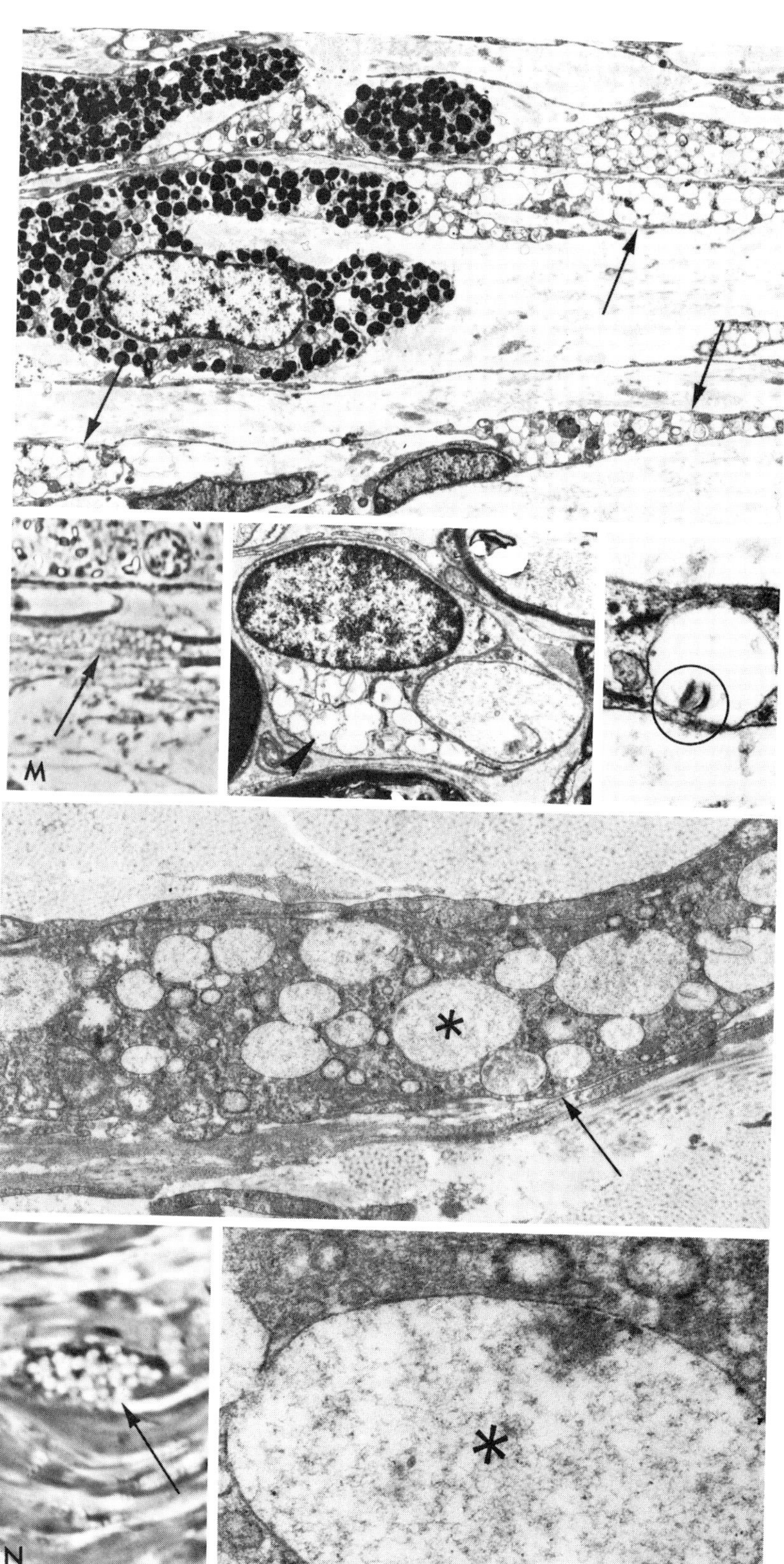

Figure 8–474 *Continued M*, Choroid with fibrocytes (arrows) distended by vacuoles (lower left inset) which, by electron microscopy, are seen to be membrane-bound inclusions containing fibrillogranular material and, rarely, membranous stacks attached to and arranged perpendicular to the limiting membrane (circle, lower right inset). A Schwann cell of a myelinated ciliary nerve within the choroid has some inclusions that contain fibrillogranular material (arrowhead, lower middle inset). × 4300; lower left inset, paraphenylenediamine, ×1250; lower middle inset, × 8750; lower right inset, ×26,000. *N*, Fibrocyte (arrows) in sclera is distended by vacuoles (lower left inset) which, by electron microscopy, are seen to be variable-sized, membrane-bound inclusions (asterisks) that contain fibrillogranular material. ×12,500; lower left inset, paraphenylenediamine, ×1250; lower right inset, ×50,000.

(From Lavery MA, Green WR, Jabs EW, et al: Ocular histopathology and ultrastructure of Sanfilippo disease, Type B. Arch Ophthalmol *100*:1263–1274, 1983.)

ithelium (Fig. 8–474,*L*); fibrocytes and Schwann cells of choroid (Fig. 8–474,*M*); and sclerocytes (Fig. 8–474,*N*).

Lamellar cytoplasmic membranous bodies of complex lipid were found in most tissues but were mainly in the retinal ganglion cells (Fig. 8–474,*K*) and the lens epithelium (Fig. 8–474,*I*). Many tissues had inclusions that were of an intermediate type and were composed of combined fibrillogranular and lamellar membranous material.

Hypopigmentation of the neuroepithelial pigment layers (iris, ciliary, and retinal) appeared to be the result of autophagocytosis with melanolysis (Fig. 8–474,*G, H, J,* and *L*). Photoreceptor cell degeneration was similar to that seen in sex-linked and autosomal dominant retinitis pigmentosa. The mechanism of photoreceptor cell degeneration is unknown, but it may be the result of metabolic dysfunction caused by the accumulation of mucopolysaccharide in the retinal pigment epithelium.

Additional types of MPS III have been described clinically: MPS III-C (Klein, Kresse, von Figura, 1978; Bartsocas, Gröbe, van de Kamp, et al, 1979) and MPS III-D (Kresse, Paschke, von Figura, et al, 1980).

Systemic Mucopolysaccharidosis IV (MPS-IV; Morquio syndrome) (Morquio, 1929). Eyes from patients with MPS-IV have not been studied.

Systemic Mucopolysaccharidosis VI (MPS VI; Maroteaux-Lamy syndrome (Maroteaux, Leveque, Marie, Lamy, 1963). There are two varieties: severe, or MPS VI-A; and mild, MPS VI-B. The light microscopic and electron microscopic features of MPS VI-A have been reported by Kenyon, Topping, Green, and Maumenee (1972) and by Naumann (1982).

Kenyon and associates (1972) observed corneal clouding that was attributed to accumulation of mucopolysaccharidosis in the corneal epithelium and histiocytes in the region of Bowman's membrane and in keratocytes (Fig. 8–475). There was near-total loss of the nerve fiber and ganglion cell layers of the retina and marked optic atrophy (Fig. 8–476). The sclera posteriorly was markedly thickened because of extensive accumulation of mucopolysaccharide (Fig. 8–477).

MPS VI-B (Di Ferrante, Hyman, Klish, et al,

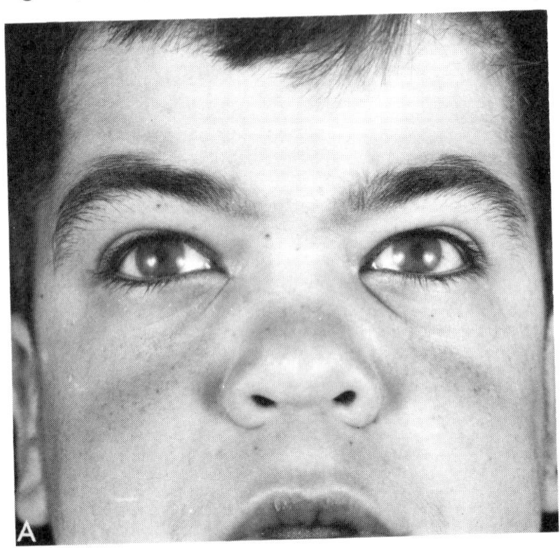

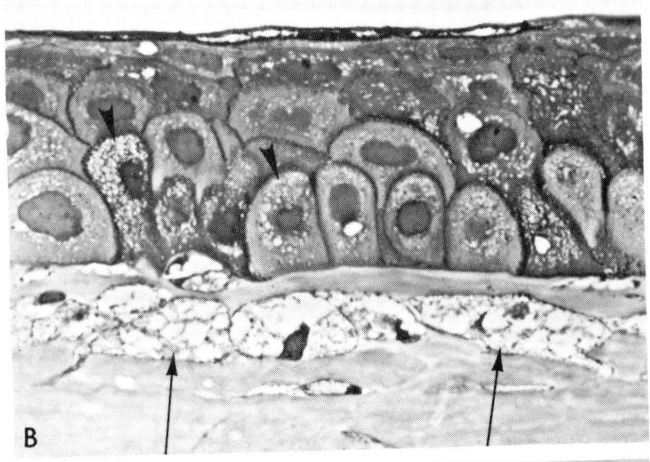

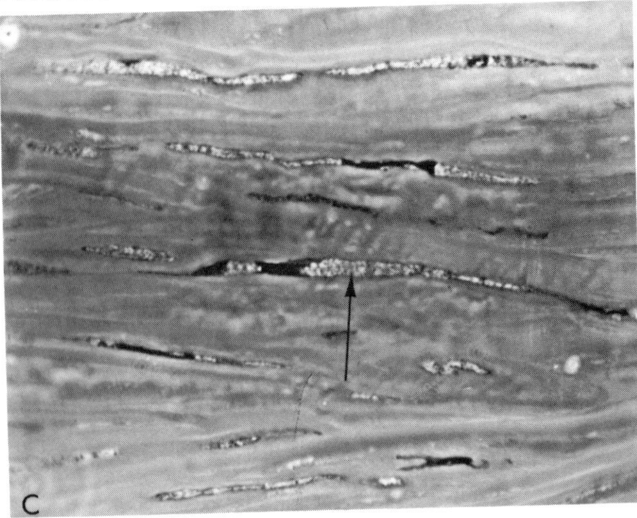

Figure 8–475. MPS-VI, Maroteaux-Lamy syndrome. *A*, Corneal clouding. *B*, Basal layer of corneal epithelium has numerous inclusions (arrowheads), which stain positively for mucopolysaccharide and have a fibrillogranular appearance by electron microscopy. Histiocytes (arrows), located in anterior stroma and in some areas having replaced Bowman's membrane, have similar inclusions. Paramethylenediamine; phase contrast, ×400. *C*, Keratocytes (arrow) contain similar inclusions. Paraphenylenediamine; phase contrast, × 400.

EP 31032. (From Kenyon, KR, Topping TM, Green WR, and Maumenee, AE: Ocular pathology of Maroteaux-Lamy syndrome (systemic mucopolysaccharidosis, Type VI); A histopathologic and ultrastructural report of two cases. Am J Ophthalmol *73*:718–741, 1972.)

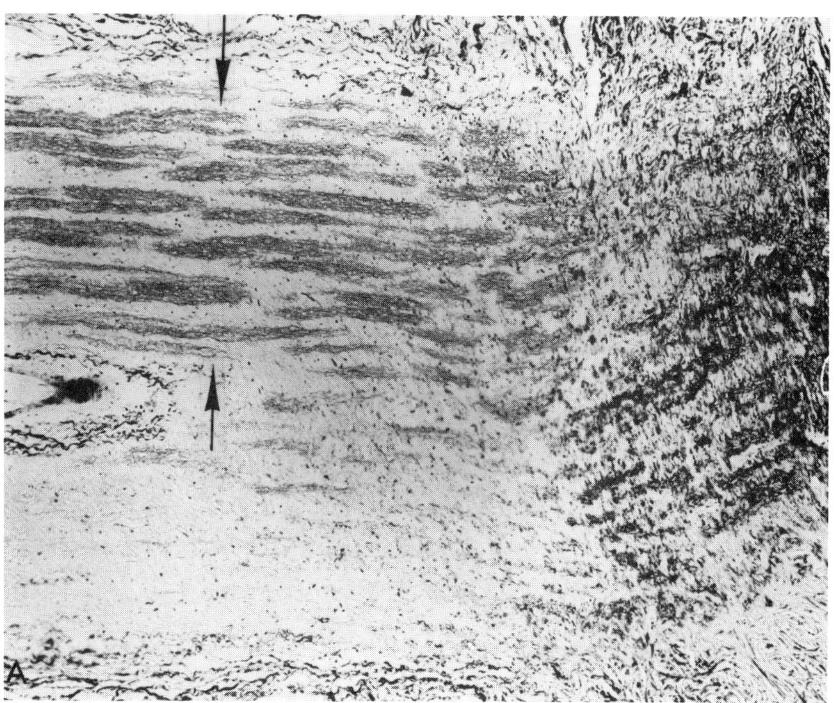

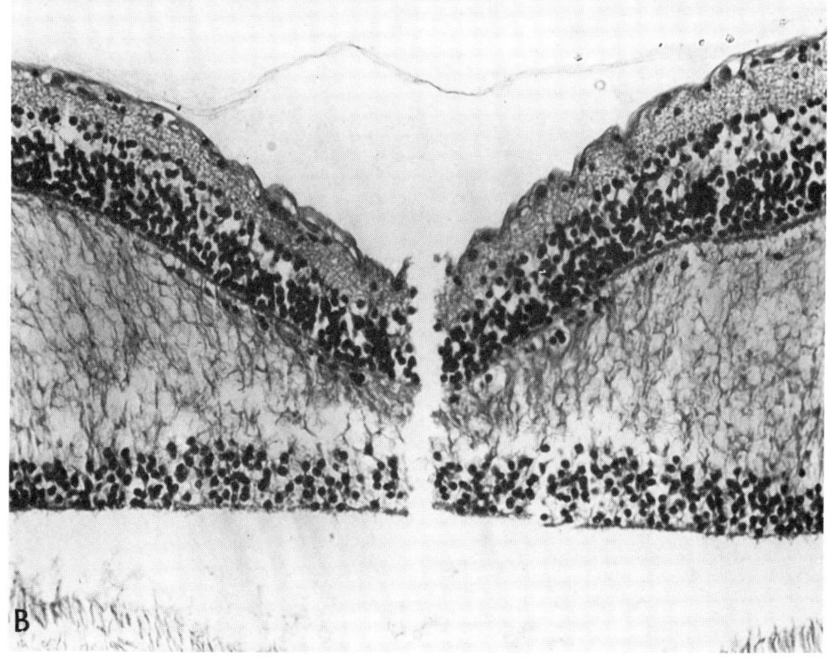

Figure 8–476. *A*, Partial optic atrophy in patient with **MPS VI-A**. Longitudinal section of nerve shows partial preservation of myelin on nasal side (between arrows). Verhoeff van Gieson, ×60. *B*, Section near foveola showing marked loss of nerve fiber and ganglion cell layers. H and E, ×200. EP 31032. (From Kenyon KR, Topping TM, Green WR, et al: Ocular pathology of the Maroteaux-Lamy syndrome (systemic mucopolysaccharidosis, Type VI); A histopathologic and ultrastructural report of two cases. Am J Ophthalmol 73:718–741, 1972.)

1974). The whole eye with this mild phenotype of MPS VI has not been studied. Quigley and Kenyon (1974) have studied corneal tissues, conjunctiva, and skin. They found that connective tissue cells from all three sites contained vacuoles and mucopolysaccharide. Occasional multimembranous inclusions were observed.

Sphingolipidoses. This group of diseases is from inborn errors of metabolism in which glycolipids having a sphingosine base accumulate in neural and, in some instances, visceral tissues. By electron microscopy, these substances are noted to form multimembranous inclusion bodies (zebra bodies) in lysosomes. In each disease entity, there is an enzymatic defect in the degradation of sphingolipid. With the exception of Fabry's disease and Krabbe's disease, the principal ocular abnormalities are caused by accumulation of glycolipid in the retinal ganglion cells and atrophy of the optic nerve. See Table 8–5 for the differential features of the sphingolipidoses.

Although biochemical analysis is the most ef-

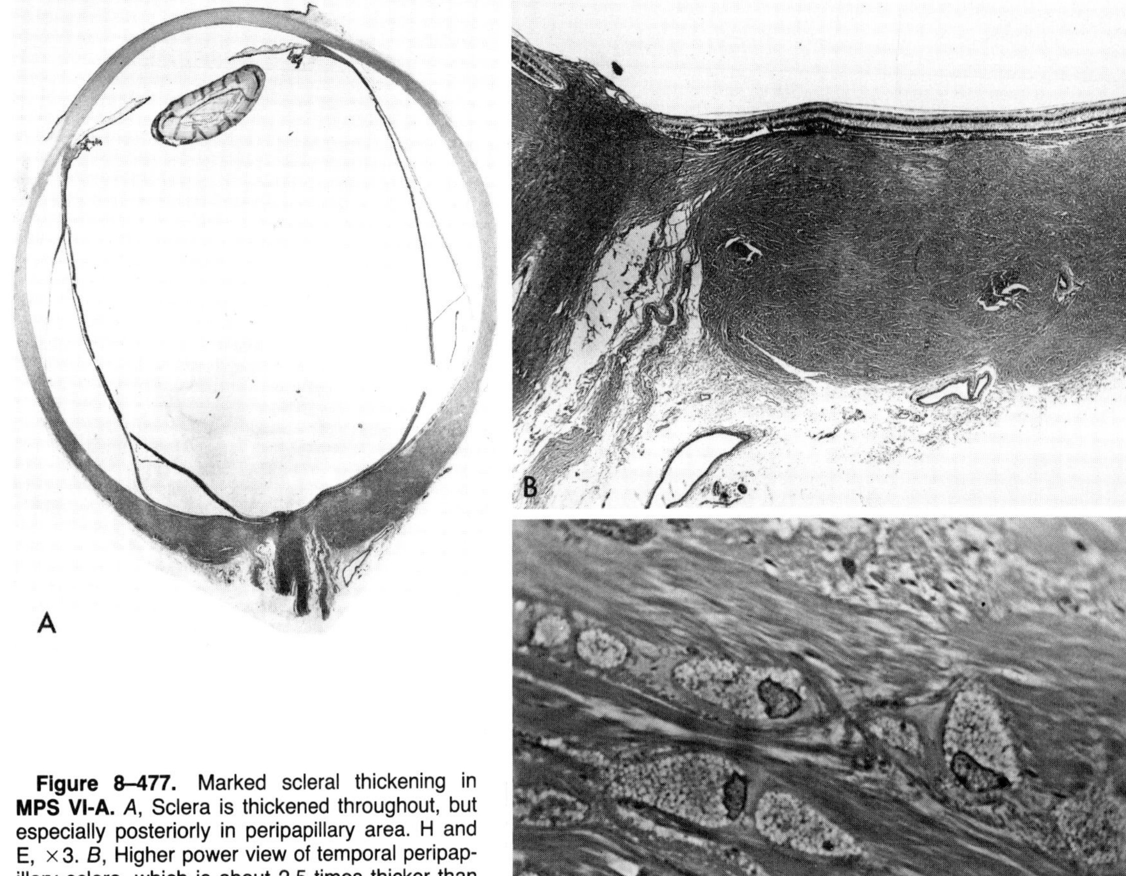

Figure 8–477. Marked scleral thickening in **MPS VI-A.** *A*, Sclera is thickened throughout, but especially posteriorly in peripapillary area. H and E, ×3. *B*, Higher power view of temporal peripapillary sclera, which is about 2.5 times thicker than usual. H and E, ×15. *C*, Sclerocytes are packed with inclusions of mucopolysaccharide. Paraphenylenediamine; phase contrast, ×1050. EP 31032. (From Kenyon KR, Topping TM, Green WR, et al: Ocular pathology of Maroteaux-Lamy syndrome (systemic mucopolysaccharidosis, Type VI): A histopathologic and ultrastructural report of two cases. Am J Ophthalmol *73*:718–741, 1972.)

Table 8–5. DIFFERENTIAL FEATURES OF THE SPHINGOLIPIDOSES

		Ocular Features				
SLS Type	**Genetics**	***Corneal Clouding***	***Macular Grayness or Cherry-Red Spot***	***Optic Atrophy***	**Storage Substance**	**Deficient Enzyme**
Tay-Sachs disease (GM_2 gangliosidosis I)	AR	—	+	+	GM_2 ganglioside	Hexosaminidase A
Sandhoff's disease (GM_2 gangliosidosis II)	AR	—	+	—	GM_2 ganglioside	Hexosaminidase A, B
Juvenile GM_2 gangliosidosis (GM_2 gangliosidosis III)	AR	—	—	+	GM_2 ganglioside	Hexosaminidase A (partial)
Niemann-Pick disease	AR	±	+	+?	Sphingomyelin and cholesterol	Sphingomyelinase
Gaucher's disease	AR	—	±	—	Glucosyl ceramide	β-Glucosidase
Fabry's disease	XR	+	—	—	Ceramide trihexoside	α-Galactosidase
Krabbe's disease	AR	—	—	+	Galactosyl ceramide	Galactocerebroside β-galactosidase
Late infantile metachromatic leukodystrophy	AR	+	+	+	Cerebroside sulfate	Arylsulfatase A
Lactosyl ceramidosis	AR	—	+	?	Lactosyl ceramide	Lactosylceramide galactosylhydrolase
Farber's lipogranulomatosis	AR	—	+	—	Ceramide GM_3 ganglioside	Ceramidase

AR, autosomal recessive; XR, X-linked recessive; —, absent; ±, variable; +, present.

After Kenyon KR: Ocular ultrastructure of inherited metabolic disease, *in* Goldberg MF (ed): Genetic and Metabolic Diseases. Boston, Little, Brown, 1974, p 161.

fective technique in establishing the diagnosis of most metabolic diseases with progressive encephalopathy, ultrastructural study of conjunctival and skin biopsy specimens is a valuable procedure in patients without detectable enzyme deficiencies (Arsenio-Nunes, Goutieres, 1978; Arsenio-Nunes, Goutieres, Aicardi, 1981).

Tay-Sachs Disease, or GM_2 Gangliosidosis, Type I. Tay-Sachs disease is caused by a deficiency of hexosaminidase A. It is characterized by the

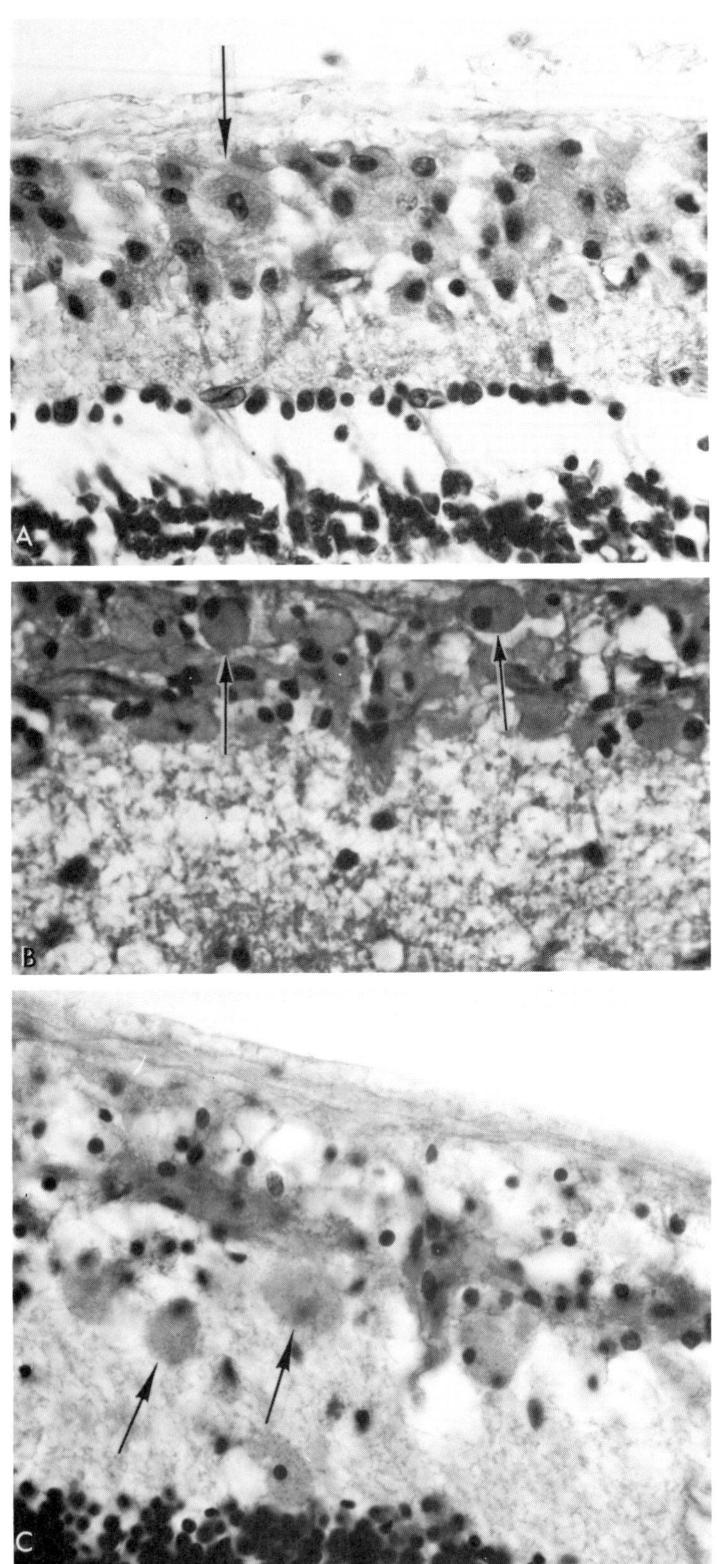

Figure 8–478. *A–C*, Distended ganglion cells (arrows) in **Tay-Sachs disease.** *A*, PAS, ×400. EP 3299. *B*, PAS, ×400. EP 15844. *C*, H and E, ×575. EP 17686.

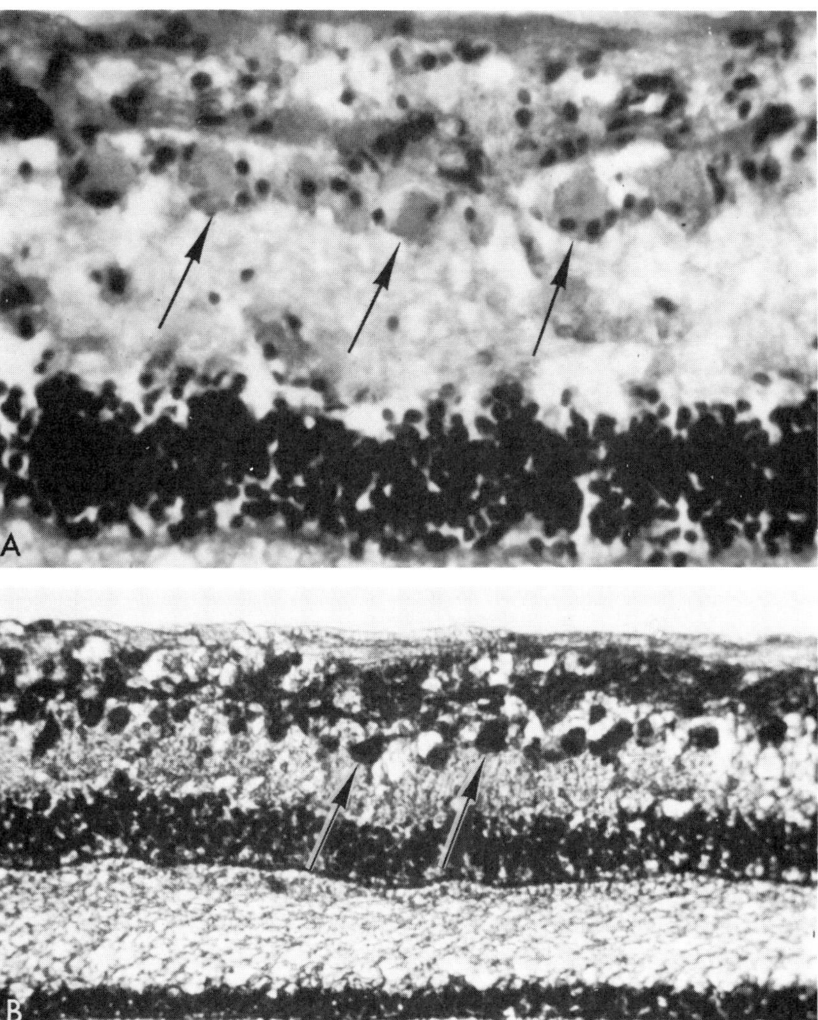

Figure 8–479. *A* and *B*, Cytoplasm of distended ganglion cell stains positively for lipid (arrows). A, Oil red O, ×250. *B*, Sudan black B, ×400. EP 17686.

onset, in infancy, of retardation and then paralysis, dementia, and blindness. Death occurs in the second or third year of life. Storage material accumulates in neuronal tissues of the brain, retina (Cogan, Kuwabara, 1959a; Dhermy, 1962), and ganglia. In the retina, the accumulation gives rise to the cherry-red spot because of the larger number of ganglion cells in the para- and perifoveal areas. These areas of numerous ganglion cells have a whitish appearance, in contrast to the foveola which is free of ganglion cells, thus allowing the normal reddish color of the choroid to be visible.

The retinal ganglion cells are distended (Fig. 8–478) and stain positively for the presence of lipids (Fig. 8–479) (Duke, Clark, 1962). Electron microscopy reveals numerous membranous inclusions in the cytoplasm of the ganglion cells (Fig. 8–480) (Harcourt, Dobbs, 1968; Cogan, Kuwabara, 1968).

Sandhoff Disease, or GM$_2$ Gangliosidosis, Type II. The clinical and pathologic features of this disease are very similar to those of Tay-Sachs disease. Both hexosaminidase A and B are deficient (Table 8–4). Garner (1973), in a study of the ocular pathology of a case of Sandhoff's disease, found that the only difference between Tay-Sachs and Sandhoff's disease was that the membranous cytoplasmic inclusions in the ganglion cells in Sandhoff's disease were more pleomorphic. Similar results were reported by Cordier, Grignon, Vidailhet, and Rasiller (1976) and Brownstein, Carpenter, Polomeno, and Little (1980). The latter found abundant pleomorphic storage cytosomes in all neurons of the retina (Fig. 8–481), including the inner segments of the photoreceptor cells (Fig. 8–482), and in glial cells of the optic nerve. These investigators also found fibrogranular and occasional membranous lamellar inclusions in keratocytes. Prenatal diagnosis using enzyme assays of amniotic fluid has been accomplished (Norby, Jansen, Schwartz, 1980).

Juvenile Tay-Sachs Disease (Juvenile GM$_2$ Gangliosidosis, Type III). This disease is due to a partial deficiency of hexosaminidase. The clinical and general pathologic features are similar to those of types I and II, but manifestations are

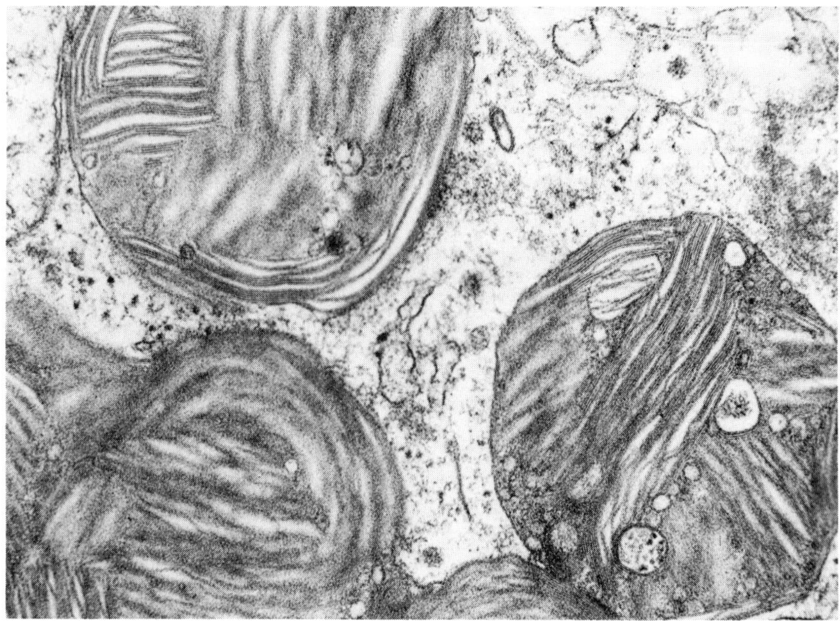

Figure 8–480. Ganglion cell with membranous cytoplasmic inclusion. ×30,000. (From Cogan DG, Kuwabara T: Sphingolipidoses and eye. Arch Ophthalmol *79*:437–452, 1968.)

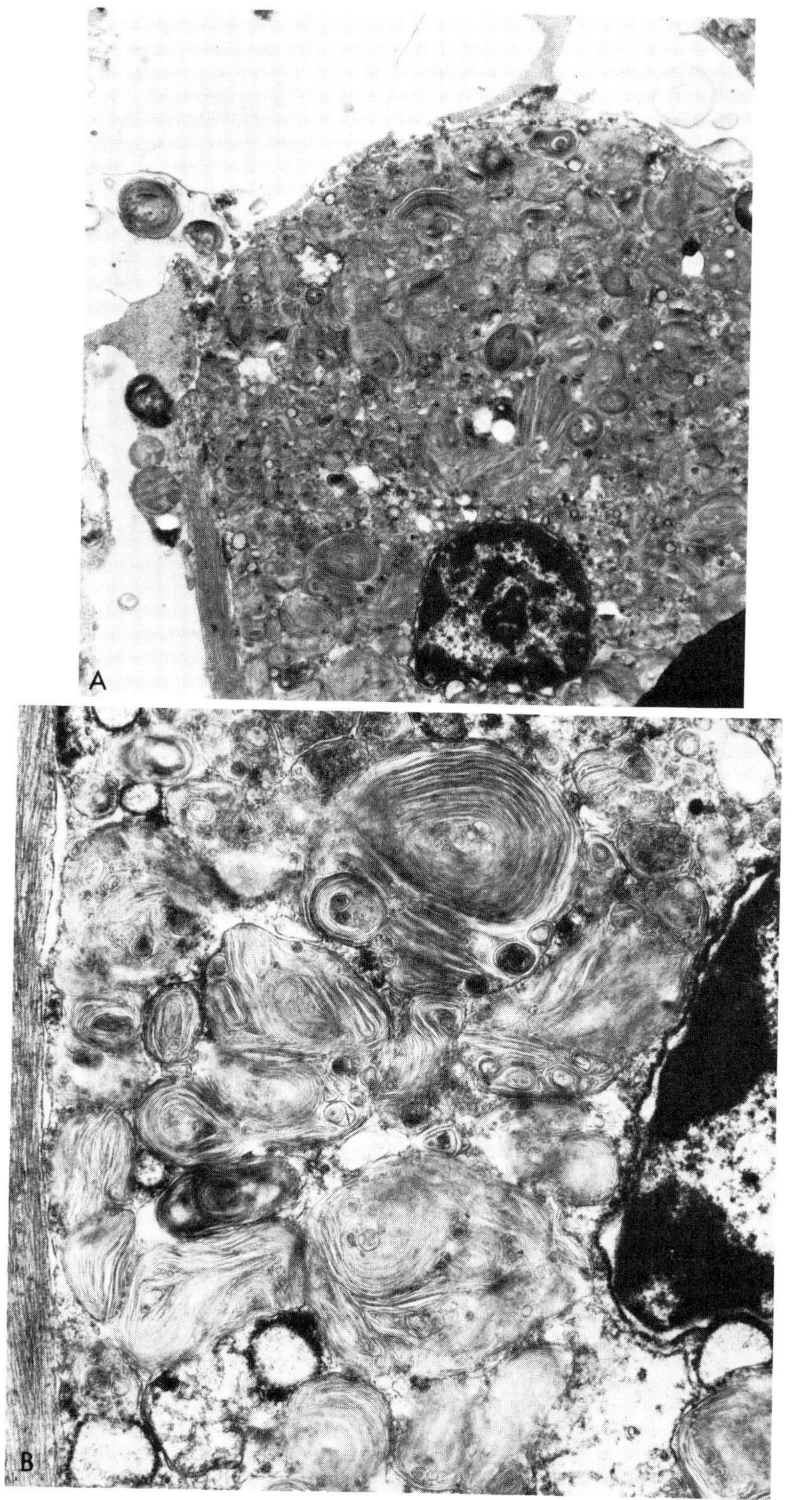

Figure 8–481. Sandhoff's disease (GM_2 gangliosidosis, type II). *A*, Ganglion cell with cytoplasm packed with membranous bodies. ×6700. *B*, Higher magnification of cytoplasm, showing concentric membranous bodies and smaller circular profiles. ×25,000. (From Brownstein S, Carpenter S, Polomeno RC, Little JM: Sandhoff's disease (GM_2 gangliosidosis, Type II): Histopathology and ultrastructure of eye. Arch Ophthalmol *98*:1089–1097, 1980.)

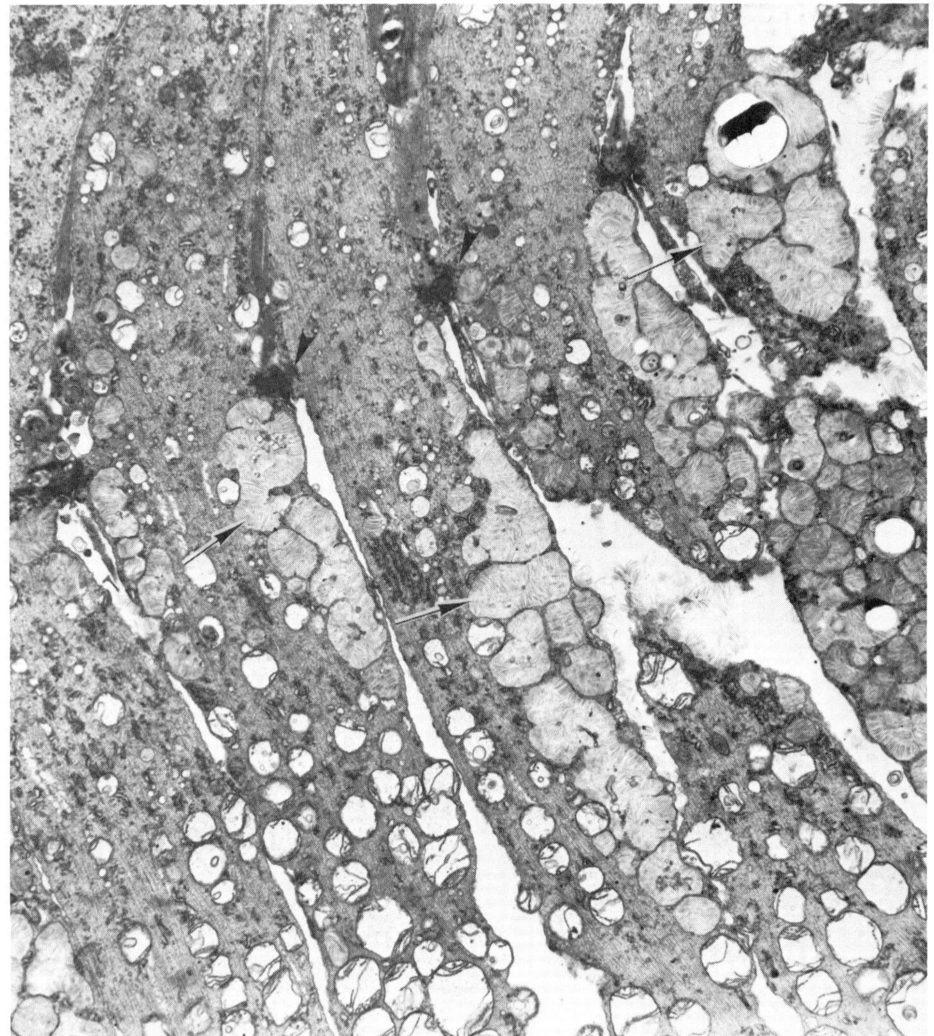

Figure 8–482. Larger storage cytosomes (arrows) in inner segments of photoreceptor cells. Mitochondria show artifactitious swelling. Intercellular junctions (arrowheads) of outer limiting membrane are evident. ×7500. (From Brownstein S, Carpenter S, Polomeno RC; Little JM: Sandhoff's disease (GM_2 gangliosidosis, Type II): Histopathology and ultrastructure of eye. Arch Ophthalmol *98*:1089–1097, 1980.)

slower in developing, and affected individuals usually die later, by the age of 15 years.

Niemann-Pick Disease (Sphingomyelin Lipidosis). Five distinct forms of this disease have been distinguished: the classic infantile form (type A of Crocker), the visceral form (type B), the subacute or juvenile form (type C), the Nova Scotia variant (type D), and the adult form (type E). Sphingomyelinase is deficient in types A, B, and C and has been reported as "attenuated" in types D and E. It is not definite that type D is a sphingomyelin storage disease (McKusick, 1978, page 618).

The enzyme deficiency causes storage of sphingomyelin and cholesterol in the brain and abdominal viscera. The accumulation of storage substances in the ganglion cells accounts for the cherry-red spot seen in most cases of type A Niemann-Pick disease (Goldstein, Wexler, 1931; Rintelan, 1936; Didion, 1950; Larsen, Ehlers, 1965; Cogan, Kuwabara, 1968). A cherry-red spot is not present in types B, C, and D. In addition to retinal ganglion cell and RPE involvement (Fig. 8–483), Robb and Kuwabara (1973) observed sphingolipid storage in keratocytes and endothelium of the cornea and lens epithelium in type A disease. These deposits explain the subtle opacities seen clinically in these structures. Those investigators also observed involvement of the iris sphincter muscle, ciliary epithelium, RPE, and vascular endothelium.

Howes, Wood, Golbus, and Hogan (1975) studied the eyes of a 23 week fetus that had been aborted after the demonstration of sphingomyelinase deficiency in cultural cells obtained by amniocentesis. They found lipid storage in the corneal epithelium, as well as in other areas previously reported.

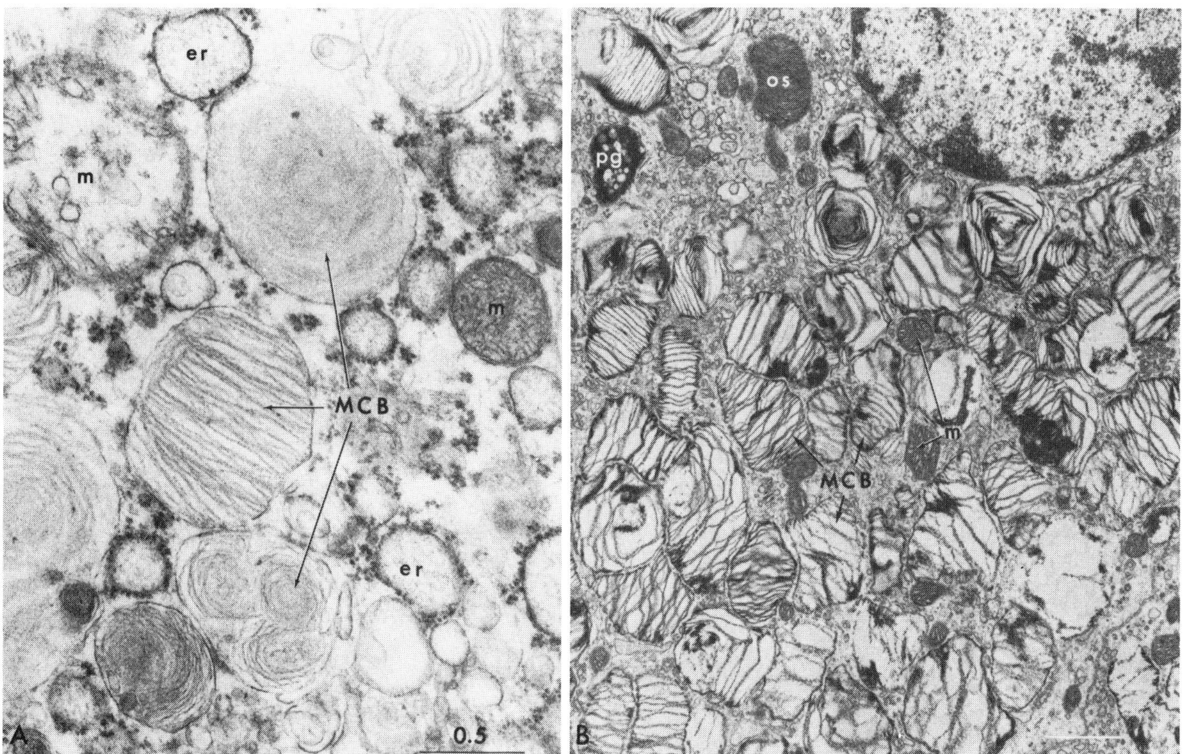

Figure 8–483. Niemann-Pick disease, Type A. *A*, Retinal ganglion cell with membranous cytoplasmic bodies (*MCB*) cut in several different planes. Mitochondria (*m*) and endoplasmic reticulum (*er*) are noted. ×42,000. *B*, Retinal pigment epithalium cell containing MCB, with lamellar material cut in various planes. What appear to be single lamellae at this magnification are actually groups of several osmiophilic and osmiophobic lines. Mitochondria (*m*), pigment granules (*pg*), and phagocytosed outer segment material (*os*) are easily distinguishable from MCB. ×15,000. (From Robb RM, Kuwabara T: Ocular pathology of Type A Niemann-Pick disease. Invest Ophthalmol *12*:366–377, 1973.)

Libert, Toussaint, and Guiselings (1975) reported finding two types of lipid inclusions. The first consisted of large, parallel or concentrically laminated membranes that resembled those seen in Tay-Sachs disease. The second type had a dense, lamellar structure that was less uniform and was round, oval, or rectangular. Those investigators suggested that the metabolism of the stored material in neurons differs from that in other cells.

Eyes of a patient with type C Niemann-Pick disease failed to show any storage material in ganglion cells (Emery, Green, Huff, 1972). Storage material was observed in visceral organs (Fig. 8–484).

Libert and Davis (1975) have reported the usefulness of conjunctival biopsy in establishing the diagnosis of type A Niemann-Pick disease.

Gaucher's Disease. Gaucher's disease is due to a deficiency of beta-glucosidase, which is a glucocerebroside-splitting enzyme found in the spleen. This disease has three forms with the same enzyme deficiency: type I (noncerebral, juvenile), type II (infantile, cerebral), and type III (juvenile and adult, cerebral). There is some question whether retinal involvement is present in Gaucher's disease (Lee, 1968).

Ueno, Ueno, Kajitani, et al (1977) studied a juvenile form of Gaucher's disease with cerebral involvement, in which they observed white patches in the posterior pole of both eyes of the patient (Fig. 8–485,*A*). Histopathologic studies disclosed lipid-laden histiocytes thoughout the choroid (Fig. 8–485,*B*) and ciliary body, and fewer numbers in the ganglion cell layer of the retina.

Further studies of the same patient (Ueno, Ueno, Matsuo, et al, 1980) showed that white patches probably correspond to clumps of histiocytes on the internal surface of the retina (Fig. 8–485,*C*). Ultrastructural study disclosed the cytoplasm of the Gaucher cells to be distended by numerous membrane-bound vacuoles containing tubular structures measuring 330 to 650 angstroms in diameter (Fig. 8–485,*D*).

Cogan, Chu, Gittinger, and Tychsen (1980) observed one patient with a macular grayness, but they found no typical cherry-red spot in an unspecified number of patients. These investigators observed white spots on the retina in three patients.

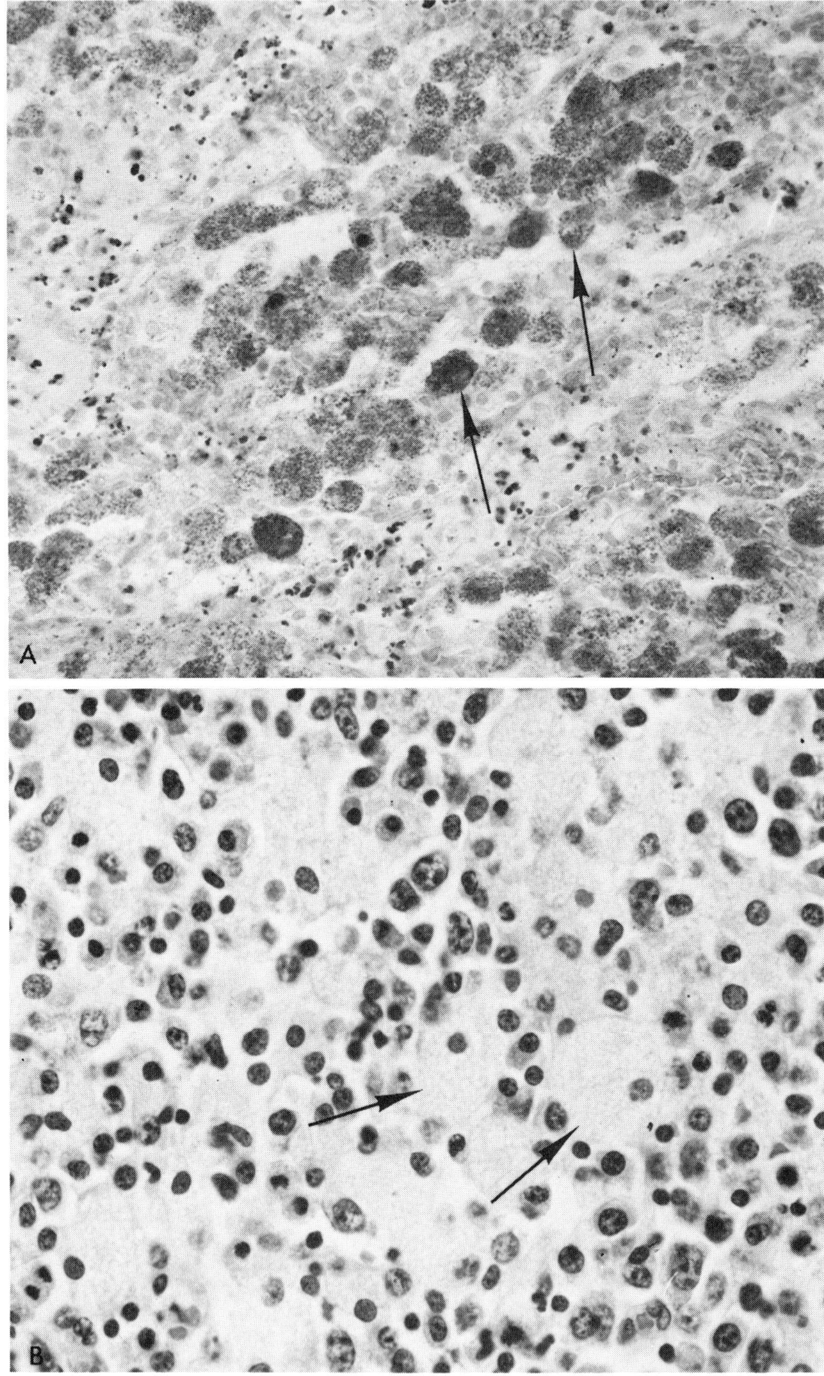

Figure 8–484. Niemann-Pick disease, type C. *A*, Lymph node with numerous lipid-laden histiocytes (arrows). Oil red O, ×500. *B*, Spleen with vacuolated, lipid-containing histiocytes (arrows). H and E, ×575. (From Emery JM, Green WR, Huff OS, Sloan HR: Niemann-Pick disease (Type C): Histopathology and ultrastructure. Am J Ophthalmol *74*:1144–1154, 1972.)

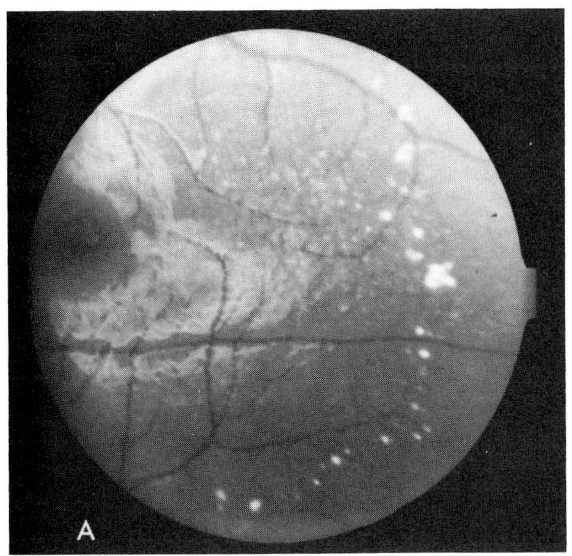

Figure 8–485. Juvenile Gaucher's disease. *A*, Ophthalmoscopic appearance of discrete deposits on the retina in a semicircular pattern temporal to the macula. *B*, Marked distension of choroid by Gaucher cells (arrowheads). Azure III, ×510. *C*, Clustered Gaucher cells (arrow) on inner surface of retina. Azure III, ×510. *D*, Electron micrograph of a lightly pigmented Gaucher cell in choroid, showing crystalline-like appearance of Gaucher bodies (arrows) containing tubules. ×6600. (From Ueno H, Ueno S, Kamitani T, et al: Clinical and histopathologic studies of a case with juvenile form of Gaucher's disease. Jap J Ophthalmol *21*:98–108, 1977.)

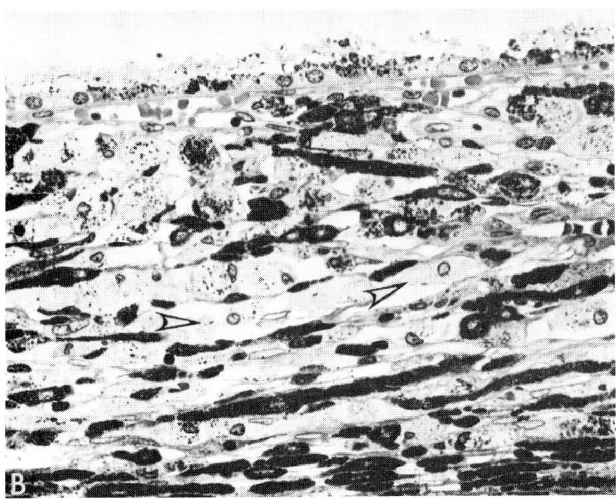

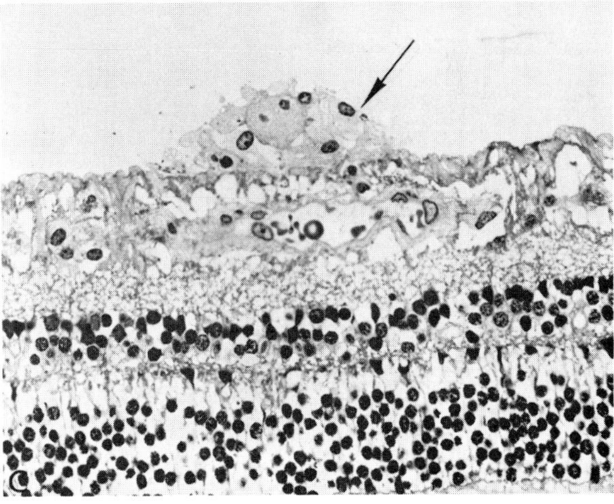

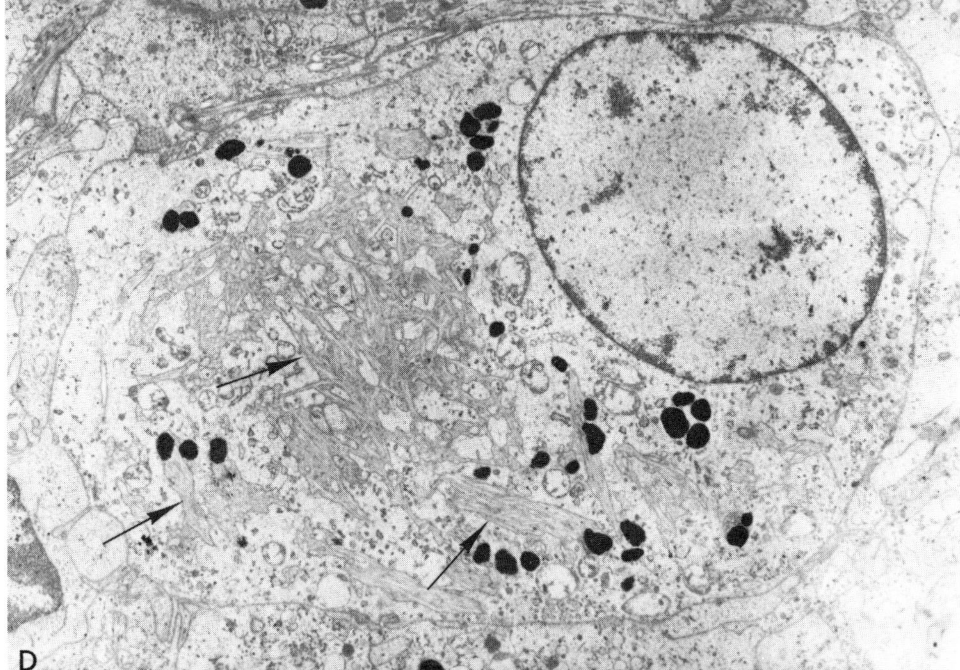

A pinguecula-like lesion caused by Gaucher-type cell infiltration has been noted in type III Gaucher disease.

Fabry's Disease (Angiokeratoma Corporus Diffusum). This condition is an inherited, sex-linked disease of males in which ceramide trihexose is stored in tissues. The syndrome consists of cutaneous angiokeratomas, painful febrile crises, renal failure, and cardiovascular disease. The ceramide trihexose accumulates, especially in blood vessels of the skin and other tissues, and leads to the clinical changes.

The ocular changes include a superficial corneal opacity in a whorl-like pattern, anterior lens capsular deposits, posterior lens capsular spoke-like opacity, conjunctival aneurysmal dilatations, and retinal vascular tortuosity (Spaeth, Frost, 1965; Velzeboer, de Groot, 1971; Sher, Letson, Desnick, 1979).

According to Sher and associates (1979), in a study of 37 hemizygous males and 35 heterozygous females, the whorl-like superficial corneal deposits were observed in almost all patients, more severe in the heterozygotes. The anterior

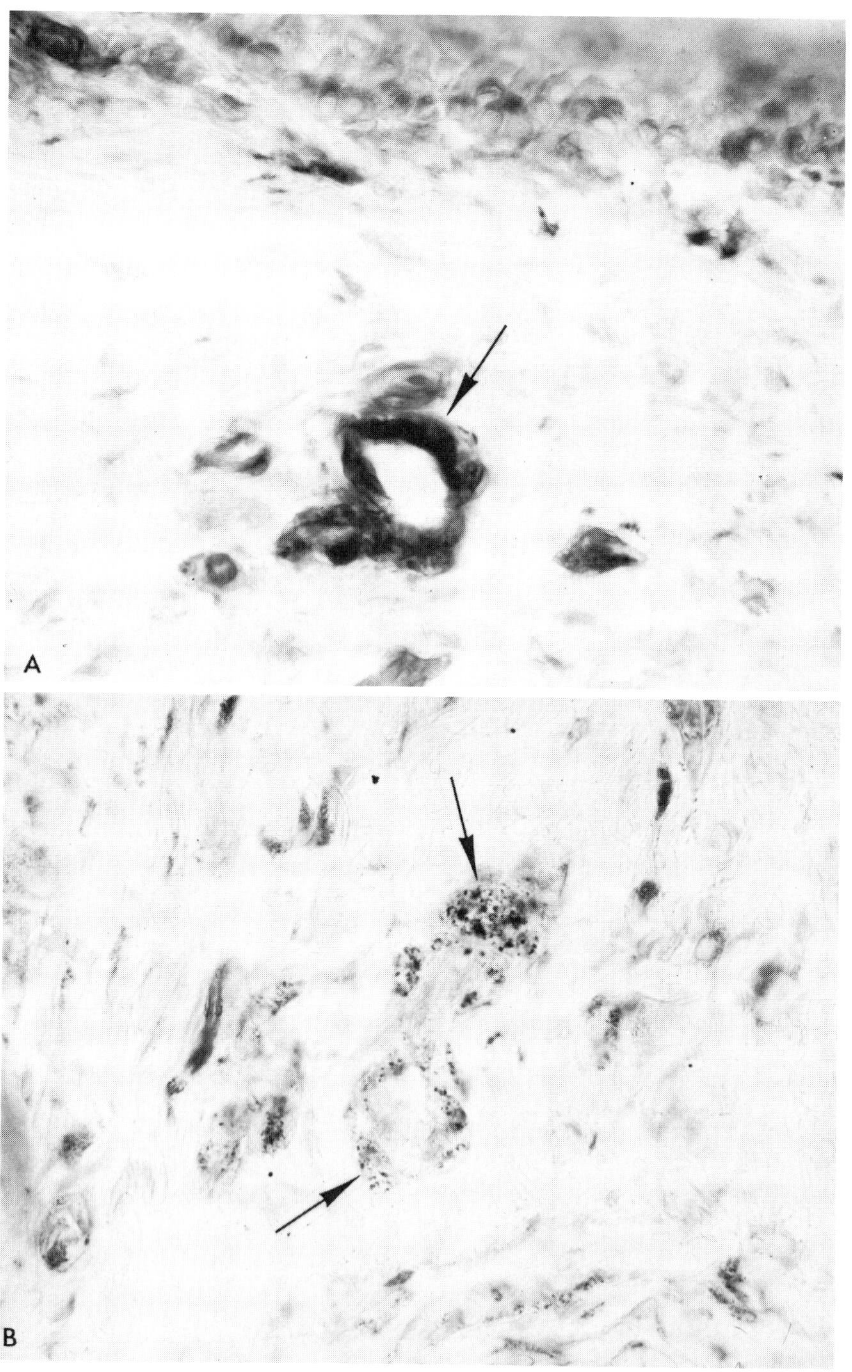

Figure 8–486. Conjunctival biopsy from patient suspected of having **Fabry's disease**. Special staining disclosed lipid in the walls of some conjunctival blood vessels (arrows). *A*, Oil red 0, ×530. *B*, Sudan black B, ×530. EP 27008.

lens capsular deposits were observed in one third of the hemizygotes and in none of the heterozygotes. The posterior lens capsular opacity was seen in 37 per cent of the hemizygotes and 14 per cent of the heterozygotes. Abnormalities of the conjunctival vessels were seen in 78 per cent of the hemizygotes and 46 per cent of the heterozygotes. Retinal vascular tortuosity was seen in 70 per cent of hemizygotes, compared with 25 per cent of heterozygotes. Sher and associates have also observed central retinal artery occlusion in two patients and a branch retinal vein occlusion in one patient with hemizygotic Fabry's disease.

Studies of conjunctival biopsy specimens have shown lipid deposition (Fig. 8–486) (Spaeth, Frost, 1965) in the vascular endothelium (Fig. 8–487,*A*), media (Fig. 8–487,*B*) and epithelium (Fig. 8–487,*C*). Enzyme analysis of tears and electron microscopic studies of conjunctival biopsy specimens have proved to be of value in establishing the diagnosis (Libert, Tondeur, Van Hoof, 1976).

Histopathologic study of an affected male (Font, Fine, 1972) revealed lipid material deposited in smooth muscle cells of the media and endothelial cells of the small and medium-sized arterioles of the choroid (Fig. 8–487,*D,E*), retina (Fig. 8–487,*F*), ciliary body, and iris (Fig. 8–487,*G*). Similar deposits were present in endothelial cells and pericytes of retinal capillaries and the choriocapillaris. Deposits of lipid also were observed in the basal cell layer of the corneal epithelium, the iris pigment epithelium (Fig. 8–487,*H*), and lens epithelium (Fig. 8–487,*I*). The ganglion cells of the retina were free of lipid storage material, but deposits were observed in the ganglion cells present in the choroid. At each of those sites, ultrastructural studies disclosed the lipid material to be composed of dense, laminated, osmiophilic inclusions.

In a histopathologic study of a female carrier, Weingeist and Blodi (1971) found similar material in the vascular endothelium, smooth muscle, and pericytes (Fig. 8–488). They also observed membranous inclusions in the apical portion of the basal layer of corneal epithelium, as well as subepithelial ridges composed of replicated basement membrane and an amorphous material between basement membrane and Bowman's membrane. The clinically observed whorl-like pattern of the superficial cornea was attributed to those ridges. The abnormal lipid may have the configuration of a Maltese cross. Such figures may be observed in urinary sediment (Fig. 8–489) and may be helpful in leading to a diagnosis in a patient suspected of having Fabry's disease.

Krabbe's Disease (Globoid Cell Sclerosis, Globoid Leukodystrophy). This is a disease caused by a deficiency of galactocerebroside beta-galactosidase, which results in the accumulation of galactosyl ceramide in cells in the white matter of the brain and optic nerves. This results in early, progressive psychomotor deterioration, blindness, and death in 2 years. There are severe loss of oligodendroglia, myelin, and axons; dense, fibrous astrocytic proliferation; and the focal accumulation of large, multinucleated globoid cells (Fig. 8–490,*A,B*), with characteristic inclusion of material with a tubular configuration (Fig. 8–480,*C*). In the optic nerve, this results in marked atrophy (Fig. 8–490,*D,E*), which is reflected in the retina by loss of the nerve fiber and ganglion cell layers (Fig. 8–490,*F*) (Emery, Green, Huff, 1972; Harcourt, Ashton, 1973; Brownstein, Meagher-Villemure, Polomeno, Little, 1978).

Metachromatic Leukodystrophy (MLD). This is an autosomal recessive disorder caused by a deficiency of sulfatase A, a lysosomal hydrolase. Histopathologically, the lesion is characterized by a degenerative process of myelin in the central and peripheral nervous systems and lysosomal storage of metachromatic glycolipids—mainly sulfatides. These lesions cause progressive symptoms of mental retardation, dementia, hypotonia, ataxia, convulsions, spastic quadriplegia, and decerebration.

Four clinical forms of MLD have been recognized on the basis of the age of onset and severity of the features.

The congenital form is lethal within the first days of life. Histopathologic features of this type apparently have not been studied but are presumed to be similar to but more severe than the late infantile form.

The late infantile form of MLD is the most common. It begins before the age of 3 years and results in death by 6 years of age or earlier. A grayness of the macular area has been described. Light microscopic studies of this type have shown enlarged retinal ganglion cells with a metachromatic substance in the cytoplasm (Cogan, Kuwabara, Richardson, Lyon, 1958; Renard, Bargeton, Dhermy, Aron, 1963; Toussaint, Conreur, Pelc, Perier, 1964).

Light and electron microscopic studies (Libert, Van Hoof, Toussaint, et al, 1979) showed the storage of metachromatic complex lipids in the retinal ganglion cells (Fig. 8–491,*A*), in the optic nerve (Fig. 8–491,*B*), and in the ciliary nerves, as well as the storage of a mucopolysaccharide-like material in the nonpigmented ciliary epithelium.

In other studies, the stored material was most marked in the ganglion cells outside the macular area (Cogan, Kuwabara, Richardson, Lyon, 1958). Electron microscopic examination disclosed laminated inclusion bodies in ganglion cells of the retina, Schwann cells, and oligodendrocytes (Cogan, Kuwabara, Moser, 1970).

Libert, Van Hoof, Toussaint, et al (1979) also have demonstrated numerous membrane-bound inclusions containing a fibrillogranular reticulum

Text continued on page 1134

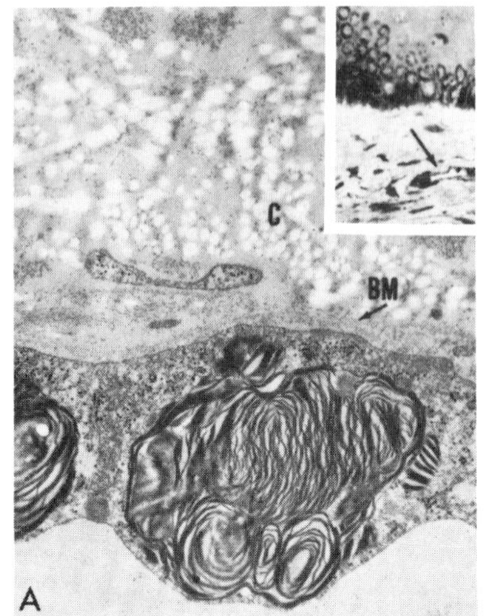

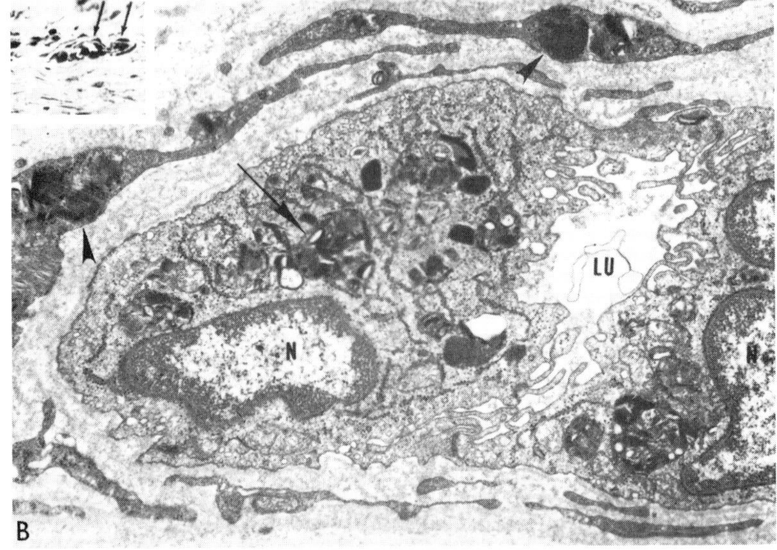

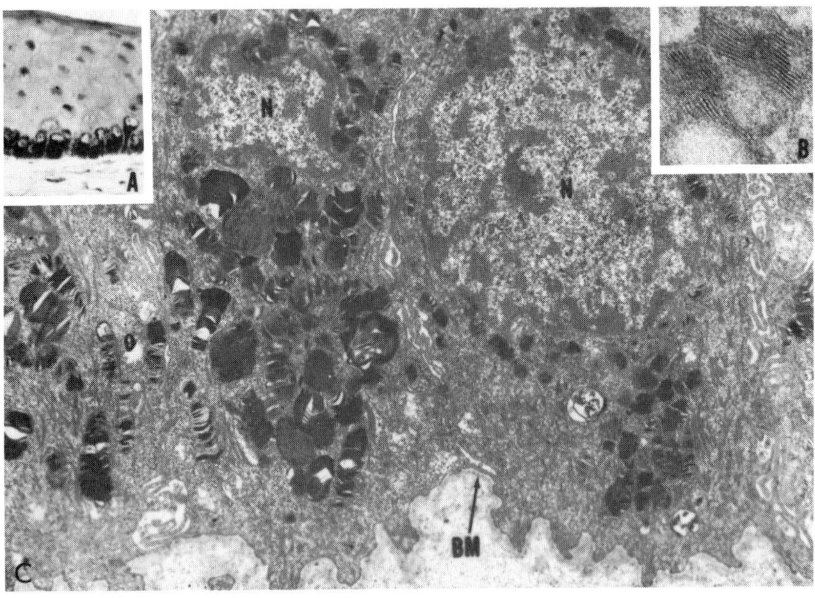

Figure 8–487. Fabry's disease. *A*, Accumulation of lamellar material within endothelial layer of limbal vessel (arrow in inset). BM, endothelial basement membrane. *C*, Collagen. ×14,000. Paraphenylenediamine, × 275. AFIP Neg. 71 1652–7. *B*, Limbal vessel (arrows in inset). A similar small vessel in the electron micrograph shows accumulated lamellar material within endothelial cells (arrow). *N*, nuclei of endothelial cells. Apical villi of endothelial cells are present in greater numbers than usual, and lumen (*LU*) of vessel is partially occluded. Adventitial cells also contain similar inclusions (arrowheads). ×15,000. Paraphenylenediamine, ×275. AFIP Neg. 71-1652-7. C. Lamellar accumulations are present within basal cells of limbal epithelium. *N*, Nuclei of basal epithelial cells; BM, basememt membrane. ×7,000). AFIP Neg. 71–1652–6. Inset *A* shows a similar region of limbal epithelium. Densely stained deposits involve most of the basal cells but only a few of the next layer of cells. Paraphenylenediamine, ×275. Inset *B* shows a fine lamellar material (like a fingerprint) at high magnification. ×80,000.

Illustration continued on opposite page

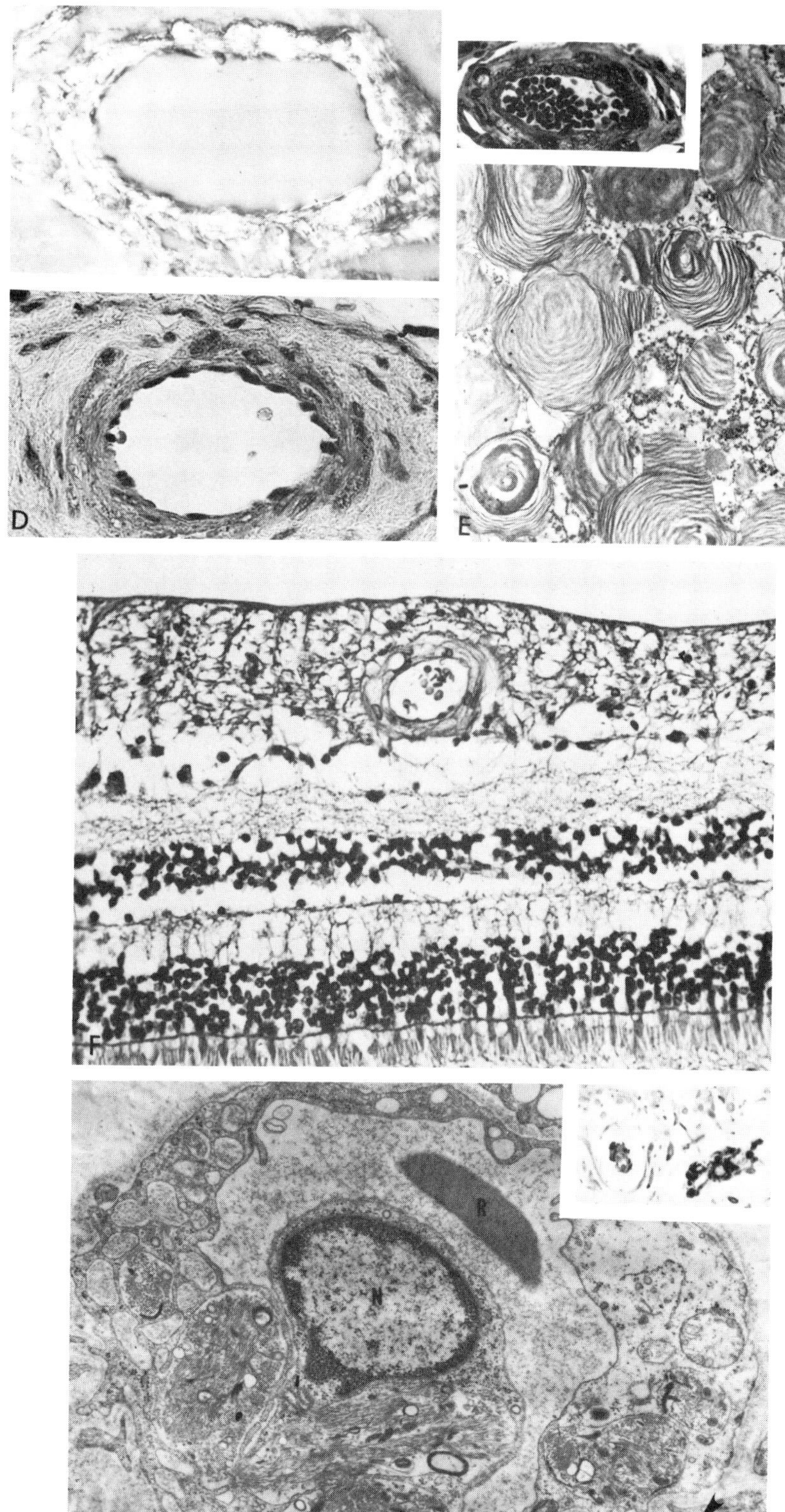

Figure 8–487. *Continued D, Top,* Under polarized light, this choroidal arteriole shows birefringent lipid in vacuolated cells of media. Frozen section, ×300. *Bottom,* Oil red O stained positively lipid granules in cells of media of adjacent choroidal vessel. ×300. AFIP Neg. 71-1652-4. *E,* Inset shows section of choroidal arteriole with many deposits within its wall. Sudan black B, ×300. Electron micrograph shows lamellar aggregates present within smooth muscle cells of media. × 12,300. AFIP Neg. 71-1652-4. *F,* Retinal vessel shows vacuolization within its wall. Otherwise, retinal architecture, except for mild autolytic changes, appears normal. H and E, ×260. AFIP Neg. 71-1652-3. *G,* Lipid deposits are present within walls of iris stromal vessels in inset (paraphenylenediamine, ×210). Endothelial cells of small vessel illustrated in electron micrograph (×16,000) contain large quantities of laminated lipid deposits (arrow). Lumen is narrowed, and a section of a red blood cell (*R*) is visible. Similar material (arrowhead) is present with pericyte (*P*). *N,* Nucleus of endothelial cell. AFIP Neg. 71-1652-8.

Illustration continued on opposite page

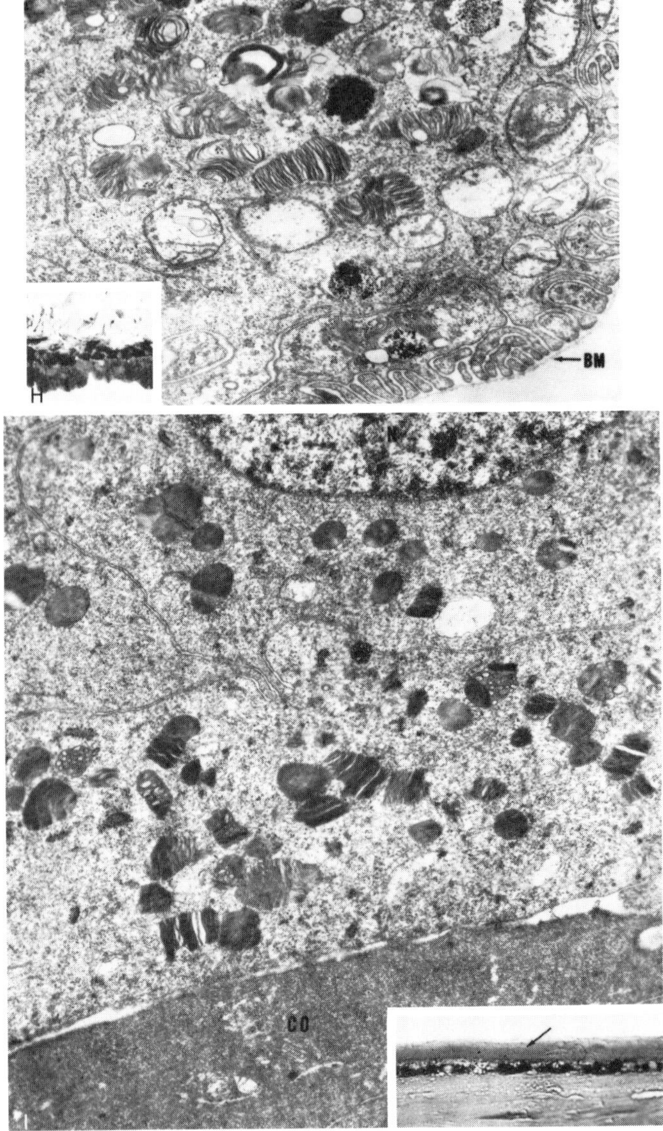

Figure 8–487 *Continued H*, Lamellar accumulations can be easily differentiated from complete and incompletely formed melanin granules by electron microscopic examination. Comparable region of pigment epithelium near root of iris in inset (paraphenylenediamine, ×210). *BM*, Basement membrane of posterior layer of iris pigment epithelium. ×14,500. AFIP Neg. 71-1652-8. *I*, Lamellar aggregates are present in large numbers within epithelial cells of lens. *N*, Nucleus. Similar bodies are not present within superficial cortical cells (*CO*). ×26,000. Inset shows heavy involvement of epithelial cells of lens with lipid material. Arrow points to capsule of lens. Sudan black B, ×300. AFIP Neg. 71-1652-5.

(From Font RL, Fine BS: Ocular pathology in Fabry's disease. Histochemical and electron microscopic observations. Am J Ophthalmol *73*:419–430, 1972.)

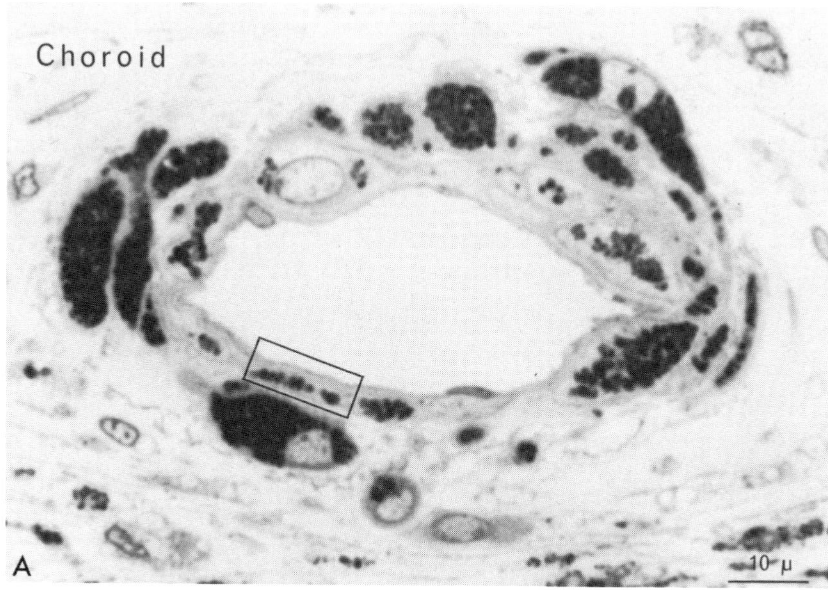

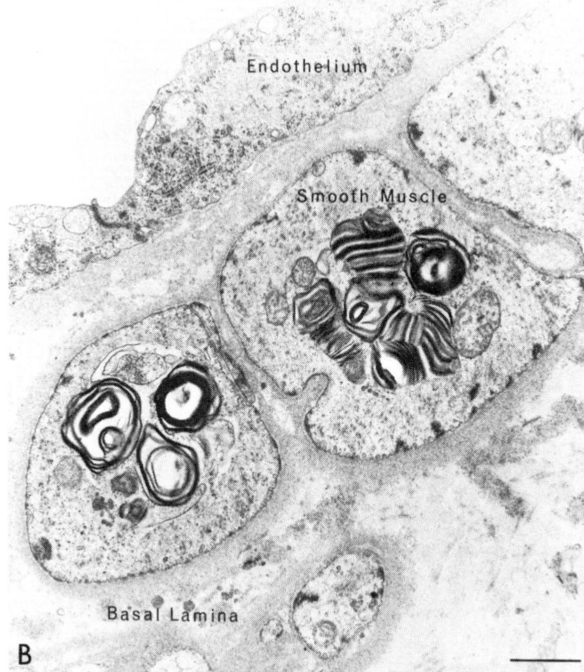

Figure 8–488. Female carrier of Fabry's disease. *A*, Light micrograph of choroidal vessel. Intracellular deposits located in smooth muscle cells of arteriole. In other sections, granules were also observed in endothelium. Rectangle encloses smooth muscle and endothelium similar to region shown by electron microscopy in *B*. Azure II stain. *B*, Membranous inclusions in cytoplasm of smooth muscle cells of choroidal arteriole. (From Weingeist TA, and Blodi FC: Fabry's disease: Ocular findings in a female carrier. Arch Opthalmol *85*:169–176, 1971.)

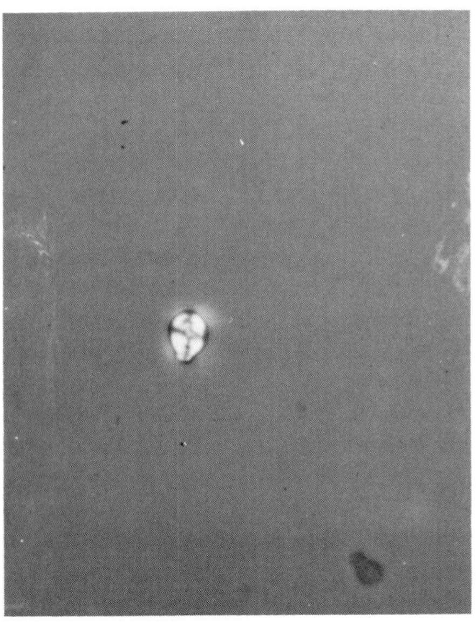

Figure 8–489. Urinary sediment of a patient with **Fabry's disease**, showing crystalline material in a Maltese Cross configuration. Unstained, ×500.

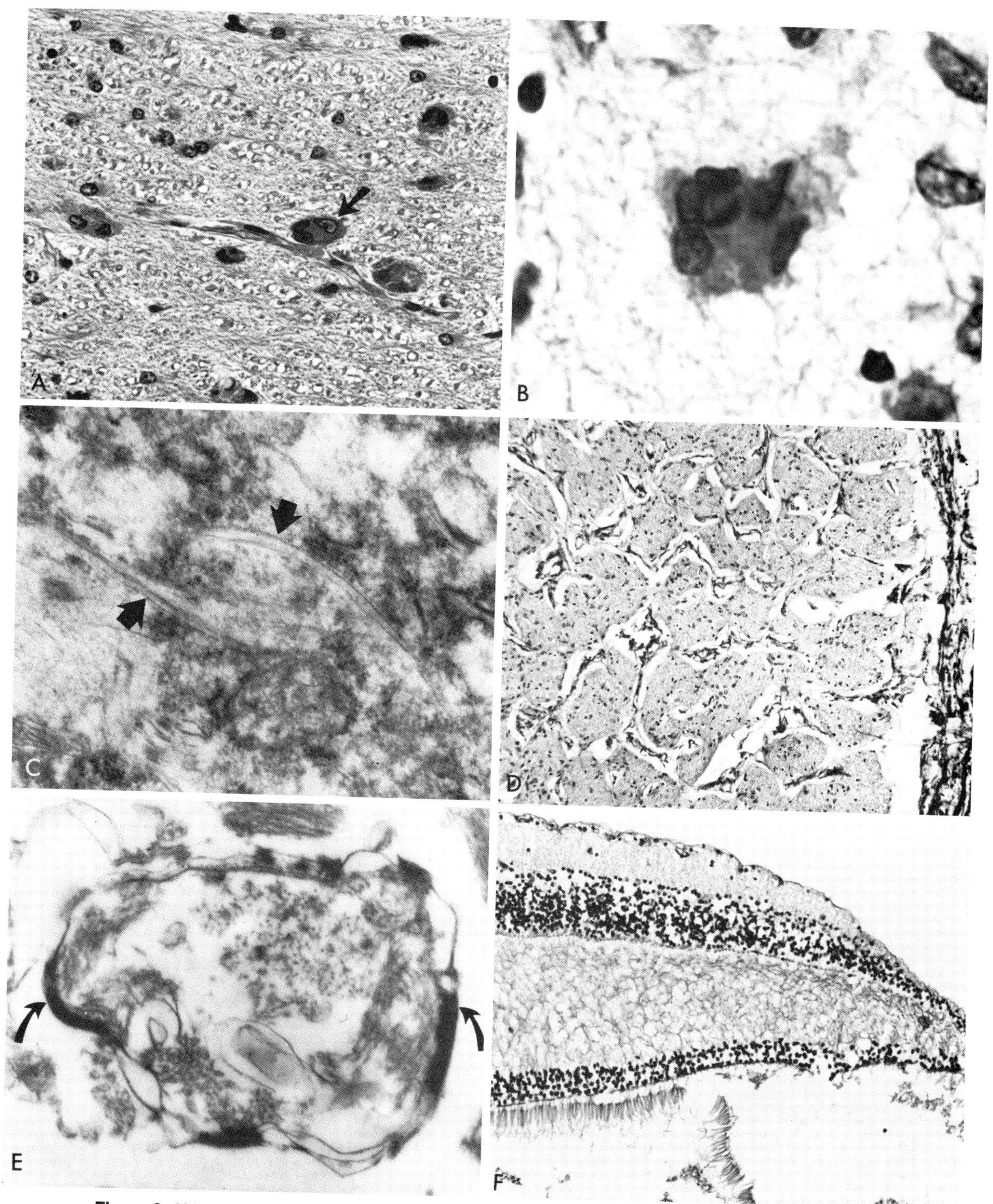

Figure 8–490. Krabbe's disease. *A*, Cerebral cortex. Multinucleated globoid cells (one indicated by arrow) in white matter. PAS, ×500. *B*, Optic nerve. Globoid cell with nuclei pushed to periphery by engorged cytoplasm. PAS, ×3,000. *C*, Optic nerve. Electron micrograph of tubular structures (arrows) in cytoplasm of globoid cell. ×61,000. *D*, Cross-section of optic nerve showing severe atrophy, with narrowing of nerve fiber bundles, gliosis, and near-total demyelinization. Verhoeff–van Gieson, ×125. *E*, Optic nerve. Electron micrograph of one of few remaining ganglion cell axons, with some partially intact myeline lamellae (arrows). ×48,500. *F*, Parafoveal area, showing marked atrophy of nerve fiber and ganglion cell layers. PAS, ×500. EP 31278. (From Emery JM, Green, WR, Huff, DS: Krabbe's disease: Histopathology and ultrastructure of eye. Am J Opthalmol *74*:400–406, 1972.)

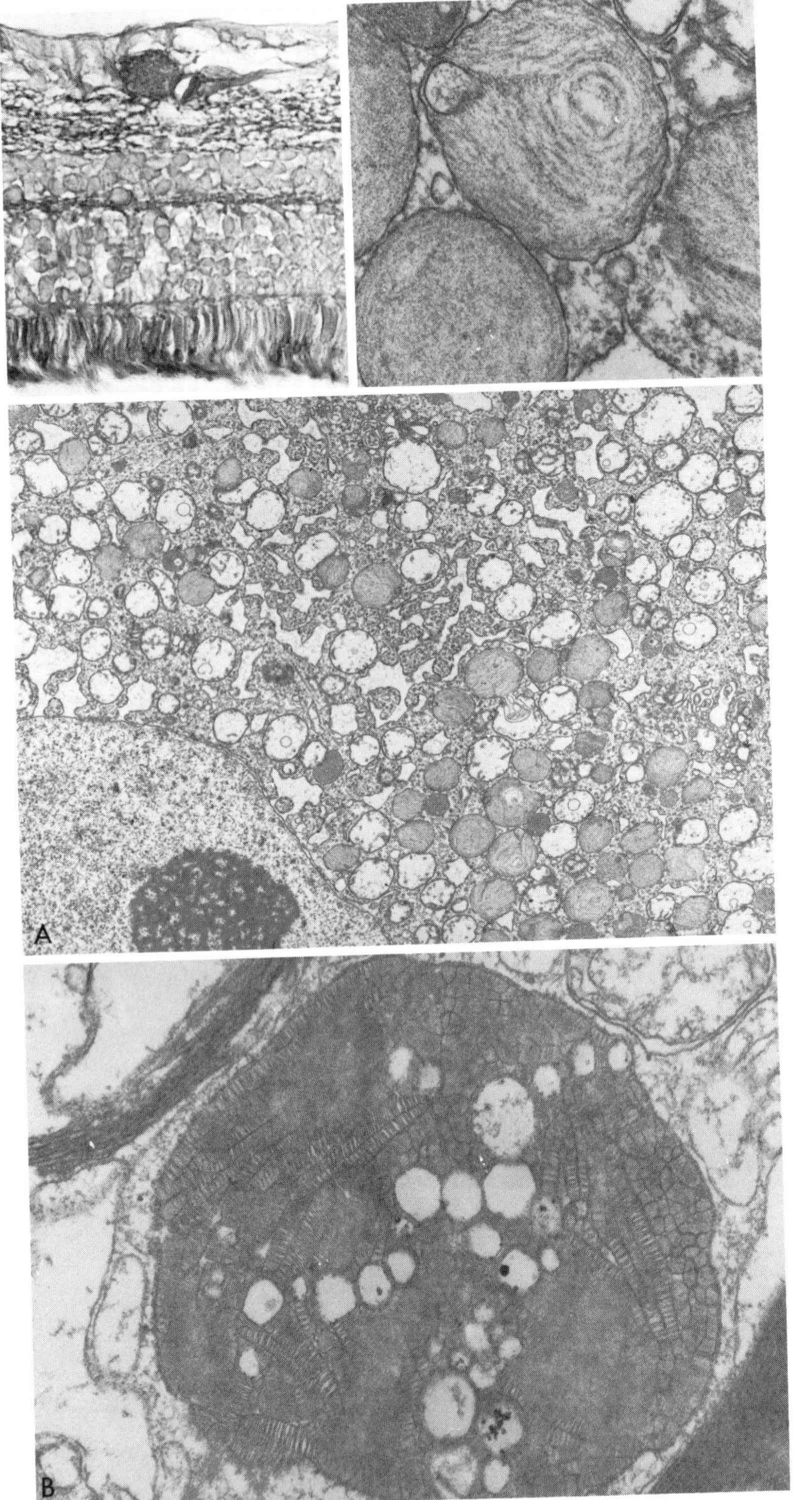

Figure 8–491. Late infantile metachromatic leukodystrophy. *A*, Top left, cytoplasm of some retinal ganglion cells shows dark red-brown metachromasia with cresyl violet stain. ×650. *Bottom*, By electron microscopy, retinal ganglion cells have many osmiophilic storage inclusions (0.2 to 1 micron). Moderate swelling of endoplasmic reticulum and mitochondria is due to post mortem autolysis. ×17,000. *Top right*, At higher magnification, inclusions, limited by unit membrane, contain irregularly stained lamellar profiles within a rather granular matrix. ×80,000. *B*, Prismatic inclusions of optic nerve glial cells are highly typical of metachromatic leukodystrophy. They contain herringbone patterns and honeycomb structures, with sometimes electron-lucent vacuoles and granular material. ×80,000.

(From Libert J, Van Hoof F, Toussaint, D et al: Ocular findings in metachromatic leukodystrophy: An electron microscopic and enzyme study in different clinical and genetic variants. Arch Ophthalmol *97*:1495–1504, 1979.)

and no lamellar lipids in the nonpigmented ciliary body epithelium. These inclusions are similar to the storage of acid mucopolysaccharides and suggest that only storage of sulfated polysaccharides occurs in the ciliary epithelium.

The juvenile form of MLD begins before the age of 10 years, and death usually occurs before the age of 20 years. Storage material is not present in the retinal ganglion cells, but optic atrophy usually occurs. Lipid inclusions are present in astrocytes and oligodendrocytes in the optic nerve and in the Schwann cells of the ciliary nerves and other peripheral nerves (Libert, Rutsaert, Toussaint, 1974). Toussaint, Conreur, Pelc, and Perier

(1964) described one patient in whom no metachromatic material was observed in retinal ganglion cells.

The adult form of MLD begins after puberty and has a more prolonged evolution. Studies of one patient showed the retinal ganglion cells to be free of inclusions, but there were large membranous inclusions in the glial cells of the optic nerve (Fig. 8–492,*A,B*). Marked optic atrophy and loss of nerve fiber and ganglion cell layers (Fig. 8–492,*C*) were present (Quigley, Green, 1976). In another study, similar inclusions were observed in the optic nerve, and an excess of residual bodies was observed in retinal ganglion cells (Goebel, Shimokawa, Argyrakis, Piez, 1978).

A variant of MLD has been described in which both lysosomal sulfatase A and B are deficient, along with the microsomal sulfatase C. This variant combines the clinical features of the mucopolysaccharidoses and late infantile metachromatic leukodystrophy (Austin, 1973) (see also the mucolipidoses in a following section).

Lactosylceramidosis. This disease is characterized by neurologic deterioration, with cerebellar ataxia, mental depression, and hypotonia. Mild redness of the macula has been observed, but no histopathologic studies of the eye have been made. Lactosylceramide accumulates in the viscera and nervous system because of a deficiency of lactosylceramide galactosyl hydrolase.

Farber's Lipogranulomatosis. This condition manifests early in life and is characterized by respiratory symptoms from nodular involvement of the larynx, swollen joints, restricted joint movements, subcutaneous nodules, and great irritability. Death usually occurs by the third year of life. The subcutaneous granulomatous lesions and the viscera contain large foamy histiocytes that have abnormal amounts of ceramide. An excess of gangliosides is also found, especially in the foam cells. Both neurons and glial cells of the nervous system are swollen and contain material characteristic of nonsulfated acid mucopolysaccharide (Abul-Haj, Martz, Douglas, Geppert, 1962). Be-

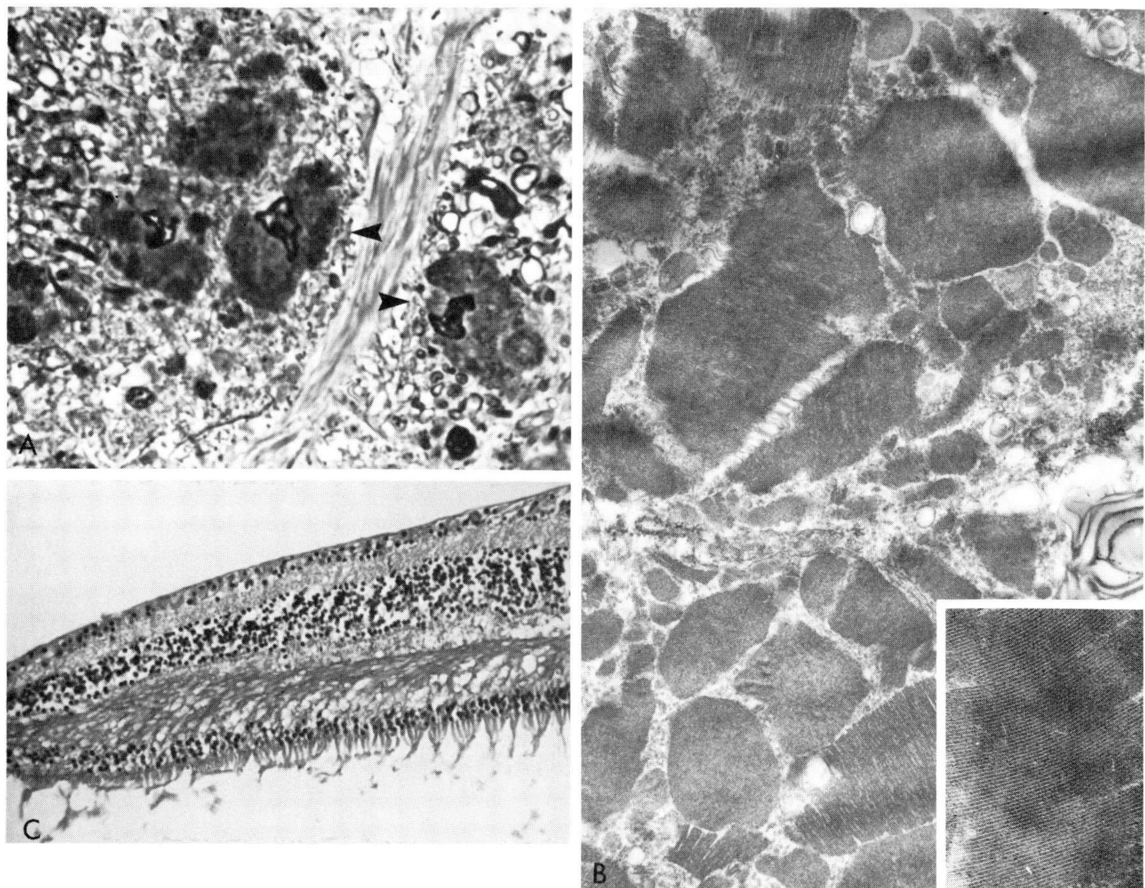

Figure 8–492. Adult metachromatic leukodystrophy. *A*, Cross-section of optic nerve, with large glial cells with dense material in distended cytoplasm (arrowheads). Epoxy-embedded, cresyl violet, ×800. *B*, Large, optic nerve glial cell with distended cytoplasm packed with lamellar inclusions. Inset shows membranous character of inclusions. ×40,000; inset, ×90,000. *C*, Parafoveal area of macula, showing marked reduction of nerve fiber and ganglion cell layers. H and E, ×500.

EP 42465. (From Quigley HA, Green WR: Clinical and ultrastructural ocular histopathologic studies of adult-onset metachromatic leukodystrophy. Am J Ophthalmol *82*:472–479, 1976.)

cause of these findings, some have placed this disease in the mucolipidosis category. The parafoveal area is gray, and there is a mild cherry-red spot.

Histopathologic studies (Cogan, Kuwabara, Moser, Hazard, 1966) have revealed an abnormal birefringent material in the ganglion cells of the retina. The ganglion cells were intact and apparently functioning despite the cytoplasmic accumulation of birefringent glycolipid. There was no optic atrophy. The substance in the ganglion cells had the staining and solubility properties of a glycolipid, but, in contrast with Tay-Sachs disease, the material did not stain with Sudan black. Also in contrast to Tay-Sachs disease, the deposited material was entirely intracellular and had not disrupted the ganglion cells.

Mucolipidoses. The mucolipidoses (MLD) are produced by a combined disorder of acid mucopolysaccharide and glycolipid metabolism. This group of diseases appears to be intermediate, in their clinical and pathologic manifestations, between the mucopolysaccharidoses and the sphingolipidoses (Spranger, Wiedemann, 1970). As with the other carbohydrate-lipid disturbances, these conditions result from a deficiency of lysosomal hydrolysis.

Affected persons are mentally retarded and have a variable degree of facial and skeletal dysmorphism but no abnormal mucopolysacchariduria. Electron microscopic studies show intracellular storage of both acid mucopolysaccharide and glycolipids within lysosomal inclusions. The eye manifestations are like those in the mucopolysaccharidoses and sphingolipid disorders and are characterized by either faint grayness of the macula or a frank cherry-red spot. In some, there are optic atrophy and corneal accumulations of stored material. Usually, there is little involvement of the RPE and photoreceptors. Classification of this group of disorders—along with the eye findings, the material stored, and the known enzyme defect—is described in Table 8–6.

Generalized Gangliosidosis (GM_1 Gangliosidosis). In this group of diseases, a deficiency in beta-galactosidase affects the metabolism of both the

Table 8–6. DIFFERENTIAL FEATURES OF THE MUCOLIPIDOSES

MLS Type	Genetics	Ocular Features: *Corneal Clouding*	Ocular Features: *Macular Grayness or Cherry-Red Spot*	Ocular Features: *Optic Atrophy*	Storage Substance	Deficient Enzyme
Generalized gangliosidosis (GM_1 gangliosidosis I)	AR	±	+	+	Keratan sulfate + GM_1 ganglioside	β-Galactosidase A, B, C
Juvenile GM^1 gangliosidosis (GM_1 gangliosidosis II)	AR	−	−	+?	Keratan sulfate + GM_1 ganglioside	β-Galactosidase B, C
Fucosidosis	AR	−	−	−	Fucose-containing AMP + ceramide oligohexoside	α-Fucosidase
Mannosidosis	AR	−	−	−	Mannose-containing glycoprotein	α-Mannosidase
Metachromatic leukodystrophy, Austin variant	AR	±	+	+	Sulfated AMP + sulfatide	Aryl sulfatase A, B, C
Mucolipidosis I (lipomucopolysaccharidosis)	AR	±	+	−	AMP + glycolipid	?
Mucolipidosis II (I-cell disease)	AR	±	−	−	AMP + glycolipid	? β-Galactosidase + ? others
Mucolipidosis III (pseudo-Hurler polydystrophy	AR	+	−	−	AMP + glycolipid	?
Mucolipidosis IV		+	−	−	AMP + glycolipid	?
Sea-blue histiocyte syndrome (chronic Niemann-Pick disease)	AR	−	+	−	? AMP + sphingomyelin	?

AR, autosomal recessive; XR, X-linked recessive; −, absent; ±, variable; +, present; AMP, acid mucopolysaccharide.
After Kenyon KR: Ocular ultrastructure of inherited metabolic disease, *in* Goldberg MF (ed): Genetic and Metabolic Diseases. Boston, Little, Brown, 1974, p 166.

mucopolysaccharides and sphingolipids, and this results in features of both the mucopolysaccharidoses and sphingolipidoses. Three types have been described on the basis of age of onset and which of the isoenzymes of beta-galactosidase are deficient.

Type I (GM_1 Gangliosidosis I) (Generalized Gangliosidosis; Norman-Landing's disease). This is the infantile form, which has variously been called "pseudo-Hurler's disease" and "Tay-Sachs disease with visceral involvement" in the past. The disease is due to deficiency of all three isoenzymes of acid beta-galactosidase (A, B, and C). The main ocular manifestations include progressive corneal clouding and cherry-red spot. Histochemical and electron microscopic studies (Emery, Green, Wyllie, Howell, 1971) have shown mucopolysaccharide deposition in the corneal epithelium, macrophages in the area of Bowman's membrane (Fig. 8–493,*A*), the keratocytes (Fig. 8–493,*B*), nonpigmented ciliary epithelium, and sclerocytes. The ultrastructural appearance of this material was in the form of fibrillogranular cytoplasmic (Fig. 8–493,*C*) inclusions, similar to those seen in the systemic mucopolysaccharides and macular corneal dystrophy. The cytoplasm of the ganglion cells was distended (Fig. 8–493,*D*) by a densely periodic acid–Schiff–positive material (Fig. 8–493,*E*) which, by electron microscopy, was seen to be composed of numerous membrane-bound multimembranous lamellar inclusions (zebra bodies) (Fig. 8–493,*F*) characteristic of most of the sphingolipidoses.

Type II (GM_1 Gangliosidosis II). This is the juvenile form; it is due to deficiency of B and C isoenzymes. Ganglioside accumulates in the brain but not in the viscera. The viscera show excessive amounts of undersulfated keratan sulfate–like mucopolysaccharide. Symptoms develop after the second year, and patients may survive up to 10 years. No corneal clouding or cherry-red spots are observed, but eyes from patients with this type have not been studied histopathologically.

Type III (GM_1 Gangliosidosis III). This is the adult form, and the phenotype has not been consistent. No ocular abnormalities have been observed.

Fucosidosis. Fucosidosis results from a deficiency of alpha-fucosidase activity in the livers of patients with a Hurler-like disorder, severe mental and physical retardation, and normal renal function. Diffuse angiokeratomas are present. Snodgrass (1976) described a patient with fucosidosis who had dilated and tortuous conjunctival vessels and a bull's-eye abnormality in the macula. Ultrastructural studies of the conjunctiva (Libert, Tondeur, Van Hoof, 1976) have shown fibrillogranular and dense granular inclusions in fibrocytes and endothelium. Eyes of patients with this disorder have not been studied.

Mannosidosis. This is a lysosomal storage disorder clinically resembling Hurler's disease. Alpha-mannosidase is deficient, and a glycoprotein containing mannose is deposited in the cerebral cortex, brain stem, spinal medulla, neurohypophysis, retina, and myenteric plexus (Ockerman, 1967).

Histopathologic study of the eyes in this condition have not been conducted. Clinical ocular findings include central corneal opacity in Bowman's membrane and corneal epithelium, dilated and tortuous conjunctival vessels with aneurysms, and dilated and tortuous conjunctival vessels with aneurysms, and dilated and tortuous retinal veins that were beaded and sausage-shaped (Snyder, Carlow, Ledman, Wenger, 1976). Opacities on the anterior surface of the lens and posterior cortical lens changes have been observed (Murphree, Beaudet, Palmer, Nichols, 1976; Arbisser, Murphree, Garcia, Howell, 1976). Biopsies of the conjunctiva have demonstrated fibroblasts, Schwann cells, and macrophages with swollen lysosomes containing fibrillogranular inclusions (Fig. 8–494) (Arbisser and associates, 1976).

Juvenile Sulfatidoses (Metachromatic Leukodystrophy, Austin Variant; Late Infantile Metachromatic Leukoencephalopathy; Metachromatic Form of Diffuse Cerebral Sclerosis). In metachromatic leukodystrophy, the enzymes aryl sulfatase A, B, and C have a defect. These enzymes are normally responsible for removal of sulfate from sulfatide, and their deficiency results in the accumulation of sulfatide in tissues throughout the body. The sulfatide tends to accumulate in the myelin sheaths, where it causes loss of normal function and eventual degeneration. The disease onset is near the age of 1 year, and there is progressive cerebral and nervous system degeneration from this time until death at about age 6 years. Optic atrophy is a common finding, but retinal lesions characterized by grayness of the macular region or a cherry-red spot have also been described.

Cogan, Kuwabara, and Moser (1970) have described the ocular findings of three patients with this disease. In all three, the disease had its onset early in life, and, in all three, the maculae showed abnormal grayness with a cherry-red spot. Metachromatic granules were found in the ganglion cells of the macular region and elsewhere in the retina. In fact, the ganglion cells away from the maculae showed a greater amount of material than those in the macular region. By electron microscopy in two cases, discrete laminated cytoplasmic inclusions were seen in the ganglion cells, corresponding to the metachromatic granules seen by light microscopy. The finding in the retina in these cases was distinct from that seen in Tay-Sachs disease. In the sulfatidosis, the glycolipid is less abundant, is

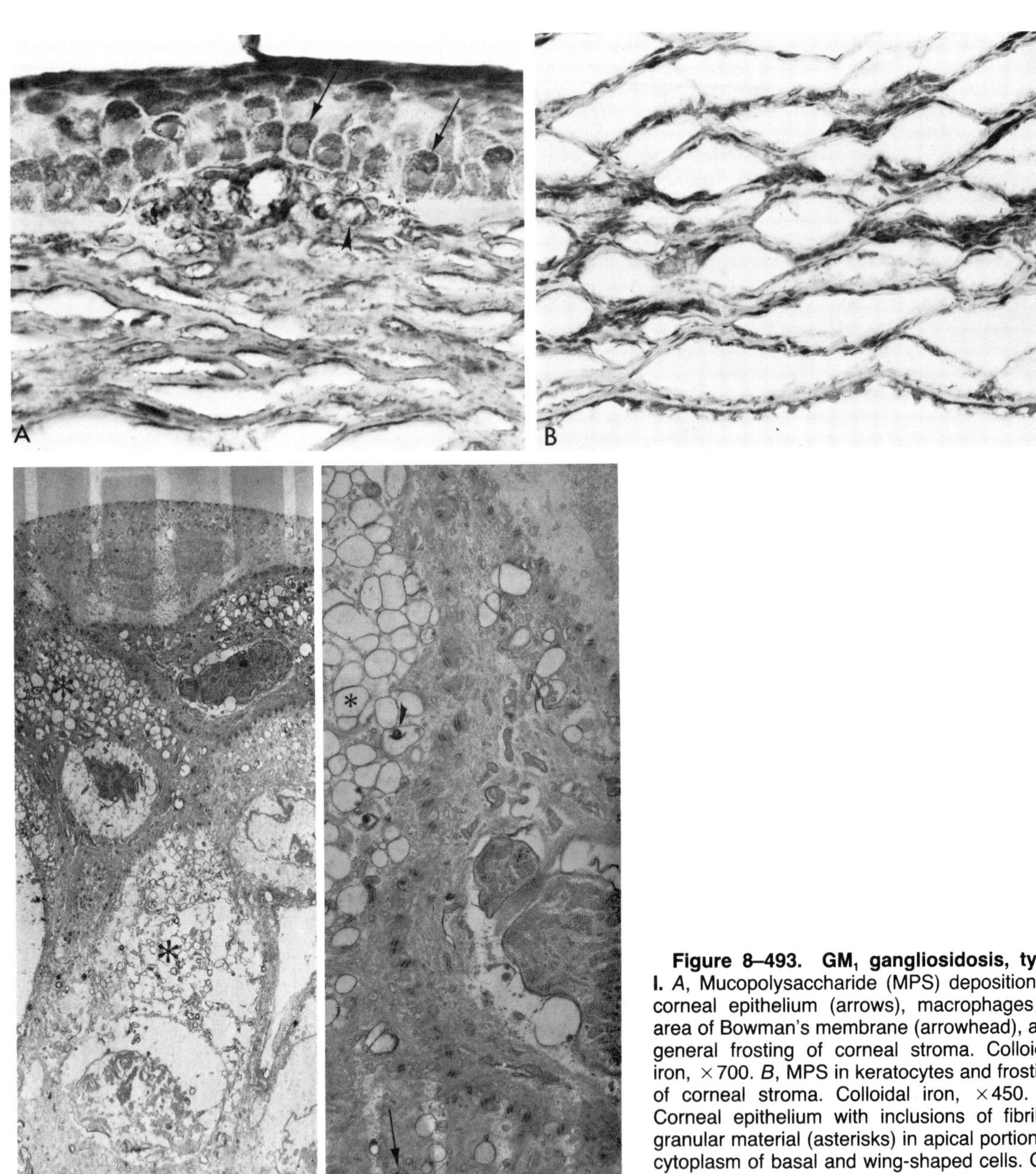

Figure 8–493. GM_1 gangliosidosis, type I. *A*, Mucopolysaccharide (MPS) deposition in corneal epithelium (arrows), macrophages in area of Bowman's membrane (arrowhead), and general frosting of corneal stroma. Colloidal iron, ×700. *B*, MPS in keratocytes and frosting of corneal stroma. Colloidal iron, ×450. *C*, Corneal epithelium with inclusions of fibrillogranular material (asterisks) in apical portion of cytoplasm of basal and wing-shaped cells. Occasional inclusion with fibrillogranular material also has laminated material (arrowhead). Rare inclusion contained only laminated material (arrow). Left, ×5,000; right, ×15,000.

Illustration continued on opposite page

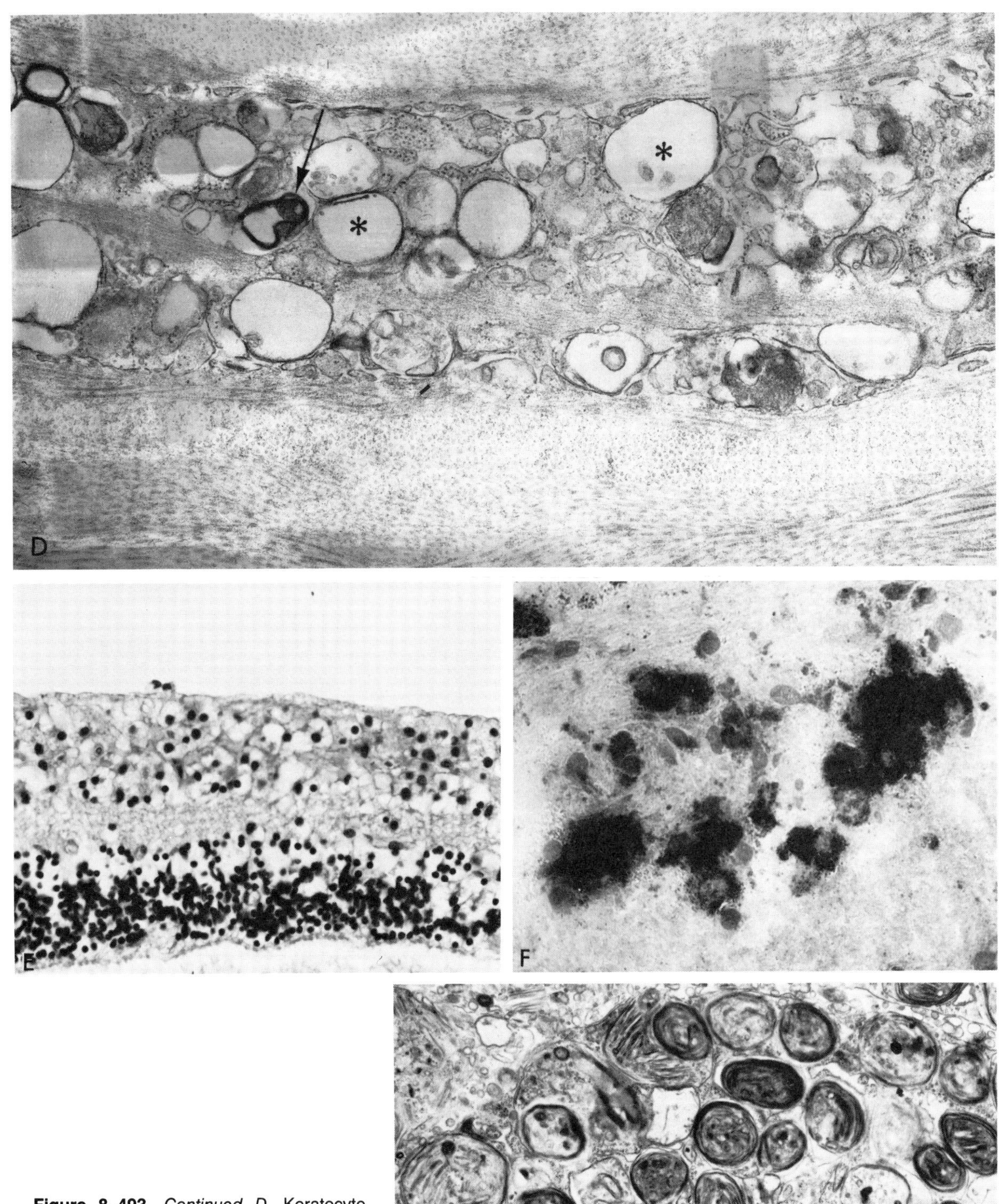

Figure 8–493 *Continued D*, Keratocyte containing cytoplasmic inclusions of fibrillogranular material (asterisks) and some concentric laminated material. ×25,000. *E*, Distended retinal ganglion cells. H and E, × 330. *F*, Cytoplasm of ganglion cell stains well with PAS. Frozen section; PAS, ×600. *G*, Electron micrograph of ganglion cell, with cytoplasm greatly distended by concentric laminated inclusions, ×7,000.

EP 30380. (From Emery JM, Green, WR, Wyllie, RG, Howell, RR: GM_1 gangliosidosis: Ocular manifestations and pathology. Arch Ophthalmol *85*:177–187, 1971.

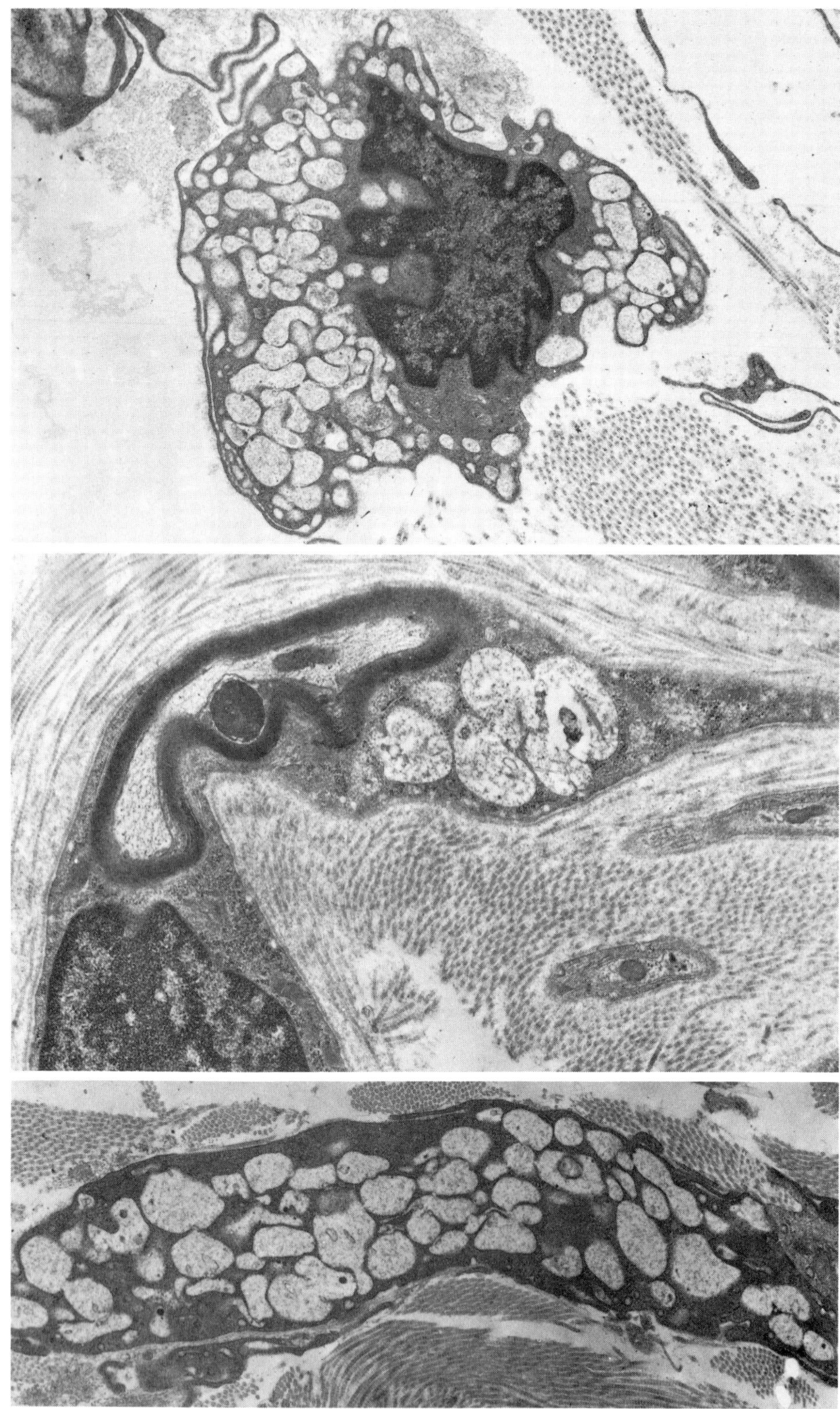

Figure 8–494. Mannosidosis. Conjunctival biopsy specimen showing fibrillogranular inclusion in macrophage (top view, ×9500); Schwann cell (middle, ×16,000); and a fibrocyte (bottom, ×11,100). EP 50176.

chiefly intracellular, and does not produce the white opacification of the entire retina as seen in Tay-Sachs disease. In a previous study, Cogan, Kuwabara, Richardson, Lyon (1958) also demonstrated metachromatic material in glial cells in the peripapillary region.

Weiter, Feingold, Kolodny, and Raghaven (1980) have observed a unique family with a leukocytic arylsulfatase-A deficiency that differed from that of patients with typical metachromatic leukodystrophy: sulfatiduria was absent and cerebroside sulfatase activity was readily detectable. Limited family studies disclosed no evidence of metachromatic leukodystrophy, and the abnormality was progressive retinal pigment epithelial degeneration in the proband.

Ultrastructural study of a conjunctival biopsy specimen showed lysosomal inclusions of both the fibrillogranular and multimembranous types within fibrocytes and epithelial cells (Fig. 8–495).

Mucolipidosis I (MLI) (Lipomucopolysaccharidosis). This genetic metabolic disorder is transmitted as an autosomal trait. Affected individuals have mild Hurler-like features, moderate mental retardation, no excess mucopolysacchariduria, and peculiar inclusions in fibroblasts. Ophthalmoscopic manifestations include variable corneal clouding and grayness of the macula.

Histopathologic studies of the entire eye with MLI have not been conducted, but conjunctival biopsies have shown fibrocytes to contain small, membrane-bound fibrillogranular and membranous inclusions (Kenyon, 1974).

Mucolipidosis II (I Cell Disease). This disease owes its name to a typical aspect of cultured fibroblasts from patients with the disease. Affected patients have a Hurler-like habitus with severe clinical and radiologic features. No excessive mucopolysacchariduria is present. Eye findings include variable corneal clouding. Ultrastructural studies of skin and conjunctiva (Kenyon, Sensenbrenner, 1971; Libert, Kenyon, Maumenee, 1977) disclosed both fibrillogranular and membranous inclusions in fibroblasts, Schwann cells, axonal processes of peripheral nerves, and vascular endothelium. Studies of the whole eye (Libert and associates, 1977), in addition, have demonstrated similar inclusions in keratocytes, sclerocytes, fibroblasts of corneoscleral trabeculum and the uveal tract, and the nonpigmented ciliary epithelium. The myoid portion of the photoreceptor cells and retinal capillary endothelium contained membrane-bound inclusions formed by numerous lamellar rings and granular material. The remaining structures of the eye were free of these inclusions.

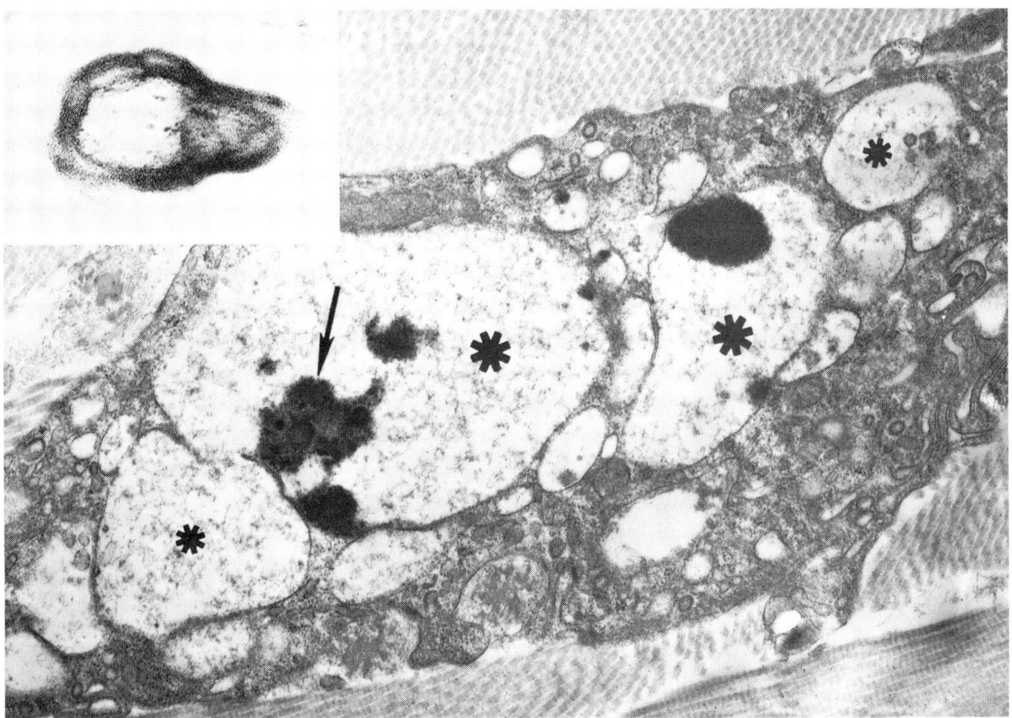

Figure 8–495. Conjunctival biopsy specimen of a patient with multiple sulfatase deficiency, showing a fibrocyte with single membrane–bound fibrillogranular material (asterisks) in which pleomorphic lipofuscin granules (arrow) are eccentrically located. Occasionally a regular laminated membranous inclusion is present (inset). ×16,000; inset, ×87,000. EP 53,449. (From Burk RD, Valle D, Thomas GH, et al: Differential diagnosis of multiple sulfatase deficiency: 2 unrelated males presenting as Hunter's syndrome (MPS II). (Manuscript in preparation.)

Mucolipidosis III (Pseudo-Hurler Polydystrophy). This disease has many features of Hurler's disease but has a much slower clinical evolution and no mucopolysacchariduria. The main ocular finding is corneal clouding. The whole eye from a patient has not been studied histopathologically, but conjunctival biopsy specimens (Quigley, Goldberg, 1971) have demonstrated fibrillogranular and multimembranous inclusions in fibrocytes. Others (Libert, Kenyon, Maumenee, 1977 have observed similar inclusions in capillary endothelial cells and occasional Schwann cells of the conjunctiva. Libert and associates suggested that MLD III may represent a mild phenotype of MLD II.

Mucolipidosis IV. A prominent clinical feature of this condition, which has been observed in children of Ashkenazi extraction, is corneal clouding from birth or early infancy. Psychomotor retardation becomes evident after the first year, but no skeletal dysplasia, facial dysmorphism, or hepatosplenomegaly is evident. Conjunctival biopsy specimens have demonstrated both fibrillogranular and membranous (Merin, Lioni, Berman, 1975; Kenyon, Maumenee, Green, et al, 1979) lamellar inclusions. In addition, studies of a corneal biopsy specimen have disclosed the predisposition for extreme inclusion storage in corneal epithelial cells, with relative sparing of the keratocytes (Kenyon and associates, 1979). The entire eye from a patient with this condition has not been studied.

Newell, Matalon, and Meyer (1975) described a 23 year old man with a new mucolipidosis characterized by the slow development of psychomotor retardation and corneal clouding. The patient developed severe optic atrophy, absence of retinal blood vessels, and an extinguished electroretinogram. Ultrastructural studies of a conjunctival biopsy specimen disclosed membranous and polymorphous inclusion material.

Sea-Blue Histiocyte Disease (Ophthalmoplegic Dystonic Lipidosis; Juvenile Dystonic Lipidosis) (Elfenbein, 1968; de Leon, Kaback, Elfenbein, et al, 1969). This disorder is characterized by splenomegaly, mild thrombocytopenia, and the finding of numerous histiocytes containing blue cytoplasmic granules as stained with the Giemsa technique (Silverstein, Ellefson, Ahern, 1970). It has similarities to Gaucher's disease and adult Niemann-Pick disease. A whitish ring around the fovea has been described.

Libert, Martin, Moser, et al (1981) noted that histopathologic studies confirm that the disease is a lysosomal storage disorder although the enzyme defect is unknown. Abnormal lysosomes contain a lamellar material with a loose arrangement or with a multivesicular pattern. The neurons and the reticuloendothelial cells are affected, but the epithelial cells, the blood and lymphatic endothelial cells, and the connective tissue cells are spared. This distribution of inclusions resembles that of Niemann-Pick disease, type C. Because of this feature and clinical similarities, these two diseases may represent different phenotypes of the same disease.

Study of the eye in this condition has revealed a mild accumulation of membranous cytoplasmic bodies in the retinal ganglion cells, similar to those seen in the brain. Skin and conjunctival biopsies may show histiocytes similar to those in bone marrow and spleen histiocytes. Ultrastructural study of bone marrow biopsy specimens appears to be the most reliable way to help establish the diagnosis (Libert, Martin, Moser, et al, 1981).

Neuraminidase Deficiency (Neuraminidase Deficiency in the Cherry-Red Spot Myoclonus Syndrome) (Rapin, Katzman, Engel, 1975; Kelly, Graetz, 1977; O'Brien, 1977). This storage disease is caused by a lysosomal enzyme deficiency, is slowly progressive, has an onset in adolescence, affects non-Jewish persons, and is inherited as an autosomal recessive trait. Persons with this disease have coarse facies, hepatosplenomegaly, and dysostosis multiplex. Patients also have increased deep tendon reflexes and may have myoclonic seizures. Dementia is not a feature. A conjunctival biopsy specimen (Sogg, Steinman, Rathjen, et al, 1979) shows fibrocytes with lysosomal inclusions of probable oligosaccharides. The Goldberg syndrome may be this same entity (McKusick, 1978, page 614).

Studies of eyes from a patient with probable cherry-red spot myoclonus syndrome (Font, personal communication, 1980) have shown lipid deposition in the retinal ganglion cells. The patient was originally considered to have Kuf's disease (Font, 1971).

Miscellaneous Systemic Diseases with Retinal Involvement

Neuronal Ceroid Lipofuscinosis (Batten-Vogt Syndrome). This group of diseases is characterized by the accumulation of lipopigments of the ceroid/lipofuscin type in neurons (Zeman, Dyken, 1969).

Zeman and Dyken (1969) have abandoned the age-dependent classification of the "amaurotic familial idiocies" and have divided them into two groups. One group is caused by abnormal ganglioside metabolism and includes GM_2 gangliosidosis, type I (Tay-Sachs disease) (see page 1118); GM_2 gangliosidosis, type II (Sandhoff's disease) (see page 1119); and GM_2 gangliosidosis, type III (juvenile Tay-Sachs disease) (see page 1119); and others.

The second group is the neuronal ceroid lipofuscinoses and includes the infantile type (Haltia-

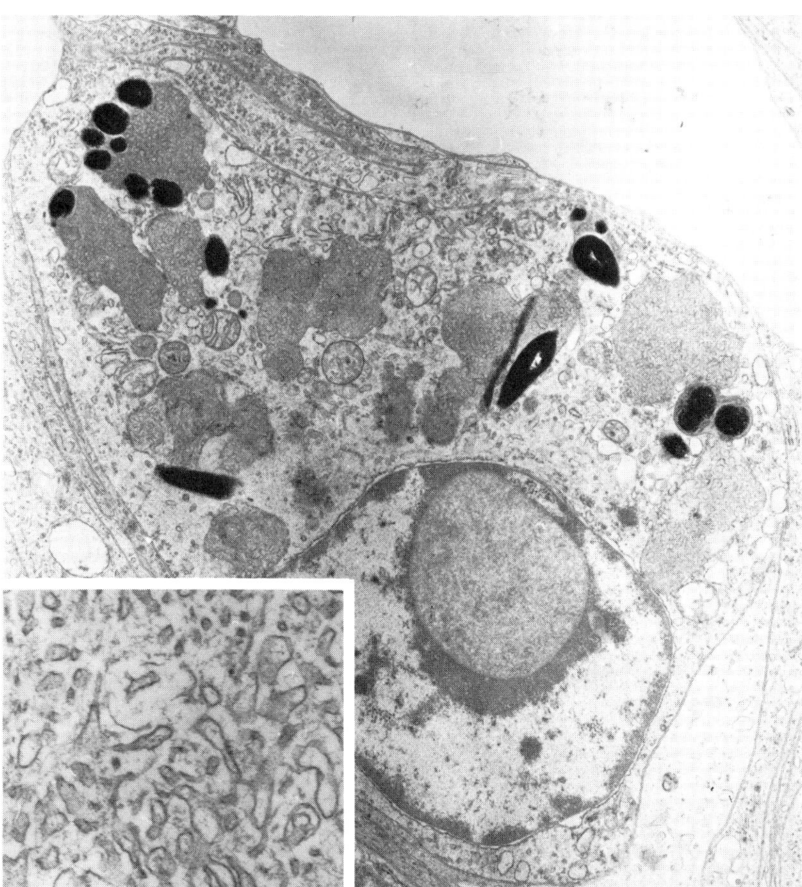

Figure 8–496. Late infantile neuronal ceroid lipofuscinosis. Retinal ganglion cell showing typical curvilinear inclusions in cytoplasm. ×15,000; inset, ×35,000. EP 37425.

Santavuori); the late infantile type (Jansky-Beilschowsky); the juvenile type (Batten's disease, Vogt-Spielmeyer, Spielmeyer-Sjögren); and the adult type (Kufs' disease). The biochemical defect in this group remains obscure. This group of diseases is characterized by the accumulation of autofluorescent lipopigments in neural, visceral, and somatic tissues. This material is present in cytosomes and has a characteristic curvilinear ultrastructural appearance (Fig. 8–496).

Infantile Type (Haltia-Santavuori Type). This disease has an early onset before the age of 2 years and is rapidly progressive, with psychomotor deterioration and blindness (Santavuori, Haltia, Rapola, 1974).

Late Infantile Type (Jansky-Bielschowsky Type). Retinal changes include variable pigmentation in the posterior pole and periphery, slowly progressive retinal vessel attenuation, and optic atrophy (Hittner, Zeller, 1975). Lipid material has been demonstrated in retinal ganglion cells (Wolter, Allen, 1964). As the disease progresses, widespread loss of the photoreceptor cells and minor migration of pigment into the outer retinal area occur (Givner, Roizin, 1944; Klien, 1954; Schochet, Font, Morris, 1980). Some cases may have a "bull's-eye" configuration in the macula, caused by the accumulation of pigmented cells in a ring configuration under the macular retina (Fig. 8–497).

Shochet, Font, and Morris (1980) observed a bull's eye macular lesion (Fig. 8–498,*A*), partial photoreceptor cell degeneration in the posterior pole (Fig. 8–498,*B*), distended ganglion cells (Fig. 8–498,*B* and *C*), and numerous membrane-bound cytosomes containing curvilinear material in retinal pigment epithelium (Fig. 8–498,*D*), inner segments of photoreceptor cells (Fig. 8–498,*E*), Müller cells (Fig. 8–498,*F*), retinal ganglion cells, (Fig. 8–498,*G*), iris pigment epithelium (Fig. 8–498,*H*), and iris dilator muscle cells (Fig. 8–498,*I*).

Juvenile Type (Spielmeyer-Sjögren Type). Severe retinal changes also occur in this form of neuronal ceroid-lipofuscinosis (Manschot, 1968c; Göttinger, Minauf, 1971). Goebel, Fix, and Zeman (1974) have observed total loss of the photoreceptor cell layer in two advanced cases, and partial preservation of the outer nuclear layer in the periphery of one patient with a shorter clinical duration. Electron microscopic studies (Goebel and associates, 1974) showed accumulation of curvilinear and occasional "fingerprint" bodies in the ganglion cells. Zebra bodies were observed in

Text continued on page 1149

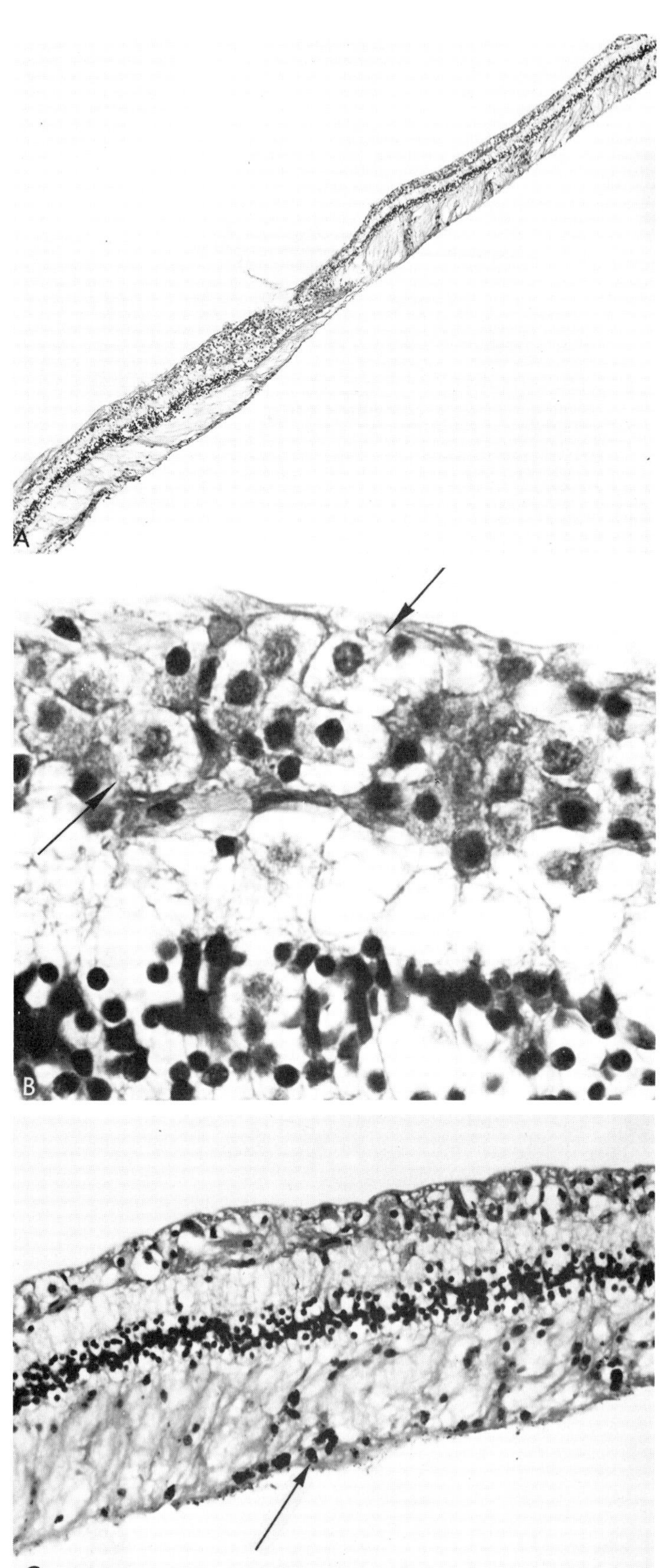

Figure 8–497. Late infantile neuronal ceroid lipofuscinosis. *A*, Section through macula shows severe atrophy of photoreceptor cell layer. H and E, ×40. *B*, Higher power view showing distended ganglion cells (arrows). H and E, ×875. *C*, Higher power view showing total loss of outer nuclear layer and migration of pigment into outer aspect of retina (arrow). Accumulation of these pigmented cells appears to correspond to "bull's-eye" pattern seen ophthalmoscopically. H and E, × 230. EP 37425.

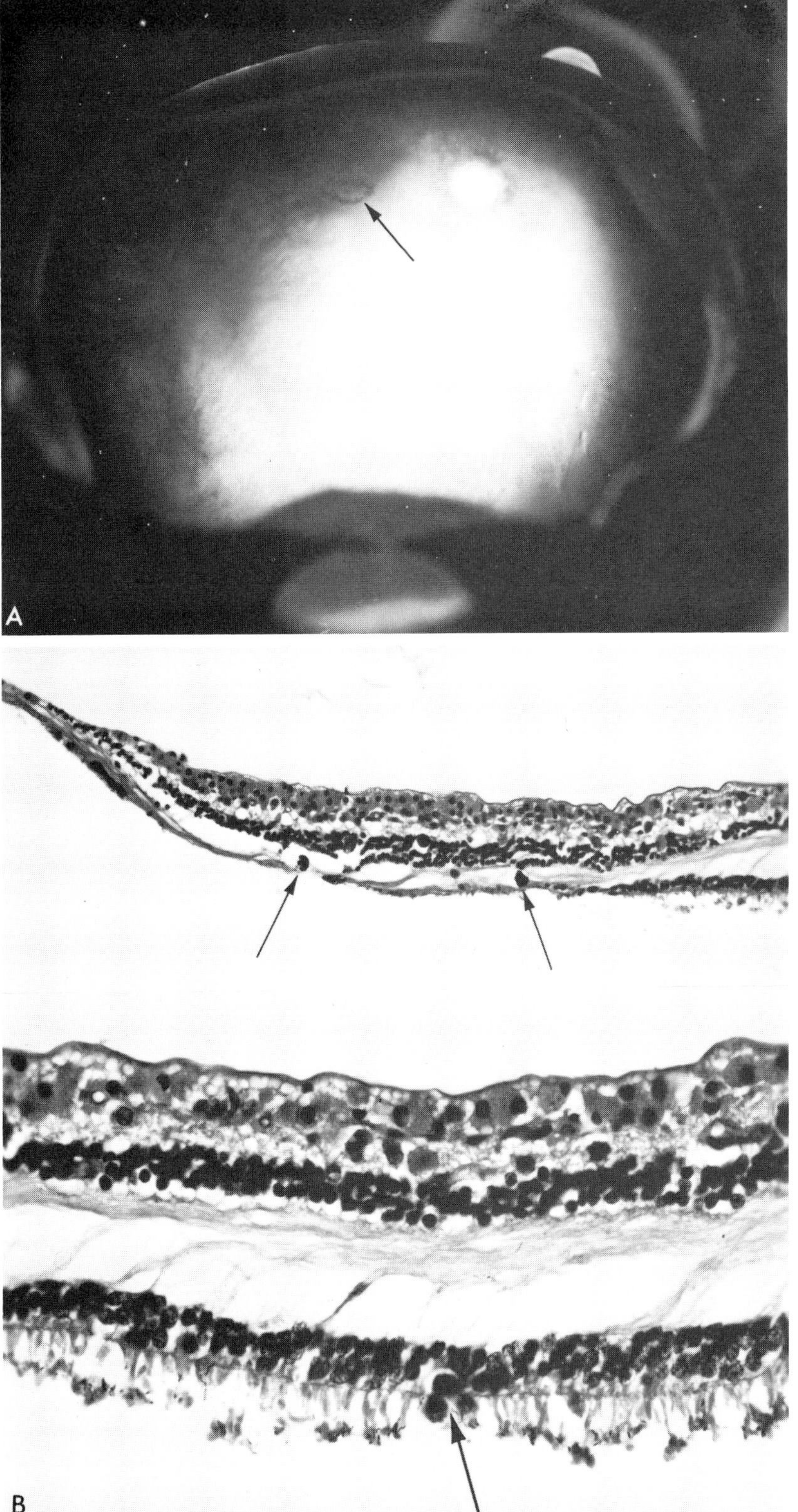

Figure 8–498. *A*, With transillumination, posterior pole of eye shows distinct ring of pigment around foveola (arrow). Pigmentation was difficult to see on direct examination. Optic disk is pale. AFIP Neg. 78-85059-1. *B*, Top, Photoreceptors and outer nuclear layer, present on right, become severely degenerated as they approach center of foveola (at left). Scattered pigment-laden macrophages cling to the outer plexiform layer of the retina (arrows). PAS, ×160. AFIP Neg. 79-11280. Bottom, Paramacular region shows good preservation of retinal architecture and many enlarged ganglion cells with distended PAS-positive granular cytoplasm and eccentric nuclei. A few PAS-positive macrophages are attached to the outer retina (arrow). PAS, ×400. AFIP Neg. 79-11281.

Illustration continued on following page

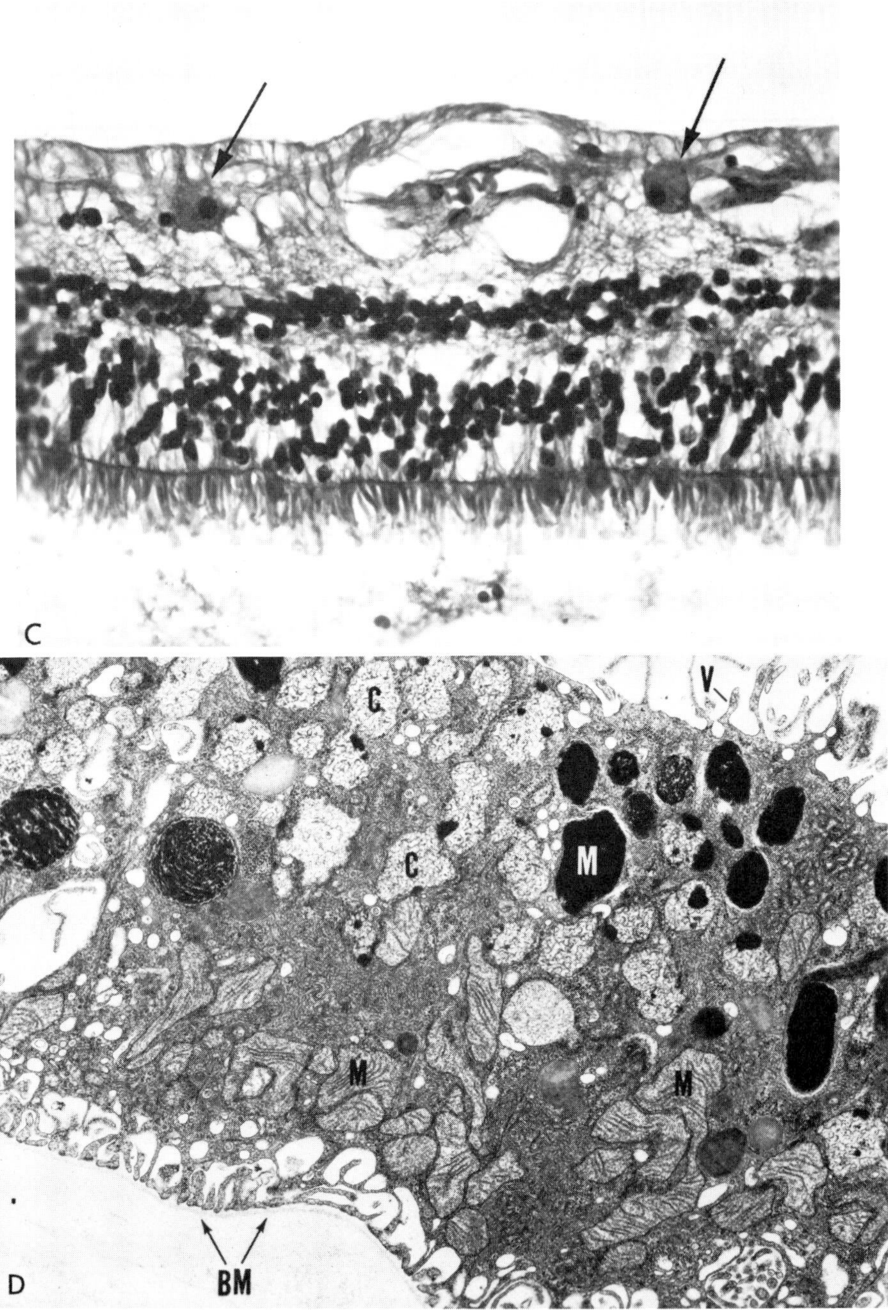

Figure 8–498 *Continued C*, Midperiphery of retina, nasally, shows relatively good preservation of architecture (except for mild postmortem autolysis of outer segments of photoreceptors). Two ganglion cells (arrows) with distended granular cytoplasm and eccentric nuclei are present. (AFIP Neg. 79-11282. H and E, ×160. *D*, Retinal pigment epithelial cells show numerous membrane-bound cytosomes (*C*) located mainly toward the middle and apical portions of cells. Mitochondria (*M*) are located toward basilar cytoplasm. White *M* indicates melanin granule; *BM* , basement membrane: *V*, villi. ×13,125. AFIP Neg. 79-12604-1.

Illustration continued on opposite page

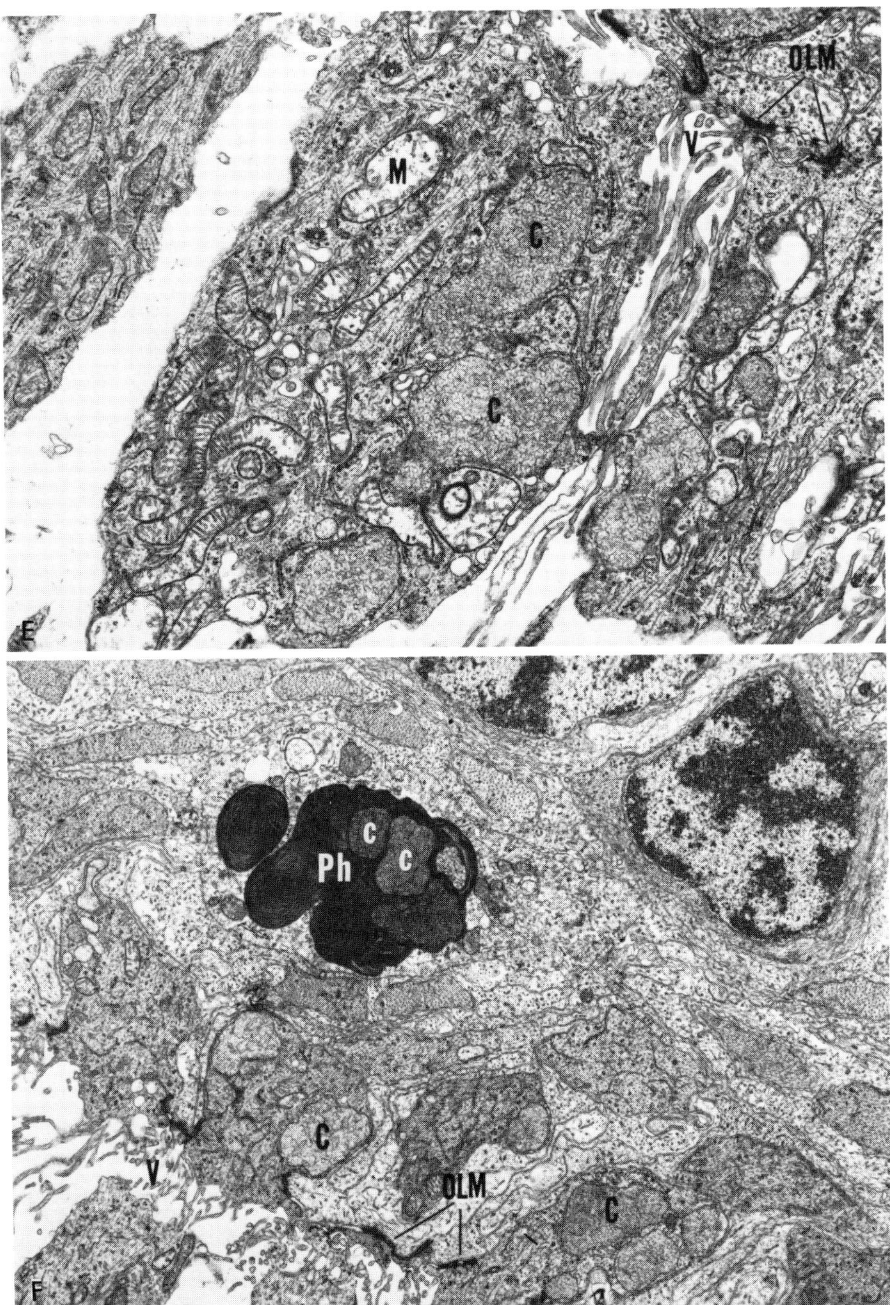

Figure 8–498 *Continued E*, Inner segment of cone cell displaying numerous mitochondria *(M)* and larger membrane-bound cytosomes (*C*) containing curvilinear structures. Numerous microvilli *(V)* from Müller cells are present. *OLM*, outer limiting membrane. ×13,125. AFIP Neg. 79-12604-2. *F*, Portion of lucent cytoplasm of Müller cell containing large phagosome *(Ph)* that has incorporated several dense, membrane-bound cytosomes (white *C*). *OLM*, outer limiting membrane; black *C*, cytosomes. Numerous microcilli *(V)* from Müller cells are present. ×8438. AFIP Neg. 79-12604-3.

Illustration continued on following page

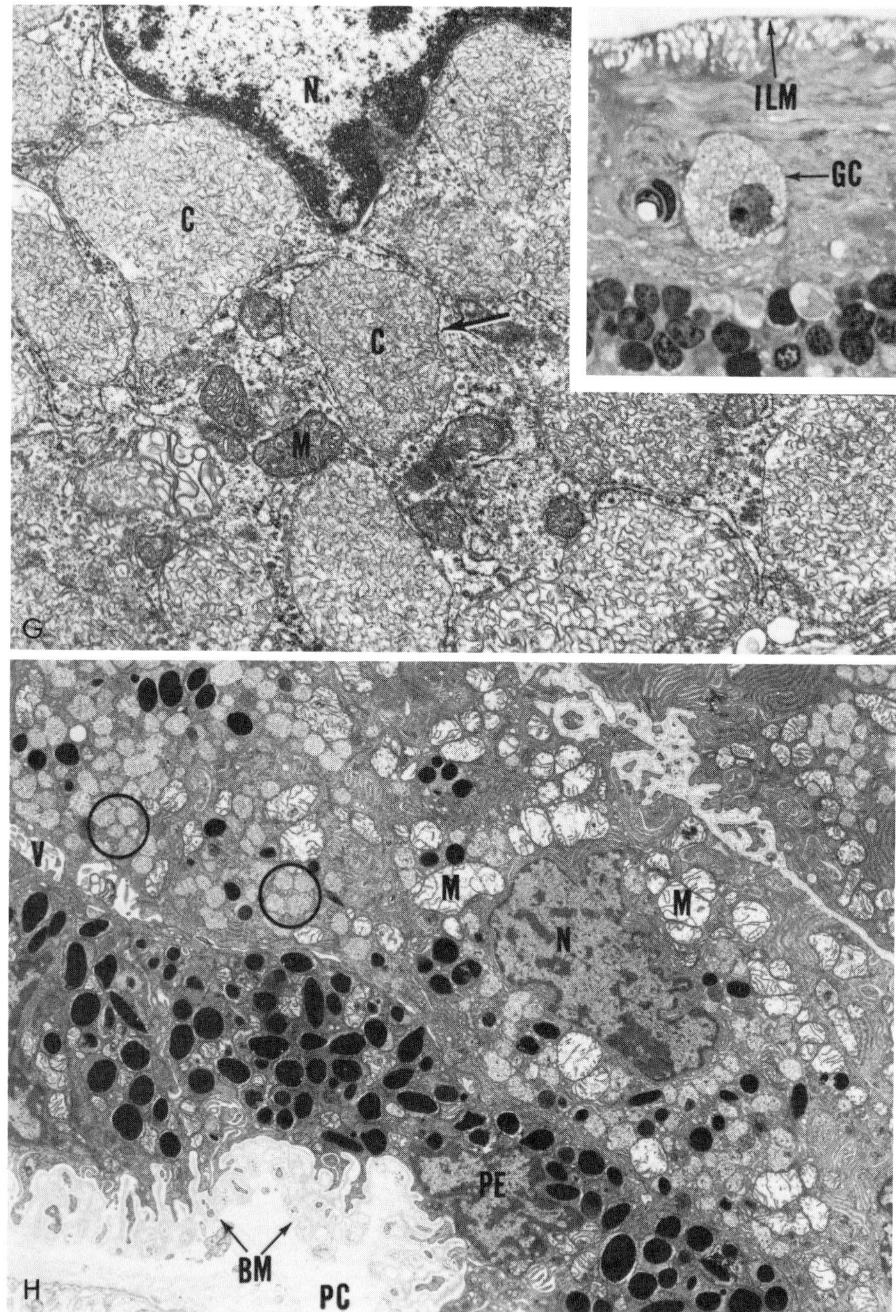

Figure 8–498 *Continued G*, Swollen ganglion cell cytoplasm with numerous cytosomes *(C)*, each surrounded by membrane (arrow) and containing curvilinear bodies. Cytosomes indent nucleus *(N)*. *M*, mitochondrium. ×18,750. AFIP Neg. 79-12604-4. Inset: Distended ganglion cell *(GC)* with finely vacuolated cytoplasm. *ILM*, internal limiting membrane. Toluidine blue, ×740. *H*, Double layer of iris pigment epithelium demonstrates large number of cytosomes (within circles) located predominantly in the anterior cell layer. *BM*, basement membrane of posterior layer; *M*, mitochondria; *PC*, posterior chamber; *PE*, nucleus of pigment epithelial cell. ×6000. AFIP Neg. 12604-5.

Illustration continued on opposite page

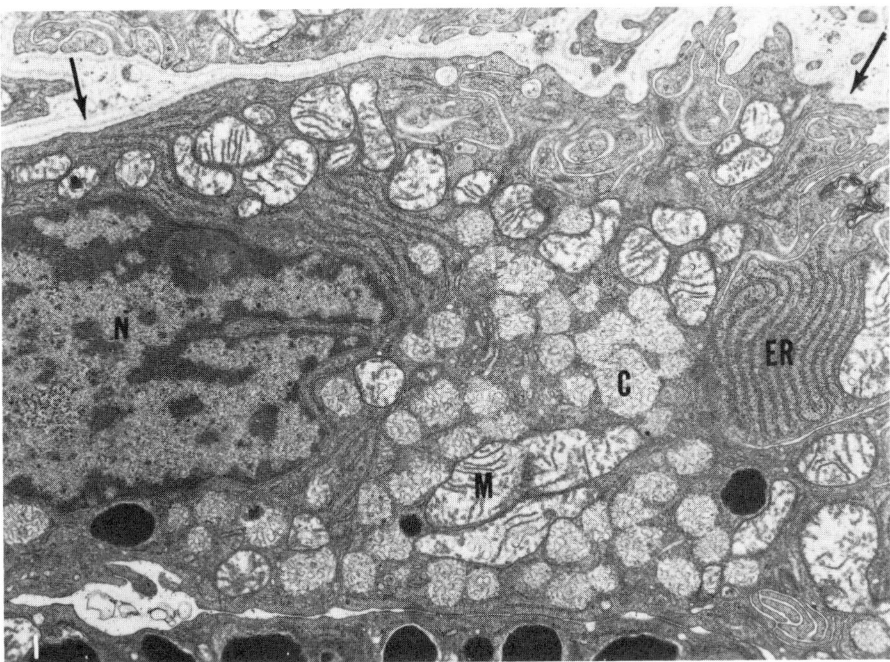

Figure 8–498 *Continued I.* Anterior cell layer of iris pigment epithelium discloses numerous membrane-bound cytosomes *(C)* intermixed with slightly swollen mitochondria *(M)*. Arrows, basement membrane; *ER*, endoplasmic reticulum; *N*, nucleus. ×14,000. AFIP Neg. 79-12604-6.

(From Schochet SS Jr, Font RL, Morris HH III: Jansky-Bielschowsky form of neuronal ceroid-lipofuscinosis. Ocular pathology of the Batten-Vogt syndrome. Arch Ophthalmol *98*:1083–1088, 1980.)

sclerocytes. The RPE was largely atrophic. Pigmented cells were present in the deeper layers of the retina.

Spalton, Taylor, and Sanders (1980) have observed that patients with the juvenile type also may have a "bull's-eye" configuration in the macula. More advanced retinal degeneration with a retinitis pigmentosa–like picture may evolve as the disease progresses. The diagnosis is supported by finding vacuolated lymphocytes and "fingerprint" (multilaminated) bodies in neurons in a retinal biopsy specimen. They suggest that phototoxicity may have a partial role in the retinal degeneration.

Adult Type (Kufs' Type). The occurrence of the juvenile and adult forms in the same family and the presence of similar anatomic characteristics suggest that these two types are probably entities that have variable ages of onset (Zeman, Hoffman, 1962). Eyes from patients with Kufs' disease have not been studied to our knowledge.

Heterozygotes and carriers of the juvenile type (Merritt, Smith, Strouth, Zeman, 1968) and the adult type (Witzleben, 1972) can be detected by the presence of inclusions in lymphocytes.

Two additional forms have been described. One is the infantile Finnish type (Hagberg, Sourander, Svennerholm, 1968), which is recessive; and the other has a late onset, is dominant, and is referred to as the Perry type (Boehme, Cottrell, Leonberg, Zeman, 1971).

Abetalipoproteinemia (Bassen-Kornzweig Syndrome). This condition is a rare familial disease characterized biochemically by absence of beta-lipoproteins. Intestinal absorption of lipids is defective, and plasma cholesterol, phospholipids, and tryglycerides are very low. In addition, there is faulty intestinal absorption of the fat-soluble vitamins. There appears to be a defect in the ability of cells to manufacture the protein component of beta-lipoprotein (Salt, Wolff, Lloyd, et al, 1960). This condition was described by Bassen and Kornzweig (1950). They found atypical retinitis pigmentosa, neuromuscular disturbances like those in Friedreich's ataxia, and abnormal-appearing red blood cells in their patients. Eye changes include xanthelasma, arcus, and retinal pigmentary degeneration.

Gouras, Carr, and Gunkel (1971) found that these patients have a severe vitamin A deficiency when maintained on a normal diet, and that this deficiency leads to the severe impairment of vision. There are abnormalities in dark adaptation and the electroretinogram that involve both the rod and cone receptor systems. Those investigators and others (Sperling, Hiles, Kennerdell, 1972) also found that massive doses of vitamin A tend to reverse these abnormalities. These and other findings suggest the possibility that the retinitis pigmentosa observed in abetalipoproteinemia is due solely to vitamin A deficiency.

Von Sallman, Gelderman, and Laster (1969) reported the light microscopic findings in the posterior segment of the eyes, from a patient with this syndrome whose vision was greatly reduced because the visual fields were markedly constricted. The main findings were those of advanced retinitis pigmentosa. In the macular area, there was slight preservation of the photoreceptor cells and the RPE (Fig. 8–499,*A*). Outside this area there were extensive-to-complete degeneration of the photoreceptor cells (Fig. 8–499,*B*) and extensive hyperplasia of the RPE, with migration into the retina in a perivascular location (Fig. 8–

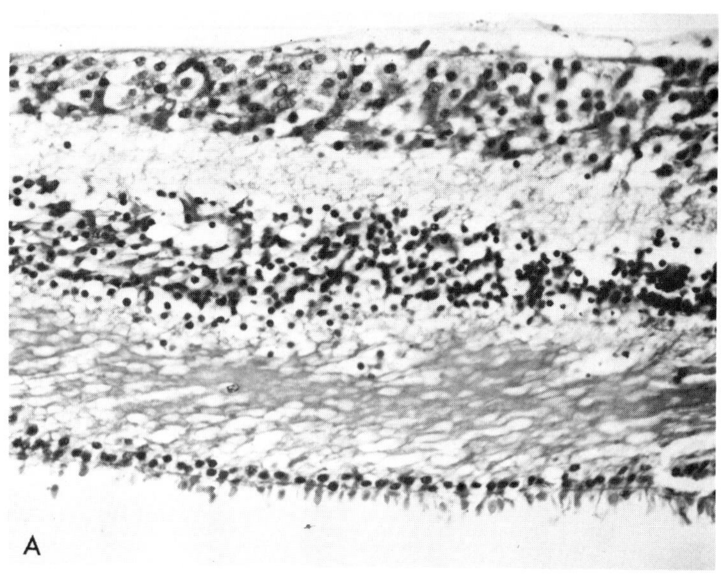

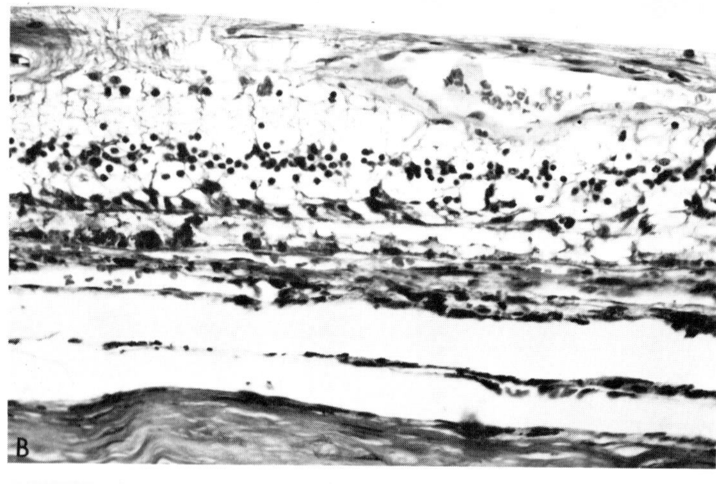

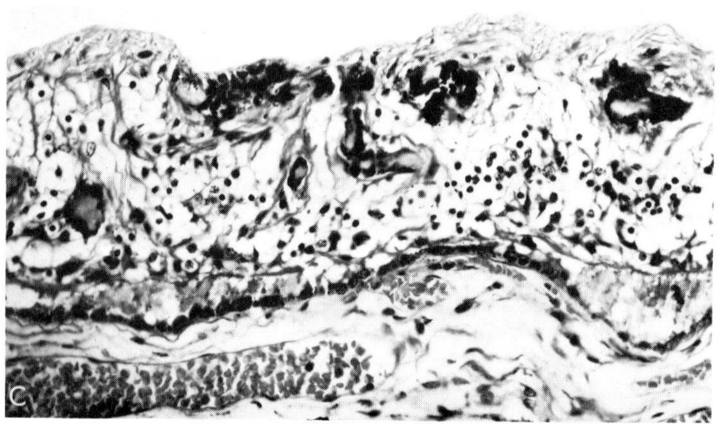

Figure 8–499. Bassen-Kornzweig syndrome. *A*, Parafoveal area showing normal ganglion cell, and inner nuclear, and plexiform layers. Outer nuclear layer is much reduced in thickness; outer segments are absent; and the remaining few inner segments are stubby. H and E, ×310. *B*, Midperiphery, showing discontinuous retinal pigment epithelium (RPE) and photorecepter cell degeneration. H and E, ×300. *C*, Equatorial area, showing total photorecepter cell atrophy and much RPE hyperplasia, with migration into retina in perivascular location. H and E, ×300. EP 34436.

499,*C*). Retinal blood vessels were markedly sclerotic, with hyalinization of their walls and reduction in lumen caliber.

Abetalipoproteinemia is one of the 35 or more systemic syndromes in which a retinitis pigmentosa–like picture is observed (see page 1220).

Maculopathy Simulating "Cherry-Red Spot" in a Patient with Crohn's Disease. Yassur, Snir, Melamed, and Ben-Sira (1981) have described the occurrence of a cherry-red spot in a patient with Crohn's disease being treated with parenteral hyperalimentation who developed copper and zinc deficiency. This appears to be an example of an acquired lipidosis secondary to the deficiency of zinc and copper.

Refsum's Disease (Refsum, 1957). This disease is characterized by a hypertrophic peripheral retinopathy of relapsing character, progressive paresis of the distal extremities, cerebellar ataxia, markedly elevated cerebrospinal fluid protein with albuminocytologic dissociation, nerve deafness, and retinitis pigmentosa (Steinberg, Vroom, Engel, et al, 1967). The underlying biochemical abnormality is a defect in oxidation of phytanic acid. Phytanic acid accumulates in the tissues throughout the body, but the main site is in the myelin sheaths of the nerves of the central and peripheral nervous systems. The disease commences in early childhood and is inherited as an autosomal recessive condition. Night blindness and progressively constricted visual fields are an important part of the clinical picture.

Histopathologic studies of the eye in Refsum's disease are few. One patient who had corneal edema and was grafted was found to have nonspecific histopathologic changes by light microscopy and no fatty acid in the cornea when analyzed by gas-liquid chromatography (Baum, Tannenbaum, Kolodny, 1965).

Levy (1970) noted photoreceptor cell loss and migration of pigmented cells into the retina.

Toussaint and Danis (1970) conducted histologic and histochemical studies of eyes from a patient with Refsum's disease. They observed the changes of retinitis pigmentosa, with atrophy of the photoreceptors and ganglion cells and decrease in the population of cells in the nuclear layers, and atrophy and disappearance of numerous areas of the RPE. Optic atrophy was secondary to degeneration of the ganglion cells and involvement of the myelin sheaths of the optic nerve behind the disk. The retinal vessel walls were generally thickened and diffusely loaded with lipid material that stained with Sudan 3 and Sudan black. There also was perivascular accumulation of pigmented cells that were infiltrated with lipid material. In addition, they observed lipid material in the remaining RPE.

Lipoid Proteinosis (Urbach-Wiethe Disease). This condition is a hereditary lipoglycoproteinosis that affects the skin and mucosae. The most characteristic ophthalmologic feature is the occurrence of multiple nodules of the lid margins. Drusen of Bruch's membrane are seen in about 50 per cent of cases (François, Bacskulin, Follmann, 1968).

The disease is transmitted as an autosomal recessive trait and becomes manifest early in life. The skin and mucosal nodules result from an accumulation of PAS-positive and sudanophilic material which has been identified as a complex of mucopolysaccharide or lipid bound to a glycoprotein. The material is deposited extracellularly in the skin of various portions of the body, including the eyelid margins. Mucous membrane may be involved, including the mouth and larynx.

Macular degeneration has been reported in this condition, and reddish-yellow drusen-like deposits have been observed in the foveal macular region.

Marquardt (1962) described similar PAS-positive deposits in the region of Bruch's membrane, and between Bruch's membrane and the RPE. In addition, a similar material involved the endothelium of the capillaries and walls of the retinal arterioles and the choriocapillaris of the choroid.

Lafora's Disease (Myoclonic Epilepsy of Unverricht and Lundborg). Unverricht (1891) described a fatal, hereditary form of diffuse neuronal disease, transmitted as an autosomal recessive trait and beginning in late childhood, with major central nervous system disturbance that ended with dementia, paralyses, blindness, and death. When this syndrome is associated with basophilic deposits that are positive with the PAS stain (Lafora bodies) in the central nervous system, retina, and other tissues, it is often known as Lafora's disease (Schwartz, Yanoff, 1965). A second form of the disease (Lundborg type) has a more benign course initially, but death occurs at a later stage.

The malady is described as a derangement of carbohydrate metabolism, with deposition of glycoprotein-S mucopolysaccharide in the affected tissues. Histologically, Lafora bodies, which are laminated, are found in the inner layers of the retina—some being intracellular and some extracellular. These bodies also may be found in the retina (Fig. 8–500,*A*), the optic nerve, and iris (Fig. 8–500,*B*). The cause of blindness in this disturbance is the combination of cortical changes, with extensive damage to the inner retinal neurons (Yanoff, Schwartz, 1965a and b).

Ultrastructural studies (Collins, Cowden, Nevis, 1968) disclose the Lafora body to contain a complex carbohydrate, of which a small portion is an acid mucopolysaccharide, and a protein, mostly sensitive to chymotrypsin and especially to pepsin. Collins and associates (1968) also observed abnormalities in neurons and glial cells in addi-

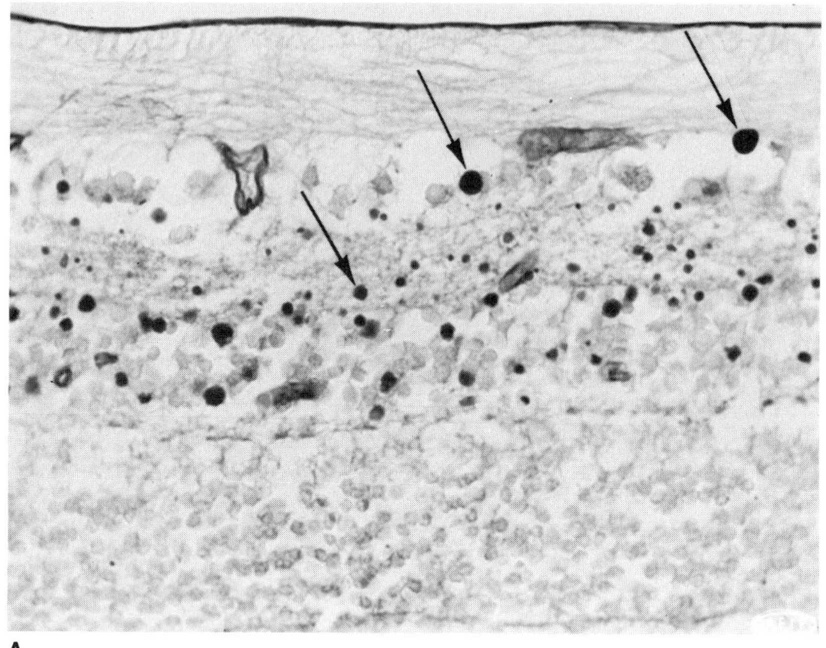

A

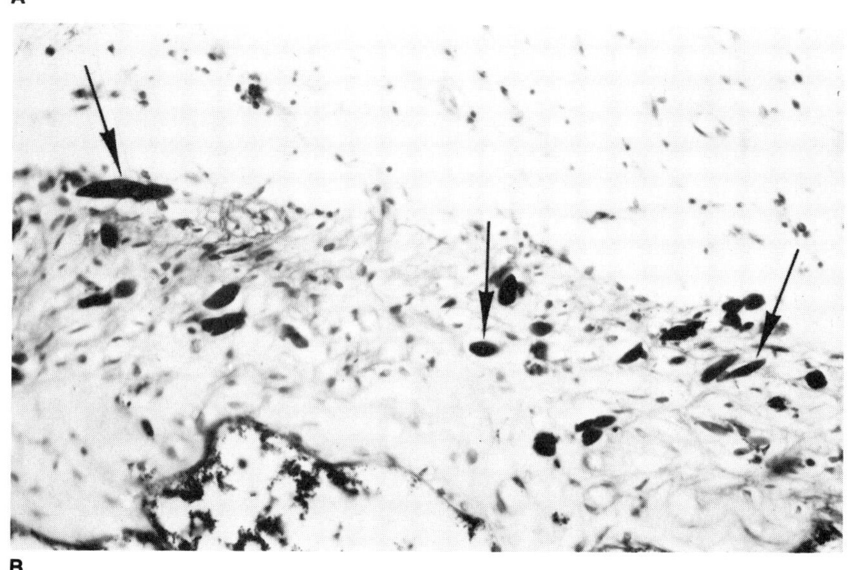

B

Figure 8–500. *A*, **Lafora bodies** (arrows) in retina. PAS, ×485. AFIP Neg. 64-6294. (From Yanoff, M, Schwartz, GA: The retinal pathology of Lafora's disease: A form of glycoprotein acid–mucopolysaccharide dystrophy. Trans Am Acad Ophthalmol Otolaryngol *69*:701–708, 1965.) *B*, Lafora bodies (arrows) in iris. (Courtesy of Dr. D.G. Cogan; case presented at combined meeting of Verhoeff Society and European Ophthalmic Pathology Society, Washington, DC, April, 1976.)

tion to the presence of Lafora bodies. The fundamental unit of the Lafora body appears to be a fibril with a diameter of 70 to 100 angstroms and occasional tubular structures that occur in association with endoplasmic reticulum and ribosomal material. Biopsy of the liver may disclose hepatocytes containing inclusions having a ground-glass appearance. This finding may be helpful in establishing a diagnosis, even with normal liver function (Nishimura, Ishak, Peddick, et al, 1980).

Von Gierke's Disease (Glycogen Storage Disease, Type I; Type I Glycogenosis). Von Gierke's disease is due to a low or absent activity of glucose-6-phosphatase and is characterized by short stature, massive hepatomegaly, hypoglycemia, lactic acidosis, and hyperlipidemia. The eyes in this disease have not been studied, but clinical studies have shown multiple bilateral and symmetric paramacular lesions that were yellowish, nonelevated, and discrete (Fine, Wilson, Donnell, 1968).

There are at least seven different types of glycogen storage diseases (McKusick, 1978: 23220, 23240, 23250, 23260, 23270, and 23280). Figure 8–501 illustrates glycogen deposits in the iris pigment epithelium and Müller cells of the retina of a 12 year old girl with probable Type I glycogenosis (von Gierke's disease).

Pompe's Disease (Glycogen Storage Disease, Type II; Type II Glycogenosis; Acid Maltase Deficiency). This recessively inherited disease re-

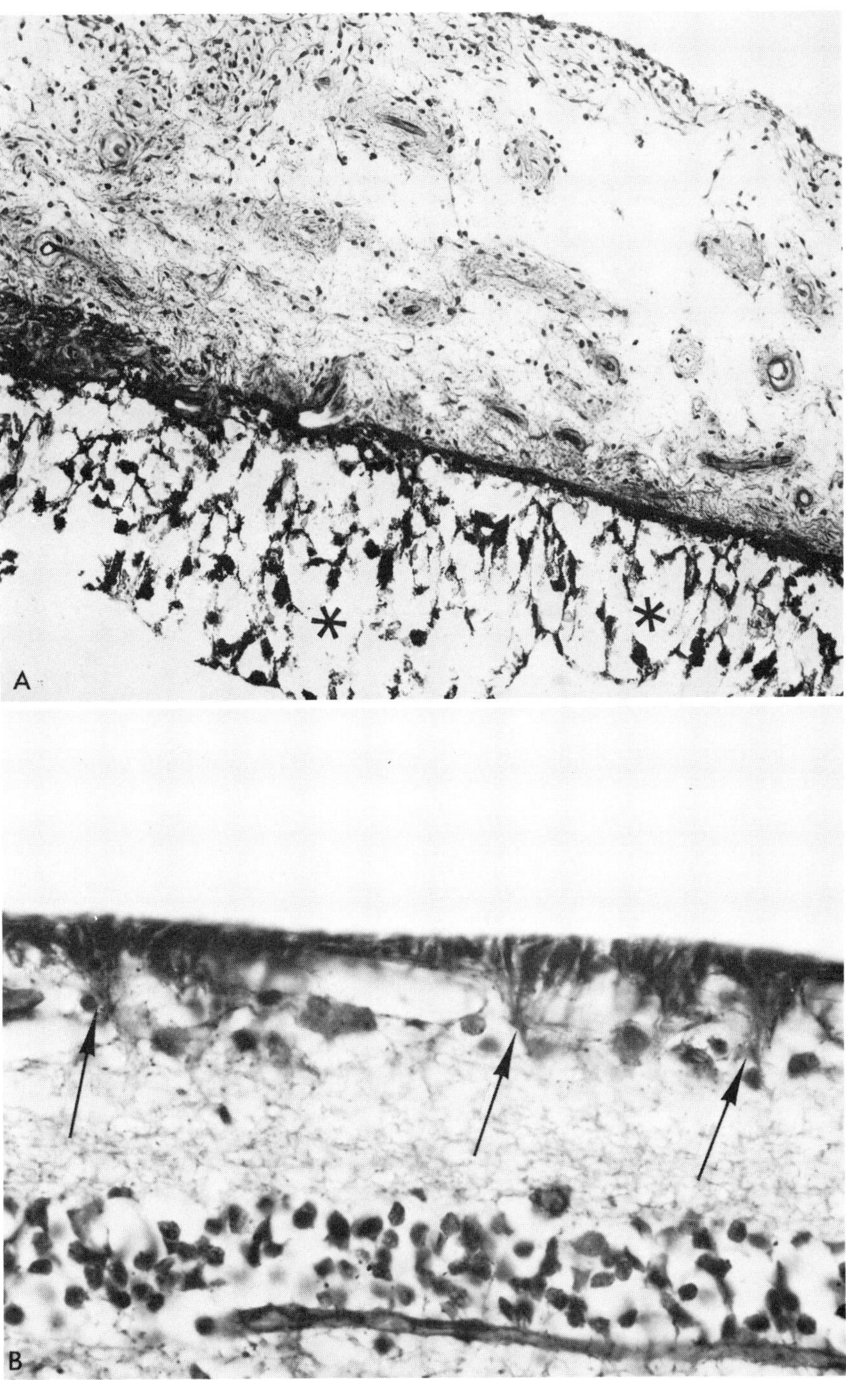

Figure 8–501. Type I glycogenosis. *A,* Iris, showing extreme vacuolization (asterisks) in pigment epithelium because of glycogen accumulation. PAS, ×185. *B,* Glycogen accumulation in footplate area of Müller cells (arrows) of retina. PAS, ×600. EP 42351.

sults from a defect of acid alpha-1,4-glucosidase, with an accumulation of glycogen throughout the body. Affected children are prostrate, appear imbecilic, are markedly hypotonic, and have enlarged hearts. In the classic cases, death occurs in the first year and cardiac involvement is prominent. Less severe forms of the disease also have been recognized, with death occurring at about age 10 years.

Glycogen was initially reported in the pericytes of the retinal vessels by Cogan (1963). A later study by Toussaint and Danis (1965) described in more detail the findings in the retina of a patient with generalized glycogenosis. The patient and her sister were both affected. Clinical symptoms developed at 4 months of age, with dyspnea, cyanosis, and lid edema. Examination showed general hypotonia, a pale, swollen skin, severe dyspnea and cyanosis, and deformation of the thorax. Biochemical studies showed elevated glycogen levels in muscles and liver. Enzymatic studies disclosed that acid maltase was absent in the liver

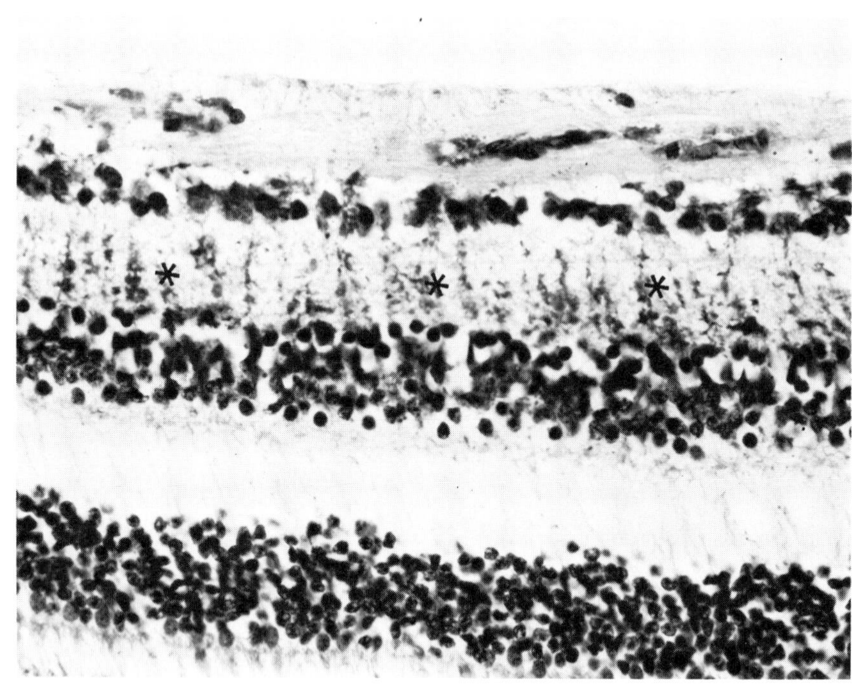

Figure 8–502. Type II glycogenosis (Pompe's disease). Accumulation of glycogen granules in inner plexiform area. PAS, ×550. EP 25863.

and in the muscles. Histologic and histochemical studies of the retina showed free glycogen granules in the form of spherules, with a diameter of approximately 10 microns, in the macular portion of the retina. The cytoplasm of the ganglion cells was intensely vacuolated and contained granules, staining like glycogen, that were sensitive to salivary amylase. Cellular vacuolation and intracytoplasmic glycogen were present throughout the retina, especially in the inner plexiform layer (Fig. 8–502) from the equator to the nerve head, and also in the muscle cells in the walls of the arteries and in the wall of the central retinal vein. The Müller cells were also involved.

Libert, Martin, Centerich, and Davis (1977) reported the ultrastructural features of an aborted fetus with type II glycogenosis. They found widespread lysosomal storage of glycogen in the viscera, the skeletal and ocular muscles, and in all ocular tissues except the RPE. Brain and heart were relatively spared. Conjunctival and skin biopsies were reported to be of importance because specific alterations are evident early in the course of the disease. Extraocular muscles also show similar changes (Smith, Reinecke, 1972).

Apparently the normal hydrolysis of glycogen to form glucose goes through the intermediary of oligosaccharides (maltose) under the influence of acid maltase (alpha-1,4-glucosidase). The deficiency of this enzyme prevents the hydrolysis of the glycogen through this portion of the cycle, but glycogenolysis can proceed in the same cell through the usual channels by mitochondrial and microsomal phosphorylase. For this reason, there are few symptoms from altered carbohydrate metabolism in this disease.

Chediak-Higashi Syndrome. This is a recessively transmitted disease characterized by a partial lack of pigmentation because of the absence of an unknown enzyme. Lymphadenopathy and organomegaly from the infiltration of immature leukocytes with granular cytoplasmic inclusions are seen. The patients lack resistance to infection, and death occurs in the second decade of life from infections (Bedoya, Grimley, Duque, 1969). Ophthalmologic features include partial albinism and photophobia. The RPE is intact, but contains little or no pigment (Fig. 8–503,*A*) and may contain giant pigment granules (Fig. 8–503,*B*) (Spencer, Hogan, 1960; Johnson, Jacobson, Toyama, Monahan, 1966). Giant pigment granules are present in the skin (Moran, Estevez, 1969). The uveal tract is also hypopigmented. Whether foveal hypoplasia is present has not been determined.

Patients apparently are prone to develop retinal detachment and to be found with leukocoria. In some cases, this picture has led to confusion with the condition of retinoblastoma.

Primary Systemic Amyloidosis. Vitreous and retinal involvement in this disorder is characteristic (see Chapter 7, Vitreous, page 573). Amyloid is observed in the wall of retinal vessels and appears to extend into the vitreous at such points (Fig. 8–504) (Schwartz, Green, Michels, et al, 1982).

Incontinentia Pigmenti (Block-Sulzberger Syndrome). This is an uncommon disorder of ecto-

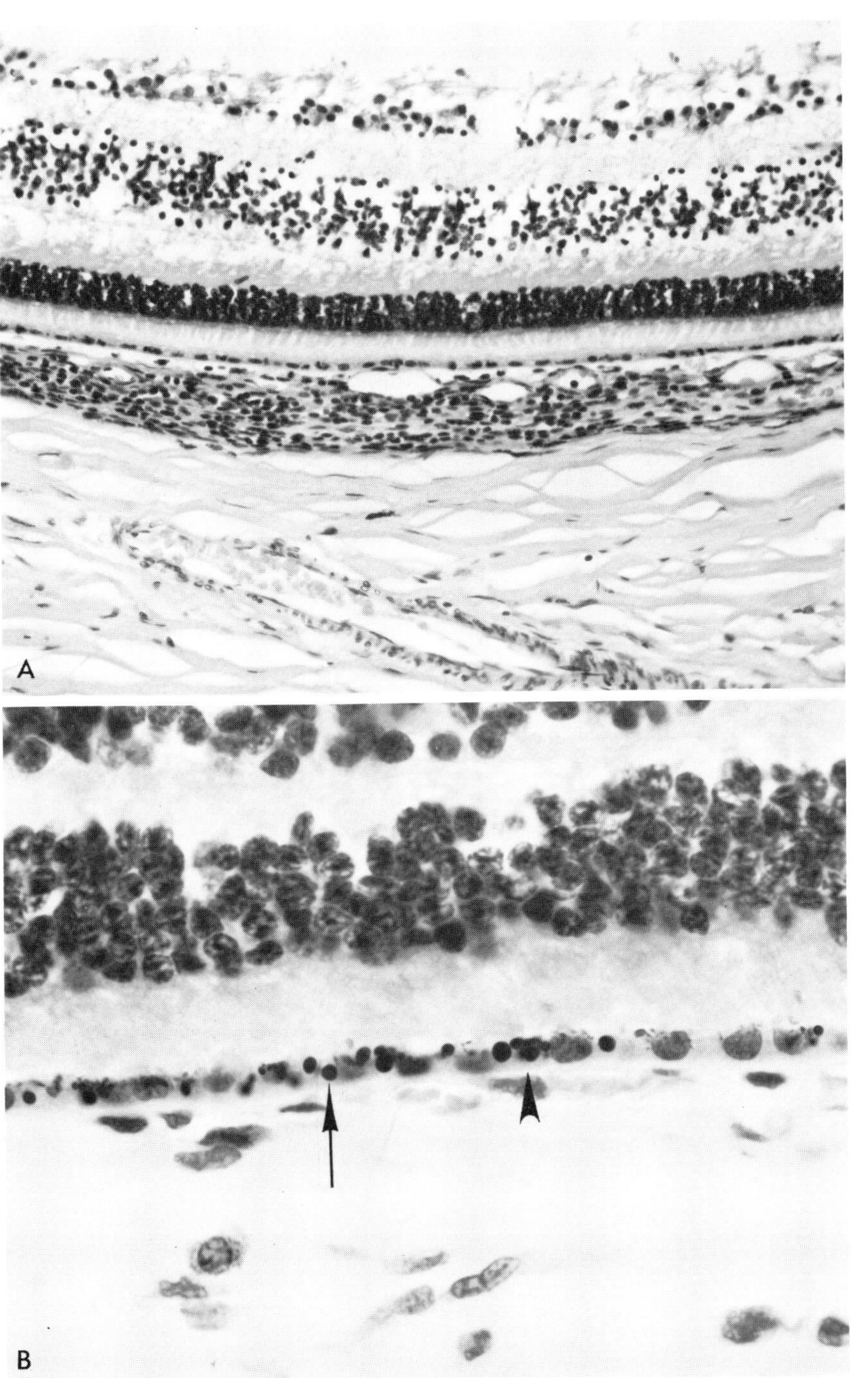

Figure 8–503. Chediak-Higashi syndrome. *A,* Hypopigmented choroid has light scattering of lymphocytes. Retinal pigment epithelium (RPE) is intact and has scant pigment. H and E, ×250. *B,* Higher power view of hypopigmented RPE shows melanin pigment granules that are large and spherical (arrow). Some of the pigment is aggregates of polymorphic melanin granules (arrowhead). H and E, ×900. EP 45769.

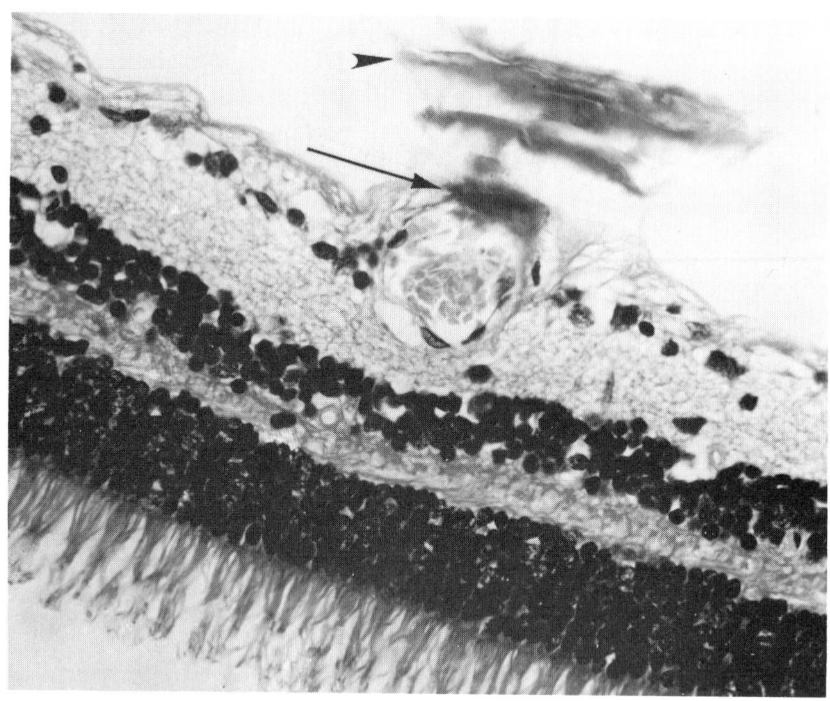

Figure 8–504. Amyloid deposit in wall of retinal vessel (arrow) and overlying vitreous (arrowhead) from patient with **nonfamilial systemic primary amyloidosis.** ×270. EP 45808. (From Schwartz MF, Green WR, Michels RG, Fogle J: An unusual case of ocular involvement in primary systemic nonfamilial amyloidosis. Ophthalmology *89*:394–401, 1982.)

dermal and mesodermal tissues, with abnormalities of the skin, hair, nails, teeth, eyes, and CNS. Characteristically, infant girls are affected; they develop recurrent vesiculobullous dermatitis that resolves spontaneously, leaving irregular, pigmented atrophic scars on the trunk and lower extremities. Ocular histopathologic studies (Zweifach, 1966; Fischbein, Schub, Lesko, 1972; Mensheha-Manhart, Rodrigues, Shields, et al, 1975; McCrary, Smith, 1968) have not elucidated the pathogenesis of the ocular findings.

A more recent study adds another possible explanation for the development of retinal detachment. Watzke, Stevens, and Carney (1976) described varied retinal vascular changes consisting of peripheral retinal nonperfusion, arteriovenous connections, preretinal tissue proliferation, and apparent neovascularization in the periphery of one patient. These vascular abnormalities also may play a role in the development of retinal detachment, and they have been compared to similar changes in Coats' disease.

Atrophy of the Maculopapillary Bundle. Many diseases of the central nervous system also affect the eye, either directly or indirectly. These are usually manifested by descending atrophy of the optic nerve, optic nerve head, and retina. Ophthalmoscopically, pallor of the optic nerve head is seen, and there may be loss of the foveal reflex. The pattern of descending atrophy of the retina includes loss of the nerve fiber and ganglion cell layers. This is the same pattern as is seen in glaucomatous atrophy. The temporal area of the optic nerve head shows loss of the nerve fiber bundles and a collapse of the columns of astrocytes. There is an apparent or real gliosis in the area of involvement.

When the atrophy involves the maculopapillary bundle, there is pallor of the temporal left half of the nerve head and a loss of the foveal reflex. Vision is reduced, and there is a central or centrocecal scotoma. Maculopapillary bundle atrophy also may be seen with multiple sclerosis, Leigh's disease, and nutritional amblyopia.

Multiple Sclerosis. Optic atrophy occurs in multiple sclerosis. However, the absence of disk pallor cannot be interpreted as absence of optic nerve fiber degeneration. Frisen and Hoyt (1974) have demonstrated that slitlike defects in the peripapillary nerve fiber layer occur frequently in multiple sclerosis, even in the absence of visual complaints. Additional ocular findings in patients with multiple sclerosis include sheathing of the retinal vein (Rucker, 1945; Möller, Hammerberg, 1963; Haarr, 1963; Porter, 1972), choroiditis (Archambeau, Hollenhorst, Rucker, 1965; Porter, 1972), and "peripheral uveitis" (Giles, 1970).

Atrophy of the maculopapillary bundle may occur in association with the retrobulbar neuritis of multiple sclerosis (Fig. 8–505). Preservation of some nerve fibers in areas of demyelinization may be observed (Fig. 8–505,*C*).

Chronic Alcoholism (Nutritional Amblyopia, Tobacco-Alcohol Amblyopia). With chronic nutritional deficiency, as seen in some alcoholic patients, atrophy of the maculopapillary bundle may occur, leading to centrocecal scotomas (Potts, 1973; Glaser, 1976). Clinical evidence suggests that a dietary deficiency of B-complex vitamins, particularly thiamine, is a greater etiologic

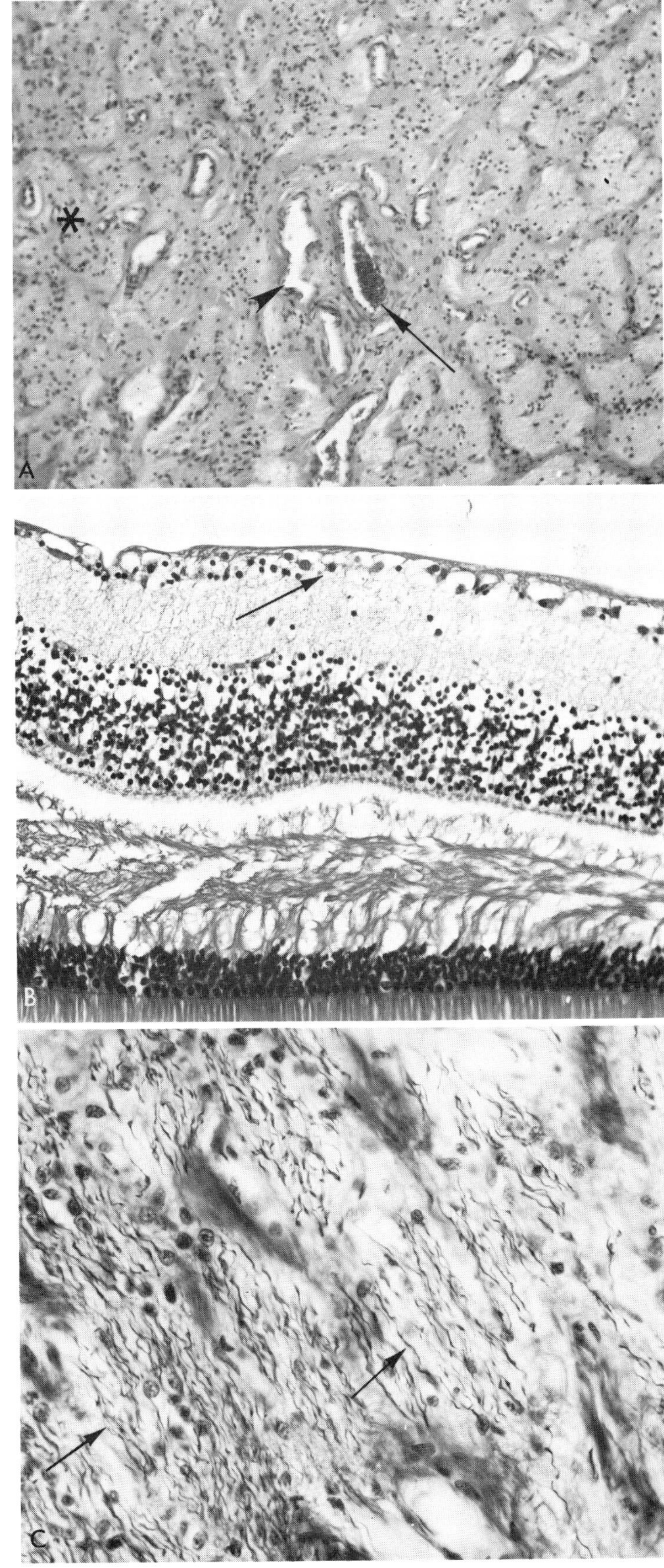

Figure 8–505. Multiple sclerosis. *A,* Cross-section of optic nerve showing central retinal artery (arrow) and vein (arrowhead) and atrophy of temporal portion of nerve (asterisk), where there are reduction of size of nerve fiber bundles, gliosis, and mild thickening of fibroglial septae. Compare with nasal side. H and E, ×110. *B,* Parafoveal area, where the ganglion cell layer is reduced to one layer (arrow). H and E, ×335. *C,* Longitudinal section of temporal portion of nerve in area of demyelinization shows preservation of some nerve fibers (arrows). Bodian, ×500. EP 48835.

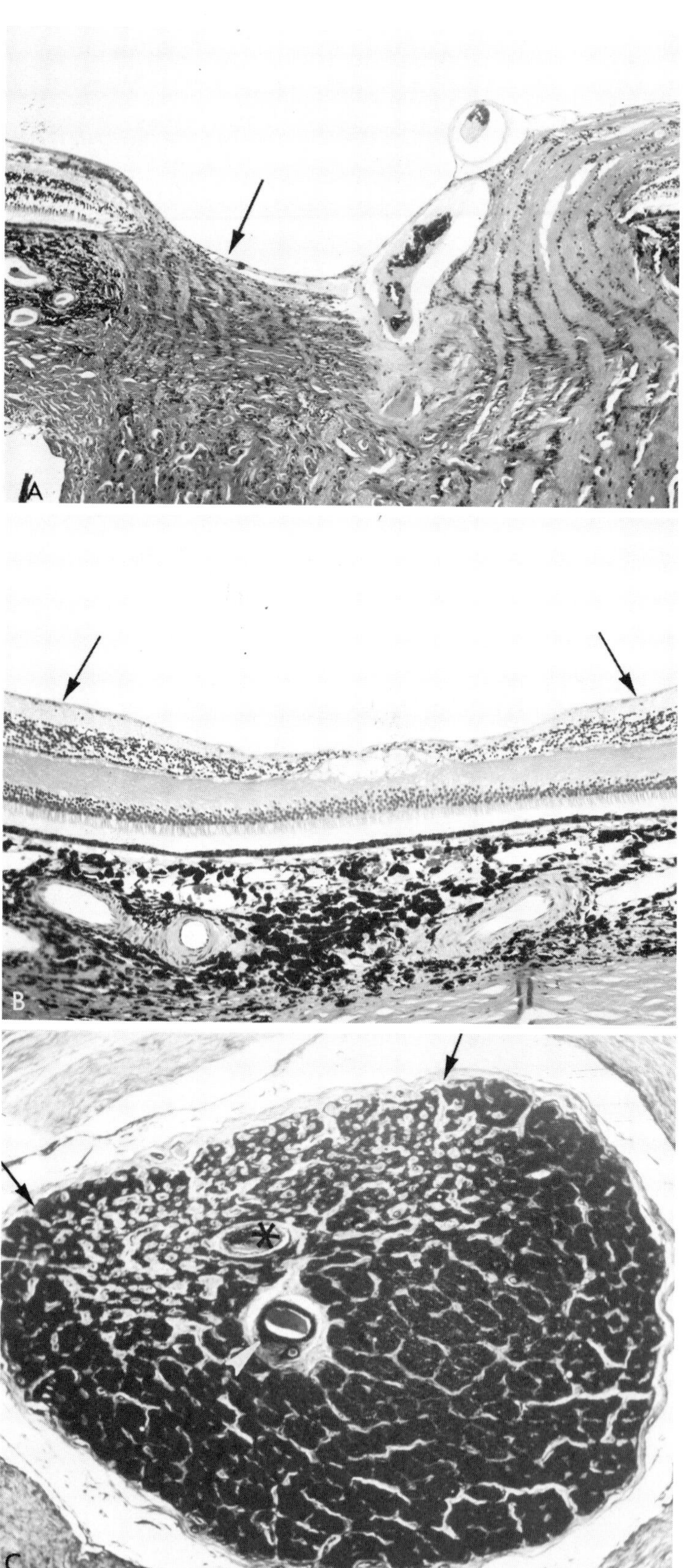

Figure 8–506. Nutritional amblyopia. *A,* Optic nerve head, showing partial atrophy of temporal side, with much reduction in size of nerve fiber bundles and closer appositon of astrocytic columns (arrow). Compare with nasal side. H and E, ×65. *B,* Section near foveola, showing much loss of ganglion cell and nerve fiber layer in parafoveal area (arrows). H and E, ×100. *C,* Thick cross-section of optic nerve stained for myelin. Artery (arrowhead) is nasal and vein (asterisk) is temporal. A sectorial area of partial atrophy is located temporally (between arrows), with partial demyelinization, thickening of fibropial septae, and narrowing of nerve fiber bundles. 12 micron- thick section, Verhoeff–van Gieson, ×35. EP 41966.

factor than are the toxic effects of alcohol or tobacco. Patients with pernicious anemia, in which there is defective absorption of vitamin B_{12}, may develop the same changes with minimal alcohol and tobacco usage. Also, thiamine improves the condition even with the continued use of alcohol and tobacco.

Knox (1978) has some preliminary evidence that indicates folic acid also may be a factor of deficiency in nutritional amblyopia.

Histopathologic studies have shown a consistent loss of the nerve fiber and ganglion cell layers in the macula and partial atrophy of the temporal aspect of the optic nerve and optic nerve head (Fig. 8–506).

Subacute Necrotizing Encephalomyelitis (Leigh's Disease; Infantile Wernicke's Disease). This genetic disorder occurs sporadically and is probably transmitted as an autosomal recessive trait. The disease manifests early, with failure to thrive, weight loss, somnolence, blindness, deafness, spasticity of limbs, and irregular respiration. The disorder is thought to result from inhibition of a thiamine-dependent enzymatic process and may be modified by increased thiamine intake. Episodes of metabolic acidosis with elevation of blood lactic and pyruvic acids are associated. Ophthalmologic disorders, such as nystagmus, ophthalmoplegia, strabismus, and optic atrophy, may precede the respiratory difficulties. A loss of

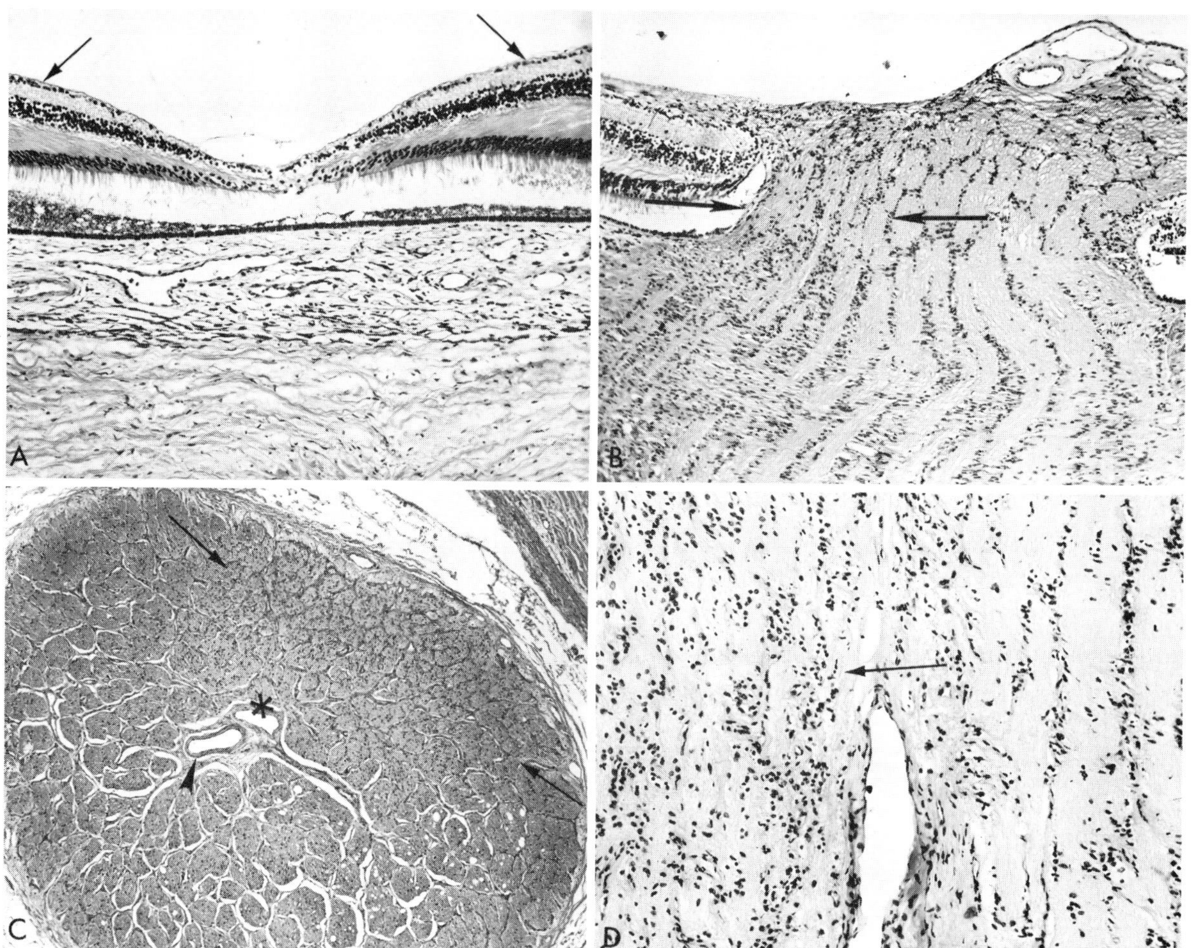

Figure 8–507. Atrophy of maculopapillary bundle in **subacute necrotizing encephalomyelitis (Leigh's disease)**. *A,* Section near center of macula, showing much atrophy of nerve fiber and ganglion cell layers in parafoveal area (arrows). H and E, ×135. *B,* Section just off center of optic nerve head, showing atrophy in temporal portion (between arrows), where nerve fiber bundles are reduced in thickness, and columns of astrocytes are more closely opposed. H and E, ×95.

C, Cross-section of optic nerve, showing temporal section of partial atrophy (arrows), with reduction in nerve fiber bundle size, mild thickening of fibrovascular pial septae, and glial hypercellularity. H and E, ×45. *D,* Longitudinal section of optic nerve behind globe, showing partial atrophy temporally (arrow), with same features as noted in *C.* Holzer, ×145.

EP 29259. (From Grover WD, Green WR, Pileggi AJ: Ocular findings in subacute necrotizing encephalomyelitis. Am J Ophthalmol *70*:599–603, 1970.)

the foveal reflex suggests that the maculopapillary bundle is involved.

Histopathologically, there is loss of the nerve fiber and ganglion cell layers in the macular area and atrophy of the temporal aspect of the optic nerve head and optic nerve (Fig. 8–507) (Grover, Green, Pileggi, 1970; Howard, Albert, 1972; Dooling, Richardson, 1977).

Behçet's Disease. Behçet's disease or syndrome (Behçet, 1937) is a systemic disease of undetermined cause characterized by recurrent iridocyclitis, with hypopyon, aphthous ulcers in the mouth and on the genitalia, and cutaneous, joint and central nervous system manifestation, all of which are attributed to a necrotizing vasculitis (Bietti, Bruna, 1966).

Behçet's disease is more prevalent in the Mediterranean area and in Japan. The prevalence of the disease is 0.6 in 100,000 in Britain and 10 in 100,000 in Japan. It affects young adults, 18 to 40 years old; men are affected twice as often as women. Associated erythema nodosum and genital ulceration are more common in women.

The most characteristic ocular feature is iritis and iritis with hypopyon. Scleritis, retinal vasculitis, uveitis, and optic neuritis also occur. Retinal involvement occurs in about 26 per cent of the patients. The frequency of Behçet's disease as a cause of uveitis is about 3 per cent in London and 20 to 30 per cent in Japan.

The earliest ocular lesion is a vasculitis with a predilection for the small peripheral retinal venules. Clinically evident vasculitis is most apparent in the retina, but it is also present in the choroid. Iris and ciliary body necrosis is probably the result of an occlusive vasculitis.

Immunofluorescent studies have demonstrated C_3 and C_9 in blood vessel walls and C_9 in basement membrane (Lehner, Batchelor, Challacombe, Kennedy, 1979).

Histocompatibility antigen studies have shown that HLA-B_5 is associated with ocular disease, HLA-B_{27} with arthritis, and HLA-B_{12} with mucocutaneous involvement. In subsequent studies, Ohno, Ohguchi, Hirose, et al (1982) found a close association of HLA-Bw51 with Behçet's disease.

Nongranulomatous uveitis, retinal vasculitis, hemorrhagic infarction of the retina, and retinal detachment are the ocular histopathologic features of eyes with a severe course leading to enucleation (Figs. 8–508 through 8–510) (Fenton and Easom, 1964; Shikano, 1966; Winter, Yukins, 1966).

In early involvement there is usually narrowing of the vessels and periarteritis. Willerson, Aaberg, and Reeser (1977) have described the clinical appearance of a necrotizing vaso-occlusive retinitis. The study of one eye of a patient with Behçet's disease disclosed a hypopyon, focal iris necrosis with neutrophils, secondary closed-angle glaucoma, rubeosis iridis, and retinal degeneration and gliosis. Little active vasculitis and perivasculitis were noted (Green, Koo, 1967). Fibrovascular and glial proliferation at the retinal periphery and pars plana area may give a pars planitis–like picture on ophthalmoscopic and gross examinations.

Acquired Immunodeficiency Syndrome (AIDS). Infectious retinitis is recognized as a complication of immunodeficiency that occurs during the course of some systemic diseases and after therapeutic immunosuppression and chemotherapy. Most have been cases of cytomegalovirus retinitis (Smith, 1964; De Venecia, Rhein, Pratt, Kisken, 1971; Aaberg, Cesarz, Rytel, 1972; Wyhinny, Apple, Guastella, Vygantas, 1973; Chumbley, Robertson, Smith, Campbell, 1975; Murray, Knox, Green, Susel, 1977; Coag, 1977; Merritt, Callender, 1978; Berger, Weinberg, Tessler, et al, 1979; Pollard, Egbert, Gallagher, Merigan, 1980; Egbert, Pollard, Gallagher, Merigan, 1980).

More recently, an acquired immunodeficient state of epidemic proportions has been recognized in male homosexuals, and these men are susceptible to ocular infections from a variety of organisms as well as Kaposi's sarcoma (Chawla, Ford, Munro, et al, 1976; Gottlieb, Schroff, Schanker, et al, 1981; Masur, Michelis, Green, et al, 1981; Siegal, Lopez, Hammer, et al, 1981; Durack, 1981; Drew, Mintz, Miner, et al, 1981). Histopathologic studies of eyes from affected homosexual males have disclosed the following infectious agents: cytomegalovirus (Friedman, 1981; Neuwirth, Gutman, Hofeldt, et al, 1982; Curtin, 1982; Cogan, 1982; Forrest, 1982; Spencer, 1982) and cryptococcal ocular infection (Spencer, 1982).

Kaposi's sarcoma in conjunctiva has been observed by Charles (1981), Curtin (1982), and Newman, Mandel, Gullett, and Fujikawa (1983). Other infectious agents recovered from various sites of these patients include herpes simplex and *Pneumocystis carinii*.

The apparently innocent ocular findings may be the first harbingers of acquired immunodeficiency (Newman, Mandel, Gullett, Fujikawa, 1983).

Retinal Degeneration as a Remote Effect of Cancer. Carcinoma has been thought to cause systemic symptoms only by direct involvement of various organ systems. Brain, Croft, and Wilkinson (1965a and b), however, observed motor neurone disease and cerebellar degeneration in association with distant neoplasm. Croft and Wilkinson (1965) observed peripheral neuropathy in association with a carcinoma. Henson, Hoffman, and Urich (1965) noted an association of encephalomyelitis, and Shy and Silverstein (1965) observed abnormalities in the cerebral motor unit associated with remote cancer. Since those reports in 1965, other organ systems, including skeletal, hematologic, vascular, and neuromuscular, also

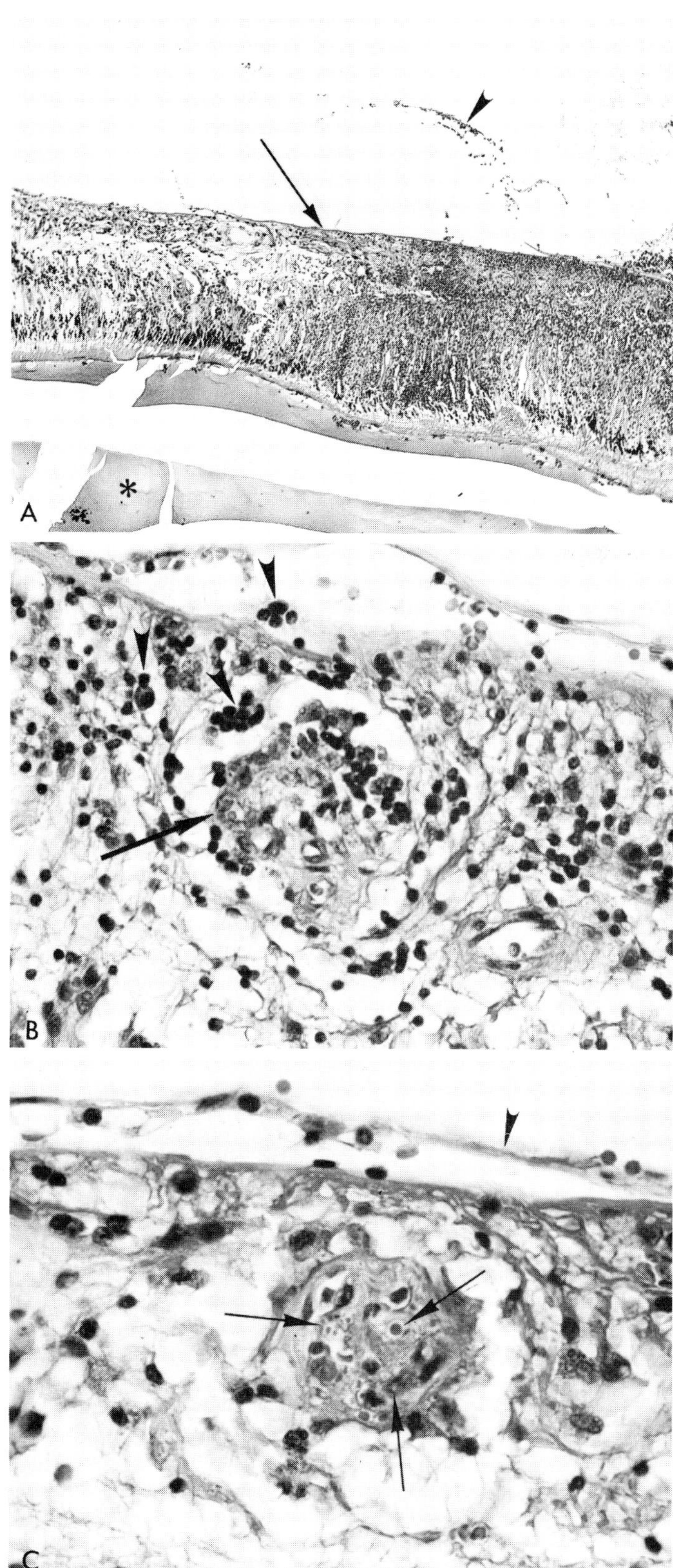

Figure 8–508. Behçet's disease. *A,* Acute necrosis and hemorrhage (arrow) of detached retina. Eosinophilic exudate and blood (asterisk) are present in subretinal spaces. Acute necrosis of retina with hemorrhage (arrow). Inflammatory cells are present in vitreous (arrowhead). H and E, ×60. AFIP Neg. 63-2453. *B,* Cellular thrombus in retinal vessel (arrow). Inflammatory cells are present in thrombus and surrounding retina (arrowheads). H and E, ×395. AFIP Neg. 63-2451. *C,* Thrombosed retinal vessel with channels of recanalization (arrows). Fibroinflammatory epiretinal membrane (arrowhead) is present.

AFIP 840404. (From Fenton RH, Eason HA: Behçet's syndrome. A histopathologic study of eye. Arch Ophthalmol *72*:71–81, 1964.)

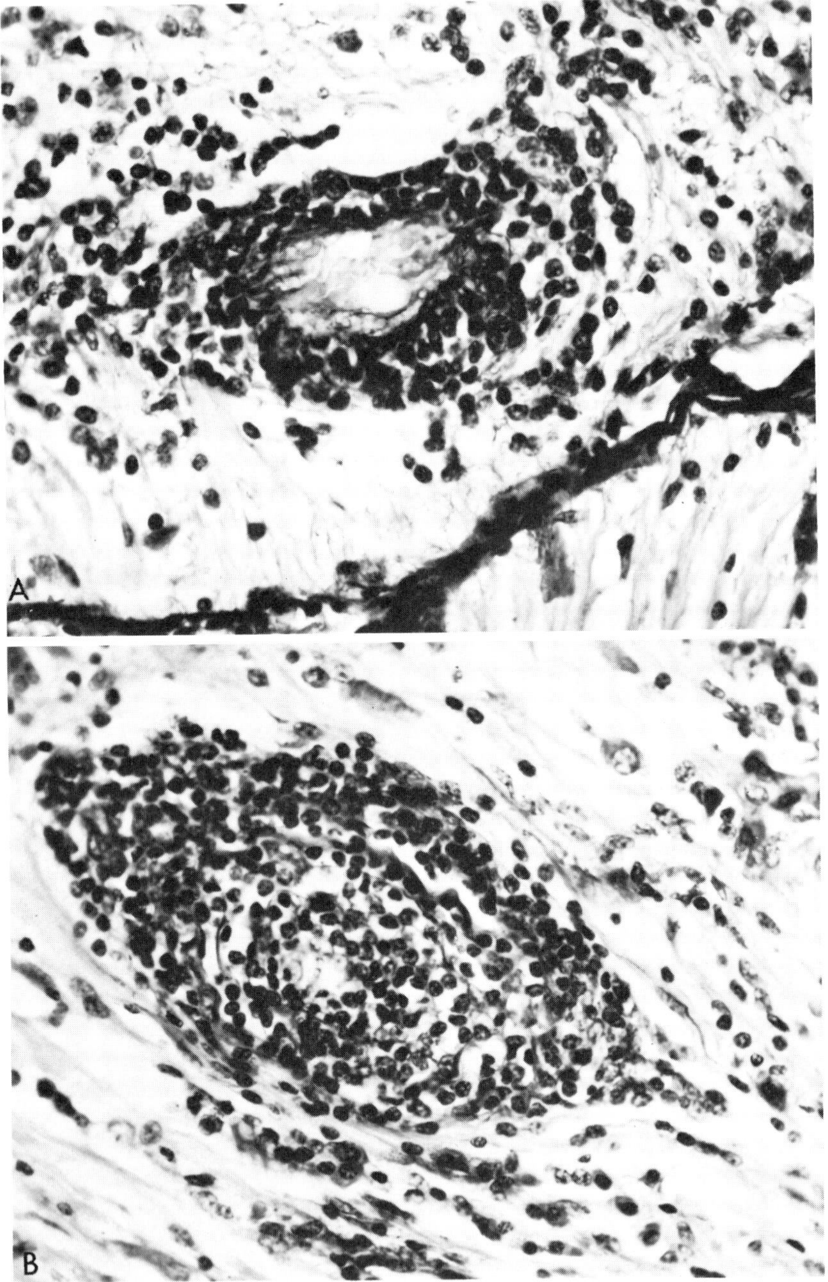

Figure 8–509. *A,* Intense lymphocytic infiltration in wall of and surrounding a retinal vessel. H and E, ×485. AFIP Neg. 63-2458. *B,* Retinal vessel with narrowed lumen from extreme inflammatory cell infiltration in its wall. H and E, ×395. AFIP Neg. 63-2457. AFIP 1065160. (From Fenton RH, Easom HA: Behçet's syndrome. A histopathologic study of eye. Arch Ophthalmol *72*:71–81, 1964.)

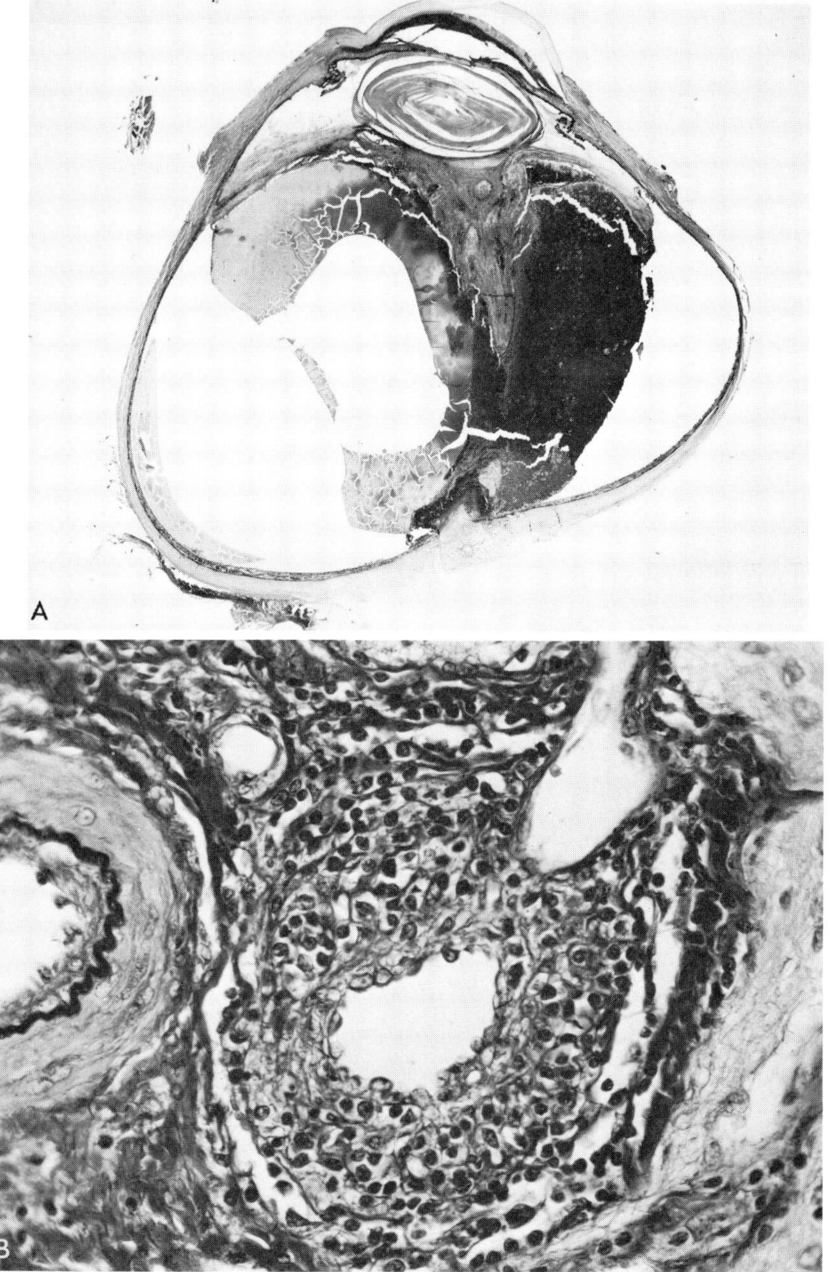

Figure 8–510. *A,* Hemorrhagic detachment of retina in **Behçet's disease**. H and E, ×2.75. AFIP Neg. 63-2741. *B,* Intense phlebitis of central retinal vein in retrolaminar area of optic nerve. Van Gieson elastica, ×350. AFIP Neg. 63-1818. AFIP 921904. (From Fenton RH, Easom HA: Behçet's syndrome. A histopathologic study of eye. Arch Ophthalmol *72*:71–81, 1964.)

have been found to be affected in some way by a distant carcinoma (Shields, 1972).

Sawyer, Selhorst, Zimmerman, and Hoyt (1976) reported three patients who became blind 1 to 4 months before or after discovery of an anaplastic tumor. Ring scotomas progressed to severe visual field loss. Retinal arteries became markedly narrowed, and the electroretinograms showed little or no response. Histopathologic studies in the three patients disclosed severe degeneration of the photoreceptor cells (Figs. 8–511 through 8–513).

Oxalosis (Hyperoxaluria). Oxalosis is characterized by high urinary oxalate excretion, oxalate urolithiasis, and nephrocalcinosis. Extrarenal deposits of oxalate may occur in the late stages. The disease has two forms (Williams, Smith, 1968), based on certain biochemical differences, including glycolic aciduria in type I and glyceric aciduria in type II. In type I primary hyperoxaluria, excessive amounts of oxalic, glycolic, and glyoxylic acid are excreted in the urine. The disease is transmitted as an autosomal recessive trait and involves a defect in glyoxalate metabolism that results in increased synthesis and excretion of oxalic acid. In type II hyperoxaluria, oxalic acid and glyceric aciduria are present, but glycolic acid is normal in the urine. Type II is

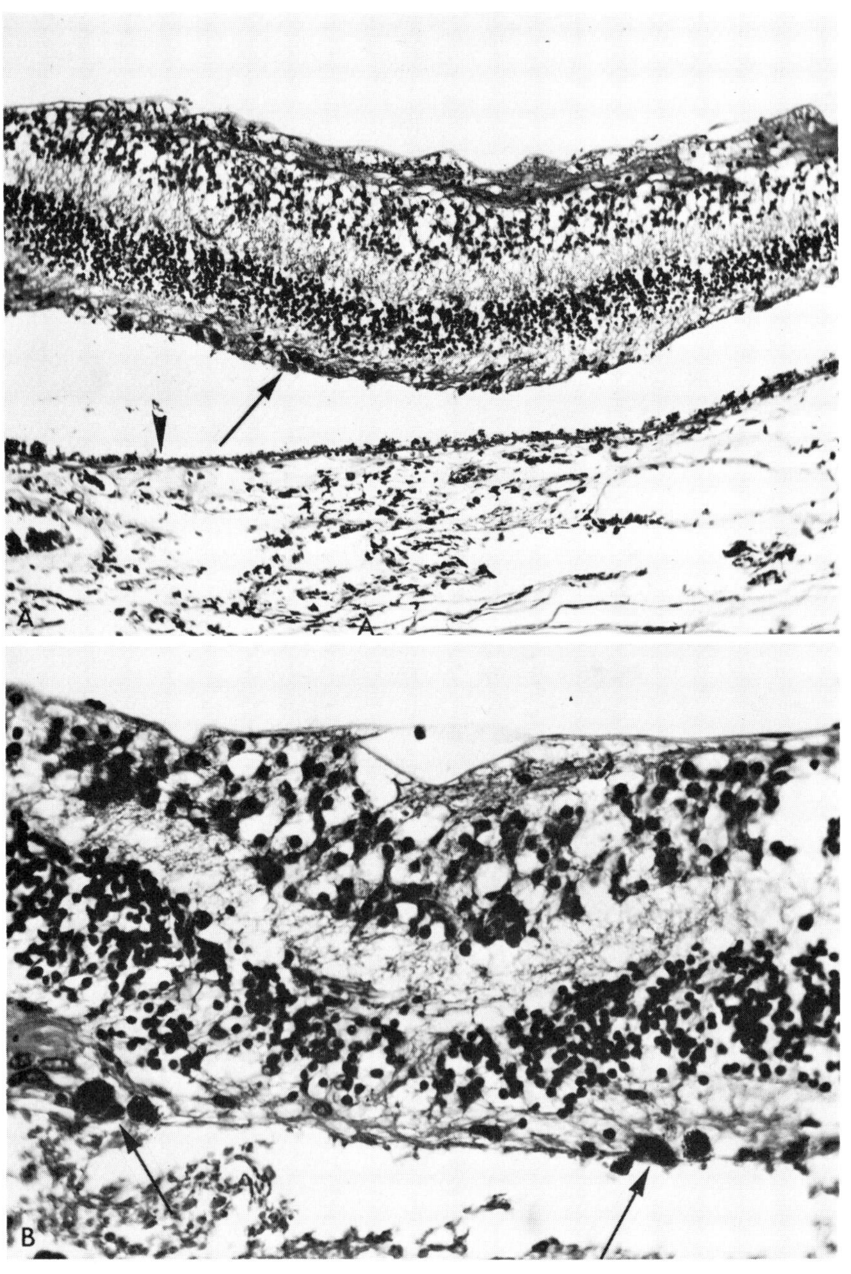

Figure 8–511. Retinal degeneration as a remote effect of cancer. *A,* Parafoveal area, showing much loss of photoreceptor cell layer and migration of pigmented cells (arrow) into outer aspect of retina. Retinal pigment epithelium (RPE) is discontinuous or artifactitiously disrupted (arrowhead). H and E, ×100. AFIP Neg. 75-1614. *B,* Higher-power view, showing loss of entire photoreceptor cell components (outer nuclear layer and inner and outer segments of the photoreceptors). Pigmented cells (arrows) are present in outer aspect of retina. H and E, ×300. AFIP Neg. 75-1611. AFIP 1477646.

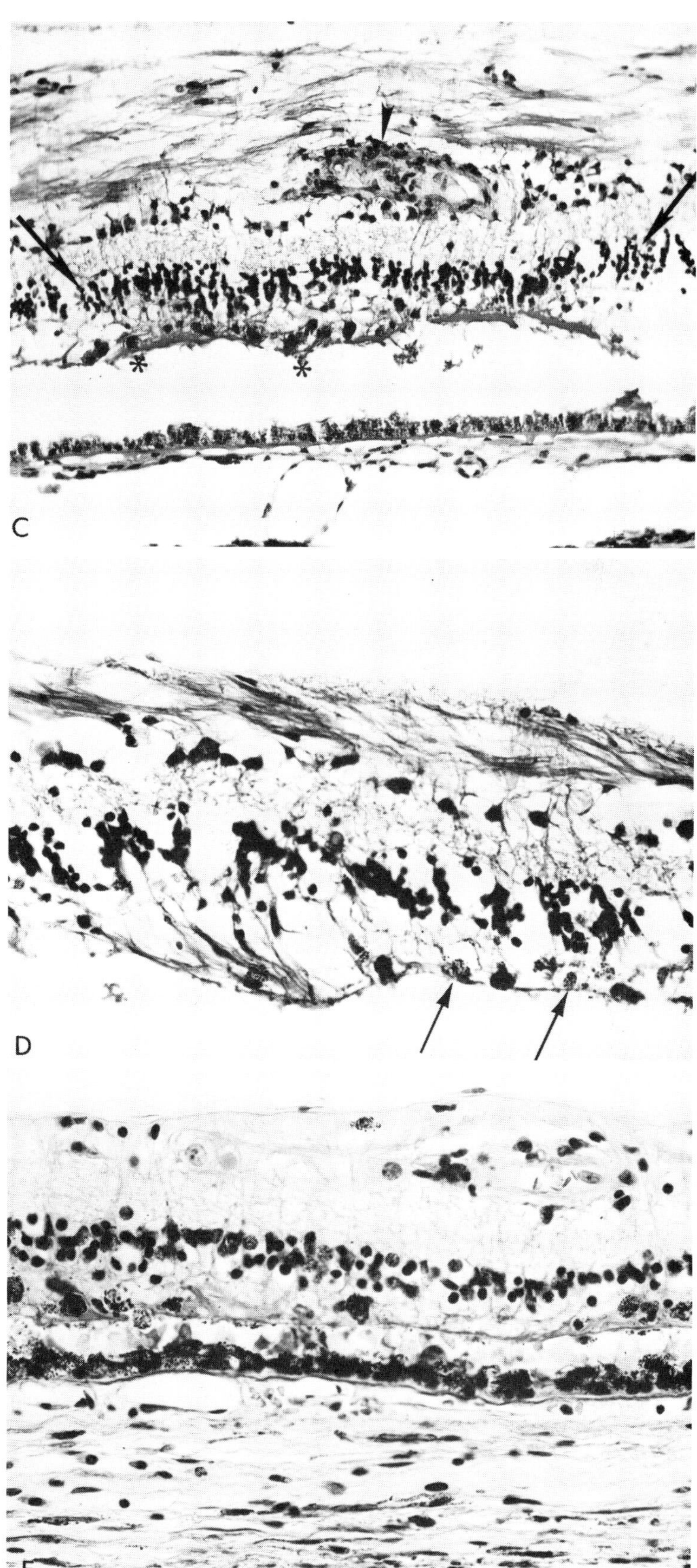

Figure 8–511 *Continued C,* Peripapillary retina, showing total photoreceptor cell degeneration, pigmented cells at outer aspect (asterisks) of retina, a mild inflammatory cell infiltrate in wall of a retinal artery (arrowhead), and an intact RPE, choriocapillaris, and inner nuclear layer (arrows). H and E, ×195. AFIP Neg. 75-2449. *D,* Peripheral retina, showing total loss of photoreceptor cell layer and pigmented cells (arrows) in outer aspect of retina. H and E, ×305. AFIP Neg. 75-2444. AFIP 1505973.

E, Complete degeneration of photoreceptor cell layer and pigmented cells is present in remains of outer plexiform layer. RPE, choriocapillaris, and inner nuclear layer are intact. H and E, ×300. AFIP Neg. 75-1603. AFIP 1500929.

(From Sawyer RA, Selhorst JB, Zimmerman LE, Hoyt WF: Blindness caused by photoreceptor degeneration as a remote effect of cancer. Am J Ophthalmol *81*:606–613, 1976.)

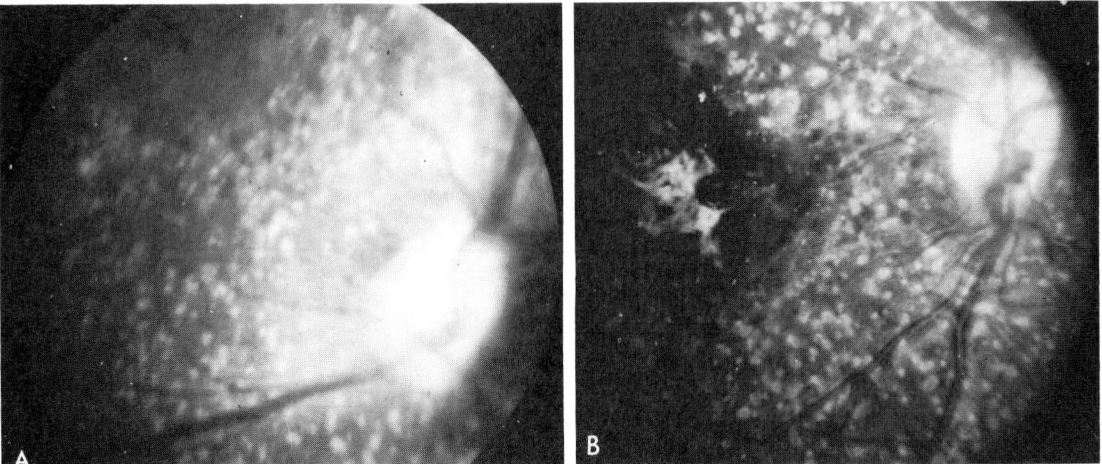

Figure 8–512. Primary oxalosis. *A.* Appearance of flecked retina in patients at 2 years of age. *B,* Appearance at age 4 years. Apparent scar in macula. (From Gottlieb RP, Ritter JA: Flecked retina: An association with primary hyperoxaluria. J Pediatr *90*:939–942, 1977.)

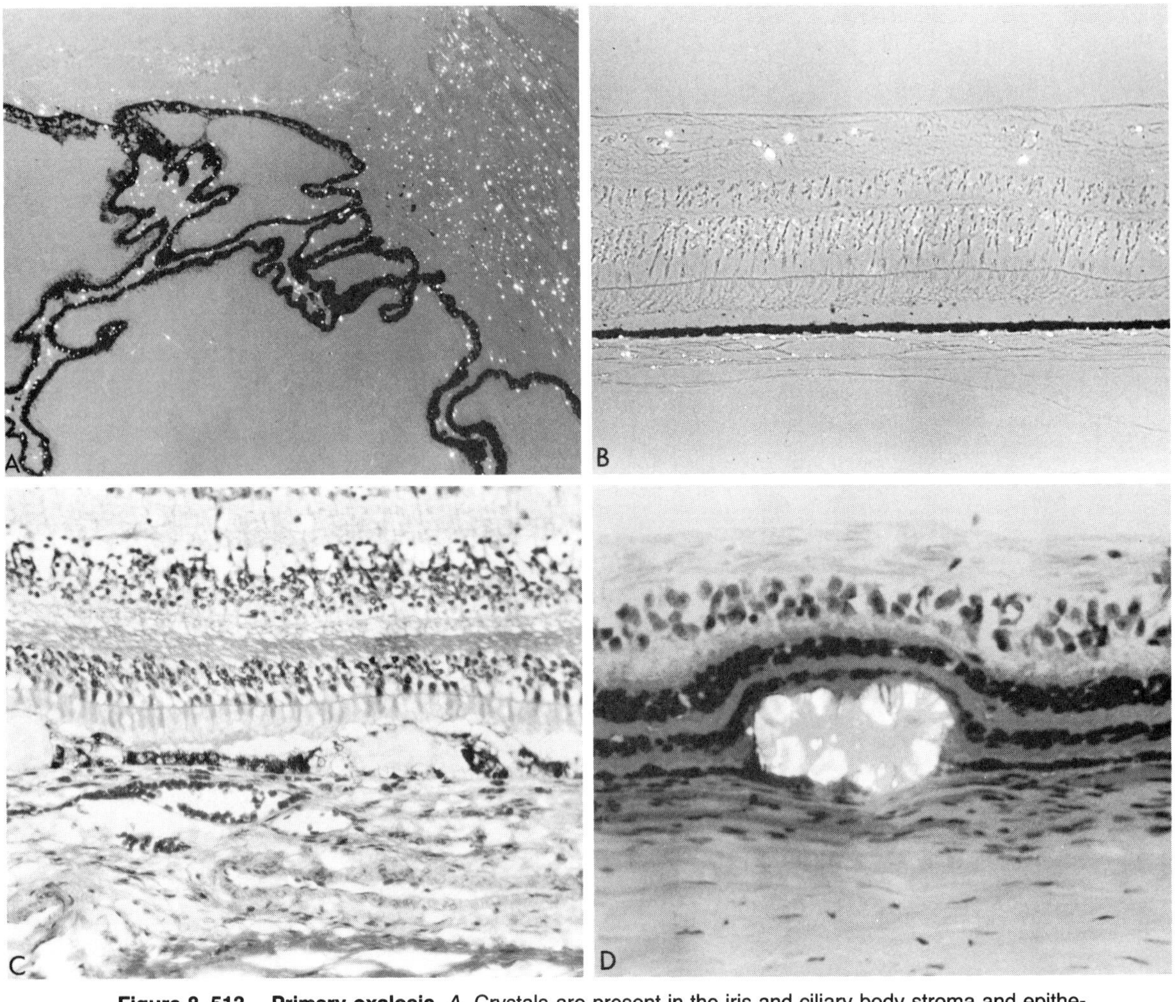

Figure 8–513. Primary oxalosis. *A,* Crystals are present in the iris and ciliary body stroma and epithelial layers, as viewed here in tissue fixed in absolute alcohol, unstained section, and partial polarization. × 25. *B,* Similar preparation shows crystals in the retina and choroid. Unstained, polarized, ×40. *C,* Calcium oxalate crystals in retinal pigment epithelium (RPE), H and E, ×50. *D,* Large calcium oxalate crystal in area of RPE, with compression of overlying outer retinal layers. H and E, partial polarization, ×100.

(From Meredith TA, Wright JD, Gammon JA, et al: Ocular involvement in primary hyperoxaluria. Arch Opthalmol *102*:584–587, 1984.)

presumed to be transmitted as an autosomal trait that results in defective hydroxypyruvate metabolism.

Buri (1962) described crystals in the macular retina of a 9 year old child with oxalosis. Gottlieb and Ritter (1977) have observed a flecked retina–like picture in a patient with probable type I hyperoxaluria (Fig. 8–512). No histopathologic studies were performed, but the features are likely to be the same as those reported by Albert, Bullock, Lahav, and Caine (1975) in a patient with flecked retina following methoxyflurane anesthesia (see page 805).

In a clinicopathologic study, Fielder, Garner, and Chambers (1980) found that oxalate crystalline deposits in the retinal pigment epithelium corresponded to the flecked retinopathy observed ophthalmoscopically in a 6 month old infant with primary oxalosis.

Meredith, Wright, Gammon, et al (1984) observed widespread deposition of calcium oxalate crystals in the iris and ciliary body (Fig. 8–513,*A*), retina and choroid (Fig. 8–513,*B*), and retinal pigment epithelium (Fig. 8–513,*C* and *D*) in a 4 month old child who died of primary oxalosis. In their review of the literature, they found eight previous reports of ocular findings in primary oxalosis.

Localized Ocular Oxalosis. Calcium oxalate crystals have been observed in the lens and in the retina. Flocks, Littwin, and Zimmerman (1955) observed these crystals in the lens nucleus of hypermature cataracts in eyes with phacolytic glaucoma. Cogan, Kuwabara, Silbert, et al (1958) observed similar crystals in the outer layers of degenerated and chronically detached retinas. Zimmerman and Johnson (1958) studied 26 eyes with retinal oxalosis and found that all had chronic retinal detachment and 77 per cent had evidence of ocular trauma. Friedman and Charles (1974) observed calcium oxalate crystals in the outer layers of the detached retina of two patients with ocular complications of diabetic retinopathy.

In mammals, the biosynthesis of oxalate is by two pathways: oxidative metabolism of ascorbic acid and oxidation of glyoxylic acid. An increase of oxalate by the glyoxylic acid pathway may be enhanced by a deficiency of pyridoxine or thiamine.

Oxidation of ascorbic acid normally accounts for about half of the daily output of oxalate (Baker, Saari, Tolbert, 1966).

Pirie (1968) has shown that napthane, which promotes oxidation of ascorbic acid, leads to the deposition of calcium oxalate in outer retinal layers when given to rabbits. Because ocular fluids have an unusually high content of ascorbic acid (Purcell, Lerner, Kinsey, 1954), Garner (1974) suggested that oxalosis that occurs in eyes with retinal detachment and hypermature cataracts may result through ascorbic metabolism.

In their review of the subject, Friedman and Charles (1974) found that calcium oxalate crystals have been observed in the following diverse pathologic conditions: nephrolithiasis; hyperoxaluria, types 1 and 2; after ingestion of ethylene glycol or oxalic acid; after methoxyflurane anesthesia; within thyroid colloid; in sarcoid crystalloids; in myocardium in uremia; and in the kidney in acute and chronic disease states.

Oxalate crystals appear round, globular, or rhomboidal, have a radial rosette pattern, are birefringent under polarized light, and can be identified by a variety of histochemical and physical techniques (Johnson, 1956; Yasue, 1969; Cogan, Kuwabara, Silvert, et al, 1958; Zimmerman and Johnson, 1958; Garner, 1974).

Vitamin A Deficiency Retinopathy. It has been well established experimentally that animals raised on a vitamin A–free diet develop night blindness and eventual degeneration of the photoreceptor cells (Dowling, Gibbons, 1961). Sommer, Tjakrasudjatma, Djunaedi, and Green (1978) reported a vitamin A retinopathy in a 25 year old woman with panocular xerophthalmia. Small, irregular, nondiscrete, whitish-yellow deposits deep to the retina were observed in the midperiphery (Figs. 8–514 and 8–515). These changes were associated with night blindness and peripheral visual field constriction. The retinal lesions, night blindness, and visual field defects disappeared after vitamin A therapy (Fig. 8–515).

Bietti's Retinal and Corneal Crystalline Dystrophy (Tapetoretinal Degeneration with Associated Corneal Deposits at the Limbus) (Bietti, 1937; Bagolini, Ioli-Spada, 1968). It has not yet been established that this is a systemic disease. It is characterized by spots with a crystalline charac-

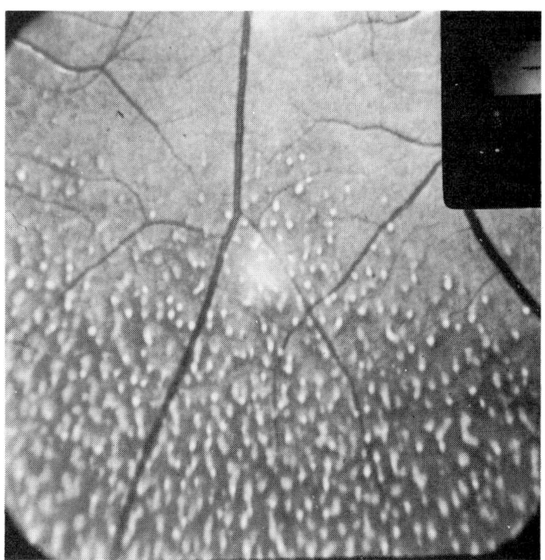

Figure 8–514. Vitamin A retinopathy with flecks deep in, or under, retina in midperiphery and periphery. (Courtesy of Dr. Alfred Sommer.)

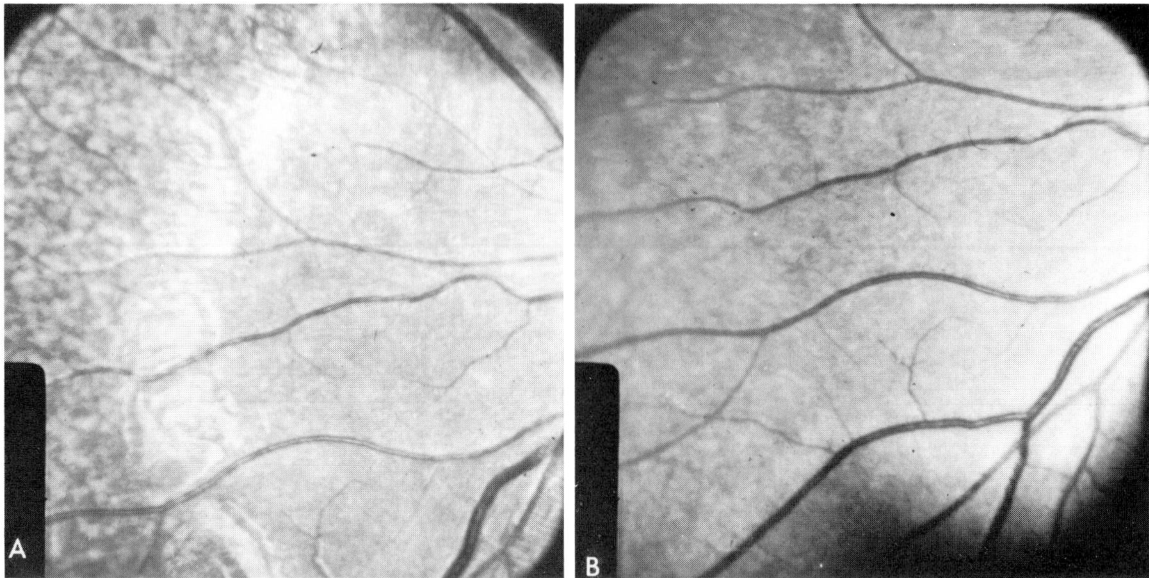

Figure 8–515. Vitamin A retinopathy. *A,* Before and *B,* after vitamin A therapy. (From Sommer A, Tjakrasudjatra S, Djunaedi E, Green WR: Vitamin A–responsive panocular xerophthalmia in a healthy adult. Arch Ophthalmol *96*:1630–1634, 1978.)

ter in the retina (Fig. 8–516) and peripheral cornea. No histopathologic studies of the retina have been conducted. Corneal and conjunctival biopsy specimens in one patient revealed lipid inclusions in both fibrocytes and the epithelium (Welch, 1977) and deposits of possible immunoprotein (Klein, Green, 1979). Extensive evaluations of those patients have failed to disclose any abnormalities of lipid metabolism, immunoprotein abnormalities, or hyperoxaluria. Grizzard, Deutman, Nijhuis, and Aan de Kerk (1978) have reviewed the reported cases.

A similar crystallin retinopathy has been observed without corneal crystals and with choroidal atrophy and pigment clumping in the periphery (François, de Laey, 1977; Noble, Carr, Siegel, 1977; Grizzard, Deutman, Nijhuis, Aan de Kerk, 1978).

Crystallin Retinopathy. Crystals or crystalline-like deposits in the retina are seen in a variety of unrelated conditions. In some instances the lesions have been clinically interpreted as having a crystallin appearance, but histopathologic confirmation is lacking. The conditions include the following, which are considered in more detail elsewhere in this chapter: Bietti's crystalline cor-

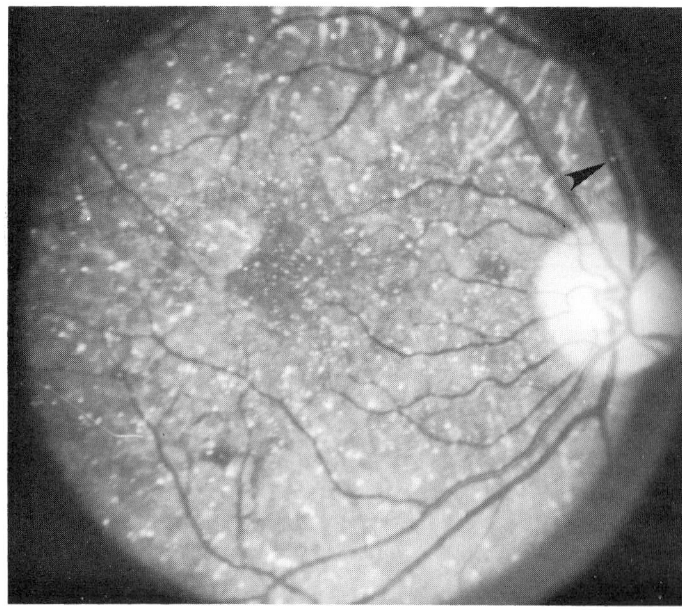

Figure 8–516. Bietti's retinal and corneal cystalline dystrophy. Ophthalmoscopic appearance of flecks in retina. Most appear deep, but some (arrowhead) are superficial to retinal blood vessels. EP 45310.

neal and retinal dystrophy, calcified drusen, primary oxalosis, secondary oxalosis due to methosyflurane toxicity, childhood cystinosis, talc retinopathy, some calcific and cholesterol emboli, tamoxifen toxicity, canthaxanthine crystallin retinopathy, gyrate atrophy with hyperornithemia, and the Sjögren-Larsson syndrome.

Retinopathy Associated with Acute Pancreatitis. The retinal lesions in acute pancreatitis are large areas of microinfarction of the nerve fiber layer in the posterior area of the eye. These lesions have been attributed to fat emboli (Inkeles, Walsh, 1975) and complement-mediated leukostasis (Jacob, Goldstein, Shapiro, et al, 1981), but these mechanisms have not been confirmed histopathologically.

In one eye studied clinically and histopathologically (Kincaid, Green, Knox, Molner, 1982), a large area of fresh, inner retinal ischemia was caused by fibrinous occlusion of a retinal arteriole (Fig. 8–517).

Olivopontocerebellar Atrophy. This disease has five forms. All are autosomal dominant, except type II, which is recessive. The various clinical features are discussed in a review by Konigsmark and Weiner (1970).

Olivopontocerebellar Atrophy, type III (OPCA III; Olivopontocerebellar Retinal Atrophy). This disease has associated retinal degeneration (Weiner, Konigsmark, Stoll, Magladery, 1967). Retinal degeneration begins in the macular area and progresses to the periphery. The macular lesion evolves to a discrete, round area of areolar RPE atrophy (Fig. 8–518). The macular lesion progresses to a discrete area of RPE and photoreceptor cell atrophy, with a generally intact choriocapillaris (Fig. 8–519) (Bessiere, Chabot, Verin, 1962; Weiner, Konigsmark, Stoll, Magladery, 1967; Ravalico, Stanig, 1972; Ryan, Knox, Green, Konigsmark, 1975).

In a clinicopathologic study of the eyes of two young siblings with this disease, Ryan and co-

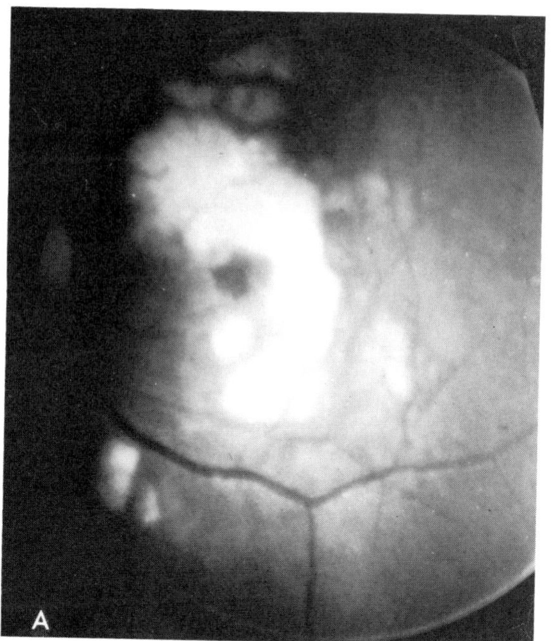

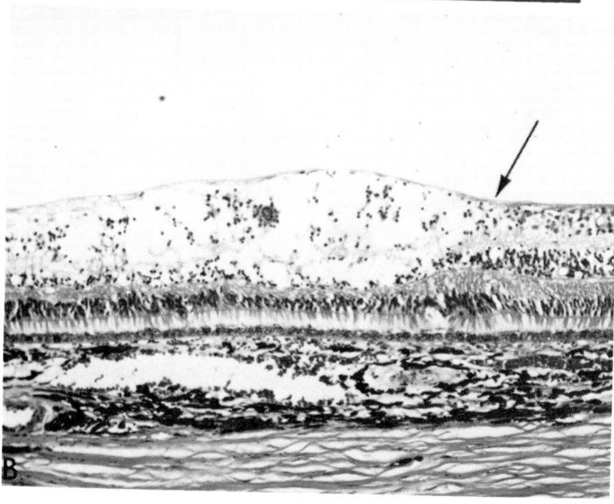

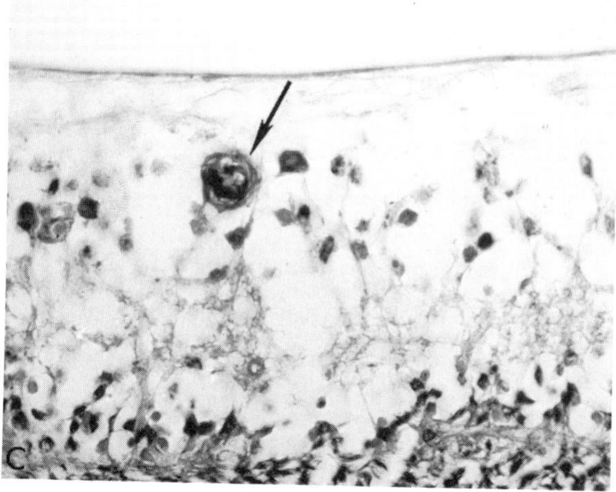

Figure 8–517. Retinopathy of acute pancreatitis. *A,* Ophthalmoscopic appearance of large areas of retinal ischemia and edema. *B,* Abrupt transition (arrow) between normal area and area of acute inner retinal ischemia, with edema and loss of inner layers. H and E, ×125. *C,* Fibrin-containing thrombus in artery at one area of infarction. Phosphotungstic acid–hematoxylin, ×530. EP 35336. (From Kincaid MC, Green WR, Knox DL, Mohler C: A clinicopathologic case report of retinopathy of pancreatitis. Br J Ophthalmol *66*:219–226, 1982.)

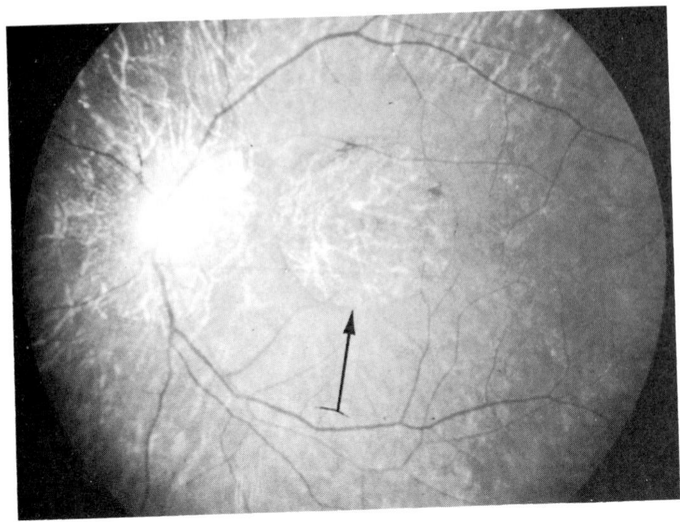

Figure 8–518. Discrete, round retinal pigment epithelium defect (arrow) in macula of patient with **olivopontocerebellar retinal degeneration**.

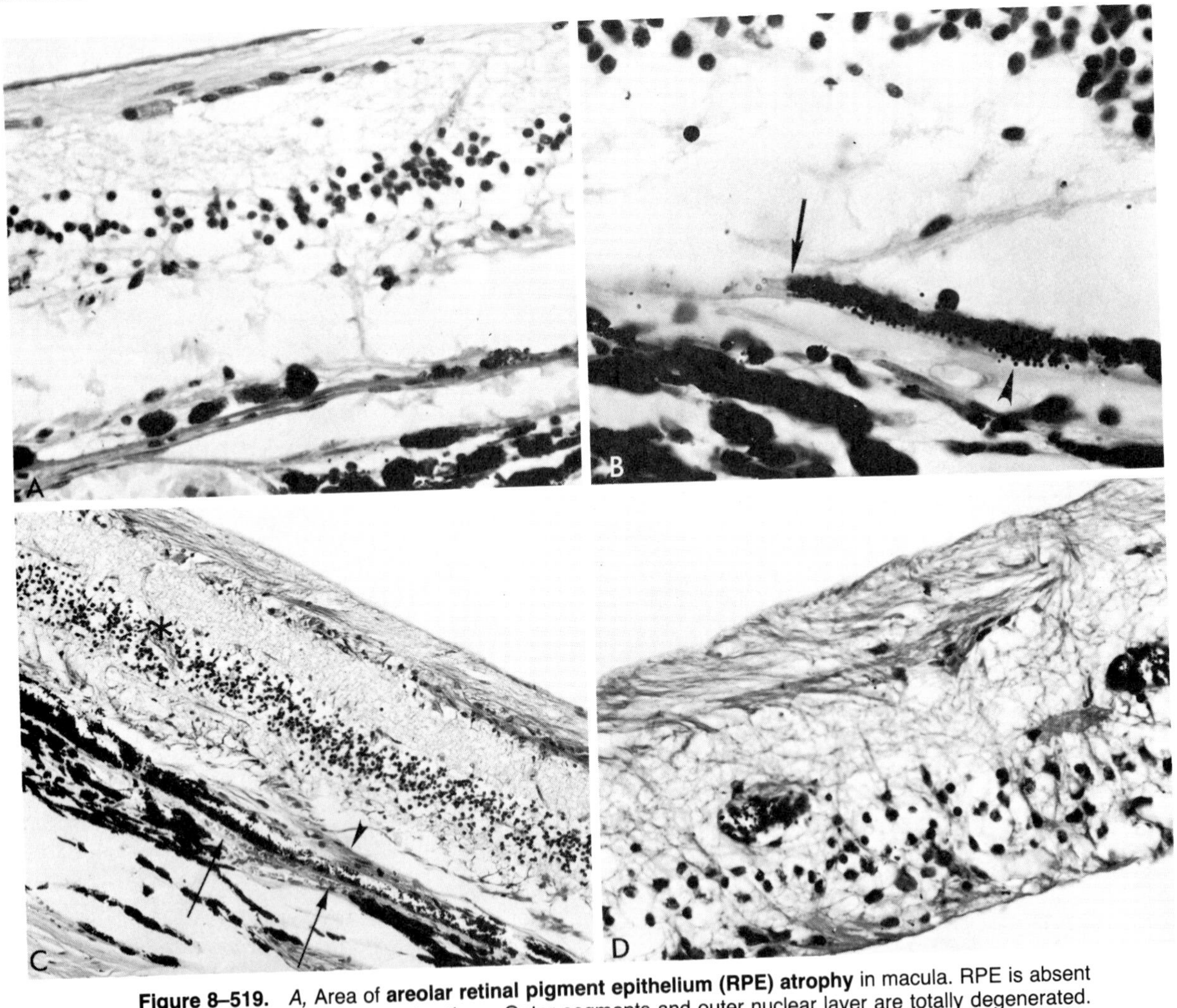

A

B

C

D

Figure 8–519. *A,* Area of **areolar retinal pigment epithelium (RPE) atrophy** in macula. RPE is absent in some areas and hypertrophic in others. Outer segments and outer nuclear layer are totally degenerated. Choriocapillaris is inconspicuous. H and E, ×490. *B,* Abrupt margin of areolar RPE atrophy (arrow). RPE at margin is hypertrophic, with large, spherical pigment granules (arrowhead). H and E, ×900. *C,* Area outside areolar RPE atrophy shows total loss of photoreceptor cell layer and hypertrophy of subjacent RPE. Minor retroretinal glial membrane (arrowhead) is present. Choriocapillaris (arrows) and inner nuclear layer (asterisk) are intact. H and E, ×200. *D,* Retina between disc and equator shows migration of pigment into retina in perivascular location. Outer nuclear layer and outer segments of photoreceptors are degenerated. H and E, ×460.

EP 24775. (From Ryan SJ, Knox DL, Green WR, Konigsmark BW: Olivopontocerebellar degeneration. Arch Ophthalmol *93*:169–172, 1975.)

workers found the RPE to be relatively intact but with alternate areas of normal or reduced pigment and areas of apparently increased pigment. The striking change was in the photoreceptor cells, which showed total loss of the outer segments, near-total loss of the inner segments, and reduction in the number of nuclei in the outer nuclear layer (Fig. 8–520). These changes account for the mottled appearance of the fundus and suggest that the primary defect is in the photoreceptor cells (de Jong, de Jong, de Jong-Ten Doeschate, Delleman, 1980).

The benign concentric annular macular dystrophy of Deutman (1974) is probably the ocular manifestation of OPCA (Duinkerke-Eerola, Cruysberg, Deutman, 1980).

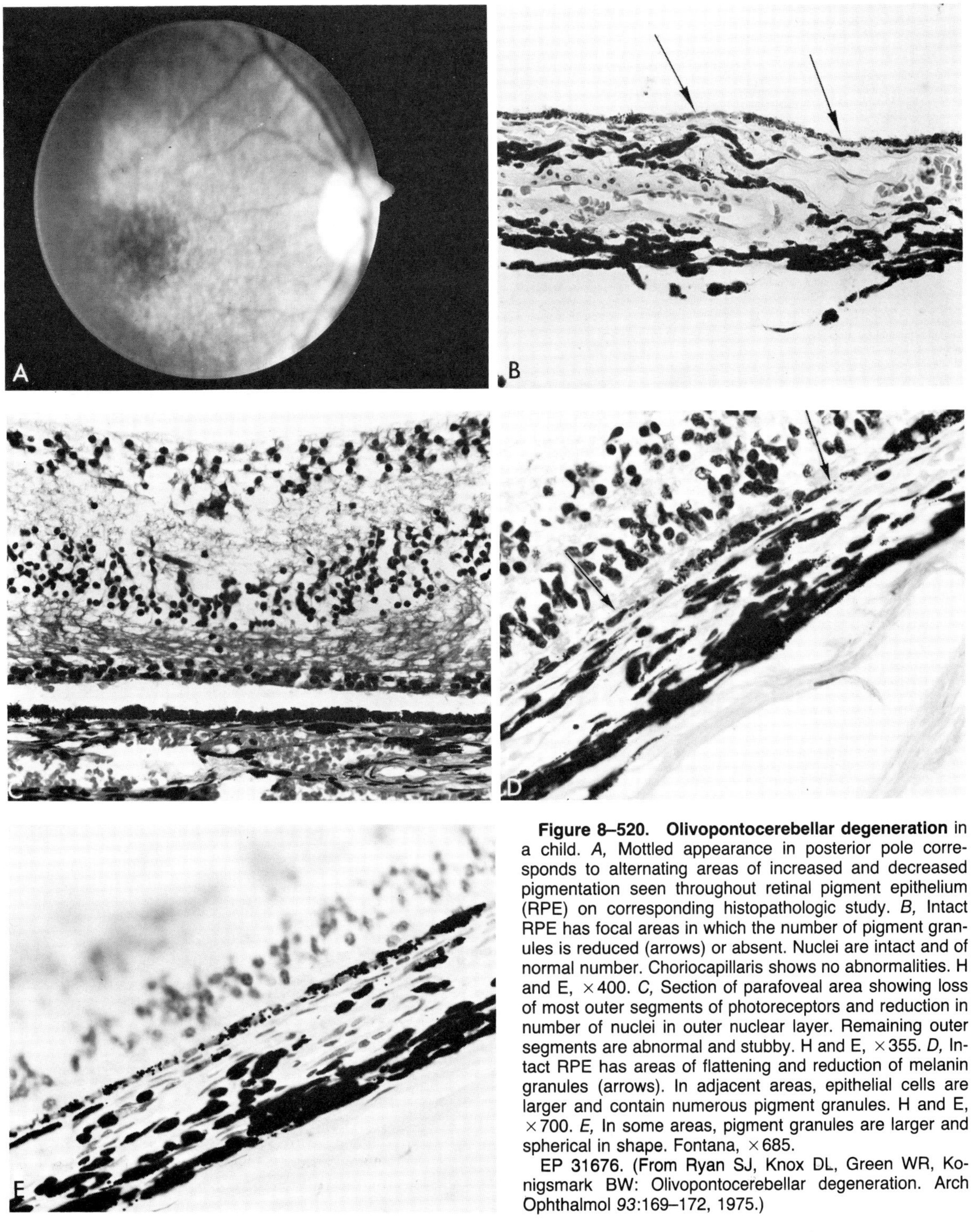

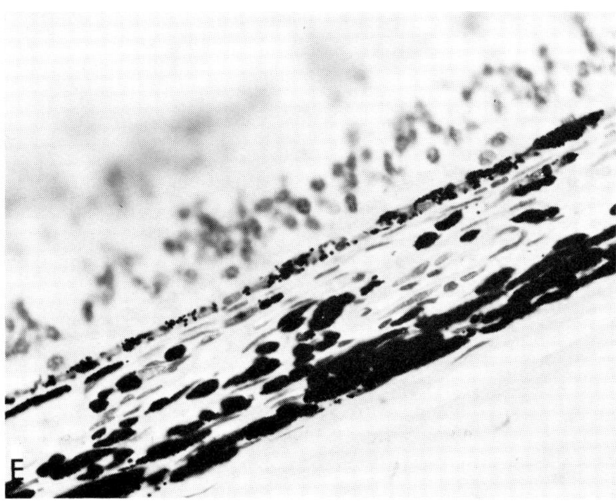

Figure 8–520. Olivopontocerebellar degeneration in a child. *A,* Mottled appearance in posterior pole corresponds to alternating areas of increased and decreased pigmentation seen throughout retinal pigment epithelium (RPE) on corresponding histopathologic study. *B,* Intact RPE has focal areas in which the number of pigment granules is reduced (arrows) or absent. Nuclei are intact and of normal number. Choriocapillaris shows no abnormalities. H and E, ×400. *C,* Section of parafoveal area showing loss of most outer segments of photoreceptors and reduction in number of nuclei in outer nuclear layer. Remaining outer segments are abnormal and stubby. H and E, ×355. *D,* Intact RPE has areas of flattening and reduction of melanin granules (arrows). In adjacent areas, epithelial cells are larger and contain numerous pigment granules. H and E, ×700. *E,* In some areas, pigment granules are larger and spherical in shape. Fontana, ×685.

EP 31676. (From Ryan SJ, Knox DL, Green WR, Konigsmark BW: Olivopontocerebellar degeneration. Arch Ophthalmol *93*:169–172, 1975.)

Myotonic Dystrophy (Steinert Disease). This dominant heredofamilial disease of the voluntary muscular system is characterized by progressive distal weakness that begins in the second or third decade. The myotonic feature consists of a sustained muscle contraction with slow relaxation, and it can be observed on mechanical testing of the thenar eminence or tongue, or reflexly on hand-shaking or forcible eyelid closure (McKusick, 1978). Ocular manifestations include cataractous changes, blepharoptosis, ophthalmoplegia, pigmentary retinopathy, and abnormalities of dark adaptation and the electroretinogram (Simon, 1962; Van Dyk, Swan, 1967).

The cataractous changes are rather characteristic when seen early; they consist of iridescent opacities in a narrow zone of the cortex. These opacities are separated from the anterior and posterior capsule by a clear zone. Light and electron microscopic studies (Dark, Streeten, 1977) have disclosed vacuoles containing whorls of multilaminated membrane that are thought to be responsible for the polychromatic appearance because of multilayer interference phenomena. The cataract may evolve to more extensive posterior, subcapsular, spokelike, cortical opacities and total cataract.

Histopathologic studies of the retina have shown degeneration of the photoreceptor cells in the midperiphery and periphery, associated hyperplasia of the RPE, and migration into the outer aspect of the retina and in some cases in a perivascular location (Figs. 8–521 and 8–522) (Manschot, 1968a; Houber, Babel, 1970; Betten, Bilchik, Smith, 1971; Ginsberg, Hamblet, Menefec, 1978). Other studies (Burns, 1969) have disclosed no retinal changes.

Studies of extraocular muscle by Kuwabara and Lessell (1970) disclosed disorganization in the arrangement of randomly distributed myofibrils. They concluded that the pathogenesis of the abnormality may be related to myofibrillogenesis and its maintenance. Other studies (Ginsberg and associates, 1978) suggest a primary disorder of mitochondria.

Cerebrohepatorenal Syndrome (Zellweger's Syndrome). This syndrome, first recognized by Bowen, Lee, Zellweger, and Lindenberg (1964), is a multisystem congenital disorder characterized by central nervous system demyelination, hepatic interstitial fibrosis, multiple renal cortical cysts, calcific stippling of the bony epiphyses, and distinctive abnormal craniofacial development.

This disorder is similar, both clinically and biochemically, to adrenoleukodystrophy (Benke, Reyes, Parker, 1981; Brown, McAdams, Cum-

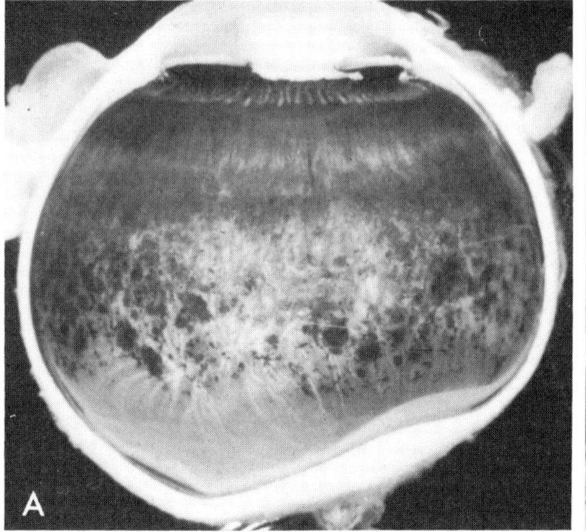

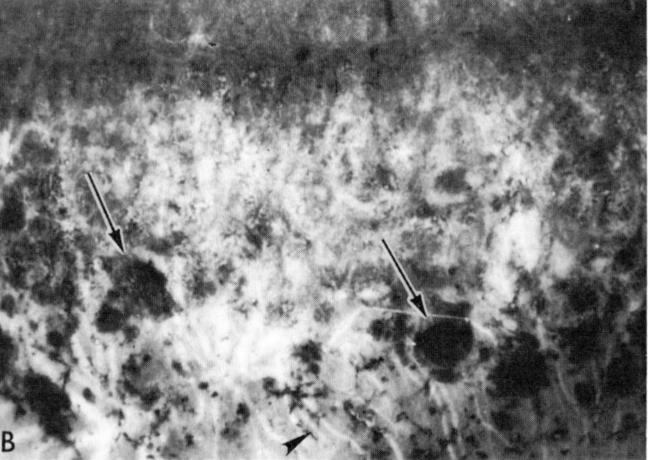

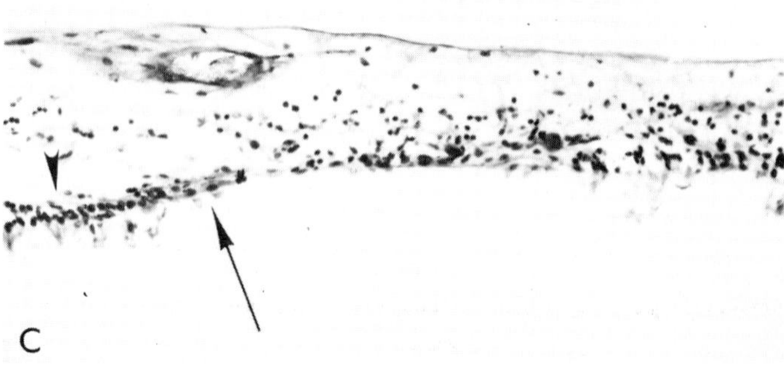

Figure 8–521. Myotonic dystrophy in 57 year old male. *A*, Gross appearance of patches of pigmentation, extending from midperiphery to ora serrata. *B*, Closer view shows patches of hypertrophic retinal pigment epithelium (RPE) (arrows). In some posterior areas (arrowhead), hyperplasia of RPE with migration into retina in perivascular location occurred. *C*, Section shows posterior junction, where outer nuclear layer becomes atrophic (arrow). Outer nuclear layer (arrowhead) with some photoreceptors is present posteriorly. PAS, ×215. EP 48440.

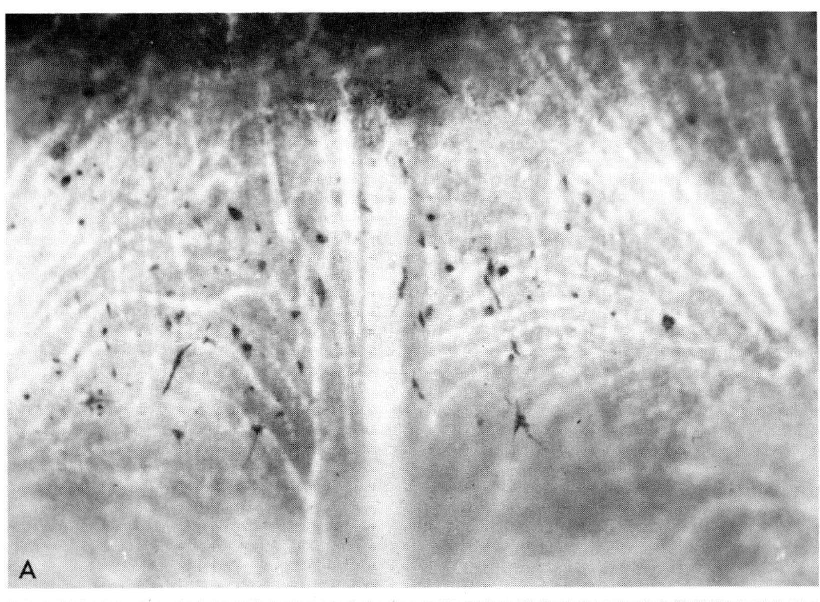

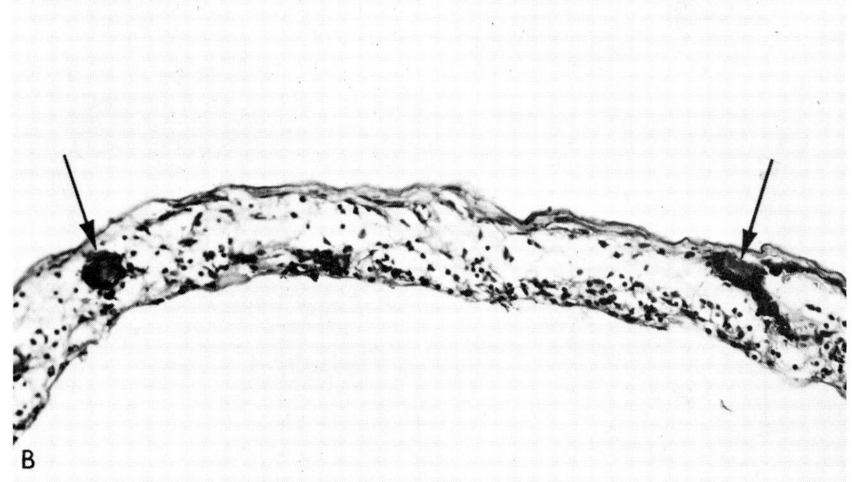

Figure 8–522. Myotonic dystrophy in 46 year old female. *A,* Gross appearance is similar to that of retinitis pigmentosa. Hyperplastic retinal pigment epithelium (RPE) has migrated into the retina in a perivascular location, and this gives a spiculate appearance. *B,* Equatorial retina showing loss of photoreceptor cell layer and hyperplastic RPE in a perivascular location (arrows). PAS, ×210. EP 49445.

mins, et al, 1982), which is a congenital neurodegenerative disorder characterized by elevated serum long-chain fatty acids.

A wide range of clinical ocular abnormalities has been described in Zellweger's syndrome, including a flat nasal bridge with apparent hypertelorism, hypoplasia of supraorbital ridges, nystagmus, microphthalmia, corneal clouding, congenital cataract, congenital glaucoma, Brushfield spots, narrowed retinal vessels, RPE changes (pigment elevations, hypopigmentation, and clumping (Fig. 8–523,*A*), and optic nerve changes. Extinguished electro-oculograms have been noted (Stanescu, Dralands, 1972; Haddad, Font, Friendly, 1976; Cohen, Brown, Martyn, et al, 1983).

Cohen and associates (1983) found ten reports of the ocular histopathology of Zellweger's syndrome. Anterior segment pathology has included corneal edema (Haddad, Font, Friendly, 1976; Cohen, Brown, Martyn, et al, 1983), posterior embryotoxin (Moser, Moser, Frayer, et al, 1981; Cohen, Brown, Martyn, et al, 1983), iridocorneal adhesions (Haddad, Font, Friendly, 1976), and lens changes (Haddad, Font, Friendly, 1976; Hittner, Kretzer, Mehta, 1981; McCormick, 1969; Cohen, Brown, Martyn, et al, 1983). In the vitreous, strands and cells have been noted (Schwartz, Green, Grover, Huff, 1971; Cohen, Brown, Martyn, et al, 1983).

In the retina, ganglion cell loss with gliosis has been noted, particularly in the midperiphery. There is marked photoreceptor degeneration (Fig. 8–523,*B* through *E*), with focal atrophy, hypertrophy, and hyperplasia of the RPE. Periodic-acid–Schiff–positive pigmented macrophages have been noted in the subretinal space admixed with degenerated photoreceptors (Fig. 8–523,*C* through *F*), and pigmented macrophages had migrated into the retina (Fig. 8–523,*H* and *I*) (Volpe, Adams, 1972; Kretzer, Hittner, Mehta, 1981; Garner, Fielder, Primavesi, Stevens, 1982; Cohen, Brown, Martyn, et al, 1983).

Text continued on page 1178

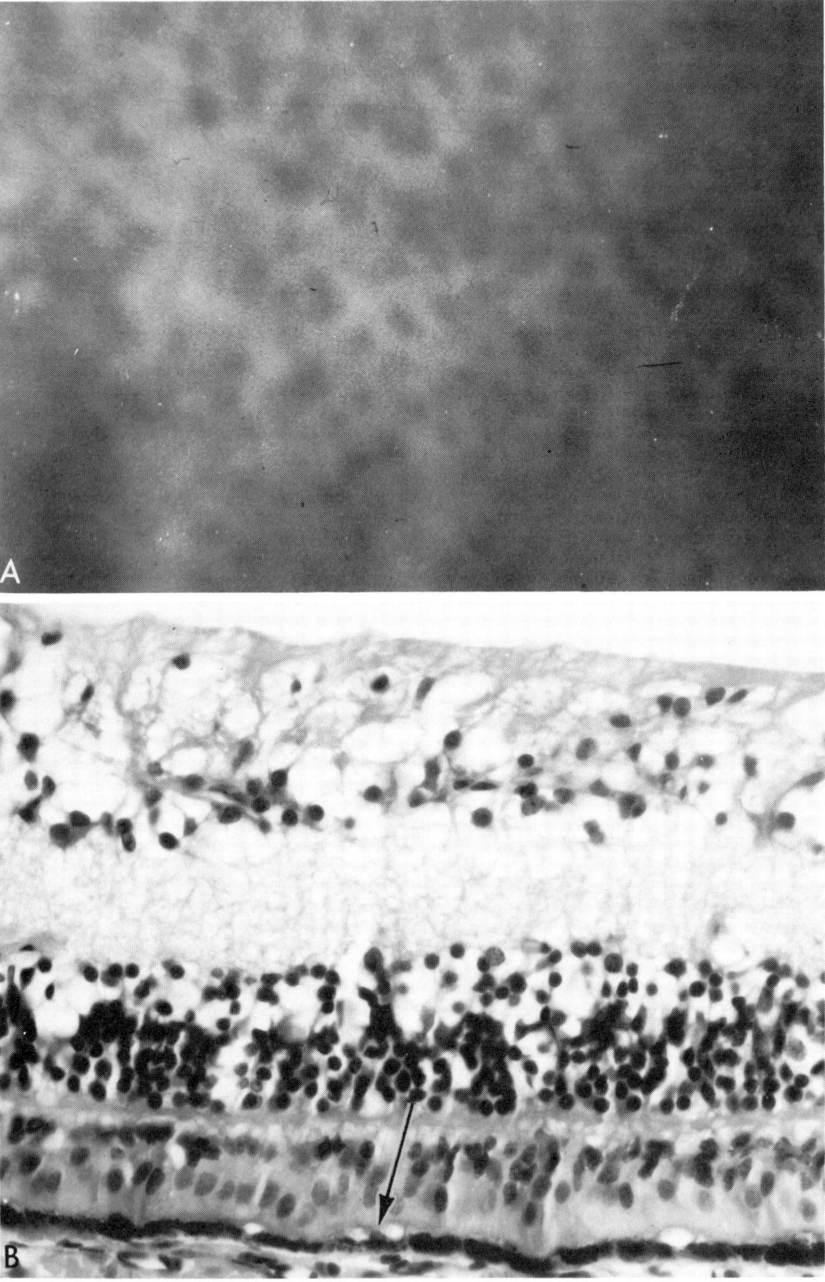

Figure 8–523. *A,* Small, multifocal hyperpigmentation of fundus in patient with **Zellweger's syndrome**. *B,* Parafoveal area, showing retinal pigment epithelium (RPE) to be intact but with areas of hypopigmentation (arrow). Outer nuclear layer is reduced in thickness. No outer or inner segments of photoreceptor cells are evident, and external limiting membrane appears to rest against RPE. EP 37155.

Illustration continued on opposite page

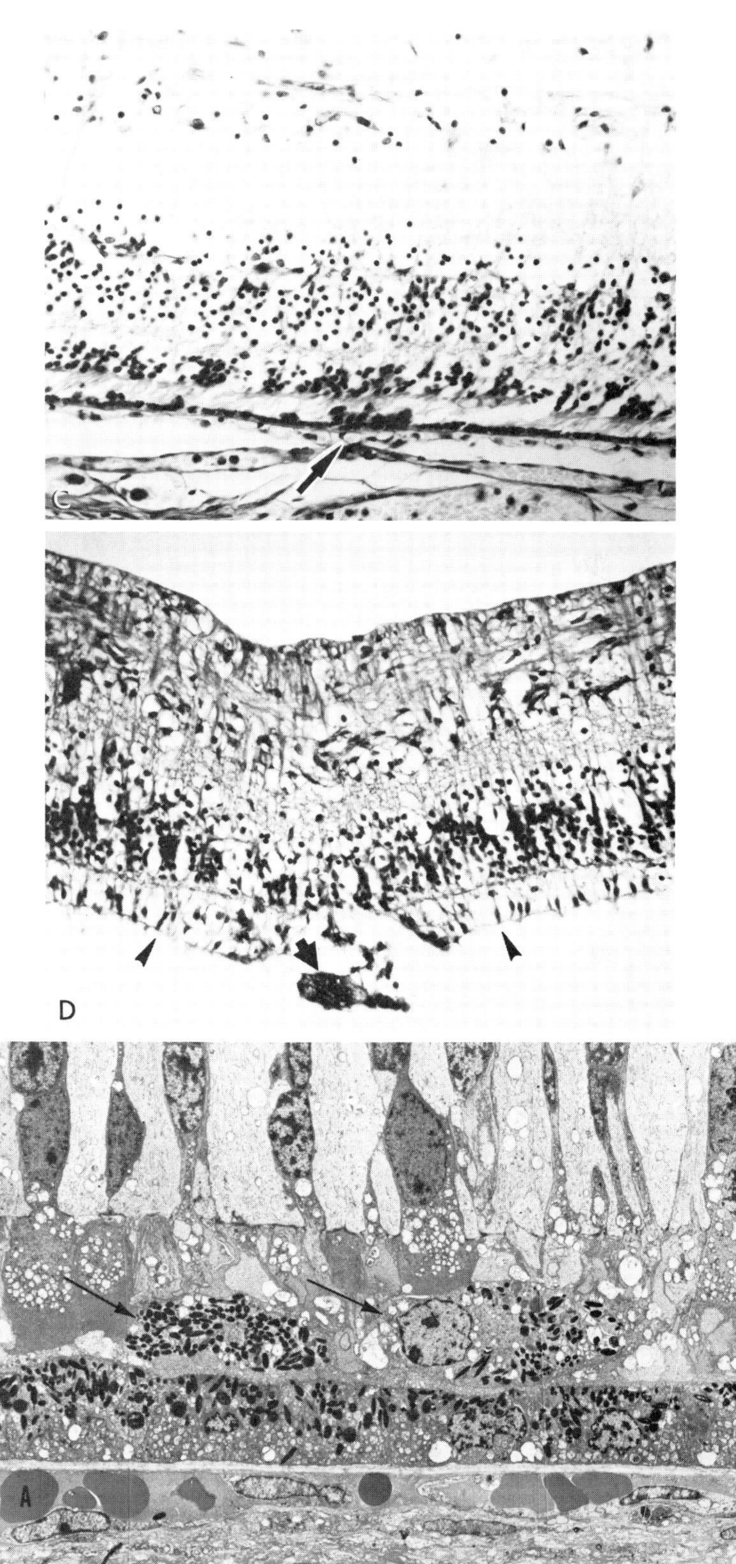

Figure 8–523 *Continued C,* Midperipheral retina showing mild thinning of the outer nuclear layer, with moderate loss of the inner and outer segments of photoreceptors. An aggregate of pigmented macrophages (arrow) is present between the RPE and retina. H and E, ×290. EP 31276.

D, Midperiphery showing marked loss of the outer nuclear layer (arrowheads), total loss of the inner and outer segments of the photoreceptors, and a nodule of pigmented cells on the posterior surface of the retina (arrow). PAS, × 280. EP 41397. *E,* Choriocapillaris *(A),* Bruch's membrane *(B),* and RPE *(C)* appear normal. No outer segments of photoreceptor cells are evident, and inner segments *(D)* are reduced in number. Remaining inner segments are shorter than normal and appear stubby. Junctional complexes of external limiting (Verhoeff's) membrane *(E)* are parallel to Bruch's membrane. Outer nuclear layer *(F)* has abnormally few nuclei. Macrophage-like cells (arrows) are located between retina and RPE. ×2500.

Illustration continued on following page

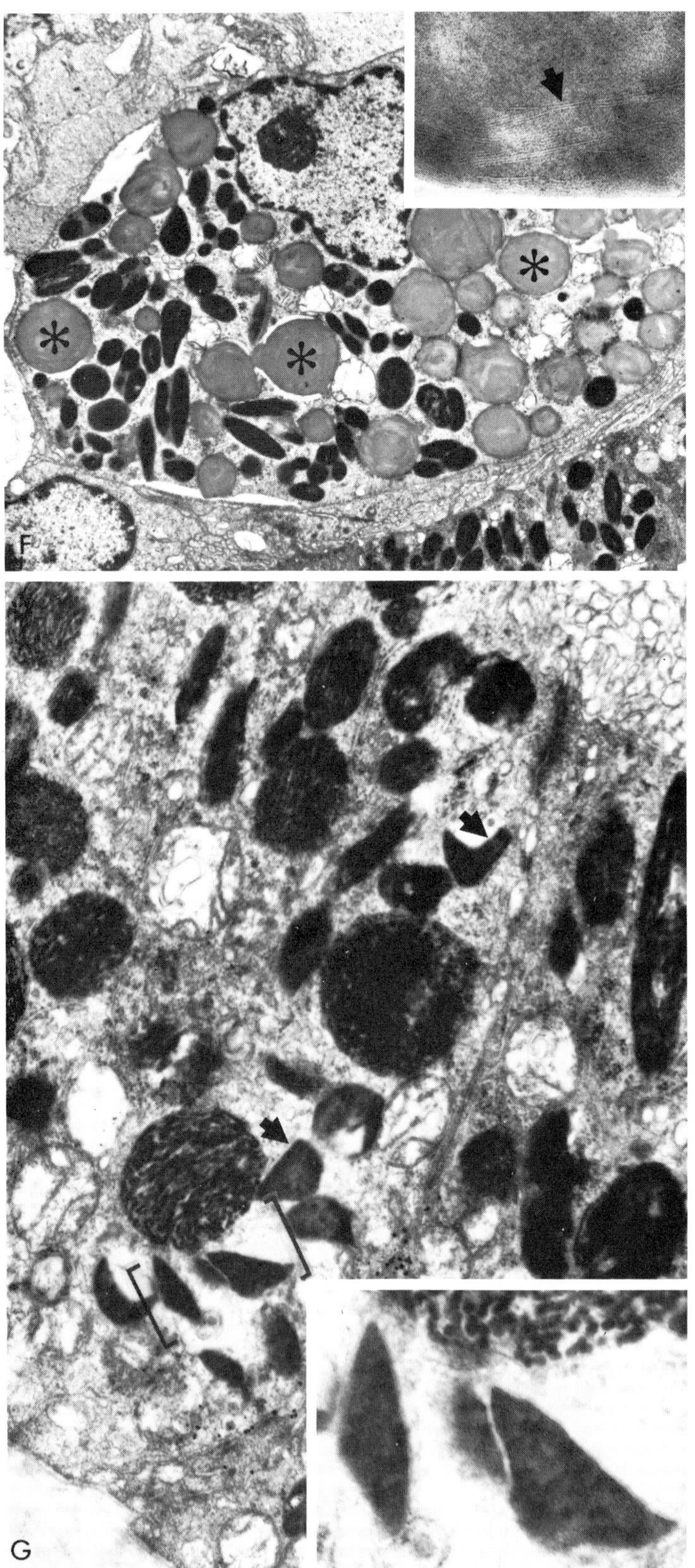

Figure 8–523 *Continued F,* Macrophage in the subretinal space from the midperiphery is densely packed with melanosomes and large, round, nonmembrane-bound bodies (asterisks). ×8000. At higher power (inset), the body is seen to consist of paired, electron-dense leaflets, 2.2 nm in diameter and separated by a 2.2 nm, electron-lucent space, intermixed with a fine granular background material. Inset, ×100,000. *G,* RPE with angulated, nonmembrane-bound inclusions (arrows and brackets), admixed with normal melanosomes.
×26,500. Higher power view of bracketed area (inset) shows angulated bodies to be composed of stacked bileaflet inclusions. Inset ×70,000. *E–G,* EP 37155.

Illustration continued on opposite page

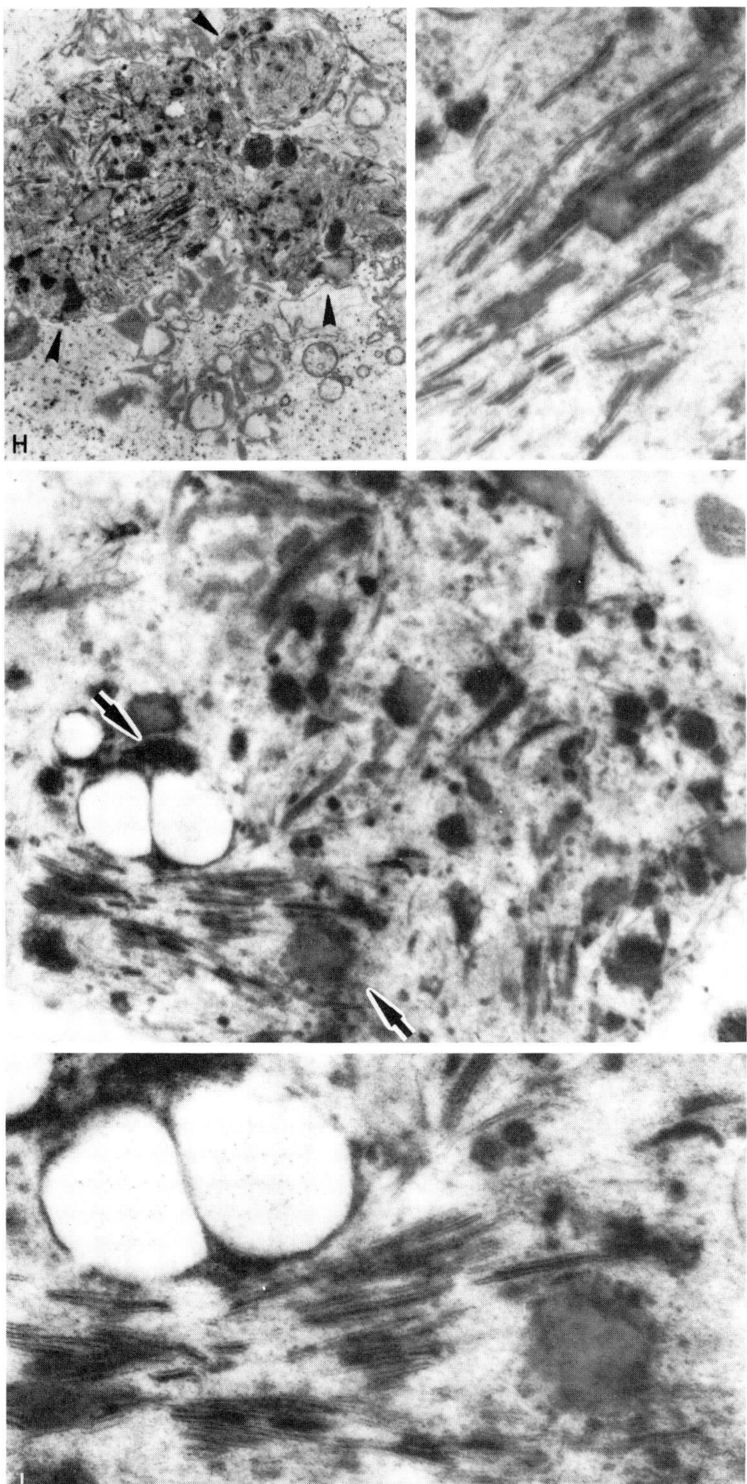

Figure 8–523 *Continued H,* Left, Macrophage in the ganglion cell layer of the peripheral retina, with multilobulated inclusion (arrowheads) admixed with lipid and melanosomes. ×10,000. Right, Higher power view of circled area shows loosely arranged bileaflet inclusions (arrows). The individual leaflets measure 3.7 nm in diameter and are separated by a 3.1 nm electron-lucent space. ×80,000. *I,* Top, Macrophage in the ganglion cell layer of the macular area has a large aggregate of heterogeneous material. ×40,000. Bottom, Higher-power view of area between arrows, showing numerous bileaflet inclusions. ×80,000.

Illustration continued on following page

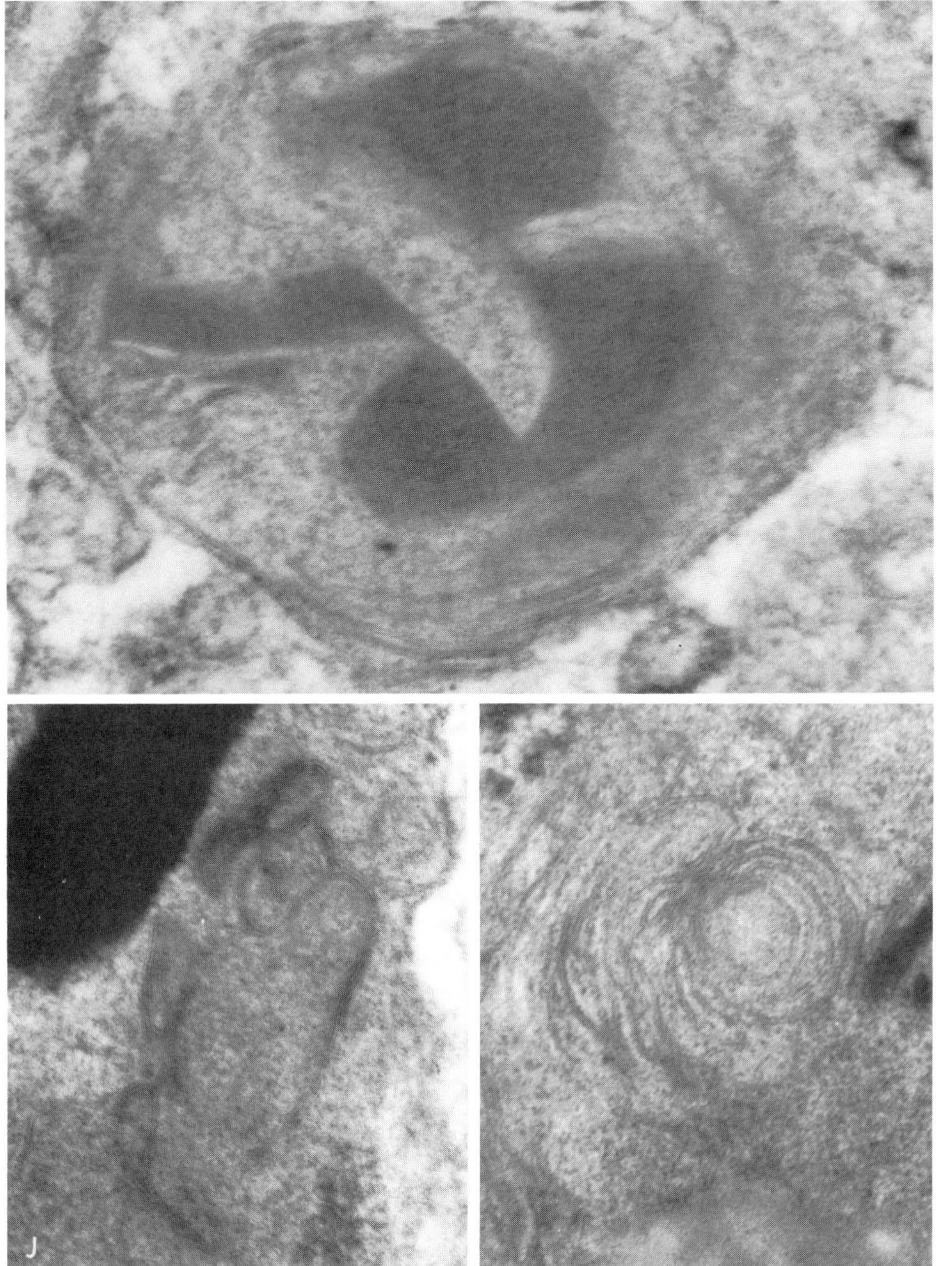

Figure 8–523 *Continued J,* Three different patterns of inclusions in macrophages from the macular area. Top, Large, nonmembrane-bound aggregate of angular dense material is surrounded by much bileaflet material. Lower left, Bileaflet material is arranged in an irregular, curved configuration and is enmeshed in a finely granular and less-defined membranous material. Lower right, Bileaflet material is arranged in a whorled pattern. All, ×90,000. *H–J,* EP 41397.

(From Cohen SMZ, Brown FR III, Martyn L, et al: Ocular histopathologic and biochemical studies of the cerebro-hepato-renal (Zellweger) syndrome and its relation to neonatal adrenoleukodystrophy. Am J Ophthalmol, accepted for publication.)

Marked atrophy and gliosis of the optic nerve are frequently present (Haddad, Font, Friendly, 1976; Kretzer, Hittner, Mehta, 1981; Garner, Fielder, Primavesi, Stevens, 1982). Cohen and associates (1983) have described two patients with optic nerve hypoplasia. Extramedullary hematopoiesis is occasionally seen (Jan, Hardwick, Lowry, McCormick, 1970; McCormick, 1969; Schwartz, Green, Grover, Huff, 1971; Cohen, Brown, Martyn, et al, 1983).

Ultrastructural studies show macrophages with melanin and electron-dense material in the subretinal space. Marked shortening of photoreceptor inner segments with absence of outer segments is noted (Fig. 8–523,*E*). Condensations of paired electron-dense bileaflet inclusions are present in pigment epithelial cells (Fig. 8–523,*G*) and also in pigment-laden macrophages in the retina (Fig. 8–523,*H* and *I*) and subretinal space (Fig. 8–523,*F*). Various inclusion patterns are noted (Fig. 8–523,*J*). These inclusions are quite similar to those found in the RPE cells, macrophages, and retinal neurons in neonatal adrenoleukodystrophy. These findings suggest a possible relationship between the Zellweger syndrome and neonatal adrenoleukodystrophy (Cohen, Green, de la Cruz, et al, 1983).

Norrie's Disease (Progressive Oculoacousticocerebral Degeneration). Persons affected with this sex-linked recessive syndrome have retinal involvement, mental retardation, and deafness (Warburg, 1966).

These patients have little or no vision and often display a retrolental mass.

Histopathologic studies have been variously interpreted. Blodi and Hunter (1969) reported serosanguineous retinal detachment, periretinal proliferation, distorted retina in a rosette-like pattern from contraction of periretinal fibrovascular tissue (Fig. 8–524), and vascular changes similar to those seen in Coats' disease. At the late stage, secondary changes are marked (Townes and Roca, 1973).

Although describing features similar to those just mentioned, Apple, Fishman, and Goldberg (1974) interpreted the changes as being an arrest in the development of the embryonic sensory retina, associated with persistence of the primary vitreous, with hypoplasia and dysplasia of the retina. They believed the changes were distinct from those of Coats' disease.

Hereditary Hemorrhagic Telangiectasis (Rendu-Osler-Weber Disease). This disease is transmitted as an autosomal dominant trait and is characterized by multiple dilations of capillaries and venules in the skin, mucous membranes, and viscera that have a tendency to bleed. Ophthalmoscopic manifestations have been caused by lid and conjunctival involvement (Wolper, Laibson, 1969), but retinal involvement has been rarely noted (François, 1938; Cuendet, Magnenat, 1953; Landau, Nelken, Davis, 1956; Roubin, 1957; Calmettes, Deodati, Bec, 1958; Massa, de Vloo, Jamotton, 1966; Meyer-Schwickerath von Barsewisch, 1968; Davis, Smith, 1971). The retinal changes have been described as being similar to those seen in diabetes (Davis, Smith, 1971). Histopathologic changes observed post mortem in the eyes of a patient with this syndrome include resolved retinal hemorrhages, branch artery occlusion, and beading of retinal arteries (Fig. 8–525). An additional patient is a 7 year old boy with Osler-Weber-Rendu disease who noted a sudden loss of vision. A large vitreous hemorrhage obscured fundus details. He subsequently developed neovascular glaucoma. Microscopic examination of the surgically enucleated eye disclosed an area of retinal neovascularization and inner ischemic atrophy (Fig. 8–526).

Hallervorden-Spatz Syndrome. This recessive disorder is characterized by progressive rigidity, first of the lower and later the upper extremities. In 1922, Hallervorden and Spatz described five sisters in a sibship of 12 who had a progressive

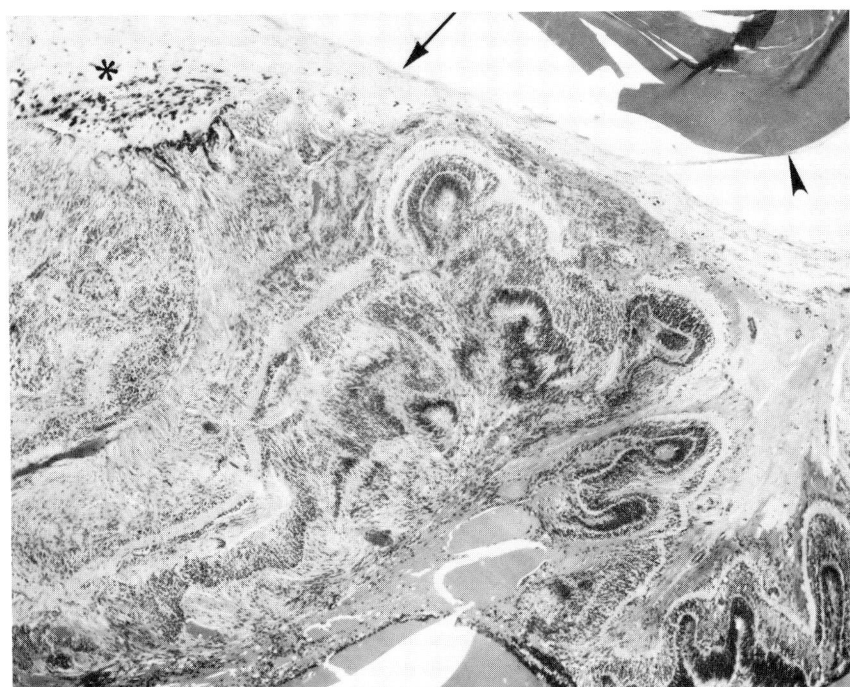

Figure 8–524. Surgically enucleated eye of 7 year old boy with **Norrie's disease**. Changes are nonspecific and include much preretinal fibrovascular proliferation (arrow), with hemosiderin depositon (arrowhead) and traction retinal detachment. Detached retina is drawn into folds, in a pseudorosette configuration, and is located behind lens (arrowhead). H and E, ×35. EP 47682.

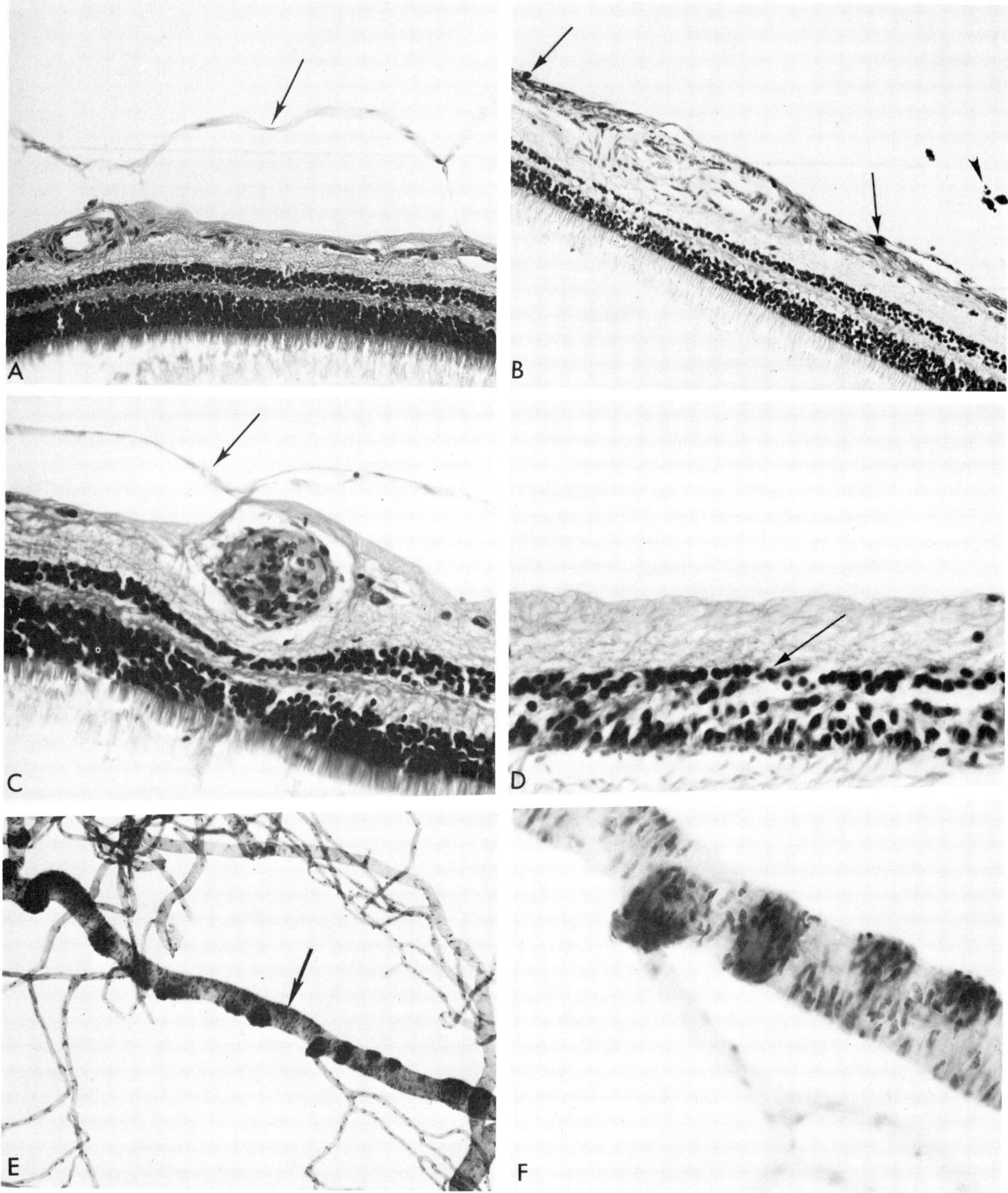

Figure 8–525. Osler-Weber-Rendu disease. *A,* Retina posteriorly is normal. Thin hypocellular epiretinal membrane (arrow) is present. H and E, ×235. *B,* Hemosiderin deposits in retina (arrows) and vitreous (arrowhead) a site of previous retinal hemorrhage. Prussian blue, ×235. *C,* Thrombosis of branch of central retinal artery (arrow). H and E, ×330.

D, Inner retinal ischemic atrophy, with loss of all inner retinal layers, including the inner portion of the inner nuclear layer. Outer portion of inner nuclear layer (arrow) remains intact. H and E, ×560. *E,* Retinal trypsin digest preparation, showing beading of an artery (arrow). Hematoxylin/PAS, ×110. *F,* Beaded areas are hypercellular and bulge slightly from surface. H and E, ×500. EP 46511.

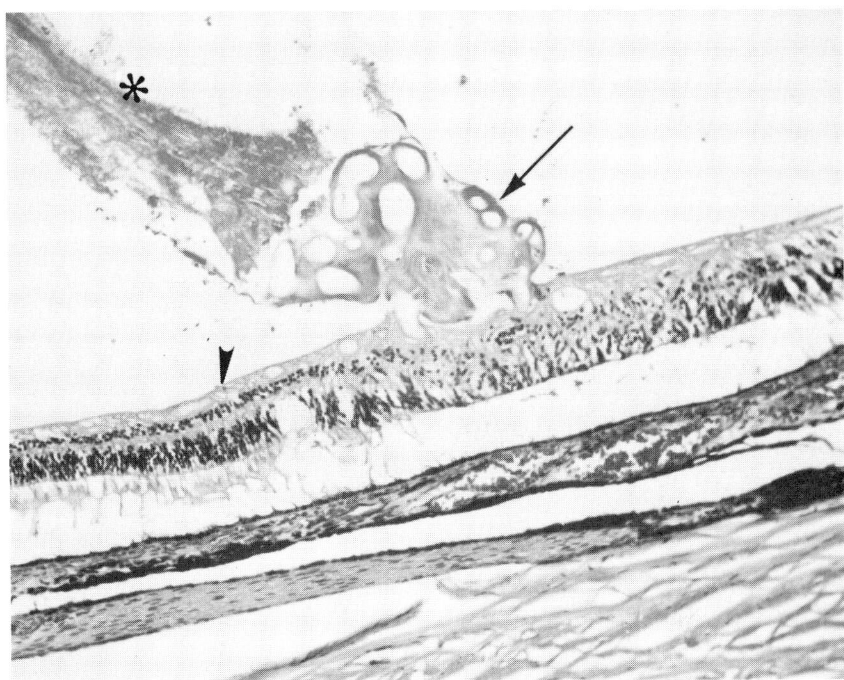

Figure 8–526. Osler-Weber-Rendu syndrome. Area of retinal neovascularization in temporal midperiphery extending into vitreous cavity (arrow). Vitreous hemorrhage (asterisk) is present. Retina peripheral to area of neovascularization shows inner ischemic atrophy (arrowhead). H and E, ×110. EP 47475. (Courtesy of Dr. F.C. Blodi; case presented at Theobald Society, Iowa City, May, 1979.)

neurodegenerative disorder characterized by extrapyramidal motor signs, dysarthria, dementia, and death.

Dooling, Schoene, and Richardson (1974) reviewed the 64 reported autopsy-proved cases, established strict clinical and histopathologic criteria, and found that 42 cases indicated a distinct clinicopathologic entity. They listed the four clinical characteristics of Hallervorden-Spatz syndrome as (1) onset at a young age, generally after earliest childhood; (2) extrapyramidal motor disorder wih dystonic posturing, muscular rigidity, chorioathetoid movements, ataxia, hyperreflexia and spasticity; (3) dementia; and (4) a relentlessly progressive course leading to death in early adulthood.

In two cases (Roth, Helper, Mukoyma, et al, 1971; Swisher, Menkes, Cancilla, Dodge, 1972), an associated acanthocytosis with normal lipid findings and normal betalipoprotein levels was noted.

The neuropathologic characteristics are (1) symmetric, partially destructive lesions of the globus pallidus, especially its internal segment, and the pars reticulata of the substantia nigra, characterized by some loss of myelinated fibers and neurons, with gliosis; (2) widely disseminated, rounded or oval non-nucleated structures ("spheroids") identifiable as swollen axons, especially numerous in the globus pallidus and pars reticulata; and (3) accumulations of pigment, much of it iron-containing, in the affected regions.

Newell, Johnson, and Huttenlocker (1979) found that almost one fourth of the 42 patients with this syndrome had retinal degeneration. They believed that such patients formed a distinct group that had a much earlier onset and a much more rapid course, with death occurring late in childhood. They observed retinal degeneration with retinal flecks and a "bull's eye" maculopathy in dizygotic twins with the Hallervorden-Spatz syndrome.

Roth, Helper, Mukoyama, et al (1971) reported the light microscopic findings of the eyes of a patient with Hallervorden-Spatz syndrome with acanthocytosis and normal levels of betalipoproteins. Clinically, that patient displayed thinning of the macula and a diffuse, gray clouding of the paramacular areas. Bone spicule pigmentation was noted in the equatorial retina, but the optic disks and vessels were normal. On light microscopy, the photoreceptors were absent, and the outer nuclear and outer plexiform layers were quite attenuated or absent in most areas. The inner retinal layers were normal, as was the optic nerve. There were accumulations of pigment, both intracellularly and extracellularly, predominantly around equatorial blood vessels. The RPE was described as irregular.

Luckenbach, Green, Miller, et al (1983) reported the clinicopathologic features of the Hallervorden-Spatz syndrome in a 10 year old girl with retinal degeneration, acanthocytosis, and normal betalipoprotein levels. The ophthalmoscopic picture was characterized initially by a flecked retina appearance (Fig. 8–527,*A*) and later by bone spicule formation and a bull's eye annular maculopathy (Fig. 8–527,*B*). Light microscopic examination disclosed extensive atrophy of the photoreceptor cell layer throughout but es-

Text continued on page 1187

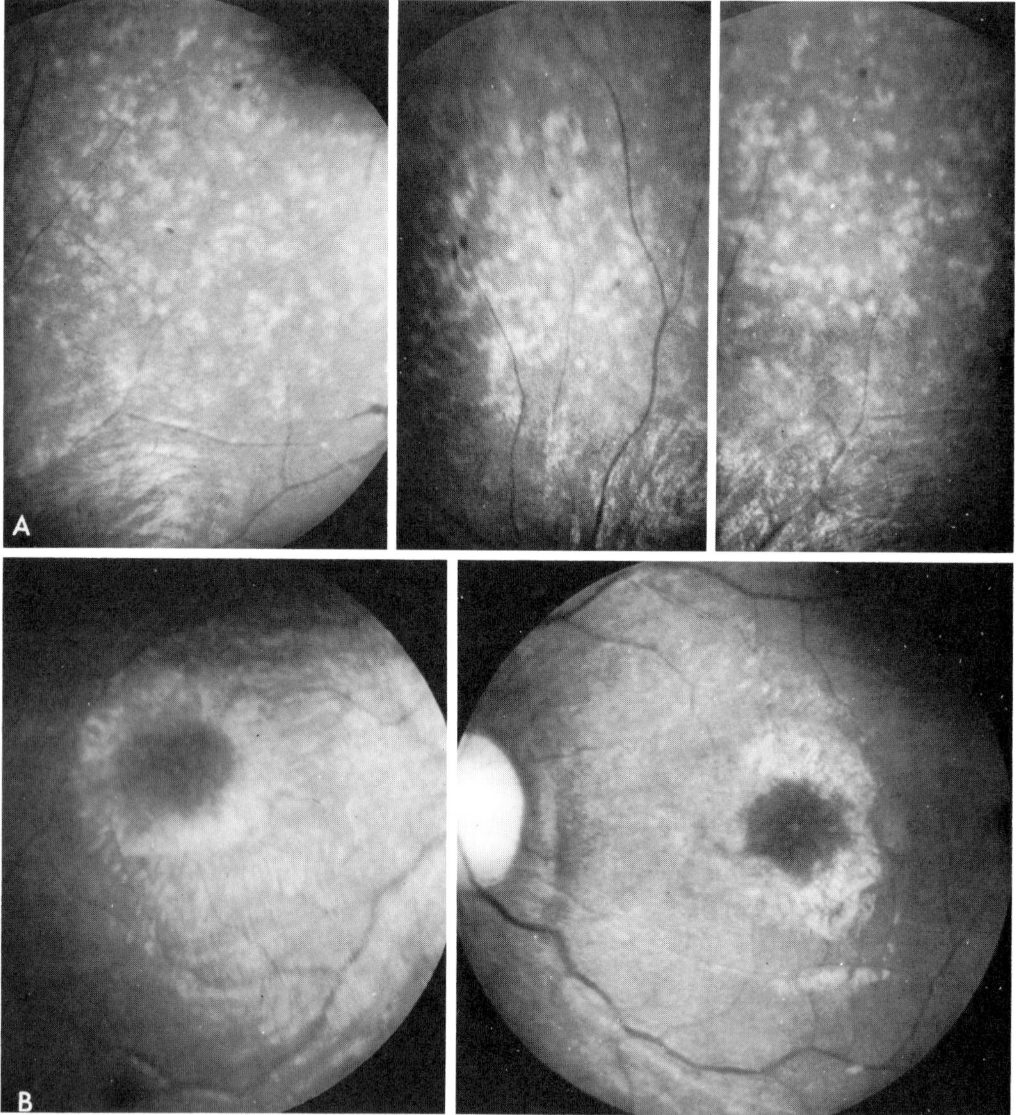

Figure 8–527. Hallervorden-Spatz syndrome with acanthocytosis and pigmentary retinopathy. *A*, Midperipheral areas of retina with many yellow-white flecks of various sizes and shapes located deep in the retinal blood vessels. *B*, Macular area of right (left) and left (right) eyes, showing bull's-eye appearance with granular hyperpigmentation of the fovea. An anular deposition of yellow material is located deep in the retinal vessels.

Illustration continued on opposite page

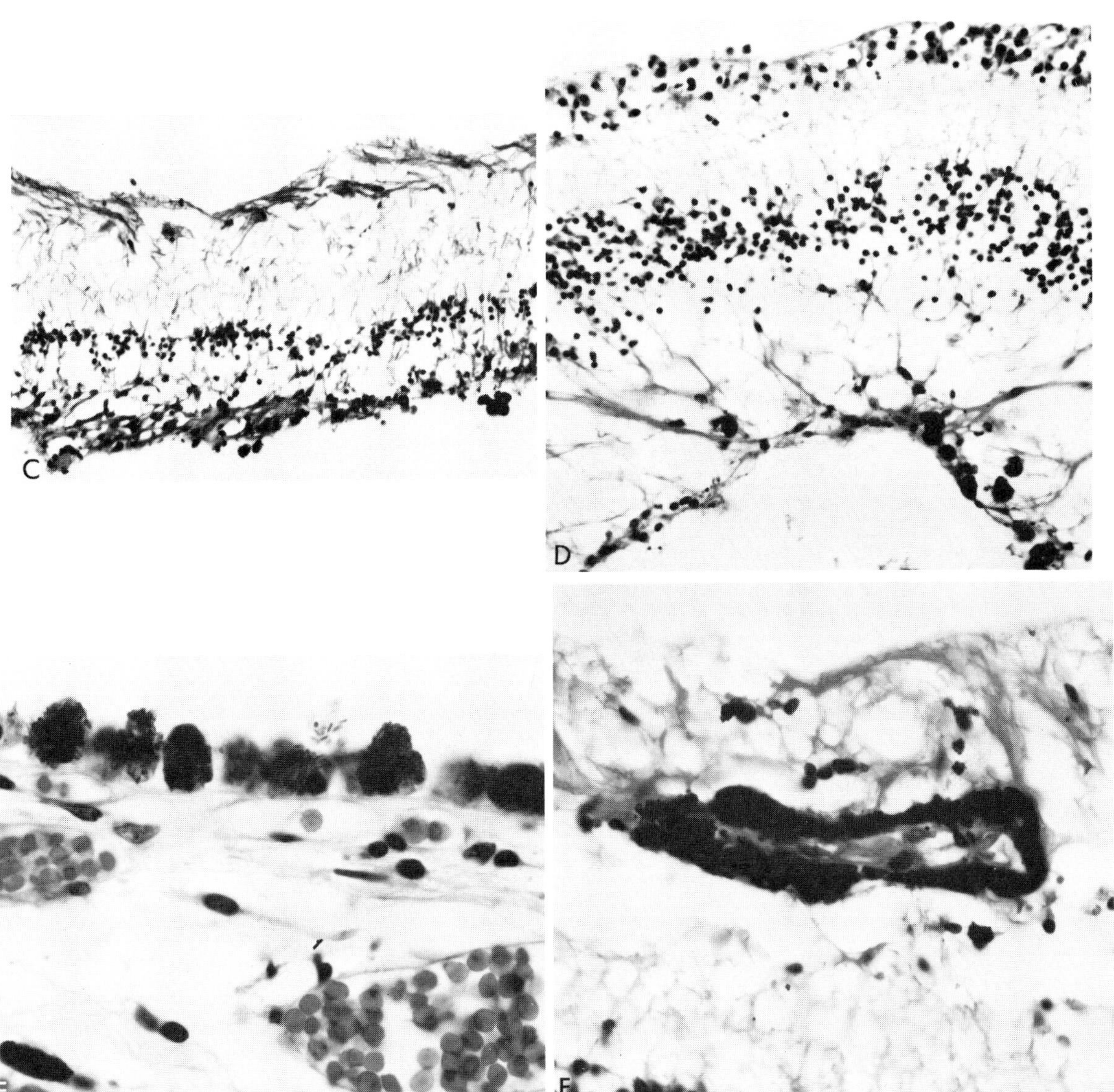

Figure 8–527 *Continued C,* Temporal midperipheral retina with total loss of the photoreceptor cell layer. Pigmented cells are present in the outer aspect of the retina. H and E, ×220. *D,* Macular area, with loss of photoreceptor cell layer and presence of pigmented cells in outer retina. PAS, ×525.

E, Posterior area showing much distension of the retinal pigment epithelial cells, which vary in size and shape and contain large, round pigment aggregates. H and E, ×900. *F,* Equatorial area, showing retinal blood vessel surrounded by pigmented cells. PAS, ×280.

Illustration continued on following page

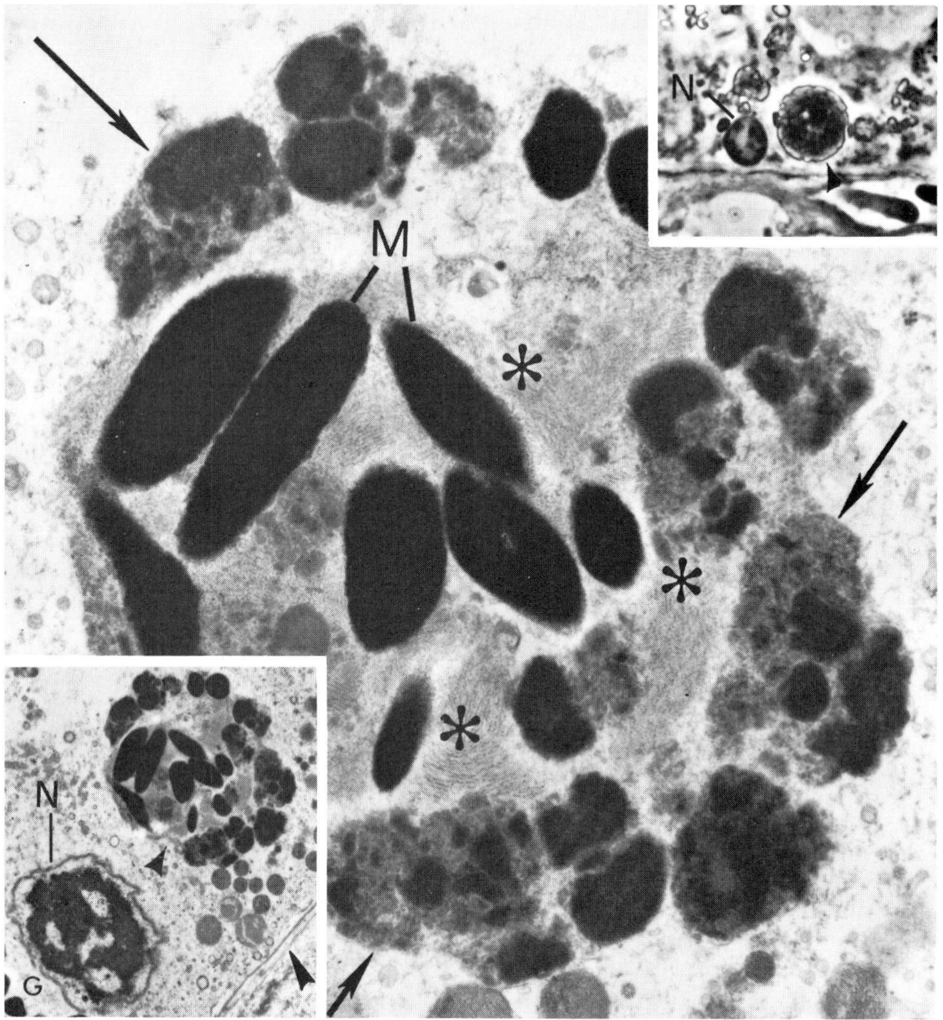

Figure 8–527 *Continued G,* Retinal pigment epithelium (RPE) with a giant, single-membrane–bound melanolipofuscin aggregate 35 μm in diameter. It is composed of cigar-shaped melanin granules *(M)* and pleomorphic lipofuscin granules (arrows) embedded in a membranous lipofuscin (asterisks) background. ×25,000. Insets: pigment aggregate (arrowhead) is larger than the nucleus *(N)* of the RPE cell. Top inset: phase-contrast, paraphenylenediamine, ×2000; bottom inset, ×6200.

Illustration continued on opposite page

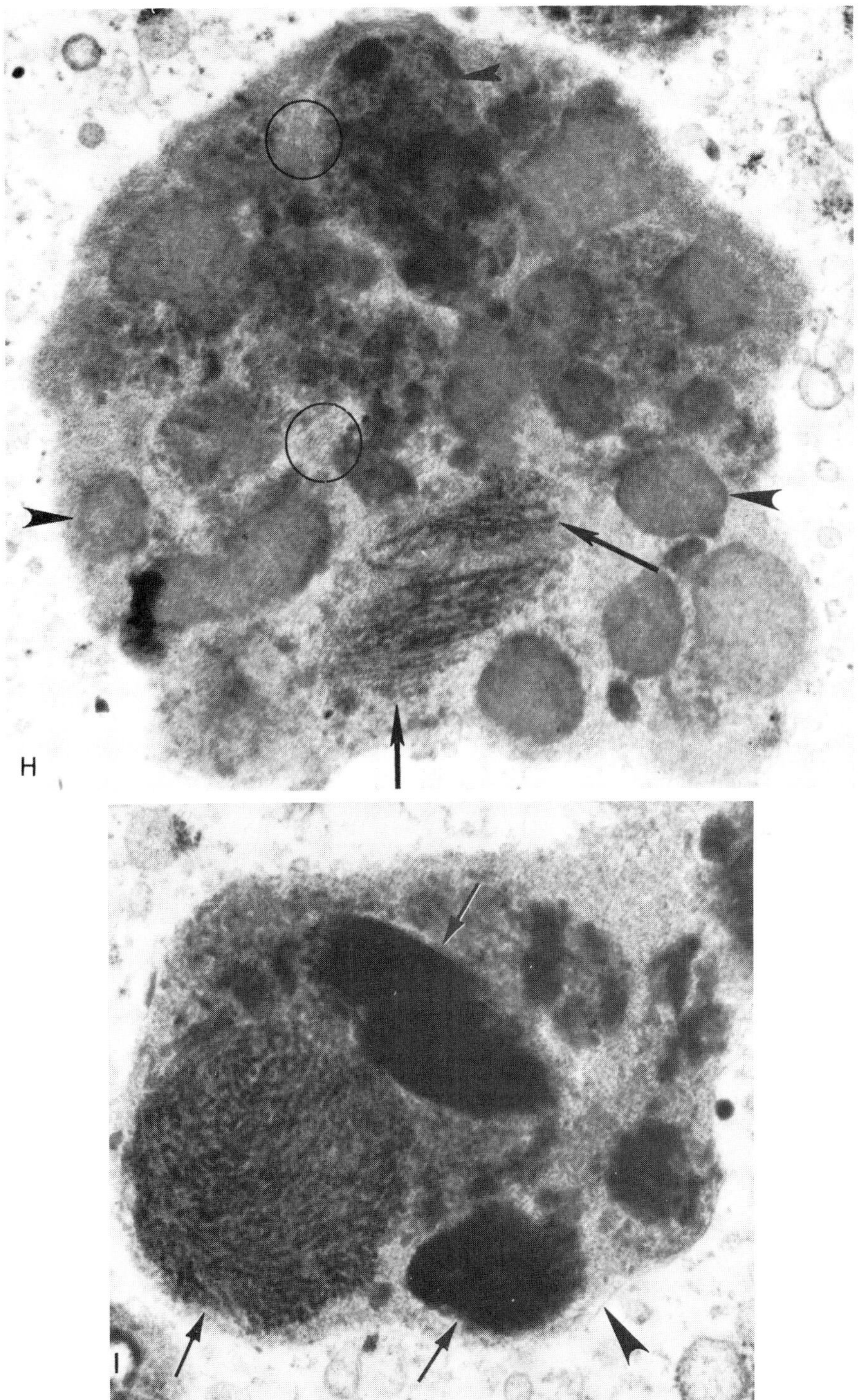

Figure 8–527 *Continued H,* RPE with pigment aggregate that measures 1.4 μm in diameter and is composed of lipofuscin in the form of membranous (circled areas), pleomorphic lipofuscin granules (arrowheads) and partially degraded melanin granules (arrows). ×40,000.

I, RPE with single-membrane–bound (arrowhead) melanolipofuscin aggregate that measures 1.4 μm in diameter and contains partially degraded melanin (arrows) in a background of finely granular lipofuscin and dense pleomorphic lipofuscin granules. ×40,000.

Illustration continued on following page

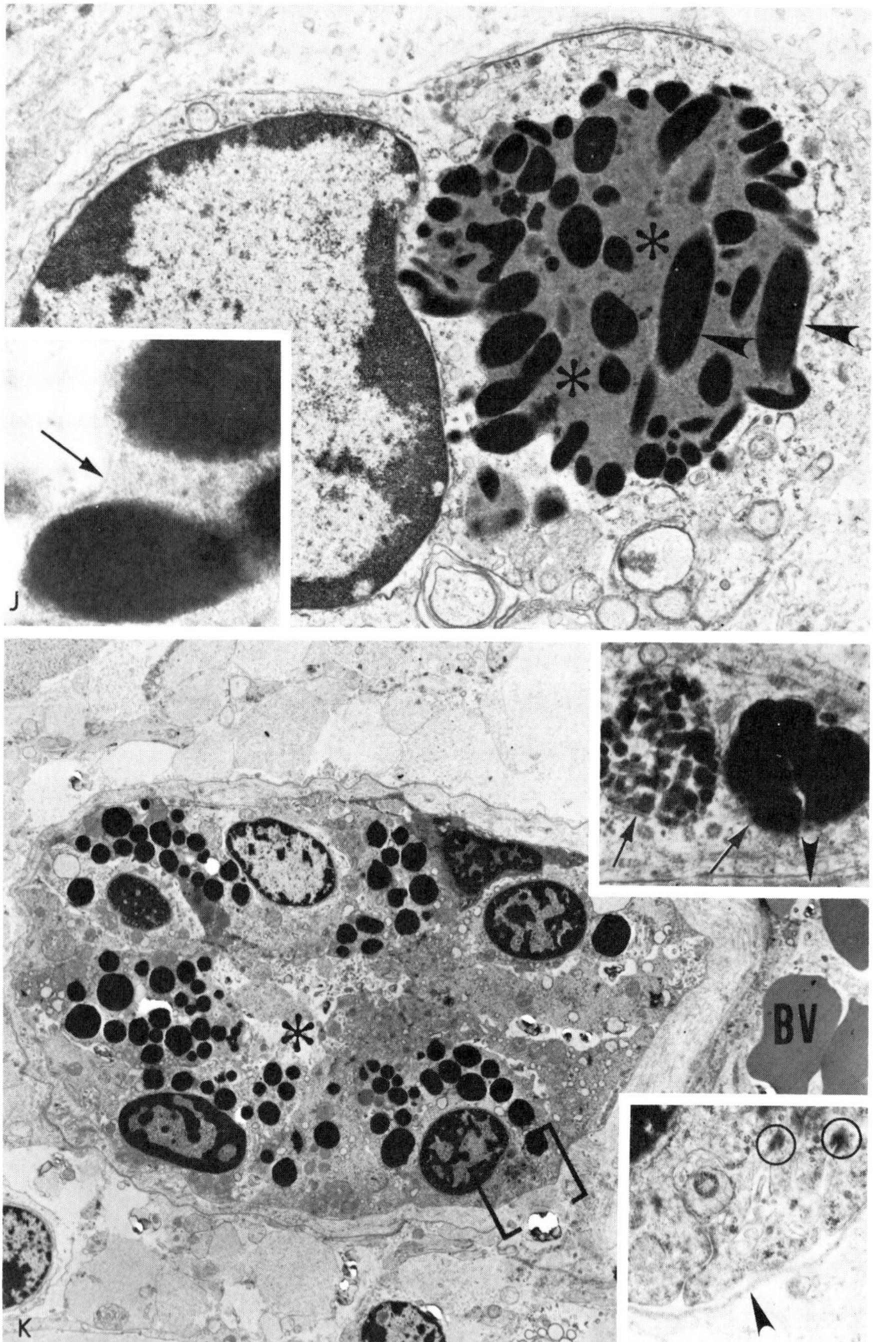

Figure 8–527 *Continued J,* Macrophage in outer retina contains a giant melanolipofuscin aggregate that measures 3.8 μm in diameter. The aggregate is composed of cigar-shaped melanin granules (arrowheads) embedded in a granular lipofuscin matrix (asterisks). ×15,300. Inset: The aggregate is bounded by a single membrane (arrow). ×60,000.

K, Hyperplastic RPE cells arranged in an acinar pattern adjacent to a retinal blood vessel *(BV)*. Cells contain round melanin granules, have microvilli at the apex facing the lumen (asterisk), have basement membrane at the base (bracketed area), and are joined by complex intercellular attachments (bracketed area). ×3,500. Top inset: Vascular pericyte is surrounded by basement membrane (arrowhead) and contains pleomorphic lipofuscin granules. ×39,170. Bottom inset: Higher-power view of the basement membrane at the base of the cells and the complex intercellular attachments (circled areas). ×17,000.

Illustration continued on opposite page

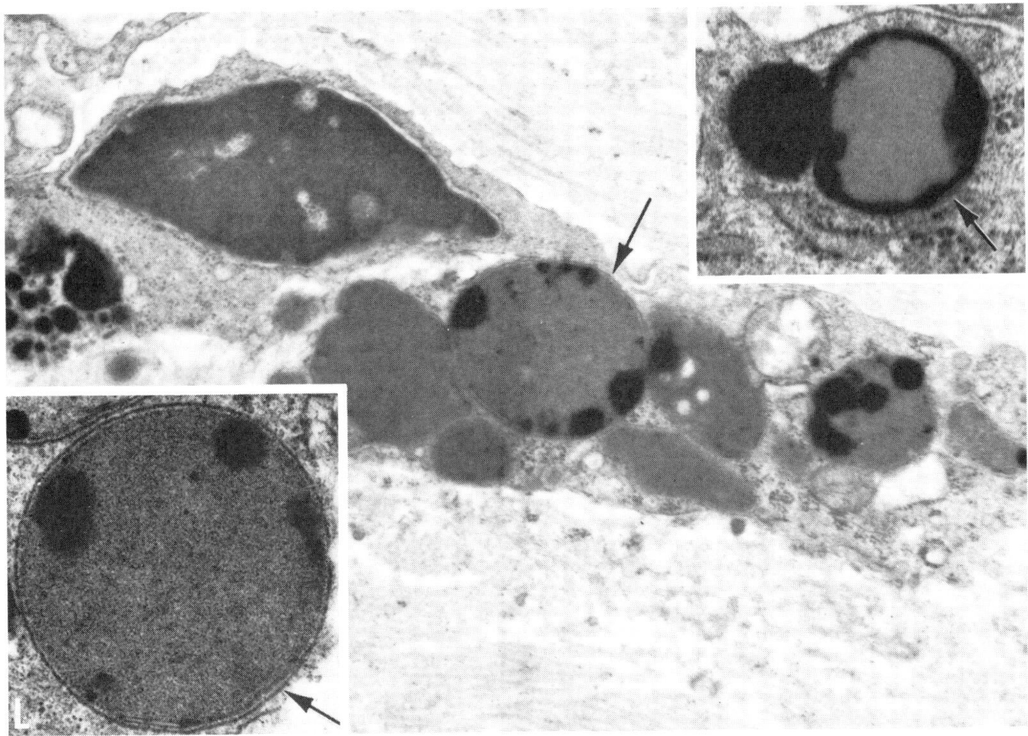

Figure 8–527 *Continued L,* Conjunctival fibrocyte contains membrane-bound (arrows) lipofuscin granules. These granules are composed of a fine granular material, with interspersed dense, homogeneous areas often located in the periphery. ×24,000. Insets: Higher power views of the lipofuscin granules. ×50,000.

(From Luckenbach MW, Green WR, Miller NR, et al: Ocular clinicopathologic correlation of Hallervorden-Spatz syndrome with acanthocytosis and pigmentary retinopathy. Am J Ophthalmol *95*:369–382, 1983.)

pecially in the posterior pole (Fig. 8–527,*C* and *D*). Pigmented cells were present in the outer aspect of the retina in an annular configuration in the parafoveal area. These cells corresponded to the bull's eye configuration seen in the macula (Fig. 8–527,*B*). The retinal pigment epithelial cells were distended and contained clumped pigment (Fig. 8–527,*E*). Hyperplastic retinal pigment had migrated into the retina in a perivascular location at the equator (Fig. 8–527,*F*).

On ultrastructural study, the retinal pigment epithelium varied in size and contained very large, round, single membrane-bound aggregates composed of complex melanolipofuscin granules (Fig. 8–527,*G* through *I*). Cells that had migrated into the outer retinal layers contained similar melanolipofuscin aggregates, were identified as macrophages (Fig. 8–527,*J*), and correlated with the flecks and macular annulus seen on ophthalmoscopy. The cells around the retinal blood vessels contained normal melanin pigment, were identified as retinal pigment epithelial cells (Fig. 8–527,*K*), and correlated with the "bone spicules" seen on ophthalmoscopic examination.

Luckenbach and associates (1983) also observed abnormal accumulation of lipofuscin in fibrocytes of the conjunctiva (Fig. 8–527,*L*).

The pathogenesis of Hallervorden-Spatz syndrome is unknown, but a common feature appears to be an abnormal accumulation of lipofuscin in certain susceptible tissues. Several investigators have conducted histochemical and ultrastructural studies and have concluded that the pigment found in the basal ganglia is primarily lipofuscin and neuromelanin (Yanagisawa, Shiraki, Minakawa, Narabayshi, 1966; Park, Netsky, Betsill, 1975; Vakili, Drew, Von Schuching, 1977).

Infantile Neuroaxonal Dystrophy. This familial disorder, probably inherited as an autosomal recessive trait, is characterized by a slowing of the rate of motor and mental development, beginning at the age of 6 months to 2 years, with a subsequent regression and loss of all previously acquired milestones. The disease is manifested by marked hypotonia, early visual disturbances, pyramidal tract signs with extensor plantar responses and exaggerated deep tendon reflexes, and terminal bulbar signs with difficulty in swallowing, dyspnea, and sphincter disturbances. The course is progressive, with decerebration, dementia, and death before the age of 10 years (Aicardi, Castelein, 1979).

Ocular involvement occurs early and may be manifested by strabismus, pendular nystagmus, incoordinate eye movements, and amaurosis. Optic atrophy occurs in 40 per cent of patients by the age of 3 years and in a further 30 per cent by age 3.5 years. When it has been performed, the electroretinogram is normal, but the visually evoked response, while sometimes unremarkable, is frequently abnormal. The mechanism of optic atrophy has not been determined as yet.

The diagnosis of infantile neuroaxonal dystrophy traditionally has been made at autopsy. In typical cases, spheroid bodies in axons, especially in their distal portions and in presynaptic terminals, are widely distributed throughout the central nervous system and are numerous in the cerebral cortex, as well as in the spinal cord, brain stem, and basal ganglia. More recently, the occurrence of spheroid bodies identical to those in the central nervous system in peripheral nerves (Duncan, Strub, McGarry, Duncan, 1970), in skin (Wisniewski, Wisniewski, 1978), and in conjunctiva (Arsenio-Nunes, Goutieres, 1978) has allowed the premortem diagnosis to be made by electron microscopic studies of peripheral nerve or skin or by conjunctival biopsy.

Ophthalmoplegia, Pigmentary Degeneration of Retina, and Cardiomyopathy (Kearns-Sayre Syndrome). The association of external ophthalmoplegia and retinal degeneration was reported by Barnard and Scholz (1944). Kearns and Sayre

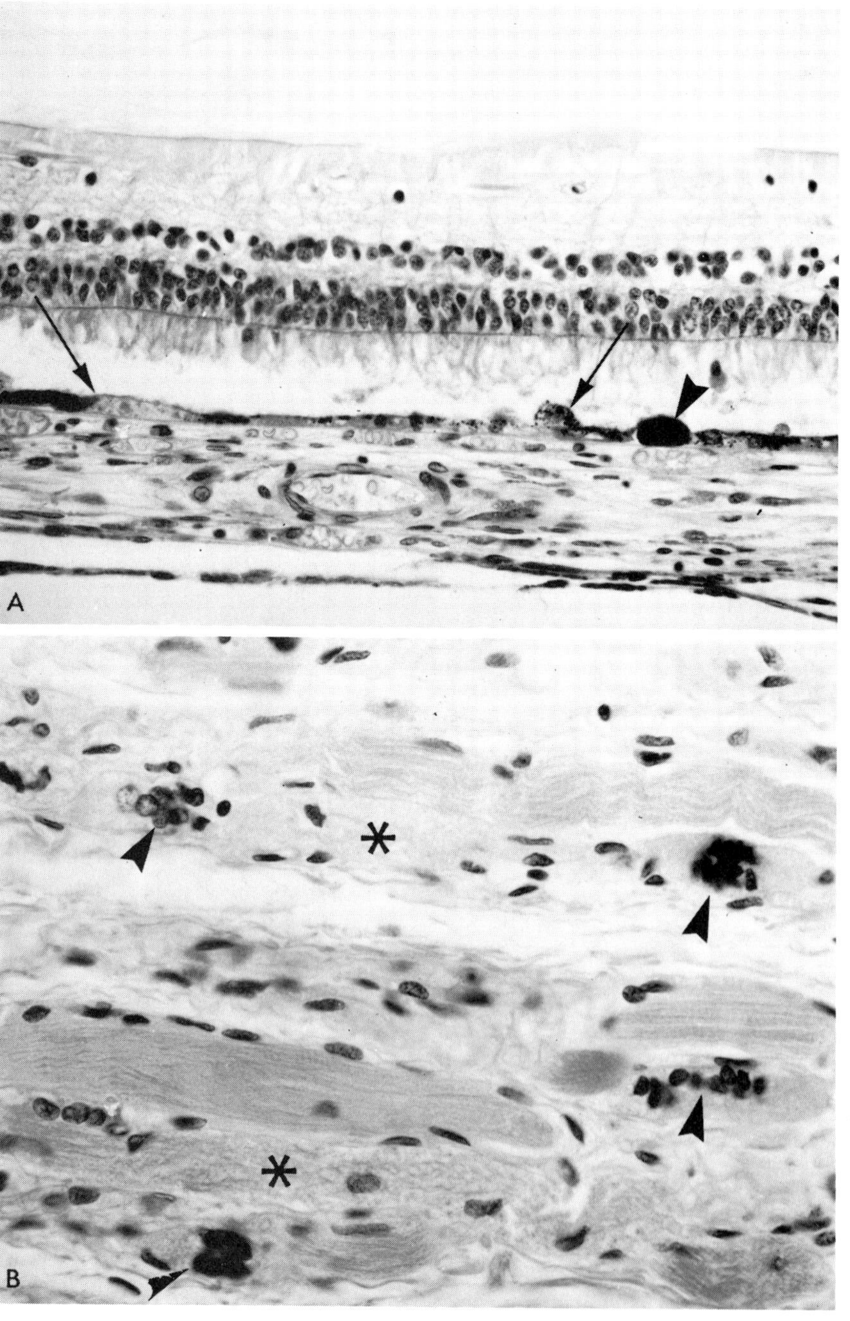

Figure 8–528. Kearns-Sayre syndrome. *A,* Midperiphery, showing old retinal layers intact. Retinal pigment epithelium (RPE) is continuous but shows areas of relative hypopigmentation (arrows) in areas where cell density is reduced and RPE cells are flattened and lose their low cuboidal configuration. An occasional larger RPE cell with denser pigmentation is present (arrowhead). Outer segments of photoreceptor cells are either degenerated or disrupted from post-mortem autolysis. H and E, ×320. *B,* Skeletal muscle, showing degeneration of some fibers (asterisks) and large aggregates of nuclei in center of fibers (arrowheads). H and E, ×310. (Courtesy of Dr. V. Curtin; case presented at Association of Ophthalmic Alumni of Armed Forces Institute of Pathology, Washington, DC, June, 1973.)

(1958) and Kearns (1965) observed the additional features of cardiomyopathy. Other, less constant features include weakness of facial and pharyngeal musculature, weakness of trunk and extremity musculature, deafness, small stature, electroencephalographic changes, and an increase in cerebrospinal fluid protein (Kearns, 1965). Autosomal dominant transmission has been observed (Leveille, Newell, 1980).

Histopathologic studies of the eyes of one patient have shown widespread loss of the retinal pigment epithelium and photoreceptor cell layer (Kearns, Sayre, 1958). The inner retinal layers and optic nerve were normal. In another study, the RPE and outer nuclear layer were intact in the posterior pole (Fig. 8–528). In the periphery, there was partial loss of the photoreceptor cell layer and migration of the RPE into the retina (Curtin, 1973).

Eagle, Hedges, and Yanoff (1982) have pointed out the differences between the retinal degeneration of the Kearns-Sayre syndrome and those of primary retinitis pigmentosa. They observed the degeneration of the retinal pigment epithelium and photoreceptor cells to be most marked in the posterior pole (Fig. 8–529,*A*). Scanning electron microscopic studies disclosed marked irregularities and enlargement of the retinal pigment epithelium (Fig. 8–529,*B* and *C*). Transmission electron microscopy showed irregular conglomerates of melanin granules (Fig. 8–529,*D*). The investigators suggest that the retinal pigment epithelium may be the site of the primary defect in the retinal degeneration.

Biopsy specimens of orbicularis oculi muscle show fibers with a subsarcolemmal accumulation of mitochondria (ragged-red fibers) (Figs. 8–528,*B* and 8–530) (Olson, Engel, Walsh, Enangler, 1972). This abnormality is a rather consistent feature in progressive external ophthalmoplegia but is not pathognomonic because it is also seen in a variety of disorders (Eshaghian, Anderson, Weingeist, et al, 1980).

Cockayne's Syndrome. This syndrome is characterized by early onset of developmental failures, skeletal dysplasia, deafness, optic atrophy, and pigmentary degeneration of the retina (Cockayne, 1936).

This autosomal recessive condition becomes manifest in early childhood, after a period of apparently normal development. The affected individual is a dwarf and appears prematurely aged, with a characteristic facies. Progressive developmental and mental retardation, partial deafness, and photosensitive dermatitis develop (Guzzetta, 1972).

A "salt-and-pepper" appearance to the retina and atrophic appearance of the optic disk are observed. Corneal ulcers, cataracts, nystagmus, and pupillary unresponsiveness to light of mydriatics have been variably reported (Levin, Green, Victor, MacLean, 1983).

No metabolic or storage defects are known in this syndrome, and its etiology is uncertain. On the basis of neuropathologic studies, Cockayne's syndrome has been generally regarded as a leukodystrophy (Peiffer, 1970). Some investigators suggest that Cockayne's syndrome may involve an abnormal aging process (Cunningham, Godfrey, Moffat, 1978). Recent attention has been given to abnormal cellular sensitivity of cultured fibrocytes and lymphocytes to ultraviolet light (Proops, Taylor, Insley, 1981).

One histologic study of the eyes demonstrated widespread atrophy of the nerve fiber layer and ganglion cell layers of the retina (Fig. 8–531,*A* and *B*) and atrophy of the optic nerve. While the inner plexiform and inner nuclear layers were normal, the outer nuclear layer had reduced numbers of cells. There was atrophy of inner and outer photoreceptor segments (Fig. 8–531). The RPE was intact but with irregular hypo- and hyperpigmentation. Pigment-laden cells were seen in the retina and subretinal space of the peripheral retina (Fig. 8–531,*C*). The capillaries of the retinal periphery were largely acellular. The vitreous showed central liquefaction and posterior detachment. Electron microscopic examination disclosed large amounts of lipofuscin in the RPE cells (Levin, Green, Victor, MacLean, 1983).

Similar retinal changes were described in another study, although attenuation of the choriocapillaris and calcification of the sclera were reported. Electron microscopy was not performed (Hijikata, Hirooka, Ohno, 1969). Dystrophic corneal disease has also been described (Brodrick, Dark, 1973).

Potter's Syndrome (Potter, 1946, 1965). The features of this condition include bilateral renal agenesis, pulmonary hypoplasia, deficiency in growth, and facial and skeletal abnormalities. Associated ocular abnormalities include microphthalmia, absence of keratocytes in the cornea centrally and posteriorly, incomplete development of the anterior chamber angle, persistent pupillary membrane cataract with retention of pyknotic nuclei in the fetal nucleus, absence of the retinal nerve fiber and ganglion cell layers, absence of retinal vasculature, and a prominent Bergmeister's papilla (Brownstein, Kirkham, Kalousek, 1976). In another case in which there was absence of retinal vasculature, a prominent vascular abnormality was noted in the optic nerve head and peripapillary retina (Crawford, 1983).

Alström's Syndrome. This recessive disease is characterized by the presence of retinitis pigmentosa, deafness, obesity, and diabetes mellitus. In contrast to Bardet-Biedl's syndrome, there is no mental defect, polydactyly, or hypogonadism (Al-

Text continued on page 1194

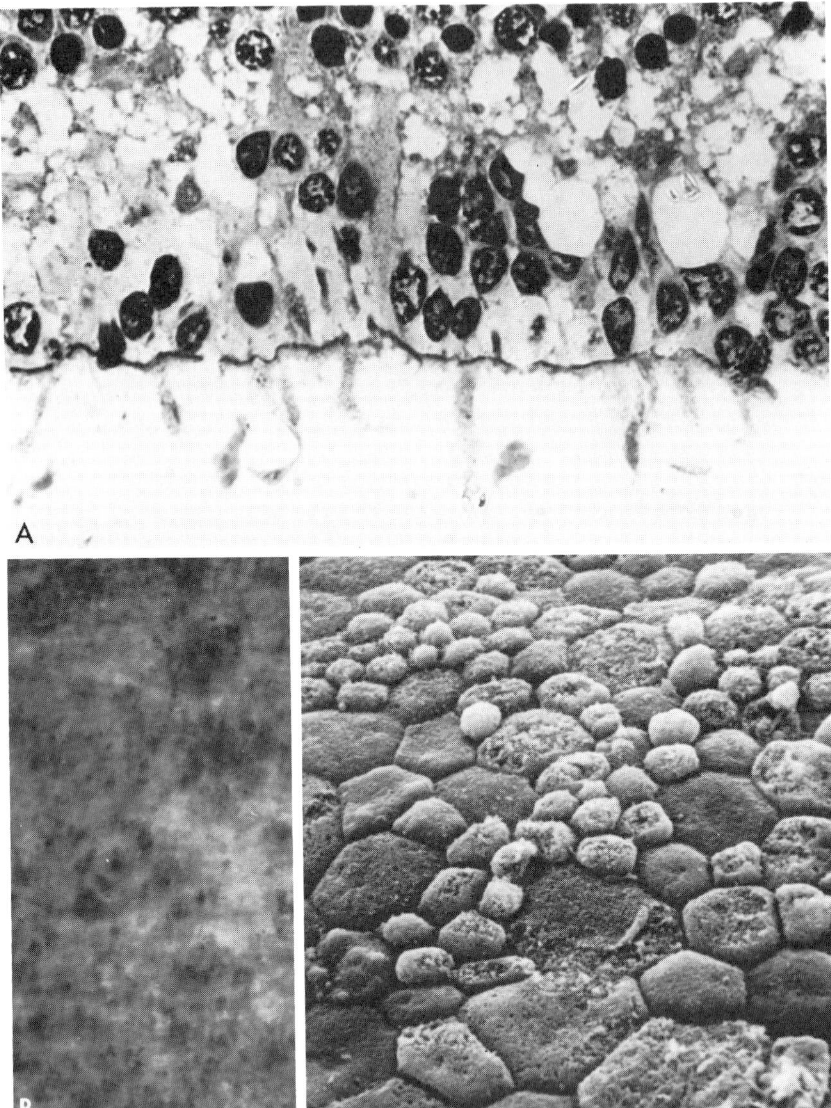

Figure 8–529. Kearns-Sayre syndrome. *A,* Paramacular retina shows extensive loss of photoreceptors and atrophy of outer nuclear layer. Toluidine blue, ×400. *B,* Left, Macrophoto of retinal pigment epithelium (RPE) flat preparation shows prominent "salt and pepper" pattern of pigment clumping and atrophy. ×60. Right, Scanning electron micrograph shows marked variation in size and shape of equatorial retinal pigment epithelial cells. ×640.

Illustration continued on opposite page

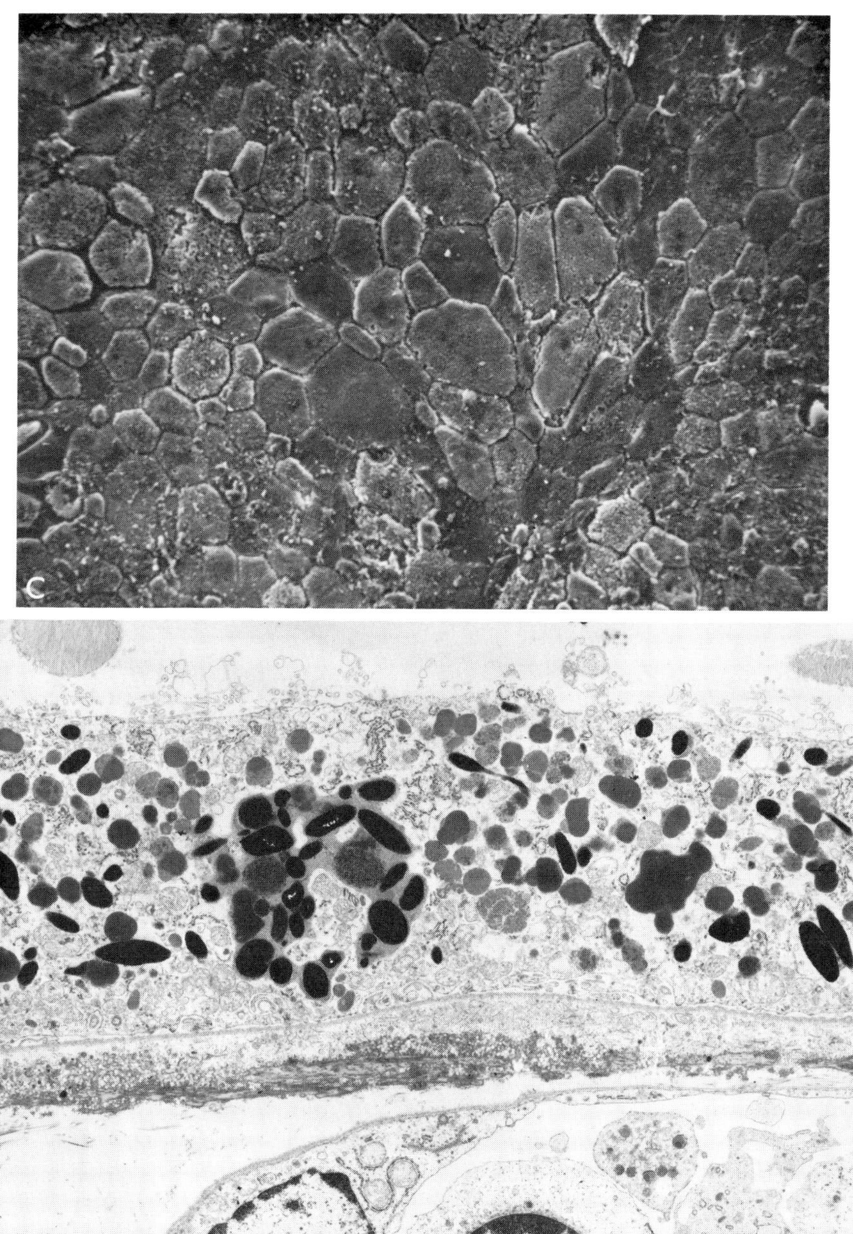

Figure 8–529 *Continued C,* Scanning electron micrograph showing flattened, irregular, polygonal RPE cells. ×460. *D,* Transmission electron micrograph of RPE, with loss of normal polarity of apical melanin and basal lipofuscin. A large, irregular conglomerate of residual melanin granules is present left of center. ×3600.

(From Eagle RC Jr, Hedges TR, Yanoff M: The atypical pigmentary retinopathy of Kearns-Sayre syndrome. A light and electron microscopic study. Ophthalmology *89*:1433–1440, 1982.)

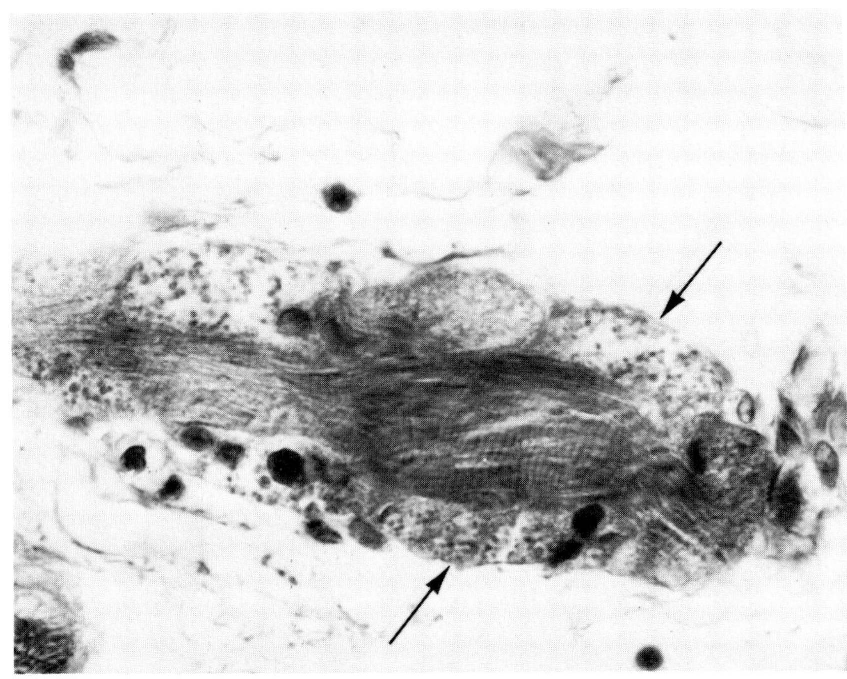

Figure 8–530. Ragged red fiber showing subsarcolemmal accumulation of fine granular material (arrows), which proved histochemically and ultrastructurally to be mitochondria. Masson, ×900. EP 46465.

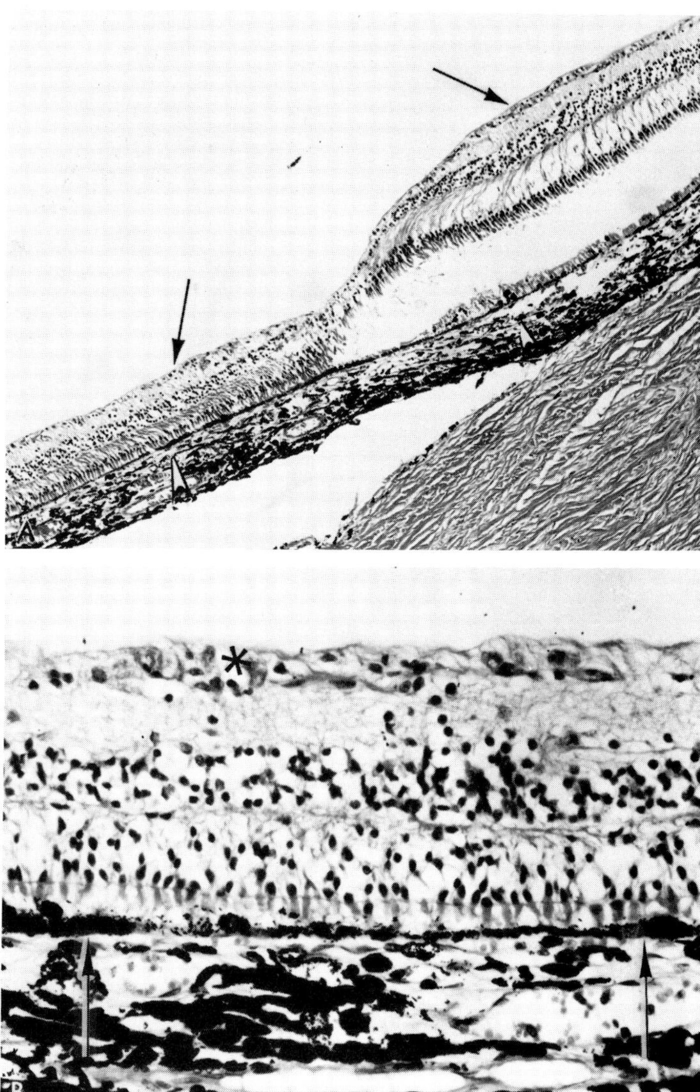

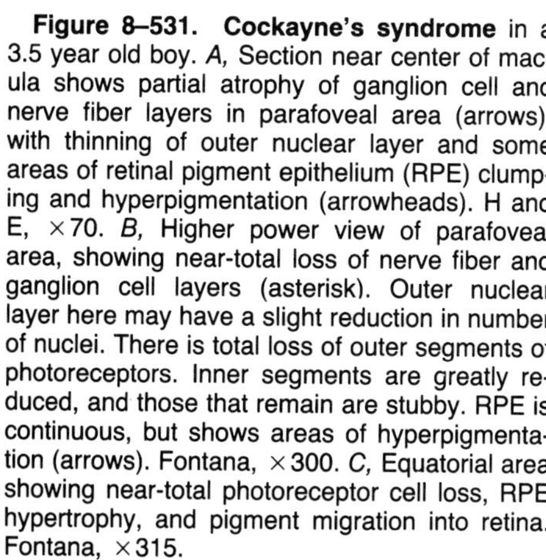

Figure 8–531. Cockayne's syndrome in a 3.5 year old boy. *A,* Section near center of macula shows partial atrophy of ganglion cell and nerve fiber layers in parafoveal area (arrows), with thinning of outer nuclear layer and some areas of retinal pigment epithelium (RPE) clumping and hyperpigmentation (arrowheads). H and E, ×70. *B,* Higher power view of parafoveal area, showing near-total loss of nerve fiber and ganglion cell layers (asterisk). Outer nuclear layer here may have a slight reduction in number of nuclei. There is total loss of outer segments of photoreceptors. Inner segments are greatly reduced, and those that remain are stubby. RPE is continuous, but shows areas of hyperpigmentation (arrows). Fontana, ×300. *C,* Equatorial area showing near-total photoreceptor cell loss, RPE hypertrophy, and pigment migration into retina. Fontana, ×315.

EP 41071. (From Levin PS, Green WR, Victor D, MacLean AL: Histopathology of the eye in Cockayne's syndrome. Arch Ophthalmol *101*: 1093–1097, 1983.)

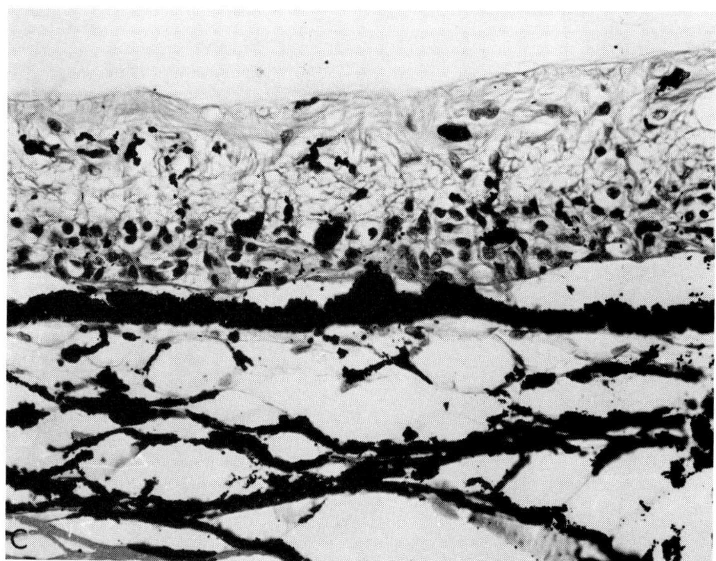

ström, Hallgren, Nilsson, Asander, 1959; Goldstein, Fialkow, 1973).

Bardet-Biedl Syndrome. This recessive syndrome is characterized by mental retardation, pigmentary retinopathy, polydactyly, obesity, and hypogenitalism. Amman (1970) pointed out that these features were present in Biedl's and Bardet's patients, but that Laurence and Moon had described a distinct entity with paraplegia and without polydactyly and obesity.

Laurence-Moon Syndrome. This recessive syndrome is characterized by mental retardation, pigmentary retinopathy, hypogenitalism, and spastic paraplegia (Bowen, Ferguson-Smith, Mosier, et al, 1965).

Ophthalmoscopic features include widespread loss of the RPE and atrophy of the choroid (Fig. 8–532), similar to that observed in choroideremia (Hutchinson, 1900). Histopathologic studies of a case on file in the Pathology Laboratory of the Wilmer Institute have shown widespread loss of the RPE, choroid, and outer retinal layers (Fig. 8–532,*B*, *C*, and *D*). An island of preserved choroid, RPE, and retina may be present in the posterior pole.

Usher's Syndrome. Pigmentary retinopathy associated with hearing loss occurs in association with various genetic disorders, including the Usher, Alström, Refsum, Cockayne, and Alport syndromes. The association of macular retinal pigment epitheliopathy and hearing loss also has been reported by Amalric (1960) as a genetic syn-

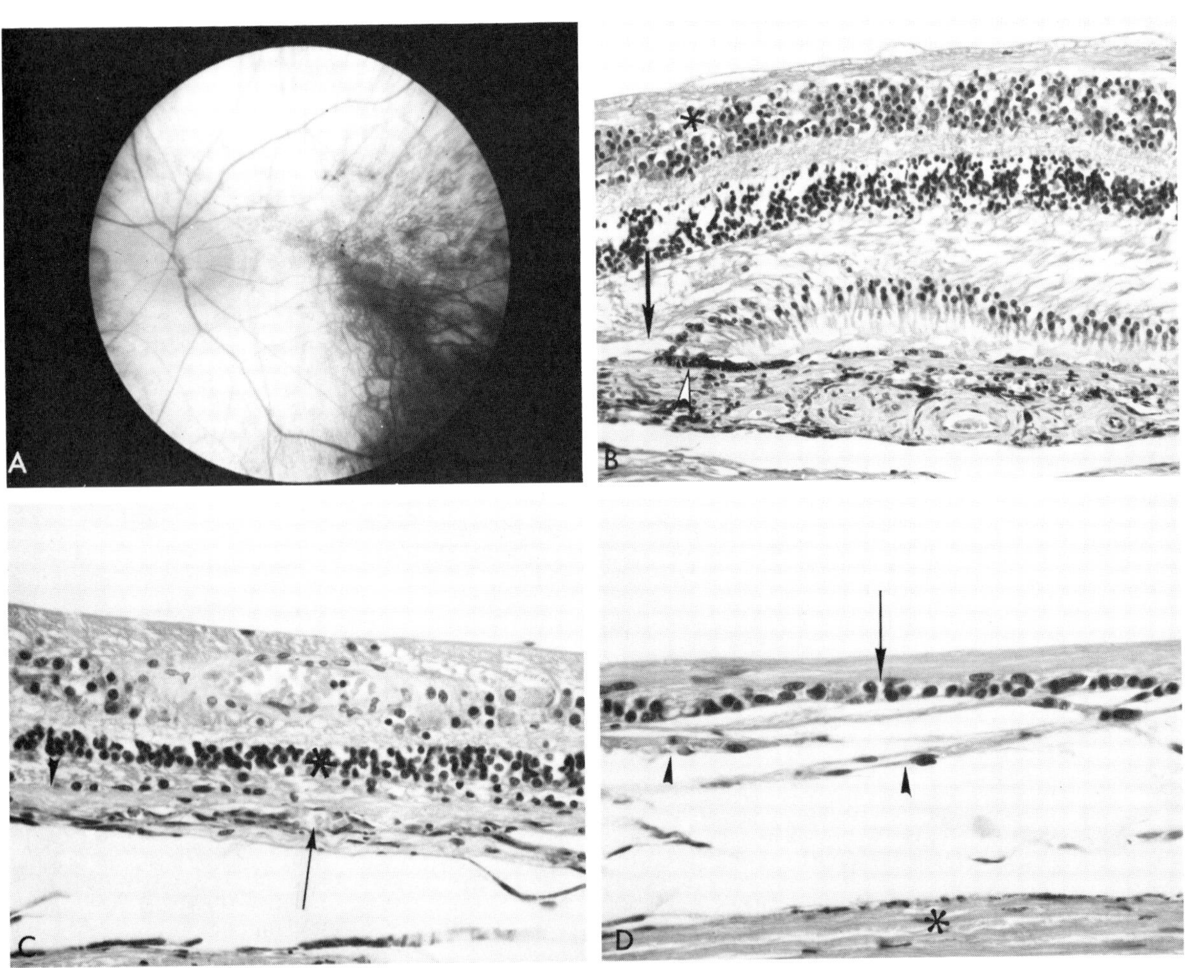

Figure 8–532. Laurence-Moon syndrome. *A,* Choroideremia-like ophthalmoscopic appearance, with extensive retinal pigment epithelium (RPE) and choroidal atrophy, attenuation of retinal vessels, and an island of remaining choroid and RPE in posterior pole. *B,* Area of relatively preserved RPE and photoreceptors in posterior pole, with abrupt margin where RPE and photoreceptor cells are lost (arrow). RPE at this margin is hypertrophic (arrowhead). Ganglion cell (asterisk) and nerve fiber layers are normal. H and E, ×240.

C, Area where a few choroidal vessels remain (arrow). RPE and photoreceptor cell layer are absent, and inner nuclear layer rests near Bruch's membrane (arrowhead). H and E, ×240. *D,* Area of near-total atrophy of choroid. Only a few fibrous strands (arrowheads) separate retina from sclera (asterisk). Bruch's membrane is ill-defined, and only some of inner nuclear (arrow) layer of retina remains. H and E, ×530. EP 26306.

drome, although the etiology of this disorder remains undecided (François, Haustrate-Gosset, Donck, 1967).

The Usher syndrome (retinitis pigmentosa and hearing impairment) is an autosomal recessive disorder with variability in the severity and progression of the ocular and audiologic manifestations. Additionally, vestibular ataxia, psychosis (Hallgren, 1959), and mental retardation (Merin, Abraham, Auervach, 1974) may occur. The hearing impairment is sensorineural.

Genetic heterogeneity was suggested by Nuutila (1970) on the basis of the age of onset of nyctalopia, with over 90 per cent of patients noting the symptom prior to age 10 years and the remainder after age 20 years. Although the majority of patients in his study had a variable but stable hearing loss, a small group of patients gave a history of progressive hearing loss. McLeod, McConnell, Sweeney, et al (1971) studied the hearing loss in a large, highly consanguineous family with six affected members and found significant intrafamilial audiologic phenotypic variability of this genotype.

Merin, Abraham, and Auervach (1974) have proposed a classification of the genetic subgroups based on the age of onset and progression of the retinitis pigmentosa, and on whether or not the hearing loss was progressive. They also reported additional subgroups with mild vestibular ataxia and mental retardation. Davenport and Omenn (1977) have suggested a different classification based on the age of onset of retinitis pigmentosa and the severity and progression of hearing impairment. They also suggested an X-linked form of the disease, although only the proband was studied (Davenport, 1980). Documented cases of progressive hearing loss in the Usher syndrome are rare (Gorlin, Tilsner, Finestein, Duvall, 1979; Morgan, Boulud, 1975; Beatty, McDonald, Colvard, 1979).

Recent experience indicates that the ophthalmologic manifestations in this disorder are variable (Bateman, Riedner, Levin, Maumenee, 1980) and may include a crystalline retinopathy or a clumped pigmentary degeneration. Additionally, enamel dysplasia has been associated with retinitis pigmentosa and hearing loss. The combination of stable maculopathy, hearing loss, and enamel dysplasia also may occur. The heritable basis for those groups is yet to be determined (Bateman, Riedner, Levin, Maumenee, 1980).

The Amalric-Diallinas syndrome of macular epitheliopathy and hearing loss also has been reported as a genetic disorder, although the etiology remains uncertain (Amalric, 1960; François, Haustrate-Gosset, Donck, 1967; Diallinas, 1959; Grimaud, Cordier, Dureux, et al, 1962). Some reported cases may be the result of rubella embryopathy.

No ocular pathologic studies have been reported on patients with Usher's syndrome. Abnormalities of axonemal microtubular structure and the presence of compound nasal cilia in patients with Usher's syndrome have been reported (Arden, Fox, 1979). Ciliated structures are common to the myoid area of photoreceptors and the organ of Corti of the ear.

As yet, methods to alter the course of the disease are not known, and prenatal diagnosis of the disorder is not feasible.

Cystinosis. This rare congenital disorder of amino acid metabolism is characterized by the widespread intracellular deposition of cystine crystals in body tissues. The precise biochemical defect is not known, but the disease is believed to be primarily lysosomal (Wong, Kuwabara, Brubaker, et al, 1970; Schulman, Wong, Olson, et al, 1970).

Three types of cystinosis have been described in the literature. The childhood type (nephropathic) is the most common form and is characterized by renal rickets, growth retardation, progressive renal failure, and death, usually before puberty (Scriver, Rosenberg, 1973). The disease is transmitted as an autosomal recessive trait (Schulman, 1975).

Cystine crystals have been found in spleen, liver, lymph nodes, bone marrow, and leukocytes, and also in iris, ciliary body, choroid, retinal pigment epithelium (Fig. 8–533,*A*), the pial septa of the optic nerve (Sanderson, Kuwabara, Stark, et al, 1974), and, rarely, in the neurosensory retina (Fig. 8–533,*B*). Crystals have been observed in the cornea since the first description by Bürki (1941) in Europe and by Guild, Walsh, and Hoover (1952) in the United States.

Additional ocular findings include patchy depigmentation of the retinal pigment epithelium in the far periphery (Fig. 8–533,*C*) (Wong, Lietman, Seegmiller, 1967; François, Hanssens, Coppieters, et al, 1972) and mottled depigmentation of the macula (Goldman, Scriver, Aaron, et al, 1971; Sanderson, Kuwabara, Stark, et al, 1974).

The second type is known as adolescent cystinosis and was first described by Goldman, Scriver, Aaron, et al (1971). This type is characterized by onset in the first or second decade, a mild nephropathy with diminished life expectancy, and the characteristic corneal and conjunctival cystine deposits but absence of retinopathy. Inheritance is believed to be autosomal recessive (Goldman, Scriver, Aaron, et al, 1971; Zimmerman, Hood, Gasset, 1974).

The third type of cystinosis (benign or adult cystinosis) was first described by Cogan, Kuwabara, Kinoshita, et al (1957). It is characterized only by mild symptoms of photophobia and is frequently diagnosed by routine ophthalmologic examination when the typical corneal crystals are

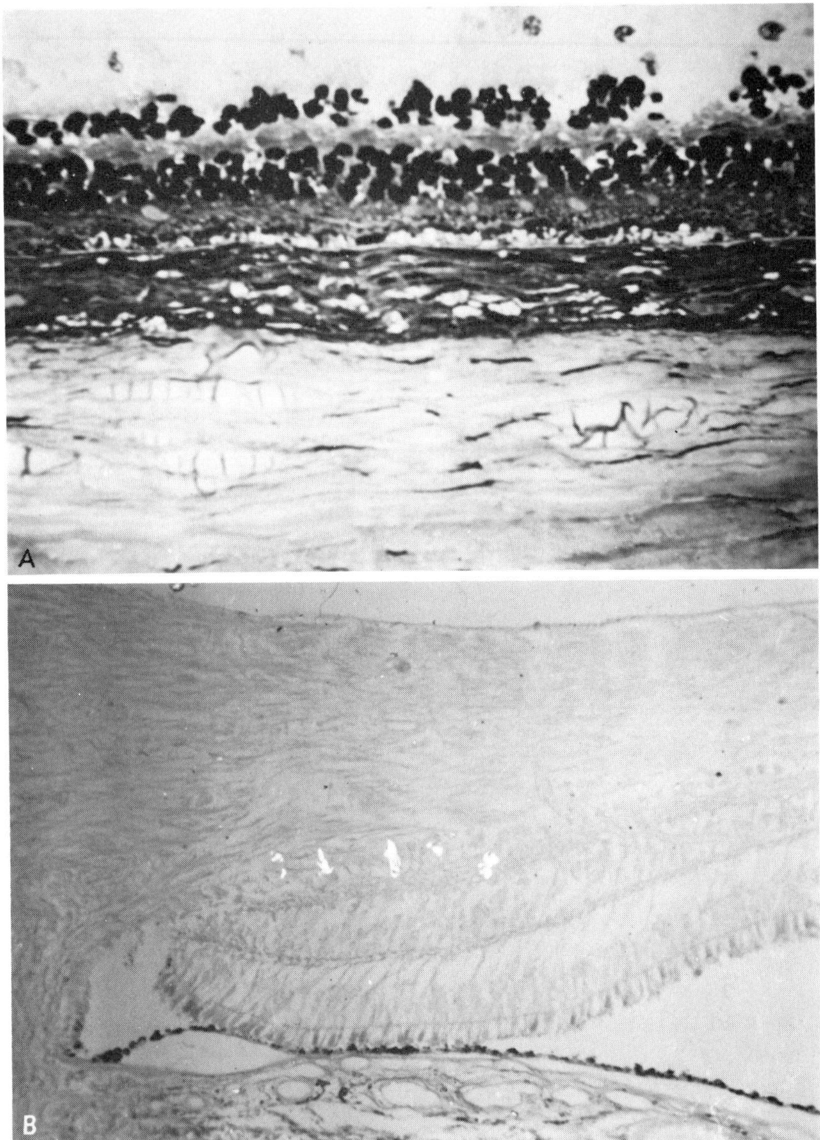

Figure 8–533. Cystinosis. *A,* Cystine crystals in retinal pigment epithelium of a patient who had the childhood form of cystinosis. 1 micron thick, epoxy resin section, ×480. (From Sanderson PA, Kuwabara T, Stark WJ, et al: Cystinosis. A clinical, histopathologic and ultrastructural study. Arch Ophthalmol *91*:270–274, 1974.) *B,* Polarized light demonstrates crystals in peripapillary retina of childhood form of cystinosis. Frozen section, unstained, ×50. EP 27737.

Illustration continued on opposite page

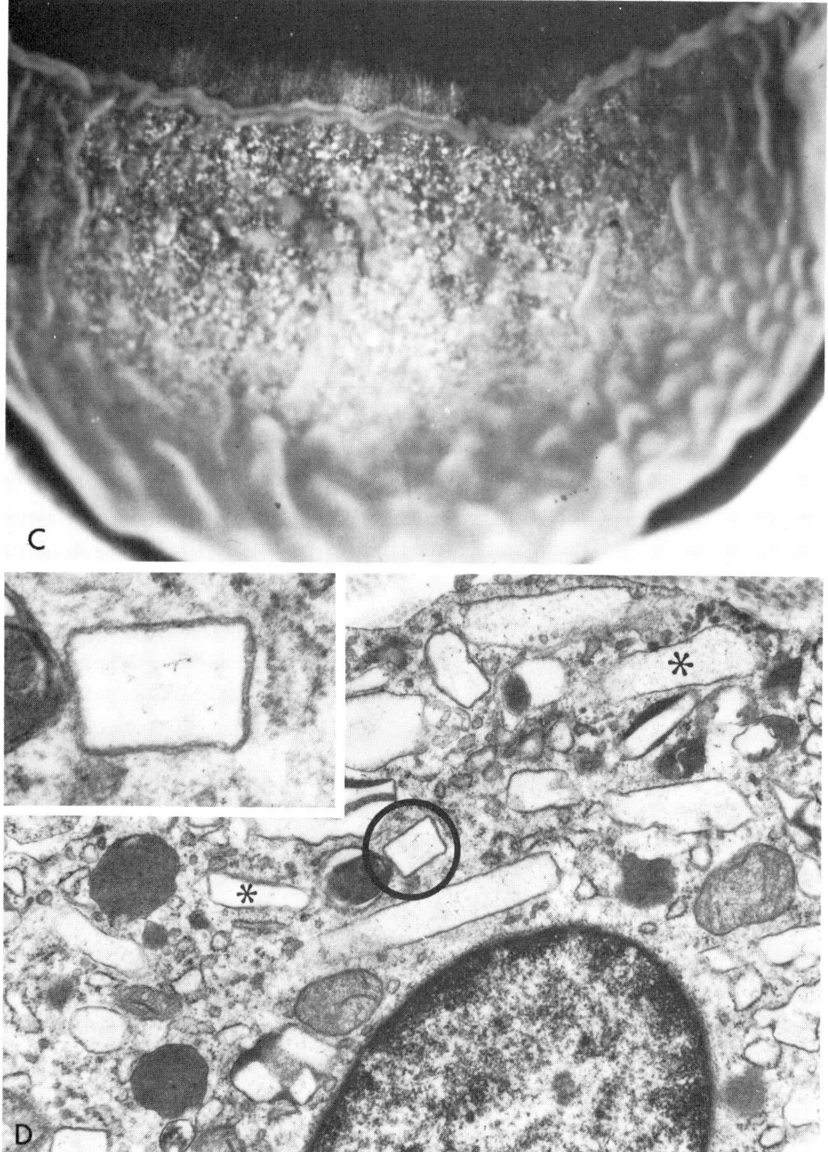

Figure 8–533 *Continued C,* Gross appearance of peripheral pigmentary change in childhood cystinosis. (Courtesy of Dr. V.G. Wong.) *D,* Conjunctival biopsy specimen from 41 year old man with cystinosis. Electron microscopic appearance of macrophage in substantia propria of conjunctiva, with numerous intracytoplasmic crystals (asterisks) bound by lysosomal membrane (circle and inset). ×24,000; inset, ×70,000. (*D* from Dodd MJ, Pusin SM, Green WR: Adult cystinosis. A case report. Arch Ophthalmol *96*:1054–1057, 1978.)

noted. There is no renal disease, and no ophthalmoscopic abnormalities have been described. The age range is from the late teens to the 50s. There is no known hereditary pattern, and life expectancy is believed to be normal (Cogan and associates, 1957; Lietman, Frazier, Wong, et al, 1966; Giles, Wong, 1969; Wong, Kuwabara, Brubaker, et al, 1970; Brubaker, Wong, Schulman, et al, 1970; Kraus, Lutz, 1971; Dodd, Pusin, Green, 1978).

Histopathologic studies of the entire eye have been conducted only in the childhood form (Garron, 1959; Cogan, Kuwabara, 1960; Wong, Lietman, Seegmiller, 1967; François, Hassens, Coppieters, et al, 1972; Sanderson, Kuwabara, Stark, et al, 1974). Most of these studies have demonstrated crystals in the cornea, conjunctiva, sclera, ciliary body, iris, and choroid. No cases have been reported in which crystals have been observed in the neurosensory retina. Crystals have been observed in the retina in an unreported case from the Wilmer Institute (Fig. 8–533,*B*). Sanderson, Kuwabara, Stark, et al (1974) did find crystals in the RPE.

Studies of conjunctival biopsy specimens in the childhood form have been reported by numerous investigators some of whom include Cogan, Kuwabara, Kinoshita, et al, 1957; Boniuk, Hill, 1966; Giles, Wong, 1969; and Kenyon and Sensenbrenner, 1974. Wong, Schulman, and Seegmiller (1970) have also established the diagnosis of cystinosis by biochemical analysis of conjunctiva using column chromatography.

A study of a conjunctival biopsy in the adolescent form of the disease has been reported by Zimmerman, Hood, and Gassett (1974).

Studies of conjunctival biopsies in the adult form of the disease have been reported by many workers, some of whom include Cogan, Kuwabara, Kinoshita, et al, 1957; Cogan, Kuwabara, Hurlbut, McMurray, 1958; Giles, Wong, 1969; Brubaker, Wong, Schulman, Seegmiller, 1970; Kraus, Lutz, 1971; Dodd, Pusin, Green, 1978 (Fig. 8–533,*D*). In addition, Cogan, Kuwabara, Hurlbut, and McMurray (1958) showed the conjunctival crystals to be cystine by x-ray diffractometry. The patients reported by Giles and Wong (1969) were children with the adult form of the disease.

Since cystine is soluble in water, the tissue should be fixed in absolute alcohol and exposed to water as little as possible. Examination of frozen sections of fresh tissue by polarized light is one way to demonstrate the crystals.

Adrenoleukodystrophy (ALD). In this degenerative metabolic disease, cholesterol esters with long-chain fatty acids (24 to 30 carbon unbranched fatty acids) accumulate in affected cells (Schaumburg, Powers, Raine, et al, 1975; Igarashi, Schaumburg, Powers, et al, 1975; Igarashi, Schaumburg, Powers, et al, 1976; Menkes, Corbo, 1977; Moser, Moser, Kawamura, et al, 1980). In its commonly described childhood form, ALD is an X-linked recessive disease with predominantly central nervous system (CNS) and adrenal dysfunction (Schaumburg, Powers, Raine, et al, 1975; Siemerling, Creutzfeldt, 1923; Blaw, 1971; Powers, Schaumburg, 1974; Powell, Tindall, Schultz, et al, 1975). The course is progressive, culminating after a few years in dementia, blindness, quadriplegia, and death.

In the less common neonatal form of ALD, the onset of symptoms is before age 1 year, with neurologic defects frequently present at birth (Jaffe, Crumrine, Hashida, Moser, 1982; Ulrich, Herschkowitz, Hertz, et al, 1978; Manz, Schuelein, McCullough, et al, 1980; Jaffe, Crumrine, Hashida, Moser, 1982; Benke, Reyes, Parker, 1981). The disorder occurs in both males and females. Development is severely delayed, and neurologic deterioration usually leads to death in early childhood. Clinical presentation includes seizures, severe mental retardation, and early loss of vision, as well as dysmorphic features (dolichocephaly, prominent and high forehead, epicanthal folds, broad nasal bridge, and low-set ears). Although the genetic details of neonatal ALD have not been fully delineated, the disease may be autosomal recessive (Jaffe, Crumrine, Hashida, Moser, 1982).

In childhood ALD, ultrastructural studies disclose linear or twisted lamellar cytoplasmic accumulations of paired electron-dense leaflets separated by an electron-lucent space in adrenal cortical cells (Schaumburg, Powers, Raine, et al, 1975), CNS macrophages (Schaumburg, Powers, Raine, et al, 1975; Powers, Schaumburg, 1974), peripheral Schwann cells (Schaumburg, Powers, Raine, et al, 1975; Powers, Schaumburg, 1974; Martin, Ceuterick, Martin, Libert, 1977; Martin, Ceuterick, Libert, 1980), Leydig's cells (Schaumburg, Powers, Raine, et al, 1975) and adrenal cortical cells (Ulrich, Herschkowitz, Hertz, et al, 1978; Manz, Schuelein, McCullough, et al, 1980). In neonatal ALD, inclusions have been found in thymus, liver, and reticuloendothelial cells (Jaffe, Crumrine, Hashida, Moser, 1982).

Visual disturbances are an early clinical feature of both neonatal and childhood ALD. In the childhood disease, gaze nystagmus, cortical blindness, and optic atrophy have been described (Wilson, 1981; Wray, Cogan, Kuwabara, et al, 1976; Cohen, Green, de la Cruz, et al, 1983). On clinical ophthalmologic examination of neonatal ALD patients, nystagmus (Manz, Schuelein, McCullough, et al, 1980), bilateral optic nerve atrophy (Jaffe, Crumrine, Hashida, Moser, 1982; Benke, Reyes, Parker, 1981; Cohen, Green, de la Cruz, et al, 1983), random eyelid movements (Ulrich, Herschkowitz, Hertz, et al, 1978), anterior polar cataracts (Cohen, Green, de la Cruz, et al, 1983), and retinal pigment epithelial changes (Manz, Schuelein, McCullough, et al, 1980) have been observed.

In childhood ALD, histopathologic abnormalities of the eye are limited to the retina and optic nerve. There is extensive atrophy of the ganglion cell and nerve fiber layers (Wray, Cogan, Kuwabara, et al, 1976; Cohen, Green, de la Cruz, et al, 1983) (Fig. 8–534,*A*). The optic nerves are quite atrophic, with reduction in size of the nerve fiber bundles, mild thickening of the fibropial septa, extensive demyelination, mild glial hypercellularity, and axonal loss (Wray, Cogan, Kuwabara, et al, 1976; Cohen, Green, de la Cruz, et al, 1983). Optic nerve macrophages (Fig. 8–534,*B*) and also a few macrophages scattered in the retina (Fig. 8–534,*C*) contained paired electron-dense leaflets measuring approximately 3 mm in diameter, separated by a 3 mm electron-lucent space (Cohen, Green, de la Cruz, et al, 1983).

In neonatal ALD, anterior subcapsular cataracts (Fig. 8–534,*D*) and also cystoid macular edema (Fig. 8–534,*E*) may occur (Cohen, Green, de la Cruz, et al, 1983).

There is extensive loss of nerve fiber and ganglion cell layers of the retina, and diffuse optic atrophy with nerve fiber bundle narrowing, glial hypercellularity, and partial demyelination (Jaffe, Crumrine, Hashida, Moser, 1982; Cohen, Green,

Text continued on page 1210

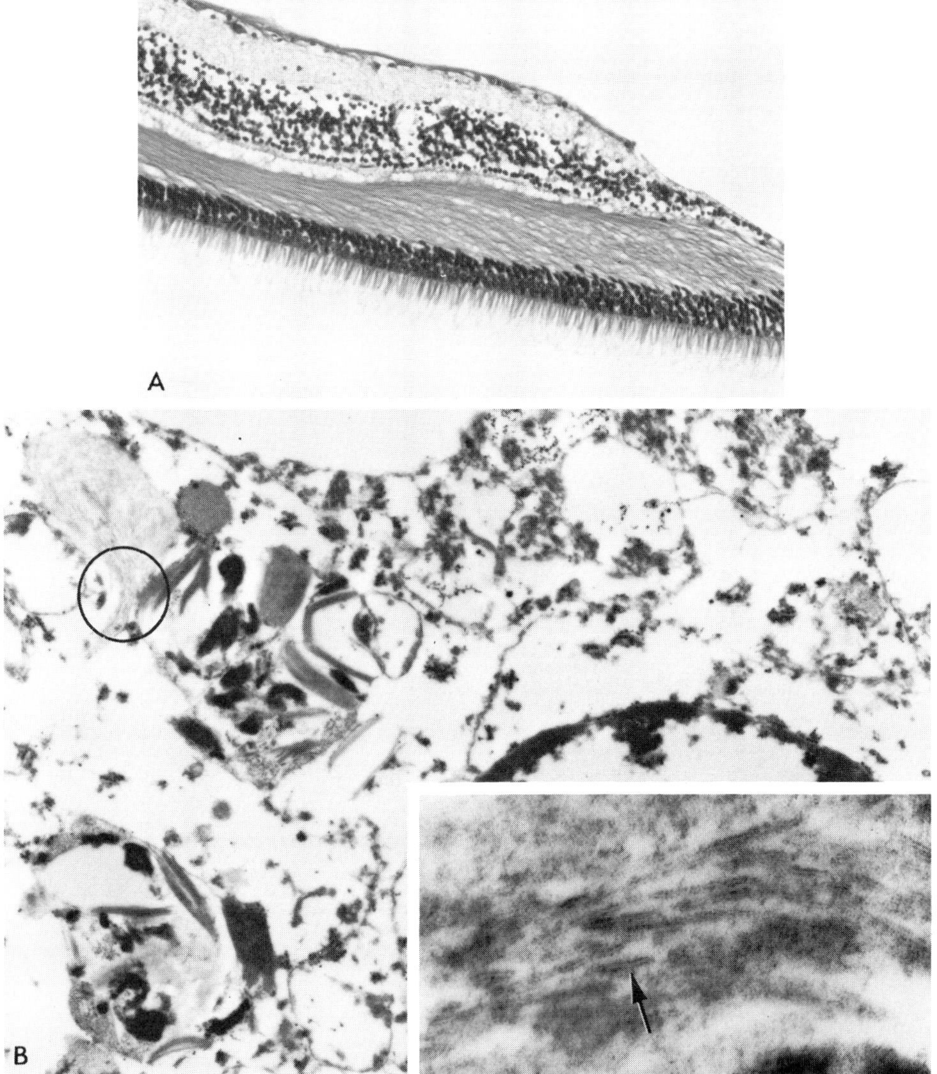

Figure 8–534. *A,* Parafoveal retina demonstrating atrophy of the ganglion cell and nerve fiber layers. H and E, ×125. *B,* Optic nerve macrophage containing aggregate of the characteristic bileaflet inclusions (circle and inset). The inclusions (arrow, inset) consist of linear paired electron-dense leaflets approximately 2.8 nm in diameter, separated by a 2.8 nm electron-lucent zone. ×117,000.

Illustration continued on following page

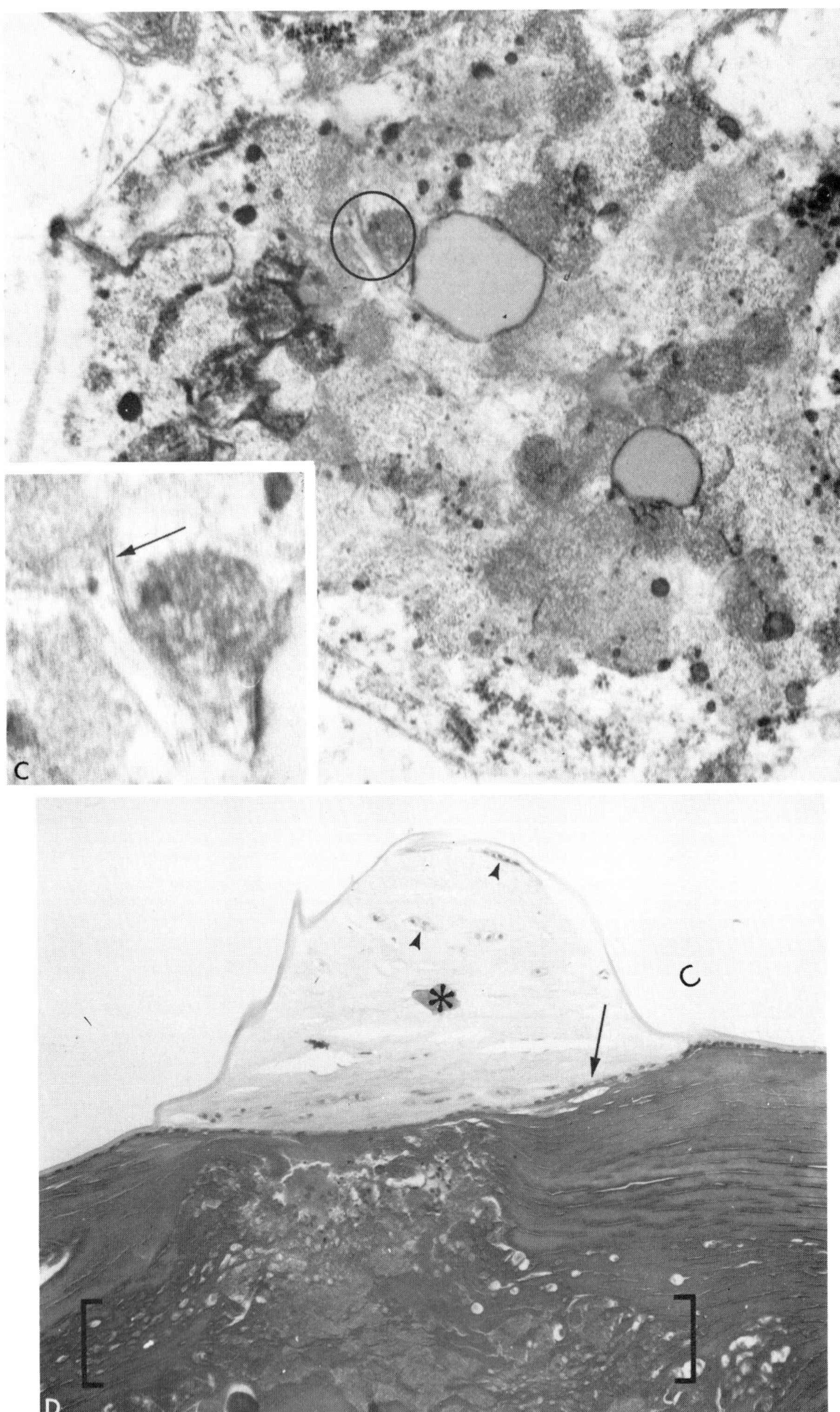

Figure 8–534 *Continued C,* Bileaflet inclusions (circle and inset) are present in macrophage within retina in macular area. At higher power (inset), the inclusion consists of electron-dense leaflets, 3.5 nm in diameter, separated by a 3.4 nm electron-lucent space (arrow). ×35,000; inset, ×86,000. *A–C,* EP 55270. *D,* Anterior subcapsular cataract. A pyramid-shaped subcapsular fibrous plaque (asterisk) containing foci of epithelium (arrowheads) is banded anteriorly by redundant anterior lens capsule and posteriorly by a single layer of epithelium (arrow) and a thin layer of basement membrane. The anterior lens cortex (brackets) shows fragmentation and liquefaction. H and E, ×125.

Illustration continued on opposite page

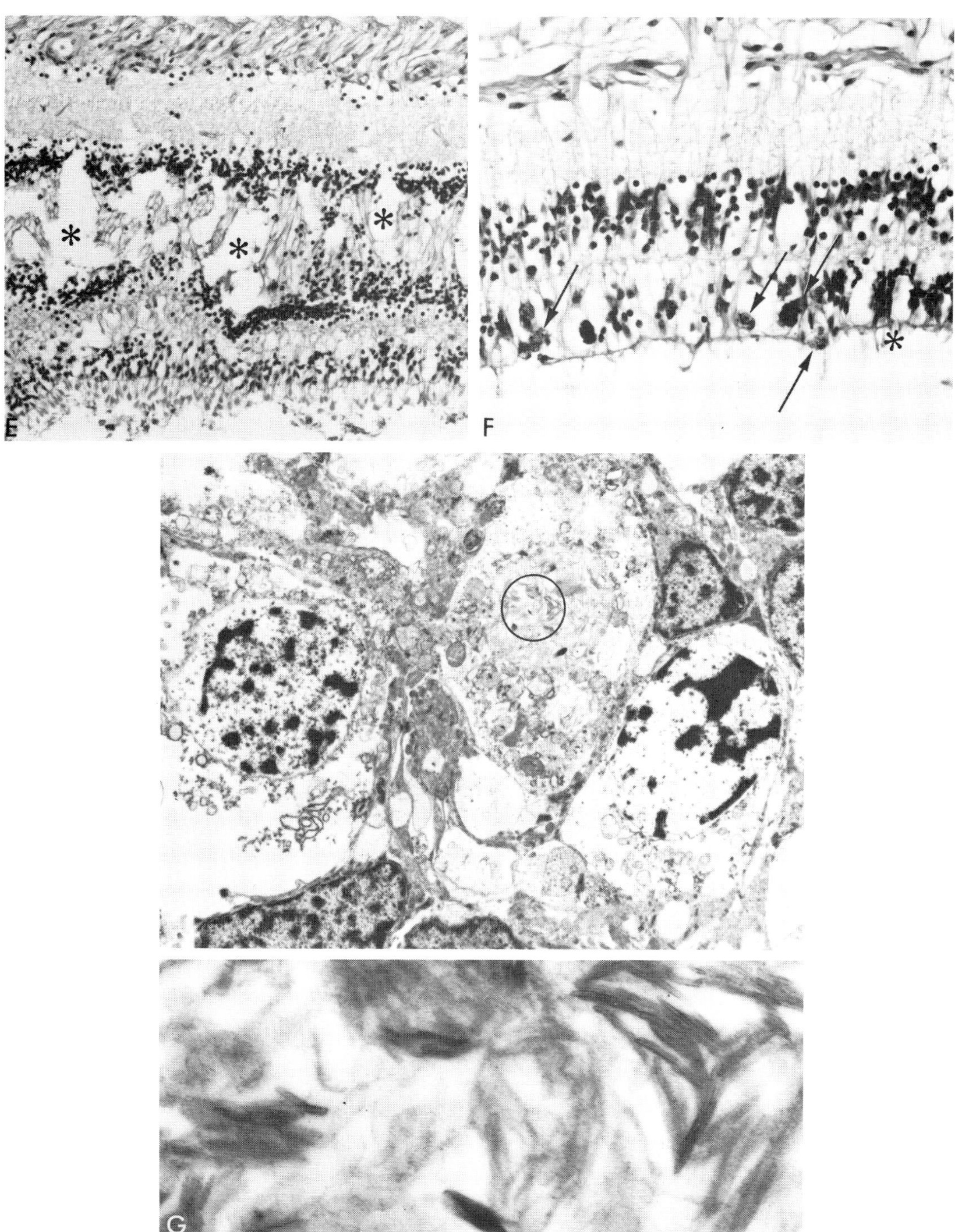

Figure 8–534 *Continued E,* Macular area demonstrating cystic edema (asterisks) in the inner and outer nuclear layers and the inner plexiform layer. The photoreceptors are partially degenerated. H and E, ×150. *F,* Peripheral retina shows total degeneration of the outer segments of the photoreceptor cells. Only a few inner segments remain (asterisk), and the outer nuclear layer shows a marked loss of nuclei. Macrophages (arrows) containing pigment and PAS-positive material are present in the outer nuclear layer. PAS, ×300.

G, Top, Inner nuclear layer of macular area with macrophage containing characteristic linear bileaflet inclusions (circled area). ×7450. Bottom, Higher-power view shows that the electron-dense leaflets measure 4.2 nm in diameter and that there is a 2.8 nm electron-lucent space between the leaflets. ×72,000.

Illustration continued on following page

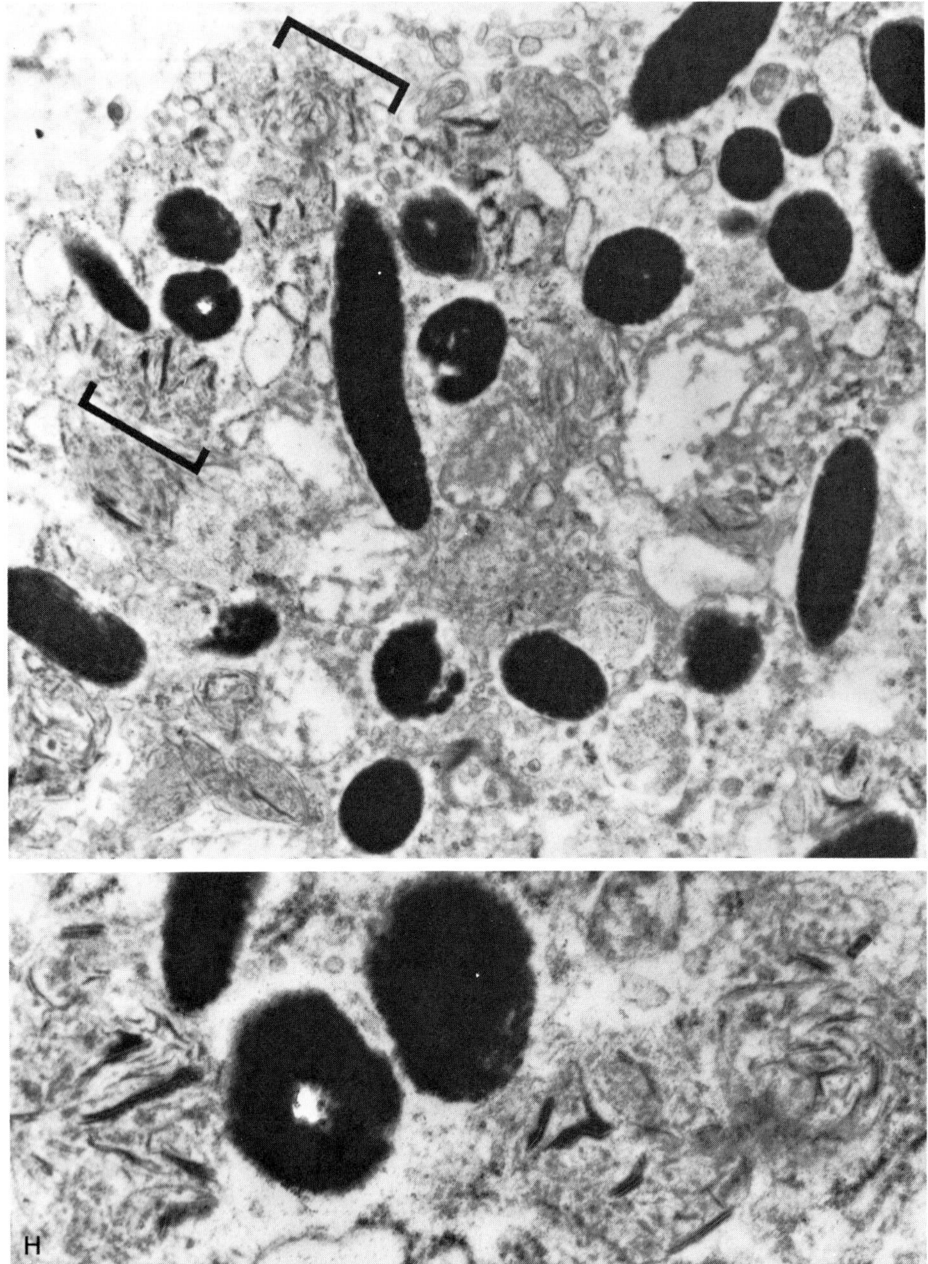

Figure 8–534 *Continued H,* Top, Peripheral retinal pigment epithelium with melanin granules admixed with aggregates of bileaflet inclusions (bracketed area). ×20,000. Bottom, Higher-power view of bracketed area shows that the inclusions are arranged in a loose, whorled configuration. ×50,000.

Illustration continued on opposite page

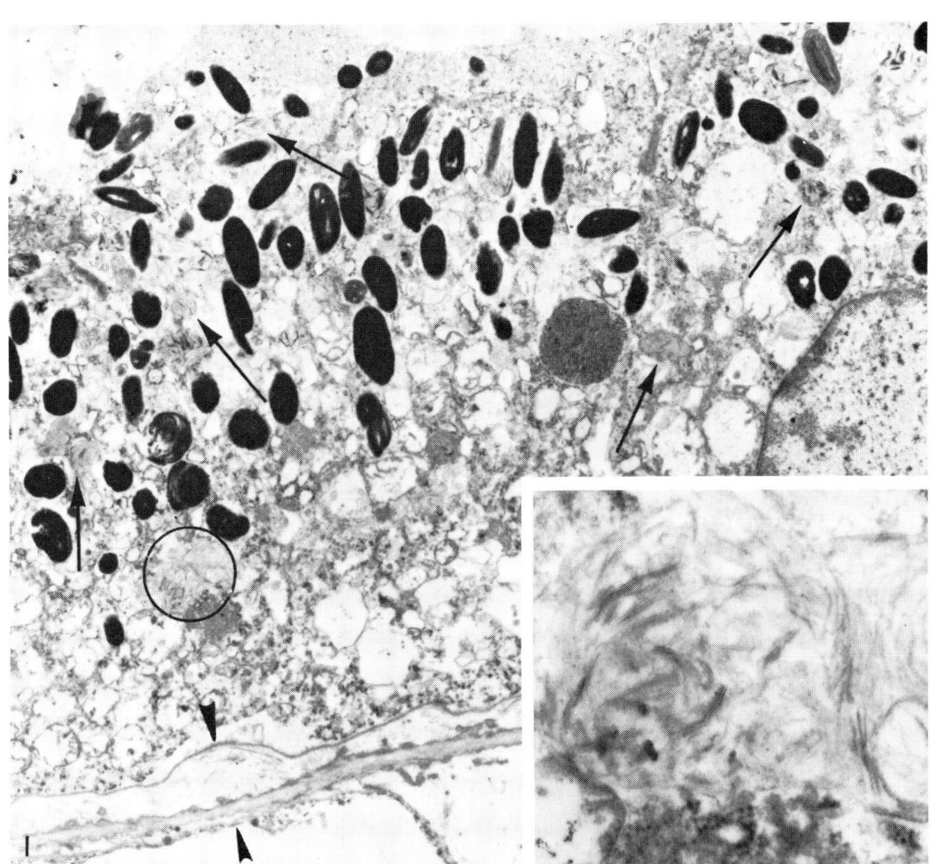

Figure 8–534 *Continued I,* Peripheral retinal pigment epithelial cell contains one large (circled area) and many smaller (arrows) aggregates of bileaflet inclusions. Bruch's membrane is shown between arrowheads. ×8000. Inset, Higher-power view of bracketed area. ×45,000.

Illustration continued on following page

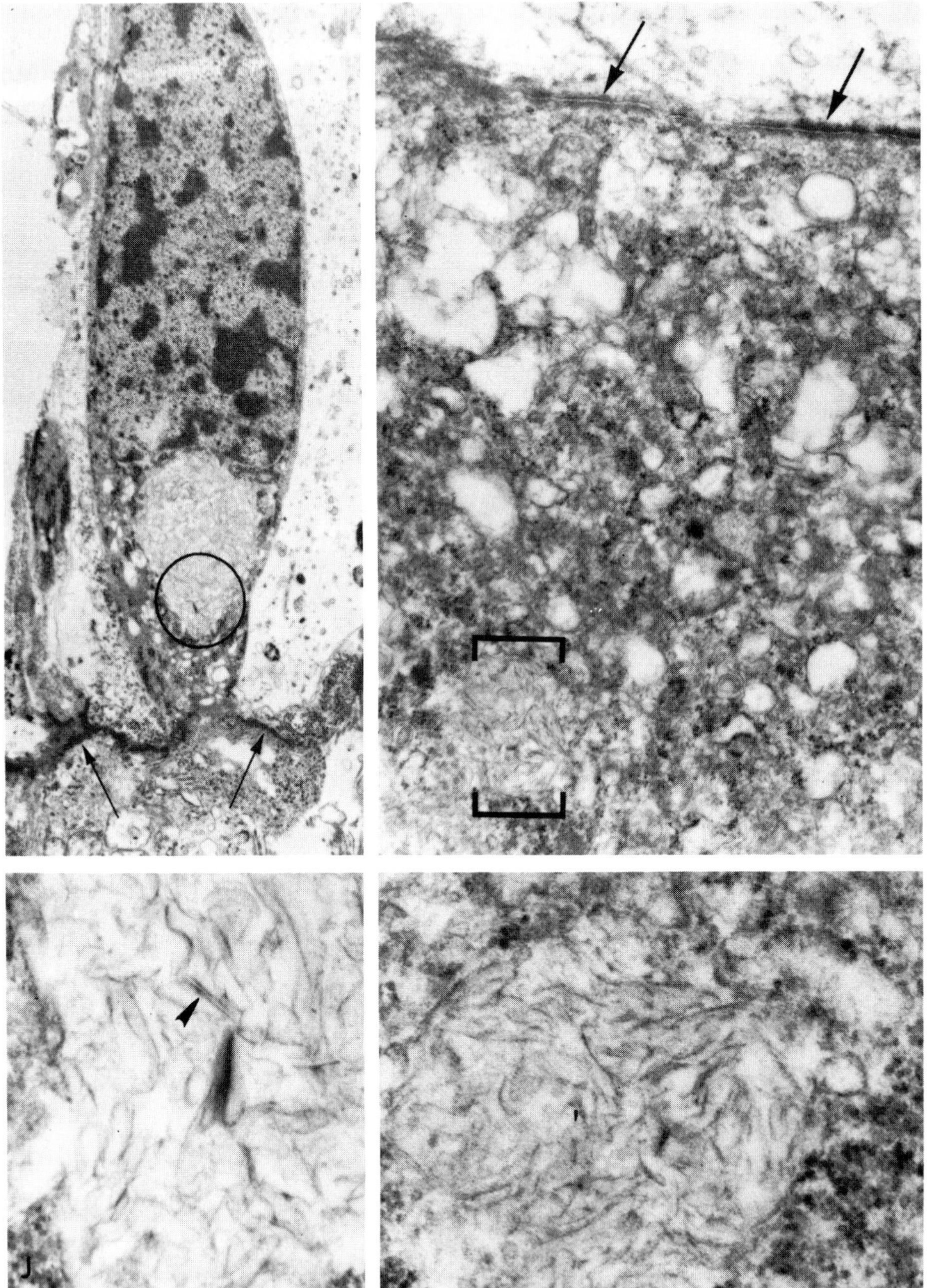

Figure 8–534 *Continued J.* Photoreceptor cells in the macular area. Upper left shows a large, whorled aggregate of inclusions in the paranuclear cytoplasm of a photoreceptor cell. Circled region of inclusion is seen at higher power in the lower left area of the figure. The leaflets of one distinct inclusion (arrowhead) measure 5.1 nm in idameter and are separated by a 3.3 nm electron-lucent zone. One inner segment contains aggregate of inclusions (bracketed, upper and lower right). Arrows mark outer limiting membrane in both photos. Upper left, ×8000; upper right, ×20,000; lower photos, ×60,000.

Illustration continued on opposite page

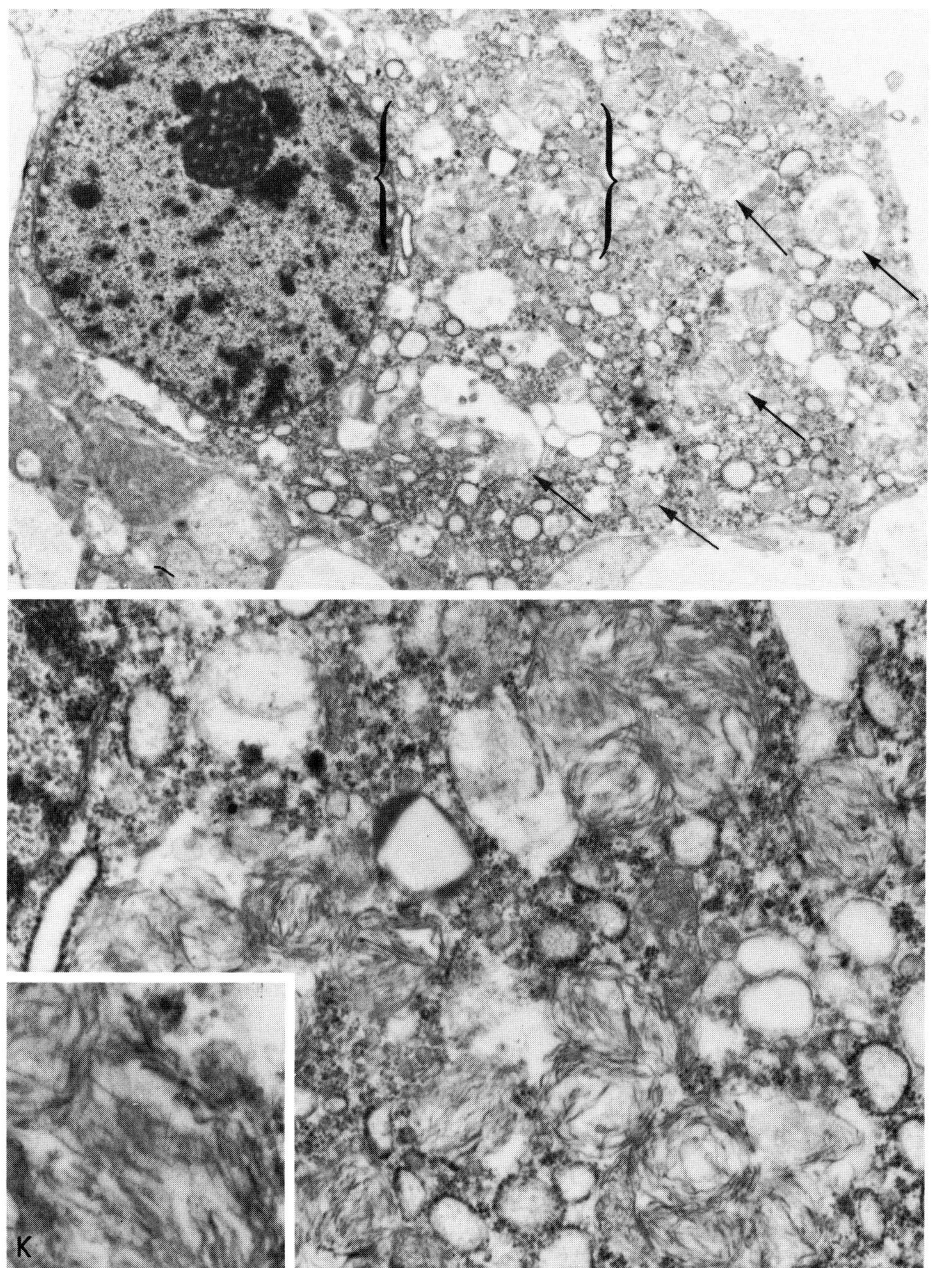

Figure 8–534 *Continued K,* Remaining ganglion cell in macular area is distended with numerous inclusions (upper photo) containing aggregates of bileaflet material (bracketed area and arrows). The bracketed area is shown at higher power in the lower photo and lower inset and demonstrates several nonmembrane-bound aggregates. Upper photo, ×10,000; lower photo, ×27,000; inset, ×72,000. *D–K,* EP 48903.

Illustration continued on following page

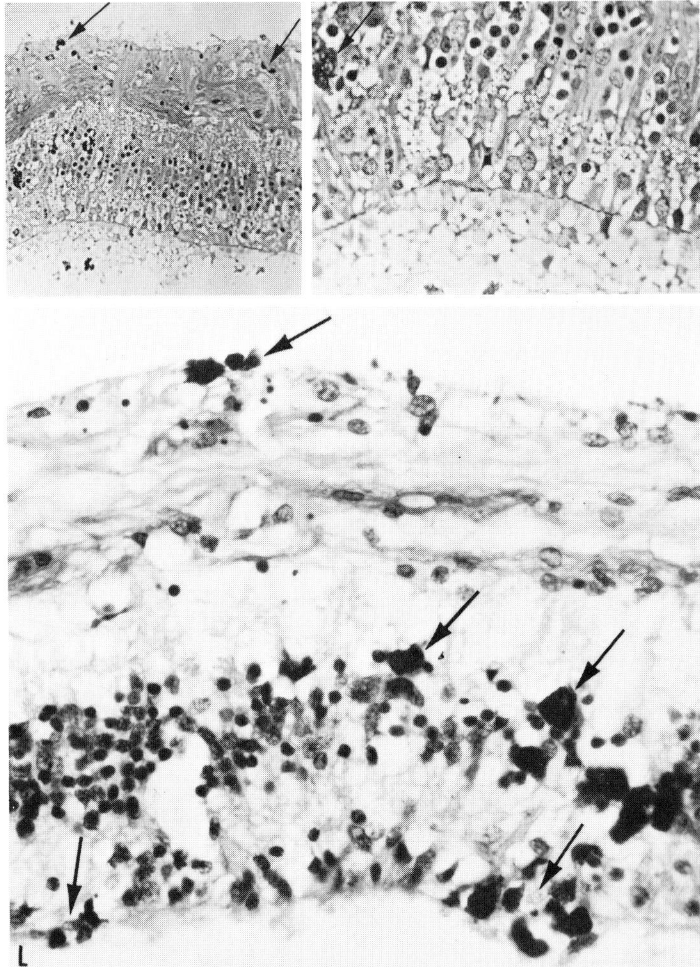

Figure 8–534 *Continued L,* Peripheral retina shows marked atrophy of nerve fiber and ganglion cell layers, total degeneration of outer and inner photoreceptor segments, and marked atrophy of the outer nuclear layer. Many macrophages (arrows) containing pigment and PAS-positive material are present throughout the retina. Top left, paraphenylenediamine, ×40; top right, paraphenylenediamine, ×150; bottom PAS, ×370.

Illustration continued on opposite page

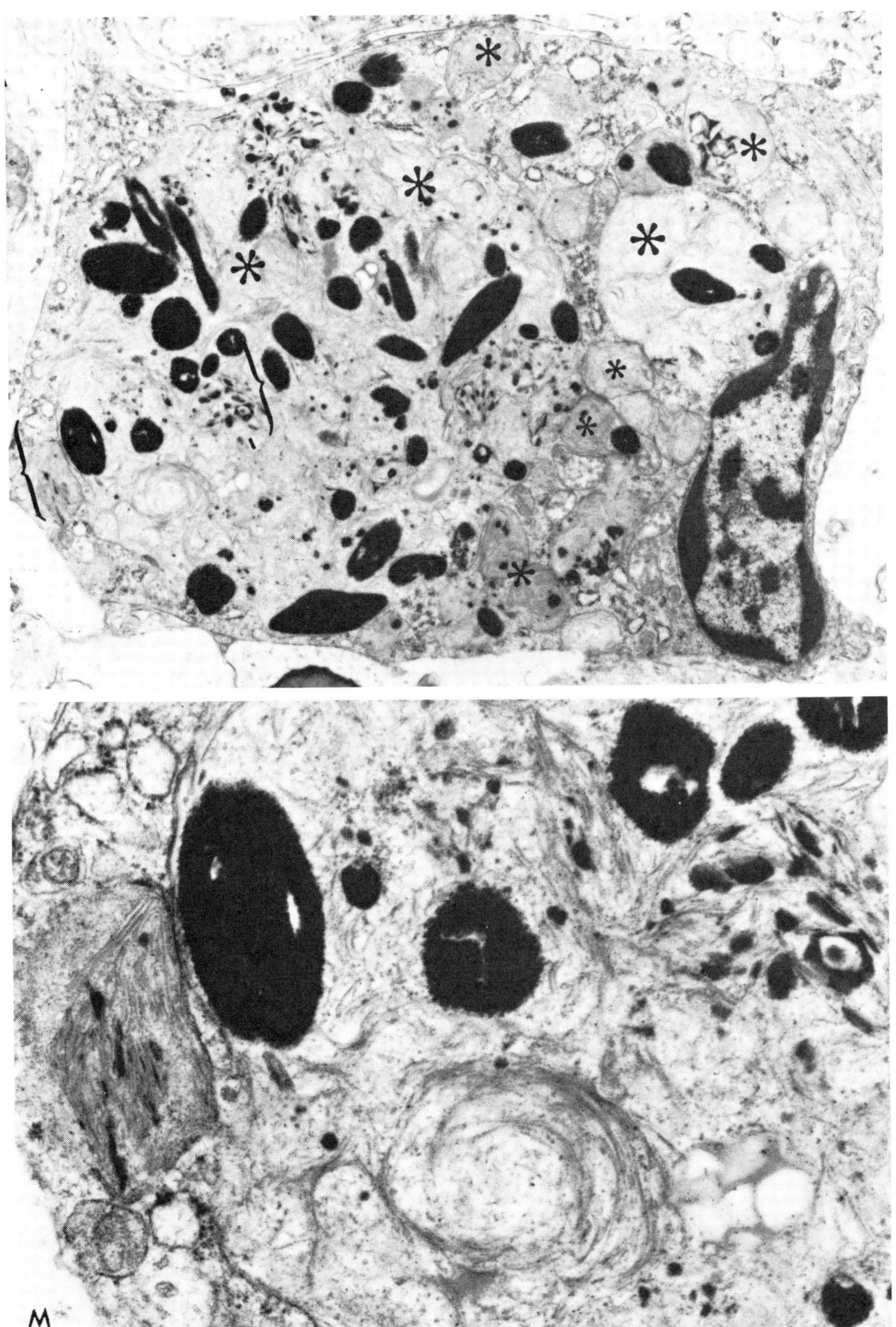

Figure 8–534 *Continued M,* Top, Macrophage in the inner nuclear layer of the peripheral retina is greatly distended by many whorled aggregates of inclusions admixed with melanin pigment. ×7500. Bottom, Higher-power view of bracketed area. ×40,000.

Illustration continued on following page

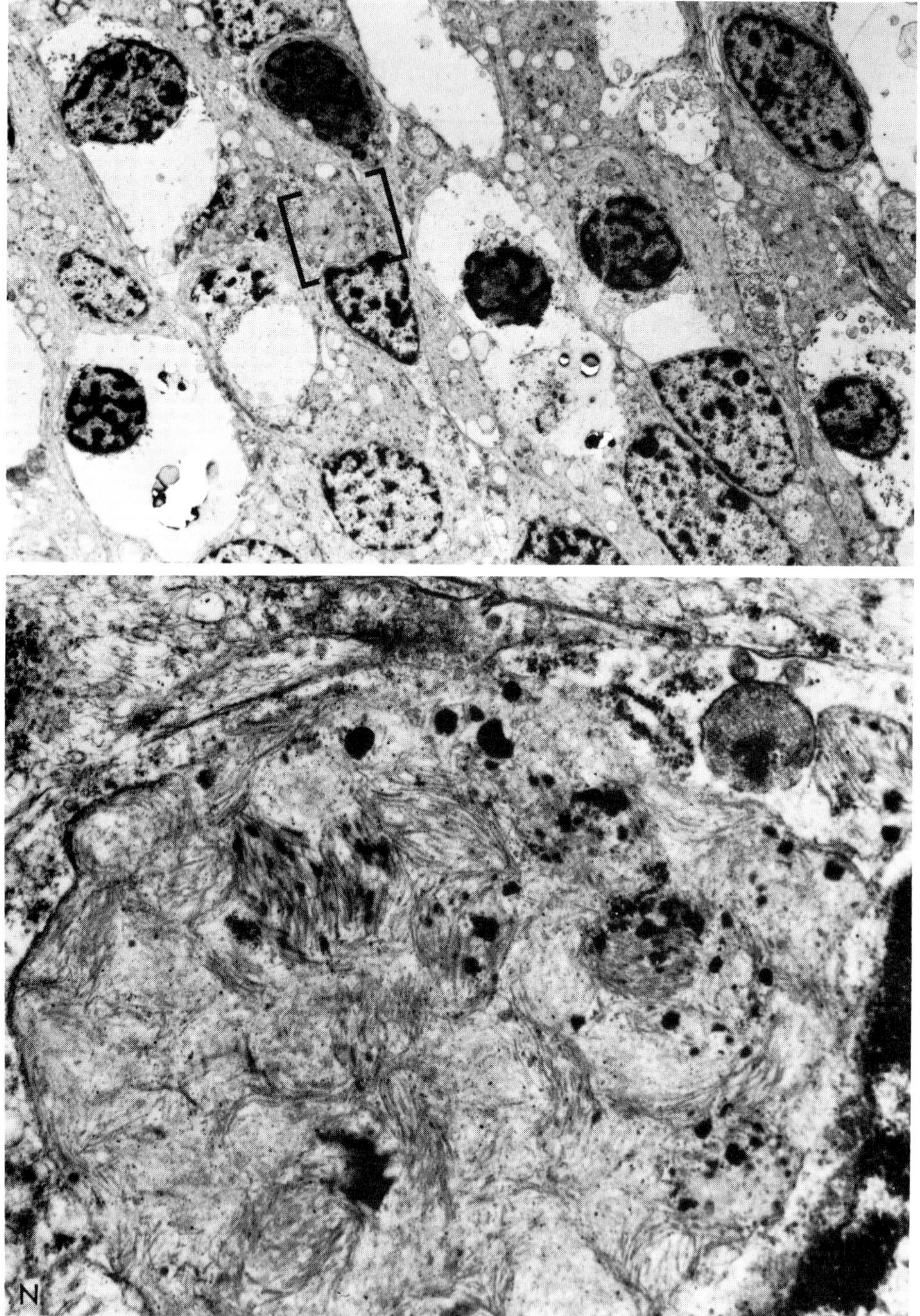

Figure 8–534 *Continued N,* Top, A large aggregate of bileaflet inclusion material in a neuron of the inner nuclear layer. ×4000. Bottom, Higher-power view of bracketed area shows whorled bileaflet inclusions admixed with electron-dense material. ×36,000.

Illustration continued on opposite page

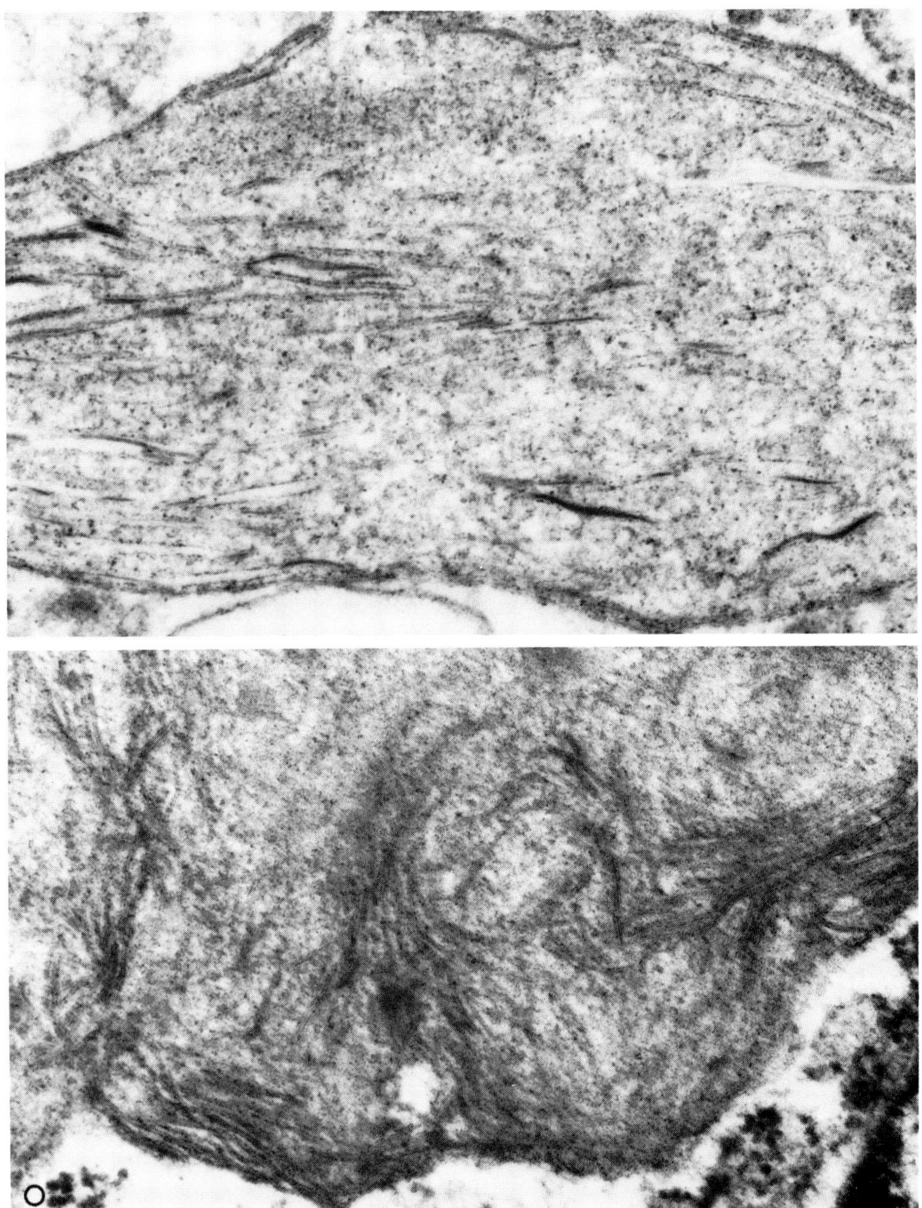

Figure 8–534 *Continued O,* High-power view of macrophages in optic nerve (upper photo) and outer nuclear layer (lower photo) of retina. Both contain whorled bileaflet inclusions on a granular background. The leaflets are 2.5 nm in diameter and are separated by a 2.5 nm electron-lucent space. Both, ×80,000. *L–O,* EP 56004.

(From Cohen SMZ, Green WR, De La Cruz ZC, et al: Ocular histopathology of neonatal and childhood adrenoleukodystrophy. Am J Ophthalmol *95*:82–96, 1983.)

de la Cruz, et al, 1983). Thinning of the outer nuclear layer with degeneration of photoreceptors is found (Fig. 8–534,*F* and *L*). Many macrophages with pigment and periodic-acid–Schiff–positive material are seen in the subretinal space and within the retina, particularly in the periphery (Fig. 8–534,*F* and *L*).

Ultrastructurally, paired electron-dense leaflet inclusions separated by an electron-lucent space were found in the retinal pigment epithelium (Fig. 8–534,*H* and *I*), in macrophages in the retina (Fig. 8–534,*G, M,* and *O*) and the optic nerve (Fig. 8–534,*0*); in photoreceptor cells (Fig. 8–534,*J*); in peripheral inner nuclear layer neurons (Fig. 8–534,*N*); and also in ganglion cells in the macular area (Fig. 8–534,*K*).

PRIMARY PIGMENTARY DEGENERATION OF THE RETINA

Primary retinal pigmentary degeneration (retinitis pigmentosa) occurs as a sporadic condition in about 39 per cent of patients, is recessive in 37 per cent, dominant in 20 per cent, and sex-linked in 4 per cent. Consanguinity is found in about 30 to 40 per cent of patients; in consanguineous marriages, the disease seems to be more severe in the offspring. Primary pigmentary degeneration of the retina is a common disease affecting about five per thousand people in the world population. All races may be affected. There is a slight preponderance of occurrence in males because of the small number of cases transmitted as a sex-linked trait. Retinitis pigmentosa may occur with or without a variety of central nervous system disorders.

Retinitis pigmentosa can be classified into typical and atypical forms. The typical form is characterized by pigmentary degeneration of the retina, attenuation of the retinal blood vessels, and pallor of the optic disk. The patients are night-blind, usually early in life, and the electroretinogram is nonrecordable. The visual field shows an annular scotoma corresponding to the area of degeneration, which spreads both peripherally and centrally until the field is small in advanced cases.

Based on evaluations of rod sensitivity relative to cone sensitivity, Massof and Finkelstein (1979, 1981) have identified two forms of each of the dominant and recessive types of retinitis pigmentosa. These findings suggest that these different forms represent different disease mechanisms, rather than different stages of disease progression.

Gradually, the central visual acuity deteriorates. Changes in the retinal vessels are found in about 80 to 90 per cent of patients, and most show retinal pigmentary degeneration, with the classic "bone spicule" migration of pigment into the inner retina around the blood vessels and in the intermediate zones. The pigmentary changes begin in an equatorial area and extend around the circumference. However, in some there is no pigmentary change, and these patients fall into the atypical groups.

Optic disk pallor is not always present—it depends on the degree of preservation of the ganglion cells and nerve fiber layers. When the inner retina is severely affected, degeneration of the axons of the ganglion cells occurs, and the typical waxy pallor of the optic disk is found. The atypical forms of primary pigmentary degeneration include occasional elderly persons with a late onset, those without pigmentary changes, the inverse (central) form, sectorial types, and rare uniocular cases. In many patients with retinitis pigmentosa, diffuse retinal vascular changes with edema (Spalton, Bird, Cleary, 1978) are observed, and sometimes these changes have a distinct inflammatory appearance.

The pathologic study of primary retinal pigmentary degeneration has been complicated by the fact that eyes are usually obtained only in the later stage of the disease and not always in the fresh state, so that some artifactual changes have occurred from delayed fixation. In occasional cases, however, the patient had a malignant melanoma of the anterior eye, and the retinal changes were less advanced than usual. The histopathologic features have been reported by numerous investigators, including Landolt, 1872; Wagenmann, 1891; Lister, 1903; Stock, 1908; Ginsberg, 1908; Suganumba, 1912; Leber, 1916; Friedenwald, 1930; Verhoeff, 1931; Ascher, 1932; Cogan, 1950; Wolter, 1957; and Gartner and Henkind, 1982.

In the initial stages, the rods are affected earlier than the cones. The outer segments seem to degenerate first, followed at a later stage by the inner segments. Concurrent with the photoreceptor degeneration, there is gradual depigmentation of the retinal epithelium with some RPE proliferation, phagocytosis of the liberated pigment by macrophages, and migration of both macrophages and RPE cells into the retina. The retina shows general atrophic changes involving the outer portion and later the inner portion.

While the degenerative changes are occurring in the outer retina, there is gliosis derived from retinal glial cells in the photoreceptor region, thus binding the retina to Bruch's membrane. The ganglion cell and nerve fiber layers may be preserved until late. In early cases observed clinically, the arteries appear narrowed, but histopathologic studies show no abnormalities of these vessels. Later, the arteries and the veins both show hyaline thickening of their walls, with narrowing of the lumen. The central retinal artery has been shown by Wolter (1957) to be reduced in caliber and the optic nerve to be atrophic in his reported case. The pigment migration into the retina may be free in the granular form, or the pigment may lie either in RPE cells or macrophages. Nodules of PAS-positive basement membrane may be produced by the hyperplastic RPE in the retina. Cogan (1950) and others have reported that in some cases the RPE cells form sheets along the inner limiting membrane, like endothelial cells. The choriocapillaris and the choroid usually show no important changes except in the later states if aging changes in the choroidal vessels cause secondary lesions. The histopathologic features in one case are illustrated in Fig. 8–535.

Gerstein and Dantzker (1969) studied the retinal vessels in a strain of rats with hereditary visual cell degeneration and found a close temporal relationship between photoreceptor cell degeneration and degeneration of retinal capillaries and

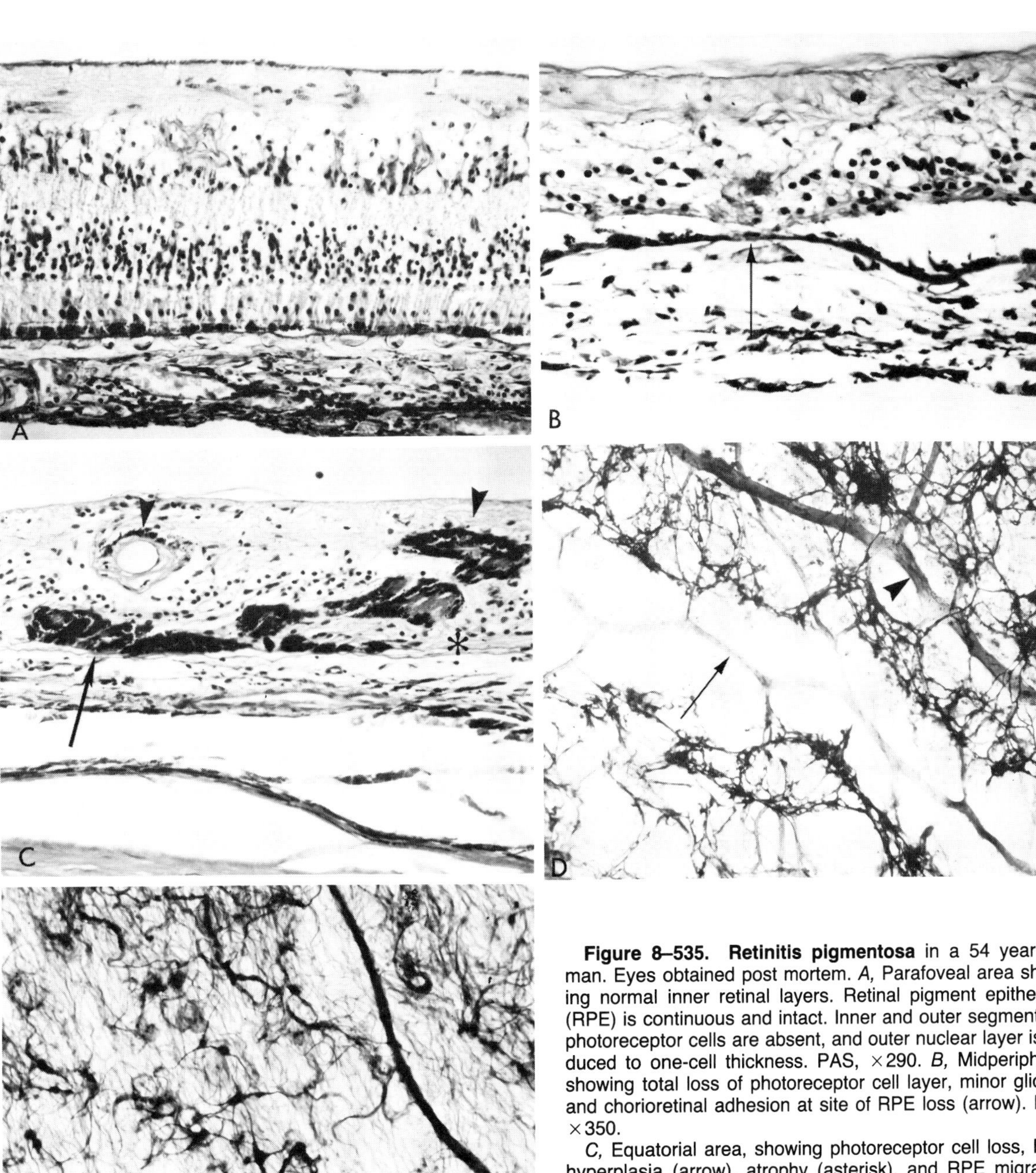

Figure 8–535. Retinitis pigmentosa in a 54 year old man. Eyes obtained post mortem. *A,* Parafoveal area showing normal inner retinal layers. Retinal pigment epithelium (RPE) is continuous and intact. Inner and outer segments of photoreceptor cells are absent, and outer nuclear layer is reduced to one-cell thickness. PAS, ×290. *B,* Midperiphery, showing total loss of photoreceptor cell layer, minor gliosis, and chorioretinal adhesion at site of RPE loss (arrow). PAS ×350.

C, Equatorial area, showing photoreceptor cell loss, RPE hyperplasia (arrow), atrophy (asterisk), and RPE migration into retina (arrowheads). PAS, ×300. *D,* Retinal trypsin digestion preparation, showing much sclerosis and acellularity of artery (arrow), vein (arrowhead), and intervening arterioles, capillaries, and venules. Hematoxylin; PAS, ×35. *E,* Peripheral retina showing curious stellate cells in trypsin digestion preparation. H and E, ×145. EP 46270.

narrowing of retinal arterioles. They postulated that thinning of the outer portion of the retina brings the retinal vascular network closer to the choroidal vessels and results in an increased oxygen tension in the retina. The increased oxygen tension appears to have a vasoconstrictive and degenerative effect on the retinal microvasculature.

Ultrastructural studies of an advanced case of autosomal dominant retinitis pigmentosa (Kolb, Gouras, 1974) disclosed loss of photoreceptor cells except for some cones in the foveal area. The outer segments of these cones were shorter and wider, and their disks were disoriented. The RPE in the foveal area contained excessive amounts of lipofuscin and reduced melanin content and and were in different stages of migration away from Bruch's membrane. Away from the foveal area, the RPE contained no lipofuscin but had large amounts of melanin.

Electron microscopic studies of a 24 year old man with sex-linked retinitis pigmentosa disclosed the foveal cones to be reduced in number by 50 per cent and to have shortened and severely distorted outer segments. Remaining cones outside the foveal area had no organized outer segments. The RPE contained large numbers of melanolysosomes and few free pigment granules in the fovea and through the midperiphery. In the far periphery, the RPE had few melanolysosomes and many free pigment granules (Szamier, Berson, Klein, Meyers, 1979).

Santos-Anderson, Tso, and Fishman (1982) have studied the ultrastructural features of the retina in two patients with X-linked recessive and one patient with autosomal dominant retinitis pigmentosa. They found the retinal pigment epithelium to be focally absent, focally proliferated, and mostly depigmented. The basement membrane of the retinal pigment epithelium was thickened. Photoreceptors were severely reduced in number, and two forms of photoreceptor cell degeneration were observed. In one form, the photoreceptor cells exhibited mitochondrial swelling, watery cytoplasm, and loss of organelles. In the other form of degeneration, the cells were dense, with shrunken cytoplasm and vacuolated mitochondria. Endothelial cell and pericyte degeneration was observed in many retinal vessels. Pigment-laden macrophages were observed in cell layers of the retina. An epiretinal membrane having features of smooth muscle cells was observed in the macular area of all six eyes.

Sector Retinitis Pigmentosa. The pigmentary features in this form of retinitis pigmentosa occur mainly in one or two quadrants. Photoreceptor cell degeneration, however, is widespread.

Rayborn, Moorhead, and Hollyfield (1982) have reported the light and electron microscopic findings of an eye from a patient with dominantly inherited sectoral retinitis pigmentosa. (Fig. 8–536,*A*). In the center of the macula, the retinal layers were intact but showed some reduction in the number of photoreceptor cells. (Fig. 8–536,*B*). Extensive degeneration of the photoreceptor cell layer was observed in all quadrants outside the central 3 to 5 mm (Fig. 8–536,*C* and *D*). These investigators observed changes in the choroidal vasculature and postulated that the RPE and retinal changes were secondary effects of alterations in the choroidal blood supply. In the fellow eye from the same patient, Bridges and Alvarez (1982) observed that the Vitamin A content was normal but that the 11-*cis* retinyl esters were extremely low in the RPE.

In some cases of central serous retinopathy, the tract of subretinal fluid inferiorly can lead to a sectoral retinitis pigmentosa–like protein (Yanuzzi, 1983).

Mizuno and Nishida (1966, 1967) found degeneration of the outer segments of cones. Remaining cones in inner segments were short and contained few mitochondria. An advanced case showed complete loss of visual cells.

Ultrastructural studies have not demonstrated whether the primary defect in retinitis pigmentosa is in the photoreceptor cells or the RPE.

In an extensive clinical study of 384 eyes of 192 patients with retinitis pigmentosa, Pruett (1983) noted that vision was often reduced by secondary changes. He observed cataractous changes in 46.4 per cent of the eyes, of which 93.6 per cent showed posterior subcapsular opacification. Vitreous degeneration and opacities were common. Electron microscopic studies of eight eyes disclosed condensed collagen fibrin and pigment granules. Retinal breaks, retinal detachment, or both were observed in only seven eyes (1.8 per cent). In seven eyes, an exudative response as in Coats' disease was observed. Changes in the macular area included striate changes with epiretinal membranes in 78 eyes (20.4 per cent); macular cystic changes in 58 (15.1 per cent); bull's eye appearance of macula in 137 (35.8 per cent); and RPE retinal degeneration in 66 (17.2 per cent). Cystoid macular edema verified by fluorescein angiography was observed in 11.9 per cent of the eyes.

Pseudoretinitis Pigmentosa. Marked pigmentary disturbance can be seen in a variety of conditions, and in some instances this can be confused with retinitis pigmentosa. Conditions that have been confused with retinitis pigmentosa in patients referred to a retina clinic include trauma, syphilis, rubella, viral encephalitis, Vogt-Koyanagi syndrome, phenothiazine and chloroquine toxicity, ophthalmic artery occlusion, postretinal detachment, and eclampsia (Carr, 1976). There are usually sufficient clinical features that allow differentiation of these conditions (Carr, 1976).

A condition that one sees more frequently in

the pathologic laboratory is pseudoretinitis pigmentosa after trauma (Cogan, 1969a). The pigmentary changes are quite diffuse and may resemble very closely those of true retinitis pigmentosa (see Figs. 8–202, 8–205, 8–208, 8–266 and 8–267), but there are always other changes of trauma, such as postcontusion deformity of the anterior chamber angle, subluxation or dislocation of the lens, scar of penetration or scars of perforation of the globe, macular hole, and so on.

Retinitis Punctata Albescens. This progressive disorder is characterized by the presence of whitish dots at the level of the RPE. They are distributed throughout the fundus but generally spare the posterior pole. The degeneration follows the pattern of retinitis pigmentosa but without the marked pigmentary change.

Light microscopic studies of eyes from a patient with this condition showed an irregular distribution of melanin pigment in the RPE, especially at the posterior pole. The RPE in the posterior pole showed vacuoles in the cytoplasm and had hyperchromatic nuclei (Wataya, 1960). No histopathologic studies of the nonprogressive form of the disease—fundus albipunctatus—have been reported.

Flecked Retina. The ophthalmoscopic appearance of flecks in or under the retina is observed in a number of unrelated conditions. These include the following and are discussed in more detail elsewhere: fundus albipunctatus (page 1213); retinitis punctata albescens (immediately above); familial drusen (page 927); Bietti's corneal and retinal crystallin dystrophy (page 1167); vitamin A retinopathy (page 1167); primary hyperoxaluria (page 1164); secondary oxalosis due to methoxyflurane toxicity (page 805); Leber's congenital amaurosis (page 1213); fundus flavimaculatus (page 1213); Hallervorden-Spatz disease (page 1179); the flecked retina of Kandori (Kandori, 1959; Kandori Tamai, Kurimoto, Fukunaga, 1972) (page 646); and tamoxifen retinopathy (page 805). In some of these conditions, the lesions may have a somewhat crystallin appearance.

Fundus Albipunctatus. See congenital night blindness, page 645.

Fundus Flavimaculatus. This bilateral, symmetric, slowly progressive disease is characterized by ill-defined, yellowish-white, round and linear "fishtail" or pisciform lesions at the level of the RPE in the posterior pole area. The size and shape of the flecks may vary, and new ones may appear as old ones fade. The condition appears early in life and is usually detected between ages 10 and 25 years. The electro-olfactogram is usually abnormal. Macular lesions (Stargardt's disease) occur in about 50 per cent of the patients with fundus flavimaculatus, leading experts in the field to consider these two conditions to be different forms of the same disease process.

In a case of fundus flavimaculatus that has been studied histopathologically (Klien, Krill, 1967), the following changes were observed diffusely and irregularly in the RPE: displacement of the nucleus from its normal location at the base of the cell, aggregation of melanin granules centrally and near the apex of the cell, accumulation of an acid mucopolysaccharide within the inner half of the cell, and variation in cell size—ranging from much larger than normal to small size, with no pigment granules or discernible nuclei. The investigators also described the accumulation of an acid mucopolysaccharide between the RPE and retina.

Eagle, Lucier, Bernardino, and Yanoff (1980) have reported the histopathologic and ultrastructural features of a 24 year old man with fundus flavimaculatus (Fig. 8–537,*A*,*B*). They found the RPE to contain a large amount of an abnormal form of lipofuscin (Fig. 8–537,*C* through *G*).

Beginning near the equator, scanning electron microscopy demonstrated a progressively marked heterogeneity in the size of the RPE cells. Enormously enlarged hypomelanotic cells measuring up to 80 microns in diameter occurred in irregular aggregates that became more prevalent posteriorly. The abnormal material within the RPE was found to be an abnormal form of lipofuscin by electron microscopic, autofluorescent, and histochemical studies. The greatest concentration of lipopigment was noted posteriorly. Stains for acid mucopolysaccharide were only mildly positive. The investigators concluded that the clinical and fluorescein angiographic manifestations of fundus flavimaculatus are consistent with accumulation of a lipofuscin-like substance in the RPE. The massive amounts of lipopigment encountered suggest that disordered lipopigment metabolism may play a major role in the pathogenesis of this retinal pigment epithelial disorder.

Histopathologic studies were also conducted on the eyes of a patient who had been followed for 40 years. When first seen, he had the typical fundus picture of fundus flavimaculatus (Fig. 8–538,*A*). He later developed widespread atrophy of the RPE (Fig. 8–536,*B*). Histopathologic study disclosed extensive loss of the RPE and photoreceptor cells (Fig. 8–538,*C*), and ganglion cell and nerve fiber layer atrophy (Maumenee, Maumenee, 1978; Frangieh, Green, Maumenee, 1982). The remaining RPE in the periphery had a large amount of abnormal pigment in the cytoplasm (Fig. 8–538,*D*,*E*).

Leber's Congenital Amaurosis. This is a major cause of congenital blindness and is probably transmitted as a recessive trait.

A striking clinicopathologic study was reported by Mizuno, Sears, Peterson, et al (1977). Ophthalmoscopic examination disclosed multiple, nondiscrete, round or oval white spots localized

Text continued on page 1219

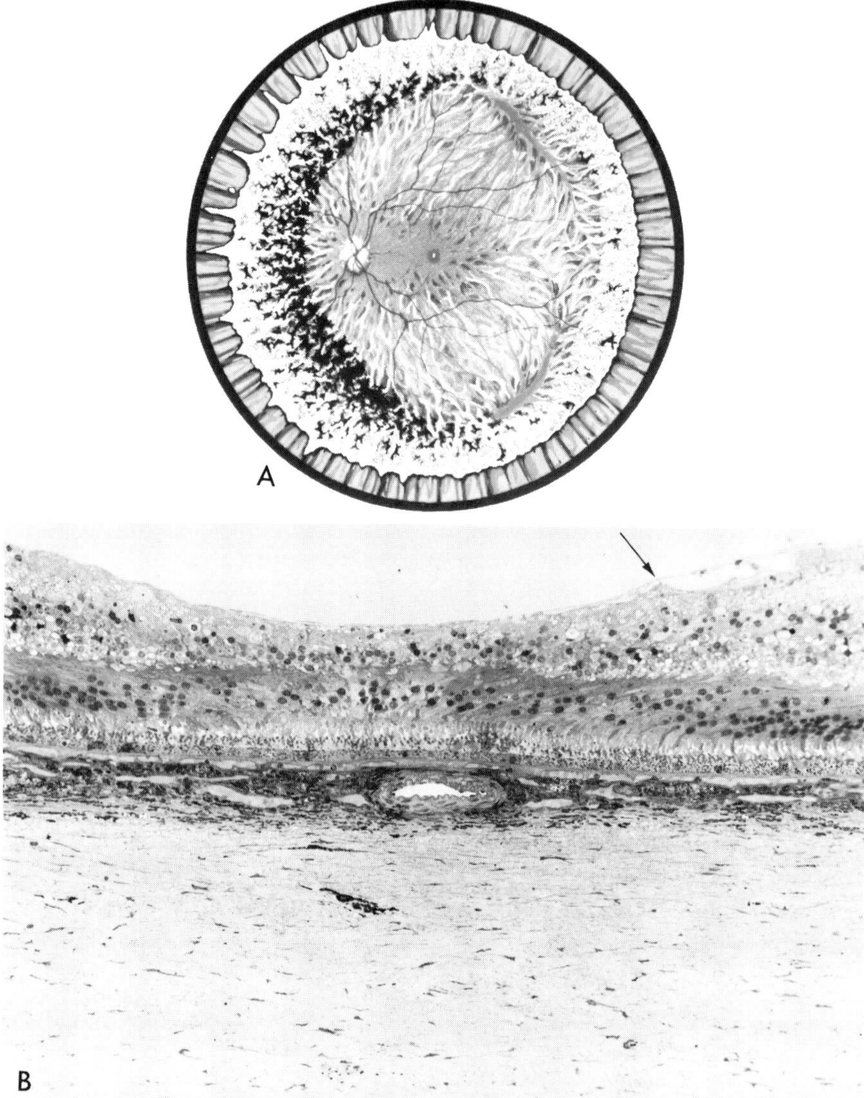

Figure 8–536. *A,* Fundus painting of the left eye of a 79 year old woman with sector retinitis pigmentosa. Bone spicule pigmentation approached the optic disk nasally. *B,* Section through the fovea shows that cone photoreceptors are present but reduced in number. A thin epiretinal membrane (arrow) is present. The retinal pigment epithelium is intact but has reduced pigmentation. The larger choroidal vessels and the choriocapillaris are normal.

Illustration continued on opposite page

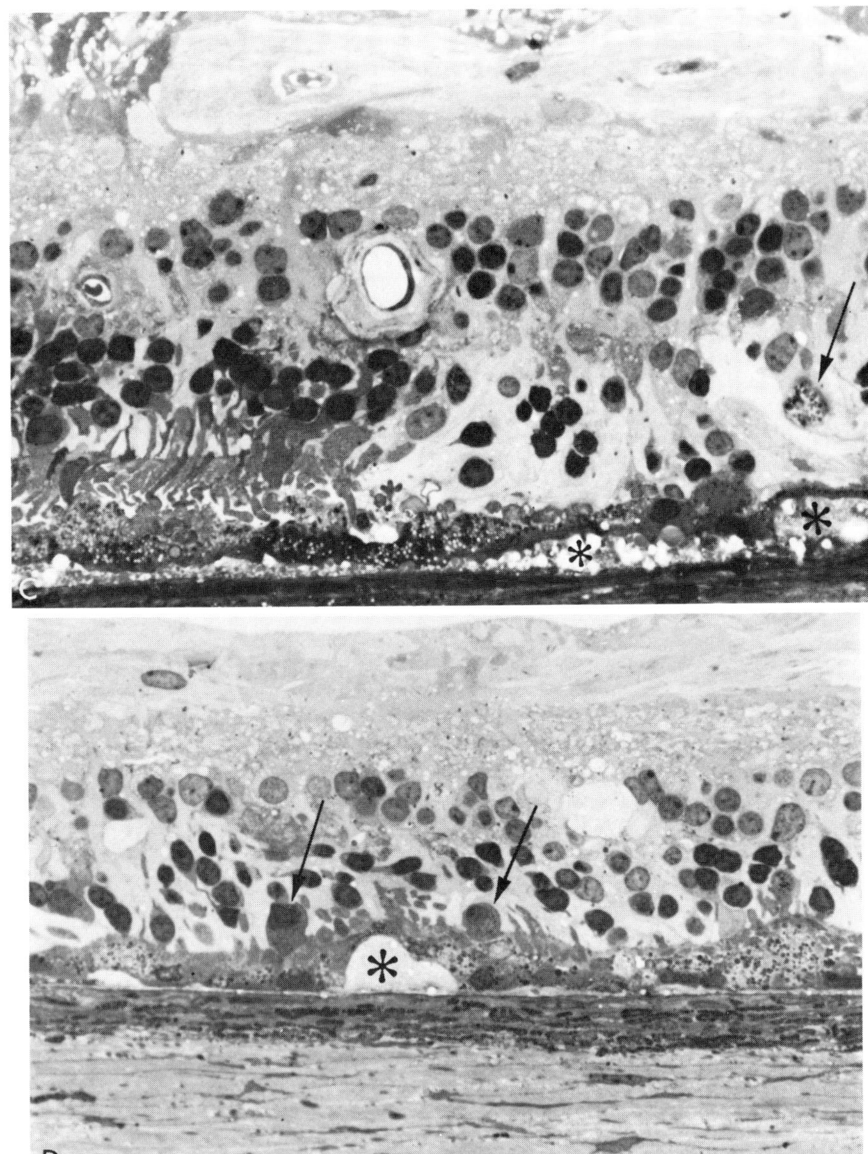

Figure 8–536 *Continued C,* Area about 5 mm temporal to the fovea shows an abrupt transition between relatively intact photoreceptors posteriorly (to left) and glial cell replacement anteriorly (to right). Drusen (asterisks) are present. A macrophage (arrow) containing pigment is present in the outer aspect of the retina. Magnification same as *D. D,* Area about 9 mm temporal to the fovea. There is disorganization of the inner and outer nuclear layers. Degenerated inner segments of rods and cones have a bulbous appearance (arrows). Drusen (asterisk) are present in this area. The choriocapillaris is obliterated, and no choroidal blood vessels are present in this section. ×160.

(From Rayborn ME, Moorhead CC, Hollyfield JG: A dominantly inherited chorioretinal degeneration resembling sectoral retinitis pigmentosa. Ophthalmology *89*:1441–1454, 1982.)

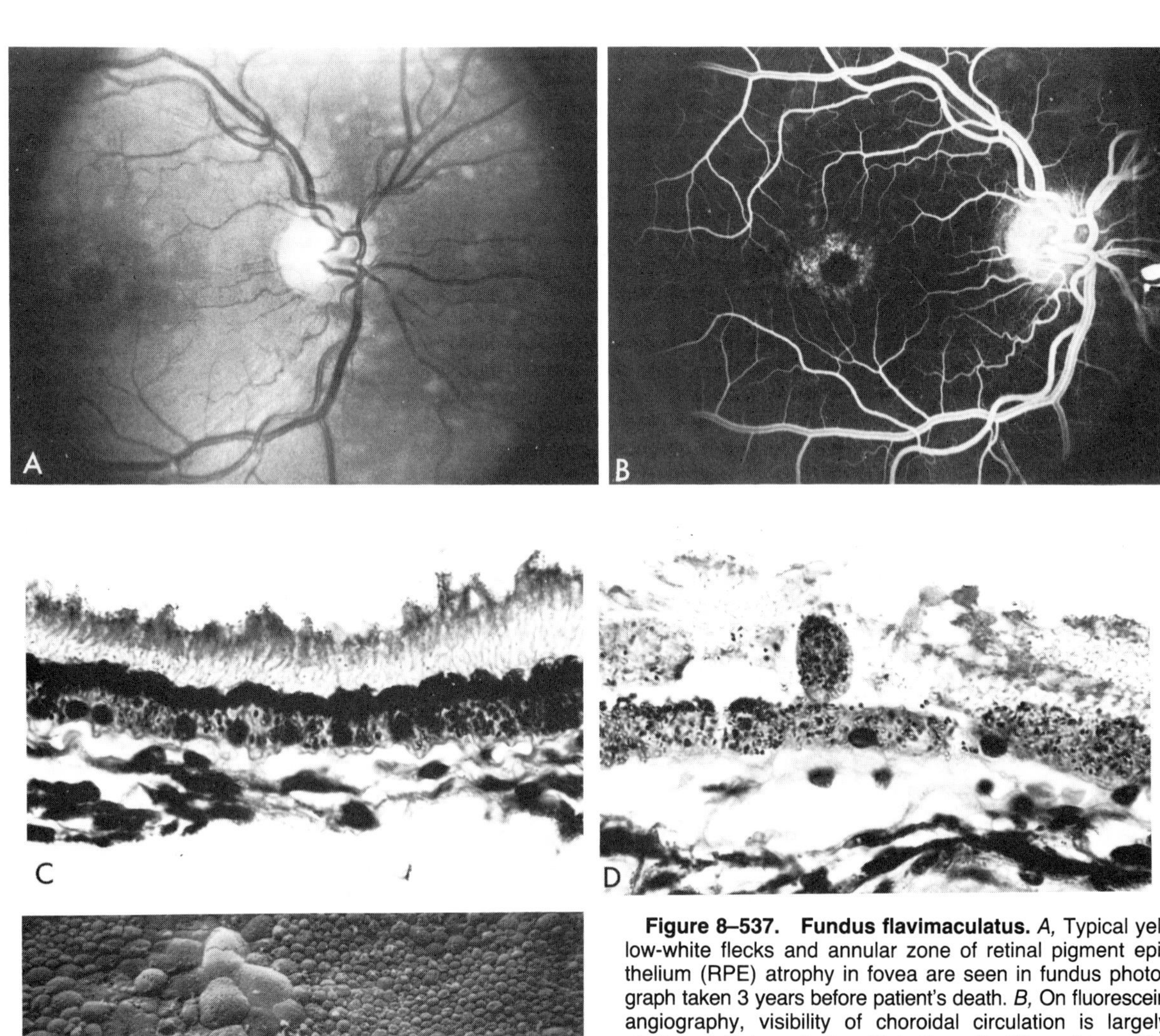

Figure 8–537. Fundus flavimaculatus. *A,* Typical yellow-white flecks and annular zone of retinal pigment epithelium (RPE) atrophy in fovea are seen in fundus photograph taken 3 years before patient's death. *B,* On fluorescein angiography, visibility of choroidal circulation is largely abolished ("sign of choroidal silence"). Ring of hyperfluorescence corresponds to foveal RPE atrophy. *C,* Peripheral RPE shows prominent line of apicalized pigment. Cells are uniform in size. Outer segments of artifactitiously disrupted retina remain adherent to RPE. H and E, ×400. *D,* Cells of posterior RPE vary much in diameter and melanin content. Retina is artifactitiously disrupted. H and E, ×400.

E, Scanning electron micrograph of midperipheral RPE shows irregular pisciform aggregate of greatly enlarged RPE cells surrounded by mosaic of smaller, relatively normal cells. ×200.

Illustration continued on opposite page

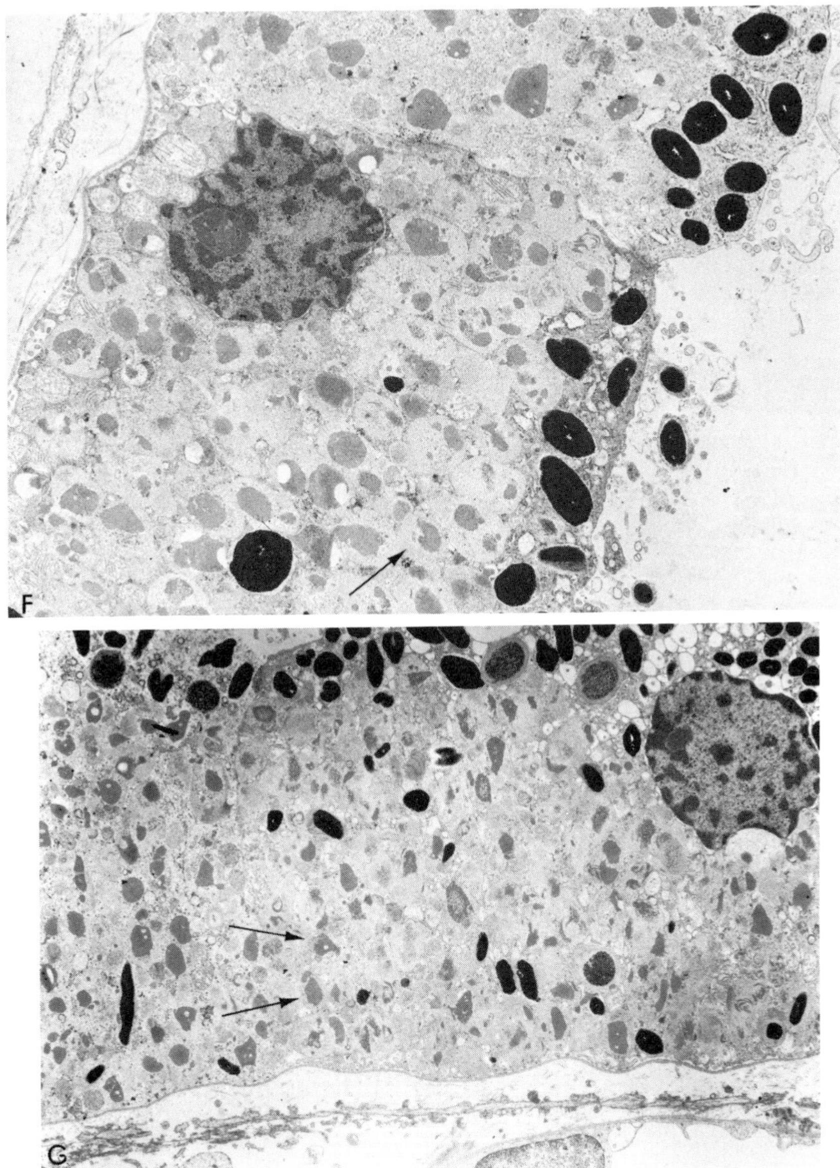

Figure 8–537 *Continued F,* Cytoplasm of peripheral RPE cell contains massive accumulation of abnormal lipofuscin (arrow), which has displaced melanin granules and other organelles. Bruch's membrane and choriocapillaris appear normal. ×8400. *G,* Larger amounts of abnormal lipofuscin are present in RPE posteriorly. Cytoplasm contains scattered melanin granules and phagosomes and numerous granules of abnormal lipofuscin (arrows). Many abnormal lipofuscin granules have several dense cores surrounded by a finely granular matrix. ×5300.

(From Eagle RC, Jr, Lucier AC, Vitaliano VG Jr, Yanoff M: RPE abnormalities in fundus flavimaculatus: A light and electron microscopic study. Ophthalmology *87*:1189–1200, 1980.)

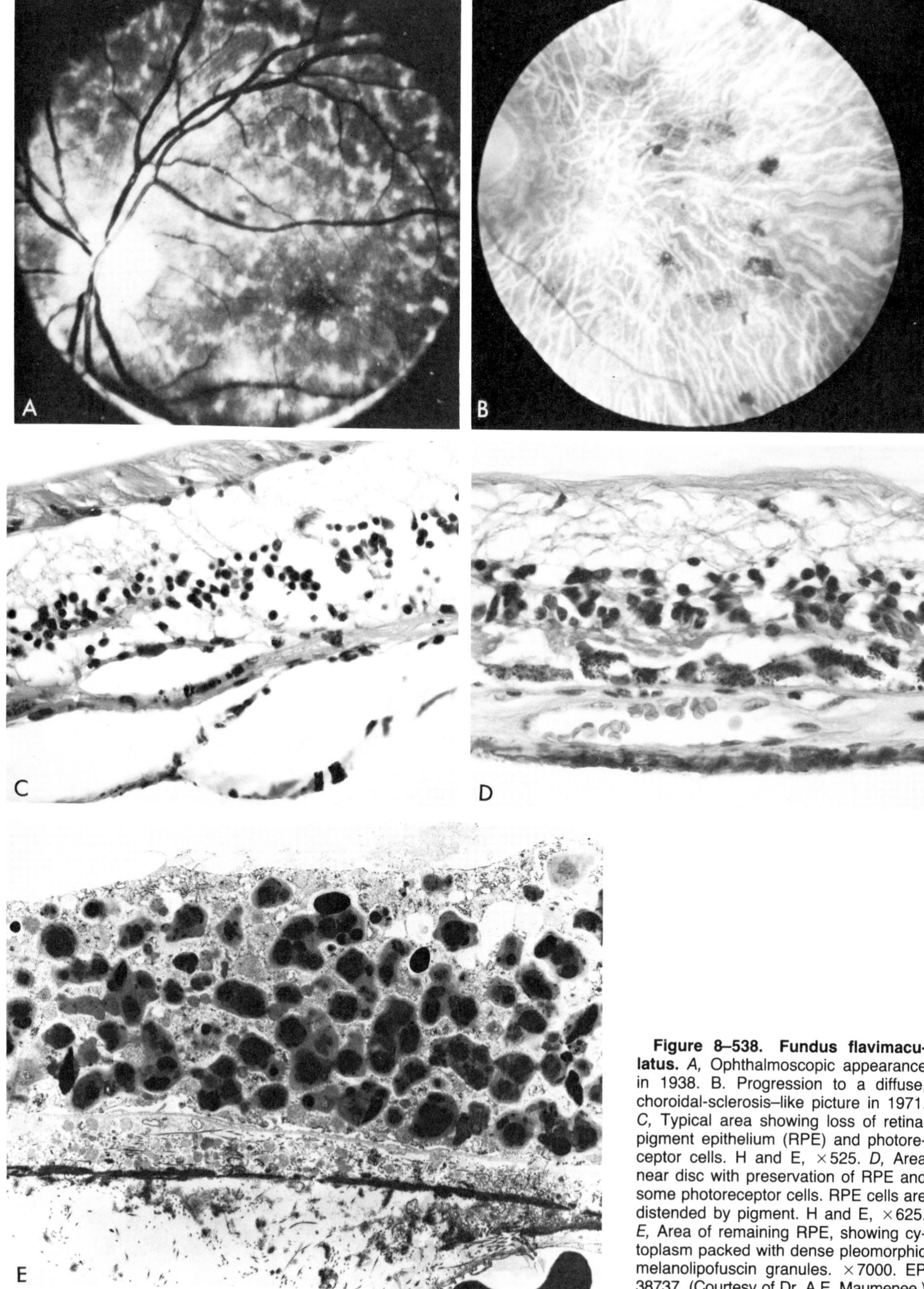

Figure 8–538. Fundus flavimaculatus. *A,* Ophthalmoscopic appearance in 1938. B. Progression to a diffuse, choroidal-sclerosis–like picture in 1971. *C,* Typical area showing loss of retinal pigment epithelium (RPE) and photoreceptor cells. H and E, ×525. *D,* Area near disc with preservation of RPE and some photoreceptor cells. RPE cells are distended by pigment. H and E, ×625. *E,* Area of remaining RPE, showing cytoplasm packed with dense pleomorphic melanolipofuscin granules. ×7000. EP 38737. (Courtesy of Dr. A.E. Maumenee.)

beneath the retinal vessels and distributed throughout the fundus except for the macular region. Light and electron microscopic studies of eyes of one child showed a selective destruction of the photoreceptor outer segments, with some macrophages in the vicinity (Fig. 8–539). The alterations that they illustrated are almost identical to those seen in monkeys blinded by experimentally induced rhodopsin sensitization (see Fig. 8–198) (Wong, Green, McMaster, Johnson, 1975).

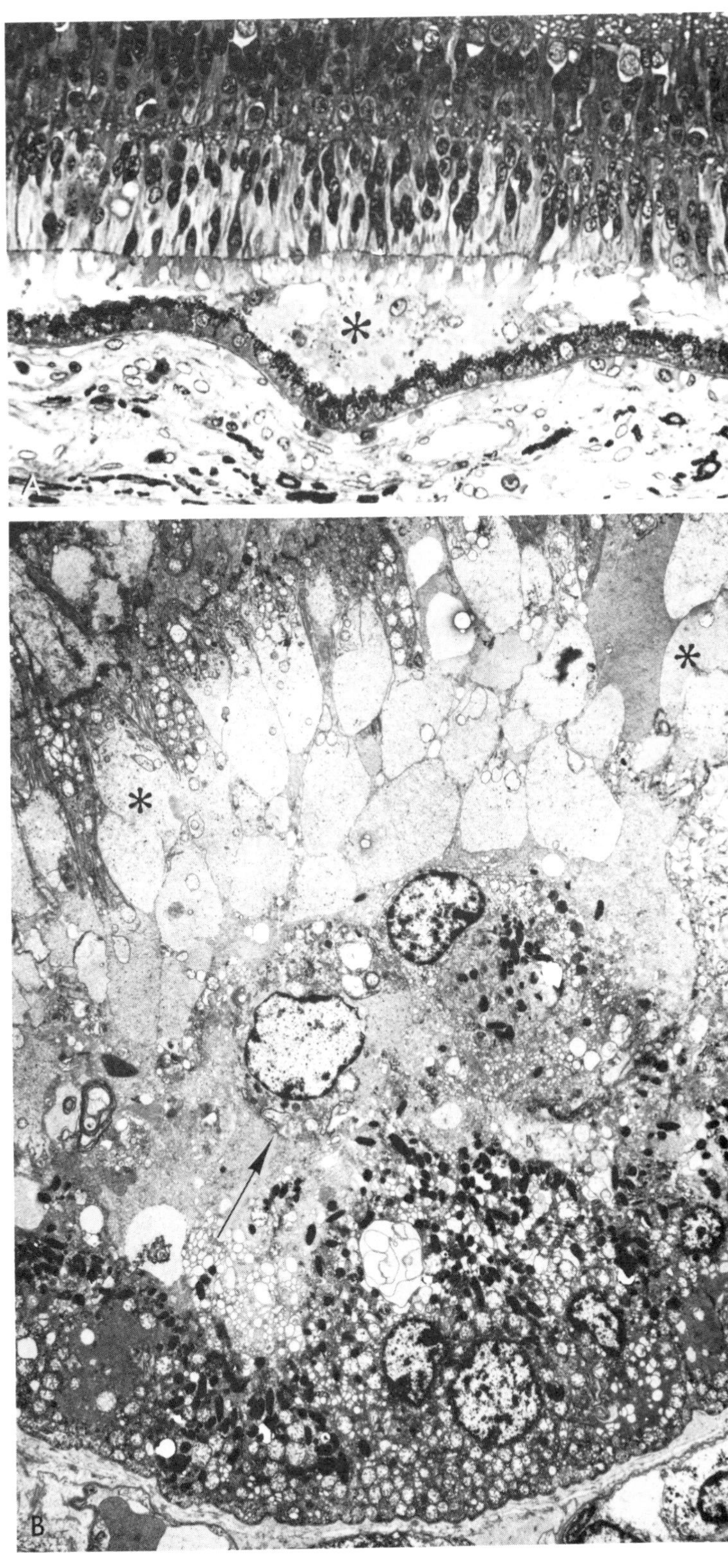

Figure 8–539. Leber's congenital amaurosis. *A,* There is destruction of outer segments of photoreceptor cells. Macrophages and cellular debris are present in subretinal space (asterisk). Toluidine blue, ×220. *B,* Electron micrograph showing loss of outer segments of photoreceptor cells. Remaining inner segments are swollen, and some are disrupted (asterisks). Macrophages (arrow) and cellular debris are present in subretinal space. ×1700. (From Mizuno K, Takei Y, Sears ML, Peterson WS, Carr RE, Jampol LM: Leber's congenital amaurosis. Am J Ophthalmol *83*:32–42, 1977.)

Other studies (Kroll, Kuwabara, 1964; François, Hanssens, 1969) showed loss of cone outer segments, shortening of the inner segments with fewer mitochondria, and large, partially pigmented inclusions in the RPE, all in the posterior region. There was total photoreceptor cell loss in the equatorial area.

Babel (1963) studied two patients. In one patient's eyes, he noted the layer of rods and cones to be absent, and in the other the rods and cones were disorganized. Some pyknosis of cells in the inner and outer nuclear layers was observed. The RPE was normal. In an additional patient (Noble, Carr, 1978), the eyes showed shortening of the outer segments of the photoreceptor cells, a reduction in the ganglion cell layer, and partial optic atrophy.

SYSTEMIC DISORDERS WITH RETINITIS PIGMENTOSA–LIKE CHANGES

Table 8–7 lists systemic disorders that have associated retinitis pigmentosa–like fundus abnormalities (Cross, 1973). Many of these conditions are discussed separately in this chapter and are listed here for grouping.

CHORIORETINAL ATROPHIES
(Choroidal Sclerosis; Choroidal Abiotrophies)

This is a group of conditions that pose a problem because of nosology and eponymity. Most have been considered primarily choroidal in origin. Primary RPE and photoreceptor cell involve-

Table 8–7. SYSTEMIC DISORDERS WITH FUNDUS ABNORMALITIES RESEMBLING RETINITIS PIGMENTOSA

Disorder	Etiology	Primary Manifestations
CENTRAL NERVOUS SYSTEM		
Bassen-Kornzweig	Autosomal recessive	Acanthocytosis Ataxia Abetalipoproteinemia
Hallervorden-Spatz	Autosomal recessive	Basal ganglia symptoms; dementia Early death
Pelizaeus-Merzbacher	X-linked recessive	Spasticity Cerebellar ataxia Dementia "Wandering eyes"
Juvenile amaurotic idiocy (Batten-Mayou) (Vogt-Spielmeyer)	Autosomal recessive	Visual loss Mental deterioration Seizures
Friedreich's ataxia	Autosomal recessive	Posterior column disease; nystagmus; ataxia
Retinitis pigmentosa with pallidal degeneration	Autosomal recessive (?)	Extrapyramidal rigidity Dysarthria
*Saldmo syndrome	Autosomal recessive (?)	Nephropathy Cerebellar ataxia Skeletal abnormalities
MUCOPOLYSACCHARIDOSES		
Type I (Hurler)	Autosomal recessive	Skeletal abnormalities Cloudy corneas Mental retardation
Type II (Hunter)	X-linked recessive	Mental retardation Skeletal abnormalities Hepatosplenomegaly
Type III (San Filippo)	Autosomal recessive	Mental retardation
Type IV (Morquio)	Autosomal recessive	Corneal clouding Skeletal abnormalities
ASSOCIATED WITH DEAFNESS		
Usher syndrome	Autosomal recessive	Deafness
Laurence-Moon syndrome	Autosomal recessive	Mental retardation Hypogenitalism Spastic paraplegia
Bardet-Biedl syndrome	Autosomal recessive	Mental retardation Polydactyly Obesity Hypogenitalism

ment may occur and then lead to secondary choroidal vascular changes.

The term *choroidal sclerosis* has been used to describe the ophthalmoscopic appearance of prominent choroidal vessels when there has been loss of the RPE. The patterns of atrophy have been considerable and have led to numerous descriptive terms—e.g., central, peripapillary, helicoid, annular, and so on. With the use of electrophysiologic methods of analysis, angiographic techniques, and histopathologic data, Krill and Archer (1971) have proposed a meritorious classification based on the location, whether the condition is primary and progressive, and whether there is choriocapillaris involvement or larger choroidal vascular involvement or involvement of both. Similarly, Carr, Mittl, and Noble (1975) have classified these conditions into three groups: central, peripapillary, and generalized. Each group has subcategories of "hereditary" and "acquired." Carr and colleagues stress the importance of determining whether there is a hereditary pattern. The choroidal vasculature has been implicated in the pathogenesis. We, however, believe that the atrophy is not ischemic and involves some abnormality in the biochemical interplay between the RPE and the photoreceptor cells.

Regional Choroidal Atrophy With Choriocapillaris Atrophy

This may be localized in the macular, peripapillary, and paramacular areas.

Table 8–7. SYSTEMIC DISORDERS WITH FUNDUS ABNORMALITIES RESEMBLING RETINITIS PIGMENTOSA *continued*

Disorder	Etiology	Primary Manifestations
ASSOCIATED WITH DEAFNESS *continued*		
Alström's syndrome	Possible autosomal recessive	Obesity Diabetes mellitus Nystagmus
Refsum's disease	Autosomal recessive	Polyneuropathy Ataxia Increased plasma phytanic acid
McGovern's syndrome	Possible autosomal recessive	Visual loss Stationary, congenital hearing loss
Cockayne syndrome	Autosomal recessive	Dwarfism Precocious senility Mental retardation
Retinitis pigmentosa with ophthalmoplegia	Unknown	May have ataxia, heart block
Flynn-Aird syndrome	Autosomal dominant	Cataracts, ataxia, Dementia, epilepsy Cutaneous changes
Retinitis pigmentosa with muscle atrophy	Unknown	Progressive muscle wasting and weakness
Retinitis pigmentosa with spastic diplegia	Autosomal recessive (?)	Spastic diplegia
MISCELLANEOUS		
Syphilis	*Treponema pallidum*	"The great imitator"
Trauma	Multiple	Variable
Retinitis pigmentosa with ophthalmoplegia	Unknown	Heart block Ophthalmoplegia
Retinitis pigmentosa with megacolon	Probably polygenic	Polar cataract Strabismus Nystagmus
Retinitis pigmentosa with muscular dystrophy	Unknown	Proximal dystrophy Cataracts
Kartagener's syndrome	Autosomal recessive	Dextrocardia Bronchiectasis Sinusitis
Retinitis pigmentosa with retinal hemorrhages	Possible autosomal recessive	One case had excess glial tissue at disk
Turner syndrome	Chromosomal aberration	Infertility, short stature, shield chest, low hairline
Imidazone aminoaciduria	Autosomal recessive	Seizures, mental deterioration, Excess carnosine and anserine excretion

*Syndrome status is uncertain.

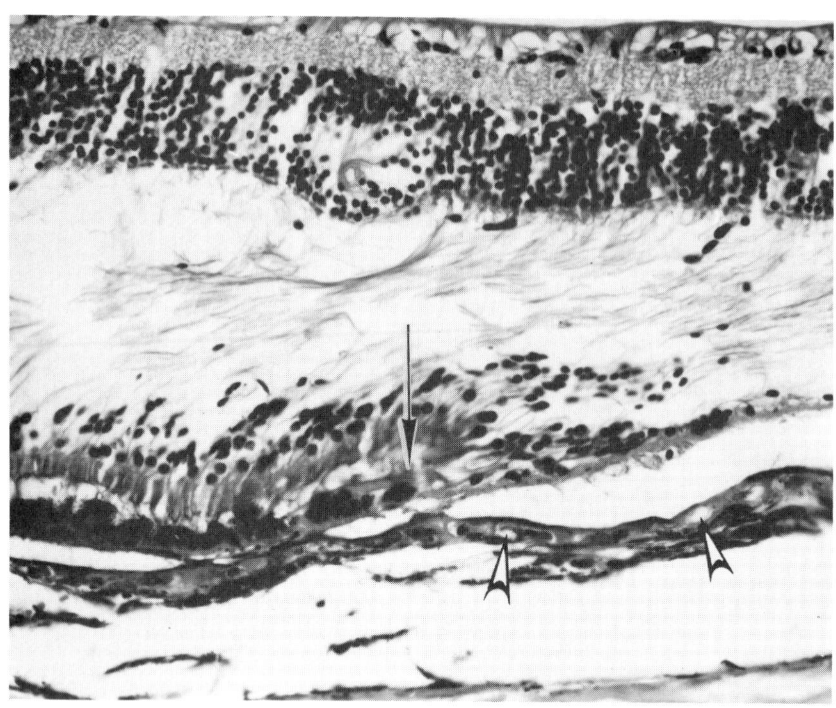

Figure 8–540. Central areolar choroidal sclerosis. An abrupt transition (arrow) is seen at point where retinal pigment epithelium (RPE) and photoreceptor cells are lost. Adjacent RPE is hypertrophic, and choriocapillaris is intact (arrowheads) in area of areolar RPE atrophy. Inner nuclear layer is intact. PAS, ×250. (Courtesy of Dr. A.P. Ferry. Case presented at Eastern Ophthalmic Pathology Society, New York, May, 1969.)

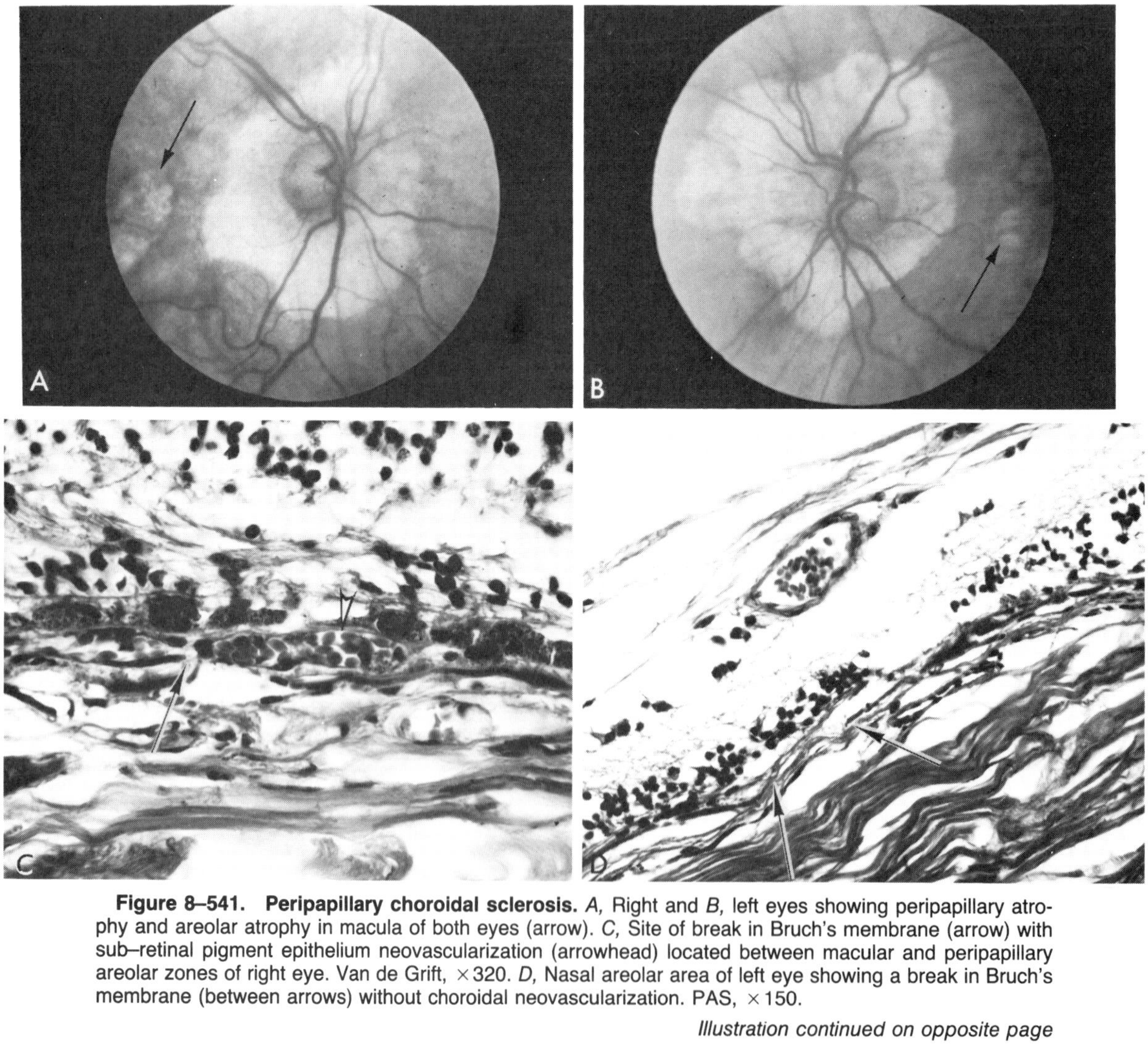

Figure 8–541. Peripapillary choroidal sclerosis. *A,* Right and *B,* left eyes showing peripapillary atrophy and areolar atrophy in macula of both eyes (arrow). *C,* Site of break in Bruch's membrane (arrow) with sub–retinal pigment epithelium neovascularization (arrowhead) located between macular and peripapillary areolar zones of right eye. Van de Grift, ×320. *D,* Nasal areolar area of left eye showing a break in Bruch's membrane (between arrows) without choroidal neovascularization. PAS, ×150.

Illustration continued on opposite page

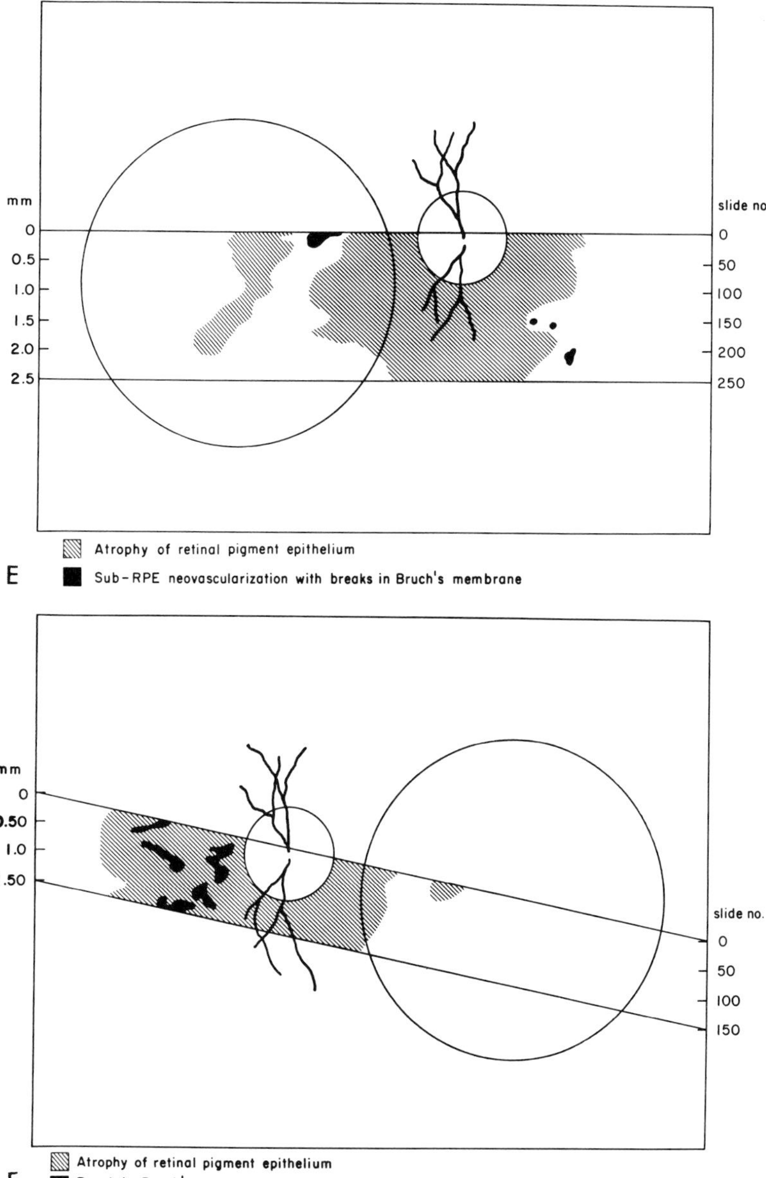

Figure 8–541 *Continued E,* Two-dimensional reconstruction of right eye, mapping macular and peripapillary lesions and breaks in Bruch's membrane. *F,* Two-dimensional reconstruction of macular and peripapillary lesions of left eye, showing size and location of macular and peripapillary areolar atrophy and breaks in Bruch's membrane nasally. EP 39896.

(From Green WR, Key SN III: Senile macular degeneration: A histopathological study. Trans Am Ophthalmol Soc *75*:180–254, 1977.)

Macular. Diseases of this type have variously been called central choroidal sclerosis, central choroidal vascular atrophy, central areolar choroidal sclerosis, central progressive areolar choroidal sclerosis, and central areolar choroidal dystrophy. This disease is transmitted in an autosomal dominant fashion (Carr, 1965). Histopathologic studies (Ashton, 1953; Babel, 1958; Howard, Wolf, 1964; Klien, 1964; Ferry, Llovera, Shafer, 1972; Sarks, 1973a) have consistently shown a sharply circumscribed area of loss of RPE and choriocapillaris and reduction of the number of photoreceptor nuclei in the outer nuclear layer (Fig. 8–540). A similar clinical and histopathologic picture is present in olivopontocerebellar degeneration (Ryan, Knox, Green, Konigsmark, 1975).

Peripapillary (Peripapillary Choroidal Sclerosis). The atrophy in this form surrounds the disk and may extend in finger-like extensions beyond the circular zone around the nerve head. The inheritance of this disease is less well established, with most cases occurring sporadically.

This pattern of choroidal atrophy is exemplified by the following case. An 84 year old man was seen with peripapillary atrophy in both eyes (Fig. 8–541). Fluorescein angiography disclosed no choriocapillaris in the center of the lesion, but there was slight staining late at the margin. Histopathologic study disclosed loss of the RPE and choriocapillaris and partial loss of the photoreceptor cell layer. The larger choroidal vessels were intact. Several breaks in the peripapillary area of Bruch's membrane were observed. One break had choroidal neovascularization extending under the RPE and was undetected either by ophthalmoscopy or fluorescein angiography (Fig. 8–539). These findings are similar to those in the one patient reported by Sarks (1973a).

The case illustrated here, like the one reported by Sarks, was late in onset and associated with drusen and breaks in Bruch's membrane. It would appear to be a senile degenerative change, compared with cases having a hereditary pattern and early onset.

Weiter and Fine (1977), in a light and electron microscopic study of the eyes of an 84 year old man, found atrophy of the choriocapillaris, RPE, and photoreceptor cells in the affected area. In addition, there was a marked decrease in the choroidal arteries and veins, breaks in Bruch's membrane in the peripapillary area, and excessive basement membrane production by the Müller's cells. These investigators postulated that the primary abnormality in this disease involves the choroidal vasculature.

Perimacular (Circinate or Annular Choroidal Sclerosis). The term was first used (Knapp, 1907) to describe a circular pattern of atrophy in both eyes of an 11 year old girl who had reduced visual acuity, an annular scotoma, and night blindness. Schocket and Ballin (1970) described two patients, aged 72 and 56 years, who had similar features. In both, dark adaptation was only moderately affected, and the electroretinogram was extinguished in one and normal in the other. Chopdar (1976) reported annular choroidal sclerosis in a 29 year old man and possible early changes of the same disorder in the patient's 7 year old daughter.

Regional Choroidal Atrophy with Total Choroidal Vascular Atrophy

Regional choroidal atrophy with total choroidal vascular atrophy may be localized to the macular, nasal, temporal, or peripapillary area. There is no uniform age of onset, and most cases are sporadic, suggesting either an environmental origin or autosomal recessive inheritance. The earliest changes include the development of a homogeneous, gray, edema-like appearance in the involved area. This is thought to be possibly due to changes in the RPE.

Macular. Total choroidal atrophy in the macular area has been known as choroidal vascular abiotrophy; helicoid, serpiginous degeneration of the choroid; and central gyrate atrophy. In the serpiginous form, the onset of atrophy has been noted between the ages of 35 and 55 years. In a study of nine patients with "serpiginous" (geographic) choroidopathy, Weiss, Annesley, Shields, et al (1979) noted inflammatory signs in two patients. One showed extensive vitreous cells and the other vitreous cells plus perivasculitis. In another study of nine patients with "serpiginous choroiditis," Laatikainen and Erkkilä (1974) considered that the features of their patients indicated that the disease is due to an immunologically induced choroiditis. Some investigators (Hamilton, Bird, 1974) stress the absence of signs of inflammation, and they believe that geographic choroidopathy is distinct from serpiginous choroidopathy. Apparently in serpiginous or geographic choroidopathy, some cases are of inflammatory origin, and others are abiotrophic.

Nasal or Temporal (Bifocal Chorioretinal Atrophy). This atrophy may begin in infancy. Autosomal dominant transmission was documented in one report of this disorder (Douglas, Waheed, Wise, 1968). The lesions are located mainly in the nasal and temporal areas. No histopathologic studies have been reported on eyes with this disorder.

Peripapillary (Helicoid Peripapillary Chorioretinal Atrophy, Choroiditis Areata, Circumpapillary Dysgenesis of RPE, Chorioretinitis Striae). This condition can become manifest between the ages of 4 and 43 years, with the majority of cases evident at around 25 years of age. X-linked transmission is suggested in some studies. Schatz, Maumenee, and Patz (1974) reported nine middle-aged adults with "geographic helicoid peripapillary choroidopathy." They noted the progressive bilateral nature of the disorder and the absence of a familial tendency or associated toxic or inflammatory signs.

A similar (but slightly different) disorder, described by Chisholm and Dudgeon (1973) and Pearlman, Kamin, Kopelow, and Saxton (1975) is characterized by a radial paravenous distribution and appears to be progressive (Pearlman, Heckenlively, Bastek, 1978).

Diffuse Choroidal Atrophy with Choriocapillaris Atrophy

The diffuse choroidal atrophies are similar to the regional forms in regard to the changes occurring in the choroidal vasculature. The diffuse atrophies are characterized by widespread involvement, with greater disturbance of peripheral retinal function. The macula may be spared or only mildly involved until the later stages of the disease.

Diffuse choroidal atrophy with primary choriocapillaris atrophy has been referred to as generalized choroidal angiosclerosis, diffuse choroidal sclerosis, and generalized choroidal sclerosis.

This condition usually becomes evident in the third to fourth decades and occasionally as early as the first and second decades. Initial manifestations include a stippled or mottled fundus appearance. The process starts in the macular or peripapillary areas and slowly extends to the equator or beyond. Hereditary transmission is usually autosomal dominant. Frequent sporadic cases appear to have an autosomal recessive transmission. Rare instances of a sex-linked mode have been noted. Central vision may or may not be involved.

The following case illustrates the features of this type of diffuse choroidal atrophy with loss of the choriocapillaris. The patient was seen first in 1951 at the age of 60 years with a history of visual loss of unknown cause since the age of 54 years. Ophthalmoscopic examination disclosed widespread RPE atrophy with quite visible choroidal vessels (Fig. 8–542,*A,B*). A small area of relatively normal-appearing RPE was present in the peripapillary area—more in the right than in the left eye. A small patch of myelinated nerve fibers was present superiorly at the left nerve head. The retinal arterioles were quite constricted. The patient was followed periodically over the next 20 years until his death in 1970 at age 80 years.

Initially, the vision was 20/30 in the right eye and 10/400 in the left eye. In 1967, the vision respectively was 20/60 and count fingers at 6 inches. The electroretinogram was extinguished in both eyes. In 1963 the vision was 20/40 in the right eye and count fingers at 3 feet, left eye. Visual fields with a 3/330 white test object showed a dense central scotoma of 30 degrees, with a moderate general constriction of the peripheral field of the left eye. The peripheral extent of the visual field of the right eye was full, but there was a 20 degree central scotoma.

Histopathologic studies disclosed widespread loss of RPE and photoreceptor cells (Fig. 8–542,*C,D*). The inner nuclear layer remained relatively intact. In many areas there was a near-total

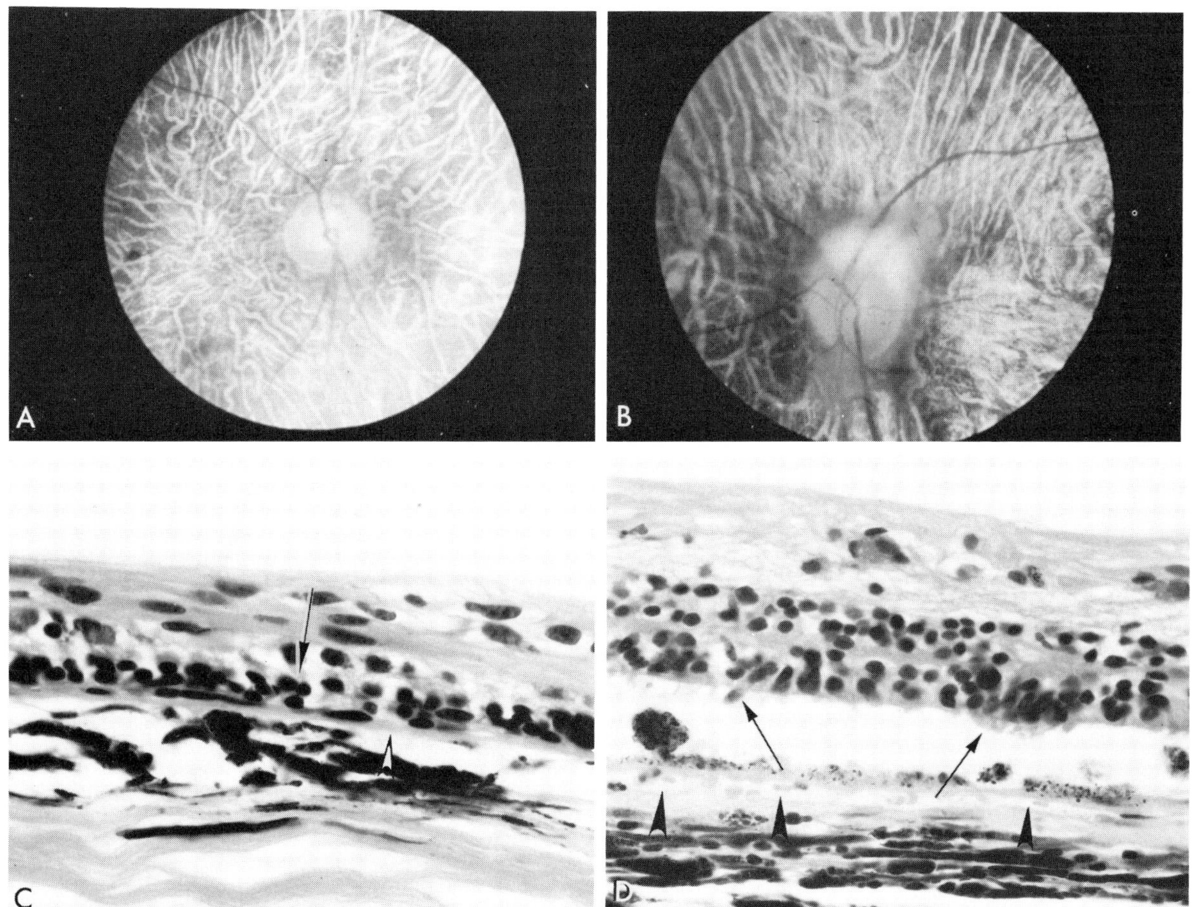

Figure 8–542. Diffuse choroidal atrophy. *A,* right eye. *B,* left eye. *C,* Typical area showing loss of retinal pigment epithelium (RPE) and outer retinal layers. Remaining inner nuclear layer (arrow) rests against Bruch's membrane (arrowhead). Choroidal vessels are not present, but melanocytes are. H and E, ×700. *D,* Area of less intense changes shows an intact choriocapillaris (arrowheads), an intact but hypopigmented RPE, and loss of outer segments of photoreceptors. A few stubby inner segments (arrows) remain. Outer nuclear layer is slightly thinned. H and E, ×600. EP 33283.

(From Green WR: Pathology of the retina, *in* Frayer WC (ed): Lancaster Course in Ophthalmic Histopathology. Unit 9. Philadelphia, F.A. Davis, 1981.)

loss of choroidal vasculature, and in other areas it was partially absent or relatively normal in appearance.

Diffuse Choroidal Atrophy with Total Vascular Atrophy

There are two well-established and recognized hereditary conditions in this category—gyrate atrophy and choroideremia.

Gyrate Atrophy. This condition is usually inherited as an autosomal recessive trait. The changes typically start in the midperiphery and extend anteriorly and posteriorly. An autosomal dominant form may have great variability in the degree of involvement. The disorder usually becomes evident between the ages of 20 and 30 years but may be detected as early as 6 years of age. Night blindness is a frequent complaint. A ring scotoma is present early. Sharply circumscribed areas of fundus atrophy with scalloped margins enlarge, become confluent, and extend anteriorly and posteriorly. The macula is usually spared until very late. The retinal vessels become markedly attenuated. Optic atrophy may ensue.

Of particular interest is the discovery by Simell and Takki (1973) of the association of hyperornithinemia with gyrate atrophy. Indeed, an ornithine loading test allows detection of heterozygous individuals with no ocular abnormalities (Takki, Simell, 1974). An extensive clinical and biochemical investigation of a 28 year old man with gyrate atrophy showed evidence of a systemic multiorgan disorder (McCulloch, Marliss, 1975). Clinical examination of the patient disclosed no abnormalities other than gyrate atrophy, visual loss and cataractous changes. The patient was hyperuremic and had an abnormal electroencephalogram. Biochemical indices of liver, renal, and muscle function were normal. Serum obtained by catheterization of an artery, the hepatic vein, a renal vein, and a deep forearm vein disclosed all these circulatory beds to be carrying ornithine. Cerebrospinal fluid and urine contained increased amounts of ornithine. Electromyography was normal, but electron microscopic study of a muscle biopsy disclosed large aggregates of a curious tubular structure.

Recently Kaiser-Kupfer, Valle, and Del Valle (1978) demonstrated the absence of ornithine aminotransferase in phytohemagglutinin-stimulated lymphocytes from a patient with gyrate atrophy. The level of enzyme activity was measured as 44 per cent of control activity in an obligate heterozygote. In other patients the level of hyperornithemia was less, and therapy with vitamin B_6 resulted in a 26 per cent reduction in plasma ornithine (Kaiser-Kupfer, Valle, Bron, 1980). Studies of additional pedigrees of patients with gyrate atrophy, however, have shown no hyperornithemia (Jaeger, Kettler, Lutz, Hilsdorf, 1979).

A symposium on this topic that included studies of dietary restructions and experimental studies was held at the 85th annual meeting of the American Academy of Ophthalmology, Chicago, November, 1980 (Ophthalmology *88*:291–336, 1981).

Choroideremia (Progressive Tapetochoroidal Dystrophy, Progessive Chorioretinal Degeneration). Choroideremia is transmitted as an X-linked recessive trait. Affected males with cho-

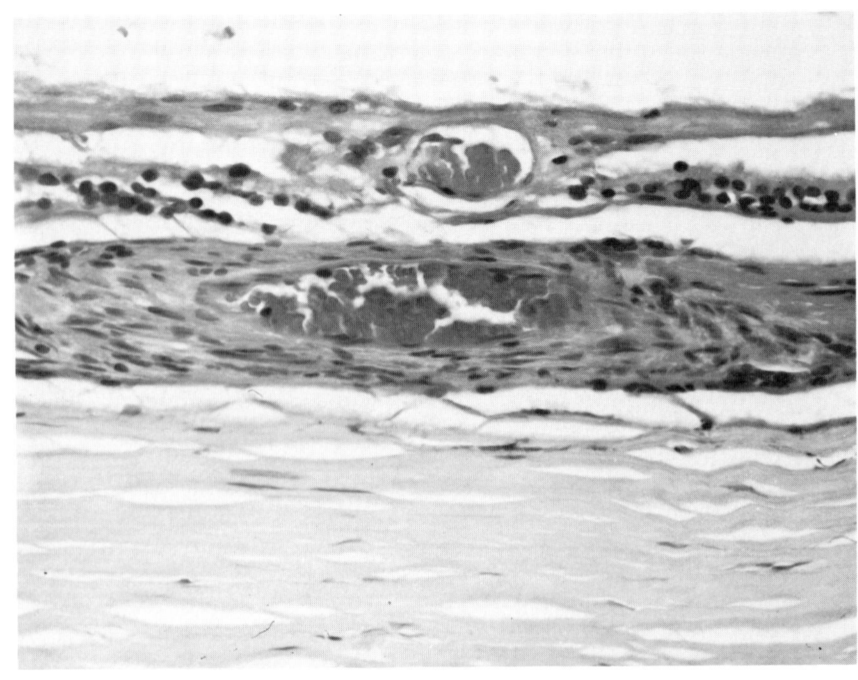

Figure 8–543. Choroideremia. Area where a single choroidal artery remains. Retinal pigment epithelium and outer retinal layers are intact, and inner nuclear layer rests against Bruch's membrane. H and E, × 330.

roideremia usually will have symptoms of night blindness within the first decade. Early changes are seen in the equatorial and paramacular areas and consist of RPE stippling and atrophy. With loss of the RPE, the choroidal vessels are at first very prominent but eventually disappear. The macula is generally spared until about age 30 years.

Some affected men in choroideremia pedigrees lose only choriocapillaries and RPE, with persistence of the larger choroidal vessels. Other men may show choriocapillaris atrophy only in one area and total choroidal vascular atrophy elsewhere. Krill and Archer (1971) note that this limited condition in men sometimes may be labeled as X-linked choroidal sclerosis, and they believe that X-linked choroidal sclerosis and choroideremia are the same condition.

Histopathologic studies (McCulloch, 1950; Rafuse, McCulloch, 1968) have revealed extensive choroidal atrophy. Minor choroidal remnants were located at the macula and near the ora serrata (Fig. 8–543).

The female carrier state usually can be detected by ophthalmologic changes, including midperipheral minor hyperplasia and migration of pigment into the deeper retinal layers; focal RPE atrophy; and peripheral radial pigment clumping. The condition is nonprogressive in women, but occasionally mild visual disturbances have been noted.

Chorioretinopathy and Pituitary Dysfunction (CPD Syndrome)

Diffuse chorioretinal degeneration in the posterior region of the eye has been described in association with trichosis and pituitary dysfunction (Oliver, McFarlane, 1965; Judisch, Lowry, Hansen, McGillivary, 1981).

SELECTED ASPECTS OF THE PATHOLOGY OF THE RETINAL PIGMENT EPITHELIUM (RPE)

The RPE is a most remarkable tissue, and it accounts in part for the ophthalmoscopic appearance of many lesions. This tissue is a single layer of hexagonal-shaped and low cuboidal epithelium. Its basement membrane forms the inner layer of Bruch's membrane, and its villous processes at the apex of the cell envelop the outer segments of the photoreceptor cells. It is a most reactive tissue, responding to various lesions either by undergoing atrophy or by hypertrophy, hyperplasia, and migration into the retina or combinations of those two processes. At about the fifth week of gestation, the primary optic vesicle invaginates to form the optic cup. The RPE is derived from the outer layer of the optic cup, which also gives rise to the pigmented ciliary epithelium and the muscles of the iris. It is the first tissue of the body to become pigmented (about the tenth week of gestation). The inner layer of the optic cup gives rise to the retina, nonpigmented ciliary epithelium, and the iris pigment epithelium.

The RPE has a high metabolic rate and is closely associated metabolically with the photoreceptor cells.

Zinn and Marmor (1979) have described the structure, function, pathophysiology, and diseases of the retinal pigment epithelium.

Hypertrophy of the Retinal Pigment Epithelium. Hypertrophic RPE cells are somewhat larger than normal and have larger spherical melanin pigment granules instead of the normal smaller, lancet- or cigar-shaped melanin granules. This change in the pigment granules gives the RPE a much darker, even black appearance. Hypertrophy of the RPE may be congenital or acquired and can have various patterns.

Congenital RPE Hypertrophy (Grouped Pigmentation, Bear Tracks). This congenital pigmentary disturbance of the RPE is nearly always unilateral, but bilateral cases have been observed. The condition is almost completely stationary, with no progression over a period of years. These lesions are discrete, dark spots that are jet-black, gray-black, or somewhat paler, and they are most often round, oval, or kidney-shaped. They have sharply defined edges, and the intervening retina is normal. Their size varies from 0.1 to 1 disk diameter or more. The largest spots are found at the periphery of the fundus and the smaller ones closer to the disc. The condition may be characterized by as few as 2 spots and up to 30, but most often there are about 4 to 10. Most often they involve only one sector of the retina, usually upper temporal or lower temporal. Occasional patients with widespread lesions have been reported.

Histopathologic studies (Shields, Tso, 1975) disclosed focal areas of increased concentrations of large oval pigment granules and taller (but otherwise normal) RPE cells (Fig. 8–544). The overlying photoreceptors showed no abnormalities.

Blair and Trempe (1980) described congenital hypertrophy of the RPE in three affected members of a kindred with Gardner's syndrome (intestinal polyps and hard and soft tissue abnormalities).

Acquired Retinal Pigment Epithelial Hypertrophy. This is a common change that is seen as a solitary lesion in the retinal periphery or peripapillary area, and it is associated with a variety of choroidal lesions.

SOLITARY HYPERTROPHY OF THE RPE. This change is usually several millimeters in diameter and may be as large as 10 millimeters. The lesion

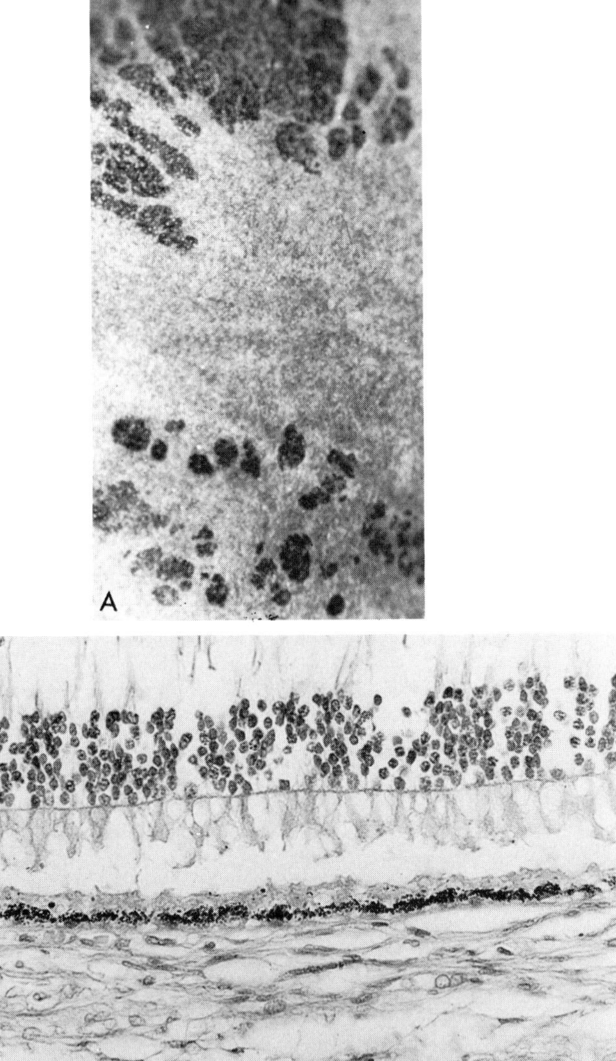

Figure 8–544. Congenital hypertrophy of retinal pigment epithelium (RPE) (grouped pigmentation). *A*, Gross appearance showing multiple, discrete, darkly pigmented areas arranged in an "animal track" configuration. AFIP Neg. 74-9230-4. *B*, Section through a normal area of RPE and retina. Compare with *C*. H and E, ×640. AFIP Neg. 74-9230-2.

Illustration continued on opposite page

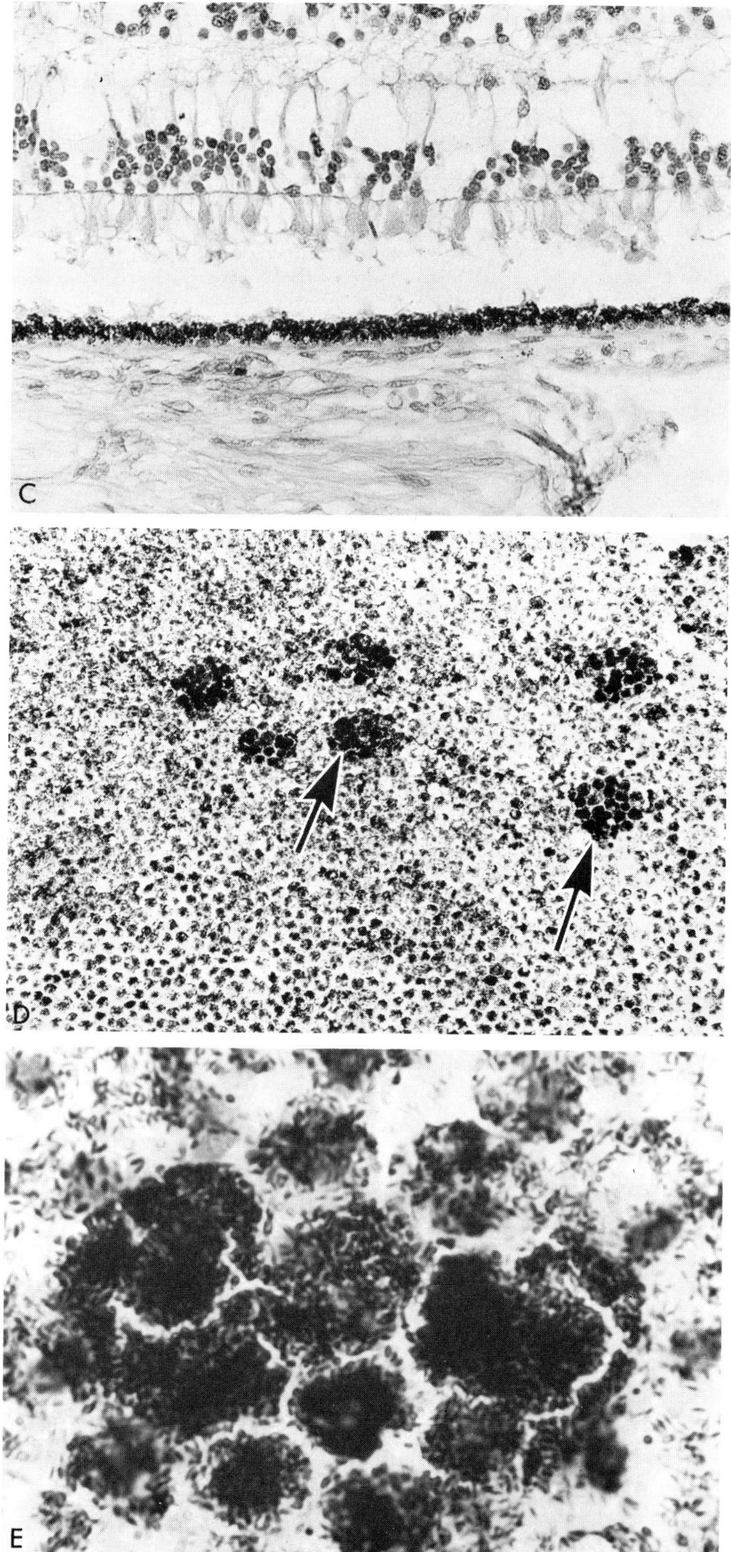

Figure 8–544 *Continued* Section through RPE lesions shows a greater concentration of pigment granules in RPE cells, H and E, ×640. AFIP Neg. 74-9230-3. *D*, Flat preparation of RPE, showing greater concentration of pigment granules in cells of grouped pigmentation (arrows). H and E, ×256. AFIP Neg. 74-9230-1. *E*, Oil immersion photomicrograph of RPE cells, showing large, oval pigment granules, H and E, ×640. AFIP Neg. 74-9230-5.

(From Shields JA, Tso MOM: Congenital grouped pigmentation of retina: Histopathologic description and report of a case. Arch Ophthalmol *93*:1153–1155, 1975.)

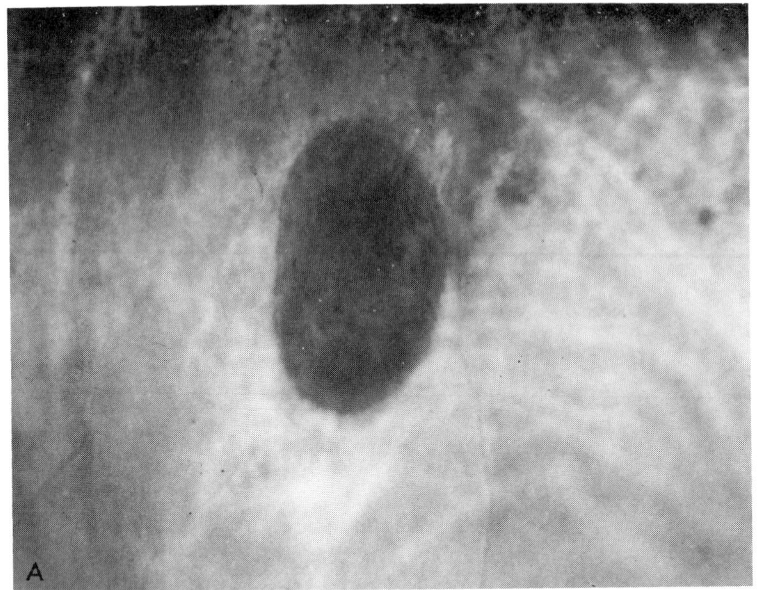

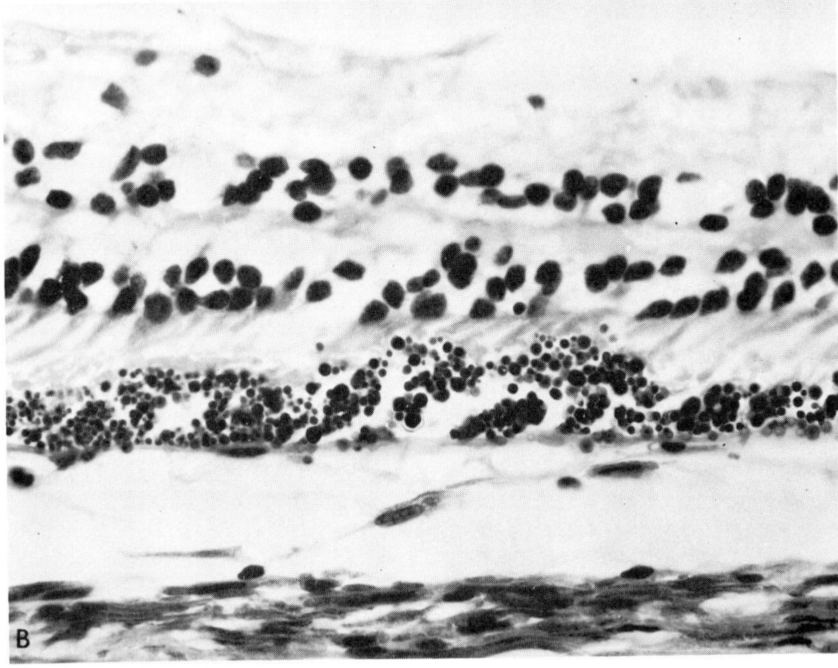

Figure 8–545. *A*, Gross appearance of discrete oval area of **retinal pigment epithalium (RPE hypertropy** in periphery. There is no central lacunar and peripheral zone of depigmentation. *B*, RPE cells are enlarged and contain many large, spherical pigment granules. Partial bleach; H and E ×650.) EP 45870.

may have characteristic central lacunae of depigmentation and a peripheral zone of less dense pigmentation. The lesions otherwise are dark or jet-black and flat (Fig. 8–545; see also Fig. 8–250).

Histopathologic studies (Kurz, Zimmerman, 1962) disclosed a focal area in the RPE in which the pigment epithelial cells are enlarged and densely packed with large spherical melanin granules, completely obscuring the nuclei (Fig. 8–546). Central lacunar areas of depigmentation are due to RPE atrophy. The overlying retina most often shows some degeneration of the photoreceptor cells and nuclei in the outer nuclear layer. Some histiocytes containing melanin granules may be found in the degenerated rod and cone area. These retinal changes may be seen in areas over intact hypertrophic RPE but are especially evident over areas of lacunar depigmentation.

In rare instances, the release of pigment by these hypertrophic cells may be striking, with migration of free pigment and pigmented macrophages into the retina (Fig. 8–547) and vitreous (Duke, Maumenee, 1959). In the area of the halo that surrounds some of these lesions, the cells are not as heavily pigmented.

Buettner (1975) also has described thickening of Bruch's membrane, granular and slightly periodic acid–Schiff–positive material in the area of photoreceptor cell degeneration, and a normal

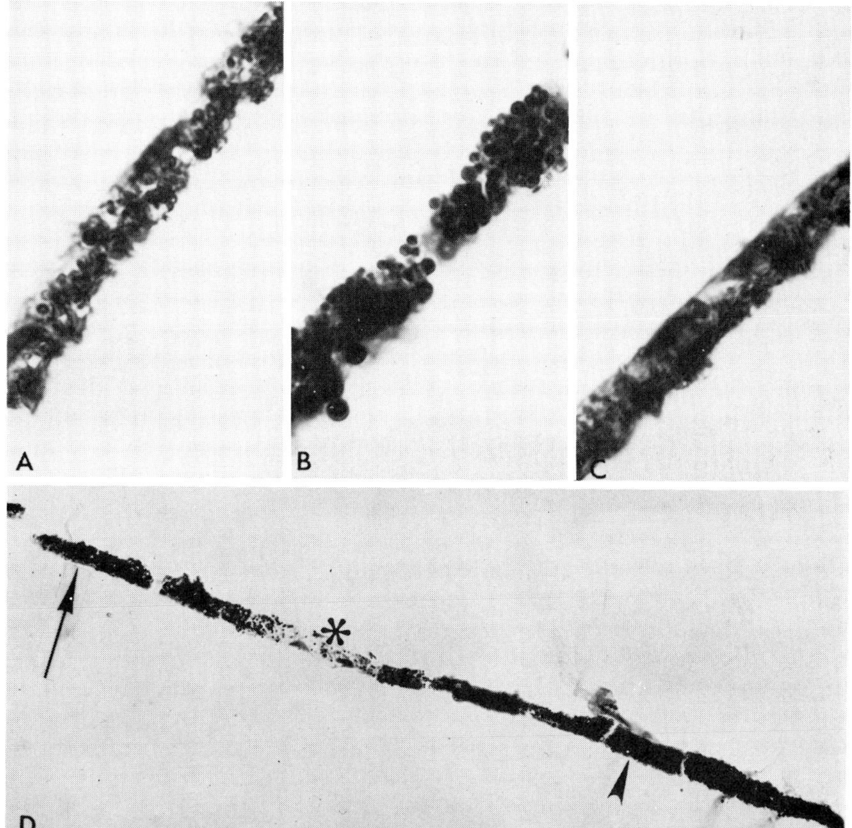

Figure 8–546. Retinal pigment epithelium (RPE) hypertrophy. *A*, Normal-appearing RPE anterior to lesion. H and E, × 990. AFIP Neg. 61–3087. *B*, Area of hypertrophy showing RPE cells to be slightly enlarged and contain large spherical pigment granules. H and E, ×990. AFIP Neg, 61–3087. *C*, Normal-appearing RPE posterior to lesion. H and E, ×990. AFIP Neg. 61–3086. *D*, Peripheral hypopigmented zone (asterisk) between hypertrophic RPE (arrowhead) and normal RPE (arrow). H and E, ×305. AFIP Neg. 61–6091.
(From Kurz, GH, Zimmerman, LE: Vagaries of retinal pigment epithelium. Intl Ophthalmol Clin 2:441–464, 1962.)

choriocapillaris. By light and electron microscopic study, he described the thickening of Bruch's membrane resulting from basement membrane elaborations by the RPE (Fig. 8–548).

Although this lesion has characteristic flat and nonprogressive features, in the past it has been confused with malignant melanoma, resulting in needless enucleation (Ferry, 1964; Shields, Zimmerman, 1973; Duke, Maumenee, 1959; Reese, Jones, 1956). Norris and Cleasby (1976) provided photographic documentation of enlargement of a solitary lesion of RPE hypertrophy in a 42 year old woman.

It is quite possible that this characteristic solitary form of RPE hypertrophy may be congenital, but observation of the lesion in an infant or young child has not been reported. In one series of ten cases, the youngest patients were 10 and 14 years (Buettner, 1975). In a clinical study of 52 patients with solitary RPE hypertrophy, Purcell and Shields (1975) reported an age range of 14 to 86 years and a mean age of 51 years.

Visual field defects were rarely demonstrated using standard clinical techniques (Purcell, Shields, 1975). Buettner (1975), using the Tübinger perimeter, demonstrated visual field defects corresponding to the location and size of the clinical lesion in all patients examined by this technique.

Miscellaneous Forms of RPE Hypertrophy. It is common in older adults to find a band of hyperpigmentation just posterior to the ora serrata that is due to hypertrophy (see Figs. 8–251, 8–252, and 8–263). This change in the RPE may precede the development of pavingstone degeneration.

A darkly pigmented crescent in the peripapillary area is a common finding and is caused by RPE hypertrophy. Figures 8–257 and 8–351 illustrate such a change associated with a vascularized druse.

Hypertrophy of the RPE is commonly seen in association with choroidal lesions, the margins of pavingstone degeneration, choroidal infarcts (see Figs. 8–91,*D*, 8–93, 8–272, 8–273, 8–275, and 8–276), and the various conditions in the choroidal sclerosis group of disease (Fig. 8–540). It may occur in a spotty configuration over sub-RPE neovascularization, serous RPE detachments, and disciform lesions and is frequently associated with vascularized (see Figs. 8–253, 8–254, 8–257, and 8–351 through 8–353) and nonvascularized drusen (see Figs. 8–255, 8–256, 8–342 through 8–344, and 8–347). Other examples of hypertrophy of the RPE are illustrated in Figures 8–170, 8–173, 8–250, 8–258, 8–270, 8–404, 8–421, 8–429, 8–519, 8–521, 8–531, and 8–532.

Hyperplasia of Retinal Pigment Epithelium. Hyperplastic RPE also has a dark appearance, because there is also hypertrophy (large, spherical pigment granules). Although hyperplastic RPE is sometimes localized only under the ret-

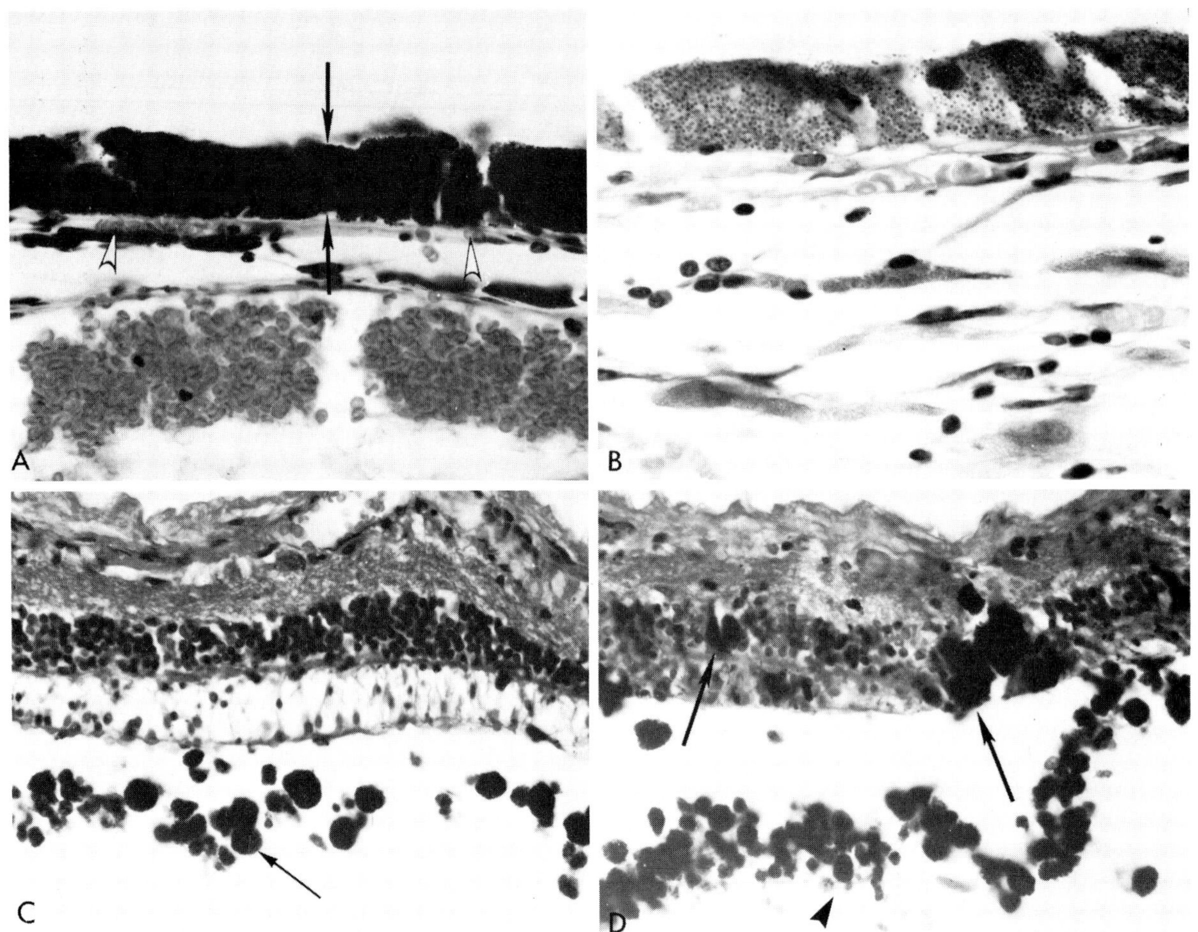

Figure 8–547. Hypertrophy of retinal pigment epithelium (RPE) that was suspected of being a malignant melanoma in a 39 year old man. *A*, Very tall RPE (between arrows) packed with melanin pigment; choriocapillaris (arrowheads) is intact. Unbleached; H and E, ×530. *B*, Hypertrophic RPE with large spherical pigment granules. Partial bleach; H and E, ×530. *C*, Area of RPE hypertrophy, with pigmented cells (arrow) in subretinal space and loss of photoreceptors and outer nuclear layer. H and E, ×330. *D*, Different area showing photoreceptor cell loss, and pigmented cells in subretinal space (arrowhead) and in retina (arrows). H and E, ×530.

EP 17656. (From Duke JR, Maumenee AR: An unusual tumor of retinal pigment epithelium in an eye with early open-angle glaucoma. Am J Ophthalmol *47*:311–317, 1959.)

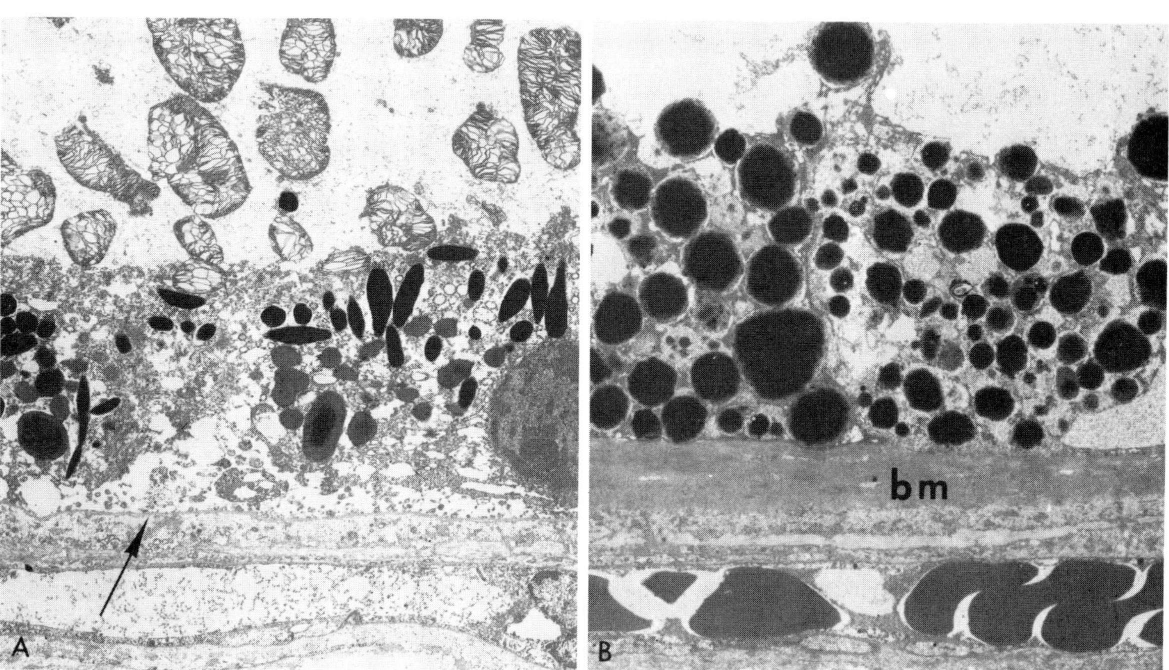

Figure 8–548. Comparison of normal and hypertrophic retinal pigment epithelium (RPE) in same eye. *A*, Normal RPE with thin, delicate basement membrane (arrow) and lancet-shaped melanin pigment granules located adjacent to area of RPE hypertrophy, ×6600. *B*, Area of RPE hypertrophy showing RPE cells that are slightly larger, contain large, spherical pigment granules, and have a very thick basement membrane *(bm)*. Choriocapillaris is intact. ×6600. (From Buettner, H: Congenital hypertrophy of retinal pigment epithelium. Am J Ophthalmol *79*:177–189, 1975.)

ina, the most reliable ophthalmoscopic feature of hyperplasia is migration into the retina, characteristically in a perivascular location. This location gives the lesion a spiculate appearance by ophthalmoscopy. Regardless of the site of RPE hyperplasia, the proliferated cells have a distinct tendency to maintain polarity in a tubuloacinar or layered configuration.

Hyperplasia of the RPE may be observed as a localized or as a diffuse process.

Localized RPE Hyperplasia. Localized hyperplastic RPE may occur unassociated with any abnormality (see Fig. 8–265). It is often observed in association with healed chorioretinal scars (see Figs. 8–161, 8–173, 8–263, 8–264, 8–265, 8–278, 8–279, and 8–411) from toxoplasmosis, cytomegalovirus retinitis, histoplasmosis, syphilis, and other diseases. Such hyperplasia often prompts the examiner to notice areas of lattice degeneration (see Figs. 8–283, 8–287, 8–289, 8–290, and 8–294). Only 9 per cent of lattice lesions have the typical lattice wicker configuration. The remaining lesions appear as retinal thinning and may well have a pigmented appearance because of RPE hypertrophy, hyperplasia, and migration into the retina.

Hyperplasia of the RPE may be a conspicuous component of the disciform lesions of senile macular degeneration (see Figs. 8–371, 8–376, 8–377, 8–378, and 8–380), angioid streaks, and ocular histoplasmosis. In the past, such hyperplasia has led to needless enucleation because of confusion with malignant melanoma, as shown in Figure 8–380, a patient from Ferry's study (1964). Hyperplasia of the RPE also may be observed in the areolar form of senile macular degeneration and migrate onto the inner surface of the retina (Fig. 8–549).

Nodular disciform lesions under the macular retina in association with Coats' disease and angiomatosis are in part derived from hyperplasia of the RPE (see Figs. 8–42 and 8–43).

Traumatic retinopathy is characterized by either localized or, more commonly, diffuse hyperplasia

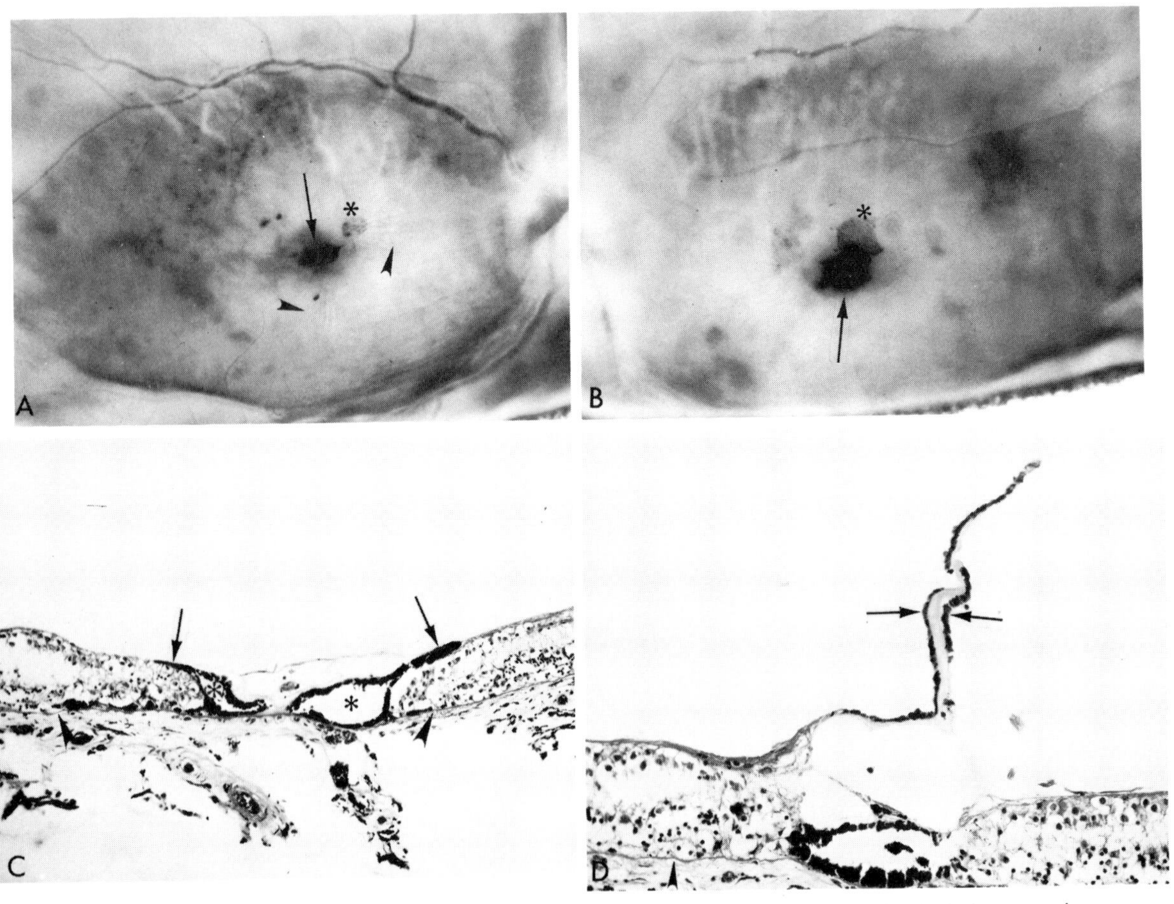

Figure 8–549. Areolar form of senile macular degeneration, with hyperplasia of retinal pigment epithelium (RPE) and migration into retina, inner surface of retina, and vitreous. Intraretinal (arrow) and preretinal (asterisk) hyperplasia of RPE in *A*, right and *B*, left eye. Wrinkling of internal limiting membrane (arrowheads) is present. *C*, RPE and photoreceptor cells are atrophic (arrowheads). Centrally, there are two cystic areas, lined by hyperplastic RPE (asterisks). RPE also extends onto inner surface of retina (arrows). H and E, ×100. *D*, Different area shows hyperplastic RPE (arrows) extending on both sides of a vitreous strand. RPE and photoreceptor cells are absent (arrowhead). H and E, ×220. EP 48647.

and migration of the RPE into the retina in perivascular locations (see Figs. 8–202, 8–205, 8–208, 8–266, and 8–267).

One of the most characteristic of the hyperplastic RPE lesions is the "black sunburst" sign of sickle cell retinopathy (see Figs. 8–262 and 8–460 through 8–462). Its pigmented, spiculate appearance is due to hyperplastic RPE that has migrated into the retina in a perivascular location.

Other examples of localized hyperplasia of the RPE include those associated with Fuch's dot (see Fig. 8–333) and lacquer cracks in myopia, some angioid streaks, ringschwiele (seen at the ora serrata in association with chronic retinal detachment and cyclitic membrane), Verhoeff streaks in choroidal detachment, subsiding uveal effusion, and Siegriest streaks (see Fig. 8–429) of hypertension and arteriosclerosis.

Vitreous traction can produce RPE hyperplasia as a localized lesion or along the vitreous base, as previously illustrated in Figures 8–259 and 8–260.

RPE hyperplasia may occur in the valleys between large, partially confluent serous detachments of the RPE in senile macular degeneration. These proliferative changes account in part for the so-called "hot cross bun" sign.

With long-standing retinal detachment, the extent of the detachment may be delineated by one or more demarcation lines. These generally represent sites of chorioretinal adhesion and often have hyperplastic RPE as a component (see Fig. 8–307,*A*). Additional conditions with associated localized RPE hyperplasia include persistent hyperplastic primary vitreous (see Fig. 8–264), choroidal infarction (see Fig. 8–91,*D*), vascular hamartoma of optic nerve head and peripapillary retina (see Figs. 8–552 through 8–554), macular holes (see Fig. 8–397), and experimental light toxicity (Fig. 8–218).

Diffuse Hyperplasia of the RPE. This change is a characteristic feature of retinitis pigmentosa (see Fig. 8–535) and the 35 or more conditions in which a retinitis pigmentosa–like picture may be associated (see Figs. 8–473, 8–519, 8–521, 8–522, 8–527,*F* and *K*, and 8–532,*C* and Table 8–6). The histopathologic picture of primary retinitis pigmentosa is quite similar to that seen in traumatic retinopathy (see Figs. 8–161, 8–202, 8–266, and 8–267). Other examples of diffuse hyperplasia of RPE include those associated with leukemia (see Fig. 8–445) and experimental rhodopsin sensitization (see Fig. 8–199,*D*).

Periretinal RPE hyperplasia has become recognized as an important complication of retinal detachment after it was noted by Machemer (Machemer, Laqua, 1975; Machemer, Van Horn, Aaberg, 1978). In an experimental retinal detachment model in the monkey, Machemer and Laqua (1975) found the RPE cell to be the main source of proliferating cells on both surfaces of the retina. Those workers proposed that this proliferative change be called massive periretinal proliferation (MPP). Figures 8–130 through 8–133 illustrate preretinal RPE proliferation, and Figures 8–141 through 8–145, and 8–427, retroretinal.

Associated Changes of RPE Hyperplasia. Hyperplasia of the RPE may occur in a tubuloacinar-like pattern that gives an adenomatous appearance. Such proliferations are called pseudoadenomatous RPE hyperplasia (see Fig. 8–265).

Hyperplastic RPE may proliferate in a laminated pattern of alternating double rows, with apices of the cells in juxtaposition with basement membrane on both sides at the bases of the cells (see Figs. 8–263 and 8–264).

Hyperplasia of the RPE can reach such size as to be confused with a tumor (Stow, 1949; Spiers, Jensen, 1963; Green, 1967; Tso, Albert, 1972).

Retinal pigment is also an apparent source of fibrous tissue, as in some disciform lesions. Collagen production by chick embryo RPE has been demonstrated in tissue culture (Newsome, Kenyon, 1973).

Hyperplastic RPE is thought to be the possible source of osseous tissue in the eye in phthisical eyes. The only evidence for this is the frequent location of bone along the inner aspect of Bruch's membrane.

Lipofuscin from the RPE is the origin of the yellow-orange color seen over choroidal lesions that chronically encroach upon the choriocapillaris (Fig. 8–550).

Partial or Complete Loss of Pigment Granules in Intact RPE. This is observed in peripheral albinotic spots (see Figs. 8–281 and 8–282), some RPE window defects (see Fig. 8–381,*C*), various forms of albinism (see Fig. 8–20), the Chediak-Higashi syndrome (see Fig. 8–503), over some drusen, and in rubella retinopathy (see Fig. 8–170). Also see Figures 8–421, 8–445,*C*, 8–446, 8–520, and 8–528.

The fluorescein angiographic features observed with partial or complete loss of pigment from localized areas of the RPE are characteristic and have been referred to as a "window defect." The lesion lights up early but does not stain or leak.

Clinicopathologic correlation of a discrete area of RPE window defect showed the RPE to be intact, but it had fewer melanin granules than did the surrounding area (Keno, Green, 1978). The RPE cells in the involved area were reduced in number, flatter, slightly elongated, and arranged more nearly parallel to Bruch's membrane. There were loss and thinning of the outer segments of photoreceptor cells and thinning of the inner segments and outer nuclear layer in the area of involvement. The subjacent choriocapillaris was intact (Fig. 8–551). This type of change may lead eventually to areas of total loss of the RPE and

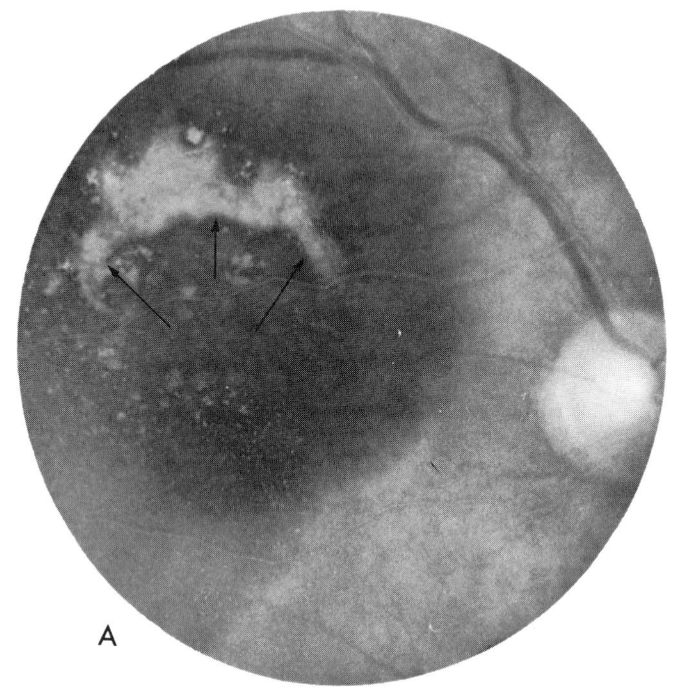

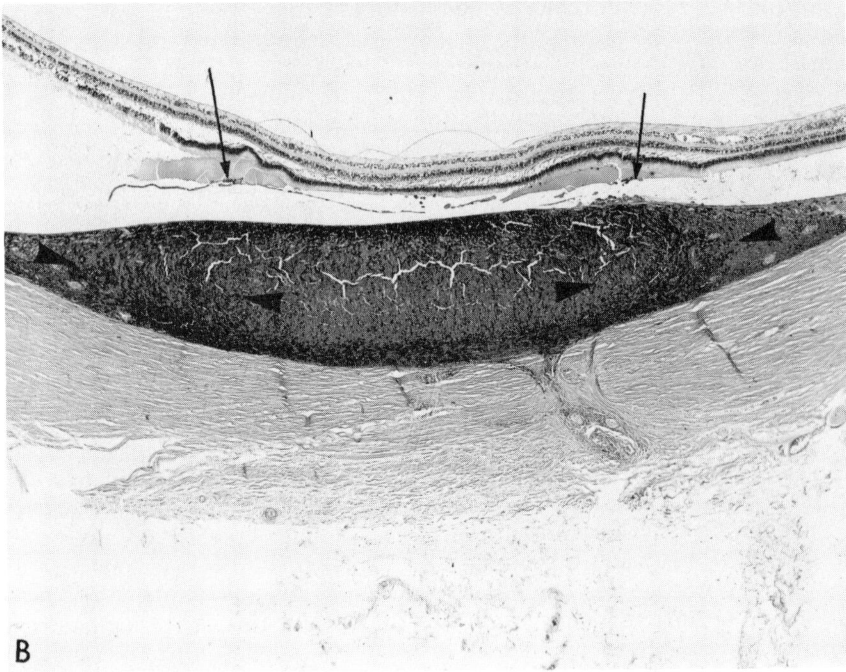

Figure 8–550. *A*, Appearance of **pigmented tumor** above macula of right eye. Yellow-orange pigment crescent is present over upper half of lesion (arrows). *B*, Section at level of lower poles of crescent-shaped yellow-orange pigment (arrows). The pigment is due to aggregates of cells with cytoplasm distended by lipofuscin granules. Retinal pigment epithelium overlying tumor is intact. H and E, ×21.

Illustration continued on opposite page

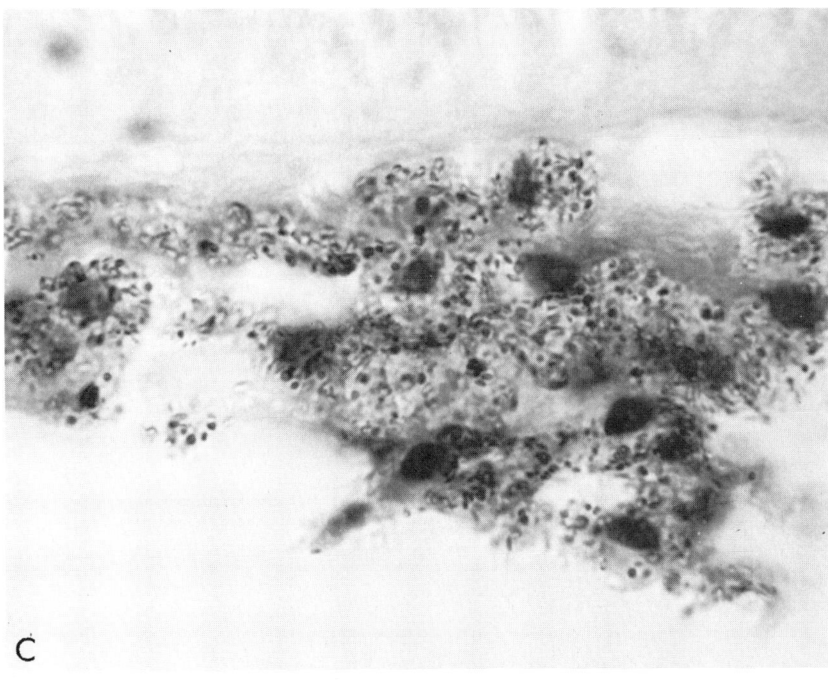

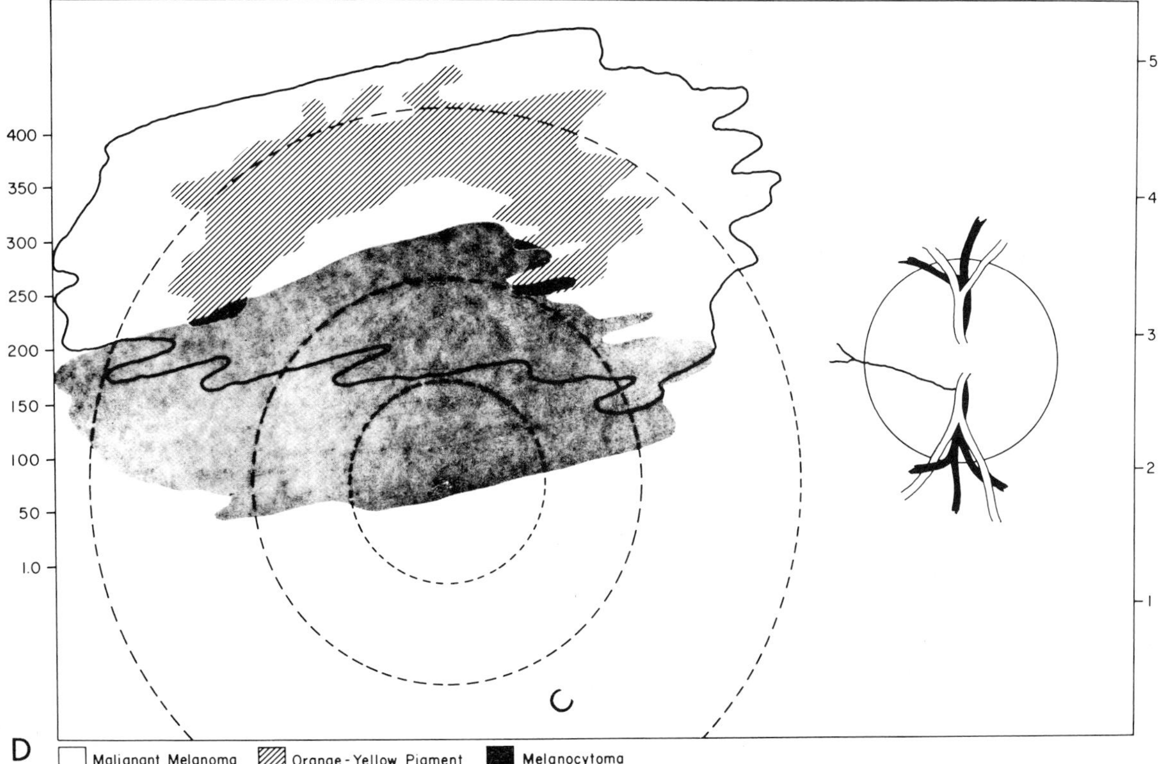

Figure 8–550. *Continued C,* Higher power view of one area of yellow-orange pigment (serial section 290) shows aggregate of cells in subretinal space. These contain abundant pigment, which fluoresced in fluorescent light. H and E, ×1200. *D,* Two-dimensional reconstruction of tumor from serial sections. Large area of melanocytoma in foveal region, with malignant melanoma in upper half and yellow-orange pigment crescent.

EP 15887. (From Barker-Griffith AE, McDonald PR, Green WR: Malignant melanoma arising in a choroidal magnacellular nevus (melanocytoma). Can J Ophthalmol *11*:140–146, 1976.)

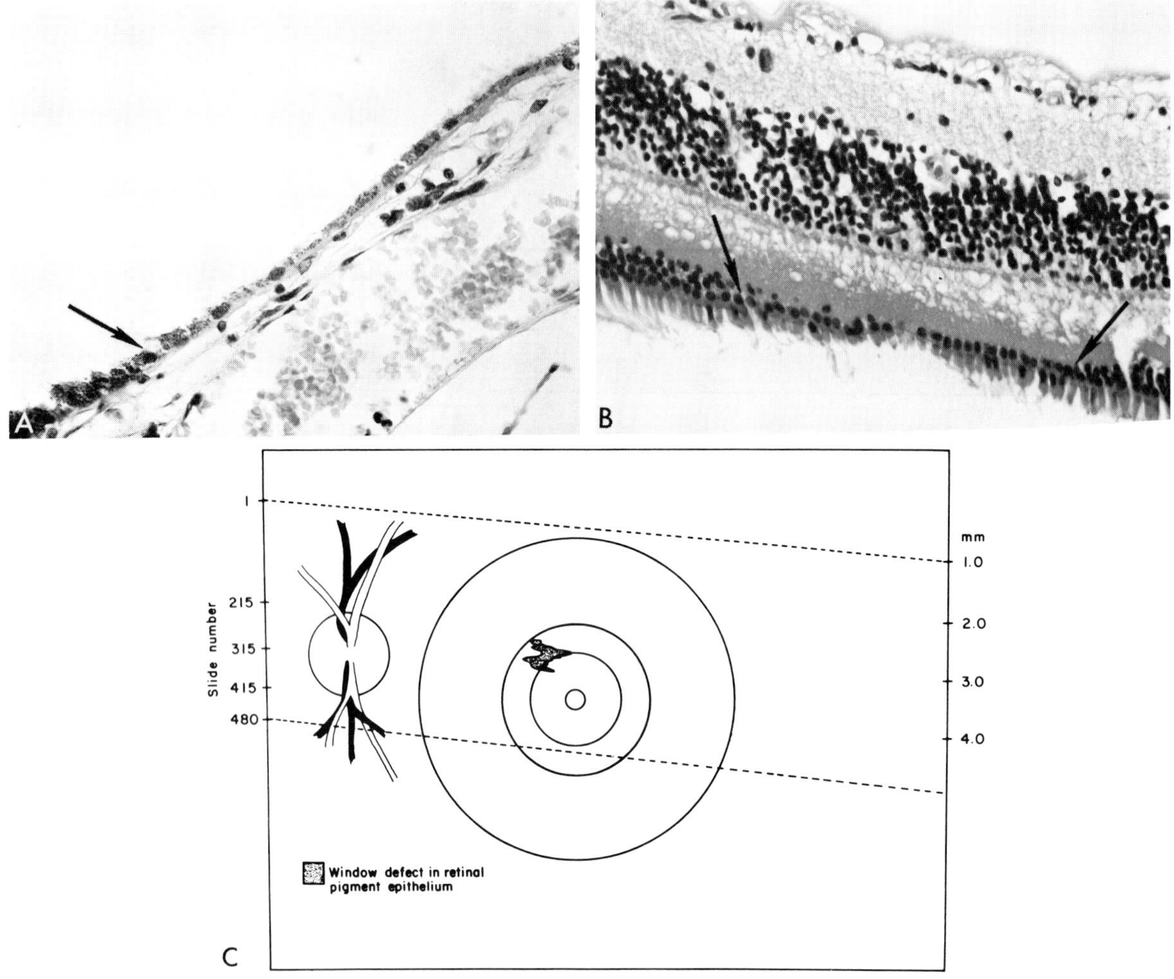

Figure 8–551. Retinal pigment epithelium (RPE) "window defect". *A*, Area near center of RPE window defect, showing flattening of epithelium, reduced number of epithelial nuclei, and partial loss of pigment granules. Arrow marks junction between relatively normal RPE (to left) and RPE window defect (to right). Bleached with potassium permanganate for 5 minutes; H and E, ×260. *B*, Area of artifactitiously detached retina corresponding to zone of RPE window defect. There is thinning of the outer nuclear layer (between arrows) and inner segments, and loss of outer segments of photorecepter cells. H and E, ×260. *C*, Two-dimensional reconstruction map from study of serial sections shows size, shape, and location of RPE defect. EP 37436. (From Keno DD, Green WR: Retinal pigment epithelial window defect. Arch Ophthalmol, *96*:854–856, 1978.)

the picture of areolar atrophy, as seen in many cases of senile macular degeneration.

Giant Pigment Granules in RPE. Conditions in which giant pigment granules are present in RPE include congenital and acquired hypertrophy (see pages 1227 to 1231), ocular and oculocutaneous albinism (see Fig. 8–22), and the Chediak-Higashi syndrome (see Fig. 8–503).

Inflammatory Lesions of the RPE. *Acute Retinal Pigment Epitheliitis* (Krill, Deutman, 1972). This condition is characterized by the development of 2 to 4 small, dark gray and sometimes black lesions at the level of the RPE in the macular area in either one or both eyes. It has not been studied histopathologically.

Acute Multifocal Placoid Pigment Epitheliopathy. This condition is characterized by a rapidly progressive, bilateral loss of central vision, caused by multifocal, yellowish-white lesions at the level of the RPE (Gass, 1968a). Other inflammatory signs may be present, and a history of a preceding virus-like illness is often elicited. Azar, Gohd, Waltman, and Gitter (1975) found the condition to be associated with an adenovirus type 5 infection in one patient. Bullock and Fletcher (1977) reported two patients with cerebrospinal fluid abnormalities. This condition is similar to Harada's disease, in which granulomatous inflammation has been observed in the choroid, with marked secondary changes in the RPE and retina.

Sigelman, Behrens, and Hilal (1979) reported a patient in whom cerebral angiography showed multiple areas of vascular narrowing compatible with vasculitis. In reviewing all 60 reported cases, those investigators found that accompanying disorders were frequent. These included papillitis, posterior uveitis, serous retinal detachment with and without vasculitis, iridocyclitis, peripheral corneal thinning, and episcleritis. Neurologic features included headache prior to or at time of onset of ocular symptoms, transient expressive aphasia with cerebral vasculitis, abnormal EEG, and CSF protein elevation and pleocytosis. Systemic manifestations included erythema multiforme and thyroiditis.

Defects in the Retinal Pigment Epithelium. Discontinuous RPE is a feature of the following: some RPE window defects, senile macular degeneration (see Figs. 8–332, 8–362, 8–363, 8–401, top, and 8–547), the choroidal atrophy (sclerosis) group of diseases (see Figs. 8–540 through 8–543), angioid streaks, and olivopontocerebellar degeneration (see Fig. 8–519). Peripheral punched-out lesions from chorioretinal scars (see Figs. 8–278 and 8–279), small choroidal infarcts (see Figs. 8–272 and 8–273), larger choroidal infarcts (Elschnig spots) (see Figs. 8–93, 8–96, and 8–274 through 8–276), pavingstone degeneration (see Figs. 8–268 through 8–271), and some drusen also have disrupted RPE.

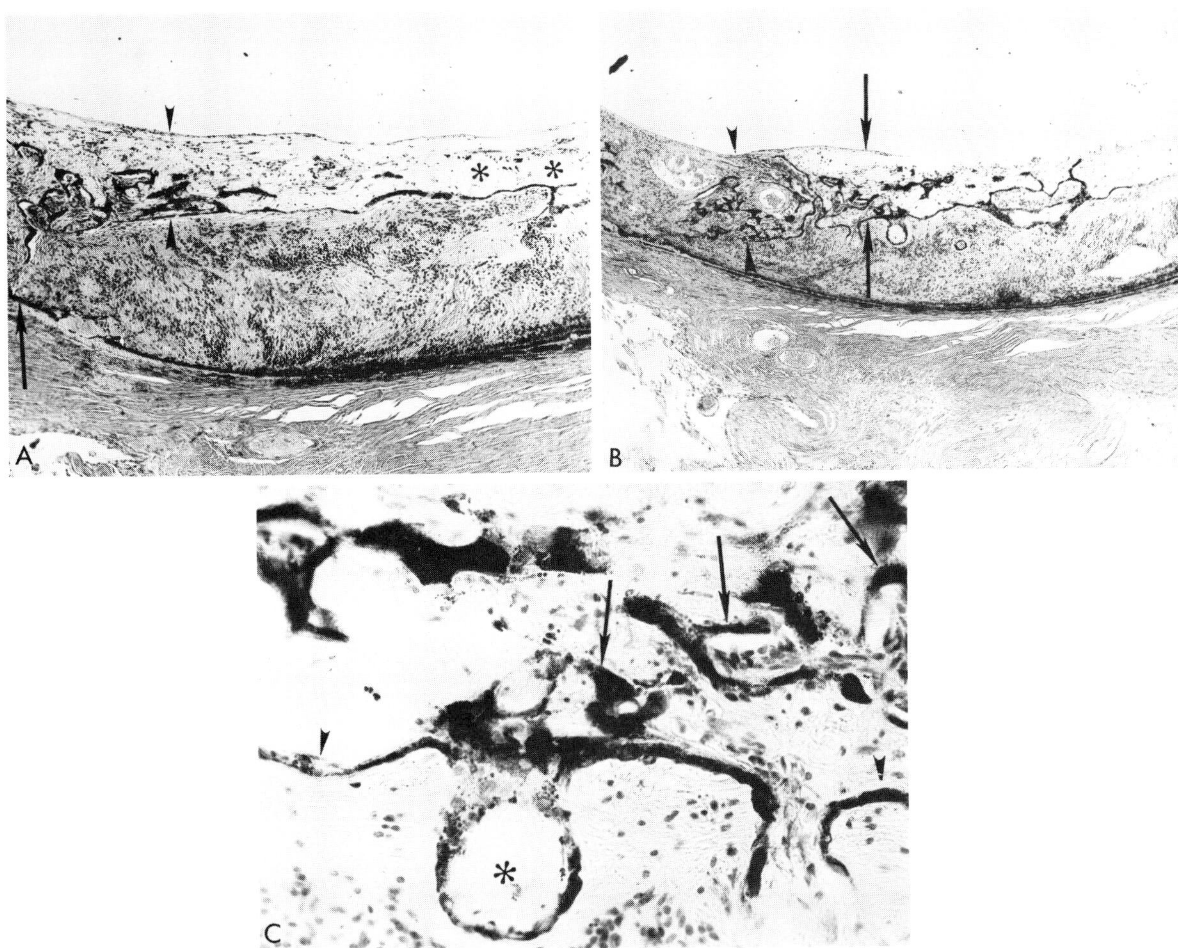

Figure 8–552. Retinal pigment epithelium (RPE) vascular hamartoma of optic nerve head. *A*, Arrow indicates margin where RPE normally terminates at temporal edge of optic nerve head. From there, RPE has migrated forward along the temporal margin of the optic nerve head and into a thick preretinal fibrovascular tissue (between arrowheads). Hyperplastic RPE extends along inner surface of retina (asterisks) and also surrounds some vessels in preretinal tissue near nerve head. H and E, ×70 AFIP Neg. 68–5969.

B, Different level, showing disorganization of retinal architecture. Hyperplastic RPE is present within retina (between arrowheads) and within extensive preretinal fibrovascular tissue (between arrows). H and E, × 45. AFIP Neg. 68–5965. *C*, Higher power view, showing hyperplastic RPE along inner surface of retina (arrowheads). At some places, RPE extends into retina and surrounds an apparently occluded vessel (asterisk). Hyperplastic RPE (arrows) surrounds vessels within preretinal fibrovascular tissue. H and E, ×265. AFIP Neg. 68–5970.

AFIP 291045. (From Vogel MH, Zimmerman LE, Gass JDM: Proliferation of juxtapapillary retinal pigment epithelium simulating malignant melanoma. Opthalmol *26*:461–481, 1969.)

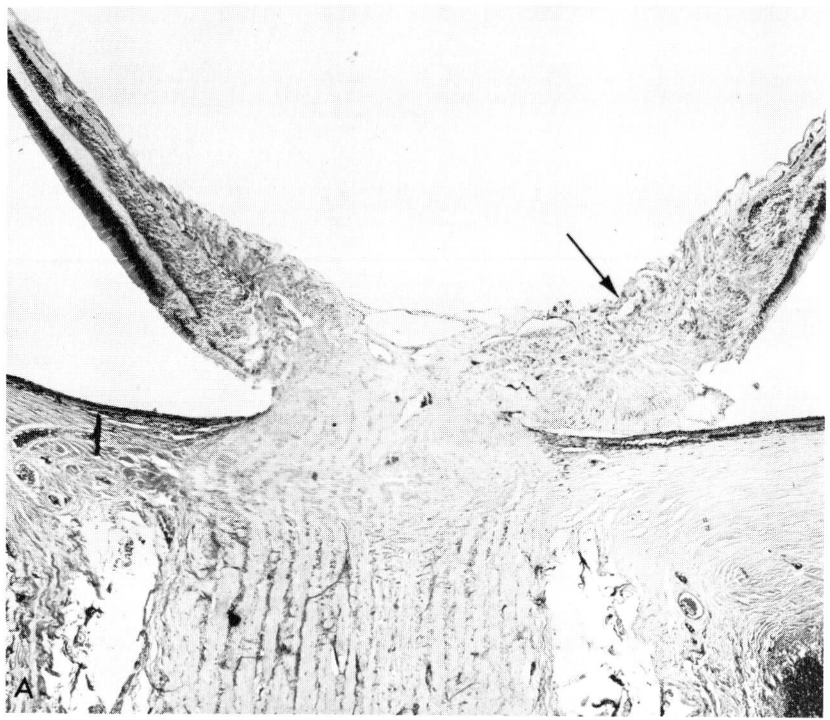

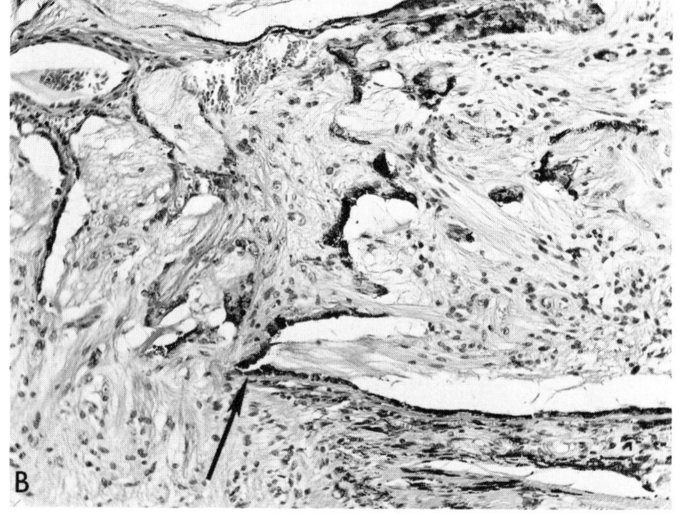

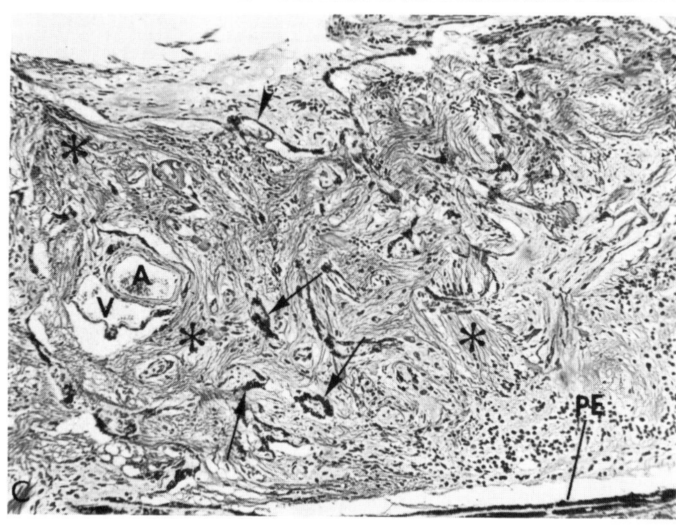

Figure 8–553. *A*, Peripapillary retina is disorganized and thickened, especially on temporal side (arrow). H and E, ×22. AFIP Neg. 68–6430. *B*, Temporal margin of optic nerve head, showing direct continuity of retinal pigment epithelium (RPE) from its normal position (arrow) into optic nerve head and peripapillary retina, Alcian blue, ×145. AFIP Neg. 68–6434.

C, Bodian stain for axis cylinders demonstrates much disorganization of nerve fiber layer. Nerve fibers (asterisks) course haphazardly in all directions. Hyperplastic RPE surrounds many small vessels (arrows) and major branches of central retinal artery *(A)* and vein *(V)*. A single layer of hyperplastic RPE (arrowhead) separates retina from a preretinal fibroglial membrane. Hyperplastic RPE in laminated pattern *(PE)* is present along the inner aspect of Bruch's membrane. Bodian stain, ×100 AFIP Neg. 67–11100.

AFIP 1127526. (From Vogel MH, Zimmerman, LE, Gass JDM: Proliferation of juxtapapillary retinal pigment epithelium simulating malignant melanoma. Doc Ophthalmol *26*:461–481, 1969.)

Other conditions in which defects in the RPE occur include malignant hypertension (see Fig. 8–427), myopia (see Figs. 8–327 through 8–332), onchocerciasis (see Fig. 8–191), disseminated intravascular coagulopathy (see Figs. 8–456 and 8–457), idiopathic thrombotic thrombocytopenia (see Fig. 8–459), Bassen-Kornzweig syndrome (see Fig. 8–499), Laurence-Moon syndrome (see Fig. 8–532), and fundus flavimaculatus (see Figs. 8–337 and 8–538).

The pinpoint RPE defect of central serous retinopathy has not been studied histopathologically.

Multiple pinpoint areas of fluorescein leakage ("Milky Way pattern") are typically seen in leukemia and metastatic carcinoma (see Figs. 8–445 and 8–446).

Detachment of the Retinal Pigment Epithelium. The various causes of RPE detachment have been discussed. One type of special interest occurs with ocular reticulum cell sarcoma. These detachments clinically may resemble multiple sites of metastatic carcinoma: small areas where necrotic and viable tumor cells collect under the RPE (see Figs. 8–450, and 8–451).

Hamartoma of the Retinal Pigment Epithelium. These lesions are characterized by a slightly elevated black or charcoal gray mass involving the retinal pigment epithelium, optic nerve head, retina, and overlying vitreous; a feathery margin; a tumor base consisting of a sheet of hyperpigmented tissue at the level of the RPE; varying amounts of thickened gray-white retinal and preretinal tissue in the tumor's inner and central portion; evidence of contraction of the tumor's inner surface, with displacement of surrounding retina and retinal blood vessels toward the tumor's center; absence of choroidal involvement, retinal detachment, exudation, hemorrhage, and inflammation; and no evidence of growth on follow-up examination (Gass, 1973a). Extension of pigment into the inner portion of the lesion may occur. The lesion may be located anywhere in the fundus but is most common in the optic nerve head and peripapillary areas.

Fluorescein angiography shows a large number of small blood vessels within the lesion. These have an aneurysmal appearance and leak dye (Gass, 1974, 1977; McLean, 1976; Schatz, Burton, Yannuzzi, Rabb, 1978; Dark, Richardson, Howe, 1978).

Histopathologic studies (Rouveda, 1952; Theobald, Floyd, Kirk, 1958; Cardell, Starbuck, 1961; Machemer, 1964; Vogel, Zimmerman, Gass, 1969; Vogel, Wessing, 1972; Laqua, Wessing, 1979) have shown rather consistent findings. There is thickening of the optic nerve head and peripapillary retina by an increased vasculature and hyperplastic RPE. The RPE has a tendency to surround blood vessels and grow onto the inner surface of the nerve head and peripapillary retina. Vitreous condensation and fibroglial tissue may be adherent to the inner surface of the nerve head and also contain hyperplastic RPE (Figs. 8–552 through 8–554).

Because the lesion is often seen in children, it has been considered to be a hamartoma. Although RPE is a conspicuous ophthalmoscopic and histologic component, fluorescein angiography and histopathologic studies have also shown a prominent vascular component. It is possible that both the pigment epithelial and vascular components are hamartomatous. It is also possi-

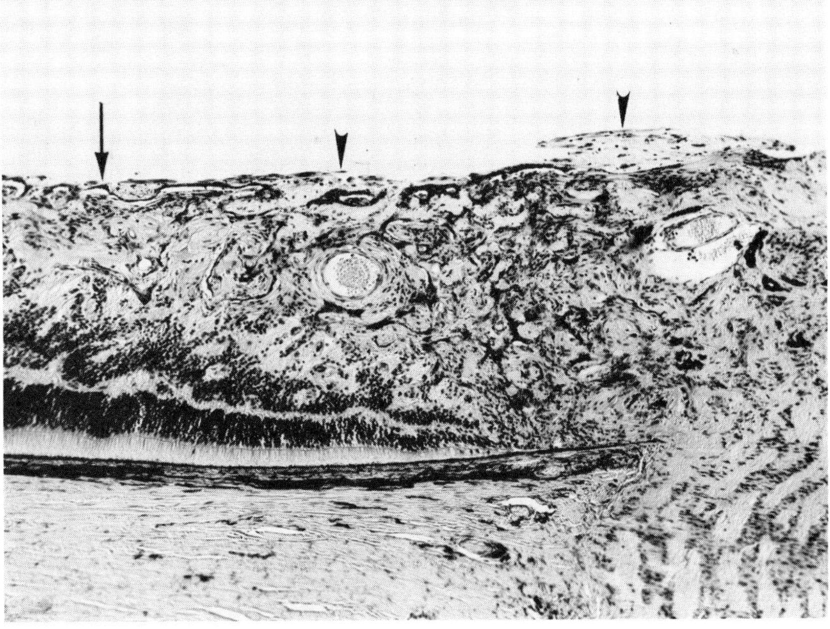

Figure 8–554. Hyperplastic retinal pigment epithelium in optic nerve head and peripapillary retina, with extension along inner surface of retina (arrow). Fibroglial epipapillary and epiretinal tissue (arrowheads) is present. H and E, ×90. AFIP Neg. 68–5963. AFIP 334475. (From Vogel MH, Zimmerman LE, Gass JDM: Proliferation of juxtapapillary retinal pigment epithelium simulating malignant melanoma. Doc Ophthalmol *26*:461–481, 1969.

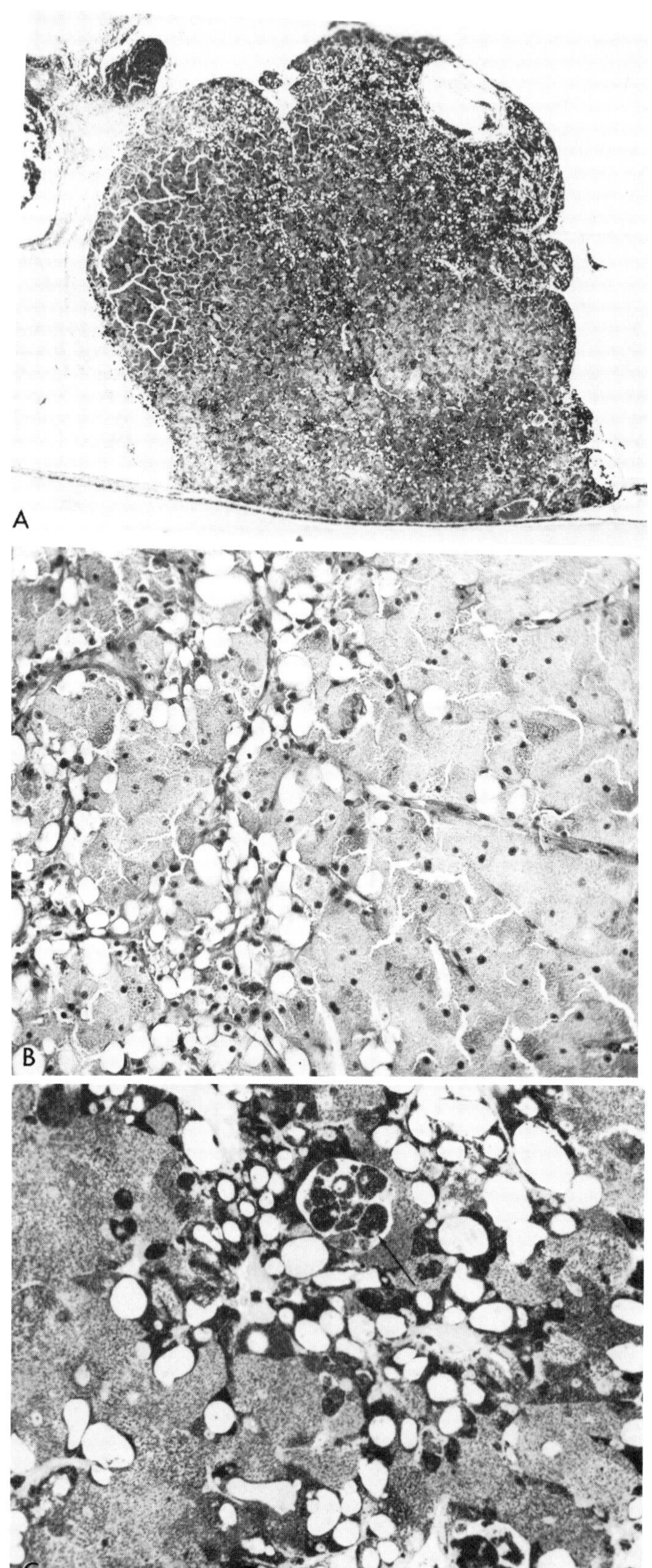

Figure 8–555. Adenoma of retinal pigment epithelium. *A*, Under low magnification, pigmented tumor has flat base toward sclera (bottom of picture). Cells with vacuolization are more numerous toward apical portion than toward base. Focal hemmorhage is present in vitreous at posterior edge of tumor. H and E, ×28. AFIP Neg. 70–7096. *B*, Bleached preparation reveals large, polyhedral cells, with eccentric round-to-oval pyknotic nuclei and abundant granular cytoplasm. Thin fibrovascular septa are present. Large intracytoplasmic vacuoles are present in many tumor cells. ×165 AFIP Neg. 70–7088.

C, Thin sections (approximately 1.5 microns) reveal presence of light and dark cells. Several melanophages are visible in cystoid space just above center of picture (arrow). Paraphenylenediamine, × 245 AFIP Neg. 70–7091.

Illustration continued on opposite page

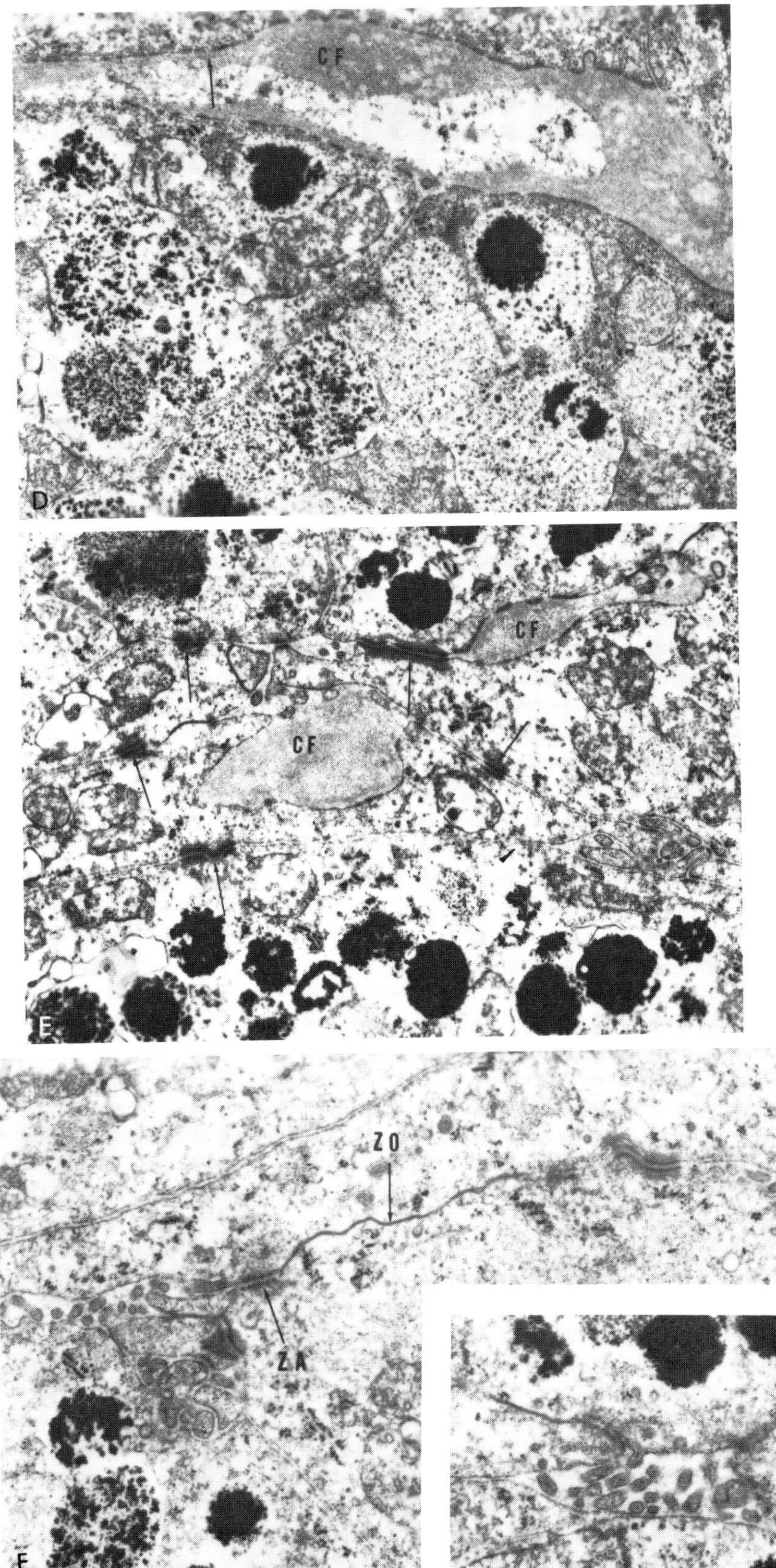

Figure 8–555. Continued *D*, A light cell has produced basement membrane (arrow) and fine collagen filaments *(CF)*. Uranyl acetate and lead citrate, ×20,000 AFIP Neg. 71–2004.

E, Tumor cells are attached to each other by desmosomes (arrows). Fine collagen filaments are present between tumor cells *(CF)*. Uranyl acetate and lead citrate, ×16,500. AFIP Neg. 71–2004. *F*, Another tumor cell shows junctional complexes containing a zonula occludens–like *(ZO)* and a zonula adherens–like *(ZA)* configuration. Numerous microvilli are present where apical portions of several cells meet (inset). Uranyl acetate and lead citrate, ×21,000. AFIP Neg. 71–2004.

AFIP 848819. (From Font, RL, Zimmerman LE, Fine BS: Adenoma of retinal pigment epithelium. Am J Ophthalmol *73*:544–554, 1972.)

ble that the vascular component is the only hamartomatous component, and the pigment epithelial component is secondary hyperplasia.

Tumors of the Retinal Pigment Epithelium. True neoplastic lesions of the RPE are rare. This is probably due to the very low rate of growth under normal circumstances, hence lack of chance for genetic mutation (Garner, 1970). In contrast, reactive hyperplasia is quite common. It may be difficult or impossible to differentiate hyperplasia from true neoplasia, since neoplastic lesions are so rare and since both types of proliferation show variable histologic characteristics. In addition, it is possible for true neoplastic proliferation to develop from reaction hyperplasia (Tso, Albert, 1972).

Clinically, adenomas and adenocarcinomas appear as jet-black masses near the optic disc (Blodi, Reuling, Sornson, 1965; Minckler, Allen, 1978) or peripherally (Font, Zimmerman, Fine, 1972), and thus are usually mistaken for malignant melanomas. Patients present with visual loss, or the tumor may be asymptomatic (Tso, Albert, 1972).

Based on their comparatively large series of 11 patients with RPE neoplasms and 6 patients with reactive hyperplasia, Tso and Albert (1972) were able to suggest criteria for differentiating the two conditions. Typically, those with reactive hyperplasia have a history or pathologic evidence of trauma or eye disease, whereas neoplastic lesions tend to be discrete tumors in otherwise normal eyes. Basement membrane elaboration is less evident in neoplastic lesions, but mitoses are more frequent and pleomorphism more evident in neoplastic lesions than in hyperplastic ones. In addition, the median age for neoplastic lesions is somewhat less (fifth decade) than that for reactive hyperplasia (seventh decade).

These tumors have a variety of histologic patterns: mosaic, tubular, papillary, vacuolated, and anaplastic. Tumors with the mosaic pattern (Fig. 8–555) are regarded as the best differentiated, the anaplastic tumor (Fig. 8–556) the least differentiated; tumors with vacuolated, tubular (Fig. 8–557), and papillary (Fig. 8–558) patterns are in the middle of the spectrum.

Adenoma of the Retinal Pigment Epithelium. Histopathologically, a variety of patterns are seen in adenomas of the RPE, as reviewed by Tso and Albert (1972). The cells may proliferate in an oval or hexagonal array with almost no fibrovascular matrix, resembling flat preparations. In other tumors the cells have large vacuoles with no evident basal or apical regions. The vacuoles contain nonsulfated, diastase-resistant, but partially hyaluronidase-sensitive mucopolysaccharide containing sialic acid (Font, Zimmerman, Fine, 1972) (Fig. 8–555). Tumors often show different histologic patterns in different regions.

The pigment granules retain their large oval configuration. Many melanosomes are immature, but no premelanosomes were noted by Font and associates. By electron microscopy, other characteristics of RPE cells are seen present, including basement membrane production, junctional complexes, and microvilli (Font, Zimmerman, Fine, 1972) (Fig. 8–557).

Blodi, Reuling, and Sornson (1965) observed an adenoma of the RPE at the optic nerve head that simulated a melanocytoma.

Adenocarcinoma of the Retinal Pigment Epithe-

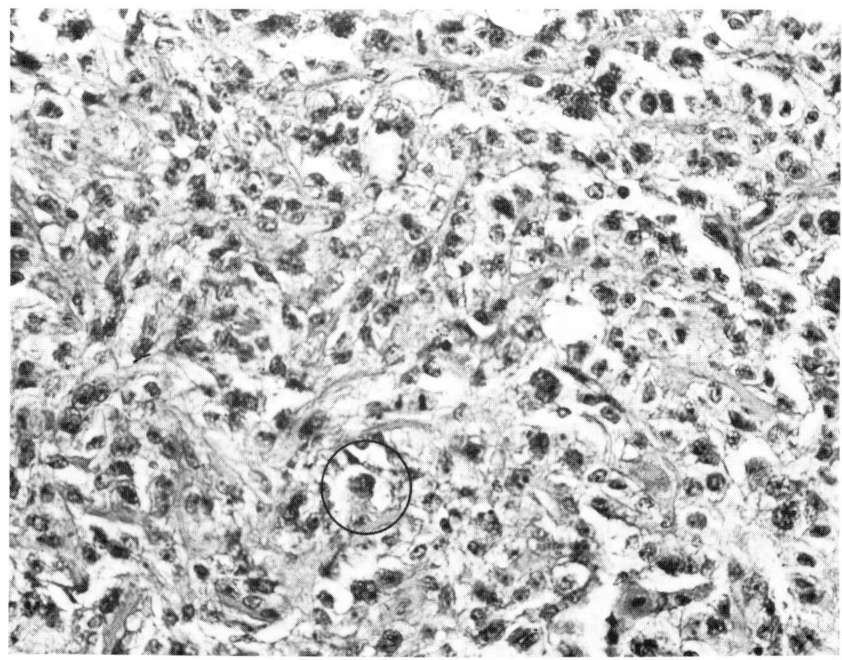

Figure 8–556. Anaplastic carcinoma of retinal pigment epithelium. A mitotic figure (circle) is present. H and E, ×300. AFIP Neg. 70–10337. AFIP 221641. (From Tso MOM, Albert DM: Pathological condition of retinal pigment epithelium. Neoplasms and nodular non-neoplastic lesions. Arch Ophthalmol *88*:27–38, 1972.)

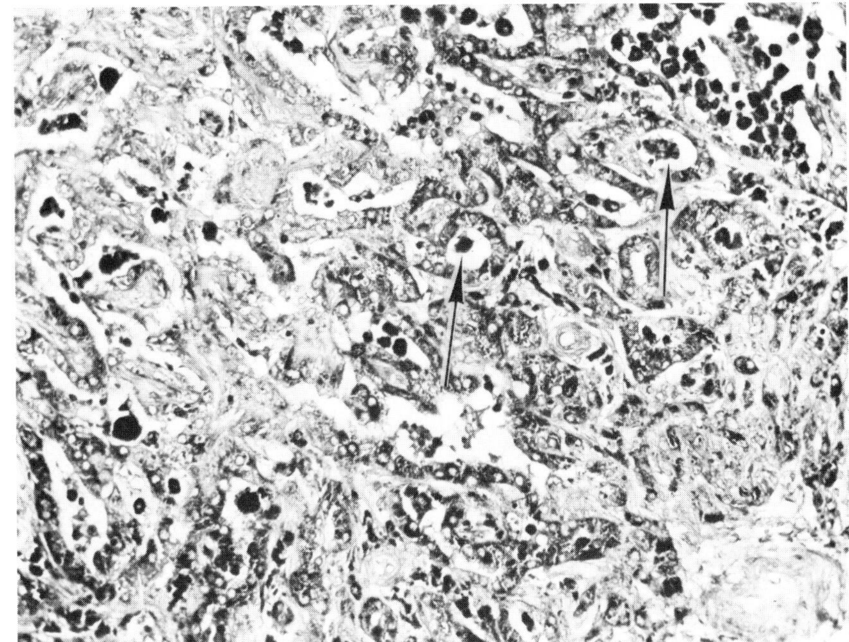

Figure 8–557. Tumor of retinal pigment epithelium showing tubular pattern. Clumps of pigment granules (arrows) are sequestered in lumens of acini. Note that pigmentation varies in different locations of tumor. H and E, ×145. AFIP Neg. 70–8471. AFIP 503113. (From Tso MOM, Albert DM: Pathological condition of retinal pigment epithelium. Neoplasms and nodular non-neoplastic lesions. Arch Ophthalmol *88*:27–38, 1972.)

lium. The name adenocarcinoma, implying malignancy, is applied to those tumors showing anaplasia, pleomorphism, and increased mitotic activity (Tso, Albert, 1972) and a tendency to local invasion of the choroid (Minckler, Allen, 1978; Kurz, Zimmerman, 1962; Fair, 1958) and optic nerve head (Fair, 1958). However, the question of distant metastases is unsettled; three tumor deaths from metastases have been cited by Garner (1970) in his review, but none had been verified histologically (Tso, Albert, 1972). In addition, no tendency for scleral invasion has been observed.

Histologically, tumors labeled malignant show more anaplastic cells with variable-sized nuclei—some large and hyperchromatic with prominent nucleoli and others with small, irregular chromatin (Fig. 8–556). Tso and Albert (1972) noted no definite basement membrane, but Minckler and Allen (1978) were able to demonstrate basement membrane production, villous processes, and junctional complexes by electron microscopy.

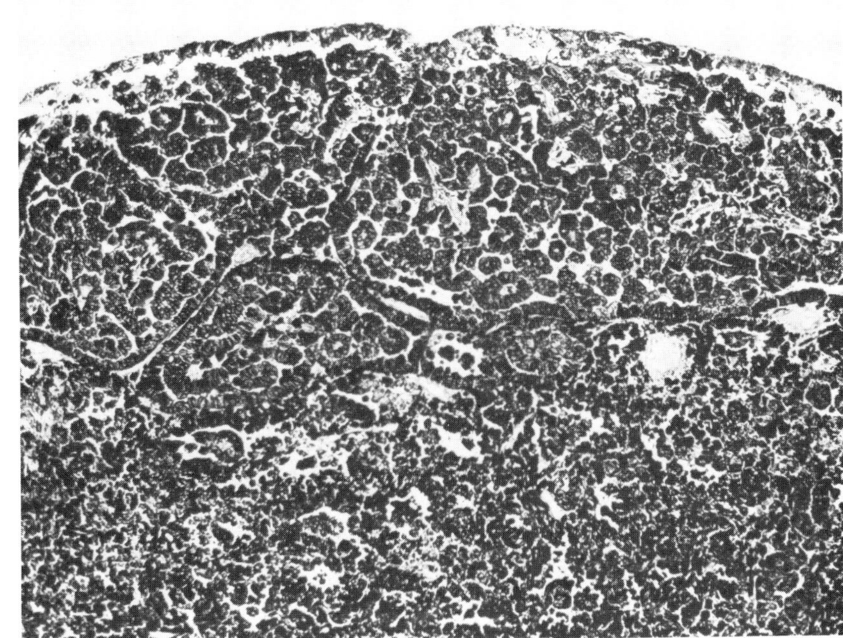

Figure 8–558. Deeply pigment papillary tumor of retinal pigment epithelium (RPE). The RPE cells are arranged in a tubuloacinar pattern. H and E, ×63. AFIP Neg. 71–7996. AFIP 848819. (From Tso MOM, Albert DM: Pathological condition of retinal pigment epithelium. Neoplasms and nodular non-neoplastic lesions. Arch Ophthalmol *88*:27–38, 1972.)

The more anaplastic tumors generally show increased mitotic activity and more pleomorphism than the benign tumors.

RPE Components of Medulloepithelioma. Embryonal medulloepithelioma, referred to as diktyoma in the past, is a rare tumor composed of tissue that looks like very early embryonal ciliary body, retina, or RPE.

NEUROEPITHELIAL TUMORS OF CILIARY BODY

(Table 8–8)

These tumors are considered in this section because of the embryologic relations of the retina, RPE, and ciliary epithelium. Zimmerman (1971) has proposed a classification of these tumors, the main categories of which are congenital and acquired. This classification is based, in some instances, on rather distinct histopathologic features and embryologic and clinical considerations. Previous classifications have been based on the presence of pigmentation and features of malignancy (Andersen, 1962; Cogan, Kuwabara, 1971). The congenital lesions are embryonic in nature and arise during embryonic or early postnatal development. The acquired lesions occur after embryologic development, and some have previously been referred to as adult diktyomas or adult medulloepitheliomas. The congenital tumors include the rare ganglioneuroma and the less rare medulloepithelioma.

Glioneuroma. This rare, benign tumor is composed of well-differentiated brain tissue containing neurons and glia (Fig. 8–559) (Kuhlenback, Haymaker, 1946; Manz, Rosen, Macklin, Willis, 1973; Spencer, Jesberg, 1973; Addison, 1977). Such tumors may be considered as choristomatous malformations in which the iris and ciliary

Table 8–8. CLASSIFICATION OF NEUROEPITHELIAL TUMORS OF THE CILIARY BODY

- I. Congenital
  - A. Glioneuroma
  - B. Medulloepithelioma
    - 1. Benign
    - 2. Malignant
  - C. Teratoid medulloepithelioma
    - 1. Benign
    - 2. Malignant
- II. Acquired
  - A. Nonpigmented
    - 1. Benign
      - a. Pseudoadenomatous hyperplasia
      - b. Adenoma
        - i. solid
        - ii. papillary
        - iii. pleomorphic
    - 2. Malignant
      - a. Glandular and papillary
      - b. Pleomorphic, low-grade
      - c. Pleomorphic with hyaline stroma
      - d. Anaplastic
  - B. Pigmented
    - 1. Benign
      - a. Adenoma
      - b. Vacuolated adenoma
    - 2. Malignant
      - a. Adenocarcinoma
  - C. Mixed pigmented and nonpigemented
    - 1. Benign
    - 2. Malignant

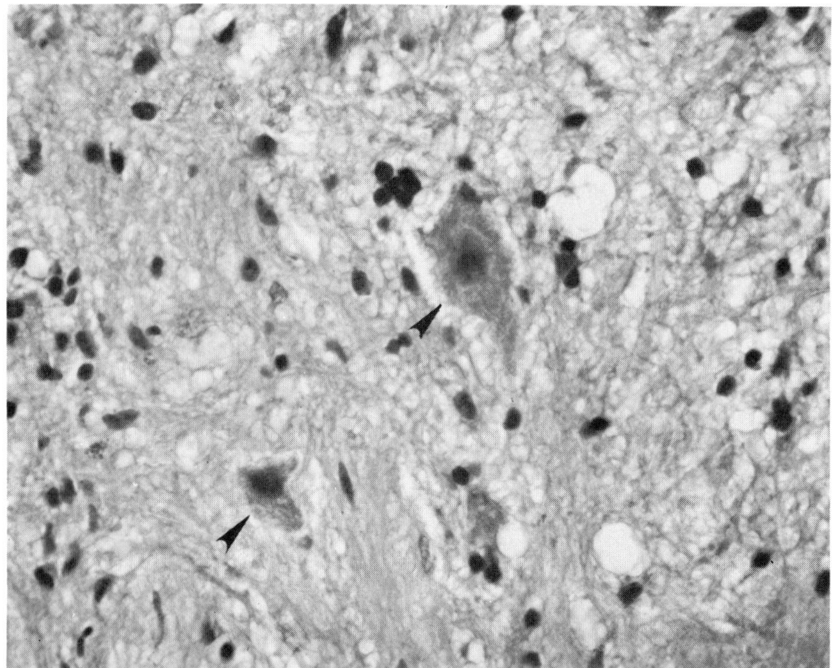

Figure 8–559. Glioneuroma of ciliary body and iris from a 20 year old woman. This choristomatous tissue consists of glial cells, neurofibrils, and ganglion cells (arrowheads). H and E, ×450. (Courtesy of Dr. D. Addison; case presented at Association of Ophthalmic Alumni of Armed Forces Institute of Pathology, June 1977.)

body fail to develop normally and instead produce masses of tissue resembling brain.

Medulloepithelioma. These tumors arise from the medullary epithelium and are also considered to be embryonic in nature. Since both benign and malignant forms occur, there is reason for considering these tumors as neoplasms rather than as choristomas. Some that occur in infancy have a conspicuous network of epithelial bands. This network led Fuchs (1908) to call these tumors *diktyomas*. Verhoeff (1904) preferred the term *teratoneuroma*.

Medulloepitheliomas contain elements that closely resemble the medullary epithelium and may contain structures resembling those derived from the optic vesicle or optic cup, RPE nonpigmented and pigmented ciliary epithelium, vitreous, and neuroglia (Andersen, 1971).

Many medulloepitheliomas contain areas in which cells are undifferentiated and resemble those seen in retinoblastoma (Fig. 8–560). Homer-Wright and Flexner-Wintersteiner-like rosettes also may be observed (Figs. 8–560,*D* and 8–561). Most rosettes in this tumor, however, have a lumen surrounded by more than a single layer of cells. The cells of those rosettes having a single layer of cells resemble primitive ciliary epithelial cells and not photoreceptor cells (Figs. 8–560 and 8–561).

Small cords of pigmented neuroepithelial cells are often present but are usually enmeshed in nonpigmented tissue, so that the tumor appears white, gray, or yellowish. In rare instances the pigmented neuroepithelial cell component may be great enough to give the tumor a pigmented appearance on clinical examination.

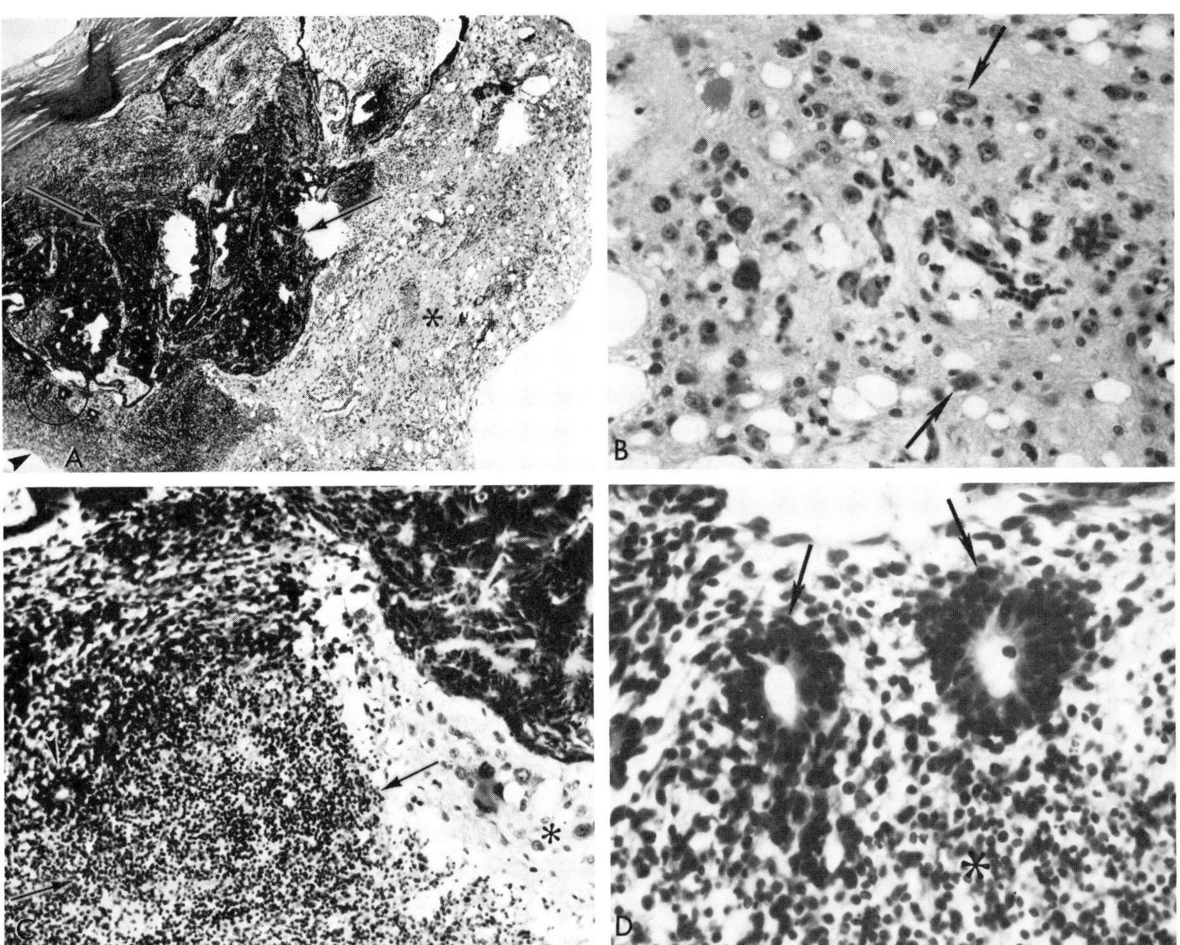

Figure 8–560. Teratoid medulloepithelioma of ciliary body from 48 year old man. *A*, Low power view showing different components: sheets and cords of medullary epithelium (between arrows), brainlike tissue (asterisk), retinoblastoma-like tissue (arrowhead), and rosettes (circle). H and E, ×30. *B*, Higher power view of brainlike tissue with ganglion cells (arrows). H and E, ×290. *C*, Higher power view of small, hyperchromic cells (between arrows), with scanty cytoplasm, that resemble retinoblastoma. A rosette (arrowhead), brainlike tissue (asterisk), and medullary epithelium are also present, H and E, ×230. *D*, Higher power view of rosettes (arrows), with two to three layers of cells and a central lumen. No distinct membrane is present, and processes extend into lumen. Retinoblastoma-like cells (asterisk) are also present. H and E, ×460. EP 20059.

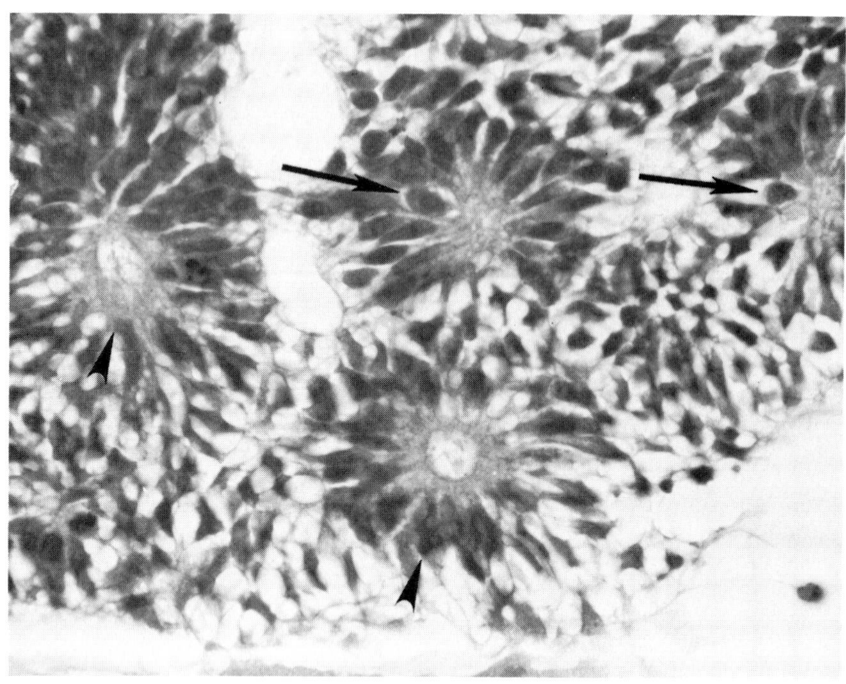

Figure 8–561. Medulloepithelioma with Homer-Wright (arrows) and Flexner-Wintersteiner–like rosettes (arrowheads) from 2.5 year old boy. H and E, ×525. EP 39760.

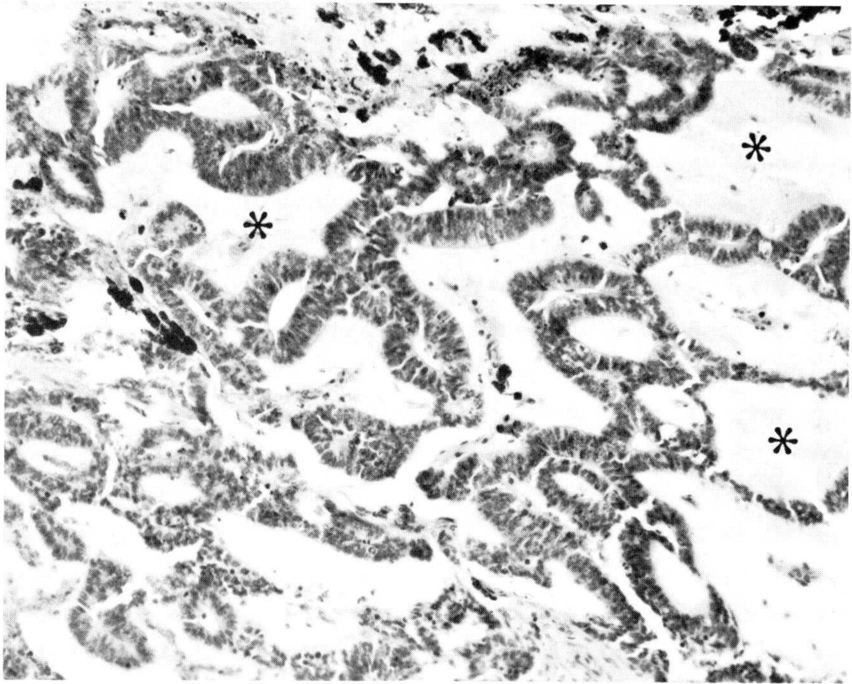

Figure 8–562. Typical cords of medullary epithelium separated by zone of vitreous-like tissue (asterisks) in medulloepithelium of optic nerve of 5 year old girl. H and E, ×380. EP 34506.

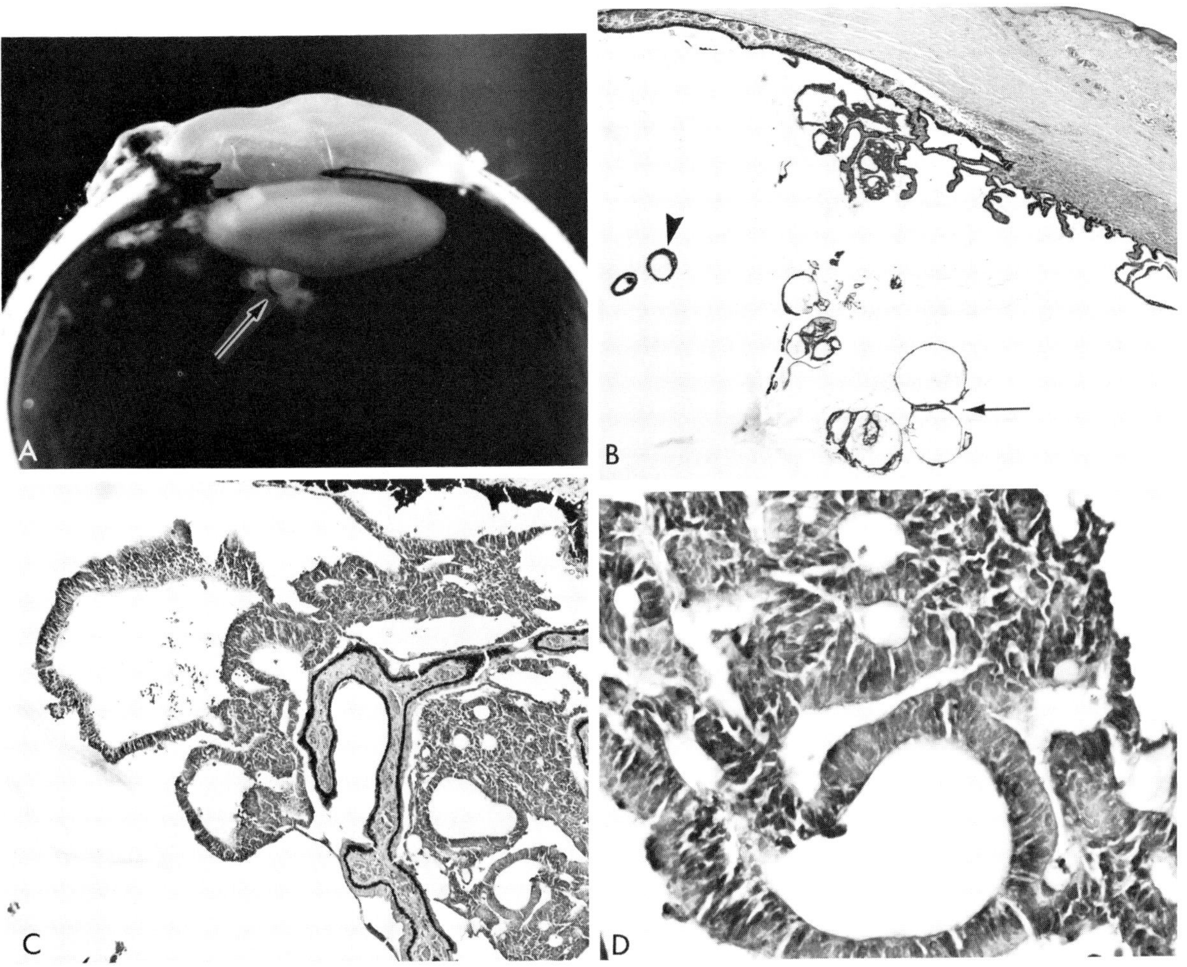

Figure 8–563. Cystic medulloepithelioma from 7 year old boy who was seen with an angioma-like iris lesion. *A*, Gross appearance of cystic lesion seeding vitreous (arrow) and posterior chamber. *B*, Medulloepithelioma cysts in vitreous (arrow) and posterior chamber (arrowhead). H and E, ×24. *C*, Medullary epithelium arranged in sheets, cords, and cysts that remain attached to pars plicata. H and E, ×105. *D*, Higher power view of medullary epithelium forming cystic structures. H and E, ×470. EP 32182.

The proliferating medullary epithelium is characteristically arranged in cords and sheets separated by cystic spaces containing hyaluronic acid (Fig. 8–562). In some instances, spherical cysts containing hyaluronic acid and lined by a single layer of epithelium are present on the surface of the tumor and may branch off and become free-floating in the vitreous (Figs. 8–563 and 8–564) and the posterior and anterior chambers (Figs. 8–565 and 8–566) (Gifford, 1966; Zimmerman, 1971; Broughton, Zimmerman, 1978). The cystic appearance of medulloepitheliomas is quite characteristic, but ciliary epithelial cysts may occur over ciliary body lesions, such as a malignant melanoma.

Malignant medulloepithelioma may not always differ appreciably from the benign tumors. Some tumors may have masses of tightly packed neuroblastic cells and mitotic activity and resemble poorly differentiated retinoblastoma (Fig. 8–560,*C*). Structures resembling Flexner-Wintersteiner rosettes may be present (Figs. 8–560,*D* and 8–561). Invasiveness and extension outside the eye are the most reliable criteria of malignancy.

Teratoid Medulloepithelioma. Medulloepitheliomas with one or more heteroplastic elements are referred to as teratoid medulloepitheliomas. The most frequently observed heterotopic tissue is hyaline cartilage (Fig. 8–567). Other, less frequent tissues are brainlike tissue (Fig. 8–560,*B*) and skeletal muscle (Fig. 8–568) (Zimmerman, Font, Andersen, 1972). Vascular elements resembling an infantile angioma may be observed rarely (Harry, Morgan, 1979).

Medulloepitheliomas of all types most commonly arise in the ciliary body area but also have been found to arise in the retina (Mullaney, 1974; Reeser, 1975) and optic nerve (Reese, 1957; Andersen, 1971; Green, Iliff, Trotter, 1974) (Fig. 8–569).

In a clinicopathologic and follow-up study of 56 intraocular medulloepitheliomas, Broughton and

Text continued on page 1254

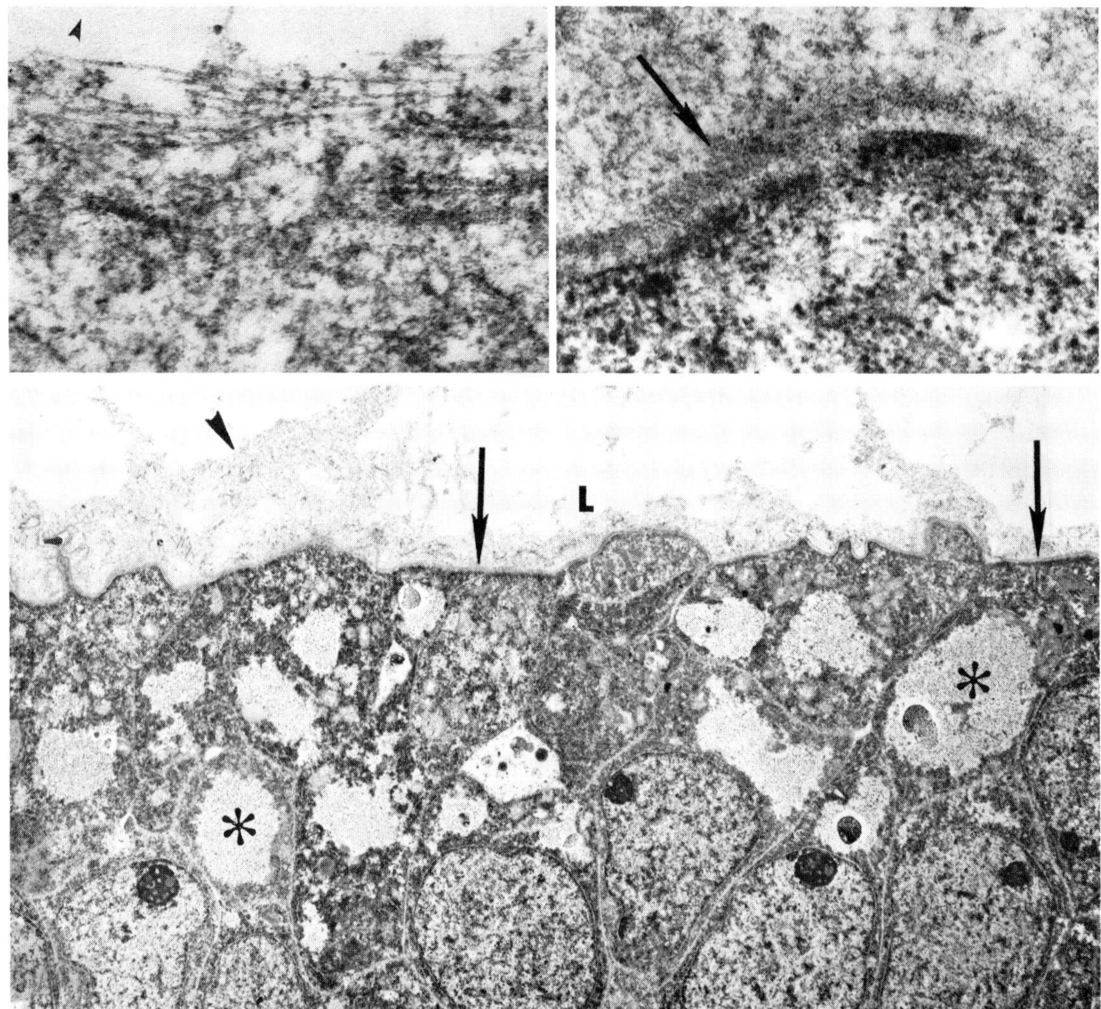

Figure 8–564. Electron microscopic appearance of portion of wall of cyst in vitreous cavity of **malignant cystic medulloepithelioma** of 21 year old man. Cyst is lined by cells with prominent nuclei, dense nucleolus, and scanty cytoplasm. These cells are closely apposed to each other, but no tight junctions are evident. Fibrillogranular inclusions (asterisks) are present in many cells. Basement membrane (arrows and upper right inset) is present on luminal *(L)* side of cells. Vitreal collagen (arrowhead and upper left inset) is present in lumen *(L)*. ×6000; insets, ×60,000. EP 50625.

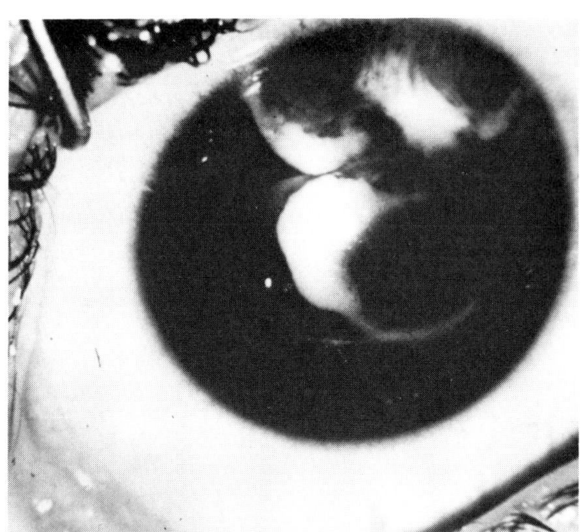

Figure 8–565. Cystic medulloepithelioma with three large cysts in anterior chamber of 2.5 year old boy. EP 39760.

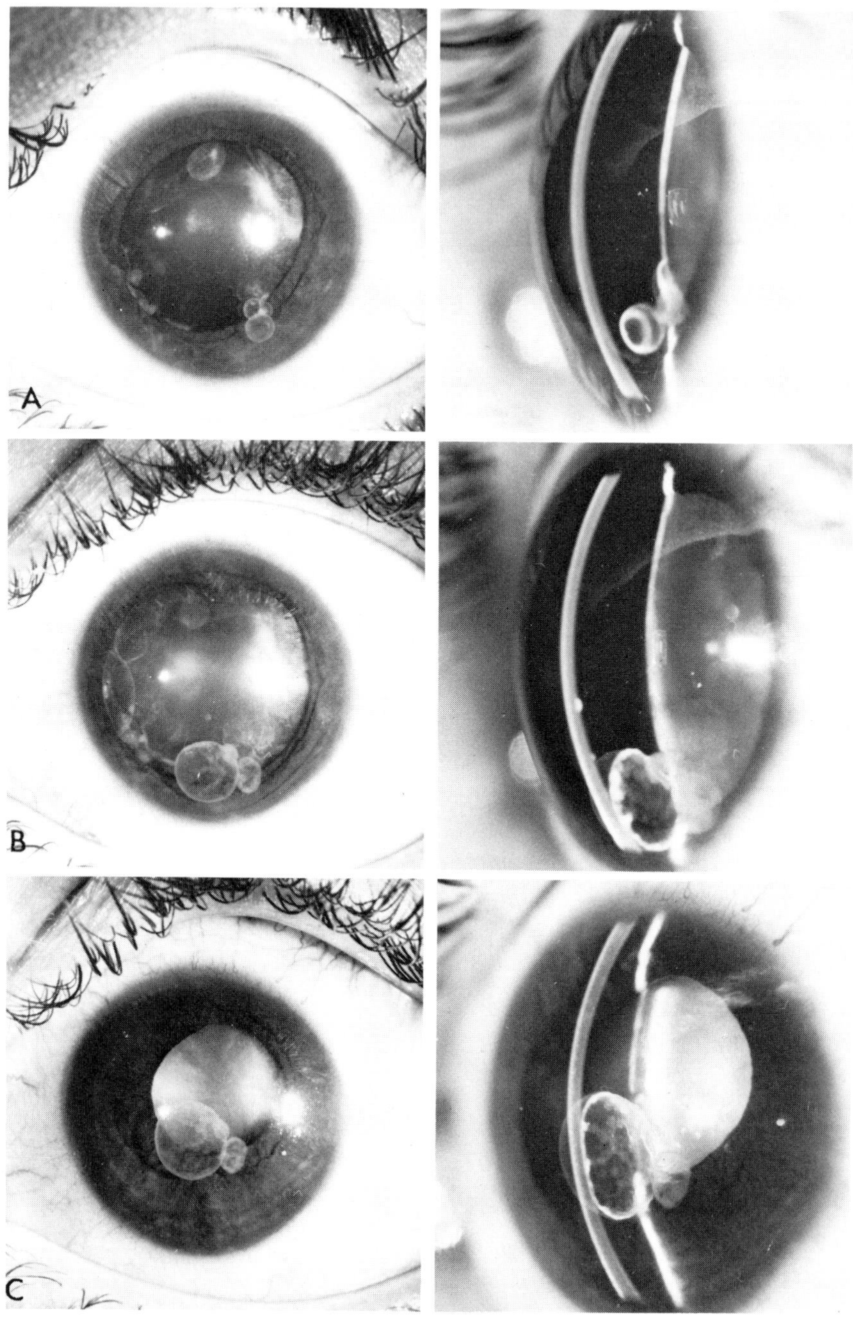

Figure 8–566. Malignant cystic medulloepithelioma in a 20 year old man. Sequence shows enlargement of cyst in anterior chamber over a 2 month period. *A*, External and split lamp appearance of cyst in anterior chamber on April 18, 1980. *B*, Appearance on June 2, 1980. Pupil is widely dilated and exposes tumor on anterior surface of lens. *C*, Appearance on June 12, 1980. Cyst in anterior chamber is about 2.5 times larger than that shown in first photograph. Smaller lesion is a more solid nodule of tumor adherent to iris.

Illustration continued on opposite page

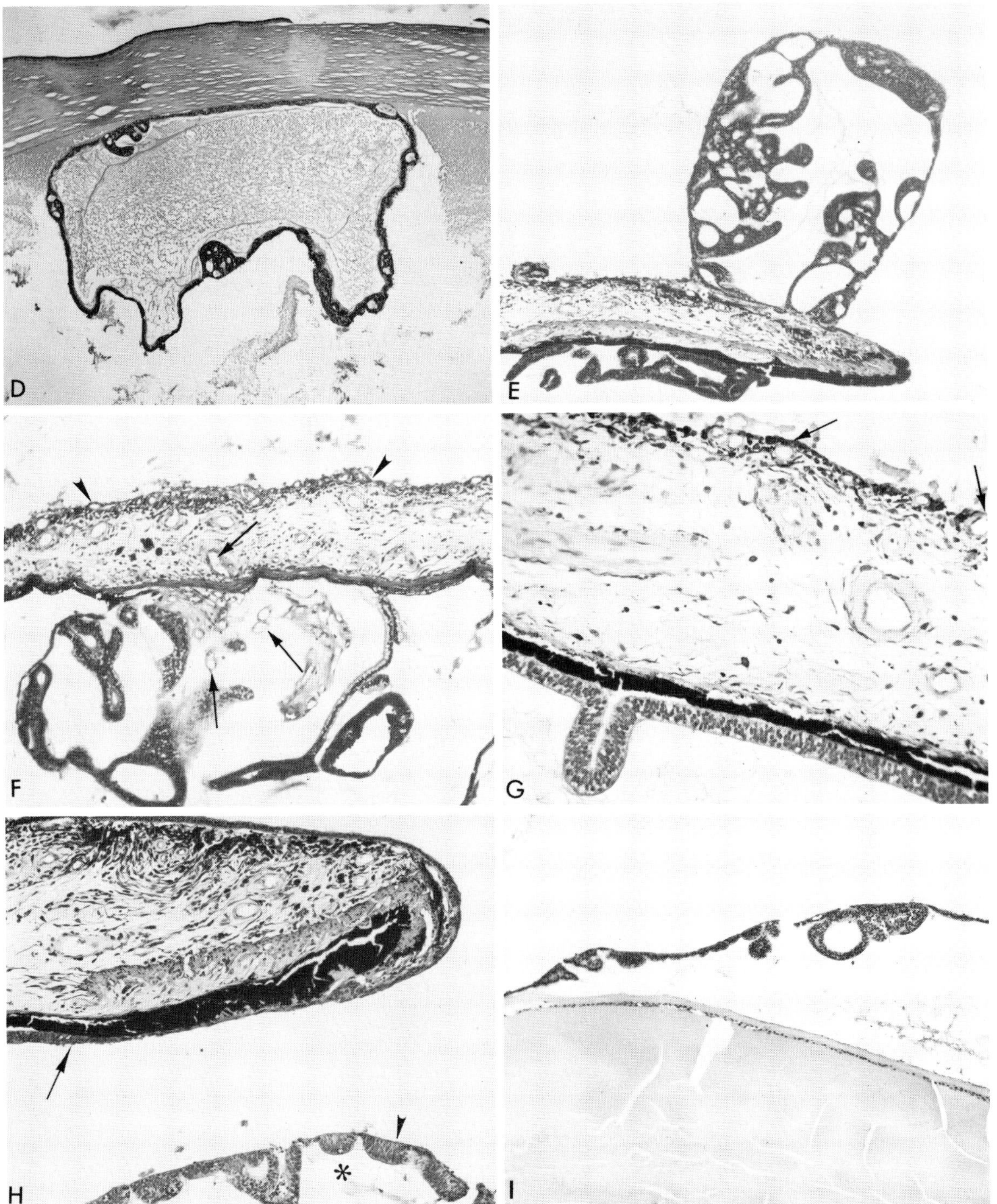

Figure 8–566 *Continued D*, Cyst is adherent to posterior surface of cornea, is lined by medullary epithelium, and contains hyaluronic acid. Alcian blue, ×35. *E*, Multilobulated cystic nodule of tumor adherent to iris. H and E, ×75. *F*, Nodule of tumor adherent to posterior surface of iris. Blood vessels (arrows) extend into tumor from iris. Extensive rubeosis iridis (arrowheads) is present. H and E, ×100.

G, Different area, showing multilayered medullary epithelium lining posterior surface of iris. Neovascularization on anterior iris surface is present (arrows) Alcian blue, ×240. *H*, Area showing tumor on posterior surface of iris (arrow), with extension around pupillary margin and onto anterior surface of iris. Cyst (asterisk) containing hyaluronic acid is bounded anteriorly by medullary epithelium (arrowhead) and lens posteriorly. Alcian blue, ×135. *I*, Sheet of tumor extends over anterior surface of lens. Alcian blue, ×100.

EP 50625. (Courtesy of Drs. Mohsen S. Samaan and Joaquin Barraquer, Barraquer Institute, Barcelona, Spain.)

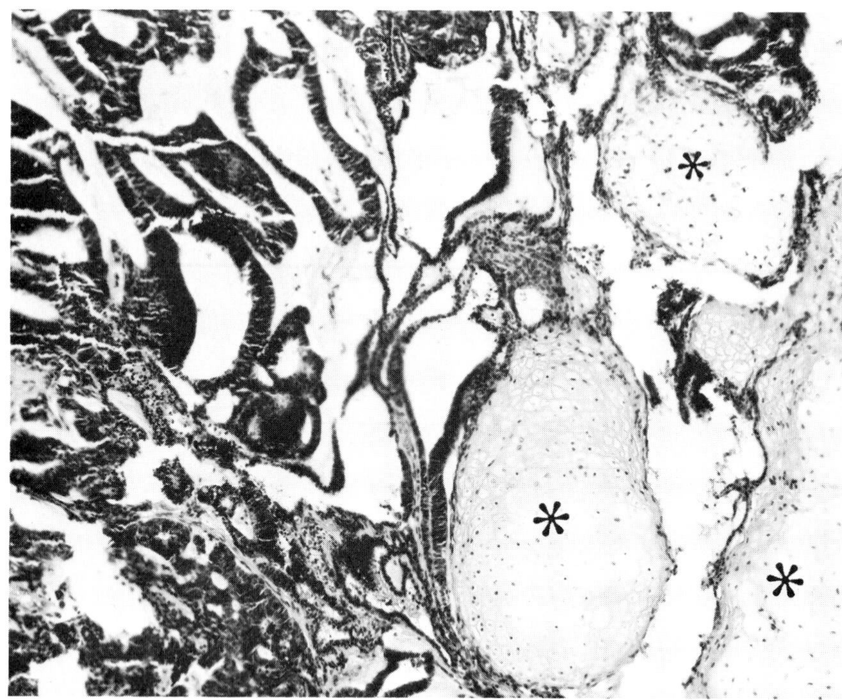

Figure 8–567. Malignant teratoid medulloepithelioma showing areas of cartilaginous differentiation (asterisks). H and E, ×115. EP 34506.

Zimmerman (1978) and Zimmerman and Broughton (1978) found that the mean age was 5 years at the time of definitive diagnosis. They found histologic evidence of malignancy in 37 (66 per cent) of the 56 cases. Follow-up was possible in 33 of the 56 cases. Four of the 33 patients (12.1 per cent) died of metastatic disease, and four additional cases with orbital involvement were lost to follow-up. Heteroplastic elements (brain tissue, cartilage, or rhabdomyoblasts) were observed in 4 benign and 17 malignant tumors. Those 21 tumors (37.5 per cent) were designated teratoid medulloepitheliomas. Extraocular extension, found in ten cases, was the most important prognostic feature of this tumor.

Acquired Neuroepithelial Tumors of the Ciliary Body. These tumors have a wide spectrum of clinical and histopathologic features and biologic

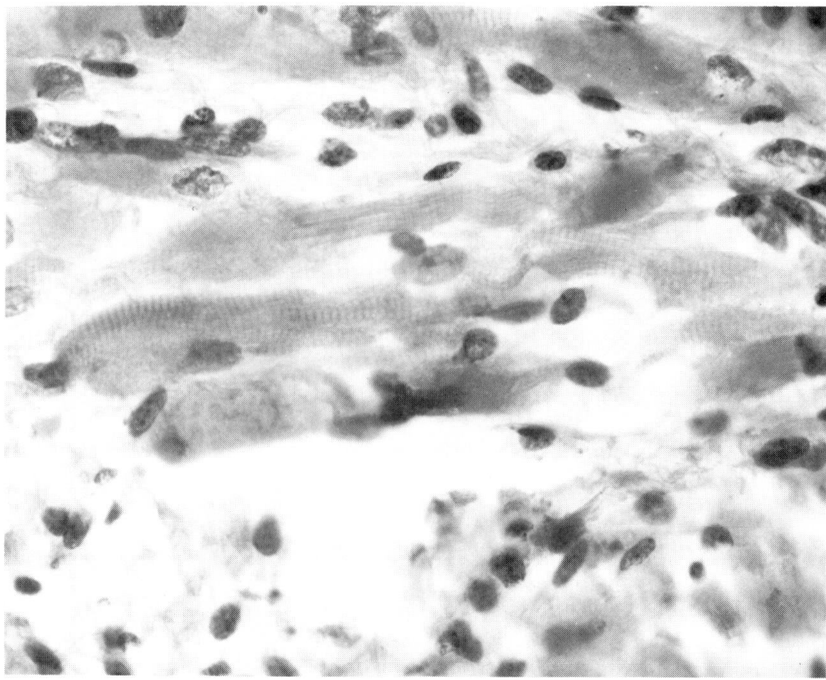

Figure 8–568. Area of skeletal muscle differentiation in a **teratoid medulloepithelioma**. H and E, × 700.

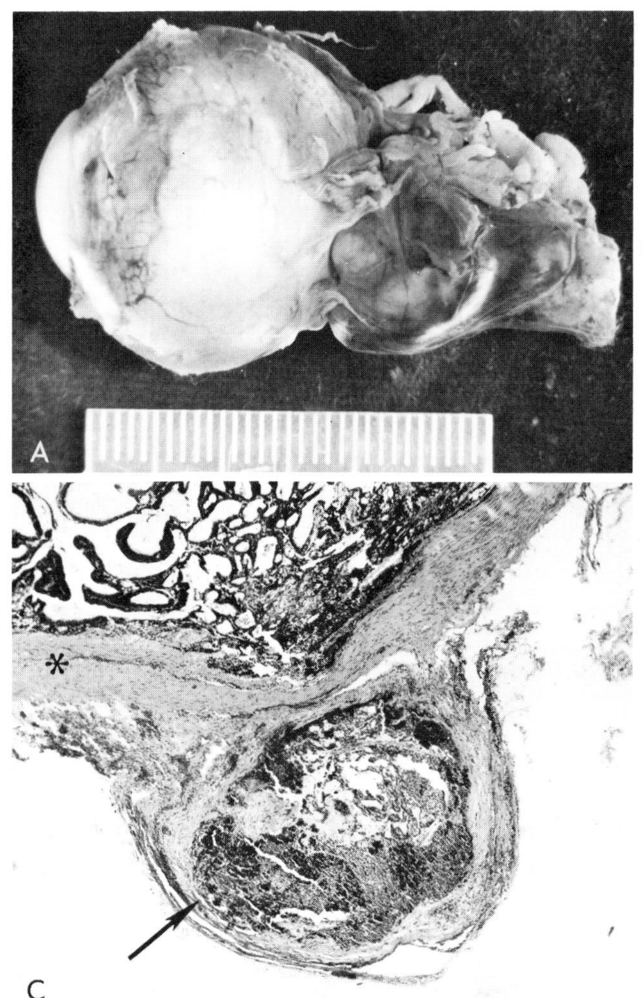

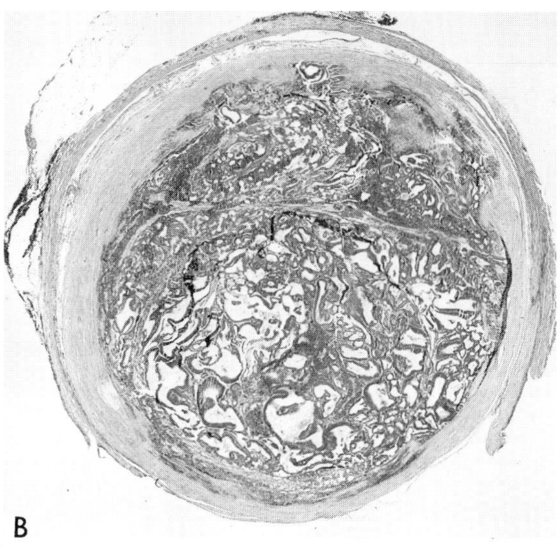

Figure 8–569. Malignant teratoid medulloepithelioma of optic nerve in a 5 year old girl considered clinically to have glioma of optic nerve. *A*, Lobulated appearance of enlarged optic nerve. *B*, Cross-section of proximal end of optic nerve, showing complete replacement by tumor. H and E, ×20. *C*, Area showing extension of tumor into orbit (arrow). Asterisk indicates dura. H and E, ×35. EP 34506. (From Green WR, Iliff WJ, Trotter RR: Malignant teratoid medulloepithelioma of optic nerve. Arch Ophthalmol *91*:451–454, 1974.)

behavior. Most are very rare, and most studies have consisted of single case reports. Classifications have been based on the presence or absence of pigmentation, the cellular patterns, and malignant behavior. The adenomas and malignant tumors in this group of acquired neoplasms have been referred to as adult medulloepitheliomas or adult diktyomas (Andersen, 1962).

A benign hyperplasia of the nonpigmented ciliary epithelium (pseudoadenomatous hyperplasia, Fuchs' adenoma, Fuchs' epithelium, coronal adenoma) is the most common acquired lesion. Grossly, these are small white nodules that measure up to 1 mm and are located on the pars plicata (Fig. 8–570,*A*). In some instances they may be covered by pigment epithelium (Fig. 8–568,*B*). In studies of eyes obtained post mortem, Fuchs' adenomas were found in 20 per cent (Iliff, Green, 1972) and in 31 per cent (Bateman, Foos, 1979) of the cases. Fuchs' adenomas were observed clinically in 57 of 320 eyes from a nonselected group of older patients (Hillemann, Naumann, 1972). These benign tumors are of no significance, except that they are age-related, may rarely incude sectoral cataracts, may simulate an iris tumor (Bateman, Foos, 1979) and may be mistaken for a ciliary body melanoma (Burch, Maumenee, 1967). Gärtner (1972) presented evidence that these lesions are a form of senile localized amyloidosis.

The lesions consist of a nodule of hyperplastic nonpigmented ciliary epithelium arranged in sheets and tubules, with alternating areas of eosinophilic, periodic acid–Schiff–positive, basement membrane–like material (Fig. 8–570,*C,D*).

Adenomas of the nonpigmented ciliary epithelium are rare and may have a solid, papillary, tubuloacinar (Fig. 8–571), or pleomorphic appearance.

Malignant acquired tumors of the nonpigmented ciliary epithelium are rare. According to Croxatto and Zimmerman (1981), there are few acceptable reports in the literature (Fuchs, 1908; Barrow, Stallard, 1932; Nordmann, 1941; Wadsworth, 1949; Wolter, James, 1958; Andersen, 1962; Timm, Fritsch, 1964; Harris, Gumucio,

Text continued on page 1260

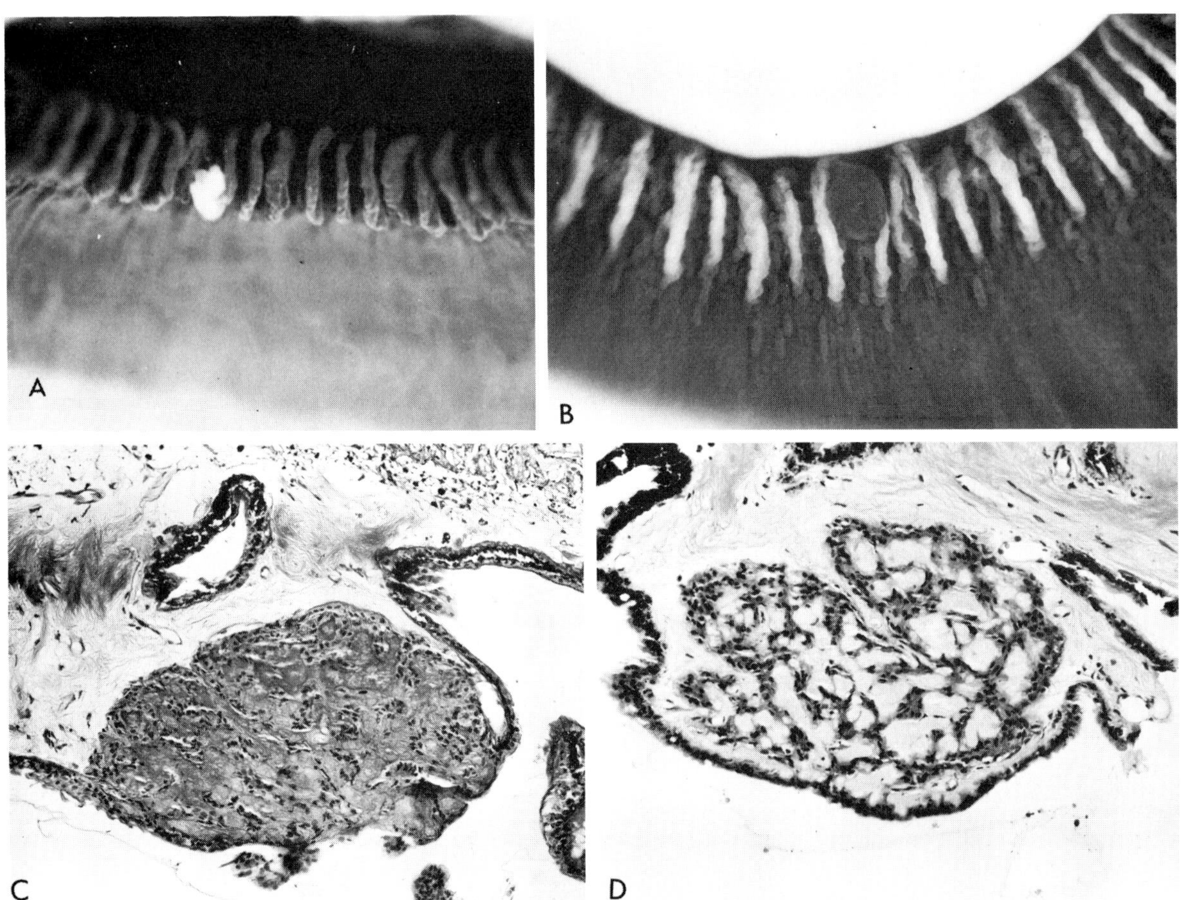

Figure 8–570. Fuchs' adenoma. *A*, Gross appearance of white nodule on pars plicata. EP 31332. *B*, Pigmented nodule on pars plicata. EP 31919. *C*, Nodule of hyperplastic, nonpigmented ciliary epithelium arranged in cords and lobules and separated by a PAS-positive hyaline material. PAS, ×150. *D*, Similar nodule of hyperplastic, nonpigmented ciliary epithelium within a ciliary process. H and E, ×185. (In part from Iliff WJ, Green WR: The incidence and histology of Fuchs' adenoma. Arch Ophthalmol *88*:249–254, 1972.)

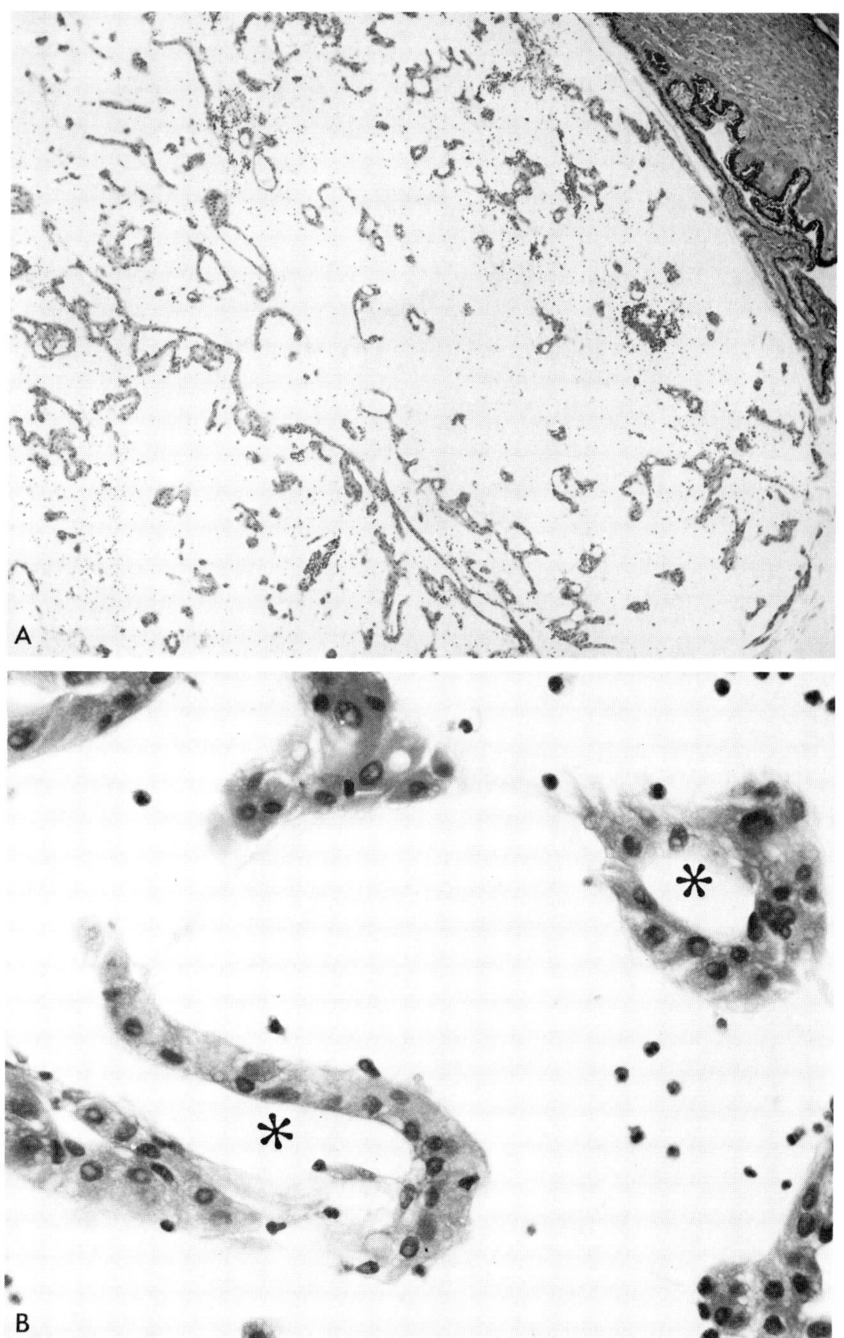

Figure 8–571. Adenoma of nonpigmented ciliary epithelium. *A*, Cords, sheets, acini, and lobules of epithelium are enmeshed in loose fibrillar and mucoid material, H and E, ×35. *B*, Higher power view illustrates the fairly uniform appearance of the epithelium and the tubuloacinar pattern (asterisks). H and E, × 350. (Courtesy of Dr. M.J. Hogan. Case presented at Verhoeff Society, Washington, DC, April, 1963.)

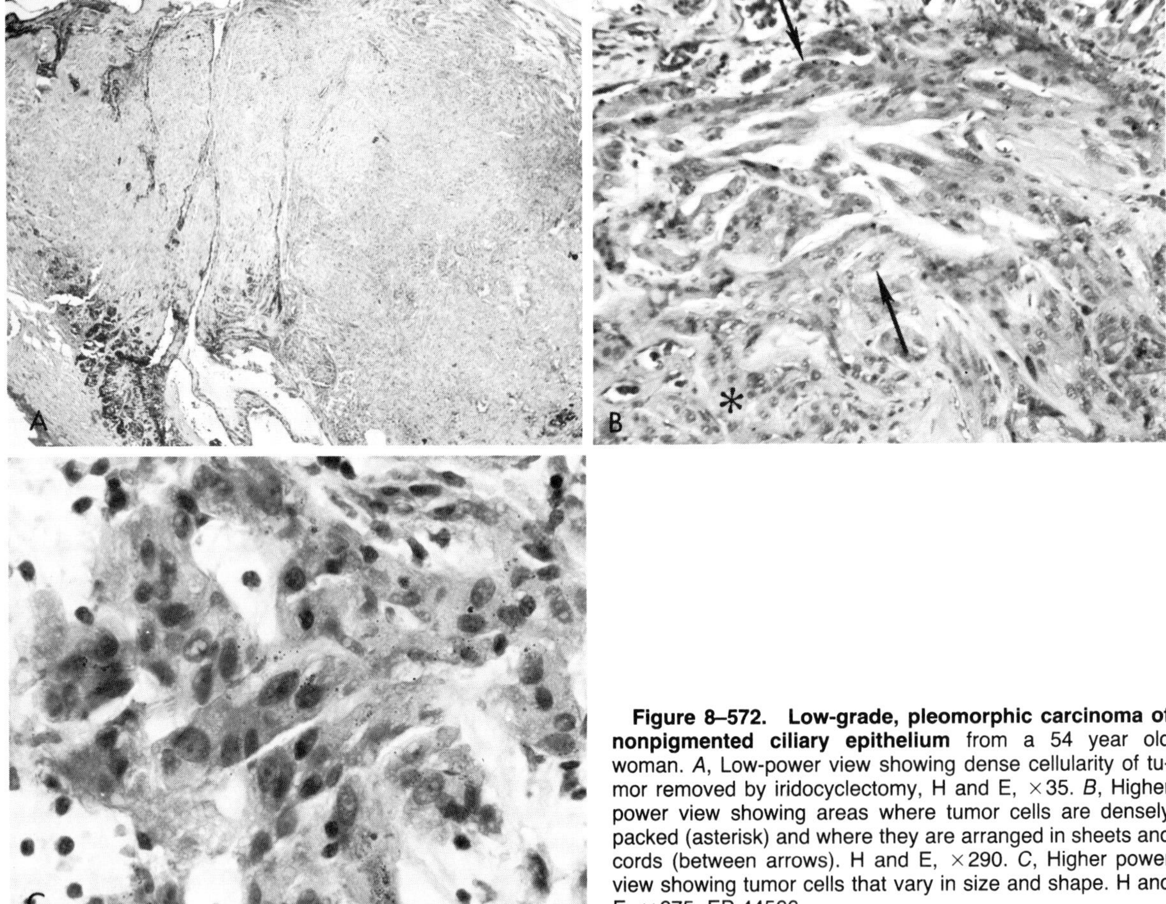

Figure 8–572. Low-grade, pleomorphic carcinoma of nonpigmented ciliary epithelium from a 54 year old woman. *A*, Low-power view showing dense cellularity of tumor removed by iridocyclectomy, H and E, ×35. *B*, Higher power view showing areas where tumor cells are densely packed (asterisk) and where they are arranged in sheets and cords (between arrows). H and E, ×290. *C*, Higher power view showing tumor cells that vary in size and shape. H and E, ×675. EP 44566.

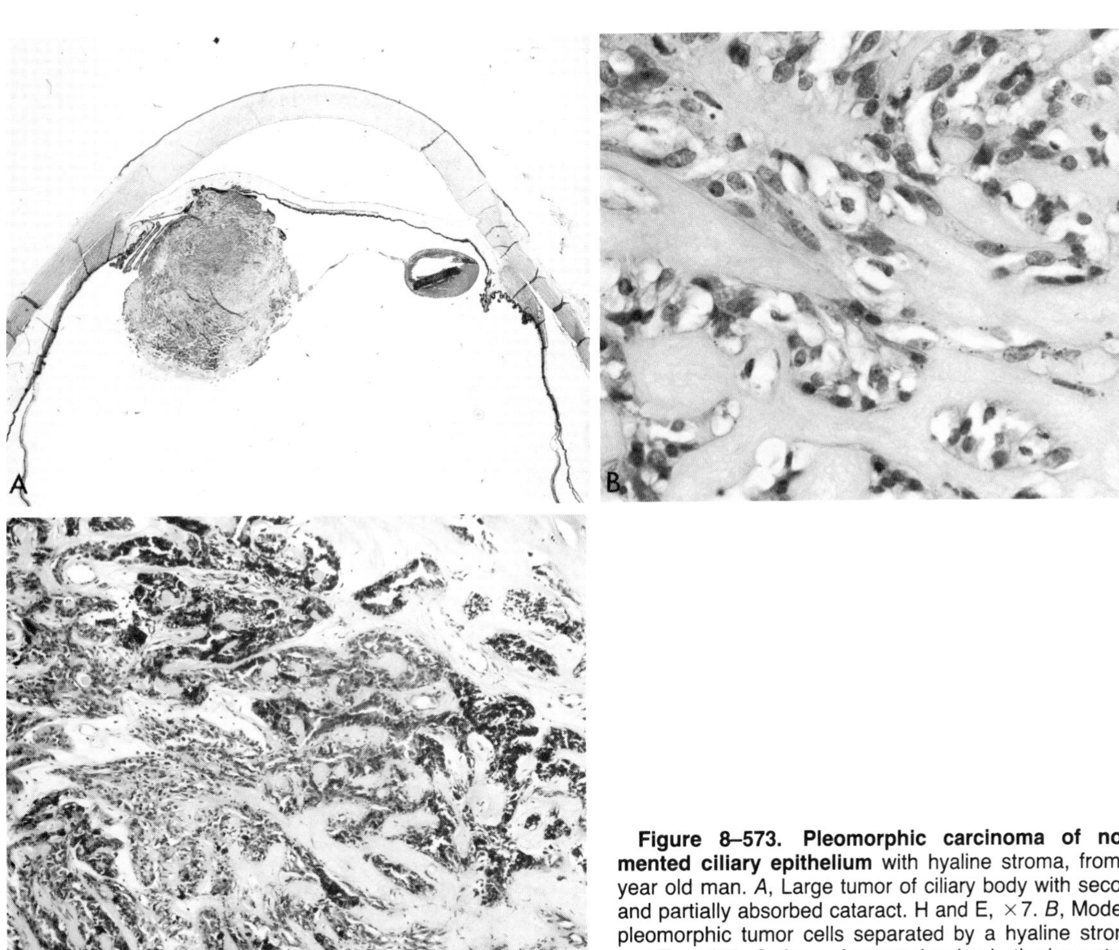

Figure 8–573. Pleomorphic carcinoma of nonpigmented ciliary epithelium with hyaline stroma, from a 56 year old man. *A*, Large tumor of ciliary body with secondary and partially absorbed cataract. H and E, ×7. *B*, Moderately pleomorphic tumor cells separated by a hyaline stroma. H and E, ×450. *C*, Area of tumor showing both pigmented and nonpigmented epithelium. H and E, ×100. EP 52748.

Ohanion, 1968; Vogel, 1974; Horie, Iwata, Tanaka, Hayashi, 1972; Kuchynka, 1979; Dryja, Albert, Horns, 1981).

No suitable classification exists. Croxatto and Zimmerman (1981), in a study of 21 cases, proposed the following categories: glandular or papillary, pleomorphic of low grade (Fig. 8–572), pleomorphic with hyaline stroma (Fig. 8–573), and anaplastic (Fig. 8–574). These tumors span a spectrum from localized, low-grade, well-differentiated, malignant neoplasms that resemble the ciliary epithelium to poorly differentiated, pleomorphic tumors, some of which resemble sarcomas.

The poorly differentiated, pleomorphic tumors usually occur in eyes that previously have been traumatized and have had long-standing inflammatory disease. These tumors appear to represent neoplastic transformation of reactive hyperplasia of the ciliary epithelium. Follow-up information is available for 16 of those 21 patients (Croxatto, Zimmerman, 1981). Eight patients

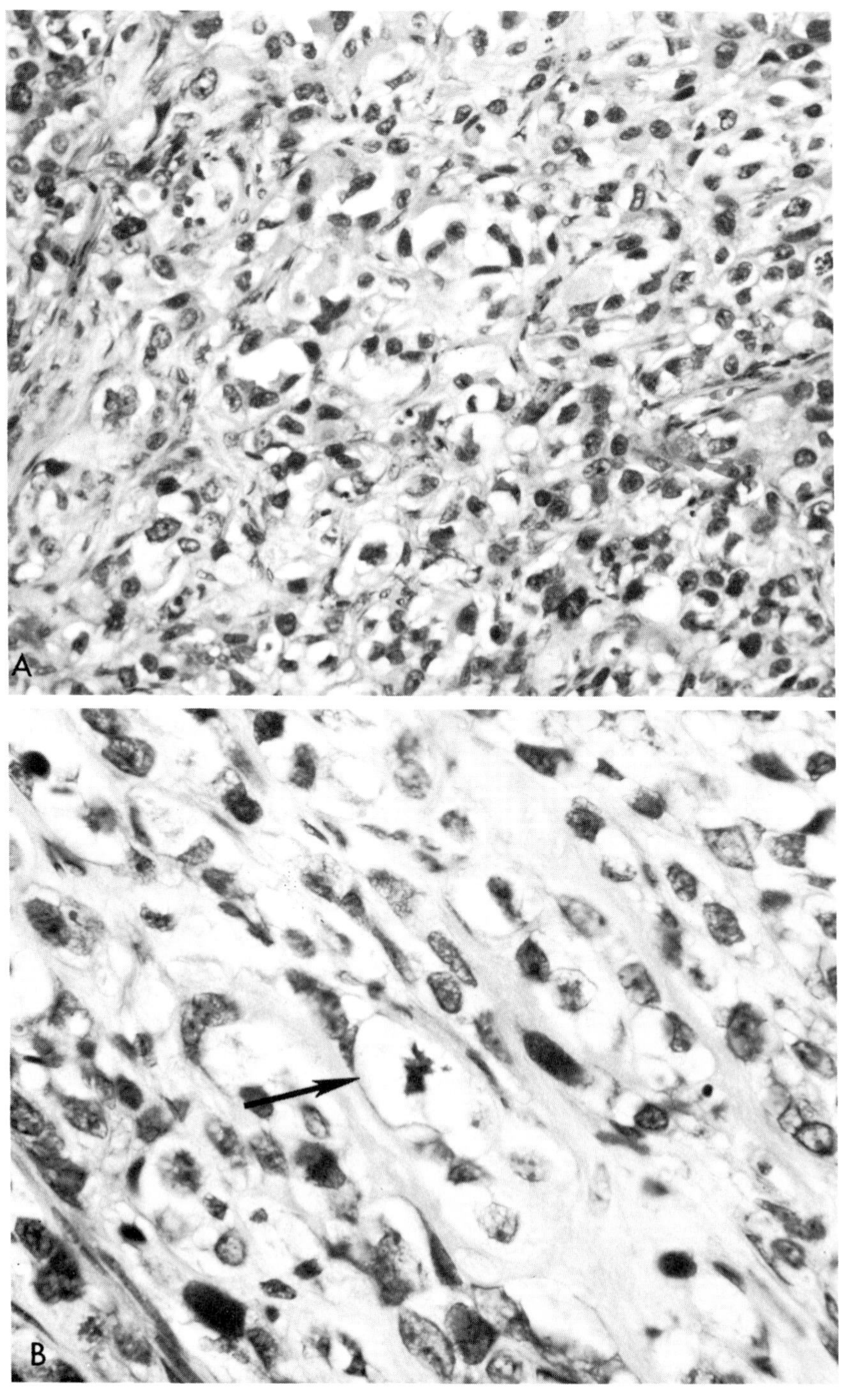

Figure 8–574. Anaplastic carcinoma of nonpigmented ciliary epithelium from a 74 year old man. *A*, Tumor cells show much pleomorphism, hyperchromatism, and no differentiating features. H and E, ×250. *B*, Higher power view showing same features and an abnormal mitotic figure (arrow). H and E, ×650. EP 52682.

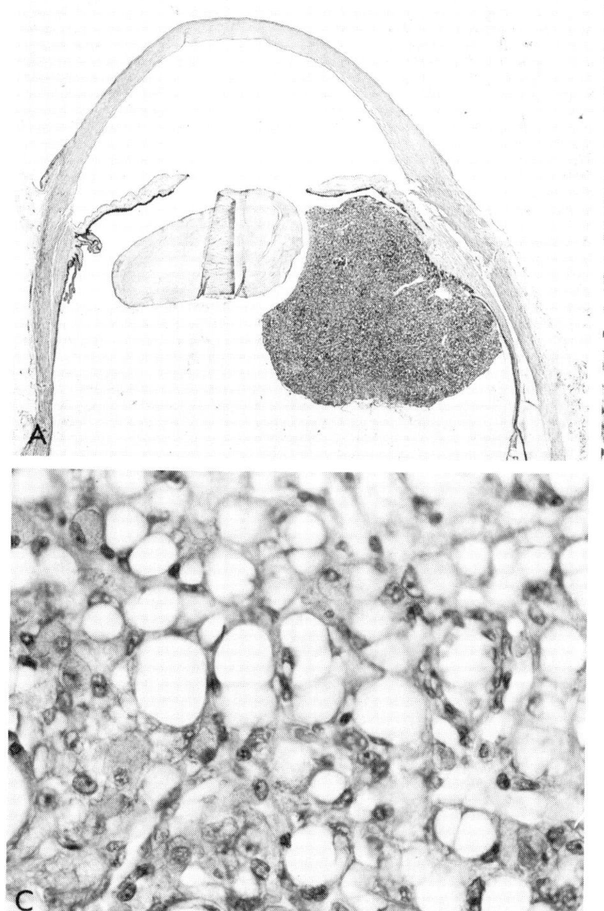

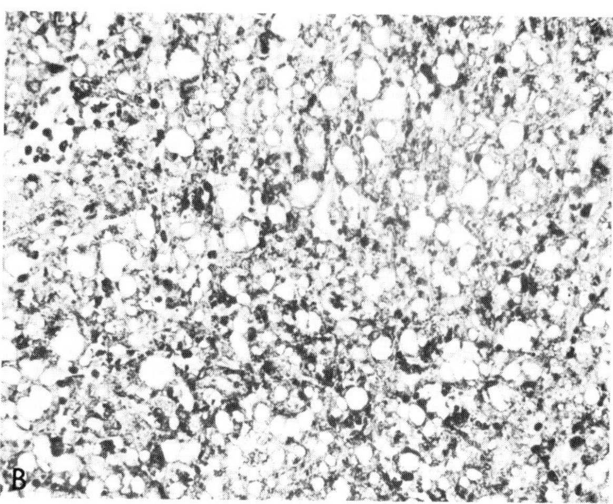

Figure 8–575. Large cystic adenoma of pigmented ciliary epithelium from a 27 year old woman. *A*, Tumor presses against lens. H and E, ×7. *B*, Tumor has numerous small cystic cavities throughout. H and E, ×120. *C*, Higher power view shows tumor cells in no particular arrangement. Bleached; H and E, ×520. EP 45996.

were alive and well with a median follow-up duration of 5.7 years. Two of those eight patients had further tumor—one an intraocular recurrence treated by iridocyclectomy and the other a metastasis to the parotid gland that was treated surgically. Five patients (31.2 per cent) died from tumor extension into the central nervous system or from widespread metastatic disease. Four of these five had opaque ocular media and extraocular extension at the time of the initial surgery, and they experienced orbital recurrence prior to central nervous system extension or metastasis.

Regarding tumors of the ciliary pigment epithelium, it is difficult to ascertain the precise number of previous cases because of inadequacies of both text and figures (Andersen, 1948, 1962; Streeten, McGraw, 1972). Similar tissues have been called adult medulloepithelioma (Hogan, Zimmerman, 1962), adenomatous hyperplasia (Keyes, Moore, 1938), and adenoma of the ciliary body (Zentmeyer, 1936).

In a study and report of 30 adult ciliary body epithelial tumors, Andersen (1962) found that 7 were of pigment epithelial origin; all were considered to be benign, although most showed some local infiltrativeness.

It is not known whether these tumors of the pigmented ciliary epithelium are hamartomatous or arise from hyperplasia, as in the case of malignant tumors of the nonpigmented ciliary epithelium. The occurrence in younger persons, the predilection for the superotemporal quadrant, and the association with some congenital abnormalities suggest a possible developmental cause (Andersen, 1962; Streeten, McGraw, 1972). The diagnosis of this tumor is usually made only after histopathologic study, with most cases being confused with malignant melanoma (Streeten, McGraw, 1972; Wilensky, Holland, 1974; Chang, Shields, Wachtel, 1979). Apparently, a variety of cellular patterns may be observed, including solid, papillary, and vacuolated.

The vacuolated or cystic variety of adenoma of the pigmented ciliary epithelium appears to be quite characteristic. The tumor is composed of large, pigmented cells arranged in nodules, lobules, and sheets. Vacuoles containing small amounts of mucopolysaccharide that is not sensitive to hyaluronidase are scattered throughout the tumor (Fig. 8–575). By electron microscopy, those vacuoles are seen to consist of intercommunicating intercellular spaces lined by cells with

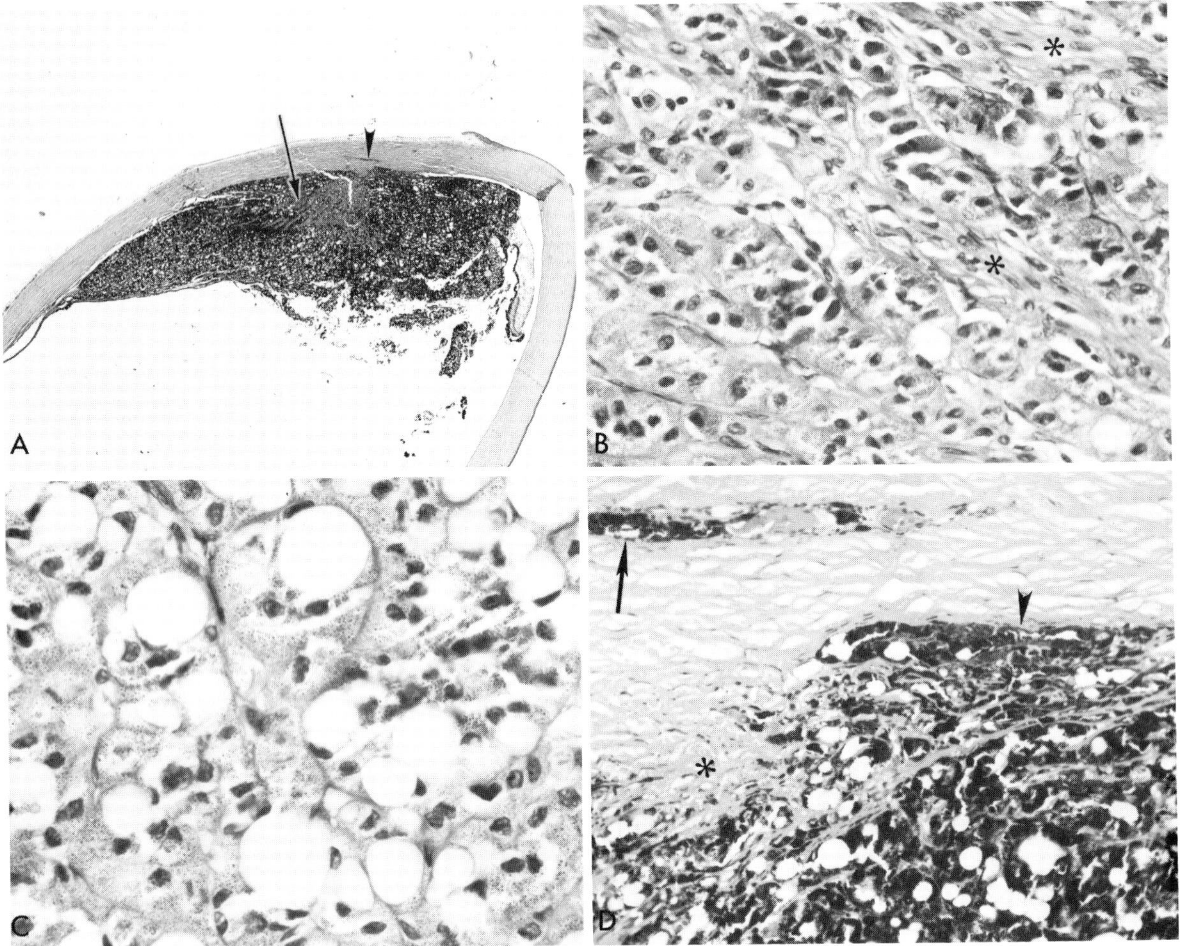

Figure 8–576. Cystic adenoma of pigmented ciliary epithelium from a 44 year old woman. *A*, Tumor infiltrates pars plana, periphery of iris, and ciliary muscles (arrow) and extends along an outflow channel (arrowhead). H and E, ×11. *B*, Bundles of smooth muscle (asterisks) are separated by tumor apparently arranged in a tubuloacinar-like pattern. Partially bleached; H and E, ×450. *C*, Higher-power view of area, showing microcysts and tumor cells with relatively large spherical pigment granules. Partially bleached; H and E, ×550. *D*, Anterior chamber angle showing extension of tumor into trabecular meshwork, Schlemm's canal (arrowhead), and outflow channel (arrow). Asterisk, scleral spur. H and E, ×205. EP 45675.

microvilli and occasional cilia (Streeten, McGraw, 1972).

These tumors are benign but may be locally invasive (Fig. 8–576). Theoretically, adenocarcinomas can occur if there are sufficient anaplastic features, mitotic activity, and invasiveness. Apparently, tumors containing both pigmented and nonpigmented cells may occur; these have cytologic features that range from a benign adenoma to adenocarcinoma.

Acknowledgments

I would like to thank the following persons for their help in the preparation of this chapter: Drs. Paul Henkind and William Spencer for critical reviews, Ms. Marcia Kelley for typing and editing, Mr. David Andrews for editorial assistance, Dr. Marilyn Kincaid for several efforts, Dr. Joseph Calkins for the light toxicity section, Drs. Rhodes Stevens and Brian Curtin for the myopia section, Dr. Bronwyn Bateman for the section on Usher's syndrome, Dr. Frank O'Donnell for the albinism section, and Mr. Peter Lund for photographic assistance.

References

Aaberg TM, Blair CJ, Gass JDM: Macular holes. Am J Ophthalmol *69*:555–562, 1970.

Aaberg TM, Cesarz TJ, Rytel MW: Correlation of virology and clinical course of cytomegalovirus retinitis. Am J Ophthalmol *74*:407–415, 1972.

Aaberg TM, Stevens TR: Snail-track degeneration of the retina. Am J Ophthalmol *73*:370–376, 1972.

Abul-Haj SK, Martz, DG, Douglas WF, Geppert LJ: Farber's disease: Report of a case with observations on its histogenesis and notes on the nature of the stored material. J Pediatr *61*:221–232, 1962.

Ackerman AL: The ocular manifestations of Waldenström's macroglobulinemia and its treatment. Arch Ophthalmol *67*:701–707, 1962.

Addison DJ: Glioneuroma of ciliary body and iris in a 20-year-old girl. Case presented at the Seventh Biennial Meeting of the Association of Ophthalmic Alumni, Armed Forces Institute of Pathology, June, 1977, Washington, DC.

Addison DJ, Font RL, Manschot WA: Proliferative retinopathy in anencephalic babies. Am J Ophthalmol *74*:967–976, 1972.

Addison DJ, Garner A, Ashton N: Degeneration of intramural pericytes in diabetic retinopathy. Br Med J *1*:264–266, 1970.

Aicardi J, Castelein P: Infantile neuroaxonal dystrophy. Brain *102*:727–748, 1979.

Akstein RB, Wilson LA, Teutsch SM: Acquired toxoplasmosis. Ophthalmology *89*:1299–1301, 1982.

Albert DM, Bullock JD, Lahav M, Caine R: Flecked retina secondary to oxalate crystals from methoxyflurane anesthesia: Clinical and experimental studies. Trans Am Acad Ophthalmol Otolaryngol *79*:817–826, 1975.

Alexander RL, Shea M: Wagner's disease. Arch Ophthalmol *74*:310–318, 1965.

Allen RA, Straatsma BR: Ocular involvement in leukemia and allied disorders. Arch Ophthalmol *66*:490–508, 1961.

Alström CH, Hallgren B, Nilsson LB, Asander H: Retinal degeneration combined with obesity, diabetes mellitus, and neurogenous deafness: A specific syndrome (not hitherto described) distinct from the Laurence-Moon-Bardet-Biedl syndrome: A clinical, endocrinological and genetic examination based on a large pedigree. Acta Psychiatr Neurol Scand *34* (Suppl 129), 1–35, 1959.

Amalric MP: Nouveau type de degénérescence tapeto-retinienne au cours de la surdimutite. Bull Soc Ophtalmol Fr *73*:196–212, 1960.

Amman F: Investigations cliniques et genetiques sur le syndrome de Bardet-Biedl en Suisse. J Genet Hum *18* (Suppl), 1–310, 1970.

Andersen SR: Medullo-epitheliomas, dictyoma and malignant epithelioma of the ciliary body. Acta Ophthalmol *26*:313–326, 1948.

Andersen SR: Medulloepithelioma of the retina, *in* Zimmerman LE (ed): Tumors of the Eye and Adnexa. Int Ophthalmol Clin *2*:483–506, 1962.

Andersen SR: Ocular pathology in hereditary (vitelliform) macular degeneration. Presented at the European Ophthalmic Pathology Society Meeting, Ghent, Belgium, May, 1970.

Andersen SR: Differentiation features in some retinal tumors and in dysplastic retinal conditions. Am J Ophthalmol *71*:231–241, 1971.

Andersen SR, Bro-Rasmussen F, Tygstrup I: Anencephaly related to ocular development and malformation. Am J Ophthalmol *64*:559–566, 1967.

Anderson JD, Lubow M: Atrial myxoma as a source of retinal embolization. Am J Ophthalmol *76*:769–772, 1973.

Annesley WH Jr: Peripheral exudative hemorrhagic chorioretinopathy. Trans Am Ophthalmol Soc *78*:321–364, 1980.

Appelbaum A: An ophthalmoscopic study of patients under treatment with thioridazine. Arch Ophthalmol *69*:578–580, 1963.

Apple DJ, Fishman GA, Goldberg MF: Ocular histopathology of Norrie's disease. Am J Ophthalmol *78*:196–203, 1974.

Apple DJ, Goldberg MF, Wyhinny GJ: Histopathology and ultrastructure of the argon laser lesion in human retinal and choroidal vasculatures. Am J Ophthalmol *75*:595–609, 1973.

Apple DJ, Wyhinny GJ, Goldberg MF, et al: Experimental argon laser photocoagulation. 1. Effects on retinal nerve fiber layer. Arch Ophthalmol *94*:137–144, 1976.

Arbisser AI, Murphree AL, Garcia CA, Howell RR: Ocular findings in mannosidosis. Am J Ophthalmol *82*:465–471, 1976.

Archambeau PL, Henderson JW: Trans-scleral freezing of the retina: An experimental study. Invest Ophthalmol *4*:885–893, 1965.

Archambeau PL, Hollenhorst RW, Rucker CW: Posterior uveitis as a manifestation of multiple sclerosis. Mayo Clin Proc *40*:544–551, 1965.

Arden GB, Fox B: Increased incidence of abnormal nasal cilia in patients with retinitis pigmentosa. Nature *279*:534–536, 1979.

Arruga J, Sanders MD: Ophthalmologic findings in 70 patients with evidence of retinal embolism. Ophthalmology *89*:1336–1347, 1982.

Arsenio-Nunes ML, Goutieres F: Diagnosis of infantile neuroaxonal dystrophy by conjunctival biopsy. J Neurol Neurosurg Psychiatry *41*:511–515, 1978.

Arsenio-Nunes ML, Goutieres F, Aicardi J: An ultramicroscopic study of skin and conjunctival biopsies in chronic neurological disorders of childhood. Ann Neurol *9*:163–173, 1981.

Artusio JF Jr, Van Poznak A, Hunt RE, et al: A clinical evaluation of methoxyflurane in man. Anesthesiology *21*:512–517, 1960.

Ascher K: Zur Histologie der Pigmentdegeneration der Netzhaut. Arch Augenheilkd *106*:585–624, 1932.

Asdourian GK, Goldberg MF, Bruce BJ: Peripheral retinal neovascularization in sarcoidosis. Arch Ophthalmol *93*:787–791, 1975.

Asdourian GK, Nagpal KC, Busse B, et al: Macular and perimacular vascular remodelling in sickling haemoglobinopathies. Br J Ophthalmol *60*:431–453, 1976.

Ashton N: Central areolar choroidal sclerosis: A histopathologic study. Br J Ophthalmol *37*:140–147, 1953.

Ashton N: Diabetic retinopathy; A new approach. Lancet *2*:625–630, 1959.

Ashton N: Larval granulomatosis of the retina due to *Toxocara*. Br J Ophthalmol *44*:129–148, 1960.

Ashton N: Pathogenesis and aetiology of Eales's disease. ACTA XIX Concilium Ophthalmologicum *2*:828–840, 1962.

Ashton N: Studies of the retinal capillaries in relation to diabetic and other retinopathies. Br J Ophthalmol *47*:521–538, 1963.

Ashton N: Pathological and ultrastructural aspect of the cotton-wool spot. Proc Roy Soc Med *62*:1271–1276, 1969.

Ashton N: Pathophysiology of retinal cotton-wool spots. Br Med Bull *26*:143–150, 1970.

Ashton N: The eye in malignant hypertension. Trans Acad Ophthalmol Otolaryngol *76*:17–40, 1972.

Ashton N, Coomes EN, Garner A, Oliver DO: Retinopathy due to progressive systemic sclerosis. J Pathol Bacteriol *96*:259–268, 1968.

Ashton N, Cunha-Vaz JG: Cytomegalic inclusion disease in the adult retina. Arch Port Oftalmol *18* (Suppl 39):39–50, 1966.

Ashton N, Dollery CT, Henkind P, et al: Focal retinal ischaemia: Ophthalmoscopic, circulatory and ultrastructural changes. Br J Ophthalmol *50*:281–384, 1966.

Ashton N, Graymore C, Pedler C: Studies on developing retinal vessels. V. Mechanism of vaso-obliteration. A preliminary report. Br J Ophthalmol *41*:449–460, 1957.

Ashton N, Harry J: The pathology of cotton-wool spots and cytoid bodies in hypertensive retinopathy and other diseases. Trans Ophthalmol Soc UK *83*:91–114, 1963.

Ashton N, Kok D'A, Foulds WS: Ocular pathology in macroglobulinaemia. J Pathol Bacteriol *86*:453–461, 1963.

Ashton N, Sorsby A: Fundus dystrophy with unusual features: A histological study. Br J Ophthalmol *35*:751–764, 1951.

Ashton N, Ward B, Serpell G: Role of oxygen in the genesis of retrolental fibroplasia. Br J Ophthalmol *37*:513–520, 1953.

Atkinson A, Sanders MD, Wong V: Vitreous haemorrhage in tuberous sclerosis: Report of two cases. Br J Ophthalmol *57*:773–779, 1973.

Audoueineix E: Les complications oculaires des richettsioses dans la Sarthe. Bull Soc Ophtalmol Fr *73*:477–490, 1960.

Austin J: Metachromatic leukodystrophy (sulfatide lipidosis), *in* Hers HO, Van Hoof F (eds): Lysosomes and Storage Disease. New York, Academic Press, 1973, pp 411–437.

Austin P, Green WR, Sallyer DC, et al: Peripheral corneal degeneration and occlusive vasculitis in Wegener's granulomatosis. Am J Ophthalmol *85*:311–317, 1978.

Avendano J, Rodrigues MM, Hackett JJ, Gaskins R: Corpora amylacea of the optic nerve and retina: A form of neuronal degeneration. Invest Ophthalmol Vis Sci *19*:550–555, 1980.

Avendano J, Tanishima T, Kuwabara T: Ocular cryptococcosis. Am J Ophthalmol *86*:110–113, 1978.

Azar P Jr, Gohd RS, Waltman D, Gitter KA: Acute posterior multifocal placoid pigment epitheliopathy associated with an adenovirus type 5 infection. Am J Ophthalmol *80*:1003–1005, 1975.

Baarsma GS: Acquired medullated nerve fibres. Br J Ophthalmol *64*:651, 1980.

Babel J: Le role de la choriocapillaire dans les affections degeneratives du pole posterieur. Bull Soc Ophtalmol Fr *71*:389–399, 1958.

Babel J: Constatations histogiques dans l'amaurose infantile de Leber et dans diverses formes d'hemeralopie [Histological findings in Leber's infantile amaurosis and in different forms of hemeralopia]. Ophthalmologica *145*:399–402, 1963.

Babel J: Retinopathie due à la chloroquine. Ophthalmologica *152*:74–79, 1966.

Babel J, Englert U: Étude experimentale de la retinopathie par chloroquine. Bull Soc Ophtalmol Fr *82*:491–505, 1969.

Badtke G, Domke H: Klinisch-histologischer Beitrag zur formalen Genese und Entwicklungsphysiologie der Ablatio falciformis congenita. Klin Monatsbl Augenheilkd *149*:593–609, 1966.

Bagan SM, Hollenhorst RW: Radiation retinopathy after irradiation of intracranial lesions. Am J Ophthalmol *88*:694–697, 1979.

Baghdassarian SA, Crawford JB, Rathbun JE Jr: Calcific emboli of the retina and ciliary arteries. Am J Ophthalmol *69*:372–375, 1970.

Bagolini B, Ioli-Spada G: Bietti's tapetoretinal degeneration with marginal corneal dystrophy. Am J Ophthalmol *65*:53–60, 1968.

Baker EM, Saari JC, Tolbert BM: Ascorbic acid metabolism in man. Am J Clin Nutr *19*:371–378, 1966.

Ball CJ: Atheromatous embolism to the brain, retina and choroid. Arch Ophthalmol *76*:690–695, 1966.

Ballowitz L, Dämmrich K: Retinaschäden bei Ratten nach einer Fototherapie. Z Kinderheilkd *113*:42–53, 1972.

Barnard RI, Scholz RO: Ophthalmoplegia and retinal degeneration. Am J Ophthalmol *27*:621–624, 1944.

Barr CC, Green WR, Payne JW, et al: Intraocular reticulum cell sarcoma: Clinicopathologic study of four cases and review of literature. Surv Ophthalmol *19*:224–239, 1975.

Barrow RH, Stallard HB: A case of primary melano-carcinoma of the ciliary body. Br J Ophthalmol *16*:98–102, 1932.

Barry DR, Kesby BR, Rubinstein K: Pathological aspects of retinal cryopexy in the rabbit. Proc Roy Soc Med *59*:1070–1072, 1966.

Bartholomew RS: Subretinal cysticercosis. Am J Ophthalmol *79*:670–673, 1975.

Bartsocas C, Gröbe H, van de Kamp JJ, et al: Sanfilippo type C disease: Clinical findings in four patients with a new variant of mucopolysaccharidosis III. Eur J Pediatr *130*:251–258, 1979.

Bassen FA, Kornzweig AL: Malformation of the erythrocytes in a case of atypical retinitis pigmentosa. Blood *5*:381–387, 1950.

Bastek JV, Siegel EB, Straatsma BR, Foos RY: Chorioretinal juncture. Pigmentary patterns of the peripheral fundus. Ophtalmology *89*:1455–1463, 1982.

Bateman JB, Foos RY: Coronal adenomas. Arch Ophthalmol *97*:2379–2384, 1979.

Bateman JB, Riedner EO, Levin LS, Maumenee IH: Heterogeneity of retinal degeneration and hearing impairment syndromes. Am J Ophthalmol *90*:755–767, 1980.

Bathrick ME, Mango CA, Mueller JF: Intraocular gnathostomiasis. Ophthalmology *88*:1293–1295, 1981.

Baum JL, Tannenbaum M, Kolodny EH: Refsum's syndrome with corneal involvement. Am J Ophthalmol *60*:699–708, 1965.

Beatty CW, McDonald TJ, Colvard DM: Usher's syndrome with unusual otologic manifestations. Mayo Clin Proc *54*:543–546, 1979.

Bec P, Arne JL, Philippot V, et al: L'uveo-retinite basale (uveite peripherique, cyclite posterieure chronique, pars planite, vitrite, hyalo-retinite) et les autres inflammations de la peripherie retinienne. Arch Ophtalmol (Paris) *37*:169–196, 1977.

Bec P, Ravault M, Arne JL, Trepsat C: La peripherie du fond d'oeil. Societé Française d'Ophtalmologie. Paris, Masson, 1979.

Bec P, Secheyron P, Arne JR, Aubry P: La neovascularisation sous-retienne peripherique et ses consequences pathologiques. J Fr Ophtalmol *2*:329–336, 1979.

Bedoya V, Grimley PM, Duque O: Chediak-Higashi syndrome. Arch Pathol *88*:340–349, 1969.

Behçet H: Über rezidivierende Aphthöse, durch ein Virus verursachte Geschwüre am Mund, am Auge und an den Genitalien. Dermatol Wochenschr *105*:1152–1157, 1937.

Behr C: Die Heredodegeneration der Makula. Klin Monatsbl Augenheilkd *65*:465–505, 1920.

Behr C: Die Anatomie der "senilen Makula" (der senilen Form der makularen Heredodegeneration). Klin Monatsbl Augenheilkd *67*:551–564, 1921.

Bellhorn RW, Friedman AH, Henkind P: Racemose (cirsoid) hemangioma in rhesus monkey retina. Am J Ophthalmol *74*:517–525, 1972.

Bellhorn RW, Friedman AH, Wise GN, Henkind P: Ultrastructure and clinicopathologic correlation of idiopathic preretinal macular fibrosis. Am J Ophthalmol *79*:366–373, 1975.

Bengtsson B, Linder B: Sex-linked hereditary juvenile retinoschisis: Presentation of two affected families. Acta Ophthalmol *45*:411–423, 1967.

Benke PJ, Reyes PF, Parker JC Jr: New form of adrenoleukodystrophy. Hum Genet *58*:204–208, 1981.

Berger BB, Weinberg RS, Tessler HH, et al: Bilateral cytomegalovirus panuveitis after high-dose corticosteroid therapy. Am J Ophthalmol *88*:1020–1025, 1979.

Bergsma DR, Kaiser-Kupfer M: A new form of albinism. Am J Ophthalmol *77*:837–844, 1974.

Berkow JW, Font RL: Disciform macular degeneration with subpigment epithelial hematoma. Arch Ophthalmol *82*:51–56, 1969.

Bernstein HN: Chloroquine ocular toxicity. Surv Ophthalmol *12*:415–447, 1967.

Bernstein HN: Some iatrogenic ocular diseeases from systemically administered drugs. Int Ophthalmol Clin *10*:553–587, 1970.

Bernstein HN, Ginsberg J: The pathology of chloroquine retinopathy. Arch Ophthalmol *71*:238–245, 1964.

Bessiere E, Chabot J, Verin P: Sur une association de maladie de Stargardt, d'atrophie optique et d'hérédodegénérescence spino-ponto-cerebelleuse. Bull Soc Ophtalmol Fr *75*:285–293, 1962.

Betten MG, Bilchik RC, Smith ME: Pigmentary retinopathy of myotonic dystrophy. Am J Ophthalmol *72*:720–723, 1971.

Bietti G: Über familiäres Vorkommen von "Retinitis punctata albescens" (verbunden mit "Dystrophia Marginalis cristallinea Corneae"), Glitzern des Glaskörpers und anderen degenerativen Augenveränderungen. Klin Mbl Augenheilk *99*:737–756, 1937.

Bietti GB, Bruna F: An ophthalmic report on Behçet's disease. International Symposium on Behçet's Disease. Basel/New York, Karger, 1966, pp 79–110.

Biglan AW, Glickman LT, Lobes LA Jr: Serum and vitreous *Toxocara* antibody in nematode endophthalmitis. Am J Ophthalmol *88*:898–901, 1979.

Birch-Hirschfeld A: Die Wirkung der ultravioletten Strahlen auf das Auges. Albrecht Von Graefes Arch Klin Exp Ophthalmol *58*:469, 1904.

Birch-Hirschfeld A: Weiterer Beitrag zur Kenntnis der Schädigung des Auges durch ultraviolettes Licht. Z Augenheilkd *20*:1–30, 1908.

Bird AC, Anderson J, Fuglsang H: Morphology of posterior segment lesions of the eye in patients with onchocerciasis. Br J Ophthalmol *60*:2–20, 1976.

Birndorf LA, Dawson WW: A normal electro-oculogram in a

patient with a typical vitelliform macular lesion. Invest Ophthalmol *2*:830–833, 1973.

Blair CJ: Geographic atrophy of the retinal pigment epithelium. A manifestation of senile macular degeneration. Arch Ophthalmol *93*:19–25, 1975.

Blair NP, Albert DM, Liberfarb RM, Hirose T: Hereditary progressive arthro-ophthalmopathy of Stickler. Am J Ophthalmol *88*:876–888, 1979.

Blair NP, Trempe CL: Hypertrophy of the retinal pigment epithelium associated with Garner's syndrome. Am J Ophthalmol *90*:661–667, 1980.

Blaw ME: Melanodermic-type leukodystrophy (adrenoleukodystrophy), *in* Vinken PJ, Bruyn GW (eds): Handbook of Clinical Neurology. Vol 10. Amsterdam, Elsevier, 1971, pp. 128–133.

Bloch FJ: Retinal tumor associated with neurofibromatosis. Arch Ophthalmol *40*:433–437, 1948.

Blodi FC: The pathology of central tapetoretinal dystrophy (hereditary macular degenerations). Trans Am Acad Ophthalmol Otolarngol *70*:1047–1053, 1966.

Blodi FC, Hervouet F: Syphilitic chorioretinitis. Arch Ophthalmol *79*:294–296, 1968.

Blodi FC, Hunter WS: Norrie's disease in North America. Doc Ophthalmol *26*:434–450, 1969.

Blodi FC, Reuling FH, Sornson ET: Pseudomelanocytoma of the optic nerve head: An adenoma of the retinal pigment epithelium. Arch Ophthalmol *73*:353–355, 1965.

Boeck J: Zur Klinik und Anatomie der gefässähnlichen Streifen im Augenhintergrund. Z Augenheilkd *95*:1–50, 1938.

Boehme DH, Cottrell JC, Leonberg SC, Zeman W: A dominant form of neuronal ceroid-lipofuscinosis. Brain *94*:745–760, 1971.

Böhringer HR, Dieterle P, Landolt E: Zur Klinik und Pathologie der Degeneratio hyaloideo-retinalis hereditaria (Wagner). Ophthalmologica *139*:330–338, 1960.

Böke W, Bäumer A: Klinische und histopathologische Augenbefunde beim akuten Lupus erythematodes disseminatus. Klin Monatsbl Augenheilkd *146*:175–187, 1965.

Böke W, Bäumer A, Müller-Limmroth W, Mludek M: Zur Frage der Chloroquinschädigung des Auges. Klin Monatsbl Augenheilkd *151*:617–633, 1967.

Bonamour G, Bonnet M: Les manifestations ocularies des rickettsioses atypiques et monosymptomatiques. Riv Ital Trac *15*:119–144, 1963.

Boniuk M, Hill LL: Ocular manifestations of de Toni-Fanconi syndrome with cystine storage disease. South Med J *59*:33–40, 1966.

Boniuk M, Zimmerman LE: Problems in differentiating idiopathic serous detachments from solid retinal detachments. Int Ophthalmol Clin *2*:411–430, 1962.

Boniuk M, Zimmerman LE: Pathological anatomy of complications, *in* Schepens CL, Regan C (eds): Controversial Aspects of the Management of Retinal Detachment. Boston, Little, Brown, 1965, pp 263–311.

Boniuk M, Zimmerman LE: Ocular pathology in the rubella syndrome. Arch Ophthalmol *77*:455–473, 1967.

Boniuk V, Boniuk M: The incidence of phthisis bulbi as a complication of cataract surgery in the congenital rubella syndrome. Trans Am Acad Ophthalmol Otolaryngol *74*:360–368, 1970.

Borley WE, Miller WW: Wegener's granulomatosis. Trans Am Acad Ophthalmol Otolaryngol *65*:316–323, 1961.

Bornstein JS, Frank MI, Radner DB: Conjunctival biopsy in the diagnosis of sarcoidosis. N Engl J Med *267*:60–64, 1962.

Bos PJM, Deutman AF: Acute macular neuroretinopathy. Am J Ophthalmol *80*:573–584, 1975.

Bourquin J: Les malformations du nouveau-né, causée par les viroses de la grossesse et plus particulierement par la rubéole (embryopathie rubéolense). Paris, Le François, 1948.

Bowen P, Ferguson-Smith MA, Mosier D, et al: The Laurence-Moon syndrome: Association with hypogonadotrophic hypogonadism and sex-chromosome aneuploidy. Arch Intern Med *116*:598–604, 1965.

Bowen P, Lee CSN, Zellweger H, Lindenberg R: A familial syndrome of multiple congenital defects. Bull Johns Hopkins Hosp *114*:402–414, 1964.

Brady HR, Israel MR, Lewin WH: Wegener's granulomatosis and corneoscleral ulcer. JAMA *193*:248, 1965.

Brain L, Croft PB, Wilkinson M: Motor neurone disease as a manifestation of neoplasm. Brain *88*:479–500, 1965.

Brain WR, Wilkinson M: Subacute cerebellar degeneration associated with neoplasms. Brain *88*:465–478, 1965.

Bresnick GH, Davis MD, Myers FL, e al: Clinicopathologic correlations in diabetic retinopathy. II. Clinical and histologic appearances of retinal capillary microaneurysms. Arch Ophthalmol *95*:1215–1220, 1977.

Bresnick GH, Engerman R, Davis MD, et al: Patterns of ischemia in diabetic retinopathy. Trans Am Acad Ophthalmol Otolaryngol *81*:694–709, 1976.

Bresnick GH, Gay AJ: Rubeosis iridis associated with branch retinal arteriolar occlusions. Arch Ophthalmol *77*:176–180, 1967.

Bresnick GH, Haight B, de Venecia G: Retinal wrinkling and macular heterotopia in diabetic retinopathy. Arch Ophthalmol *97*:1890–1895, 1979.

Bridges CDB, Alvarez RA: Selective loss of 11-*cis* vitamin A in an eye with hereditary chorioretinal degeneration similar to sector retinitis pigmentosa. Retina *2*:256–260, 1982.

Brihaye-Van Geertruyden M: Discussion. Bull Mem Soc Fr Ophtalmol *75*:291–292, 1962.

Brihaye-Van Geertruyden M, Danis P, Toussaint C: Fundus lesions with disseminated lupus erythematosus. Arch Ophthalmol *51*:799–810, 1954.

Brindley GS: The effects on colour vision of adaptation to very bright lights. J Physiol *122*:332–350, 1953.

Brockhurst RJ: Optic pits and posterior retinal detachment. Trans Am Ophthalmol Soc *73*:264–291, 1975.

Brockhurst RJ, Albert DM, Zakov ZN: Pathologic findings in familial exudative vitreoretinopathy. Arch Ophthalmol *99*:2143–2146, 1981.

Brockhurst RJ, Chishti MI: Cicatricial retrolental fibroplasia: Its occurrence without oxygen administration and in full-term infants. Albrecht Von Graefes Arch Klin Exp Ophthalmol *195*:113–128, 1975.

Brockhurst RJ, Schepens CL, Okamura ID: Uveitis. III. Peripheral uveitis: Pathogenesis, etiology and treatment. Am J Ophthalmol *51*:19–26, 1961.

Brodrick JD, Dark AJ: Corneal dystrophy in Cockayne's syndrome. Br J Ophthalmol *57*:391–399, 1973.

Broughton WL, Zimmerman LE: A clinicopathologic study of 56 cases of intraocular medulloepithelioma. Am J Ophthalmol *85*:407–418, 1978.

Brown FR III, McAdams AJ, Cummins JW, Cerebro-hepato-renal (Zellweger) syndrome and neonatal adrenoleukodystrophy: Similarities in phenotype and accumulation of very long chain fatty acids. Johns Hopkins Med J *151*:344–351, 1982.

Brown DH: Ocular *Toxocara canis*. J Pediatr Ophthalmol *7*:182–191, 1970.

Brown GC, Magargal LE, Shields JA, et al: Retinal arterial obstruction in children and young adults. Ophthalmology *88*:18–25, 1981.

Brown GC, Shields JA, Goldberg RE: Congenital pits of the optic nerve head. II. Clinical studies in humans. Ophthalmology *87*:51–65, 1980.

Brown GC, Shields JA, Patty E, Goldberg RE: Congenital pits of the optic nerve head. I. Experimental studies in collie dogs. Arch Ophthalmol *97*:1341–1344, 1979.

Brown GC, Shields JA, Sanborn G, et al: Radiation retinopathy. Ophthalmology *89*:1494–1501, 1982.

Brownstein S, Carpenter S, Polomeno RC, Little JM: Sandhoff's disease (GM_2 gangliosidosis, Type 2); Histopathology and ultrastructure of the eye. Arch Ophthalmol *98*:1089–1097, 1980.

Brownstein S, Font RL, Alper MG: Atheromatous plaques of the retinal blood vessels. Arch Ophthalmol *90*:49–52, 1973.

Brownstein S, Jannotta FS: Sarcoid granulomas of the optic nerve and retina: Report of a case. Can J Ophthalmol *9*:372–378, 1974.

Brownstein S, Kirkham TH, Kalousek DK: Bilateral renal agenesis with multiple congenital ocular abnormalities. Am J Ophthalmol *82*:770–774, 1976.

Brownstein S, Meagher-Villemure K, Polomeno RC, Little JM: Optic nerve in globoid leukodystrophy (Krabbe's disease). Arch Ophthalmol *96*:864–870, 1978.

Brubaker RF, Wong VG, Schulman JD, et al: Benign cystinosis. Am J Med *49*:546–550, 1970.

Brucker AJ: Disk and peripheral retinal neovascularization secondary to talc and cornstarch emboli. Am J Ophthalmol *88*:864–867, 1979.

Buettner H: Congenital hypertrophy of the retinal pigment epithelium. Am J Ophthalmol *79*:177–189, 1975.

Bullock JD, Fletcher RL: Cerebrospinal fluid abnormalities in acute posterior multifocal placoid pigment epitheliopathy. Am J Ophthalmol *84*:45–49, 1977.

Burch PG, Maumenee AE: Iridocyclectomy for benign tumors of the ciliary body. Am J Ophthalmol *63*:447–452, 1967.

Burde RM, Smith ME, Black JT: Retinal artery occlusion in absence of a cherry red spot. Surv Ophthalmol *27*:181–186, 1982.

Buri JR: L'oxalose. Helv Paediatr Acta *17*(Suppl 11):1–126, 1962.

Bürki E: Ueber die Cystinkrankheit im Kleinkindesalter unter besonderer Berüchsichtigung des Augenbefundes. Ophthalmologica *101*:257–272, 1941.

Burns CA: Ocular histopathology of myotonic dystrophy. Am J Ophthalmol *68*:416–422, 1969.

Burns CA, Blodi CA, Williamson BK: Acute lymphocytic leukemia and central serous retinopathy. Trans Am Acad Ophthalmol Otolaryngol *69*:307–309, 1965.

Burns RP: Cytomegalic inclusion disease uveitis: Report of a case with isolation from aqueous humor of the virus in tissue culture. Arch Ophthalmol *61*:376–387, 1959.

Burns RP, Feeney-Burns L: Clinicomorphologic correlations of drusen of Bruch's membrane. Trans Am Ophthalmol Soc *78*:206–225, 1980.

Burns RP, Lovrien EW, Cibis AB: Juvenile sex-linked retinoschisis: Clinical and genetic studies. Trans Am Acad Ophthalmol Otolaryngol *75*:1011–1021, 1971.

Buzney SM, Frank RN, Varma SD, et al: Aldose reductase in retinal mural cells. Invest Ophthalmol *16*:392–396, 1977.

Byer NE: Clinical study of lattice degeneration of the retina. Trans Am Acad Ophthalmol Otolaryngol *69*:1064–1081, 1965.

Byer NE: Clinical study of retinal breaks. Trans Am Acad Ophthalmol Otolaryngol *71*:461–473, 1967.

Byer NE: Changes in and prognosis of lattice degeneration of the retina. Trans Am Acad Ophthalmol Otolaryngol *78*:114–125, 1974a.

Byer NE: Prognosis of asymptomatic retinal breaks. Arch Ophthalmol *92*:208–210, 1974b.

Byers B, Kimura SJ: Uveitis after death of a larva in the vitreous cavity. Am J Ophthalmol *77*:63–66, 1974.

Caine R, Albert DM, Lahav M, Bullock J: Oxalate retinopathy: An experimental model of a flecked retina. Invest Ophthalmol *14*:359–363, 1975.

Calkins JL, Hochheimer BF: Retinal light exposure during ophthalmoscopy and photography: Comparison with laser safety standards. Presented at the 36th Clinical Meeting of the Residents Association of the Wilmer Ophthalmological Institute, Baltimore, April, 1977.

Calkins JL, Hochheimer BF: Retinal light exposure from operation microscopes. Arch Ophthalmol *97*:2363–2367, 1979.

Calkins JL, Hochheimer BF, D'Anna SA: Potential hazards from specific ophthalmic devices. Vision Res *20*:1039–1053, 1980.

Calmettes MM, Deodati F, Bec P: Les hemorrhages retiniennes dans la maladie de Rendu-Osler. Bull Soc Ophthalmol Fr *58*:482–483, 1958.

Cambiaggi A: Eredofamiliarta della degenerazione a graticciata della retina. Boll Oculist *48*:36–45, 1969.

Cameron ME, Greer CH: Congenital arteriovenous aneurysm of the retina: A postmortem report. Br J Ophthalmol *52*:768–772, 1968.

Campbell FW: The influence of a low atmospheric pressure on the development of the retinal vessels in the rat. Trans Ophthalmol Soc UK *71*:287–300, 1951.

Canny CLB, Oliver GL: Fluorescein angiographic findings in familial exudative vitreoretinopathy. Arch Ophthalmol *94*:1114–1120, 1976.

Cardell BS, Starbuck MJ: Juxtapapillary hamartoma of retina. Br J Ophthalmol *45*:672–677, 1961.

Carr RE: Central areolar choroidal dystrophy. Arch Ophthalmol *73*:32–35, 1965.

Carr RE: Congenital stationary nightblindness. Trans Am Ophthalmol Soc *72*:448–487, 1974.

Carr RE: Primary retinal degenerations, *in* Duane TD (ed): Clinical Ophthalmology. Vol 3. Hagerstown, Md, Harper & Row, 1976, p 14.

Carr RE, Henkind P: Retinal findings associated with serum hyperviscosity. Am J Ophthalmol *56*:23–31, 1963.

Carr RE, Mittl RN, Noble KG: Choroidal abiotrophies. Trans Am Acad Ophthalmol Otolaryngol *79*:796–816, 1975.

Carr RE, Noble KG, Nasaduke I: Pseudoinflammatory macular dystrophy. Trans Am Ophthalmol Soc *75*:255–271, 1977.

Casini F: Il metabolismo respiratorio della retina nell'intossicazione sperimentale da chinino. Arch Ottal *46*:263–279, 1939.

Chaine G, Davies J, Kohner EM, et al: Ophthalmologic abnormalities in the hypereosinophilic syndrome. Ophthalmology *89*:1348–1356, 1982.

Chamberlain WP Jr: Ocular findings in scrub typhus. Arch Ophthalmol *48*:313–321, 1952.

Chan CC, Fishman M, Egbert PR: Multiple ocular anomalies associated with maternal LSD ingestion. Arch Ophthalmol *96*:282–284, 1978.

Chan CC, Green WR, Maumenee IH, Sack GH Jr: Ocular ultrastructural studies of two cases of the Hurler syndrome (systemic mucopolysaccharidosis I-H). Ophthalmol Paediatr Genet *2*:3–19, 1983.

Chan CC, Little HL: Infrequency of retinal neovascularization following central retinal vein occlusion. Ophthalmology *66*:256–262, 1979.

Chang M, Shields JA, Wachtel DL: Adenoma of the pigment epithelium of the ciliary body simulating a malignant melanoma. Am J Ophthalmol *88*:40–44, 1979.

Charles N: Kaposi's sarcoma of palpebral conjunctiva in a homosexual. Case presented at Eastern Ophthalmic Pathology Society, Bermuda, October, 1981.

Chawla HB, Ford MJ, Munro JF, et al: Ocular involvement in cytomegalovirus infection in a previously healthy adult. Br Med J *2*:281–282, 1976.

Chee PHY: Radiation retinopathy. Am J Ophthalmol *66*:860–865, 1968.

Chisholm IA, Dudgeon J: Pigmented paravenous retinochoroidal atrophy: Helicoid retinochoroidal atrophy. Br J Ophthalmol *57*:584–587, 1973.

Chopdar A: Annular choroidal sclerosis. Br J Ophthalmol *60*:512–516, 1976.

Christensen L, Beeman HW, Allen A: Cytomegalic inclusion disease. Arch Ophthalmol *57*:90–99, 1957.

Chumbley LC, Kearns TP: Retinopathy of sarcoidosis. Am J Ophthalmol *73*:123–131, 1972.

Chumbley LC, Robertson DM, Smith TF, Campbell RJ: Adult cytomegalovirus inclusion retinouveitis. Am J Ophthalmol *80*:807–816, 1975.

Cibis GW: Neonatal herpes simplex retinitis. Albrecht Von Graefes Arch Klin Exp Ophthalmol *196*:39–47, 1975.

Cibis GW, Flynn JT, Davis EB: Herpes simplex retinitis. Arch Ophthalmol *96*:299–302, 1978.

Cibis PA: Vitreoretinal Pathology and Surgery in Retinal Detachment. St. Louis, C.V. Mosby, 1965, p 113.

Clarkson JG: A review of angioid streaks. Personal communication, July, 1976.

Clarkson JG, Green WR: Endogenous fungal endophthalmitis, *in* Duane TD (ed): Clinical Ophthalmology. Vol 3. Hagerstown, Md, Harper & Row, 1976, pp 1–44.

Clarkson JG, Green WR, Massof D: A histopathological review of 168 cases of preretinal membrane. Am J Ophthalmol *84*:1–17, 1977.

Clayman HM, Flynn JT, Koch K, Israel C: Retinal pigment epithelial abnormalities in leukemic disease. Am J Ophthalmol *74*:416–419, 1972.

Cleasby GW, Fung WE, Shekter WB: Astrocytoma of the retina: Report of two cases. Am J Ophthalmol *64*:633–637, 1967.

Clifton F, Greer CH: Ocular changes in acute systemic lupus erythematosus. Br J Ophthalmol *39*:1–10, 1955.

Coats G: Forms of retinal disease with massive exudation. Royal London Ophthal Hosp Rep *17*:440–525, 1907/1908.

Coats G: Über Retinitis exsudativa (Retinitis haemorrhagica externa). Graefes Arch Ophthalmol *81*:275–327, 1912.

Cockayne EA: Dwarfism with retinal atrophy and deafness. Arch Dis Child *11*:1–8, 1936.

Cogan DG: Primary chorioretinal aberrations with night blindness: Pathology (Symposium). Trans Am Acad Ophthalmol Otolaryngol *54*:629–661, 1950.

Cogan DG: Development and senescence of the human retinal vasculature. Doyne Memorial Lecture. Trans Ophthalmol Soc UK *83*:465–491, 1963.

Cogan DG: Pseudoretinitis pigmentosa: Report of two traumatic cases of recent origin. Arch Ophthalmol *81*:45–53, 1969a.

Cogan DG: Retinal and papillary vasculitis, *in* Cant JS (ed): The William MacKenzie Centenary Symposium on the Ocular Circulation in Health and Disease. St. Louis, C.V. Mosby, 1969b, pp 247–270.

Cogan DG: Ocular involvement in disseminated intravascular coagulopathy. Arch Ophthalmol *93*:1–8, 1975.

Cogan GD: Immunosuppression and eye disease. First Vail lecture. Am J Ophtholmol *83*:777–788, 1977.

Cogan DG: Cytomegalic retinopathy in a homosexual. Case presented at the Verhoeff Society, Washington, DC, April, 1982.

Cogan DG, Chu FC, Gittinger J, Tychsen L: Fundal abnormalities of Gaucher's disease. Arch Ophthalmol *98*:2202–2203, 1980.

Cogan DG, Kuwabara T: Histochemistry of the retina in Tay-Sachs disease. Arch Ophthalmol *61*:414–423, 1959a.

Cogan DG, Kuwabara T: Tetrazolium studies on the retina. II. Substrate dependent patterns. J Histochem Cytochem *7*:334–341, 1959b.

Cogan DG, Kuwabara T: Ocular pathology of cystinosis. Arch Ophthalmol *63*:51–57, 1960.

Cogan DG, Kuwabara T: Capillary shunts in the pathogenesis of diabetic retinopathy. Diabetes *12*:293–300, 1963.

Cogan DG, Kuwabara T: Ocular pathology of the 13–15 trisomy syndrome. Arch Ophthalmol *72*:246–253, 1964.

Cogan DG, Kuwabara T: The sphingolipidoses and the eye. Arch Ophthalmol *79*:437–452, 1968.

Cogan DG, Kuwabara T: Tumors of the ciliary body. Int Ophthalmol Clin *2*:27–56, 1971.

Cogan DG, Kuwabara T, Hurlbut CS Jr, McMurray V: Further observations on cystinosis in the adult. JAMA *166*:1725–1726, 1958.

Cogan DG, Kuwabara T, Kinoshita J, et al: Cystinosis in an adult. JAMA *164*:394–396, 1957.

Cogan DG, Kuwabara T, Moser H: Fat emboli in the retina following angiography. Arch Ophthalmol *71*:308–313, 1964.

Cogan DG, Kuwabara T, Moser H: Metachromatic leukodystrophy. Ophthalmologica *160*:2–17, 1970.

Cogan DG, Kuwabara T, Moser H, Hazard GW: Retinopathy in a case of Farber's lipogranulomatosis. Arch Ophthalmol *75*:752–757, 1966.

Cogan DG, Kuwabara T, Richardson EP, Lyon G: Histochemistry of the eye in metachromatic leukoencephalopathy. Arch Ophthalmol *60*:397–402, 1958.

Cogan DG, Kuwabara T, Silbert J, et al: Calcium oxalate and calcium phosphate crystals in detached retina. Arch Ophthalmol *60*:366–371, 1958.

Cogan DG, Kuwabara T, Young GF, Knox DL: Herpes simplex retinopathy in an infant. Arch Ophthalmol *72*:641–645, 1964.

Cogan DG, Toussaint D, Kuwabara T: Rettnal vascular patterns. IV. Diabetic retinopathy. Arch Ophthalmol *66*:366–378, 1961.

Cogan DG, Wray SH: Vascular occlusions in the eye from cardiac myxomas. Am J Ophthalmol *80*:396–403, 1975.

Cohen SMZ, Brown FR, Martyn L, et al: Ocular histopathologic and biochemical studies of the cerebrohepatorenal (Zellweger) syndrome and its relationship to neonatal adrenoleukodystrophy. Am J Ophthalmol 96488–501, 1983.

Cohen SMZ, Green WR, de la Cruz ZC, et al: Ocular histopathologic studies of neonatal and childhood adrenoleukodystrophy. Am J Ophthalmol *95*:82–96, 1983.

Cole MP, Jones CTA, Todd IDH: A new anti-oestrogenic agent in late breast cancer. An early clinical appraisal of ICI 46474. Br J Cancer *25*:270–275, 1971.

Collins ET: A pathological report upon a case of Doyne's choroiditis ("honeycomb" or "family" choroiditis). Ophthalmoscope *11*:537–538, 1913.

Collins GH, Cowden RR, Nevis AH: Myoclonus epilepsy with Lafora bodies. Arch Pathol *86*:239–254, 1968.

Collis WJ, Cohen DN: Rubella retinopathy: A progressive disorder. Arch Ophthalmol *84*:33–35, 1970.

Colvard DM, Robertson DM, Trautmann JC: Cavernous hemangioma of the retina. Arch Ophthalmol *96*:2042–2044, 1978.

Condon PI, Serjeant GR: Ocular findings in elderly cases of homozygous sickle-cell disease in Jamaica. Br J Ophthalmol *60*:361–364, 1976.

Conn H, Green WR, De La Cruz Z: Scleropachynis maculopathy. Arch Ophthalmol *100*:793–799, 1982.

Connell MM, Poley BJ, McFarlane JR: Chorioretinopathy associated with thioridazine therapy. Arch Ophthalmol *71*:816–821, 1964.

Connor DH, Morrison NE, Kerdel-Vegas F: Onchocerciasis: Onchocercal dermatitis, lymphodermatitis and elephantiasis in the Ubangi Territory. Hum Pathol *1*:553–579, 1970.

Constable IJ: Pathology of vitreous membrane and effect of haemorrhage and new vessels on the vitreous. Trans Ophthalmol Soc UK *95*:382–386, 1975.

Constable IJ, Tolentino FI, Donovan RH, Schepens CL: Clinico-pathologic correlation of vitreous membranes, *in* Pruett RC, Regan CDJ (eds): Retina Congress. New York, Appleton-Century-Crofts, 1974, pp 245–257.

Cook GR, Knobloch WH: Autosomal recessive vitreoretinopathy and encephaloceles. Am J Ophthalmol *94*:18–25, 1982.

Coppeto J, Lessel S: Retinopathy in systemic lupus erythematosus. Arch Ophthalmol *95*:794–797, 1977.

Cordes FC: A type of foveomacular retinitis observed in the U.S. Navy. Am J Ophthalmol *27*:803–816, 1944.

Cordier J, Grignon G, Vidailhet M, Rasiller A: Une forme particuliere d'idiotie amaurotique du premier age: La maladie de Sandhoff au gangliosidose à GM_2 de Type 2. Bull Mem Soc Ophtalmol *87*:238–242, 1976.

Cortin P, Corriveau LA, Rousseau AP, et al: Maculopathie en paillettes d'or. Can J Ophthalmol *17*:103–106, 1982.

Cox F, Meyer D, Hughes WT: Cytomegalovirus in tears from patients with normal eyes and with acute cytomegalovirus chorioretinitis. Am J Ophthalmol *80*:817–824, 1975.

Cox MS, Schepens CL, Freeman HM: Retinal detachment due to ocular contusion. Arch Ophthalmol *76*:679–685, 1966.

Craig EL, Suie T: *Histoplasma capsulatum* in human ocular tissue. Arch Ophthalmol *91*:285–289, 1974.

Crandell WB, Pappas SG, McDonald A: Nephrotoxicity associated with methoxyflurane anesthesia. Anesthesiology *27*:591–607, 1966.

Crawford JB: Potter's syndrome. Case presented at Verhoeff Society meeting, Silver Spring, Md, April 1983.

Criswick VG, Schepens CL: Familial exudative vitreoretinopathy. Am J Ophthalmol *68*:578–594, 1969.

Croft PB, Wilkinson M: The incidence of carcinomatous neu-

romyopathy in patients with various types of carcinoma. Brain *88*:427–434, 1965.
Cross H: Personal communication, 1973.
Crouch ER Jr, Goldberg MF: Retinal periarteritis secondary to syphilis. Arch Ophthalmol *93*:384–387, 1975.
Croxatto JO, Zimmerman LE: Malignant nonpigmented intraocular tumors of neuroectodermal origin in adults: A review of 21 cases. Personal communication, April, 1981.
Cuendet JF, Magnenat P: Symptomatologie oculaire de la maladie de Rendu-Osler. Schweiz Med Wochenschr *83*:1531–1533, 1953.
Culbertson WW, Blumenkranz MS, Haines H, et al: The acute retinal necrosis syndrome. Part 2: Histopathology and etiology. Ophthalmology *89*:1317–1325, 1982.
Culler AM: Fundus changes in leukemia. Trans Am Ophthalmol Soc *49*:445–473, 1951.
Cunningham M, Godfrey S, Moffat WMV: Cockayne's syndrome and emphysema. Arch Dis Child *53*:722–725, 1978.
Curran RE, Robb RM: Isolated foveal hypoplasia. Arch Ophthalmol *94*:48–50, 1976.
Curtin BJ: Myopia: A review of its etiology, pathogenesis, and treatment. Surv Ophthalmol *15*:1–17, 1970.
Curtin BJ: The posterior staphyloma of pathologic myopia. Trans Am Ophthalmol Soc *75*:67–86, 1977.
Curtin BJ: Personal communication, February, 1981.
Curtin BJ, Iwamoto T, Renaldo DP: Normal and staphylomatous sclera of high myopia: An electron microscopic study. Arch Ophthalmol *97*:912–915, 1979.
Curtin BJ, Karlin DB: Axial length measurements and fundus changes of the myopic eye. Am J Ophthalmol *71*:42–53, 1971.
Curtin BJ, Teng CC: Scleral changes in pathological myopia. Trans Am Acad Ophthalmol Otolaryngol *62*:777–790, 1958.
Curtin VT: Subretinal *Cysticercus*. Case presented at Verhoeff Society, Washington, DC, April, 1970.
Curtin VT: Case presentation at Association of Ophthalmic Alumni of the Armed Forces Institute of Pathology, June, 1973.
Curtin VT: Kaposi's sarcoma and cytomegalic retinitis. Case presented at the Verhoeff Society, Washington, DC, April, 1982.
Curtin VT, Fujino T, Norton EWD: Comparative histopathology of cryosurgery and photocoagulation. Observations on the advantages of cryosurgery in retinal detachment operations. Arch Ophthalmol *75*:674–682, 1966.
Cutler WM, Blatt IM: The ocular manifestations of lethal midline granuloma (Wegener's granulomatosis). Am J Ophthalmol *41*:21–35, 1956.
Cypress RH, Karol MH, Zidian JL, et al: Larva-specific antibodies in patients with visceral larva migrans. J Infect Dis *135*:633–640, 1977.
Dahrling BE II: The histopathology of early central retinal artery occlusion. Arch Ophthalmol *73*:506–510, 1965.
Daicker B: Lineare Degenerationen des peripheren retinalen Pigmentepithels. Albrecht Von Graefes Arch Klin Exp Ophthalmol *186*:1–12, 1973.
Daicker B, Eisner G: Pearls of the ora serrata, their clinical and pathological anatomy [Die Drusen der Ora serrata, ihre Klinik und pathologische Anatomie]. Albrecht Van Graefes Arch Klin Exp Ophthalmol *174*:336–343, 1968.
Daily L: Biomicroscopic protrusions and irregularities of the inner retinal surface. Excerpta Medica International Congress Series No. 222, Ophthalmology. Proceedings of XXI International Congress, Mexico, DF, March, 1970a.
Daily L: Foveolar splinter and macular wisps. Arch Ophthalmol *83*:406–411, 1970b.
Daily L: Further observations on foveolar splinter and macular wisps. Arch Ophthalmol *90*:102–103, 1973.
Danis P, Toussaint D: Alterations histologiques retiniennes dans la mucopolysaccharidose type Hunter (note preliminaire). Bull Soc Belge Ophtalmol *157*:365–373, 1971.
Dark AJ, Streeten BW: Ultrastructural study of cataract in myotonia dystrophica. Am J Ophthalmol *84*:666–674, 1977.
Dark AJ, Richardson J, Howe JW: Retinal harartoma in childhood. J Pediatr Ophthalmol Strabis *15*:273–277, 1978.
Davenport SLH: Personal communication to Dr. J. Bronwyn Bateman, 1980. University of Missouri, Columbia, Mo.
Davenport SLH, Omenn GA: The heterogeneity of Usher syndrome. Abstract, Fifth International Conference on Birth Defects. Amsterdam, Excerpta Medica, 1977, pp 87–88.
David NJ, Klintworth GK, Friedberg SJ, Dillon M: Fetal atheromatous cerebral embolism associated with bright plaques in the retinal arterioles. Neurology *13*:708–713, 1963.
Davidorf FH: Thioridazine pigmentary retinopathy. Arch Ophthalmol *90*:251–255, 1973.
Davidson C, Green WR, Wong VG: Retinal atrophy induced by intravitreous colchicine. Invest Ophthalmol Vis Sci *24*:301–311, 1983.
Davies WS, Thumin M: Cavernous hemangioma of the optic disc and retina. Trans Am Acad Ophthalmol Otolaryngol *60*:217–218, 1956.
Davis DG, Smith JL: Retinal involvement in hereditary hemorrhagic telangiectasia. Arch Ophthalmol *85*:618–623, 1971.
Davis MD: Natural history of retinal breaks without detachment. Arch Ophthalmol *92*:183–194, 1974.
Davis MD, Myers FL, Engerman RL, et al: Clinical observations concerning the pathogenesis of diabetic retinopathy, *in* Goldberg MF, Fine SL (eds): Symposium on the Treatment of Diabetic Retinopathy. Public Health Service Publication 1890. Washington, DC, US Government Printing Office, 1969, pp 47–53.
Dayton GO Jr, Straatsma BR: Eales' disease and photocoagulation. Trans Pac Coast Otoophthalmol Soc Annu Meet *43*:129–148, 1962.
de Jong PTVM, de Jong JGY, de Jong–Ten Doeschate JMM, Delleman JW: Olivopontocerebellar atrophy with visual disturbances: An ophthalmologic investigation into four generations. Ophthalmology *87*:793–804, 1980.
de Juan E, Green WR, Rice TR, Erozan YS: Optic disc neovascularization associated with ocular involvement in acute lymphocytic leukemia. Retina *2*:61–64, 1982.
Delaney WV Jr: Presumed ocular chalcosis: A reversible maculopathy. Ann Ophthalmol *7*:378–380, 1975.
de Leon GA, Kaback MM, Elfenbein IB, et al: Juvenile dystonic lipidosis. Johns Hopkins Med J *125*:62–77, 1969.
Del Monte M, Maumenee IH, Green WR, Kenyon KR: Clinical and ocular histopathologic studies of mucopolysaccharidosis type III-A: The Sanfilippo syndrome. Arch Ophthalmal *101*:1255–1262, 1983.
Delong SL, Poley BJ, McFarlane JR: Ocular changes associated with long-term chlorpromazine therapy. Arch Ophthalmol *73*:611–617, 1965.
D'Epinay SL, Reme CE: Kongenitales Glaukom bei einem Hurler-Syndrom und einem Lowe-Syndrom: Klinische und elektronmikroskopische Befunde. Adv Ophthalmol *36*:80–89, 1978.
Desmonts G, Couvreur J, Ben Rachid MS: Le toxoplasme, la mère et l'enfant. Arch Pediatr *22*:1183–1200, 1965.
Deutman A: Benign concentric annular macular dystrophy. Am J Ophthalmol *78*:384–396, 1974.
Deutman AF, Grizzard WS: Rubella retinopathy and subretinal neovascularization. Am J Ophthalmol *85*:82–87, 1978.
Deutman AF, Jansen LMAA: Dominantly inherited drusen of Bruch's membrane. Br J Ophthalmol *54*:373–382, 1970.
Deutman AF, Klomp HJ: Rift Valley fever retinitis. Am J Ophthalmol *92*:38–42, 1981.
Deutschmann R: Über die Blendung der Netzhaut durch direktes Sonnenlicht. von Graefes Arch Ophthalmol *26*(2):241–254, 1882.
de Venecia G, Davis M, Engerman R: Clinicopathologic correlations in diabetic retinopathy. I. Histology and fluorescein angiography of microaneurysms. Arch Ophthalmol *94*:1766–1773, 1976.
De Venecia G, Zu Rhein GM, Pratt MV, Kisken W: Cytomegalic inclusion retinitis in an adult: A clinical, histopathologic, and ultrastructural study. Arch Ophthalmol *86*:44–57, 1971.
Devoe AG: Ocular fat embolism. Trans Am Ophthalmol Soc *47*:254–262, 1949.

Dhermy P: Histological study of the retina in the course of Tay-Sachs disease. Bull Soc Ophthalmol *62*:41–45, 1962 (in French).

Diabetic Retinopathy Study Research Group: Preliminary report on effects of photocoagulation therapy. Am J Ophthalmol *81*:383–396, 1976.

Diabetic Retinopathy Study Research Group: Photocoagulation treatment of proliferative diabetic retinopathy. The second report of diabetic retinopathy study findings. Ophthalmology *85*:82–106, 1978.

Diabetic Retinopathy Study Research Group: Four risk factors for severe visual loss in diabetic retinopathy. The third report from the diabetic retinopathy study. Arch Ophthalmol *97*:654–655, 1979.

Diabetic Retinopathy Study Research Group: Report 6. Design, methods, and baseline results. Invest Ophthalmol Vis Sci *21*:149–209, 1981a.

Diabetic Retinopathy Study Research Group: Report 7. A modification of the Airlie House classification of diabetic retinopathy. Invest Ophthalmol Vis Sci *21*:210–226, 1981b.

Diallinas NP: Les alterations oculaires chez les sourd-muets. J Genet Hum *8*:225–262, 1959.

Diaz D: Mas subre miopia y hipertension ocular. Arch Soc Oftalmol Hisp-AM *26*:935–941, 1966.

Diddie KR, Aronson AJ, Ernest JT: Chorioretinopathy in a case of systemic lupus erythematosus. Trans Am Ophthalmol Soc *75*:122–131, 1975.

Diddie KR, Ernest JT: The effect of photocoagulation on the choroidal vasculature and retinal oxygen tension. Am J Ophthalmol *84*:62–66, 1977.

Diddie KR, Schanzlin DJ, Mausolf FA, et al: Necrotizing retinitis caused by opportunistic virus infection in a patient with Hodgkin's disease. Am J Ophthalmol *88*:668–673, 1979.

Didion H: Die anatomischen Veränderungen des Augenhintergrundes bei der Niemann-Pickschen Krankheit. Klin Monatsbl Augenheilkd *116*:131–135, 1950.

Di Ferrante N, Hyman BH, Klish W, et al: Mucopolysaccharidosis VI (Maroteaux-Lamy disease). Clinical and biochemical study of a mild variant case. Johns Hopkins Med J *135*:42–54, 1974.

Di Sant'Agnese PA, Davis PB: Research in cystic fibrosis. N Engl J Med *295*:481–485, 535–541, 597–602, 1976.

Dixon JM, Winkler CH, Nelson JH: Ophthalmomyiasis interna caused by *Cuterebra* larva. Trans Am Ophthalmol Soc *67*:110–115, 1969.

Dodd MJ, Pusin SM, Green WR: Adult cystinosis: A case report. Arch Ophthalmol *96*:1054–1057, 1978.

Doden W: Zur Semiologie der Periphlebitis retinae. Klin Monatsbl Augenheilkd *137*:328–334, 1960.

Doft BH, Clarkson JG, Rebell G, Forster RK: Endogenous *Aspergillus* endophthalmitis in drug abusers. Arch Ophthalmol *98*:859–862, 1980.

Dollery CT: Circulatory, clinical and pathological aspects of the cotton-wool spots: Microcirculatory changes and the cotton-wool spot. Proc Roy Soc Med *62*:1267–1269, 1969.

Dollery CT, Henkind P, Paterson JW, et al: Focal retinal ischaemia. I. Ophthalmoscopic and circulatory changes in focal retinal ischaemia. Br J Ophthalmol *50*:285–324, 1966.

Dominguez-Vazquez A, Taylor HR, Greene BM, et al: Comparison of flubendazole and diethylcarbamazine in treatment of onchocerciasis. Lancet *1*:139–142, 1983.

Donders PC: Eales' disease. Doc Ophthalmol *12*:1–21, 1958.

Dooling EC, Richardson EP Jr: Ophthalmoplegia and Ondine's curse. Arch Ophthalmol *95*:1790–1793, 1977.

Dooling EC, Schoene WC, Richardson EP, Jr: Hallervorden-Spatz syndrome. Arch Neurol *30*:70–83, 1974.

Douglas AA, Waheed I, Wyse CT: Progressive bifocal chorioretinal atrophy: A rare familial disease of the eyes. Br J Ophthalmol *52*:742–751, 1968.

Dowling JE, Gibbons IR: The effect of vitamin A deficiency on the fine structure of the retina, *in* The Structure of the Eye. New York, Academic Press, 1961, pp 85–99.

Dowling JL Jr, Smith TR: An ocular study of pulseless disease. Arch Ophthalmol *64*:236–243, 1960.

Drew WL, Mintz L, Miner RC, et al: Prevalence of cytomegalovirus infection in homosexual men. J Infect Dis *143*:188–192, 1981.

Dreyer R, Green WR: The pathology of angioid streaks: A study of 21 cases. Trans Pa Acad Ophthalmol Otolaryngol *31*:158–167, 1978.

Dryden RM: Central retinal vein occlusions and chronic simple glaucoma. Arch Ophthalmol *73*:659–663, 1965.

Dryja TP, Albert DM, Horns D: Adenocarcinoma arising from the epithelium of the ciliary body. Ophthalmology *88*:1290–1292, 1981.

Duane TD: Valsalva hemorrhagic retinopathy. Am J Ophthalmol *75*:637–642, 1973.

Duane TD, Osher RH, Green WR: White centered hemorrhages: Their significance. Ophthalmology *87*:66–69, 1980.

Dubois EL (ed): Lupus Erythematosus. New York, McGraw-Hill, Blakiston Div, 1966.

Dubois EL: Primer on the rheumatic diseases. Section 8: Systemic lupus erythematosus. JAMA *224*:701–711, 1973.

Duinkerke-Eerola KU, Cruysberg JRM, Deutman AF: Atrophic maculopathy associated with hereditary ataxia. Am J Ophthalmol *90*:597–603, 1980.

Duke JR, Clark DB: Infantile amaurotic familial idiocy (Tay-Sachs disease) in the Negro race. Am J Ophthalmol *53*:800–805, 1962.

Duke JR, Maumenee AE: An unusual tumor of the retinal pigment epithelium, in an eye with early open-angle glaucoma. Am J Ophthalmol *47*:313–317, 1959.

Duke JR, Wilkinson CP, Sigelman S: Retinal microaneurysms in leukemia. Br J Ophthalmol *52*:368–374, 1968.

Duke-Elder S: System of Ophthalmology. Vol 10, Diseases of the Retina. St. Louis, C.V. Mosby, pp 373–408.

Duke-Elder S, Abrams D: Pathological myopia, *in* Duke-Elder S (ed): System of Ophthalmology. Vol 5, Ophthalmic Optics and Refraction. St. Louis, C.V. Mosby, 1970, pp 300–362.

Dumas J, Schepens CL: Chorioretinal lesions predisposing to retinal breaks. Am J Ophthalmol *61*:620–630, 1966.

Duncan C, Strub R, McGarry P, Duncan D: Peripheral nerve biopsy as an aid to diagnosis in infantile neuroaxonal dystrophy. Neurology *20*:1024–1032, 1970.

Durack DT: Opportunistic infections and Kaposi's sarcoma in homosexual men (editorial). N Engl J Med *305*:1465–1467, 1981.

Eagle RC Jr, Hedges TR, Yanoff M: The atypical pigmentary retinopathy of Kearns-Sayre. A light and electron microscopic study. Ophthalmology *89*:1433–1440, 1982.

Eagle RC Jr, Lucier AC, Bernardino VB Jr, Yanoff M: Retinal pigment epithelial abnormalities in fundus flavimaculatus. Ophthalmology *87*:1189–1200, 1980.

Edwards JE, Foos RY, Montgomerie JZ, Guze LB: Ocular manifestations of Candida septicemia: Review of seventy-six cases of hematogenous Candida endophthalmitis. Medicine *53*:47–75, 1974.

Egbert PR, Chan CC, Winter FC: Flat preparations of the retinal vessels in Coats' disease. J Pediatr Ophthalmol *13*:336–339, 1977.

Egbert PR, Pollard RB, Gallagher JG, Merigan TC: Cytomegalovirus retinitis in immunosuppressed hosts. II. Ocular manifestations. Ann Intern Med *93*:664–670, 1980.

Elfenbein IB: Dystonic juvenile idiocy without amaurosis: A new syndrome. Johns Hopkins Med J *123*:205–221, 1968.

Elliot AJ: Recurrent intraocular hemorrhage in young adults (Eales's disease): A report of 31 cases. Trans Am Ophthalmol Soc *52*:811–875, 1954.

Elliot AJ: Thirty-year observation of patients with Eales' disease. Am J Ophthalmol *80*:404–408, 1975.

Elliot JH, in discussion of Nichols CW, Eagle RC Jr, Yanoff M, Menocal NG: Conjunctival biopsy as an aid in the evaluation of the patient with suspected sarcoidosis. Ophthalmology *87*:287–291, 1980.

Elschnig A: Die diagnostiche und prognostische Bedeutung

der Netzhauterkrankungen bei Nephritis. Wien Med Wehr *54*:436, 1904.

Elwyn H: Heredodegenerations and heredoconstitutional defects of the retina. Arch Ophthalmol *53*:619–633, 1955.

Emery JM, Green WR, Huff DS: Krabbe's disease: Histopathology and ultrastructure of the eye. Am J Ophthalmol *74*:400–406, 1972.

Emery JM, Green WR, Wyllie RG, Howell RR: GM_1 gangliosidosis: Ocular and pathological manifestations. Arch Ophthalmol *85*:177–187, 1971.

Engel H, De La Cruz ZC, Jimenez-Abalahin BS, et al: Cytopreparatory techniques for eye fluid specimens obtained by vitrectomy. Acta Cytol (Baltimore), *26*:551–560, 1982.

Engel HM, Green WR, Michels RG, et al: Diagnostic vitrectomy. Retina *1*:121–149, 1981.

Epstein DL: Cystoid macular edema occurring 13 years after cataract extraction. Am J Ophthalmol *83*:501–503, 1977.

Epstein GA, Rabb MF: Adult vitelliform macular degeneration: Diagnosis and natural history. Br J Ophthalmol *64*:733–740, 1980.

Eshaghian J, Anderson RL, Weingeist TA, et al: Orbicularis oculi muscle in chronic progressive external ophthalmoplegia. Arch Ophthalmol *98*:1070–1073, 1980.

Estimated Statistics on Blind and Visual Problems. New York, National Society for Prevention of Blindness, 1966, p 44.

Evans DE, Zahorchak JA, Kennerdell JS: Visual loss as a result of primary optic nerve neuropathy after intranasal corticosteroid injection. Am J Ophthalmol *90*:641–644, 1980.

Everett WG: A family study of lattice degeneration and retinal detachment. Trans Am Ophthalmol Soc *65*:128–135, 1967.

Fair JR: Tumors of the retinal pigment epithelium. Am J Ophthalmol *45*:495–505, 1958.

Falls HF: Hereditary congenital macular degeneration. Am J Hum Genet *1*:96–104, 1949.

Faris B, Tolentino FI, Freeman HM, et al: Retrolental fibroplasia in the cicatricial stage. Arch Ophthalmol *85*:661–668, 1971.

Farkas TG: Drusen of the retinal pigment epithelium. Surv Ophthalmol *16*:75–87, 1971.

Farkas TG, Krill AE, Sylvester VM, Archer D: Familial and secondary drusen: Histologic and functional correlations. Trans Am Acad Ophthalmol Otolaryngol *75*:333–343, 1971.

Farkas TG, Sylvester V, Archer D: The choroidopathy of progressive systemic sclerosis (scleroderma). Am J Ophthalmol *74*:875–886, 1972.

Farkas TG, Sylvester V, Archer D, Altona M: The histochemistry of drusen. Am J Ophthalmol *71*:1206–1215, 1971.

Farnan P: Whipple's disease: The clinical aspects. Q J Med *28*:163–182, 1959.

Fastenberg DM, Fetkenhour CL, Choromokos E, Shoch DE: Choroidal vascular changes in toxemia of pregnancy. Am J Ophthalmol *89*:362–368, 1980.

Favre M: À propos de deux cas de degenerescence hyaloideoretinienne. Ophthalmologica (Basel) *135*:604–609, 1958.

Feeney-Burns L: The pigments of the retinal pigment epithelium, *in* Current Topics in Eye Research. New York, Academic Press, 1980, pp 119–178.

Fenton RH, Easom HA: Behçet's syndrome: A histopathologic study of the eye. Arch Ophthalmol *72*:71–81, 1964.

Ferry AP: Macular detachment associated with congenital pit of the optic nerve head: Pathologic findings in two cases simulating malignant melanoma of the choroid. Arch Ophthalmol *70*:346–357, 1963.

Ferry AP: Lesions mistaken for malignant melanoma of the posterior uvea: A clinicopathologic analysis of 100 cases with ophthalmoscopically visible lesions. Arch Ophthalmol *72*:463–469, 1964.

Ferry AP: Retinal cotton-wool spots and cytoid bodies. Mt Sinai J Med (NY) *39*:604–609, 1972.

Ferry AP: *Cysticercus cellulosae* extracted from vitreous body. Case presentation at Verhoeff Society, Washington, DC, April, 1980.

Ferry AP, Leopold IH: Marginal (ring) corneal ulcer as presenting manifestation of Wegener's granuloma: A clinicopathologic study. Trans Am Acad Ophthalmol Otolaryngol *74*:1276–1282, 1970.

Ferry AP, Llovera IL, Shafer DM: Central areolar choroidal dystrophy. Arch Ophthalmol *88*:39–43, 1972.

Fichte C, Streeten BW, Friedman AH: A histopathologic study of retinal arterial aneurysms. Am J Ophthalmol *85*:509–518, 1978.

Fielder AR, Garner A, Chambers TL: Ophthalmic manifestations of primary oxalosis. Br J Ophthalmol *64*:782–788, 1980.

Fine BS: Lipoidal degeneration of the retinal pigment epithelium. Am J Ophthalmol *91*:469–473, 1981.

Fine RN, Wilson WA, Donnell GN: Retinal changes in glycogen storage disease Type I. Am J Dis Child *115*:328–331, 1968.

Finkelstein D, Clarkson J, Diddie K, et al: Branch vein occlusion: Retinal neovascularization outside the involved segment. Ophthalmology *89*:1357–1361, 1982.

Fischbein FI: Ischemic retinopathy following amniotic fluid embolization. Am J Ophthalmol *67*:351–357, 1969.

Fischbein FI, Schub M, Lesko WS: Incontinentia pigmenti, pheochromocytoma, and ocular abnormalities. Am J Ophthalmol *73*:961–964, 1972.

Fisher JP, Lewis ML, Blumenkranz M, et al: The acute retinal necrosis syndrome: Part 1. Clinical manifestations. Ophthalmology *89*:1309–1316, 1982.

Fishman GA, Jampol LM, Goldberg MF: Diagnostic features of the Favre-Goldmann syndrome. Br J Ophthalmol *60*:345–353, 1976.

Fishman GA, Trimble S, Rabb MF, Fishman M: Pseudovitelliform macular degeneration. Arch Ophthalmol *95*:73–76, 1977.

Fitzgerald CR, Rubin ML: Intraocular parasite destroyed by photocoagulation. Arch Ophthalmol *91*:162–164, 1974.

Flick JJ: Ocular lesions following the atomic bombing of Hiroshima and Nagasaki. Am J Ophthalmol *31*:137–154, 1948.

Flocks M, Littwin CS, Zimmerman LE: Phacolytic glaucoma: Clinicopathologic study of 138 cases of glaucoma associated with hypermature cataract. Arch Ophthalmol *54*:37–45, 1955.

Flower RW: Personal communication, 1980.

Fogle JA, Green WR: Ciliochoroidal effusion, *in* Duane TD (ed): Clinical Ophthalmology. Vol 4. Hagerstown, Md, Harper & Row, 1976, pp 1–32.

Fogle JA, Welch RB, Green WR: Retinitis pigmentosa and exudative vasculopathy. Arch Ophthalmol *96*:696–702, 1978.

Font RL: Case presentation at combined meeting of Verhoeff Society and European Ophthalmic Pathology Society, London, England, April, 1971.

Font RL, Ferry AP: The phakomatoses. Int Ophthalmol Clin *12*:1–50, 1972.

Font RL, Fine BS: Ocular pathology in Fabry's disease: Histochemical and electron microscopic observations. Am J Ophthalmol *73*:419–430, 1972.

Font RL, Jenis EH, Tuck KD: Measles maculopathy associated with subacute sclerosing panencephalitis. Arch Pathol *96*:168–174, 1973.

Font RL, Naumann G: Ocular histopathology in pulseless disease. Arch Ophthalmol *82*:784–788, 1969.

Font RL, Rao NA, Issarescu S, McEntee WJ: Ocular involvement in Whipple's disease. Arch Ophthalmol *96*:1431–1436, 1978.

Font RL, Zimmerman LE, Fine BS: Adenoma of retinal pigment epithelium. Am J Ophthalmol *73*:544–554, 1972.

Fontan P, Barbancon S: Alterations vasculaires retiniennes de l'adulte jeune. Role possible des rickettsies. Bull Soc Ophtalmol Fr *73*:521–539, 1960.

Foos RY: Zonular traction tufts of the peripheral retina in cadaver eyes. Arch Ophthalmol *82*:620–632, 1969.

Foos RY: Senile retinoschisis: Relationship to cystoid degeneration. Trans Am Acad Ophthalmol Otolaryngol *74*:33–51, 1970.

Foos RY: Postoral peripheral retinal tears. Ann Ophthalmol *6*:679–687, 1974a.

Foos RY: Vitreoretinal juncture: Simple epiretinal membranes. Albrecht Von Graefes Arch Klin Exp Ophthalmol *189*:231–250, 1974b.

Foos RY: Regional ischemic infarcts of the retina. Albrecht Von Graefes Arch Klin Exp Ophthalmol *200*:183–194, 1976.

Foos RY: Surface wrinkling retinopathy, *in* Freeman HM, Hirose T, Shepens CL (eds): Vitreous Surgery and Advances in Fundus Diagnosis and Treatment. New York, Appleton-Century-Crofts, 1977, pp 23–38.

Foos RY: Retinal holes. Am J Ophthalmol *86*:354–358, 1978.

Foos RY, Allen RA: Retinal tears and lesser lesions of the peripheral retina in autopsy eyes. Am J Ophthalmol *64*:643–655, 1967.

Foos RY, Feman SS: Reticular cystoid degeneration of the peripheral retina. Am J Ophthalmol *69*:392–403, 1970.

Forni S, Babel J: Étude clinique et histologique de la malattia leventinese: Affection appartenant au groupe des dégénérescences hyalines du pole posterior [Clinical and histological study of the disease of Leventina. Disease belonging to the group of hyaline degenerescences of the posterior pole]. Ophthalmologica *143*:313–322, 1962.

Forrest A: Cytomegalic virus retinitis. Case presented at the Verhoeff Society, Washington, DC, April, 1982.

Forsius H, Eriksson AW: Ein neues Augensyndrom mit X-chromosomaler Transmission: Eine Sippe mit Fundusalbinismus, Foveahypoplasie, Nystagmus, Myopie, Astigmatismus und Dyschromatopsie. Klin Monatsbl Augenheilkd *144*:447–457, 1964.

Forsius H, Eriksson AW, Vainio-Mattila B: Geschlechtsgebundene erbliche Retinoschisis in zwei Familien in Finnland. Klin Monatsbl Augenheilkd *143*:806–816, 1963.

Fraga A, Mintz G, Valle L, Flores-Izquierdo G: Takayasu's arteritis: Frequency of systemic manifestations (study of 22 patients) and favorable response to maintenance steroid therapy with adrenocorticosteroids (12 patients). Arthritis Rheum *15*:617–624, 1972.

Franceschetti A: Ueber tapeto-retinale Degenerationen im Kindesalter, *in* Sautter H (ed): Entwicklung und Fortschritt in der Augenheilkunde. Stuttgart, Enke Verlag, 1963, pp 107–120.

Franceschetti A, François J, Babel J: Chorioretinal Heredodegenerations. Springfield, Ill, Charles C Thomas, 1974.

François J: L'angiomatose hemorragique familiale et ses complications oculaires. Arch Ophthalmol (Paris) *2*:425–432, 1938.

François J: Rickettsiae in ophthalmology. Ophthalmologica *156*:459–472, 1968.

François J, Bacskulin J, Follmann P: Manifestations oculaires du syndrome d'Urbach-Wiethe: Hyalinosis cutis et mucosae. Ophthalmologica *155*:433–448, 1968.

François J, De Becker L: Ocular manifestations of chloroquine intoxication. Ann Oculist (Paris) *198*:513–544, 1965.

François J, de Laey JJ: Biettische kristalline Fundusdystrophie. Klin Mbl Augenheilkd *170*:353–362, 1977.

François J, De Rouck A, Cambie E: Degenerescence hyaloideo-tapeto-retinienne de Goldmann-Favre. Ophthalmologica *168*:81–96, 1974.

François J, Hanssens M: A histopathological study of two cases of Leber's congenital tapetoretinal degeneration. Ann Oculist (Paris) *202*:127–155, 1969.

François J, Hanssens M, Coppieters R, et al: Cystinosis: A clinical and histopathologic study. Am J Ophthalmol *73*:643–650, 1972.

François J, Haustrate-Gosset F, Donck D: Macular dystrophy in deaf mutism. Acta Genet Med Gemellol (Rome) *16*:63–70, 1967.

François J, Mandgal MC; Experimentally induced chloroquine retinopathy. Am J Ophthalmol *64*:886–893, 1967.

François J, Rabaez M: Histopathologic examination of a bilateral symmetrical cyst of the retina. Br J Ophthalmol *37*:601–608, 1953.

Frandsen E: Hereditary hyaloideo-retinal degeneration (Wagner) in a Danish family. Acta Ophthalmol *44*:223–232, 1966.

Frangieh GT, Green WR, Barraquer-Somers E, Finkelstein D: Histopathologic study of nine branch retinal vein occlusions. Arch Ophthalmol *100*:1132–1140, 1982.

Frangieh GT, Green WR, Engel HM: A histopathologic study of macular cysts and holes. Retina, *1*:311–336, 1981.

Frangieh GT, Green WR, Engel HM: A clinicopathologic study of Best's macular dystrophy: Arch Ophthalmol *100*:1115–1121, 1982.

Frangieh GT, Green WR, Maumenee IH, et al: Fundus flavimaculatus: Clinical observations of two brothers during 38 years, and histopathologic studies in one brother. Poster at the XXIV International Congress of Ophthalmology, San Francisco, October-November, 1982.

Frank KE, Purnell EW: Subretinal neovascularization following rubella retinopathy. Am J Ophthalmol *86*:462–466, 1978.

Frank RN, Green WR, Pollack IP: Senile macular degeneration: Clinicopathologic correlations of a case in the predisciform stage. Am J Ophthalmol *75*:587–594, 1973.

Frank RN, Ryan SJ Jr: Peripheral retinal neovascularization with chronic myelogenous leukemia. Arch Ophthalmol *87*:585–589, 1972.

Fraunfelder FT, Hanna C: Electric cataracts. I. Sequential changes, unusual and prognostic findings. Arch Ophthalmol *87*:179–183, 1972.

Frenkel JK: Toxoplasmosis: Mechanisms of infection, laboratory diagnosis, and management. Curr Top Pathol *54*:28–75, 1971.

Frenkel JK, Dubey JP, Miller NL: *Toxoplasma gondii* in cats: Fecal stages identified as coccidian oocysts. Science *167*:893–896, 1970.

Friberg TR, Gragoudas ES, Regan CD: Talc emboli and macular ischemia in intravenous drug abuse. Arch Ophthalmol *9*:1089–1091, 1979.

Friedenwald JS: Massive gliosis of the retina, *in* Crisp WH and Finnoff WC (eds): Contributions to Ophthalmic Science. Dedicated to Dr. Edward Jackson. Menasha, Wis, George Banta, 1926, pp 23–28.

Friedenwald JS: Pathology of the Eye. Baltimore, Williams & Wilkins, 1929, p 187.

Friedenwald, JS: In discussion of Verhoeff FH: Microscopic observations in a case of retinitis pigmentosa. Arch Ophthalmol *4*:767–768, 1930.

Friedman AH: Cytomegalic inclusion disease in a homosexual male. Case presented at Eastern Ophthalmic Pathology Society, Bermuda, October, 1981.

Friedman AH, Charles NC: Retinal oxalosis in two diabetic patients. Am J Ophthalmol *78*:189–195, 1974.

Friedman AH, Marchevsky A, Odel JG, et al: Immunofluorescent studies of the eye in Waldenström's macroglobulinemia. Arch Ophthalmol *98*:743–746, 1980.

Friedman E, Kuwabara T: The retinal pigment epithelium. IV. The damaging effects of radiant energy. Arch Ophthalmol *80*:265–279, 1968.

Friedman E, Smith TR: Symposium: Macular Diseases. Senile changes of the choriocapillaries of the posterior pole. Trans Am Acad Ophthalmol Otolaryngol *69*:625–661, 1965.

Friedman E, Smith TR: Clinical and pathological study of choroidal lipid globules. Arch Ophthalmol *75*:334–336, 1966.

Friedman E, T'so MOM: The retinal pigment epithelium. II. Histologic changes associated with age. Arch Ophthalmol *79*:315–320, 1968.

Friedman Z, Neumann E, Hyams S: Vitreous and peripheral retina in aphakia: A study of 200 non-myopic aphakic eyes. Br J Ophthalmol *57*:52–57, 1973.

Frisen L, Hoyt WF: Insidious atrophy of the retinal nerve fibers in multiple sclerosis: Funduscopic identification in patients with and without visual complaints. Arch Ophthalmol *92*:91–97, 1974.

Fritz MH, Hogan MJ: Fat embolization involving the human eye. Am J Ophthalmol *31*:527, 1948.

Fry WE, Spaeth EB: Subacute circumscribed macular retinochoroiditis simulating intraocular tumor. Trans Am Acad Ophthalmol *59*:346–355, 1955.

Fuchs E: Über Erythropsie. Arch Ophthalmol *42*:207, 1896.

Fuchs E: Der centrale schwarze Fleck bei Myopie. Z Augenheilkd *5*:171–178, 1901.
Fuchs E: Wucherungen und Geschwülste des Ciliarepithels. Albrecht Von Graefe's Arch Ophthalmol *68*:534–587, 1908.
Fuchs E: Text-Book of Ophthalmology (translation by A. Duane). Philadelphia, J. B. Lippincott, 1923, p 705.
Fuller B, Gitter KA: Traumatic choroidal rupture with late serous detachment of macula. Arch Ophthalmol *89*:354–355, 1973.
Fulton, AB, Albert DM, Craft JL: Human albinism: Light and electron microscopic study. Arch Ophthalmol *96*:305–310, 1978.
Gabbay KH, Merola LO, Field RA: Sorbitol pathway: Presence in nerve and cord with substrate accumulation in diabetes. Science *151*:209–210, 1966.
Ganley JP, Streeten BW: Glial nodules of the inner retina. Am J Ophthalmol *71*:1109–1103, 1971.
Garner A: Tumours of the retinal pigment epithelium. Br J Ophthalmol *54*:715–723, 1970.
Garner A: Ocular pathology of GM_2 gangliosidosis Type II (Sandhoff's disease). Br J Ophthalmol *57*:514–520, 1973.
Garner A: Retinal oxalosis. Br J Ophthalmol *58*:613–619, 1974.
Garner A: Pathology of ocular onchocerciasis: Human and experimental. Trans Roy Soc Trop Med Hygiene *70*:374–377, 1976.
Garner A, Ashton N: Ultrastructure of hypertensive retinopathy. Part I. Transactions XXI Congress of Ophthalmology, Mexico, DF, 1970, 583.
Garner A, Ashton N, Tripathi R, et al: Pathogenesis of hypertensive retinopathy: An experimental study in the monkey. Br J Ophthalmol *59*:3–44, 1975.
Garner A, Fielder AR, Primavesi R, Stevens A: Tapetoretinal degeneration in the cerebro-hepato-renal (Zellweger's) syndrome. Br J Ophthalmol *66*:422–431, 1982.
Garron LK: Cystinosis. Trans Am Acad Ophthalmol Otolaryngol *63*:99–108, 1959.
Garron LK: The ultrastructure of the retinal pigment epithelium, with observations on the choriocapillaris and Bruch's membrane. Trans Am Ophthalmol Soc *61*:545, 1963.
Gärtner J: Fine structure of pars plana cysts. Am J Ophthalmol *73*:971–984, 1972.
Gartner S, Henkind P: Neovascularization of the iris (rubeosis iridis). Surv Ophthalmol *22*:291–312, 1978.
Gartner S, Henkind P: Aging and degeneration of the human macula. I. Outer nuclear layer and photoreceptors. Br J Ophthalmol *65*:23–28, 1981a.
Gartner S, Henkind P: Lange's folds: A meaningful ocular artifact. Ophthalmology *88*:1307–1310, 1981b.
Gartner S, Henkind P: Pathology of retinitis pigmentosa. Ophthalmology *89*:1425–1432, 1982.
Gass JDM: Acute posterior multifocal placoid pigment epitheliopathy. Arch Ophthalmol *80*:177–185, 1968a.
Gass JDM: A fluorescein angiographic study of macular dysfunction secondary to retinal vascular disease. V. Retinal telangiectasis. Arch Ophthalmol *80*:592–605, 1968b.
Gass JDM: Serous detachment of the macula: Secondary to congenital pit of the optic nerve head. Am J Ophthalmol *67*:821–841, 1969.
Gass JDM: Drusen and disciform macular detachment and degeneration. Trans Am Ophthalmol Soc *70*:409–436, 1972a.
Gass JDM: Options in the treatment of macular diseases. Trans Ophthalmol Soc UK *92*:449, 1972b.
Gass JDM: An unusual hamartoma of the pigment epithelium and retina simulating choroidal melanoma and retinoblastoma. Trans Am Ophthalmol Soc *71*:171–185, 1973a.
Gass JDM: Drusen and disciform macular detachment and degeneration. Arch Ophthalmol *90*:206, 1973b.
Gass JDM: Nicotinic acid maculopathy. Am J Ophthalmol *76*:500–510, 1973c.
Gass JDM: Tumors of the retinal pigment epithelium, *in* Differential Diagnosis of Intraocular Tumors: A Stereoscopic Presentation. St. Louis, C.V. Mosby, 1974a, pp 221–224.
Gass JDM: Tumors of the retinal pigment epithelium, *in* Differential Diagnosis of Intraocular Tumors: A Stereoscopic Presentation. St. Louis, C. V. Mosby, 1974b, pp 234–246.
Gass, JDM: A clinicopathologic study of a peculiar foveomacular dystrophy. Trans Am Ophthalmol Soc *72*:139–156, 1974c.
Gass JDM: Lamellar macular hole. Arch Ophthalmol *94*:793–800, 1976.
Gass JDM: Stereoscopic Atlas of Macular Disease: A Funduscopic and Angiographic Presentation. St. Louis, C.V. Mosby, 1977.
Gass JDM, Clarkson JG: Angioid streaks and disciform macular detachment in Paget's disease (osteitis deformans). Am J Ophthalmol *75*:576–586, 1973.
Gass JDM, Gilbert WR Jr, Guerry RK, Scelfo R: Diffuse unilateral subacute neuroretinitis. Trans Am. Acad Ophthalmol Otolaryngol *85*:521–545, 1978.
Gass JDM, Norton EWD: Cystoid macular edema and papilledema following cataract extraction. Arch Ophhthalmol *76*:646–661, 1966.
Gass JDM, Olson CL: Sarcoidosis with optic nerve and retinal involvement. Trans Am Acad Ophthalmol Otolaryngol *77*:739–750, 1973.
Gautier-Smith PC, Sanders MD, Sanderson KV: Ocular and nervous system involvement in angioma serpiginosum. Br J Ophthalmol *55*:433–443, 1971.
Geeraets WJ, Ham WT, Williams HA, et al: Laser vs. light coagulator: A funduscopic and histologic study of chorioretinal injury as a function of exposure time. Fed Proc *24*:S48–S61, 1965.
Genley JP, Streeten, BW: Glial nodules of the inner retina. Am J Ophthalmol *71*:1099–1103, 1971.
Gerde LS: Angioid streaks in sickle cell trait hemoglobinopathy. Am J Ophthalmol *77*:462–464, 1974.
Gerstein DD, Dantzker DR: Retinal vascular changes in hereditary visual cell degeneration. Arch Ophthalmol *81*:99–105, 1969.
Gifford H: A cystic diktyoma. Surv Ophthalmol *11*:557–561, 1966.
Gilchrist KW, Gilbert EF, Shahidi NT, et al: The evaluation of infants with Zellweger (cerebro-hepato-renal) syndrome. Clin Genet *7*:413–416, 1975.
Giles CL: Peripheral uveitis in patients with multiple sclerosis. Am J Ophthalmol *70*:17–19, 1970.
Giles CL, Wong VG: Occurrence of adult cystinosis in childhood. J Pediat Ophthalmol *6*:195–197, 1969.
Ginsberg J, Hamblet J, Menefec M: Ocular abnormality in myotonic dystrophy. Ann Ophthalmol *10*:1021–1028, 1978.
Ginsberg S: Über Retinitis pigmentosa. Klin Monatsbl Augenheilkd *46*:1, 1908.
Gipson IK: Cytoplasmic filaments: Their role in motility and cell shape. Invest Ophthalmol Vis Sci *16*:1081–1084, 1977.
Gitter KA, Rothschild H, Waltman DD, et al: Dominantly inherited peripheral retinal neovascularization. Arch Ophthalmol *96*:1601–1605, 1978.
Givner I, Roizin L: Juvenile amaurotic familial idiocy: Its ocular pathology. Arch Ophthalmol *32*:39–47, 1944.
Glaser JS: Topical diagnosis: Prechiasmal visual pathways, *in* Duane TD (ed): Clinical Ophthalmology. Vol 2. Hagerstown, Md, Harper & Row, 1976, pp 39–40.
Glatt HJ, Henkind P: Aging changes in the retinal capillary bed of the rat. Microvasc Res *18*:1–17, 1979.
Goebel HH, Fix JD, Zeman W: The fine structure of the retina in neuronal ceroid-lipofuscinosis. Am J Ophthalmol *77*:25–39, 1974.
Goebel HH, Shimokawa K, Argyrakis A, Pilz H: The ultrastructure of the retina in adult metachromatic leukodystrophy. Am J Ophthalmol *85*:841–849, 1978.
Gold D, Feiner L, Henkind P: Retinal arterial occlusive disease in systemic lupus erythematosus. Arch Ophthalmol *95*:1580–1585, 1977.
Gold D, Friedman A, Wise GN: Predisciform senile macular degeneration. Am J Ophthalmol *76*:763–768, 1973.
Gold D, La Piana F, Zimmerman LE: Isolated retinal arterial aneurysms. Am J Ophthalmol *82*:848–857, 1976.

Goldberg MF: Classification and pathogenesis of proliferative sickle retinopathy. Am J Ophthalmol *71*:649–665, 1971.
Goldberg MF, Duke JR: Ocular histopathology in Hunter's syndrome (systemic mucopolysaccharidosis type II). Arch Ophthalmol *77*:503–512, 1967.
Goldberg MF, Duke JR: Von Hippel–Landau disease: Histopathological finding in a treated and an untreated eye. Am J Ophthalmol *66*:693–705, 1968.
Goldberg MF, Pollack I, Green WR: Familial retinal arteriolar tortuosity with retinal hemorrhage. Am J Ophthalmol *73*:183–191, 1972.
Goldberg RE, Pheasant TR, Shield JA: Cavernous hemangioma of the retina: A four-generation pedigree with neurocutaneous manifestations and an example of bilateral retinal involvement. Arch Ophthalmol *97*:2321–2324, 1979.
Goldfischer S, Moore CL, Johnson AB, et al: Peroxisomal and mitochondrial defects in the cerebro-hepato-renal syndrome. Science *182*:62–64, 1973.
Goldman H, Scriver CR, Aaron K, et al: Adolescent cystinosis: Comparisons wth infantile and adult forms. Pediatrics *47*:979–988, 1971.
Goldmann M: Biomicroscopie due corps vitre et du fond de l'oeil. Bull Mem Soc Fr Ophtalmol *70*:265–272, 1957.
Goldschmidt E: On the Etiology of Myopia: An Epidemiological Study. Copenhagen, Munksgaard, 1968.
Goldstein I, Wexler D: Niemann-Pick's disease with cherry-red spots in the macula: Ocular pathology. Arch Ophthalmol *5*:704, 1931.
Goldstein JL, Fialkow PJ: The Alström syndrome: Report of three cases with further delineation of the clinical, pathophysiological and genetic aspects of the disorder. Medicine *52*:53–71, 1973.
Gonin J: La pathogenie du decollement spontane de la retine. Ann Oculist *32*:30–55, 1904.
Gonin J: Examen anatomique d'un oeil atteint de retinite pigmentaire avec scotome zonulaire. Ann Ocul *29*:24, 1930.
Gonin J: Le Decollement de la Retine: Pathogenie, Traitement. Lausanne, Librairie Payot, 1934, p 1.
Gorlin RJ, Tilsner TJ, Finestein S, Duvall A: Usher's syndrome, Type III. Arch Otolaryngol *105*:333–354, 1979.
Gorn RA, Kuwabara T: Retinal damage by visible light. Arch Ophthalmol *77*:115–118, 1967.
Göttinger W, Minauf M: Netzhautveränderungen bei juveniler amaurotischer Idiotie. Ophthalmoskopisch und histopathologische Befunde. Klin Monatsbl Augenheilkd *159*:532, 1971.
Gottlieb MS, Schroff R, Schanker HM, et al: *Pneumocystis carinii* pneumonia and mucosal candidiasis in previously healthy homosexual men: Evidence of a new acquired cellular immunodeficiency. N Engl J Med *305*:1425–1431, 1981.
Gottlieb RP, Ritter JA: "Flecked retina"—an association with primary hyperoxaluria. J Pediatr *90*:939–942, 1977.
Gould H, Kaufman HE: Sarcoid of the fundus. Arch Ophthalmol *65*:453, 1961.
Gouras P, Carr RE, Gunkel RD: Retinitis pigmentosa in abetalipoproteinemia: Effect of vitamin A. Invest Ophthalmol *10*:784–793, 1971.
Gow J, Oliver GL: Familial exudative vitreoretinopathy. Arch Ophthalmol *86*:150–155, 1971.
Gragoudas ES, Zakov NZ, Albert DM, Constable IJ: Long-term observations of proton-irradiated monkey eyes. Arch Ophthalmol *97*:2184–2191, 1979.
Granato JE, Abben RP, May WS: Familial association of giant cell arteritis. Arch Intern Med *141*:115–117, 1981.
Grant WM: Toxicology of the Eye. 2nd ed. Springfield IL, Charles C Thomas, 1974, pp 39–47.
Green WR: Bilateral Coats' disease: Massive gliosis of the retina. Arch Ophthalmol *77*:378–383, 1967.
Green WR: Retinal and optic nerve atrophy induced by intravitreous vincristine in the primate. Trans Am Ophthalmol Soc *73*:389–416, 1975.
Green WR: Clinicopathologic studies of senile macular degeneration, *in* Nicholson D (ed): Ocular Pathology Update. New York, Masson, 1980.
Green WR, Chan CC, Hutchins GM, Terry JM: Central retinal vein occlusion: A prospective histopathologic study of 29 eyes of 28 patients. Trans Am Ophthalmol Soc, *79*:371–422, 1981 and Retina *1*:27–55, 1981.
Green WR, Gass JDM: Senile disciform degeneration of the macula: Retinal arterialization of the fibrous plaque demonstrated clinically and histopathologically. Arch Ophthalmol *86*:487–494, 1971.
Green WR, Iliff WJ, Trotter RR: Malignant teratoid medulloepithelioma of the optic nerve. Arch Ophthalmol *91*:451–454, 1974.
Green WR, Kenyon KR, Michels RG, et al: Ultrastructure of epiretinal membranes causing macular pucker after retinal re-attachment surgery. Trans Ophthalmol Soc UK *99*:63–77, 1979.
Green WR, Key SN III: Senile macular degeneration: A histopathologic study. Trans Am Ophthalmol Soc *75*:180–254, 1977.
Green WR, Kincaid MC, Michels RG, et al: Study of the vitreous in pars planitis. Unpublished data, 1981.
Green WR, Koo BS: Behçet's disease. A report of ocular histopathology of one case. Surv Ophthalmol *12*:324–332, 1967.
Green WR, Quigley HT, de la Cruz Z, Cohen B: Parafoveal retinal telangiectasis. Trans Ophthalmol Soc UK *100*:162–170, 1980.
Gregory MH, Rutty DA, Wood RD: Differences in the retinotoxic action of chloroquine and phenothiazine derivatives. J Pathol *102*:97–108, 139–150, 1970.
Grey RHB: Foveo-macular retinitis, solar retinopathy, and trauma. Br J Ophthalmol *62*:543–546, 1978.
Grimaud R, Cordier J, Dureux JB, et al: Les altérations chorio-rétiniennes chez les sourds-muets. Rev Otoneuroophthalmol *34*:59–63, 1962.
Grizzard WS, Deutman AF, Nijhuis F, Aan de Kerk A: Crystalline retinopathy. Am J Ophthalmol *86*:81–88, 1978.
Grover WD, Green WR, Pileggi AJ: Ocular findings in subacute necrotizing encephalomyelitis. Am J Ophthalmol *70*:599–603, 1970.
Guild HG, Walsh FB, Hoover RE: Ocular cystinosis. Am J Ophthalmol *35*:1241–1248, 1952.
Gunning AJ, Pickering GW, Robb-Smith AHT, Russell RR: Mural thrombosis of internal carotid artery and subsequent embolism. Q J Med *33*:155–195, 1964.
Gutman FA, Zegarra H: The natural course of temporal retinal branch vein occlusion. Trans Am Acad Ophthalmol Otolaryngol *78*:178–192, 1974.
Guzzetta F: Cockayne-Neill-Dingwall syndrome, *in* Vinken PJ, Bruyn GW (eds): Handbook of Clinical Neurology. Vol 13. Amsterdam, Elsevier, 1972, pp 431–440.
Haarr M: Retinal periphlebitis in multiple sclerosis. Acta Neurol Scand (Suppl 4) *39*:270–272, 1963.
Haddad R, Font RL, Friendly DS: Cerebro-hepato-renal syndrome of Zellweger: Ocular histopathologic findings. Arch Ophthalmol *94*:1927–1930, 1976.
Hagberg B, Sourander P, Svennerholm L: Late infantile progressive encephalopathy with disturbed polyunsaturated fat metabolism. Acta Paediatr Scand *57*:495–499, 1968.
Hagedoorn A: Angioid streaks. Arch Ophthalmol *21*:746–774, 1939.
Hagler WS, Crosswell, HH Jr: Radial perivascular chorioretinal degeneration and retinal detachment. Trans Am Acad Ophthalmol Otolaryngol *72*:203–216, 1968.
Hagler WS, Walters PV, Nahmias AJ: Ocular involvement in neonatal herpes simplex virus infection. Arch Ophthalmol *82*:169–176, 1969.
Hallervorden J, Spatz H: Eigenartige Erkrankung im extrapyramidalen System mit besonderer Beteiligung des Globus pallidus und der Substantia nigra: Ein Beitrag zu den Beziehungen zwischen diesen beiden Zentren. Z Ges Neurol Psychiat *79*:254–302, 1922.
Hallgren B: Retinitis pigmentosa combined with congenital deafness, with vestibulocerebellar ataxia and mental abnormality in proportion of cases: A clinical and genetico-statis-

tical study. Acta Psychiatr Neurol Scand *34*(Suppl 138):1–101, 1959.
Haltia M, Tarkkanen A, Vaheri A, et al: Measles retinopathy during immunosuppression. Br J Ophthalmol *62*:356–360, 1978.
Ham WT Jr, Mueller HA, Ruffolo JJ Jr, Clarke AM: Sensitivity of the retina to radiation damage as a function of wavelength. Photochem Photobiol *29*:735–743, 1979.
Hamidi-Toosi S, Maumenee IH: Vitreoretinal degeneration in spondyloepiphyseal dysplasia congenita. Arch Ophthalmol *100*:1104–1107, 1982.
Hamilton AM, Bird AC: Geographical choroidopathy. Br J Ophthalmol *58*:784–797, 1974.
Hamm H: Zentralskotom nach Sonnenblendung. Dissertation, Hamburg, 1947.
Hansen RI, Friedman AH, Gartner S, Henkind P: The association of retinitis pigmentosa with preretinal macular gliosis. Br J Ophthalmol *61*:597–600, 1977.
Harcourt B, Ashton N: Ultrastructure of the optic nerve in Krabbe's leucodystrophy. Br J Ophthalmol *57*:885–891, 1973.
Harcourt B, Dobbs RH: Ultrastructure of the retina in Tay-Sachs disease. Br J Ophthalmol *52*:898–902, 1968.
Harley RD, Grover WD: Tuberous sclerosis: Description and report of 12 cases. Ann Ophthalmol *1*:477–481, 1970.
Harley RD, Huang NN, Macri CH, Green WR: Optic neuritis and optic atrophy following chloramphenicol in cystic fibrosis patients. Trans Am Acad Ophthalmol Otolaryngol *74*:1011–1031, 1970.
Harms C: Anatomisches über die senile Maculaaffektion. Klin Monatsbl Augenheilkd *42*:448–461, 1904.
Harris JL, Gumucio CC, Ohanion MB: Adenocarcinoma of the ciliary epithelium. Arch Ophthalmol *80*:217–219, 1968.
Harry J, Ashton N: The pathology of hypertensive retinopathy. Trans Ophthalmol Soc UK *83*:71–90, 1963.
Harry J, Morgan G: Pathology of a unique type of teratoid medulloepithelium. Br J Ophthalmol *63*:132–134, 1979.
Hart CD, Sanders MD, Miller SJH: Benign retinal vasculitis. Br J Ophthalmol *55*:721–733, 1971.
Harwerth RS, Sperling HG: Prolonged color blindness induced by intense spectral lights in rhesus monkeys. Science *174*:520–523, 1971.
Hayreh SS: Post-radiation retinopathy. A fluorescence fundus angiographic study. Br J Ophthalmol *54*:705–714, 1970.
Hayreh SS: Optic disc vasculitis. Br J Ophthalmol *56*:652–670, 1972.
Hayreh SS, Kolder HE, Weingeist TA: Central retinal artery occlusion and retinal tolerance time. Ophthalmology *87*:75–78, 1980.
Hedges TR Jr: Ophthalmoscopic findings in internal carotid artery occlusion. Am J Ophthalmol *55*:1007–1012, 1963.
Hedges TR: The aortic arch syndromes. Arch Ophthalmol *71*:28–34, 1964.
Henkind P: Personal communication, Nov, 1980.
Henkind P, Bellhorn RW, Schall B: Retinal edema: Postulated mechanism(s), *in* Cunha-Vaz JG (ed): The Blood-Retinal Barriers. New York, Plenum Press, 1980, pp 251–268.
Henkind P, Carr RE, Siegel IM: Early chloroquine retinopathy: Clinical and functional findings. Arch Ophthalmol *71*:157–165, 1964.
Henkind P, Morgan G: Peripheral retinal angioma with exudative retinopathy in adults (Coats's lesion). Br J Ophthalmol *50*:2–11, 1966.
Henkind P, Rothfield NF: Ocular abnormalities in patients treated with synthetic antimalarial drugs. N Engl J Med *269*:433–439, 1963.
Henkind P, Wise GN: Retinal neovascularization, collaterals, and vascular shunts. Br J Ophthalmol *58*:413–422, 1974.
Henry MM, Henry LM, Henry LM: A possible cause of chronic cystic maculopathy. Ann Ophthalmol *9*:455–457, 1977.
Henson RA, Hoffman HL, Urich H: Encephalomyelitis with carcinoma. Brain *88*:449–464, 1965.
Hermann J, France TD, Spranger JW, et al: The Stickler syndrome (hereditary arthro-ophthalmopathy). Birth Defects *11*:76–103, 1975.
Herrmann MK, Hunziker JA, Szymanski CM, et al: Peripheral retinal albinotic spots in three dogs. J Am Vet Med Assoc *163*:1175–1176, 1973.
Hersh PS, Green WR, Thomas JV: Tractional venous loops in diabetic retinopathy. Am J Ophthalmol *92*:661–671, 1981.
Hervouët F, Baron A, Lenoir A: Anatomie pathologique de la rétinose hespéranopie. Arch Ophthalmol (Paris) *15*:263–284, 1955.
Heshe J, Engelstoft FH, Kirk L: Retinal injury developing under thioridazine treatment. Nord Psykiatr Tidskr *15*:442–447, 1961
Hijikata F, Hirooka M, Ohno T, et al: Cockayne's syndrome: A histopathological study of the ocular tissues. Rinsho Ganka *23*:187–194, 1969.
Hiles DA, Font RL: Bilateral intraocular cryptococcosis with unilateral spontaneous regression: Report of a case and review of the literature. Am J Ophthalmol *65*:98–108, 1968.
Hillemann J, Naumann G: Beitrag zum benignen Epitheliom (Fuchs) des Zilarkörpers. Ophthalmologica *164*:321–335, 1972.
Hilton GF: Late serosanguineous detachment of the macular after traumatic choroidal rupture. Am J Ophthalmol *79*:997–1000, 1975.
Hilton GF, Machemer R, Michels RG, et al (The Retina Society Terminology Committee): The classification of retinal detachment with proliferative vitreoretinopathy. Ophthalmology *90*:121–125, 1983.
Hirose T, Lee KY, Schepens CL: Wagner's hereditary vitreoretinal degeneration and retinal detachment. Arch Ophthalmol *89*:176–185, 1973.
Hirose T, Lee KY, Schepens CL: Snowflake degeneration in hereditary vitreoretinal degeneration. Am J Ophthalmol *77*:143–153, 1974.
Hitchings RA: Aphakic macular oedema: A two-year follow-up study. Br J Ophthalmol *61*:628–630, 1977.
Hitchings RA, Chisholm IH: Incidence of aphakic macular oedema: A prospective study. Br J Ophthalmol *59*:444–450, 1975.
Hittner HM, Kretzer FL, Mehta RS: Zellweger syndrome: Lenticular opacities indicating carrier status and lens abnormalities characteristic of homozygotes. Arch Ophthalmol *99*:1977–1982, 1981.
Hittner HM, Zeller RS: Ceroid-lipofuscinosis (Batten disease). Fluorescein angiography, electrophysiology, histopathology, ultrastructure, and a review of amaurotic familial idiocy. Arch Ophthalmol *93*:178–183, 1975.
Hoare GW: Traumatic retinal angiopathy resulting from chest compression by safety belt. Br J Ophthalmol *54*:667–669, 1970.
Hobbs HE, Sorsby A, Freedman A: Retinopathy following chloroquine therapy. Lancet *2*:478–480, 1959.
Hoefnagels KLJ, Pijpers PM: Histoplasma capsulatum in a human eye. Am J Ophthalmol *63*:715–723, 1967.
Hogan MJ, Alvarado JA: Studies on the human macula. IV. Aging changes in Bruch's membrane. Arch Ophthalmol *77*:410–420, 1967.
Hogan MJ, Alvarado JA, Weddell JE: Histology of the Human Eye. Philadelphia, W.B. Saunders Company, 1971, pp 344–363, 491–498.
Hogan MJ, Kimura SJ: Cyclitis and peripheral chorioretinitis. Arch Ophthalmol *66*:667–677, 1961.
Hogan MJ, Kimura SJ, Spencer WH: Visceral larva migrans and peripheral retinitis. JAMA *194*:1345–1347, 1965.
Hogan MJ, Zimmerman LE: Ophthalmic Pathology. 2nd ed. Philadelphia, W.B. Saunders Company, 1962, p 439.
Horie A, Iwata Y, Tanaka K, Hayashi F: Electron microscopic study on the so-called malignant medullo-epithelioma (ciliary epithelial carcinoma). Virchows Arch [Pathol Anat] *355*:284–289, 1972.
Horiuchi T, Gass JDM, David NJ: Arteriovenous malformation in the retina of a monkey. Am J Ophthalmol *82*:896–904, 1976.

Horowitz P: Von Hippel-Lindau disease, *in* Tasman W (ed): Retinal Diseases in Children. New York, Harper & Row, 1971, pp 78–91.

Horta-Barbosa L, Fuccillo DA, London WT, et al: Isolation of measles virus from brain cell cultures of two patients with subacute sclerosing panencephalitis. Proc Soc Exp Biol Med *132*:272–277, 1969.

Houber JP, Babel J: Les lesions uveo-rétiniennes de la dystrophie myotonique. Étude histologique. Ann Oculist *203*:1067–1076, 1970.

Howard GM, Wolf E: Central choroidal sclerosis: A clinical and pathologic study. Trans Am Acad Ophthalmol Otolaryngol *68*:647–660, 1964.

Howard RO, Albert DM: Ocular manifestations of subacute necrotizing encephalomyelitis (Leigh's disease). Am J Ophthalmol *74*:386–393, 1972.

Howes EL Jr, Wood IS, Golbus M, Hogan MJ: Ocular pathology of infantile Niemann-Pick disease. Arch Ophthalmol *93*:494–500, 1975.

Hunt EW Jr: Unusual case of ophthalmomyiasis interna posterior. Am J Ophthalmol *70*:978–980, 1970.

Hunter C: A rare disease in two brothers. Proc Roy Soc Med *10*:104–121, 1917.

Hunter WS, Zimmerman LE: Unilateral retinal dysplasia. Arch Ophthalmol *74*:23–30, 1965.

Hurler G: Über einen Typ multipler Abartungen, vorwiegend am Skelettsystem. Sischr Kinderheilkd *24*:220–234, 1919.

Hutchinson J: Slowly progressive paraplegia and disease of the choroid with defective intellect and arrested sexual development. Arch Surg (London) *11*:118–122, 1900.

Hutchison WM, Dunachie JF, Work K, et al: The life cycle of the coccidian parasite *Toxoplasma gondii* in the domestic cat. Trans Roy Soc Trop Med Hyg *65*:380–399, 1971.

Hutton WL, Snyder WB, Fuller D, Vaiser A: Focal parafoveal retinal telangiectasis. Arch Ophthalmol *96*:1362–1367, 1978.

Hutton WL, Vaiser A, Snyder WB: Pars plana vitrectomy for removal of intravitreous cysticerus. Am J Ophthalmol *81*:571–573, 1976.

Hyams SW, Meir E, Ivry M, et al: Chorioretinal lesions predisposing to retinal detachment. Am J Ophthalmol *78*:429–437, 1974.

Igarashi M, Schaumburg HH, Powers J, et al: Fatty acid abnormality in adrenoleukodystrophy. J Neurochem *26*:851–860, 1976.

Ikui H: Histological studies of vascular changes in the retina in hypertension. Acta Soc Ophthalmol Jpn *67*:562–590, 1963.

Ikui H: Histological examination of central serous retinopathy. Folia Ophthalmol Jpn *20*:1035–1043, 1969.

Ikui H, Tominaga Y, Inomata H, et al: A concept of "capillarosclerosis retinae." Report 1. Pathological changes of the capillaries in the retina and optic nerve head occurring in senescence and in benign hypertension. Acta Soc Ophthalmol Jpn *72*:553–562, 1968.

Iliff WJ, Green WR: The incidence and histology of Fuchs' adenoma. Arch Ophthalmol *88*:249–254, 1972.

Inkeles DM, Walsh JB: Retinal fat emboli as a sequela to acute pancreatitis. Am J Ophthalmol *80*:935–938, 1975.

Inomata H, Ikui H, Kimura K: Fine structure of cytoid bodies. Jap J Ophthalmol *11*:1–14, 1967.

Irvine AR: Cystoid maculopathy. Surv Ophthalmol *21*:1–17, 1976.

Irvine AR, Spencer WH, Hogan MJ, et al: Presumed chronic ocular histoplasmosis syndrome: A clinical-pathologic case report. Trans Am Ophthalmol Soc *74*:91–106, 1976.

Irvine SR: A newly defined vitreous syndrome following cataract surgery: Interpreted according to recent concepts of the structure of the vitreous: The Seventh Francis I. Proctor Lecture. Am J Ophthalmol *36*:599–619, 1953.

Israel H, Park CH, Mansfield CM: Gallium scanning in sarcoidosis. Ann NY Acad Sci *278*:514–516, 1976.

Jabbour JT, Duenas DA, Sever JL, et al: Epidemiology of subacute sclerosing panencephalitis (S.S.P.E.); A report of the S.S.P.E. Registry. JAMA *220*:959–962, 1972.

Jack MK: Central serous retinopathy with optic pit treated with photocoagulation. Am J Ophthalmol *67*:519–521, 1969.

Jacob HS, Goldstein IM, Shapiro I, et al: Sudden blindness in acute pancreatitis: Possible role of complement-induced retinal leukoembolization. Arch Intern Med *141*:134–137, 1981.

Jaeger W, Kettler JV, Lutz P, Hilsdorf C: Differential diagnosis of gyrate atrophy of the choroid and retina: (Gyrate atrophy of choroid and retina with and without hyperornithinemia). Metab Pediat Ophthalmol *3*:189–191, 1979.

Jaffe R, Crumrine P, Hashida Y, Moser HW: Neonatal adrenoleukodystrophy in a brother and sister. J Neuropathol Exp Neurol *40*:308, 1981.

Jaffe R, Crumrine P, Hashida Y, Moser HW: Neonatal adrenoleukodystrophy: Clinical, pathologic, and biochemical delineation of a syndrome affecting both males and females. Am J Pathol *108*:100–111, 1982.

Jakobiec FA, Font RL, Johnson FB: Angiomatosis retinae: An ultrastructural study and lipid analysis. Cancer *38*:2042–2056, 1976.

James DG, Anderson R, Langley D, Ainslie D: Ocular sarcoidosis. Br J Ophthalmol *48*:461–470, 1964.

James DG, Neville E, Langley DA: Ocular sarcoidosis. Trans Ophthalmol Soc UK *96*:133–139, 1976.

Jampol LM, Goldberg MF, Busse B: Peripheral retinal microaneurysms in chronic leukemia. Am J Ophthalmol *80*:242–248, 1975.

Jampol LM, Wong AS, Albert DM: Atrial myxoma and central retinal artery occlusion. Am J Ophthalmol *75*:242–249, 1973.

Jampol LM, Woodfin W, McLean EB: Optic nerve sarcoidosis. Arch Ophthalmol *87*:355–360, 1972.

Jan JE, Hardwick DF, Lowry RB, McCormick AQ: Cerebrohepato-renal syndrome of Zellweger. Am J Dis Child *119*:274–277, 1970.

Jansen LMAA: Degeneratio hyaloideo-retinalis hereditaria. Ophthalmologica *144*:458–464, 1962.

Jarrett WH, Brockhurst RJ: Unexplained blindness and optic atrophy following retinal detachment surgery. Arch Ophthalmol *73*:782–791, 1965.

Jensen OA: Mucopolysaccharidosis type III (Sanfilippo's syndrome). Histochemical examination of the eyes and brain with a survey of the literature. Acta Pathol Microbiol Scand (Sec A) *79*:257–273, 1971.

Johnson BL: Proteinaceous cysts of the ciliary epithelium. II. Their occurrence in nonmyelomatous hypergammaglobulinemic conditions. Arch Ophthalmol *84*:171–175, 1970.

Johnson BL, Storey JD: Proteinaceous cysts of the ciliary epithelium. I. Their clear nature and immunoelectrophoretic analysis in a case of multiple myeloma. Arch Ophthalmol *84*:166–170, 1970.

Johnson BL, Wisotzkey HM: Neuroretinitis associated with herpes simplex encephalitis in an adult. Am J Ophthalmol *83*:481–489, 1977.

Johnson DL, Jacobson LW, Toyama R, Monahan RH: Histopathology of eyes in Chediak-Higashi syndrome. Arch Ophthalmol *75*:84–88, 1966.

Johnson FB: A method for demonstrating calcium oxalate in tissue sections. J Histochem Cytochem *4*:404–405, 1956.

Jones SE, Fuks Z, Bull M, et al: Non-Hodgkin's lymphomas. IV. Clinicopathologic correlation in 405 cases. Cancer *31*:806–823, 1973.

Judisch GF, Lowry B, Hansen JW, McGillivary BC: Chorioretinopathy and pituitary dysfunction. Arch Opthalmol *99*:253–256, 1981.

Kaiser-Kupfer MI, Kupfer C, Rodrigues MM: Tamoxifen retinopathy: A clinicopathologic report. Ophthalmology *88*:89–93, 1981.

Kaiser-Kupfer MI, Lippman ME: Tamoxifen retinopathy. Cancer Treat Rep *62*:315–320, 1978.

Kaiser-Kupfer MI, Valle D, Bron AJ: Clinical and biochemical heterogeneity in gyrate atrophy. Am J Ophthalmol *89*:219–222, 1980.

Kaiser-Kupfer MI, Valle D, Del Valle LA: A specific enzyme defect in gyrate atrophy. Am J Ophthalmol *85*:200–204, 1978.

Kalina RE: A histopathologic postmortem and clinical study of peripheral retinal folds in infant eyes. Am J Ophthalmol *71*:446–448, 1971.

Kalina RE: Treatment of retrolental fibroplasia. Surv Ophthalmol *24*:229–236, 1980.

Kaluzny J: Myopia and retinal detachment. Pol Med J *9*:1544–1549, 1970.

Kampik A, Green WR, Michels RG, Nase PK: Ultrastructural features of progressive idiopathic epiretinal membrane removed by vitreous surgery. Am J Ophthalmol *90*:797–809, 1980.

Kampiik A, Green WR, Michels RG, Rice TA: Epiretinale Membranen nach Photokoagulation (postkoagulative Maculopathie). Ber Dtsch Ophthalmol Ges *78*:593–598, 1981.

Kampik A, Kenyon KR, Michels RG, et al: Epiretinal and vitreous membranes: A comparative study of 56 cases. Arch Ophthalmol *99*:1445–1454, 1981.

Kanchanaranya C, Prechanond A, Punyagupta S: Removal of living work in retinal *Angiostrongylus cantonensis*. Am J Ophthalmol *74*:456–458, 1972.

Kandori F: Very rare cases of congenital cases of nonprogressive nightblindness with flecked retina. Jpn J Ophthalmol *13*:384, 1959.

Kandori F, Tamai A, Kurimoto S, Fukunaga K: Flecked retina. Am J Ophthalmol *73*:673–685, 1972.

Karlin DB, Curtin BJ: Peripheral chorioretinal lesions and axial length of the myopic eye. Am J Ophthalmol *81*:625–635, 1976.

Karlsberg RC, Green WR, Patz A: Congenital retrolental fibroplasia. Arch Ophthalmol *89*:122–123, 1973.

Kaufer G, Zimmerman LE: Direct rupture of the choroid. Arch Ophthalmol *75*:384–385, 1966.

Kaufman SJ, Goldberg MF, Orth DH, et al: Autosomal dominant vitreoretinochoroidopathy. Arch Ophthalmol *100*:272–278, 1982.

Kean BH, Kimball AC, Christenson WN: An epidemic of acute toxoplasmosis. JAMA *208*:1002–1004, 1969.

Kearns TP: Fat embolism of the retina: Demonstrated by a flat retinal preparation. Am J Ophthalmol *41*:1–2, 1956.

Kearns TP: External ophthalmoplegia, pigmentary degeneration of the retina, and cardiomyopathy: A newly recognized syndrome. Trans Am Ophthalmol Soc *63*:559–625, 1965.

Kearns TP, Hollenhorst RW: Venous-stasis retinopathy of occlusive disease of the carotid artery. Mayo Clin Proc *38*:304–312, 1963.

Kearns TP, Sayre GP: Retinitis pigmentosa, external ophthalmoplegia, and complete heart block. Unusual syndrome with histologic study in one of two cases. Arch Ophthalmol *60*:280–289, 1958.

Kearns TP, Young BR, Piepgras DB: Resolution of venous-stasis retinopathy after carotid artery bypass surgery. Mayo Clin Proc *55*:342–346, 1980.

Kelley JS: Purtscher's retinopathy related to chest compression by safety belts: Fluorescein angiographic findings. Am J Ophthalmol *74*:278–283, 1972.

Kelley JS, Green WR: Sarcoidosis involving the optic nerve head. Arch Ophthalmol *89*:486–488, 1973.

Kelley JS, Hoover RE, George T: Whiplash maculopathy. Arch Ophthalmol *96*:834–835, 1978.

Kelly TE, Graetz G: Isolated acid neuraminidase deficiency: A distinct lysosomal storage disease. Am J Med Genet *1*:31–46, 1977.

Keno DD, Green WR: Retinal pigment epithelial window defect. Arch Ophthalmol *96*:854–856, 1978.

Kenyon KR: Ocular ultrastructure of inherited metabolic disease, *in* Goldberg MF (ed): Genetic and Metabolic Eye Diseases. Boston, Little, Brown, 1974, pp 139–185.

Kenyon KR: Ocular manifestations and pathology of systemic mucopolysaccharidoses, *in* Birth Defects. Original Article Series, Vol XII, No 3. New York, The National Foundation, 1976, pp 133–144.

Kenyon KR, Maumenee IH, Green WR, et al: Mucolipidosis IV: Histopathology of conjunctiva, cornea, and skin. Arch Ophthalmol *97*:1106–1111, 1979.

Kenyon KR, Michels RG: Ultrastructure of epiretinal membrane removed by pars plana vitreoretinal surgery. Am J Ophthalmol *83*:815–823, 1977.

Kenyon KR, Pederson JE, Green WR, Maumenee AE: Fibroglial proliferation in pars planitis. Trans Ophthalmol Soc UK *95*:391–397, 1975.

Kenyon KR, Quigley HA, Hussels IE, Wyllie RG: The systemic mucopolysaccharidoses. Ultrastructural and histochemical studies of conjunctiva and skin. Am J Ophthalmol *73*:811–833, 1972.

Kenyon KR, Sensenbrenner JA: Mucolipidosis II (I-cell disease): Ultrastructural observations of conjunctiva and skin. Invest Ophthalmol *10*:555–567, 1971.

Kenyon KR, Sensenbrenner JA: Electron microscopy of cornea and conjunctiva in childhood cystinosis. Am J Ophthalmol *78*:68–76, 1974.

Kenyon KR, Topping TM, Green WR, Maumenee AE: Ocular pathology of the Maroteaux-Lamy syndrome (systemic mucopolysaccharidosis type VI). Histologic and ultrastructural report of two cases. Am J Ophthalmol *73*:718–741, 1972.

Key SN III, Green WR, Maumenee AE: Pathology of macular lesion of ocular histoplasmosis: Its pathogenetic and therapeutic implications, *in* Brockhurst RJ, Boruchoff SA, Hutchinson BT, Lessell S (eds): Controversy in Ophthalmology. Philadelphia, W.B. Saunders Company, 1977, pp 732–747.

Keyes JEL, Moore PG: Adenomatous hyperplasia of the epithelium of the ciliary body. Arch Ophthalmol *19*:39–45, 1938.

Khan SG, Frenkel M: Intravitreal hemorrhage associated with rapid increase in intracranial pressure (Terson's syndrome). Am J Ophthalmol *80*:37–43, 1975.

Khodadoust AA, Payne JW: Cryptococcal (torular) retinitis: A clinicopathologic case report. Am J Ophthalmol *67*:745–750, 1969.

Kielar RA: Exudative retinal detachment and scleritis in polyarteritis. Am J Ophthalmol *82*:694–698, 1976.

Kim EW, Zakov N, Albert DM, et al: Intraocular reticulum cell sarcoma: A case report and literature review. Albrecht Von Graefes Arch Klin Exp Ophthalmol *209*:167–178, 1979.

Kimura SJ, Carriker FR, Hogan MJ: Retinal vasculitis with intraocular hemorrhage: Classification and results of special studies. Arch Ophthalmol *56*:361–374, 1956.

Kimura SJ, Hogan MJ: Chronic cyclitis. Trans Am Ophthalmol Soc *61*:397–417, 1963.

Kimura T: Studies on fine structure of retinal blood vessels in arteriolar sclerosis of the human retina (Report 1). Jpn Ophthalmol Soc. *69*:284–301, 1965a.

Kimura T: Studies on the fine structure of retinal blood vessels in arteriolar sclerosis of the human retina. Acta Soc Ophthal Jpn *69*:1140–1157, 1965b.

Kimura T: Studies on the fine structure of the retinal blood vessels in arteriolar sclerosis of the human retina. Acta Soc Ophthal Jpn *70*:1442–1454, 1966.

Kimura T: Studies on the fine structure of retinal blood vessels in arteriolar slcerosis of the human retina (Report II). Jpn Ophthalmol Soc. *70*:356–368, 1967a.

Kimura T: Studies on the fine structure of retinal blood vessels in arteriolar sclerosis of the human retina. Jpn J Ophthalmol *11*:39–49, 1967b.

Kimura T: Light and electron microscopic studies on the sclerotic changes in human central retinal arteries. I. The "crossing phenomenon." Acta Soc Ophthal Jpn *74*:987–998, 1970a.

Kimura T: Light and electron microscopic studies on the sclerotic changes in human central retinal arteries. II. Observation comparing ophthalmoscopic and histologic findings. Acta Soc Ophthal Jpn *74*:1494–1508, 1970b.

Kincaid MC, Green WR: Ocular and orbital involvement in leukemia. Surv Ophthalmol *27*:211–232, 1983.

Kincaid MC, Green WR, Kelley JS: Acute ocular leukemia. Am J Ophthalmol *87*:698–702, 1979.

Kincaid MC, Green WR, Knox DL, Molner C: A clinicopathological case report of retinopathy of pancreatitis. Br J Ophthalmol *66*:219–226, 1982.

Kingham JD, Lochen GP: Vitelliform macular degeneration. Am J Ophthalmol *84*:526–531, 1977.

Kini MH, Leibowitz HM, Colton T, et al: Prevalence of senile cataract, diabetic retinopathy, senile macular degeneration, and open-angle glaucoma in the Framingham Eye Study. Am J Ophthalmol *85*:28–34, 1978.

Kinoshita JH: Mechanisms initiating cataract formation. Invest Ophthalmol *13*:713–724, 1974.

Kinsey VE, Arnold HJ, Kalina RE, et al: PaO_2 levels and retrolental fibroplasia: A report of the cooperative study. Pediatrics *60*:655–668, 1977.

Kirker GEM, McDonald DJ: Peripheral retinal degeneration in high myopia. Can J Ophthalmol *6*:58–61, 1971.

Klein M, Green WR: Unpublished data, 1979.

Klein RM, Curtin BJ: Lacquer crack lesions in pathologic myopia. Am J Ophthalmol *79*:386–392, 1975.

Klein RM, Yannuzzi L: Cystoid macular edema in the first week after cataract extraction. Am J Ophthalmol *81*:614–615, 1976.

Klein U, Kresse H, von Figura K: Sanfilippo syndrome type C: Deficiency of acetyl-CoA:alpha-glucosaminide *N*-acetyltransferase in skin fibroblasts. Proc Natl Acad Sci USA *75*:5185–5189, 1978.

Klien BA: The heredodegeneration of the macula lutea: Diagnostic and differential diagnostic considerations and a histopathologic report. Am J Ophthalmol *33*:371–379, 1950.

Klien BA: Late infantile amaurotic idiocy: A clinico-histopathologic study. Am J Ophthalmol *38*:470–475, 1954.

Klien BA: Macular and extramacular serous chorioretinopathy. With remarks upon the role of an extrabulbar mechanism in its pathogenesis. Am J Ophthalmol *51*:231–242, 1961.

Klien BA: Some aspects of classification and differential diagnosis of senile macular degeneration. Am J Ophthalmol *58*:927–939, 1964.

Klien BA: Ischemic infarcts of the choroid (Elschnig spots). A cause of retinal separation in hypertensive disease with renal insufficiency. A clinical and histopathologic study. Am J Ophthalmol *66*:1069–1074, 1968.

Klien BA, Krill AE: Fundus flavimaculatus: Clinical, functional, and histopathologic observations. Am J Ophthalmol *64*:3–23, 1967.

Klingele TG, Hogan MJ: Ocular reticulum cell sarcoma. Am J Ophthalmol *79*:39–47, 1975.

Klintworth GK, Hollingsworth AS, Lusman PA, Bradford WD: Granulomatous choroiditis in a case of disseminated histoplasmosis: Histologic demonstration of *Histoplasma capsulatum* in choroidal lesions. Arch Ophthalmol *90*:45–48, 1973.

Knapp JW: Isolated macular infarction in sickle cell (SS) disease. Am J Ophthalmol *73*:857–859, 1972.

Knapp P: Ein seltener Augenspiegelbefund: Sclerosis choroidea circinata. Klin Monatsbl Augenheilkd *45*:171–177, 1907.

Knobloch WH, Layer JM: Retinal detachment and encephalocele. J Pediatr Ophthalmol *8*:181–184, 1971.

Knox DL: Ischemic ocular inflammation. Am J Ophthalmol *60*:995–1002, 1965.

Knox DL: Ocular aspects of cervical vascular disease. Surv Ophthalmol *13*:245–262, 1969.

Knox DL: Personal communication, 1978.

Knox DL, Bayless TM, Yardley JH, Charache P: Whipple's disease presenting with ocular inflammation and minimal intestinal symptoms. Johns Hopkins Med J *123*:175–182, 1968.

Knox DL, King JT Jr: Retinal arteritis, iridocyclitis, and giardiasis. Ophthalmology *89*:1303–1308, 1982.

Kohner EM, Dollery CT, Bulpitt CJ: Cotton-wool spots in diabetic retinopathy. Diabetes *18*:691–704, 1969.

Kohner EM, Henkind P: Correlation of fluorescein angiogram and retinal digest in diabetic retinopathy. Am J Ophthalmol *69*:403–414, 1970.

Kolb H, Gouras P: Electron microscopic observations of human retinitis pigmentosa, dominantly inherited. Invest Ophthalmol *13*:487–498, 1974.

Kollaritis CR, Lubow M, Hissong SL: Retinal strokes. I. Incidence of carotid atheromata. JAMA *222*:1273–1275, 1972.

Konigsmark BW, Weiner LP: The olivopontocerebellar atrophies: A review. Medicine *49*:227–242, 1970.

Kornzweig AL: The eye in old age. V. Disease of the macula: A clinicopathologic study. Am J Ophthalmol *60*:835–843, 1965.

Kornzweig AL, Eliasoph I, Feldstein M: Retinal vasculature in the aged. Bull NY Acad Med *40*:116–129, 1964.

Kornzweig AL, Eliasoph I, Feldstein M: The retinal vasculature in macular degeneration. Arch Ophthalmol *75*:326–333, 1966.

Kornzweig AL, Feldstein M, Schneider J: The pathogenesis of senile macular degeneration. Am J Ophthalmol *48*:22–28, 1959.

Kranenburg E: Crater-like holes in the optic disc and central serous retinopathy. Arch Ophthalmol *64*:912–924, 1960.

Kraus E, Lutz P: Ocular cystine deposits in an adult. Arch Ophthalmol *85*:690–694, 1971.

Kresca LJ, Goldberg MF, Jampol LM: Talc emboli and retinal neovascularization in a drug abuser. Am J Ophthalmol *87*:334–339, 1979.

Kresse H, Paschke E, von Figura K, et al: Sanfilippo disease type D: Deficiency of *N*-acetylglucosamine-6-sulfate sulfatase required for heparan sulfate degradation. Proc Natl Acad Sci USA *77*:6822–6826, 1980.

Kretzer FL, Hittner HM, Mehta R: Ocular manifestations of Conradi and Zellweger syndromes. Metab Pediatr Ophthalmol *5*:1–11, 1981.

Krill AE: Hereditary Retinal and Choroidal Diseases. Vol II. Clinical Characteristics. Hagerstown, Md, Harper & Row, 1977, pp 636–643.

Krill AE, Archer D: Classification of the choroidal atrophies. Am J Ophthalmol *72*:562–585, 1971.

Krill AE, Deutman AF: Acute retinal pigment epitheliitis. Am J Ophthalmol *74*:193–205, 1972.

Kroll AJ, Kuwabara T: Electron microscopy of a retinal abiotrophy. Arch Ophthalmol *71*:683–690, 1964.

Kroll AJ, Machemer R: Experimental retinal detachment and reattachment in the Rhesus monkey: Electron microscopic comparison of rods and cones. Am J Ophthalmol *68*:58–77, 1969.

Kruecke HW, Stochdorph O: Über Veränderungen in Zentralnervensystem bei Whipplescher Krankheit [On changes in the central nervous system in Whipple's disease]. Verh Deutsch Ges Pathol *46*:198–202, 1962.

Krug EF, Samuels B: Venous angioma of the retina, optic nerve, chiasm and brain. A case report with postmortem observations. Arch Ophthalmol *8*:871–879, 1932.

Kuchynka P: Malignant epithelioma of the ciliary body. Ophthalmologica (Basel) *178*:190–193, 1979.

Kuhlenbeck H, Haymaker W: Neuroectodermal tumors containing neoplastic neuronal elements: Ganglioneuroma, spongioneuroblastoma and glioneuroma. Mil Surgeon *99*:273–304, 1946.

Kurz GH, Zimmerman LE: Vagaries of the retinal pigment epithelium. Int Ophthalmol Clin *2*:441–464, 1962.

Kushner BJ, Essner D, Cohen IJ, Flynn JT: Retrolental fibroplasia. II. Pathologic correlation. Arch Ophthalmol *95*:29–38, 1977.

Kuwabara T: Retinal recovery from exposure to light. Am J Ophthalmol *70*:187–198, 1970.

Kuwabara T, Aiello L: Leukemic miliary nodules in the retina. Arch Ophthalmol *72*:494–497, 1964.

Kuwabara T, Cogan DG: Tetrazolium studies on the retina. I. Introduction and technique. J Histochem Cytochem *7*:329–333, 1959.

Kuwabara T, Cogan DG: Retinal vascular patterns. VI. Mural cells of the retinal capillaries. Arch Ophthalmol *69*:492–502, 1963.

Kuwabara T, Cogan DG: Retinal vascular patterns. VII. Acellular change. Invest Ophthalmol *4*:1049–1064, 1965.

Kuwabara T, Gorn RA: Retinal damage by visible light: An electron microscopic study. Arch Ophthalmol *79*:69–78, 1968.

Kuwabara T, Ishihara K, Akiya S: Histopathological and electron-microscopic studies of the retina in Oguchi's disease. Acta Soc Ophthalmol Jpn *67*:1323–1351, 1963.

Kuwabara T, Lessell S: Electron microscopic study of extraocular muscles in myotonic dystrophy. Am J Ophthalmol *82*:303–309, 1976.

Laatikainen L, Erkkilä H: Serpiginous choroiditis. Br J Ophthalmol *58*:777–783, 1974.

Laatikainen L, Kohner EM: Fluorescein angiography and its prognostic significance in central retinal vein occlusion. Br J Ophthalmol *60*:411–418, 1976.

Lahav M, Albert DM, Wyand S: Clinical and histopathologic classification of retinal dysplasia. Am J Ophthalmol *75*:648–667, 1973.

Landau J, Nelken E, Davis E: Hereditary hemorrhagic telangiectasia with retinal and conjunctival lesions. Lancet *271*:230–231, 1956.

Landers MB III, Klintworth GK: Subacute sclerosing panencephalitis (S.S.P.E.). Arch Ophthalmol *86*:156–163, 1971.

Landolt E: Anatomische Untersuchungen über typische Retinitis pigmentosa. Von Graefes Arch Ophthalmol *18*:325, 1872.

Lanum J: The damaging effects of light on the retina: Empirical findings, theoretical and practical implications. Surv Ophthalmol *22*:221–249, 1978.

Laqua H, Machemer R: Clinical-pathological correlation in massive periretinal proliferation. Am J Ophthalmol *80*:913–929, 1975a.

Laqua H, Machemer R: Glial cell proliferation in retinal detachment (massive preretinal proliferation). Am J Ophthalmol *80*:602–618, 1975b.

Laqua H, Wessing A: Congenital retinopigment epithelial malformation, previously described as hamartoma. Am J Ophthalmol *87*:34–42, 1979.

Larsen HW, Ehlers N: Ocular manifestations of Tay-Sachs and Niemann-Pick diseases: A clinical, pathological, histochemical and biochemical investigation. Acta Ophthalmol *43*:285–293, 1965.

Laties AM, Scheie HG: Sarcoid granuloma of the optic disk: Evolution of multiple small tumors. Trans Am Ophthalmol Soc *68*:219–233, 1970.

Lavery MA, Green WR, Jabs EW, et al: Ocular histopathology and ultrastructure of Sanfilippo's syndrome, Type III-B. Arch Ophthalmol *101*:1263–1274, 1983.

Leber T: Über eine durch Vorkommen multipler Miliaraneurysmen charakterisierte Form von Retinaldegeneration. Arch f Ophthalmol *81*:1–14, 1912.

Lee RE: The fine structure of the cerebroside occurring in Gaucher's disease. Proc Natl Acad Sci *61*:484–489, 1968.

Lehner T, Batchelor JR, Challacombe SJ, Kennedy L: An immunogenetic basis for tissue involvement in Behçet's syndrome. Immunology *37*:895–900, 1979.

Lerman S: Radiant Energy and the Eye. Functional Ophthalmology Series, Vol. 1. New York, Macmillan Publishing Company, 1980, p 286.

Leveille AS, Newell FW: Autosomal dominant Kearns-Sayre syndrome. Ophthalmology *87*:99–108, 1980.

Levene R, Horton G, Gorn R: Flat-mount studies of human retinal vessels. Am J Ophthalmol *61*:283–289, 1966.

Levin PS, Green WR, Victor DL, MacLean AL: Histopathology of the eye in Cockayne's syndrome. Arch Ophthalmol *101*:1093–1097, 1983.

Levy IS: Refsum's syndrome. Trans ophthalmol Soc UK *90*:181–186, 1970.

Levy JH, Pollack HM, Curtin BJ: The Fuchs' spot: An ophthalmoscopic and fluorescein angiographic study. Ann Ophthalmol 9:1433–1443, 1977.

Lewis RA, Cohen MH, Wise GM: Cavernous haemangioma of the retina and optic disc: A report of three cases and a review of the literature. Br J Ophthalmol *59*:522–534, 1975.

Lewis RA, Falls HF, Troyer DO: Ocular manifestations of hypercupremia associated with multiple myeloma. Arch Ophthalmol *93*:1050–1053, 1975.

Lewkonia I, Davies MS, Salmon JD: Lattice degeneration in a family, with retinal detachment and cataract. Br J Ophthalmol *57*:566–571, 1973.

Libert J: Personal communication, 1977.

Libert J, Davis P: Diagnosis of Type A Niemann-Pick's disease by conjunctival biopsy. Pathol Eur *10*:233–239, 1975.

Libert J, Kenyon KR, Maumenee IH: Mucolipidosis III (pseudo-Hurler polydystrophy); Ultrastructure of conjunctival biopsies. Metab Ophthalmol *1*:145–148, 1977.

Libert J, Martin JJ, Centerich C, Davis P: Ocular ultrastructure in a fetus with Type II glycogenosis. Br J Ophthalmol *61*:476–482, 1977.

Libert J, Martin JJ, Moser HW, et al: Ultrastructural studies in opthalmoplegic dystonic lipidoses, *in* Huber A, Klein D (eds): Neurogenetics and Neuro-ophthalmology. Amsterdam, Elsevier/North Holland Biomedical Press, 1981, pp 317–321.

Libert J, Rutsaert J, Toussaint D: Ultrastructure oculaire d'un cas de leucodystrophie metachromatique juvenile. Bull Soc Belge Ophtalmol *167*:655–663, 1974.

Libert J, Tondeur M, Van Hoof F: The use of conjunctival biopsy and enzyme analysis in tears for the diagnosis of homozygotes and heterozygotes with Fabry disease, *in* Birth Defects. Original Article Series, Vol XII, No 3. New York, The National Foundation, 1976, pp 221–239.

Libert J, Toussaint D, Guiselings R: Ocular findings in Niemann-Pick disease. Am J Ophthalmol *80*:991–1002, 1975.

Libert J, Van Hoof F, Farriaux JP, Toussaint D: Ocular findings in I-cell disease (mucolipidosis type II). Am J Ophthalmol *83*:617–628, 1977.

Libert J, Van Hoof F, Toussaint D, et al: Ocular findings in metachromatic leukodystrophy. Arch Ophthalmol *97*:1495–1504, 1979.

Lieberman J: Elevation of serum angiotensin–converting enzyme (ACE) level in sarcoidosis. Am J Med *59*:365–372, 1975.

Lietman PS, Frazier PD, Wong VG, et al: Adult cystinosis: A benign disorder. Am J Med *40*:511–517, 1966.

Lincoff HA, Kreissig I: The mechanism of the cryosurgical adhesion. 4. An electron microscopy. Am J Ophthalmol *71*:674–689, 1971.

Lister WT: A case of retinitis pigmentosa with pathological report. Roy London Ophthalmol Hosp Rep *15*:254, 1903.

Lobes LA Jr, Folk JC: Syphilitic phlebitis simulating branch vein occlusion. Ann Ophthalmol *13*:825–827, 1981.

Lonn LI: Neonatal cytomegalic inclusion disease chorioretinitis. Arch Ophthalmol *88*:434–438, 1972.

Lonn LI, Hoyt WF: Papillophlebitis: A cause of protracted yet benign optic disc edema. Eye Ear Nose Throat Monthly *45*:62–passim, 1966.

Lonn LI, Smith TR: Ora serrata pearls: Clinical and histological correlation. Arch Ophthalmol *77*:809–813, 1967.

Lubin JR, Rennie D, Hackett P, Albert DM: High altitude retinal hemorrhage: A clinical and pathological case report. Ann Ophthalmol *14*:1071–1076, 1982.

Luckenbach MW, Green WR, Miller NR et al: Ocular clinicopathologic correlation of Hallervorden-Spatz syndrome with acanthocytosis and pigmentary retinopathy. Am J Ophthalmol *95*:369–382, 1983.

Lyle TK, Wybar K: Retinal vasculitis. Br J Ophthalmol *45*:778, 1961.

Mabie WC, Ober RR: Fluorescein angiography in toxemia of pregnancy. Br J Ophthalmol *64*:666–671, 1980.

MacFaul PA, Bedford MA: Ocular complications after therapeutic irradiation. Br J Ophthalmol *54*:237–247, 1970.

Machemer R: Die primäre retinale Pigment-epithelhyperplasie. Albrecht Von Graefes Arch Ophthalmol *167*:284–295, 1964.

Machemer R, Kroll AJ: Experimental retinal detachment in the owl monkey. VII. Photoreceptor protein renewal in normal and detached retina. Am J Ophthalmol *71*:690–695, 1971.

Machemer R, Laqua H: Pigment epithelium proliferation in

retinal detachment (massive periretinal proliferation). Am J Ophthalmol *80*:1–23, 1975.

Machemer H, van Horn D, Aaberg TM: Pigment epithelial proliferation in human retinal detachment with massive periretinal proliferation. Am J Ophthalmol *85*:181–191, 1978.

MacLean A, Victor D, Green WR: Cockayne's disease: Clinical-pathologic studies of 2 cases. Unpublished data, 1978.

Macular Photocoagulation Study Group: Argon laser photocoagulation for senile macular degeneration. Results of a randomized clinical trial. Arch Ophthalmol *100*:912–918, 1982.

MacVicar JE, Wilbrandt HR: Hereditary retinoschisis and early hemeralopia. Arch Ophthalmol *83*:629–636, 1970.

Macy JI, Baerveldt G: Pseudophakic serous maculopathy. Arch Ophthalmol *101*:228–231, 1983.

Maggiore L: Contributo sperimentale alle alterazioni retiniche nell'occhio umano esposto a luce intensa. Anna Ottal Clin Ocul *61*:81–98, 1933.

Mahneke A, Videboek A: On changes in the optic fundus in leukemia. Aetiology; diagnostic and prognostic role. Acta Ophthalmol *42*:201–210, 1964.

Makley TA, Craig EL, Long JW: Histopathology of presumed ocular histoplasmosis. Palest Oftal Panamer *1*:72–82, 1977.

Malinow MR, Feeney-Burns L, Peterson LH, et al: Diet-related macular anomalies in monkeys. Invest Ophthalmol Vis Sci *19*:857–863, 1980.

Manschot WA: Persistent hyperplastic primary vitreous. Arch Ophthalmol *59*:188–203, 1958.

Manschot WA: Embolism of the central retinal artery originating from an endocardial myxoma. Am J Ophthalmol *48*:381–385, 1959.

Manschot WA: Generalized scleroderma with ocular symptoms. Ophthalmologica *149*:131–137, 1965.

Manschot WA: Histological findings in a case of dystrophia myotonica. Ophthalmologica *155*:294–296, 1968a.

Manschot WA: Intraocular cysticercus. Arch Ophthalmol *80*:772–774, 1968b.

Manschot WA: Retinal histology in amaurotic idiocies and tapeto-retinal degenerations. Ophthalmologica *156*:28–37, 1968c.

Manschot WA: Juxtapapillary retinal angiomatosis. Arch Ophthalmol *80*:775–776, 1968d.

Manschot WA: Pathology of hereditary juvenile retinoschisis. Arch Ophthalmol *88*:131–138, 1972.

Manschot WA: *Coenurus* infestation of eye and orbit. Arch Ophthalmol *94*:961–964, 1976.

Manz HJ, Rosen DA, Macklin RD, Willis WE: Neuroectodermal tumor of anterior lip of optic cup. Arch Ophthalmol *89*:382–386, 1973.

Manz HJ, Schuelein M, McCullough DC, et al: New phenotypic variant of adrenoleukodystrophy. Pathologic, ultrastructural, and biochemical study in two brothers. J Neurol Sci *45*:245–260, 1980.

Marak GE Jr: Recent advances in sympathetic ophthalmia. Surv Ophthalmol *24*:141–156, 1979.

Margolis L, Fraser R, Lichter A, Char DH: The role of radiation therapy in the management of ocular reticulum cell sarcoma. Cancer *45*:688–692, 1980.

Marlor RL, Blais BR, Preston FR, Boyden DG: Foveomacular retinitis, an important problem in military medicine: Epidemiology. Invest Ophthalmol *12*:5–16, 1973.

Marmor MF: "Vitelliform" lesions in adults. Ann Ophthalmol *11*:1705–1712, 1979.

Maroteaux, P, Leveque B, Marie J, Lamy M: Une nouvelle dypostose avec elimination urinaire de chondroitine-sulfate B. Presse Med *71*:1849–1852, 1963.

Marquardt R: Manifestation der Hyalinosis cutis et mucosae (Lipoidproteinose Urbach-Wiethe) am Auge. Klin Monatsbl Augenheilkd *140*:684–692, 1962.

Marquardt R: Vergleichende klinische und morphologische Untersuchungen am Augenhintergrund bei cronisch-progressiver Hypertonie. Albrecht Von Graefes Arch Klin Exp Ophthalmol *179*:20–31, 1969.

Marr WG, Marr EG: Some observations on Purtscher's disease: Traumatic retinal angiopathy. Am J Ophthalmol *54*:693–705, 1962.

Marshall J, Mellerio J: Pathological development of retinal laser photocoagulations. Exp Eye Res *6*:303–308, 1967.

Martin JJ, Ceuterick C, Libert J: Skin and conjunctival nerve biopsies in adrenoleukodystrophy and its variants. Ann Neurol *8*:291–295, 1980.

Martin JJ, Ceuterick C, Martin L, Libert J: Skin and conjunctival biopsies in adrenoleukodystrophy. Acta Neuropathol (Berlin) *38*:247–250, 1977.

Martin NF, Green WR, Martin LW: Retinal phlebitis in the Irvine-Gass syndrome. Am J Ophthalmol *83*:377–386, 1977.

Martyn LJ, Knox DL: Glial hamartoma of the retina in generalized neurofibromatosis (von Recklinghausen's disease). Br J Ophthalmol *56*:487–491, 1972.

Mass JM, de Vloo N, Jamotton L: Les manifestations oculaires des hemopathies. Bull Soc Belge Ophthalmol *142*:1–413, 1966 (see pp 317–338).

Massof RW, Finkelstein D: Rod sensitivity relative to cone sensitivity in retinitis pigmentosa. Invest Ophthalmol Vis Sci *18*:263–272, 1979.

Massof RW, Finkelstein D: Subclassification of retinitis pigmentosa from two-color scotopic static perimetry. Doc Ophthalmol *24*:219–225, 1981.

Masur H, Michelis MA, Greene JB, et al: An outbreak of community-acquired *Pneumocystis carinii* pneumonia: Initial manifestation of cellular immune dysfunction. N Engl J Med *305*:1431–1438, 1981.

Matsuda H, Satake Y, Katsumata H: Ultrastructural observation on the cornea of Hurler syndrome. Jpn J Ophthalmol *14*:237–246, 1970.

Maumenee AE: Retinal lesions in lupus erythematosus. Am J Ophthalmol *23*:971–981, 1940.

Maumenee AE: Serous and hemorrhagic disciform detachment of the macula. Trans Pacif Coast Oto-Ophthalmol Soc *40*:139–160, 1959.

Maumenee IH: The effect of plasma and plasma derivative infusion in the mucopolysaccharidoses. Acta Soc Ophthalmol Jpn *77*:1422–1433, 1973.

Maumenee IH: Vitreoretinal degeneration as a sign of generalized connective tissue diseases. Am J Ophthalmol *88*:432–449, 1979.

Maumenee IH, Maumenee AE: Fundus flavimaculatus—clinical, genetic, and pathologic observations, *in* François J: Proceedings from the 5th Congress of the European Society of Ophthalmology. Hamburg, 1976; Stuttgart, Ferdinand Enke Verlag, 1978.

Maumenee IH, Stoll HU, Mets MB: The Wagner syndrome versus hereditary arthro-ophthalmopathy. Trans Am Ophthalmol Soc *80*:349–365, 1982.

Mazow ML, Ruiz RS: Eccentric disciform degeneration. Trans Am Ophthalmol Otolaryngol *77*:68–73, 1973.

McBrien DJ, Bradley RD, Ashton N: The nature of retinal emboli in stenosis of the internal carotid artery. Lancet *1*:697–699, 1963.

McCormick AQ: Ocular findings in a case of stippled epiphyses with cystic kidneys. Presented at the Verhoeff Society Meeting, Washington, DC. April, 1969.

McCrary JA III, Smith JL: Conjunctival and retinal incontinentia pigmenti. Arch Ophthalmol *79*:417, 1968.

McCulloch JC: The pathologic findings in two cases of choroideremia. Trans Am Acad Ophthalmol Otolaryngol *54*:565–572, 1950.

McCulloch C, Marliss EB: Gyrate atrophy of the choroid and retina with hyperorinithinemia. Am J Ophthalmol *80*:1047–1057, 1975.

McDonnell PJ, Fine SL, Hillis AI: Clinical features of idiopathic macular cysts and holes. Am J Ophthalmol *93*:777–786, 1982.

McFarland CB: Heredodegeneration of the macula luten. Arch Ophthalmol *53*:224–228, 1955.

McKibbin DW, Bulkley BH, Green WR, et al: Fatal cerebral

atheromatous embolization after cardiopulmonary bypass. J Thorac Cardiovasc Surg *71*:741–745, 1976.

McKusick VA: Mendelian Inheritance in Man: Catalogs of Autosomal Dominant, Autosomal Recessive, and X-Linked Phenotypes. 5th ed. Baltimore, Johns Hopkins University Press, 1978, pp 268, 528, 618–619.

McLean EB: Hamartoma of the retinal pigment epithelium. Am J Ophthalmol *82*:227–231, 1976.

McLean JM: Astrocytoma (true glioma) of the retina. Arch Ophthalmol *18*:255–262, 1937.

McLeod AC, McConnell FE, Sweeney A, et al: Clinical variations in Usher's syndrome. Arch Otolaryngol *94*:321–334, 1971.

McLeod D, Marshall J, Kohner EM, Bird AC: The role of axoplasmic transport in the pathogenesis of cotton-wool spots. Br J Ophthalmol *61*:177–191, 1977.

Meier-Ruge W: Experimental investigation of the morphogenesis of chloroquine retinopathy. Arch Ophthalmol *73*:540–544, 1965.

Menezo JL, Suarez-Reynolds R, Francés J, Vila E: Shape, number and localization of retinal tears in myopia over 8D, aphakic, and traumatic cases of retinal detachment: An experience report. Ophthalmologica *175*:10–18, 1977.

Menkes JH, Corbo LM: Adrenoleukodystrophy. Accumulation of cholesterol esters with very long chain fatty acids. Neurology *27*:928–932, 1977.

Mensheha-Manhart O, Rodrigues MM, Shields JA, et al: Retinal pigment epithelium in incontinentia pigmenti. Am J Ophthalmol *79*:571–577, 1975.

Meredith TA, Green WR, Key SN III, et al.: Ocular histoplasmosis: Clinicopathologic correlation of 3 cases. Surv Ophthalmol *22*:189–205, 1977.

Meredith TA, Kenyon KR, Singerman LJ, et al: Perifoveal vascular leakage and macular aedema after intracapsular cataract extraction. Br J Ophthalmol *60*:765–769, 1976.

Meredith TA, Wright JD, Gammon JA, et al: Ocular involvement in primary hyperoxaluria. Arch Ophthalmol *102*:584–587, 1984.

Merin S, Abraham FS, Auervach E: Usher's and Hallgren's syndromes. Acta Genet Med Gemellol (Rome) *23*:49–55, 1974.

Merin S, Livni N, Berman ER, Yatziv S: Mucolipidosis IV: Ocular, systemic, and ultrastructural findings. Invest Ophthalmol *14*:437–448, 1975.

Merrian GR Jr, Szechter A, Focht EF: The effects of ionizing radiations on the eye, *in* Vaeth JM (ed): Frontiers of the Radiation Therapy and Oncology. Vol 6. Baltimore, University Park Press, 1972, pp 346–385.

Merritt AD, Smith SA, Strouth JC, Zeman W: Detection of heterozygotes in Batten's disease. Ann NY Acad Sci *155*:860–867, 1968.

Merritt JC, Callender CO: Adult cytomegalic inclusion retinitis. Ann Ophthalmol *10*:1059–1063, 1978.

Messner KH, Kammerer WS: Intraocular cysticercosis. Arch Ophthalmol *97*:1103–1105, 1979.

Messner KH, Maisels MJ, Leure-DuPree AE: Phototoxicity to the newborn primate retina. Invest Ophthalmol Vis Sci *17*:178–182, 1978.

Meyer E, Kurz GH: Retinal pits: A study of pathologic findings in two cases. Arch Ophthalmol *70*:640–646, 1963.

Meyer KT, Heckenlively JR, Spitznas M, Foos RY: Dominant retinitis pigmentosa. A clinicopathologic correlation. Ophthalmology *89*:1414–1424, 1982.

Meyer-Schwickerath G: Koagulation der Netzhaut mit Sonnenlicht. Ber Dtsch Ophthalmol Ges (Heidelberg) *55*:256–259, 1950.

Meyer-Schwickerath G, von Barsewisch B: Gefässveränderungen an Haut und Retina. Ber Dtsch Ophthalmol Ges *68*:525–530, 1968.

Meyers SM: The incidence of fundus lesions in septicemia. Am J Ophthalmol *88*:661–667, 1979.

Michels RG, Gass JDM: The natural course of retinal branch vein obstruction. Trans Am Acad Ophthalmol Otolaryngol *78*:166–177, 1974.

Michels RG, Knox DL, Erozan YS, Green WR: Intraocular reticulum cell sarcoma: Diagnosis by pars plana vitrectomy. Arch Ophthalmol *93*:1331–1335, 1975.

Michelson JB, Whitcher JP, Wilson S, O'Connor GR: Possible foreign body granuloma of the retina associated with intravenous cocaine addiction. Am J Ophthalmol *87*:278–280, 1979.

Michelson PE, Knox DL, Green WR: Ischemic ocular inflammation: A clinicopathologic case report. Arch Ophthalmol *86*:274–280, 1971.

Michelson PE, Stark WJ, Reeser F, Green WR: Endogenous *Candida* endophthalmitis: Report of thirteen cases and sixteen from the literature. Int Ophthalmol Clin *2*:125–147, 1971.

Miller FS III, Bunt-Milam AH, Kalina RE: Clinical-ultrastructural study of thioridazine retinopathy. Ophthalmology *89*:1478–1488, 1982.

Miller M, Robbins J, Fishman R, et al: A chromosomal anomaly with multiple ocular defects, including retinal dysplasia. Am J Ophthalmol *55*:901–910, 1963.

Mimatsu T: A histological study of retinal blood vessels in Japanese hypertensive patients. Acta Soc Ophthalmol Jpn *67*:1463–1480, 1963.

Minckler D, Allen AW Jr: Adenocarcinoma of the retinal pigment epithelium. Arch Ophthalmol *96*:2252–2254, 1978.

Minckler DS, Font RL, Zimmerman LE: Uveitis and reticulum cell sarcoma of brain with bilateral neoplastic seeding of vitreous without retinal or uveal involvement. Am J Ophthalmol *80*:433–439, 1975.

Minckler DS, McLean EB, Shaw CM, Hendrickson A: *Herpesvirus hominis* encephalitis and retinitis. Arch Ophthalmol *94*:89–95, 1976.

Miyake K: Prevention of cystoid macular edema after lens extraction by topical indomethacin. II. A control study in bilateral extractions. Jpn J Ophthalmol *22*:80–94, 1978.

Mizuno K, Nishida S: Pathology and electron microscopy of retinitis pigmentosa. Rinsho Ganka *20*:949–965, 1966.

Mizuno K, Nishida S: Electron microscopic studies of human retinitis pigmentosa. Part 1. Am J Ophthalmol *63*:791–803, 1967.

Mizuno K, Sears ML, Peterson WS, et al: Leber's congenital amaurosis. Am J Ophthalmol *83*:32–42, 1977.

Möller PM, Hammerberg PE: Retinal periphlebitis in multiple sclerosis. Acta Neurol Scand (Suppl 4) *39*:263–269, 1963.

Monahan RH, Horns RC: The pathology of chloroquine in the eye. Trans Am Acad Ophthalmol Otolaryngol *68*:40–44, 1964.

Moon ME, Clarke AM, Ruffolo JJ Jr, et al: Visual performance in the Rhesus monkey after exposure to blue light. Vis Res *18*:1573–1577, 1978.

Moran TJ, Estevez JM: Chediak-Higashi disease: Morphologic studies of a patient and her family. Arch Pathol *88*:329–339, 1969.

Morax PV, Saraux H, Moday S, Coscas G: Les manifestations oculaires des rickettsioses et des neorickettsioses. Ann Oculist *194*:929–956, 1961.

Morgan A, Boulud B: Evolutivité de syndrome d'Usher. J Fr Otorhinolaryngol *24*:614–620, 1975.

Moron-Salas J: Obliteracion de los desgarros retinianos por quemadura con luz. Arch Soc Oftal Hispano-Am *10*:566–578, 1950.

Morquio L: Sur une forme de dystrophie osseuse familiale. Bull Soc. Pediatr (Paris) *27*:145–152, 1929.

Morris DA, Henkind P: Pathological responses of the human retinal pigment epithelium, *in* Zinn KM, Marmor MF (eds): The Retinal Pigment Epithelium. Cambridge, Mass, Harvard University Press, 1979, pp 247–266.

Morse PH: Elschnig's spots and hypertensive choroidopathy. Am J Ophthalmol *66*:844–852, 1968.

Morse PH, McCready JL: Peripheral retinal neovascularization in chronic myelocytic leukemia. Am J Ophthalmol *72*:975–978, 1971.

Moser HW, Moser AB, Frayer KK, et al: Adrenoleukodystrophy: Increased plasma content of saturated, very long chain fatty acids. Neurology *31*:1241–1249, 1981.

Moser HW, Moser AB, Kawamura N, et al: Adrenoleukodystrophy; Studies of the phenotype, genetics and biochemistry. Johns Hopkins Med J *147*:217–224, 1980.

Mueller H: Anatomische Beiträge zur Ophthalmologie. Arch Ophthalmol *2*:1–69 (Part 2), 1855.

Mueller-Jensen K, Machemer R, Azarnia R: Autotransplantation of retinal pigment epithelium in intravitreal diffusion chamber. Am J Ophthalmol *80*:530–537, 1975.

Mullaney J: Primary malignant medulloepithelioma of the retinal stalk. Am J Ophthalmol *77*:499–504, 1974.

Murphree AL, Beaudet AL, Palmer EA, Nichols BL: Cataract in mannosidosis. Birth Defects *12*:319–334, 1976.

Murphy RP, Patz A: The natural history and management of nonproliferative diabetic retinopathy, *in* Little H, Patz A (eds): Diabetic Retinopathy. New York, Thieme-Stratton, 1983, pp 225–241.

Murray HW, Knox DL, Green WR, Susel RM: Cytomegalovirus retinitis in adults: A manifestation of disseminated viral infection. Am J Med *63*:574–584, 1977.

Nadel AJ, Gupta KK: Macroaneurysms of the retinal arteries. Arch Ophthalmol *94*:1092–1096, 1976.

Nagel A: Hochgradige Amblyopie, bedingt durch glashäutige Wucherungen und krystallinische Kalkablagerungen an der innenfläche der Aderhaut. Klin Monatsbl Augenheilkd *13*:338–351, 1875.

Naidoff MA, Green WR: Endogenous *Aspergillus* endophthalmitis occurring after kidney transplant. Am J Ophthalmol *79*:502–509, 1975.

Naidoff MA, Kenyon KR, Green WR: Iris hemangioma and abnormal retinal vasculature in a case of diffuse congenital hemangiomatosis. Am J Ophthalmol *72*:633–644, 1971.

Naiman J, Green WR, Patz A: Retrolental fibroplasia in hypoxic newborn. Am J Ophthalmol *88*:55–58, 1979.

Nakao K, Ikeda M, Kimata SI, et al: Takayasu's arteritis: Clinical report of eighty-four cases and immunological studies of seven cases. Circulation *35*:1141–1155, 1967.

Nasu K: Studies on drug-induced retinal degeneration. Part I. Early stages of experimental chloroquine retinopathy. Acta Soc Ophthalmol Jpn *73*:1663–1673, 1969.

Naumann G, Gass JDM, Font RL: Histopathology of herpes zoster ophthalmicus. Am J Ophthalmol *65*:533–541, 1968.

Naumann GOH: Maroteaux-Lamy syndrome (mucopolysaccharidosis type VI) in two sisters. Case presented at European Ophthalmic Pathology Society, Göttingen, Germany, May, 1982.

Naumann GOH, Lerche W, Schroeder W: Foveola-Aplasie bei Tyrosinase-posivitem oculocutanen Albinismus. Albrecht Von Graefes Arch Ophthal *200*:39–50, 1976.

Nelson DA, Weiner A, Yanoff M, de Peralta J: Retinal lesions in subacute sclerosing panencephalitis. Arch Ophthalmol *84*:613–621, 1970.

Nessan VJ, Jacoway JR: Biopsy of minor salivary glands in the diagnosis of sarcoidosis. N Engl J Med *301*:922–924, 1979.

Neufeld EF, Cantz MJ: Corrective factors for inborn errors of mucopolysaccharide metabolism. Ann NY Acad Sci *179*:580–587, 1971.

Neumann E, Gunders AE: The posterior segment lesion of ocular onchocerciasis. Isr J Med Sci *8*:1158–1162, 1972.

Neumann E, Gunders AE: Pathogenesis of the posterior segment lesion of ocular onchocerciasis. Am J Ophthalmol *75*:82–89, 1973.

Neuwirth J, Gutman I, Hofeldt AJ, et al: Cytomegalovirus retinitis in a young homosexual male with acquired immunodeficiency. Ophthalmology *89*:805–808, 1982.

Newell FW, Johnson RO II, Huttenlocher PR: Pigmentary degeneration of the retina in the Hallervorden-Spatz syndrome. Am J Ophthalmol *88*:467–471, 1979.

Newell FW, Koistinen A: Lipochondrodystrophy (gargoylism). Pathologic findings in five eyes of three patients. Arch Ophthalmol *53*:45–62, 1955.

Newell FW, Matalon R, Meyer S: A new mucolipidosis with psychomotor retardation, corneal clouding, and retinal degeneration. Am J Ophthalmol *80*:440–449, 1975.

Newman NM, Hoyt WF, Spencer WH: Macula-sparing monocular blackouts. Clinical and pathologic investigations of intermittent choroidal vascular insufficiency in a case of periarteritis nodosa. Arch Ophthalmol *91*:367–370, 1974.

Newman NM, Mandel MR, Gullett J, Fujikawa L: Clinical and histologic findings in opportunistic ocular infections. Part of a new syndrome of acquired immunodeficiency. Arch Ophthalmol *101*:386–401, 1983.

Newman NM, Smith ME, Gay AJ: An unusual case of leukemia involving the eye: A clinicopathological study. Surv Ophthalmol *16*:316–321, 1972.

Newsome DA, Kenyon KR: Collagen production in vitro by the retinal pigmented epithelium of the chick embryo. Dev Biol *32*:387–400, 1973.

Nicholls JVV: The effect of section of the posterior ciliary arteries in the rabbit. Br J Ophthalmol *22*:672–687, 1938.

Nichols CW, Eagle RC Jr, Yanoff M, Menocal NG: Conjunctival biopsy as an aid in the evaluation of the patient with suspected sarcoidosis. Ophthalmology *87*:287–291, 1980.

Nichols RL: The etiology of visceral larva migrans: Diagnostic morphology of infective second-stage *Toxocara* larvae. J Parasitol *42*:349–362, 1956.

Nicholson DH, Green WR, Kenyon KR: Light and electron microscopic study of early lesions in angiomatosis retinae. Am J Ophthalmol *82*:193–204, 1976.

Nicholson DH, Wolchok EB: Ocular toxoplasmosis in an adult receiving long-term corticosteroid therapy. Arch Ophthalmol *94*:248–254, 1976.

Nishimura RN, Ishak KG, Reddick R, et al: Lafora disease: Diagnosis by liver biopsy. Ann Neurol *8*:409–415, 1980.

Noble KG, Carr RE: Leber's congenital amaurosis: A retrospective study of 33 cases and a histopathological study of one case. Arch Ophthalmol *96*:818–821, 1978.

Noble KG, Carr RE, Siegel IM: Fluorescein angiography of the hereditary choroidal dystrophies. Br J Ophthalmol *61*:43–53, 1977.

Noell WK, Walker VS, Kang BS, Berman S: Retinal damage by light in rats. Invest Ophthalmol *5*:450–473, 1966.

Nørby S, Jansen OA, Schwartz M: Retinal and cerebellar changes in early fetal Sandhoff disease (GM_2-gangliosidosis, Type 2). Metab Pediatr Ophthalmol *4*:115–119, 1980.

Nordmann J: Les tumeurs de la rétine ciliare. Ophthalmologica (Basel) *102*:257–274, 1941.

Norris JL, Cleasby GW: An unusual case of congenital hypertrophy of the retinal pigment epithelium. Arch Ophthalmol *94*:1910–1911, 1976.

Nosal A, Schleissner LA, Mishkin FS, Lieberman J: Angiotensin I–converting enzyme and gallium scan in noninvasive evaluation of sarcoidosis. Ann Intern Med *90*:328–331, 1979.

Novak M, Green WR, Miller NR: Ophthalmologic manifestations in a case of familial giant cell arteritis, in preparation.

Nuutila A: Dystrophia retinae pigmentosa—dysacusis syndrome (DRD): A study of the Usher or Hallgren syndrome. J Genet Hum *18*:57–88, 1970.

Obenauf CD, Shaw HE, Sydnor CF, Klintworth GK: Sarcoidosis and its ophthalmic manifestations. Am J Ophthalmol *86*:648–655, 1978.

Ober RR, Bird AC, Hamilton AM, et al: Autosomal dominant exudative vitreoretinopathy. Br J Ophthalmol *64*:112–120, 1980.

Oberman J, Cohn H, Grand M: Retinal complications of gas myelography. Arch Ophthalmol *97*:1905–1906, 1979.

O'Brien JS: Neuraminidase deficiency in the cherry-red-spot myoclonus syndrome. Biochem Biophys Res Commun *79*:1136–1141, 1977.

Ockerman PA: A generalised storage disorder resembling Hurler's syndrome. Lancet *2*:239–241, 1967.

O'Donnell FE Jr, Green WR: The Eye in albinism, *in* Duane

TD (ed): Clinical Ophthalmology. Vol 4. New York, Harper & Row, 1979, pp 1–23 (see pp 13–19).
O'Donnell FE Jr, Green WR, Fleischman JA, Hambrick GW Jr: X-linked ocular albinism in blacks. Arch Ophthalmol *96*:1189–1192, 1978.
O'Donnell FE Jr, Green WR, McKusick VA, et al: Forsius-Eriksson syndrome: Its relation to the Nettleship-Falls X-linked ocular albinism. Clin Genet *17*:403–408, 1980.
O'Donnell FE Jr, Hambrick GW, Green WR, et al: X-linked ocular albinism. Arch Ophthalmol *94*:1883–1892, 1976.
O'Donnell FE Jr, King RA, Green WR, Witkop CJ Jr: Autosomal recessively inherited ocular albinism. Arch Ophthalmol *96*:1621–1625, 1978.
O'Donnell FE Jr, Schaltz H, Reid P, Green WR: Autosomal dominant dystrophy of the retinal pigment epithelium. Arch Ophthalmol *97*:680–683, 1979.
Ohnishi K, Kagoshima M: Discussion. Acta Soc Ophthalmol Jpn *12*:555–556, 1908.
Ohno S, Ohguchi M, Hirose S, et al: Close association of HLA-Bw51 with Behçet's disease. Arch Ophthalmol *100*:1455–1458, 1982.
Okun E: Retinal detachment. JAMA *174*:2218–2220, 1960.
Okun E: Gross and microscopic pathology in autopsy eyes. III. Retinal breaks without detachment. Am J Ophthalmol *51*:369–391, 1961a.
Okun E: Gross and microscopic pathology in autopsy eyes. IV. Pars plana cysts. Am J Ophthalmol *51*:1221–1228, 1961b.
Oliver GL, McFarlane DC: Congenital trichomegaly: With associated pigmentary degeneration of the retina, dwarfism and mental retardation. Arch Ophthalmol *74*:169–171, 1965.
Oliver M, Uchenik D: Bilateral exudative retinal detachment in eclampsia without hypertensive retinopathy. Am J Ophthalmol *90*:792–796, 1980.
Olson W, Engel WK, Walsh GO, Enangler R: Oculocraniosomatic neuromuscular disease with "ragged-red" fibers: Histochemical and ultrastructural changes in limb muscles of a group of patients with idiopathic progressive external ophthalmoplegia. Arch Neurol *26*:193–211, 1972.
O'Malley PF, Allen RA: Peripheral cystoid degeneration of the retina: Incidence and distribution in 1,000 autopsy eyes. Arch Ophthalmol *77*:769–776, 1967.
O'Malley PF, Allen RA, Straatsma BR, O'Malley CC: Pavingstone degeneration of the retina. Arch Ophthalmol *73*:169–182, 1965.
Opitz JM: Ocular anomalies in malformation syndromes. Trans Am Acad Ophthalmol Otolaryngol *76*:1193–1202, 1972.
Opitz JM, France TD, Hermann J, Spranger JW: The Stickler syndrome. N Engl J Med *286*:546–547, 1972.
Orth DH, Fine BS, Fagman W, Quirk TC: Clarification of foveomacular nomenclature and grid for quantitation of macular disorders. Trans Am Acad Ophthalmol Otholaryngol *83*:506–514, 1977.
Orth DH, Fishman GA, Segall M, et al: Rubella maculopathy. Br J Ophthalmol *64*:201–205, 1980.
O'Steen WK, Anderson KV, Shear CR: Photoreceptor degeneration in albino rats: Dependency on age. Invest Ophthalmol *13*:334–339, 1974.
Pahwa JM, Garg MP: Eales's disease: Its clinical course and treatment by photocoagulation. A review of 100 cases. EENT Monthly *47*:174–180, 1968.
Parelhoff ES, Wood WJ, Green WR, Kenyon KR: Radial perivascular lattice degeneration of the retina. Ann Ophthalmol *12*:25–32, 1980.
Park BE, Netsky MG, Betsill WL Jr: Pathogenesis of pigment and spheroid formation in Hallervorden-Spatz syndrome and related disorders. Neurology *25*:1172–1178, 1975.
Parver LM, Font RL: Malignant lymphoma of the retina and brain. Initial diagnosis by cytologic examination of vitreous aspirate. Arch Ophthalmol *97*:1505–1507, 1979.
Paton D: The significance of angioid streaks. Middle East Med J *1*:301–338, 1962.
Paton D: The Relation of Angioid Streaks to Systemic Disease. Springfield, Ill, Charles C Thomas, 1972, pp 58–61.
Patrinely JR, Green WR, Randolph ME: Retinal phlebitis with chorioretinal emboli. Am J Ophthalmol *94*:49–57, 1982.
Paufique L, Hervouet F: Anatomie pathologique d'un cas de maladie de Stargardt. Bull Soc Ophtalmol Fr *76*:108–114, 1963.
Paufique L, Ravault MP, Bonnet M, Istre M: L'angiomatose miliaire rétinienne de Leber. Ann Oculist (Paris) *197*:937–955, 1964.
Paul EV, Zimmerman LE: Some observations on the ocular pathology of onchocerciasis. Hum Pathol *1*:581–594, 1970.
Payne FE, Baublis JV, Itabashi HH: Isolation of measles virus from cell cultures of brain from a patient with subacute sclerosing panencephalitis. N Engl J Med *281*:585–589, 1969.
Pearlman JT, Heckenlively JR, Bastek JV: Progressive nature of pigmented paravenous retinochoroidal atrophy. Am J Ophthalmol *85*:215–217, 1978.
Pearlman JT, Kamin DF, Kopelow SM, Saxton J: Pigmented paravenous retinochoroidal atrophy. Am J Ophthalmol *80*:630–635, 1975.
Pears MA, Pickering GW: Changes in the fundus oculi after haemorrhage. Q J Med *29*:153–178, 1960.
Pederson JE, Kenyon KR, Green WR, Maumenee AE: Pathology of pars planitis. Am J Ophthalmol *86*:762–774, 1978.
Peiffer J: The pure leucodystrophic forms of orthochromatic leucodystrophies (simple type, pigment type), *in* Vinken PJ, Bruyn GW (eds): Handbook of Neurology. Vol 10. Amsterdam, Elsevier, 1970, pp 105–119.
Penner R, Font RL: Retinal embolism from calcified vegetations of aortic valve. Arch Ophthalmol *81*:565–568, 1969.
Perkins ES: Ocular toxoplasmosis. Br J Ophthalmol *57*:1–17, 1973.
Perraut LE, Zimmerman LE: The occurrence of glaucoma following occlusion of the central retinal artery. Arch Ophthalmol *61*:845–865, 1959.
Perry HD, Zimmerman LE, Benson WE: Hemorrhage from isolated aneurysm of a retinal artery. Arch Ophthalmol *95*:281–283, 1977.
Peyman GA, Fishman GA, Sanders DR, et al: Histopathology of Goldmann-Favre syndrome obtained by full-thickness eye-wall biopsy. Ann Ophthalmol *9*:479–484, 1977.
Pfaffenbach DD, Hollenhorst RW: Morbidity and survivorship of patients with embolic cholesterol crystals in the ocular fundus. Trans Am Ophthalmol Soc *70*:337–349, 1972.
Phelps DL, Rosenbaum AL: Vitamin E in kitten oxygen-induced retinopathy. II. Blockage of vitreal neovascularization. Arch Ophthalmol *97*:1522–1526, 1979.
Pinkham RA: The ocular manifestations of the pulseless syndrome. Acta XVII Congress Ophthalmology, New York and Montreal, 1954. Vol 1. Toronto, University of Toronto Press, 1955, pp 348–366.
Pirie A: Pathology in the eye of the naphthalene-fed rabbit. Exp Eye Res *7*:354–357, 1968.
Pitta CG, Steinert RF, Gragoudas ES, Regan CDJ: Small unilateral foveal hemorrhages in young adults. Am J Ophthalmol *89*:96–102, 1980.
Pluth JR, Danielson GK: Poppet embolization in cloth-covered Silastic poppet valves. Mayo Clin Proc *49*:811–814, 1974.
Pollard RB, Egbert PR, Gallagher JG, Merigan TC: Cytomegalovirus retinitis in immunosuppressed hosts. I. Natural history and effects of treatment with adenine arabinoside. Ann Intern Med *93*:655–664, 1980.
Pollard ZF: Ocular *Toxocara* in siblings of two families. Arch Ophthalmol *97*:2319–2320, 1979.
Pollard ZF, Jarrett WH, Hagler WS, et al: ELISA for diagnosis of ocular toxocariasis. Ophthalmology *86*:743–749, 1979.
Popkin JS, Polomeno RC: Stickler's syndrome (hereditary progressive arthro-ophthalmopathy). Can Med Assoc J *111*:1071–1076, 1974.

Porter R: Uveitis in association with multiple sclerosis. Br J Ophthalmol *56*:478–481, 1972.

Potter EL: Facial characteristics of infants with bilateral renal agenesis. Am J Obstet Gynecol *51*:885–888, 1946.

Potter EL: Bilateral absence of ureters and kidneys. A report of 50 cases. Obstet Gynecol *25*:3–12, 1965.

Potts AM: Uveal pigment and phenothiazine compounds. Trans Am Ophthalmol Soc *60*:517–552, 1962.

Potts AM: Tobacco amblyopia. Surv Ophthalmol *17*:313–339, 1973.

Pouliquen Y, Faure JP, Bisson J, et al: Ultrastructure de la cornee dans un cas de polydystrophie de Hurler. Arch Ophthalmol (Paris) *27*:495–512, 1967.

Powell MB, Tindall R, Schultz P, et al: Adrenoleukodystrophy: Electron microscopic findings. Arch Neurol *32*:250–260, 1975.

Powers JM, Schaumburg HH: Adrenoleukodystrophy (sex-linked Schilder's disease): A pathogenetic hypothesis based on ultrastructural lesions in adrenal cortex, peripheral nerve and testis. Am J Pathol *76*:481–491, 1974.

Presley, GD: Fundus changes in Rocky Mountain spotted fever. Am J Ophthalmol *67*:263–267, 1969.

Price FW Jr, Schlaegel TF Jr: Bilateral acute retinal necrosis. Am J Ophthalmol *89*:419–424, 1980.

Price JA Jr, Wadsworth JAC: An intraretinal worm. Arch Ophthalmol *83*:768–770, 1970.

Priluck IA, Buettner H, Robertson DM: Acute macular neuroretinopathy. Am J Ophthalmol *86*:775–778, 1978.

Primer on Rheumatic Diseases. 8. Systemic Lupus Erythematosus. JAMA (Suppl 5) *224*:701–710, 1973.

Pringle JA: A case of multiple aneurysms of the retinal arteries . Br J Ophthalmol *1*:87–92, 1917.

Proops R, Taylor AMR, Insley J: A clinical study of a family with Cockayne's syndrome. J Med Genet *18*:288–293, 1981.

Pruett RC: Retinitis pigmentosa: Clinical observations and correlations. Trans Am Ophthalmol Soc *81*:693–735, 1983.

Pruett RC, Brockhurst J, Letts NF: Fluorescein angiography of peripheral uveitis. Am J Ophthalmol *77*:448–453, 1974.

Pruett RC, Carvalho ACA, Trempe CL: Microhemorrhagic maculopathy. Arch Ophthalmol *99*:425–432, 1981.

Purcell EF, Lerner LH, Kinsey VE: Ascorbic acid in aqueous humor and serum of patients with and without cataract. Arch Ophthalmol *51*:1–16, 1954.

Purcell JJ Jr, Shields JA: Hypertrophy with hyperpigmentation of the retinal pigment epithelium. Arch Ophthalmol *93*:1122–1126, 1975.

Quigley HA: Gap junctions between optic nerve head astrocytes. Invest Ophthalmol *16*:582–585, 1977.

Quigley HA, Goldberg MF: Conjunctival ultrastructure in mucolipidosis III (pseudo-Hurler polydystrophy). Invest Ophthalmol *10*:568–580, 1971.

Quigley HA, Green WR: Clinical and ultrastructural ocular histopathologic studies of adult-onset metachromatic leukodystrophy. Am J Ophthalmol *82*:472–479, 1976.

Quigley HA, Kenyon KR: Ultrastructural and histochemical studies of a newly recognized form of systemic mucopolysaccharidosis (Maroteaux-Lamy syndrome, mild phenotype). Am J Ophthalmol *77*:809–818, 1974.

Quigley HA, Maumenee AE, Stark WJ: Acute glaucoma in systemic mucopolysaccharidosis I-S. Am J Ophthalmol *80*:70–72, 1975.

Raab EL, Leopold IH, Hodes HL: Retinopathy in Rocky Mountain spotted fever. Am J Ophthalmol *68*:42–46, 1969.

Rabinowicz IM, Litman S, Michaelson IC: Branch venous thrombosis: A pathological report. Trans Ophthalmol Soc UK *88*:191–210, 1968.

Radtke ND, Tano Y, Chandler D, Machemer R: Simulation of massive periretinal proliferation by autotransplantation of retinal pigment epithelial cells in rabbits. Am J Ophthalmol *91*:76–87, 1981.

Rafuse EV, McCulloch C: Choroideremia: A pathological report. Can J Ophthalmol *3*:347–352, 1968.

Raistrick ER, Hart JCD: Ocular toxocariasis in adults. Br J Ophthalmol *60*:365–370, 1976.

Ramsey HJ: Ultrastructure of corpora amylacea. J Neuropathol Exp *24*:25–39, 1965.

Ramsey MS, Fine BS: Chloroquine toxicity in the human eye: Histopathologic observations by electron microscopy. Am J Ophthalmol *73*:229–235, 1972.

Ramsay RC, Kinyoun JL, Hill CW, et al: Retinal astrocytoma. Am J Ophthalmol *88*:32–36, 1979.

Rao NA, T'so MOM, Rosenthal AR: Chalcosis in the human eye. A clinicopathologic study. Arch Ophthalmol *94*:1379–1384, 1976.

Rao NA, Wacker WB, Marak GE Jr: Experimental allergic uveitis: Clinicopathologic features associated with varying doses of S antigen. Arch Ophthalmol *97*:1954–1958, 1979.

Rapin I, Katzman R, Engel J Jr: Cherry-red spots and progressive myoclonus without dementia: A distinct syndrome with neuronal storage. Trans Am Neurol Assoc *100*:39–42, 1975.

Rappaport H: Tumors of the hematopoietic system, *in* Atlas of Tumor Pathology. Section III, Fascicle 8. Washington, DC, Armed Forces Institute of Pathology, 1966, pp 99–101.

Rasteiro A: Sindroma de Scheie (mucopolisacaridose I-S). Exp Ophthal (Coimbra) *3*:62–64, 1977.

Ravalico G, Stanig L: Degenerazione olivo-ponto-cerebellare associata ad atrofia corioretinica. Soc Oftalmol Ital *28*:3–11, 1972.

Rayborn ME, Moorhead LC, Hollyfield JG: A dominantly inherited chorioretinal degeneration resembling sectoral retinitis pigmentosa. Ophthalmology *89*:1441–1454, 1982.

Raymond LA, Gutierrez Y, Strong LE, et al: Living retinal nematode (filarial-like) destroyed with photocoagulation. Ophthalmology *85*:944–949, 1978.

Raymond LA, Sacks JG, Choromokos E, Khodadad G: Short posterior ciliary artery insufficiency with hyperthermia (Uhthoff's symptom). Am J Ophthalmol *90*:619–623, 1980.

Reeh MJ: Toxoplasmosis in an immunosuppressed host. Presented at the Verhoeff Society Meeting, Washington, DC, May, 1973.

Reese AB: Telangiectasis of the retina and Coats' disease. The Eleventh Sanford R. Gifford Lecture. Am J Ophthalmol *42*:1–8, 1956.

Reese AB: Medullo-epithelioma (dictyoma) of the optic nerve. Am J Ophthalmol *44*:4–6, 1957.

Reese AB, Blodi FC: Retinal dysplasia. Am J Ophthalmol *33*:23–32, 1950.

Reese AB, Jones IS: Benign melanomas of the retinal pigment epithelium. Am J Ophthalmol *42*:207–212, 1956.

Reese AB, Jones IS: Hematomas under the retinal pigment epithelium. Trans Am Ophthalmol Soc *59*:43–79, 1961 and Am J Ophthalmol *53*:897–910, 1962.

Reese AB, Stepanik J: Cicatricial stage of retrolental fibroplasia. Am J Ophthalmol *38*:308–316, 1954.

Reese AB, Straatsma BR: Retinal dysplasia. Am J Ophthalmol *45*:199–211, 1958.

Reeser F: Medulloepithelioma. Case presented at the Sixth Biennial Meeting of the Association of Ophthalmic Alumni of the Armed Forces Institute of Pathology, Washington, DC, June, 1975.

Reeser FH, Aaberg TM, Van Horn DL: Astrocytic hamartoma of the retina not associated with tuberous sclerosis. Am J Ophthalmol *86*:688–698, 1978.

Refsum S: Heredopathia atactica polyneuritiformis. Acta Genet (Basel) *7*:344–347, 1957.

Regenbogen L, Godel V: Hereditary vitreoretinal degeneration, cleft lip and palate, deafness, and skeletal dysplasia. Am J Ophthalmol *89*:414–418, 1980.

Reid AM, Jones DWE: *Porocephalus armillatus* larvae presenting in the eye. Br J Ophthalmol *47*:169–172, 1963.

Reim H, Rohen JW, Dittrich JK: Klinische, histologische und electronen-mikroskopische Augenbefunde bei einem Säugling mit Mukopolysaccharidose Typ Pfaundler-Hurler. Klin Mbl Augenheilkd *159*:444–456, 1971.

Remington JS: The present status of the IgM fluorescent antibody technique in the diagnosis of congenital toxoplasmosis. J Pediatr *75*:1116–1124, 1969.

Remington JS, Melton ML, Jacobs L: Chronic *Toxoplasma* infection in the uterus. J Lab Clin Med *56*:879–883, 1960.
Renard G, Bargeton E, Dhermy P, Aron JJ: A histological study of the changes in the retina and optic nerve in metachromatic leucodystrophy (Scholz-Greenfield's disease). Bull Soc Ophtal Fr *76*:40–58, 1963 (in French).
Reynolds ES, Walls KW, Pfeiffer RI: Generalized toxoplasmosis following renal transplantation. Arch Intern Med *118*:401–405, 1966.
Ricci A: Clinique et transmission genetique des differentes formes de degenerescences vitreo-retiniennes. Ophthalmologica (Basel) *139*:338–343, 1960.
Ridley ME, Shields JA, Brown GC, Tasman W: Coats' disease. Evaluation of management. Ophthalmology *89*:1381–1387, 1982.
Riehl JL: Paradoxes of Takayasu's disease. Calif Med *102*:185–193, 1965.
Riehl JL, Brown WJ: Takayasu's arteritis: An auto-immune disease. Arch Neurol *12*:92–97, 1965.
Riise D: The nasal fundus ectasia. Acta Ophthalmol [Suppl] (Copenh) *126*:5–106, 1975.
Rintelan F: Die Histopathologie der Augenhintergrundsveränderungen bei Niemann-Pick-schen Lipoidose: Zugleich ein Beitrag zur Frage der Beziehungen zwischen Tay-Sachs-scher Idiotie and Niemann-Pickschen Lipodose. Arch Augenheilkd *109*:332, 1936.
Robb RM, Ervin LD, Sallan SE: A pathological study of eye involvement in acute leukemia of childhood. Trans Am Ophthalmol Soc *76*:90–101, 1978.
Robb RM, Kuwabara T: The ocular pathology of Type-A Niemann-Pick disease: A light and electron microscopic study. Invest Ophthalmol *12*:366–377, 1973.
Robertson DM: Macroaneurysms of the retinal arteries. Trans Am Acad Ophthalmol Otolaryngol *77*:55–67, 1973.
Robertson DM, Ilstrup D: Direct, indirect, and sham laser photocoagulation in the management of central serous chorioretinopathy. Am J Ophthalmol *95*:457–466, 1983.
Robertson DM, Link TP, Rostvold JA: Snowflake degeneration of the retina. Ophthalmology *89*:1513–1517, 1982.
Roggenbau C, Wetthauer A: Zur Frage der Erwärmbarkeit der einzelnen licht-brechenden Teile des Auges nach Bestrahlung durch einen leuchtenden Körper. Z Augenheilkd *64*:143–149, 1928.
Romayananda N, Goldberg MF, Green WR: Histopathology of sickle cell retinopathy. Trans Am Acad Ophthalmol Otolaryngol *77*:652–676, 1973.
Rones B: Senile changes and degenerations of the human eye. Am J Ophthalmol *21*:239–255, 1938.
Rosen DA, Haust MD, Yamashita T, et al: Keratoplasty and electron microscopy of the cornea in systemic mucopolysaccharidosis (Hurler's disease). Can J Ophthalmol *3*:218–230, 1968.
Rosenthal AR, Appleton B: Histochemical localization of intraocular copper foreign bodies. Am J Ophthalmol *79*:613–625, 1975.
Rosenthal AR, Appleton B, Hopkins JL: Intraocular copper foreign bodies. Am J Ophthalmol *78*:671–678, 1974.
Rosenthal AR, Appleton B, Zimmerman R, Hopkins JL: Intraocular copper foreign bodies: Use of Dexamethasone to suppress inflammation. Arch Ophthalmol *94*:1571–1576, 1976.
Rosenthal AR, Kolb H, Bergsma D, et al: Chloroquine retinopathy in the rhesus monkey. Invest Ophthalmol Vis Sci *17*:1158–1175, 1978.
Rosenthal AR, Marmor MF, Leuenberger P, Hopkins JL: Chalcosis: A study of natural history. Ophthalmology *86*:1956–1969, 1979.
Ross WH, Sutton HFS: Acquired syphilitic uveitis. Arch Ophthalmol *98*:496–498, 1980.
Roth AM, Foos RY: Surface wrinkling retinopathy in eyes enucleated at autopsy. Trans Am Acad Ophthalmol Otolaryngol *75*:1047–1058, 1971.
Roth AM, Foos RY: Surface structure of the optic nerve head: 1. Epipapillary membranes. Am J Ophthalmol *74*:977–985, 1972.
Roth AM, Helper RS, Mukoyama M, et al: Pigmentary retinal dystrophy in Hallervorden-Spatz disease: Clinicopathological report of a case. Surv Ophthalmol *16*:24–35, 1971.
Roth M: Über Netzhantaffekstionen bei Wundfiebrin. Dtsch A Chir *1*:471–484, 1872.
Rothkoff L, Kushelevsky A, Blumenthal M: Solar retinopathy: Visual prognosis in 20 cases. Isr J Med Sci *14*:238–243, 1978.
Rothstein T: Bilateral, central retinal vein closure as the initial manifestation of polycythemia. J Ophthalmol *74*:256–260, 1972.
Roubin IV: Telangiectasis of the disc in Osler's disease. Vestn Oftalmol *3*:29–30, 1957 (in Russian).
Rouveda JM: Melanosis de la papila. Arch Ophtalmol (Buenos Aires) *27*:61–64, 1952.
Rubenstein RA, Yanoff M, Albert DM: Thrombocytopenia, anemia, and retinal hemorrhage. Am J Ophthalmol *65*:435–439, 1968.
Rubin ML, Kaufman HE, Tierney JP, Lucas HC: An intraretinal nematode. Trans Am Acad Ophthalmol Otolaryngol *72*:855–866, 1968.
Rucker CW: Sheathing of retinal veins in multiple sclerosis. JAMA *127*:970–973, 1945.
Ruiz RS: Giant cyst of the pars plana. Am J Ophthalmol *72*:481–482, 1971.
Rundles WZ, Falls HF: Congenital arteriovenous (racemose) aneurysm of the retina: Report of three cases. Arch Ophthalmol *46*:408–418, 1951.
Rush JA: Acute macular neuroretinopathy. Am J Ophthalmol *83*:490–494, 1977.
Rush JA, Kearns TP, Danielson GK: Cloth-particle emboli from artificial cardiac valves. Am J Ophthalmol *89*:845–850, 1980.
Ruskin J, Remington JS: Toxoplasmosis in the compromised host. Ann Intern Med *84*:193–199, 1976.
Rutnin U, Schepens CL: Fundus appearance in normal eyes. III. Peripheral degenerations. Am J Ophthalmol *64*:1040–1062, 1967a.
Rutnin U, Schepens CL: Fundus appearance in normal eyes. IV: Retinal breaks and other findings. Am J Ophthalmol *64*:1063–1078, 1967b.
Ryan SJ Jr: Occlusion of the macular capillaries in sickle cell hemoglobin C disease. Am J Ophthalmol *77*:459–461, 1974.
Ryan SJ Jr, Goldberg MF: Anterior segment ischemia following scleral buckling in sickle cell hemoglobinopathy. Am J Ophthalmol *72*:35–50, 1971.
Ryan SJ Jr, Knox DL, Green WR, Konigsmark BW: Olivopontocerebellar degeneration: Clinicopathologic correlation of the associated retinopathy. Arch Ophthalmol *93*:169–172, 1975.
Sabates R, Pruett RC, Hirose T: Pseudovitelliform macular degeneration. Retina *2*:197–205, 1982.
Salt HB, Wolff OH, Lloyd JK, et al: On having no beta-lipoprotein: A syndrome comprising a-beta-lipoproteinaemia, acanthocytosis, and steatorrhoea. Lancet *2*:325–329, 1960.
Samuels B, Fuchs A: Clinical Pathology of the Eye: A Practical Treatise of Histopathology. New York, P.B. Hoeber, 1952.
Sanderson PA, Kuwabara T, Cogan DG: Optic neuropathy presumably caused by vincristine therapy. Am J Ophthalmol *81*:146–150, 1976.
Sanderson PA, Kuwabara T, Stark WJ, et al: Cystinosis: A clinical, histopathologic, and ultrastructural study. Arch Ophthalmol *91*:270–274, 1974.
Sanfilippo SJ, Podosin R, Langer L, Good RA: Mental retardation associated with acid mucopolysaccharidura (heparitin sulfate type). J Pediat *63*:837–838, 1963.
Santavuori P, Haltia M, Rapola J: Infantile type of so-called neuronal ceroid-lipofuscinosis. Dev Med Child Neurol *16*:644–653, 1974.
Santos-Anderson RM, Tso MOM, Fishman GA: A histopath-

ologic study of retinitis pigmentosa. Ophthalmol Paediatr Genet *1*:151–168, 1982.

Sarin LK, Green WR, Dailey EG: Juvenile retinoschisis. Congenital vascular veils and hereditary retinoschisis. Am J Ophthalmol *57*:793–796, 1964.

Sarin LK, McDonald PR: Changes in the posterior pole following successful reattachment of the retina. Trans Am Acad Ophthalmol Otolaryngol *74*:75–79, 1970.

Sarks SH: Senile choroidal sclerosis. Br J Ophthalmol *57*:98–109, 1973a.

Sarks SH: New vessel formation beneath the retinal pigment epithelium in senile eyes. Br J Ophthalmol *57*:951–965, 1973b.

Sarks SH: Ageing and degeneration in the macular region: A clinicopathological study. Br J Ophthalmol. *60*:324–341, 1976.

Sarks SH: Drusen and their relationship to senile macular degeneration (Council Lecture). Aust J Ophthalmol *8*:117–130, 1980.

Sawyer RA, Selhorst JB, Zimmerman LE, Hoyt WF: Blindness caused by photoreceptor degeneration as a remote effect of cancer. Am J Ophthalmol *81*:606–613, 1976.

Schachat AP, Miller NR: Atrophy of myelinated retinal nerve fibers after acute optic neuropathy. Am J Ophthalmol *92*:854–856, 1981.

Schatz H: Fundus Fluorescein Angiography; A Composite Slide Collection. New York, Appleton-Century-Crofts, 1975, pp 26–28.

Schatz H, Burton TC, Yannuzzi LA, Rabb MF: Interpretation of fundus fluorescein angiography. St. Louis, C.V. Mosby, 1978, pp 426–428.

Schatz H, Drake M: Self-injected retinal emboli. Ophthalmology *86*:468–483, 1979.

Schatz H, Glitter K, Yannuzzi L, Irvine A: Retinal arterial macroaneurysms: A large collaborative study. Presented at the American Academy of Ophthalmology, Chicago, Nov, 1980.

Schatz H, Maumenee AE, Patz A: Geographic helicoid peripapillary choroidopathy. Trans Am Acad Ophthalmol Otolaryngol *78*:747–761, 1974.

Schatz H, Patz A: Exudative senile maculopathy: I. Results of argon laser treatment. II. Complications of argon laser treatment. Arch Ophthalmol *90*:183–202, 1973.

Schaumburg HH, Powers JM, Raine CS, et al: Adrenoleukodystrophy: A clinical and pathological study of 17 cases. Arch Neurol *32*:577–591, 1975.

Scheie HG: Ocular changes associated with scrub typhus. Arch Ophthalmol *40*:245–267, 1948.

Scheie HG: Evaluation of ophthalmoscopic changes of hypertension and arteriolar sclerosis. Arch Ophthalmol *49*:117–138, 1953.

Scheie HG, Hambrick GW Jr, Barness LA: A newly recognized forme fruste of Hurler's disease (gargoylism). J Ophthalmol *53*:753–769, 1962.

Schepens CL: L'inflammation de la region de l'ora serrata et ses sequelles. Bull Mem Soc Fr Ophtalmol *63*:113–125, 1950.

Schepens CL, Marden D: Data on the natural history of retinal detachment: Further characterization of certain unilateral nontraumatic cases. Am J Ophthalmol *61*:213–226, 1966.

Scherbel AL, Mackenzie AH, Nousek JE, Atdjian M: Ocular lesions in rheumatoid arthritis and related disorders with particular reference to retinopathy. N Engl J Med *273*:360–366, 1965.

Schlaegel TF Jr: Toxoplasmosis, *in* Duane TD (ed): Clinical Ophthalmology. Vol 4. Hagerstown, Md, Harper & Row, 1976, rev 1981.

Schlernitzauer DA, Green WR: Peripheral retinal albinotic spots. Am J Ophthalmol *72*:729–732, 1971.

Schmidt JGH: Angiopathia retinae traumatica (Purtscher) and Fettembolie. Klin Monatsbl Augenheilkd *152*:672–679, 1968.

Schnabel J: Zur Lehre von den Ursachen der Kurzsichtigkeit. Albrecht Von Graefes Arch Ophthalmol *20*:1–70 (Part 2), 1874.

Schochet SS, Ballin N: Circinate choroidal sclerosis. Trans Am Acad Ophthalmol Otolaryngol *74*:527–533, 1970.

Schochet SS, Font RL, Morris HH: Ocular pathology of Jansky-Bielschowsky form of neuronal ceroid-lipofuscinosis (Batten-Vogt syndrome). Arch Ophthalmol *98*:1083–1088, 1980.

Scholz RO: Epivascular choroidal pigment streaks, their pathology and possible prognostic significance. Bull Johns Hopkins Hosp *77*:345–371, 1945.

Schreiner RL, McAlister WH, Marshall RE, et al: Stickler syndrome in a pedigree of Pierre Robin syndrome. Am J Dis Child *126*:86–90, 1973.

Schulman JD: Cystinosis: A review. Scott Med J *20*:5–18, 1975.

Schulman J, Jampol LM, Schwartz H: Peripheral proliferative retinopathy without oxygen therapy in a full-term infant. Am J Ophthalmol *90*:509–514, 1980.

Schulman JD, Wong VG, Olson WH, et al: Lysosomal site of crystalline deposits in cystinosis as shown by ferritin uptake. Arch Pathol *90*:259–264, 1970.

Schwartz GA, Yanoff M: Lafora's disease: Distinct clinicopathologic form of Unverricht's syndrome. Arch Neurol *12*:172–188, 1965.

Schwartz JN, Cashwell F, Hawkins HK, et al: Necrotizing retinopathy with herpes zoster ophthalmicus: A light and electron microscopical study. Arch Pathol Lab Med *100*:386–391, 1976.

Schwartz MF, Green WR, Grover WD, Huff D: Zellweger's syndrome: Report of a case and pathological correlation. Presented at Wilmer Residents Association Meeting, Baltimore, April, 1971.

Schwartz MF, Green WR, Michels RG, et al: An unusual case of ocular involvement in primary systemic nonfamilial amyloidosis. Ophthalmology *89*:394–401, 1982.

Scott AW: Retinal pigmentation in a patient receiving thioridazine. Arch Ophthalmol *70*:775–778, 1963.

Scriver CR, Rosenberg LE: Amino Acid Metabolism and Its Disorders. Philadelphia, W.B. Saunders Company, 1973, pp 222–224.

Segal P, Mrzyglod S, Smolarz-Dudarewicz J: Subretinal cysticercosis in the macular region. Am J Ophthalmol *57*:655–664, 1964.

Seitz R: Die Genese und Ätiologie des Kreuzungsphänomens und seine Bedeutung für die Diagnostik von Netzhautgefässerkrankungen. Klin Monatsbl Augenheilkd *139*:491–512, 1961.

Seitz R: The Retinal Vessels (translated by Blodi FC). St. Louis, C.V. Mosby, 1964, pp 60–61.

Sergovich F, Madronich JS, Barr ML, et al: The D trisomy syndrome: A case report with a description of ocular pathology. Can Med Assoc J *89*:151–157, 1963.

Shakib M, Ashton N: Focal retinal ischaemia: Part II. Ultrastructural changes in focal retinal ischaemia. Br J Ophthalmol *50*:325–384, 1966.

Shea M, Dickson D: Thermoelectric retinal cryosurgery. Can J Ophthalmol *1*:138–146, 1966.

Shea M, Maberley AL, Walters J, et al: Intraocular *Taenia crassiceps* (Cestoda). Trans Am Acad Ophthalmol Otolaryngol *77*:778–783, 1973a.

Shea M, Maberley AL, Walters J, et al: Intraretinal larval trematode. Trans Am Acad Ophthalmol Otolaryngol *77*:784–791, 1973b.

Shea M, Schepens CL, Von Pirquet SR: Retinoschisis. I. Senile type: A clinical report of one hundred seven cases. Arch Ophthalmol *63*:1–9, 1960.

Sheffer A, Green WR, Fine SL, Kincaid M: Presumed ocular histoplasmosis syndrome: A clinicopathologic correlation of a treated case. Arch Ophthalmol *98*:335–345, 1980.

Sher NA, Letson RD, Desnick RJ: The ocular manifestations in Fabry's disease. Arch Ophthalmol *97*:671–676, 1979.

Shields JA, Lerner HA, Felberg NT: Aqueous cytology and

enzymes in nematode endophthalmitis. Am J Ophthalmol *84*:319–322, 1977.

Shields JA, T'so, MOM: Congenital grouped pigmentation of the retina: Histopathologic description and report of a case. Arch Ophthalmol *93*:1153–1155, 1975.

Shields JA, Zimmerman LE: Lesions simulating malignant melanoma of the posterior uvea. Arch Ophthalmol *89*:466–471, 1973.

Shields TW (ed): Carcinoma of the Lung, *in* General Thoracic Surgery. Philadelphia, Lea & Febiger, 1972, p 813.

Shikano S: Ocular pathology of Behçet's syndrome, *in* International Symposium on Behçet's Disease. Basel, Rome, Karger, 1966, pp 111–136.

Shimizu K, Ujiie K: Structure of Ocular Vessels. Tokyo and New York, Igaku-Shoin, 1978, pp 9–10.

Shultz WT, Swan KC: Pulsatile aneurysms of the retinal arterial tree. Am J Ophthalmol *77*:304–309, 1974.

Shy GM, Silverstein I: A study of the effects upon the motor unit by remote malignancy. Brain *88*:515–528, 1965.

Siam AL, Meegan JM, Gharbawi KF: Rift Valley fever ocular manifestations: Observations during the 1977 epidemic in Egypt. Br J Ophthalmol *64*:366–374, 1980.

Siegal FP, Lopez C, Hammer GS, et al: Severe acquired immunodeficiency in male homosexuals, manifested by chronic perianal ulcerative herpes simplex lesions. N Engl J Med *305*:1439–1444, 1981.

Siemerling E, Creutzfeldt HG: Bronze-krankheit und sklerosierende Encephalomyelitis. Arch Psychiat *68*:217–244, 1923.

Sigelman J, Behrens M, Hilal S: Acute posterior multifocal placoid pigment epitheliopathy associated with cerebral vasculitis and homonymous hemianopia. Am J Ophthalmol *88*:919–924, 1979.

Silverstein AM: Retinal dysplasia and rosettes induced by experimental intrauterine trauma. Am J Ophthalmol *77*:51–58, 1974.

Silverstein AM, Parshall CJ Jr, Osburn BI, Prendergast RA: An experimental, virus-induced retinal dysplasia in the fetal lamb. Am J Ophthalmol *72*:22–34, 1971.

Silverstein MN, Ellefson RD, Ahern EJ: The syndrome of the sea-blue histiocyte. N Engl J Med *282*:1–4, 1970.

Simell O, Takki K: Raised plasma-ornithine and gyrate atrophy of the choroid and retina. Lancet *1*:1031–1033, 1973.

Simon KA: Diabetes and lens changes in myotonic dystrophy. Arch Ophthalmol *67*:312–315, 1962.

Sipperley JO, Quigley HA, Gass JDM: Traumatic retinopathy in primates: The explanation of commotio retinae. Arch Ophthalmol *96*:2267–2273, 1978.

Sisson TRC, Glauser SC, Glauser EM, et al: Retinal changes produced by phototherapy. J Pediatr *77*:221–227, 1970.

Skalka HW: Vitelliform macular lesions. Br J Ophthalmol *65*:180–183, 1981.

Skikano S: Ocular pathology of Behçet's syndrome. International Symposium on Behçet's Disease. New York, Karger, 1966, pp 111–136.

Slusher MM, Hutton WE: Familial exudative vitreoretinopathy. Am J Ophthalmol *87*:152–156, 1979.

Smiddy WE, Green WR: Retinal dialysis. Pathology and pathogenesis. Retina *2*:94–116, 1982.

Smith ME: Retinal involvement in adult cytomegalic inclusions disease. Arch Ophthalmol *72*:44–49, 1964.

Smith ME: Congenital toxoplasmosis; Case presentation at the Association of Ophthalmic Alumni of the Armed Forces Institute of Pathology, June, 1973.

Smith ME, Zimmerman LE, Harley RD: Ocular involvement in congenital cytomegalic inclusion disease. Arch Ophthalmol *76*:696–699, 1966.

Smith PH, Greer CH: Unusual presentation of ocular *Toxocara* infestation. Br J Ophthalmol *55*:317–320, 1971.

Smith RE, Ganley JP: Ophthalmic survey of a community. I. Abnormalities of the ocular fundus. Am J Ophthalmol *74*:1126–1130, 1972.

Smith RE, Kelley JS, Harbin TS: Late macular complications of choroidal ruptures. Am J Ophthalmol *77*:650–658, 1974.

Smith RE, Macy JI, Parrett C, Irvine J: Variations in acute multifocal histoplasmic choroiditis in the primate. Invest Ophthalmol Vis Sci *17*:1005–1018, 1978.

Smith RS, Berson EL: Acute toxic effects of chloroquine on the cat retina: Ultrastructural changes. Invest Ophthalmol *10*:237–246, 1971.

Smith RS, Reinecke RD: Electron microscopy of ocular muscle in type II glycogenosis (Pompe's disease). Am J Ophthalmol *73*:965–970, 1972.

Smith RS, van Heuven WAJ, Streeten B: Vitreous membranes: A light and electron microscopical study. Arch Ophthalmol *95*:1556–1560, 1976.

Smith TW, Burton TC: The retinal manifestations of Rocky Mountain spotted fever. Am J Ophthalmol *84*:259–262, 1977.

Snip RC, Michels RG: Pars plana vitrectomy in the management of endogenous *Candida* endophthalmitis. Am J Ophthalmol *82*:699–704, 1976.

Snodgrass MB: Ocular findings in a case of fucosidosis. Br J Ophthalmol *60*:508–511, 1976.

Snyder C: Helmholtz at Columbia University. Arch Ophthalmol *72*:573–576, 1964.

Snyder RD, Carlow TJ, Ledman J, Wenger DA: Ocular findings in fucosidosis. Birth Defects *12*:241–256, 1976.

Sogg RL, Steinman L, Rathjen B, et al: Cherry-red spot: Myoclonus syndrome. Ophthalmology *86*:1861–1870, 1979.

Somerset EJ, Sen NR: Leprosy lesions of the fundus oculi. Br J Ophthalmol *40*:167–172, 1956.

Sommer A, Tjakrasudjatma S, Djunaedi E, Green WR: Vitamin A–responsive panocular xerophthalmia in a healthy adult. Arch Ophthalmol *96*:1630–1634, 1978.

Soomsawasdi B, Romayananda N, Kanchanaranya D: Ocular cysticercosis. Orient Arch Ophthalmol *1*:153–158, 1963.

Sorsby A, Mason EEJ, Gardener N: A fundus dystrophy with unusual features. Br J Ophthalmol *33*:67–97, 1949.

Spaeth GL, Frost P: Fabry's disease: Its ocular manifestations. Arch Ophthalmol *74*:760–769, 1965.

Spalter HF: Abnormal serum proteins and retinal vein thrombosis. Arch Ophthalmol *62*:868–881, 1959.

Spalton DJ, Bird AC, Cleary PE: Retinitis pigmentosa and retinal oedema. Br J Ophthalmol *62*:174–182, 1978.

Spalton DJ, Taylor DSI, Sanders MD: Juvenile Batten's disease: An ophthalmological assessment of 26 patients. Br J Ophthalmol *64*:726–732, 1980.

Speiser P, Gittelsohn AM, Patz A: Studies on diabetic retinopathy. III. Influence of diabetes on intramural pericytes. Arch Ophthalmol *80*:332–337, 1968.

Spellacy E, Kennerley-Bankes JL, Crow J, et al: Glaucoma in a case of Hurler disease. Br J Ophthalmol *64*:773–778, 1980.

Spencer LM, Foos RY: Paravascular vitreoretinal attachments: Role in retinal tears. Arch Ophthalmol *84*:557–564, 1970.

Spencer LM, Foos RY, Straatsma BR: Meridional folds, meridional complexes, and associated abnormalities of the peripheral retina. Am J Ophthalmol *70*:697–714, 1970.

Spencer R, Tolentino FI, Doyle GJ: Takayasu's arteritis: Case report and review emphasizing ocular manifestations. Ann Ophthalmol *12*:935–938, 1980.

Spencer WH: Macular Diseases; Pathogenesis: Light microscopy (Symposium). Trans Am Acad Ophthalmol Otolaryngol *69*:662–667, 1965.

Spencer WH: Combined cytomegalovirus retinitis and cryptococcus uveitis and meningitis. Case presented at Verhoeff Society, Washington, DC, April, 1982.

Spencer WH, Hogan MJ: Ocular manifestations of Chediak-Higashi syndrome: Report of a case with histopathologic examination of ocular tissues. Am J Ophthalmol *50*:1197–1203, 1960.

Spencer WH, Jesberg DO: Glioneuroma (choristomatous malformation of the optic cup margin): A report of two cases. Arch Ophthalmol *89*:387–392, 1973.

Sperduto RD, Seigel D, Roberts J, Rowland M: Prevalence of myopia in the United States. Arch Ophthalmol *101*:405–407, 1983.

Sperling HG: Functional changes and cellular damage associated with two regimes of moderately intense blue light exposure in Rhesus monkey retina. Presented at Association for Research in Vision and Ophthalmology, April, 1978, Sarasota, Florida.

Sperling MA, Hiles DA, Kennerdell JS: Electroretinographic responses following vitamin A therapy in abetalipoproteinemia. Am J Ophthalmol *73*:342–351, 1972.

Spiers F, Jensen OA: Pseudoepitheliomatous hyperplasia of the retinal pigment epithelium. Report of a case with complete serial sections. Acta Ophthalmol *41*:722–727, 1963.

Spitznas M: Personal communication, July, 1977.

Spranger JW, Wiedemann HR: The genetic mucolipidoses: Diagnosis and differential diagnosis. Humangenetik *9*:113–139, 1970.

Stanescu B, Dralands L: Cerebro-hepato-renal (Zellweger's) syndrome: Ocular involvement. Arch Ophthalmol *87*:590–592, 1972.

Stargardt K: Ueber familiäre, progressive Degeneration in der Maculagegend des Auges. Graefes Arch Ophthalmol *71*:534–550, 1909, and Z Augenheilkd *30*:95–116, 1913.

Stefani FH, Ehalt H: Non-oxygen-induced retinitis proliferans and retinal detachment in full-term infants. Br J Ophthalmol *58*:490–513, 1974.

Steinberg D, Vroom FQ, Engel WK, et al: Refsum's disease: A recently characterized lipidosis involving the nervous system. Ann Intern Med *66*:365–395, 1967.

Sternberg P Jr, Knox DL, Finkelstein D, et al: Acute retinal necrosis syndrome. Retina *2*:145–151, 1982.

Stevens TS, Busse B, Lee CB, et al: Sickling hemoglobinopathies: Macular and perimacular vascular abnormalities. Arch Ophthalmol *92*:455–463, 1974.

Stickler GB, Belau PG, Farrell FJ, et al: Hereditary progressive arthro-ophthalmopathy. Mayo Clin Proc *40*:433–455, 1965.

Stickler GB, Pugh DG: Hereditary progressive arthro-ophthalmopathy. 2. Additional observations on vertebral abnormalities, a hearing defect, and a report of a similar case. Mayo Clin Proc *42*:495–500, 1967.

Stock W: Über eine bis jetzt noch nicht beschriebene Form der familiär auftretenden Netzhautdegeneration bei gleichzeitiger Verblödung und über typische Pigmentdegeneration der Netzhaut. Klin Monatsbl Augenheilkd *46*:225–244, 1908.

Stow MN: Hyperplasia of the pigment epithelium of the retina simulating a neoplasm. Trans Am Acad Ophthalmol Otolaryngol *52*:674–677, 1949.

Straatsma BR: Ocular manifestations of Wegener's granulomatosis. Am J Ophthalmol *44*:789–799, 1957.

Straatsma BR, Allen RA: Lattice degeneration of the retina. Trans Am Acad Ophthalmol Otolaryngol *66*:600–613, 1962.

Straatsma BR, Foos RY: Typical and reticular degenerative retinoschisis. XXVI Francis I. Proctor Memorial Lecture. Am J Ophthalmol *75*:551–575, 1973.

Straatsma BR, Foos RY, Feman SS: Degenerative diseases of the peripheral retina, *in* Duane TD (ed): Clinical Ophthalmology. Vol 3, rev ed. Hagerstown, Md, Harper & Row, 1979, Chapter 26.

Straatsma BR, Foos RY, Heckenlively JR, Taylor GN: Myelinated retinal nerve fibers. Am J Ophthalmol *91*:25–38, 1981.

Straatsma BR, Zeegan PD, Foos RY, et al: Lattice degeneration of the retina. Trans Am Acad Ophthalmol Otolaryngol *78*:87–113, 1974.

Strachan RW: The natural history of Takayasu's arteriopathy. Q J Med *33*:57–69, 1964.

Streeten BF, McGraw JL: Tumor of the ciliary pigment epithelium. Am J Ophthalmol *74*:420–429, 1972.

Streeten BW: Development of the human retinal pigment epithelium and the posterior segment. Arch Ophthalmol *81*:383–384, 1969.

Streeten BW, Bert M: The retinal surface in lattice degeneration of the retina. Am J Ophthalmol *74*:1201–1209, 1972.

Suganumba S: Ein Beitrag zur Kenntnis der Pathologie der Pigmentdegeneration der Netzhaut. Klin Monatsbl Augenheilkd *50*:175–184, 1912.

Sugar HS: An explanation for the acquired macular pathology associated with congenital pits of the optic disc. Am J Ophthalmol *57*:833–835, 1964.

Sugar HS, Mandell GH, Shalev J: Metastatic endophthalmitis associated with injection of addictive drugs. Am J Ophthalmol *71*:1055–1058, 1971.

Sullivan SF, Dallow RL: Intraocular reticulum cell sarcoma: Its dramatic response to systemic chemotherapy and its angiogenic potential. Ann Ophthalmol *9*:401, 1977.

Swanson D, Rush P, Bird AC: Visual loss from retinal-oedema in autosomal dominant exudative vitreoretinopathy. Br J Ophthalmol *66*:627–629, 1982.

Swisher CN, Menkes JH, Cancilla PA, Dodge PR: Coexistence of Hallervorden-Spatz disease with acanthocytosis. Trans Am Neurol Assoc *97*:212–216, 1972.

Switz DM, Casey TR, Bogaty GV: Whipple's disease and papilledema. Arch Intern Med *123*:74–77, 1969.

Szamier RB, Berson EL, Klein R, Meyers S: Sex-linked retinitis pigmentosa: Ultrastructure of photoreceptors and pigment epithelium. Invest Ophthalmol *18*:145–160, 1979.

Szirmai JA, Balazs EA: Studies on the structure of the vitreous body. III. Cells in the cortical layer. Arch Ophthalmol *59*:34–48, 1958.

Takayasu H: Case report of a peculiar abnormality of the retinal central vessels. Acta Soc Ophthalmol Jpn *12*:554–556, 1908.

Takki K, Simell O: Genetic aspects in gyrate atrophy of the choroid and retina with hyperornithinaemia. Br J Ophthalmol *58*:907–916, 1974.

Tarkkanen A, Merenmies L, Mäkinen J: Embolism of the central retinal artery secondary to metastatic carcinoma. Acta Ophthalmol *51*:25–33, 1973.

Tashiro M: A study of the hemorrhagic tendency in leukemic eyes. Acta Soc Ophthalmol Jpn *70*:1724–1728, 1966.

Taylor HR: Onchocerciasis, *in* Dawson CR, O'Connor GR (eds): Infections and Inflammatory Diseases of the Eye. Philadelphia, WB Saunders, in preparation.

Teeters VW, Bird AC: The development of neovascularization of senile disciform macular degeneration. Am J Ophthalmol *76*:1–18, 1973.

Teng CC, Katzin HM: An anatomic study of the peripheral retina: II. Peripheral cystoid degeneration of the retina; formation of cysts and holes. Am J Ophthalmol *36*:29–39, 1953.

Terson A: Le syndrome de l'hematome du corps vitre et de l'hemorragie intracranienne spontanes. Ann Oculist *163*:666–673, 1926.

Theobald GD, Floyd G, Kirk HQ: Hyperplasia of the retinal pigment epithelium simulating a neoplasm: Report of two cases. Am J Ophthalmol *45*:235–240, 1958.

Theodossiadis G: Fluorescein angiography in Eales's disease. Am J Ophthalmol *69*:271–277, 1970.

Theodossiadis G: Evolution of congenital pit of the optic disk with macular detachment in photocoagulated and nonphotocoagulated eyes. Am J Ophthalmol *84*:620–631, 1977.

Thomas C, Cordier J, Algan B: Altérations vasculaires rétiniennes d'origine rickettsienne. Bull Soc Ophtalmol Fr *72*:621–634, 1959.

Thomas EL, Michels RG, Rice TA, et al: Idiopathic progressive unilateral vitreous fibrosis and secondary traction retinal detachment. Retina *2*:134–144, 1982.

Thomas EL, Olk RJ, Markman M, et al: Irreversible visual loss in Waldenström's macroglobulinaemia. Br J Ophthalmol *67*:102–106, 1983.

Thomas JV, Green WR: Endophthalmitis, *in* Mandell GL, Douglas RG, Bennett JE (eds): Principles and Practice of Infectious Diseases. New York, John Wiley & Sons, 1979, pp 1023–1035.

Thomas JV, Green WR: Fungus infections of the orbit, *in* Garner A, Klintworth G (eds): Pathobiology of Ocular Disease. New York, Marcel Dekker, 1981, Chapter 12.

Tillery WV, Lucier AC: Round atrophic holes in lattice degeneration: An important cause of phakic retinal detachment. Trans Am Acad Ophthalmol Otolaryngol *81*:509–518, 1976.

Timm G: Zur pathologischen Anatomie des Auges bei der

Makroglobinämie Waldenström. Klin Monatsbl Augenheilkd *137*:772–781, 1960.
Timm G, Fritsch S: Über epitheliale tumoren des ciliarkörpers. Frankfurter Z Pathol *73*:401–417, 1964.
Tolentino FI, Schepens CL, Freeman HM: Massive preretinal retraction. A biomicroscopic study. Arch Ophthalmol *78*:16–22, 1967.
Tomlinson A, Phillips CI: Ratio of optic cup to optic disc in relation to axial length of eyeball and refraction. Br J Ophthalmol *53*:765–768, 1969.
Topping TM, Kenyon KR, Goldberg MF, Maumenee AE: Ultrastructural ocular pathology of Hunter's syndrome: Systemic mucopolysaccharidosis Type II. Arch Ophthalmol *86*:164–177, 1971.
Toussaint D, Conreur L, Pelc S, Perier O: Les lesions oculaires de la leucodystrophie metachromatique. Bull Soc Belge Ophtalmol *138*:579–586, 1964.
Toussaint D, Danis P: Ocular histopathology in generalized glycogenosis (Pompe's disease). Arch Ophthalmol *73*:342–349, 1965.
Toussaint D, Danis P: Étude histologique d'un cas de syndrome de Refsum. Bull Soc Belge Ophtalmol *155*:532–540, 1970.
Toussaint D, Danis P: An ocular pathologic study of Refsum's disease. Am J Ophthalmol *72*:342–347, 1971.
Toussaint D, Dustin P: Electron microscopy of normal and diabetic retinal capillaries. Arch Ophthalmol *70*:96–108, 1963.
Toussaint MD: Étude anatomique des altérations vasculaires rétiniennes dans certaines dysglobulinémies. Bull Soc Belge Ophtalmol *143*:685–701, 1966.
Townes PL, Roca PD: Norrie's disease (hereditary oculo-acoustic-cerebral degeneration). Am J Ophthalmol *76*:797–803, 1973.
Tredici TJ, Fenton RH: Hematoma beneath the retinal pigment epithelium. Report of a case mistaken clinically for a malignant melanoma of the choroid. Arch Ophthalmol *72*:796–799, 1964.
Trese M: Retinal hemorrhage caused by overdose of methaqualone (Quaalude). Am J Ophthalmol *91*:201–203, 1981.
Trier JS, Phelps PC, Eidelman S, Rubin LE: Whipple's disease: Light and electron microscopic correlation of jejunal mucosal histology with antibiotic treatment and clinical status. Gastroenterology *48*:684–707, 1965.
Tripathi R, Ashton N: Electron microscopical study of Coats's disease. Br J Ophthalmol *55*:289–301, 1971.
Tse DT, Ober RR: Talc retinopathy. Am J Ophthalmol *90*:624–640, 1980.
Tso MOM: Photic maculopathy in rhesus monkey: A light and electron microscopic study. Invest Ophthalmol *12*:17–34, 1973.
Tso MOM, Albert DM: Pathologic conditions of the retinal pigment epithelium: Neoplasms and nodular nonneoplastic lesions. Arch Ophthalmol *88*:27–38, 1972.
Tso MOM, Cunha-Vaz JG, Shih CV, Jones CW: Clinicopathologic study of blood-retinal barrier in experimental diabetes mellitus. Arch Ophthalmol *98*:2032–2040, 1980.
Tso MOM, Fine BS: Repair and late degeneration of the primate foveola after injury by argon laser. Invest Ophthalmol Vis Sci *18*:447–461, 1979.
Tso MOM, Fine BS, Zimmerman LE: Photic maculopathy produced by the indirect ophthalmoscope: I. Clinical and histopathologic study. Am J Ophthalmol *73*:686–699, 1972.
Tso MOM, Jampol LM: Pathophysiology of hypertensive retinopathy. Ophthalmology *89*:1132–1145, 1982.
Tso MOM, Wallow IHL, Elgin S: Experimental photocoagulation of the human retina. 1. Correlation of physical, clinical, and pathologic data. Arch Ophthalmol *95*:1035–1040, 1977.
Tudor RC, Blair E: Gnathostoma spinigerum: An unusual cause of ocular nematodiasis in the Western Hemisphere. Am J Ophthalmol *72*:185–190, 1971.
Turner G: The Stickler syndrome in a family with the Pierre-Robin syndrome and severe myopia. Aust Pediatr J *10*:103–108, 1974.
Tyner GS: Wegener's granulomatosis: A case report. Am J Ophthalmol *50*:1203–1207, 1960.
Uemura J, Morizane H: The fundus anomalies in high hypermetropic eyes: The interpapillomacular retinal fold. Jpn J Clin Ophthalmol *24*:961, 1970.
Ueno H, Ueno S, Kajitani T, et al: Clinical and histopathological studies of a case with juvenile form of Gaucher's disease. Jpn J Ophthalmol *21*:98–108, 1977.
Ueno H, Ueno S, Matsuo N, et al: Electron microscopic study of Gaucher cells in the eye. Jpn J Ophthalmol *24*:75–81, 1980.
Ulrich J, Herschkowitz N, Heitz P, et al: Adrenoleukodystrophy: Preliminary report of a connatal case. Light and electron microscopical, immunohistochemical and biochemical findings. Acta Neuropathol (Berlin) *43*:77–83, 1978.
Unverricht H: Die Myoklonie. Leipzig, Wien, Franz Deuticke, 1891, p 128.
Urbanek J: Ueber Fettembolie des Auges. Arch Ophthalmol *131*:147–173, 1933.
Vaghefi HA, Green WR, Kelley JS, et al: Correlation of clinicopathologic findings in a patient: Congenital night blindness, branch retinal vein occlusion, cilioretinal artery, drusen of the optic nerve head, and intraretinal pigmented lesion. Arch Ophthalmol *96*:2097–2104, 1978.
Vail D, Shoch D: Hereditary degeneration of the macula. II. Follow-up report and histopathologic study. Trans Am Ophthalmol Soc *63*:51–63, 1965.
Vakili S, Drew AL, Von Schuching S, et al: Hallervorden-Spatz syndrome. Arch Neurol *34*:729–738, 1977.
Van der Hoeve J: Die optische Heterogenität der Linse. Arch Ophthalmol *98*:39–48, 1919.
Van Dyk HJL, Swan KC: The cataract patient with myotonic dystrophy. Trans Am Acad Ophthalmol Otolaryngol *71*:838–846, 1967.
Van Hoof F, Hers HG: L'ultrastructure des cellules hepatiques dans la maladie de Hurler (gargoylisme). Conte Rend Acad Sci (Paris) *259*:1281–1283, 1964.
Van Horn DL, Aaberg TM, Machemer R, Fenzl R: Glial cell proliferation in human retinal detachment with massive periretinal proliferation. Am J Ophthalmol *84*:383–393, 1977.
Velzeboer CMJ, de Groot WP: Ocular manifestations in angiokeratoma corporis diffusum (Fabry). Br J Ophthalmol *55*:683–692, 1971.
Verhoeff FH: A rare tumor arising from the pars ciliaris retinae (terato-neuroma), of a nature hitherto unrecognized, and its relation to the so-called glioma retinae. Trans Am Ophthalmol Soc *10*:351–377, 1904.
Verhoeff FH: Microscopic observations in a case of retinitis pigmentosa. Arch Ophthalmol *5*:392–407, 1931.
Verhoeff FH: Histological findings in a case of angioid streaks. Br J Ophthalmol *32*:531–544, 1948.
Verhoeff FH, Bell L, Walker CB: The pathological effects of radiant energy on the eye. Proc Am Acad Arts Sci *51* (No 13), July, 1916.
Verhoeff FH, Sisson RJ: Basophilic staining of Bruch's membrane. Arch Ophthalmol *55*:125–127, 1926.
Vine AK, Schatz H: Adult-onset foveomacular pigment epithelial dystrophy. Am J Ophthalmol *89*:680–691, 1980.
Virgi MA: Medulloepithelioma (diktyoma) presenting as a perforated, infected eye. Br J Ophthalmol *61*:229–232, 1977.
Vogel MH: Tumoren des Ziliarkörperepithels. Klin Monatsbl Augenheilkd *165*:458–469, 1974.
Vogel MH, Font RL, Zimmerman LE, Levine RA: Reticulum cell sarcoma of the retina and uvea: Report of six cases and review of literature. Am J Ophthalmol *66*:205–215, 1968.
Vogel MH, Müller KM, Witting C: Ocular histopathology in mucopolysaccharidosis III (Sanfilippo). Ophthalmologica *169*:311–319, 1974.
Vogel MH, Wessing A: Die Proliferation des juxtapapillären retinalen Pigmentepithels. Klin Mbl Augenheilkd *162*:736–743, 1972.
Vogel MH, Zimmerman LE, Gass JDM: Proliferation of the juxtapapillary retinal pigment epithelium simulating malignant melanoma. Doc Ophthalmol *26*:461–481, 1969.

Volpe JJ, Adams RD: Cerebro-hepato-renal syndrome of Zellweger: An inherited disorder of neuronal migration. Acta Neuropathol (Berlin) *20*:175–198, 1972.

Von Hippel E: Über diffuse Gliose der Netzhaut und ihre Beziehungen zu der Angiomatosis retinae. Albrecht Von Graefes Arch Ophthal *95*:173–183, 1918.

Von Noorden GK, Khodadoust A: Retinal hemorrhage in newborns and organic amblyopia. Arch Ophthalmol *89*:91–93, 1973.

Von Sallmann L, Gelderman AH, Laster L: Ocular histopathologic changes in a case of a-beta-lipoproteinemia (Bassen-Kornzweig syndrome). Doc Ophthalmol *26*:451–460, 1969.

Vosgien I: Le cercus cellulosae chez l'homme et chez les animaux. Bull Soc Centr Vet *12*:270–277, 1912.

Wacker WB, Donoso LA, Kalsow CM, et al: Experimental allergic uveitis: Isolation, characterization, and localization of a soluble uveitopathogenic antigen from bovine retina. J Immunol *119*:1949–1958, 1977.

Wacker WB, Lipton MM: Experimental allergic uveitis: Homologous retina as uveitogenic antigen. Nature *206*:253–254, 1965.

Wadsworth JAC: Epithelial tumors of the ciliary body. Am J Ophthalmol *32*:1487–1501, 1949.

Wagenmann A: Beitrag zur Kenntniss der pathologischen Anatomie der Retinitis pigmentosa. Albrecht Von Graefes Arch Ophthalmol *37*:230–242, 1891.

Wagner H: Ein bisher unbekanntes Erbleiden des Auges (Degeneratio hyaloideo-retinalis hereditaria), beobachtet im Kanton Zurich. Klin Mbl Augenheilkd *100*:840–857, 1938.

Wallow IHL, Davis MD: Clinicopathologic correlation of xenon arc and argon laser photocoagulation. Procedure in human diabetic eyes. Arch Ophthalmol *97*:2308–2315, 1979.

Wallow IHL, Greaser ML, Stevens TS: Actin filaments in diabetic fibrovascular preretinal membrane. Arch Ophthalmol *99*:2175–2181, 1981.

Wallow IHl, Lund OE, Gable VP, et al: A comparison of retinal argon laser lesions in man and in cynomolgus monkey. Albrecht von Graefes Arch Klin Exp Ophthalmol *189*:159–164, 1974.

Wallow IHL, Miller SA: Preretinal membrane by retinal pigment epithelium. Arch Ophthalmol *96*:1643–1646, 1978.

Wallow IHL, T'so MOM: Proliferation of the retinal pigment epithelium over malignant choroidal tumors: A light and electron microscopic study. Am J Ophthalmol *73*:914–926, 1972.

Wallow IHL, Tso MOM: Repair after xenon arc photocoagulation. 2. A clinical and light microscopic study of the evolution of retinal lesions in the rhesus monkey. Am J Ophthalmol *75*:610–626, 1973a.

Wallow IHL, Tso MOM: Repair after xenon arc photocoagulation. 3. An electron microscopic study of the evolution of retinal lesions in rhesus monkeys. Am J Ophthalmol *75*:957–972, 1973b.

Wallow IHL, Tso MOM, Elgin S: Experimental photocoagulation of the human retina. 2. Electron microscopic study. Arch Ophthalmol *95*:1041–1050, 1977.

Wallow IHL, Tso MOM, Fine BS: Retinal repair after experimental xenon arc photocoagulation. 1. A comparison between rhesus monkey and rabbit. Am J Ophthalmol *75*:32–52, 1973.

Wallyn RH, Hilton GF: Subretinal fibrosis in retinal detachment. Arch Ophthalmol *97*:2128–2129, 1979.

Walsh FB, Sloan LL: Idiopathic flat detachment of the macula. Am J Ophthalmol *19*:195–208, 1936.

Wang FM, Henkind P: Visual system involvement in giant cell (temporal) arteritis. Surv Ophthalmol *23*:264–271, 1979.

Warburg M: Norrie's disease: A congenital, progressive oculo-acoustico-cerebral degeneration. Acta Ophthalmol (Suppl.) *89*:1–145, 1966.

Warwick R: Eugene Wolff's Anatomy of the Eye and Orbit. 7th ed. London, H.K. Lewis, and Philadelphia, W.B. Saunders Company, 1976, pp 137–142.

Wataya T: A histopathological study of retinitis punctata albescens. Clin Ophthalmol *14*:552–556, 1960.

Watzke RC, Folk JC, Lang RM: Pattern dystrophy of the retinal pigment epithelium. Ophthalmology *89*:1400–1406, 1982.

Watzke RC, Stevens TS, Carney RG Jr: Retinal vascular changes of incontinentia pigmenti. Arch Ophthalmol *94*:743–746, 1976.

Weekley RD, Potts AM, Reboton J, May RH: Pigmentary retinopathy in patients receiving high doses of a new phenothiazine. Arch Ophthalmol *64*:65–76, 1960.

Weiner LP, Konigsmark BW, Stoll J Jr, Magladery JW: Hereditary olivopontocerebellar atrophy with retinal degeneration: Report of a family through six generations. Arch Neurol *16*:364–376, 1967.

Weingeist TA, Blodi FC: Fabry's disease: Ocular findings in a female carrier. Arch Ophthalmol *85*:169–176, 1971.

Weingeist TA, Kobrin JL, Watzke RC: Histopathology of Best's macular dystrophy. Arch Ophthalmol *100*:1108–1114, 1982.

Weinreb RN, Barth R, Kimura SJ: Limited gallium scans and angiotensin-converting enzyme in granulomatous uveitis. Ophthalmology *87*:202–206, 1980.

Weinreb RN, Kimura SJ: Uveitis associated with sarcoidosis and angiotensin-converting enzyme. Am J Ophthalmol *89*:180–185, 1980.

Weinreb RN, O'Donnell JJ, Sandman R, et al: Angiotensin-converting enzyme in sarcoid uveitis. Invest Ophthalmol Vis Sci *18*:1285–1287, 1979.

Weiss H, Annesley WJ Jr, Shields JA, et al: The clinical course of serpiginous choroidopathy. Am J Ophthalmol *87*:133–142, 1979.

Weiter JJ, Feingold M, Kolodny EH, Raghaven SS: Retinal pigment epithelial degeneration associated with leucocytic arylsulfatase A deficiency. Am J Ophthalmol *90*:768–772, 1980.

Weiter JJ, Fine BS: A histologic study of regional choroidal dystrophy. Am J Ophthalmol *83*:741–750, 1977.

Welch RB: Von Hippel–Lindau disease: The recognition and treatment of early angiomatosis retinae and the use of cryosurgery as an adjunct to therapy. Trans Am Ophthalmol Soc *68*:367–424, 1970.

Welch RB: Bietti's tapetoretinal degeneration with marginal corneal dystrophy: Crystalline retinopathy. Trans Am Ophthalmol Soc *75*:164–179, 1977.

Welch RB, Maumenee AE, Wahlen HE: Peripheral posterior segment inflammation, vitreous opacities, and edema of the posterior pole: Pars planitis. Arch Ophthalmol *64*:540–549, 1960.

Wendenberg D: Schädigungen des Sehorgans durch Blendung bei Sonnenfinsternis Boebachtungen. Berlin, S. Karger, 1914.

Wetterholm DH, Winter FC: Histopathology of chloroquine retinal toxicity. Arch Ophthalmol *71*:82–87, 1964.

Whipple GH: A hitherto undescribed disease characterized anatomically by deposits of fat and fatty acids in the intestinal and mesenteric lymphatic tissues. Bull Johns Hopkins Hosp *18*:382–391, 1907.

Whiteman DW, Rosen DA, Pinkerton RMH: Retinal and choroidal microvascular embolism after intranasal corticosteroid injection. Am J Ophthalmol *89*:851–853, 1980.

Widmark EJ: Über den Einfluss des Lichtes auf die vordern Medien des Auges und Haut: Über die Durchlässigkeit der Augen für ultravioletten Strahlen. Leipzig, Beiträge zur Ophthalmologie, 1891, pp. 355–502.

Wiesinger H, Schmidt FH, Williams RC, et al: The transmission of light. Am J Ophthalmol *42*:907–910, 1956.

Wilder HC: Nematode endophthalmitis. Trans Am Acad Ophthalmol Otolaryngol *55*:99–109, 1950.

Wilder HC: *Toxoplasma* chorioretinitis in adults. Arch Ophthalmol *48*:127–136, 1952.

Wilensky JT, Holland MG: A pigmented tumor of the ciliary body. Arch Ophthalmol *92*:219–220, 1974.

Wilkinson CP, Welch RB: Intraocular *Toxocara*. Am J Ophthalmol *71*:921–930, 1971.

Willerson D Jr, Aaberg TM: Senile macular degeneration and geographic atrophy of the retinal pigment epithelium. Br J Ophthalmol *62*:551–553, 1978.

Willerson D Jr, Aaberg TM, Reeser FH: Necrotizing vaso-occlusive retinitis. Am J Ophthalmol *84*:209–219, 1977.
Williams HE, Smith LH Jr: L-Glyceric aciduria: New genetic variant of primary hyperoxaluria. N Engl J Med *278*:233–239, 1968.
Williams PH, Templeton AC: Infection of the eye by tapeworm *Coenurus*. Br J Ophthalmol *55*:766–769, 1971.
Wilson WB: The visual system manifestations of adrenoleukodystrophy. Neuro-ophthalmology *1*:175–183, 1981.
Winter FC, Yukins RE: The ocular pathology of Behçet's disease. Am J Ophthalmol *62*:257–262, 1966.
Wise GN: Retinal neovascularization. Trans Am Ophthalmol Soc *54*:729–826, 1956.
Wise GN, Dollery CT, Henkind P: The Retinal Circulation. New York, Harper & Row, 1971, pp 294–297.
Wise GW: Arteriosclerosis secondary to retinal vein obstruction. Trans Am Ophthalmol Soc *56*:361–382, 1958.
Wisniewski K, Wisniewski HM: Diagnosis of infantile neuroaxonal dystrophy by skin biopsy. Ann Neurol *7*:377–379, 1978.
Witkop CJ Jr: Albinism, *in* Harris H, Hirschhorn K (eds): Advances in Human Genetics. Vol 2. New York, Plenum Press, 1971, pp 61+.
Witzleben CL: Lymphocyte inclusions in late-onset amaurotic idiocy: Value as a diagnostic test and genetic marker. Neurology *22*:1075–1078, 1972.
Wolff SM, Fauci AS, Horn RG, Dale DC: Wegener's granulomatosis. Ann Intern Med *81*:513–525, 1974.
Wolper J, Laibson PR: Heriditary hemorrhagic telangiectasis (Rendu-Osler-Weber disease) with filamentary keratitis. Arch Ophthalmol *81*:272–277, 1969.
Wolter JR: Retinitis pigmentosa: A histopathologic study with a new technique. Arch Ophthalmol *57*:539–553, 1957.
Wolter JR: Hyaline bodies of ganglion-cell origin in the human retina. Arch Ophthalmol *61*:127–134, 1959a.
Wolter JR: Pathology of a cotton-wool spot. Am J Ophthalmol *48*:473–485, 1959b.
Wolter JR: Pores in the internal limiting membrane of the human retina. Acta Ophthalmol *42*:971–974, 1964.
Wolter JR: Axonal enlargements in the nerve-fiber layer of the human retina. Am J Ophthalmol *65*:1–12, 1968.
Wolter JR: Double embolism of the central retinal artery and one long posterior ciliary artery followed by secondary hemorrhagic glaucoma. Am J Ophthalmol *73*:651–657, 1972.
Wolter JR, Allen RJ: Retinal neuropathology of late infantile amaurotic idiocy. Br J Ophthalmol *48*:277–284, 1964.
Wolter JR, Benz CA, Roth FD: Early disciform degeneration of the macula: Simulating choroidal melanoma. Am J Ophthalmol *59*:870–875, 1965.
Wolter JR, Falls HF: Bilateral confluent drusen. Arch Ophthalmol *68*:219–226, 1962.
Wolter JR, James BR: Adult type of medullo-epithelioma of the ciliary body. Am J Ophthalmol *1*:19–26, 1958.
Wolter JR, Liss RL: Hyaline bodies of the human optic nerve: Histopathologic study of a case of advanced syphilitic optic atrophy. Arch Ophthalmol *61*:780–788, 1959.
Wolter JR, Mertus JM: Exophytic retinal astrocytoma in tuberous sclerosis. J Pediatr Ophthalmol *6*:186–191, 1969.
Wolter JR, Pfister RR: Tumors of the pars ciliaris retinae. Am J Ophthalmol *52*:659–672, 1961.
Wolter JR, Ryan RW: Atheromatous embolism of the central retinal artery: Secondary hemorrhagic glaucoma. Arch Ophthalmol *87*:301–304, 1972.
Wong L, O'Donnell FE Jr, Green WR: Giant pigment granules in the retinal pigment epithelium of a fetus with X-linked ocular albinism. Ophthal Paediat Genet *2*:47–65, 1983.
Wong VG: Focal choroidopathy in experimental ocular histoplasmosis. Trans Am Ophthalmol Soc *70*:615–630, 1972.
Wong VG, Collins E: Optic atrophy in cystic fibrosis of the pancreas. Am J Ophthalmol *59*:763–769, 1965.
Wong VC, Green WR, Kuwabara T, et al: Homologous retinal outer segment immunization in primates: A clinical and histopathological study. Trans Am Ophthalmol Soc *72*:184–195, 1974.
Wong VG, Green WR, McMaster PRB: Rhodopsin and blindness. Trans Am Ophthalmol Soc *75*:272–284, 1977.
Wong VG, Green WR, McMaster PRB, Johnson DK: Rhodopsin and autoimmune blindness in primates. Trans Pa Acad Ophthalmol Otolaryngol *28*:135–137, 1975.
Wong VG, Kuwabara T, Brubaker R, et al: Intralysosomal cystine crystals in cystinosis. Invest Ophthalmol *9*:83–88, 1970.
Wong VG, Lietman PS, Seegmiller JE: Alterations of pigment epithelium in cystinosis. Arch Ophthalmol *77*:361–369, 1967.
Wong VG, Schulman JD, Seegmiller JE: Conjunctival biopsy for the biochemical diagnosis of cystinosis. Am J Ophthalmol *70*:278–281, 1970.
Wood CGR: Choroidal sclerosis. Ophthalmoscope (London) *13*:374–376, 1915.
Woodford B, Tso MOM: An ultrastructural study of the corpora amylacea of the optic nerve head and retina. Am J Ophthalmol *90*:492–502, 1980.
Wray SH, Cogan DG, Kuwabara T, et al: Adrenoleukodystrophy with disease of the eye and optic nerve. Am Ophthalmol *82*:480–485, 1976.
Wyburn-Mason R: Arteriovenous aneurysm of mid-brain and retina, facial naevi and mental changes. Brain *66*:163–203, 1943.
Wyhinny GJ, Apple DJ, Guastella FR, Vygantas CM: Adult cytomegalic inclusion retinitis. Am J Ophthalmol *76*:773–781, 1973.
Yamanaka M: Histologic study of Oguchi's disease: Its relationship to pigmentary degeneration of the retina. Am J Ophthalmol *68*:19–26, 1969.
Yanagisawa N, Shiraki H, Minakawa M, Narabayshi H: Clinico-pathological and histochemical studies of Hallervorden-Spatz disease with torsion dystonia, with special reference to diagnostic criteria of the disease from the clinico-pathological viewpoint. Prog Brain Res *21*:373–425, 1966.
Yanko L, Behar A: Teratoid intraocular medulloepithelioma. Am J Ophthalmol *85*:850–853, 1978.
Yanoff M: Diabetic retinopathy. N Engl J Med *274*:1344–1349, 1966.
Yanoff M: In discussion of Diddie KR, Aronson AJ, Ernest JT: Chorioretinopathy in a case of systemic lupus erythematosus. Trans Am Ophthalmol Soc *75*:122–131, 1977.
Yanoff M: Case presentation at Eastern Ophthalmic Pathology Society, New York, Oct, 1979.
Yanoff M, Frayer WC, Scheie HG: Ocular findings in a patient with 13–15 trisomy. Arch Ophthalmol *70*:372–375, 1963.
Yanoff M, Rahn EK, Zimmerman LE: Histopathology of juvenile retinoschisis. Arch Ophthalmol *79*:49–53, 1968.
Yanoff M, Schaffer DB, Scheie HG: Rubella ocular syndrome: Clinical significance of viral and pathologic studies. Trans Am Acad Ophthalmol Otolaryngol *72*:896–902, 1968.
Yanoff M, Schwartz GA: Lafora's disease: A distinct, genetically determined form of Unverricht's syndrome. J Genet Hum *14*:235–244, 1965a.
Yanoff M, Schwartz GA: The retinal pathology of Lafora's disease: A form of glycoprotein acid-mucopolysaccharide dystrophy. Trans Am Acad Ophthalmol Otolaryngol *69*:701–708, 1965b.
Yanoff M, Zimmerman LE, Davis RL: Massive gliosis of the retina, *in* Smith ME (ed): Ocular Pathology. Int Ophthalmol Clin *11*:211–229, 1971.
Yanuzzi LA: Some observations on central serous retinopathy. Presented at the Macula Society, Orlando, Florida, March, 1983.
Yanuzzi LA, Landan AN, Klein RM: Topical indomethacin: One per cent suspension in the prevention of aphakic cystoid macular edema. Presented at the Annual Meeting of the American Academy of Ophthalmology, Nov, 1980.
Yardley JH, Hendrix TR, Brown GD: Combined electron and

light microscopy in Whipple's disease: Demonstration of "bacillary bodies" in the intestine. Bull Johns Hopkins Hosp *109*:80–98, 1961.

Yassur Y, Shir M, Melamed S, Ben-Sira I: Bilateral maculopathy: "Cherry-red-spot" in a patient with Crohn's disease. Br J Ophthalmol *65*:184–188, 1981.

Yasue T: Histochemical identification of calcium oxalate. Acta Histochem Cytochem *2*:83–95, 1969.

Yimoyines DJ, Topilow HW, Abedin S, McMeel JW: Bilateral peripapillary exophytic retinal hemangioblastomas. Ophthalmology *89*:1388–1392, 1982.

Yoshioka H: Clinical studies on macular holes. III. On the pathogenesis of the senile macular hole. Acta Soc Ophthalmol Jpn *72*:575–584, 1968.

Yoshioka H, Katsume Y: Experimental central serous chorioretinopathy. III. Ultrastructural findings. Jpn J Ophthalmol *26*:397–409, 1982.

Yoshioka H, Katsume Y, Akune H: Experimental central serous chorioretinopathy. I. Clinical findings. Jpn J Ophthalmol *25*:112–118, 1981.

Yoshioka H, Katsume Y, Akune H: Experimental central serous chorioretinopathy in monkey eyes: Fluorescein angiographic findings. Ophthalmologica (Basel) *185*:168–178, 1982.

Yoshizumi MO, Thomas JV, Hirose T: Foveal hypoplasia and bilateral 360-degree peripheral retinal rosettes. Am J Ophthalmol *87*:186–192, 1979.

Young L: Clinicopathologic studies of Zellweger's syndrome. Unpublished data, 1973.

Young NJA, Baird AC: Bilateral acute retinal necrosis. Br J Ophthalmol *62*:581–590, 1978.

Young NJA, Hitchings RA, Sehmi K, and Bird AC: Stickler's syndrome and neovascular glaucoma. J Ophthalmol *63*:826–831, 1979.

Young RW: A theory of central retinal disease, *in* Sears ML (ed): Future Directions in Ophthalmological Research. New Haven, Conn, Yale University Press, 1981, pp 237–270.

Young RW: The Bowman Lecture, 1982. Biological renewal: Application to the eye. Trans Ophthalmol Soc UK *102*:42–75, 1982.

Young RW, Droz B: The renewal of protein in retinal rods and cones. J Cell Biol *39*:169–184, 1968.

Zanen J, Meunier A: L'amaurose post-hemorrhagique. Bull Soc Belge Ophtalmol *127*:235–244, 1961.

Zauberman H, Merin S: Unilateral high myopia with bilateral degenerative fundus changes. Am J Ophthalmol *67*:756–759, 1969.

Zeman W, Dyken P: Neuronal ceroid-lipofuscinosis (Batten's disease): Relationship to amaurotic familial idiocy? Pediatrics *44*:570–583, 1969.

Zeman W, Hoffman J: Juvenile and late forms of amaurotic idiocy in one family. J Neurol Neurosurg Psychiatry *25*:352–362, 1962.

Zentmeyer W: A case of hyperplasia of the epithelium of the ciliary processes. Arch Ophthalmol *16*:677, 1936.

Zimmerman LE: Embolism of central retinal artery secondary to myocardial infarction with mural thrombosis. Arch Ophthalmol *73*:822–826, 1965.

Zimmerman LE: Histopathologic basis for ocular manifestations of congenital rubella syndrome. The Eighth William Hamlin Wilder Memorial Lecture. Am J Ophthalmol *65*:837–862, 1968.

Zimmerman LE: Case presentation at the Ophthalmic Pathology Club, Washington, DC, 1969.

Zimmerman LE: Verhoeff's "terato-neuroma": A critical reappraisal in light of new observations and current concepts of embryonic tumors. The Fourth Frederick H. Verhoeff Lecture. Am J Ophthalmol *72*:1039–1057, 1971.

Zimmerman LE, Broughton WL: A clinicopathologic and follow-up study of fifty-six intraocular medulloepitheliomas, *in* Jakobiec FA (ed): Ocular and Adnexal Tumors. Birmingham, Ala, Aesculapius, 1978, pp 181–195.

Zimmerman LE, Font RL, Andersen SR: Rhabdomyosarcomatous differentiation in malignant intraocular medulloepitheliomas. Cancer *30*:817–835, 1972.

Zimmerman LE, Johnson FB: Calcium oxalate crystals within ocular tissues. A clinicopathologic and histochemical study. Arch Ophthalmol *60*:372–383, 1958.

Zimmerman LE, Maumenee AE: Ocular aspects of sarcoidosis. Am Rev Resp Dis *84* (Suppl 5):38–44, 1961.

Zimmerman LE, Naumann G: The pathology of retinoschisis, *in* McPherson A (ed): New and Controversial Aspects of Retinal Detachment. New York, Hoeber, 1968, pp 400–423.

Zimmerman LE, Spencer WH: The pathologic anatomy of retinoschisis: With a report of two cases diagnosed clinically as malignant melanoma. Arch Ophthalmol *63*:10–19, 1960.

Zimmerman TJ, Hood CI, Gasset AR: "Adolescent" cystinosis. Arch Ophthalmol *92*:265–268, 1974.

Zinn KM, Benjamin-Henkind JV: Anatomy of the human retinal pigment epithelium, *in* Zinn KM, Marmor MF (eds): The Retinal Pigment Epithelium. Cambridge, Mass, Harvard University Press, 1979, pp 3–31.

Zinn KM, Guillory SL, Friedman AH: Removal of intravitreous cysticerci from surface of the optic nerve head. A pars plana approach. Arch Ophthalmol *98*:714–716, 1980.

Zinn KM, Marmor MF (eds): The Retinal Pigment Epithelium. Cambridge, Mass, Harvard University Press, 1979.

Zion VM, Burton TC: Retinal dialysis. Arch Ophthalmol *98*:1971–1974, 1980.

Zscheile FP: Recurrent toxoplasmic retinitis with weakly positive methylene blue dye test. Arch Ophthalmol *71*:645–648, 1964.

Zweifach PH: Incontinentia pigmenti: Its association with retinal dysplasia. Am J Ophthalmol *62*:716–722, 1966.

Retinoblastoma and Retinocytoma

Lorenz E. Zimmerman

DEFINITIONS AND TERMINOLOGY

Retinoblastoma, the most important primary tumor of the retina, has a long and interesting history. The retinoblastoma story provides not only a model for what can be achieved in the conquest of cancer through research and education, but recently it has also provided a model of oncogenesis with exciting insights into the specific genetic alterations required to transform normal cells into cancerous cells. James Wardrop, the great Edinburgh ophthalmologist, is credited as the one who in 1809 established retinoblastoma as an entity and reached the then radical and subsequently controversial decision that early enucleation might save the patient's life (Albert, Robinson, 1974; Duke-Elder, Dobree, 1967; Dunphy, 1964; Sang, Albert, 1977). Although he never achieved a cure, Wardrop steadfastly maintained that his failures were attributable to the advanced stage of the disease at the time of enucleation and to the fact that the optic nerve had always been involved. Duke-Elder and Dobree (1967) provide an excellent summary of the early history.

The famous Rudolph Virchow considered the tumor a glioma of the retina, and because of his influence, this remained its most widely used name for many years. Flexner in 1881 and Wintersteiner in 1897 described and illustrated the characteristic and almost pathognomonic rosettes, which have been given their names. Influenced by these rosettes, Flexner suggested that the tumor be called neuroepithelioma of the retina, which is also the term used by Wintersteiner in the title of his monumental monograph. Over the years, many names have been proposed but under the profound influence of Frederick H. Verhoeff of Boston, the American Ophthalmological Society in 1926 adopted retinoblastoma, which he had suggested in 1922 (Verhoeff, Jackson, 1926). Verhoeff, recognizing that the tumor was basically an undifferentiated neuroblastic neoplasm derived from hypothetic retinoblasts, coined the logical name, which has gradually replaced virtually all others that have been proposed from time to time.

According to Offret, Dhermy, Brini, and Bec (1974), retinocytoma has been used in the French literature to designate the most highly differentiated forms of retinoblastoma ever since Mawas introduced the term in the early 1920s, and in their book these authors recommend continued use of this valuable term. They divided retinocytomas into two groups—one characterized by large numbers of highly differentiated Flexner-Wintersteiner rosettes, the other featuring fleurettes.

Parkhill and Benedict (1941) also proposed different names to reflect varying degrees of differentiation—retinoblastoma for undifferentiated tumors and neuroepithelioma for tumors containing rosettes. This nomenclature has not enjoyed great popularity for two reasons. First, it is difficult to classify tumors by the presence or absence of rosettes. The degrees of differentiation vary greatly. Most retinoblastomas show some attempts to form Flexner-Wintersteiner rosettes, but the rosettes may not be present in many sections or they may be poorly formed. Well-differentiated rosettes may be numerous in some foci but totally absent in others. Another problem is necrosis. Some tumors are so extensively necrotic and calcified that the absence of rosettes is meaningless. A second reason for not favoring the Parkhill-Benedict classification is that in advocating the term neuroepithelioma for tumors containing rosettes, they were fostering the concept that these are glial neoplasms that have differentiated by forming structures (rosettes) that represent the primitive neuroepithelium of the neural tube. Verhoeff and many subsequent investigators, including myself, have favored the concept that these are not glial tumors but neuroblastic neoplasms that are almost unique to the retina and that the formation of rosettes is an attempt to produce photoreceptor cells. Some electron microscopic observations support this concept (Tso, Fine, Zimmerman, 1969, 1970). The presence of acid mucopolysaccharide resistant to hyaluronidase (similar to that which normally coats the outer surface of photoreceptors) along the luminal surface of the cells forming rosettes (Zimmerman, 1958) provides additional support for the belief that Flexner-Wintersteiner rosettes represent a uniquely retinal type of differentiation with attempts to form photoreceptor cells.

It has long been appreciated that retinoblastomas vary greatly in their degrees of differentiation and this is in part responsible for so many different names having been proposed for them. Until 1970, it was believed that a great number of very well-differentiated rosettes represented the highest degree of differentiation. Then Tso, Zimmerman, and Fine (1970) described an even higher degree of differentiation characterized by the formation of benign-appearing cells that individually or in small, bouquet-like clusters ("fleurettes") exhibit photoreceptor differentiation. In most instances, such areas of benign-appearing tumor cells represented only a small component within an otherwise typical retinoblastoma, but in rare cases the entire tumor was observed to have a similarly benign cytologic makeup. In a subsequent communication, Tso, Zimmerman, Fine, and Ellsworth (1970) postulated that such cytologically benign-appearing portions of retinoblastomas are much less sensitive to radiation, and that some therapeutic failures following radiation are attributable to the presence of a less radiosensitive, more highly differentiated tumor.

Tso and coworkers did not give any new name to those tumors composed entirely of viable, benign-appearing tumor cells exhibiting photoreceptor differentiation. Recently, however, Margo, Hidayat, Kopelman, and Zimmerman (1983) have reintroduced the term *retinocytoma* for such tumors that histologically appear to be composed entirely of benign, well-differentiated tumor cells. In proposing this term, they follow the neuropathologic classification of the neural tumors of the pineal: pineoblastoma for the malignant group and pineocytoma for the more highly differentiated and comparatively benign group (Rubinstein, 1982). Inasmuch as retinoblastoma is already the accepted name for the common malignant tumor of the retina, it seemed appropriate to name its very rare, totally benign counterpart retinocytoma. This terminology is not inconsistent with the original use of the name by Mawas and his French followers (Offret, Dhermy, Brini, Bec 1974), but it does restrict use of the name retinocytoma to those tumors that adequate histologic sampling has shown to be completely benign.

Independently, based on careful, long-term clinical observations, Gallie and her coworkers, Ellsworth, Abramson, and Phillips (1982) introduced a new name, retinoma, for small, often partially calcified but viable retinal tumors exhibiting no growth. While conceptually they considered these to be benign variants of retinoblastoma, they wanted a new name to differentiate them clearly from retinoblastoma. Although they studied clinically 36 eyes with such lesions, none was examined histologically, so they had no pathologic material from which to base a cytologic designation for these tumors. It seems clear, however, that the tumors they studied clinically are identical to the retinocytomas of Margo and coworkers. Retinocytoma is described and illustrated on page 1320 and in Figures 8–605 through 8–608, and discussed further in relation to the subject of spontaneous regression of retinoblastomas on pages 1326 to 1328.

EPIDEMIOLOGY AND GENETICS

Retinoblastoma is the most common malignant intraocular tumor of infancy and early childhood. It is worldwide in distribution, affecting all racial groups. Evidence documents a higher incidence in some black populations as in Haiti, Jamaica, Nigeria, and South Africa (Abiose, Adido, 1984; Freedman, Goldberg, 1976; Sang, Albert, 1977, 1982). In Africa, Asia, and certain parts of Latin America where uveal melanomas are seen much less frequently, retinoblastoma is the most common of all primary intraocular malignancies regardless of age. Its frequency has been calculated to range from 1 in 34,000 to 1 in 15,000 live births; in Holland and Finland, a significant increase in incidence has been reported over the 50 year period between 1915 and 1965 (Schappert-Kimmijser Hemmes, Nijland, 1966; Tarkkanen, Tuovinen, 1971; Sang, Albert, 1977).

Explanations offered for the increased incidence include the improving survival rate of patients with heritable forms and a greater pollution of the environment by ambient radiation and other mutagenic agents. A more recent and very thorough analysis of the Dutch Retinoblastoma Registry showed that since 1950 the frequency of retinoblastoma in The Netherlands has become stabilized at around an average of 1 in 15,560 persons for the period 1950 through 1969 (Schipper, 1980). From the study it was also deduced that what had previously been interpreted as an increasing occurrence was really attributable to a decreasing number of untraced cases and, consequently, to a more complete registration. This new study also showed that from 1920 through 1969 there was no increase in the proportion of bilateral cases. The percentage of bilateral cases remained at about 33 per cent.

The incidence of retinoblastoma decreases with age, with the great majority of cases being diagnosed before age 4 years. Retinoblastoma has been observed in premature babies as well as in infants born at term (Warburg, 1974). In a series of 760 cases on file in the Registry of Ophthalmic Pathology, only five patients were over 10 years of age (Zimmerman, 1969). The tumor, however, has been documented as occurring in adults. I have studied sections of the tumors in adults recorded by Verhoeff (1966) and by Takahashi, Tamara, Inoue, and coworkers (1983) and can attest to the validity of the histologic diagnosis in those cases as well as in several others in the Registry of Ophthalmic Pathology. In their review of the literature, Takahashi and colleagues found only 11 histologically confirmed retinoblastomas in patients older than 20 years.

There is no significant sex prevalence for the occurrence of retinoblastoma.

Warburg (1974) collected data on the occurrence of retinoblastoma in 25 pairs of twins. She found that among monozygotic twins almost invariably both were affected, whereas among dizygotic twins there was only one report of the tumor occurring in both twins. While in most twins with retinoblastoma the tumors were bilateral, there was a surprisingly large proportion with unilateral retinoblastoma (9 of 29).

The median age at the time of diagnosis of bilateral retinoblastoma is significantly less than that for unilateral retinoblastoma (Warburg, 1974). Knudson (1971) and Gallie and Phillips (1982) have plotted the ages of patients with unilateral and bilateral retinoblastomas versus the logarithm of the proportion in each category not yet diagnosed and found significant differences in the shapes of the two curves. For bilateral retinoblastoma, the curve fits a simple exponential, implying that a single event in addition to the germline mutation is required to produce the tumors, whereas the shape of the curve for unilateral cases suggests that tumorigenesis involves more than one event. From such data, Knudson formulated his "2 hit hypothesis." He postulated that the development of any retinoblastoma requires two complementary tumor-inducing, presumably genetic events to convert a normal retinal cell into a neoplastic cell. In the case of bilateral retinoblastoma, the initial event is a germinal or inherited mutation, so all retinal cells, like all other somatic cells, require only one more tumor-inducing event for oncogenesis. By contrast in the great majority of unilateral retinoblastoma cases, there is no constitutional genetic abnormality, and the developing retinal cells must sustain both genetic alterations to become converted to a neoplastic cell.

This theory is attractive as it provides a rational explanation to account for both the similarities and the differences between heritable and nonheritable retinoblastomas. These tumors are almost indistinguishable clinically and histologically. One sees the same variations in degrees of differentiation, in growth characteristics, in ocular complications, and in lethality. Two major clinicopathologic differences between the two groups are the earlier age at time of diagnosis (13 to 16 months earlier according to Schipper, 1980) and the multicentricity of heritable retinoblastoma. Since in nonheritable retinoblastoma a normal retinal cell must sustain two separate genetic events for it to become neoplastic, a longer period is required for these two events to take place—hence the older age of the affected children (mean age, 20 to 27 months). In a genetically normal child it is statistically improbable that more than a single retinal cell would ever sustain the two genetic events required to transform it into a retinoblastoma cell; this accounts for the lack of multicentricity and bilaterality in nongenetic cases. While documentation of the genetic implications of bilaterality is reasonably well established, the same cannot be claimed for multicentricity in cases of unilateral retinoblastoma (Schipper, 1980).

There is one additional major difference between patients with heritable and those with nonheritable retinoblastoma: survivors of heritable retinoblastoma (Abramson, Ellsworth, Zimmerman, 1976; Abramson, Ronner, Ellsworth, 1979; Abramson, Ellsworth, Kitchin, 1980) and other family members (Gordon, 1974; Chan, Pratt, 1977) are highly susceptible to the development of other nonocular cancers. They are especially vulnerable to development of sarcomas of bone and other neoplasms at sites of irradiation used in the treatment of retinoblastoma. They are also much more likely to have bone tumors at sites remote from portals of irradiation. It has been estimated that osteosarcoma of the lower extremities occurs 500-fold more frequently in survivors of bilateral retinoblastoma than in other children. Separate tumors, which may resemble retinoblastoma very closely, have recently been recognized as occurring far more frequently in the pineal gland or in a parasellar location in patients with heritable retinoblastoma than in other retinoblastoma patients (Bader, Miller, Meadows, et al, 1980; Bader, Meadows, Zimmerman, et al, 1982) (see discussion of trilateral retinoblastoma, pages 1345 to 1347). Abramson, Ellsworth, Kitchin, and Tung (1984) estimated that within 20 years of treatment for bilateral retinoblastoma, about half the patients will have developed another cancer.

The Knudson hypothesis, of course, does not postulate what the specific etiologic factors or genetic events might be that are required to produce retinoblastomas. It seems clear, however, that whatever they may be, they are operational in utero, as the occurrence of congenital or neonatal retinoblastoma is well documented (Fig. 8–577). It is also clear that with increasing age after birth, the vulnerability of the retina to the specific etiologic factors decreases even in the genetically predisposed patients. It is assumed, therefore, that incompletely differentiated retinal cells ("retinoblasts") are the most vulnerable. On the other hand, the rare occurrence of typical retinoblastoma in adults is established.

In 1970, before Knudson's theory had been presented, I postulated in a lecture on "Changing Concepts Concerning the Pathogenesis of Infectious Diseases" that what is inherited as a mendelian dominant characteristic is a special sus-

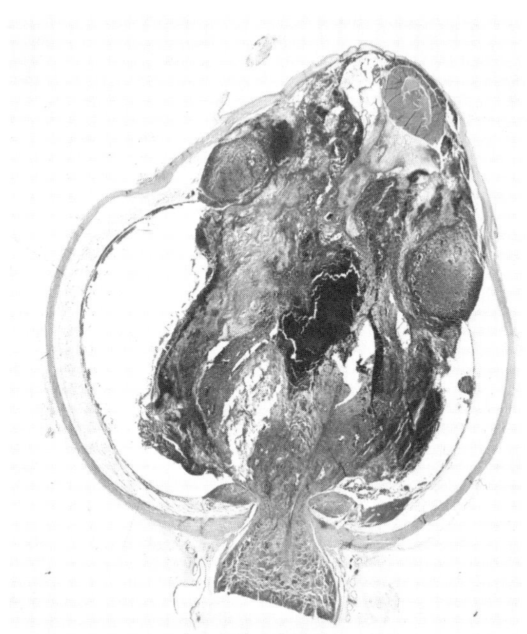

Figure 8–577. Congenital retinoblastoma that led to rupture of cornea and enucleation on the second day after birth. At the time of delivery the cornea appeared thin and ectatic, and bloody fluid was observed to drain from the site of rupture. The section shows the eye to be almost filled by the huge retinoblastoma that has totally replaced the retina, largely destroyed the internal architecture of the globe, and massively invaded the optic nerve and uvea. × 4. AFIP Neg. 68-9151. (From Zimmerman, LE: Retinoblastoma, including a report of illustrative cases. Med Ann Dist Columbia *38*:366–374, 1969.)

ceptibility of the retina to an oncogenic agent, perhaps a ubiquitous virus, to which the retina and other tissues of normal individuals are very resistant. As in the case of congenital rubella, the "retinoblastoma virus" could be transmitted in utero by asymptomatic mothers to their babies and the latter could become infected without showing any clinical manifestations. Such a ubiquitous subclinical viral infection could be the etiologic factor responsible for either the second or both mutagenic events postulated by Knudson. Reid and Albert (1972) and Albert and Reid (1973) and their colleagues have presented evidence of RNA-directed DNA polymerase activity in retinoblastomas and in retinoblastoma cell lines grown in culture for more than 30 months.

One way of categorizing retinoblastoma cases is based on whether there is a known family history. Familial cases account for less than 10 per cent, and in some underdeveloped countries where there are virtually no survivors, there are no familial cases (Kodilinye, 1967). The remainder are called sporadic, but this is a heterogeneous group: about one fourth of the sporadic group are heritable tumors arisen in patients with new germinal mutations; the remainder are nonheritable tumors derived from somatic mutations in retinal cells.

For genetic considerations, a more useful classification that is rapidly replacing the foregoing is as follows:

Chromosomal Deletion Retinoblastoma. In children who typically have various somatic and mental developmental abnormalities and a partial deletion of the long arm of chromosome 13 (13q− syndrome) (Figure 8–578,*A*), there has been a significant occurrence of retinoblastoma associated with a deletion that includes the q14 band (Schipper, 1980; Vogel, 1979; Weichselbaum, Zakov, Albert, et al, 1979; Yunis, Ramsay, 1978). When the q14 band is not included in the deleted segment, there is no retinoblastoma. This observation directed attention to the 13q14 band as the possible locus for the "retinoblastoma gene." This is also the locus of the gene responsible for esterase D activity (Fig. 8–578,*B*) (Sparkes, Sparkes, Wilson, et al, 1980) and possibly of the gene associated with the ability of tissues to repair DNA after exposure to radiation (Gallie, 1980; Weichselbaum, Zakov, Albert, et al, 1979); Arlett, Harcourt, 1980; Paterson, Torben Bech-Hansen, 1983). Patients who have a deletion that includes the 13q14 band have only half normal levels of esterase D activity in their tissues because they have only one functioning esterase D allele, whereas patients who have a 13 trisomy have a 50 per cent increase in the level of esterase D because they possess three esterase D alleles.

Fewer than 5 per cent of retinoblastoma patients have a deletion of 13q14 (Dryja, Bruns, Gallie, et al, 1983; Matsunaga, 1980).

Heritable Retinoblastoma. This is synonymous with genetically determined retinoblastoma and includes familial cases, in which the genetic abnormality has been passed on from one of the parents, and sporadic cases, in which a new genetic mutation is responsible for the initial appearance of the tumor in a given family. In affected families, retinoblastoma is passed on as a mendelian dominant trait with incomplete penetrance and variable expressivity. Typically, multiple discrete tumors are present in one or both retinas. Rarely are both retinas completely replaced by the tumors, and in about one third of familial cases only one eye is affected (Vogel, 1979). Some 10 to 15 per cent of sporadic unilateral retinoblastoma cases are also heritable (Murphree, Benedict, 1984; Nielson, Goldschmidt, 1968). Variable expressivity, therefore, includes total sparing of both retinas, total sparing of one retina, and the sparing of variable portions of the retinas in eyes with bilateral multicentric tumors. Statements made to the effect that the penetrance is 80 per cent (Klein, 1962) imply that at least one tumor in one eye will be found in 80 per cent of the genotypically affected individuals.

In this group, chromosomal studies made with

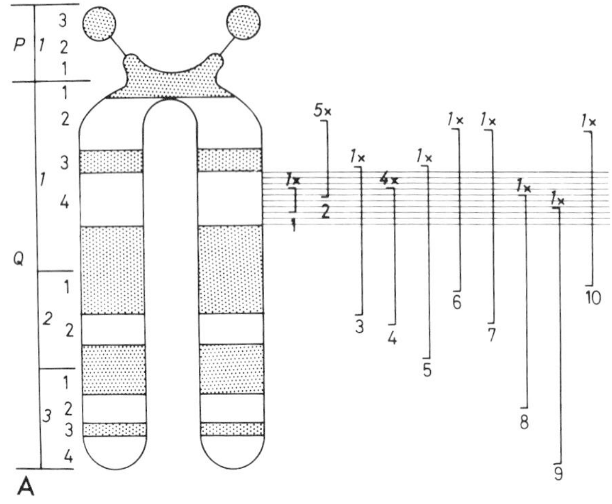

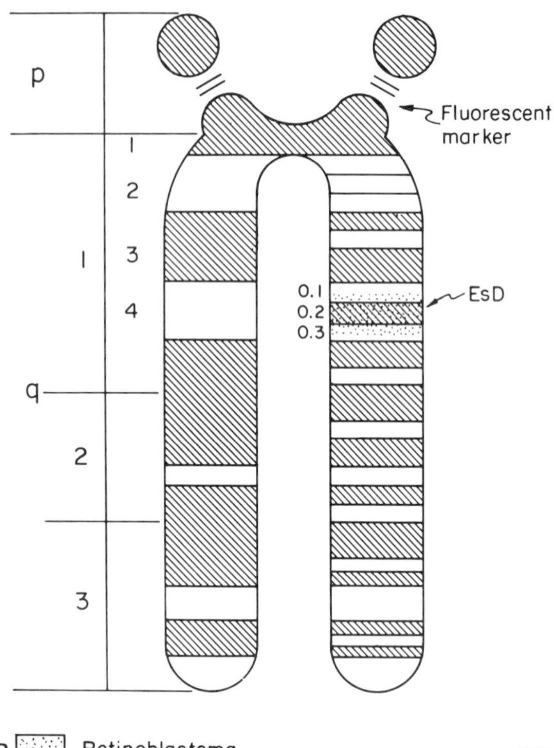

Figure 8–578. *A*, **Normal chromosome 13** and, indicated by vertical bars, the probable locations of the deleted segments in 17 patients who had retinoblastoma. In each case, the deletion included q14. AFIP Neg. 84-6977 from original provided by Dr. J. Schipper from his 1980 monograph. *B*, **Chromosome 13 and its markers.** The left chromatid shows Giemsa-stained bands observed in metaphase; on the right, the sub-bands are depicted as seen in late prophase. The genetic abnormality associated with retinoblastoma is believed to be located between sub-bands q14.1 and q14.3 in close proximity to the locus of the gene for esterase D. AFIP Neg. 84-7422, from original provided by Dr. Brenda Gallie, modified from her publication of 1980. (The locus for radiation repair in q14 has been deleted, as confirmation for its existence in 13q14 has not been obtained.)

the best banding techniques currently available typically fail to reveal any morphologically recognizable alterations. However, in one recently recorded case of bilateral retinoblastoma in which repeated studies of peripheral blood lymphocytes, fibroblasts, and lymphoblastoid cell lines had failed to disclose any morphologic abnormalities in chromosome 13, a submicroscopic deletion in 13q14 must have been present because the esterase D activity was about one half of normal levels in red blood cells, fibroblasts, and lymphoblastoid lines (Benedict, Murphree, Banerjee, et al, 1983). Current thought is that despite the typically normal karyotype, a chromosomal abnormality resulting from a submicroscopic deletion or some other alteration is undoubtedly present in the region of q14 of one of the two chromosomes 13, and that it may be equated with the "first hit" of Knudson's 2 hit hypothesis. To date, however, documentation has been provided in only the case reported by Benedict and coworkers (1983).

Nonheritable Retinoblastoma. In these cases, there is a single tumor in one eye of a child with no family history of retinoblastoma. Chromosomal studies reveal no abnormalities. Survivors do not pass on the disease to their offspring.

A further discussion of esterase D is necessary. This is a polymorphic enzyme of unknown function found in most tissues. By deletion mapping and somatic hybridization studies, its gene has been localized to chromosomal region 13q14, the same location as that of the "retinoblastoma gene" (Benedict, Murphree, Banerjee, et al, 1983; Murphree, Gomez, Doiron, Benedict, 1982; Mukai, Rapaport, Shields, et al, 1984; Sparkes, Sparkes, Wilson, et al, 1980; Sparkes, Murphree, Lingua, et al, 1983; Yunis, Ramsay, 1978). Electrophoretically, there are two common allelic forms of the enzyme, types 1 and 2. By genetic linkage analysis in several retinoblastoma families, a close linkage of the tumor gene with the genetic locus for esterase D has been reported (Connolly, Payne, Johnson, et al, 1983; Sparkes, Murphree, Lingua, et al, 1983). To be informative for linkage analysis, the affected parent must be heterozygous for esterase D types 1 and 2. Thus, in informative families, determination of the esterase D type may have predictive value in prenatal amniocentesis examinations and placental biopsies, as well as in the evaluation of neonates whose fundi may appear to be uninvolved (Mukai, Rapaport, Shields, et al, 1984). Unfortunately, only 10 to 15 per cent of families have an informative set of esterase D alleles. Dryja, Rapaport, Weichselbaum, and Bruns (1984), in an effort to improve predictability of the occurrence of retinoblastoma, have cloned DNA fragments that identify restriction length polymorphisms on chromosome 13.

The activity of esterase D in various tissues is related to the "dose" of the gene (Benedict, Murphree, Banerjee, et al, 1983; Sparkes, Sparkes, Wilson, et al, 1980). Thus, when there is a deletion involving 13q14 of one of the alleles, the tissue level of esterase D will be about half the normal level. Conversely, when one finds half-normal values of esterase D, one expects the karyotype to reveal a deletion involving 13q14. When half-normal levels of esterase D are found in patients whose chromosomes appear to be normal, the assumption may be made that there has been a submicroscopic deletion within the 13q14 band.

Although the genes related to retinoblastoma and esterase D are believed to lie in close proximity, the gene for esterase D activity is not affected in the great majority of patients who have heritable retinoblastoma (Dryja, Bruns, Gallie, et al, 1983).

Following Knudson's proposal of his two-mutation theory of tumorigenesis for retinoblastoma, alternative suggestions and modifications were introduced. One hypothesis launched by Hashem and Khalifa in 1975 postulated that a specific region on the long arm of one of the D chromosomes, most likely chromosome 13, is the site of a locus essential for sustained differentiation of specialized retinal tissue and perhaps the site of other loci essential for maturation of other embryonic tissues. Fragility of this region and its potentiality for breakage under the influence of various environmental insults was suggested as the basic cytologic event leading to the development of sporadic retinoblastomas.

Comings (1973) outlined a general theory of carcinogenesis that involved the concept of diploid pairs of suppressor regulatory genes. He postulated that in autosomal dominant hereditary tumors, one inactive suppressor allele leads to tumor formation by allowing the expression of a "transforming gene." Sporadic tumors were thought to result from somatic mutations in both alleles at the regulatory locus releasing the cell from restraints on growth.

Ten years later Benedict and coworkers (1983) recorded a case in which there was a morphologically undetectable deletion at 13q14 associated with half-normal levels of esterase D in constitutional cells, while the retinoblastoma cells exhibited a missing chromosome 13 and a total absence of esterase D. They logically concluded that the one normal allele for esterase D that was present in the patient's constitutional cells was contained in the chromosome that was missing in the tumor and proposed, therefore, that the second event in oncogenesis of retinoblastoma involves the loss of the remaining functional locus in 13q14. Balaban, Gilbert, Nichols, et al (1982) had already found that in five of six retinoblastomas there was a demonstrable deletion at the 13q14 locus in the tumor cells. Then in 1983 Godbout, Dryja, Squire, and coworkers, who studied six retinoblastoma patients who were heterozygous for esterase D types 1 and 2, found that in four cases the tumor cells expressed enzyme of only one type. This observation led them to the tentative conclusion that induction of a retinoblastoma requires somatic inactivation of genes near but not identical to the gene for esterase D, including the remaining normal gene at the retinoblastoma locus. Soon afterward Cavenee, Dryja, Phillips, et al (1983) presented the most convincing support for this new concept. Using cloned DNA segments homologous to arbitrary loci for human chromosome 13 and which revealed polymorphic restriction endonuclease fragments, they looked for somatic genetic events that might occur during tumorigenesis and presented evidence that the development of homozygosity for the mutant allele at the retinoblastoma locus leads to tumorigenesis.

Drawing upon these new developments, Murphree and Benedict (1984) have again focused attention on Comings' theory of 1973 that the "retinoblastoma gene" is a model for a class of human cancer genes that have a "suppressor" or "regulatory" function.

A summary of other new investigations aimed at testing the hypothesis that the normal allele at the retinoblastoma locus probably regulates differentiation whereas its absence leads to uncontrolled neoplastic transformations was presented by Gallie and Phillips (1984). Among the various possible mechanisms for the development of homozygosity of recessive alleles in 13q14, the following four have been documented in retinoblastoma (Dryja, Cavenee, White, et al, 1984): loss of entire chromosome 13 (Benedict, Murphree, Banerjee, et al, 1983; Cavenee, Dryja, Phillips, et al, 1983); loss of one chromosome 13 homolog with reduplication of the remaining chromosome 13 homolog (Cavenee and coworkers; 1983); somatic recombination with subsequent segregation resulting in homozygosity at all loci distal to the recombination site (Cavenee et al, 1983); and deletion of a segment of chromosome 13, including 13q14 (Balaban, Gilbert, Nichols, et al, 1982). Other possible mechanisms include localized gene conversion in the neighborhood of the retinoblastoma locus and point mutations (Dryja et al, 1984).

Current thought about the retinoblastoma gene and genetic alterations involved in tumorigenesis for retinoblastoma may be summarized as follows:

1. A single locus common to heritable, nonheritable, and 13-deletion retinoblastoma exists within

chromosomal band 13q14, and a deletion, point mutation, or rearrangement affecting that locus in both homologous chromosomes is common to the tumor cells in all three forms of retinoblastoma.

2. The normal (so-called wild type) allele at the retinoblastoma locus somehow tends to prevent the formation of tumors, especially retinoblastomas. A mutant allele at this locus (often referred to as the retinoblastoma gene) predisposes cells to tumorigenesis, but a normal allele at the homologous locus is sufficient to prevent malignant change.

3. Only when a given cell acquires mutant alleles at both homologous retinoblastoma loci in q14 (that is, there is a complete loss of the normal or wild type of allele) does the cell develop the capacity to undergo malignant transformation. The two separate alterations affecting each normal homologous allele at the retinoblastoma locus represent the "hits" of Knudsen's 2 hit hypothesis. The requirement that a cell become homozygous for the mutant, tumor-producing allele for retinoblastoma to develop implies that the mutant allele ("Rb gene") is recessive to the normal ("wild type") allele.

4. In heritable retinoblastoma, there is a constitutional abnormality in that all cells of the body are heterozygous at the retinoblastoma locus: one chromosome 13 contains the normal allele while the homologous chromosome contains the tumor-predisposing allele. Any chromosomal alteration that inactivates or causes a loss of the normal allele creates a state of homozygosity characterized by a complete loss of the normal allele that prevents the formation of retinoblastoma and probably other tumors as well.

In summary, the normal allele at the retinoblastoma locus behaves as a mendelian dominant, whereas the abnormal, tumor-predisposing mutant allele is recessive. Thus, the presence of a

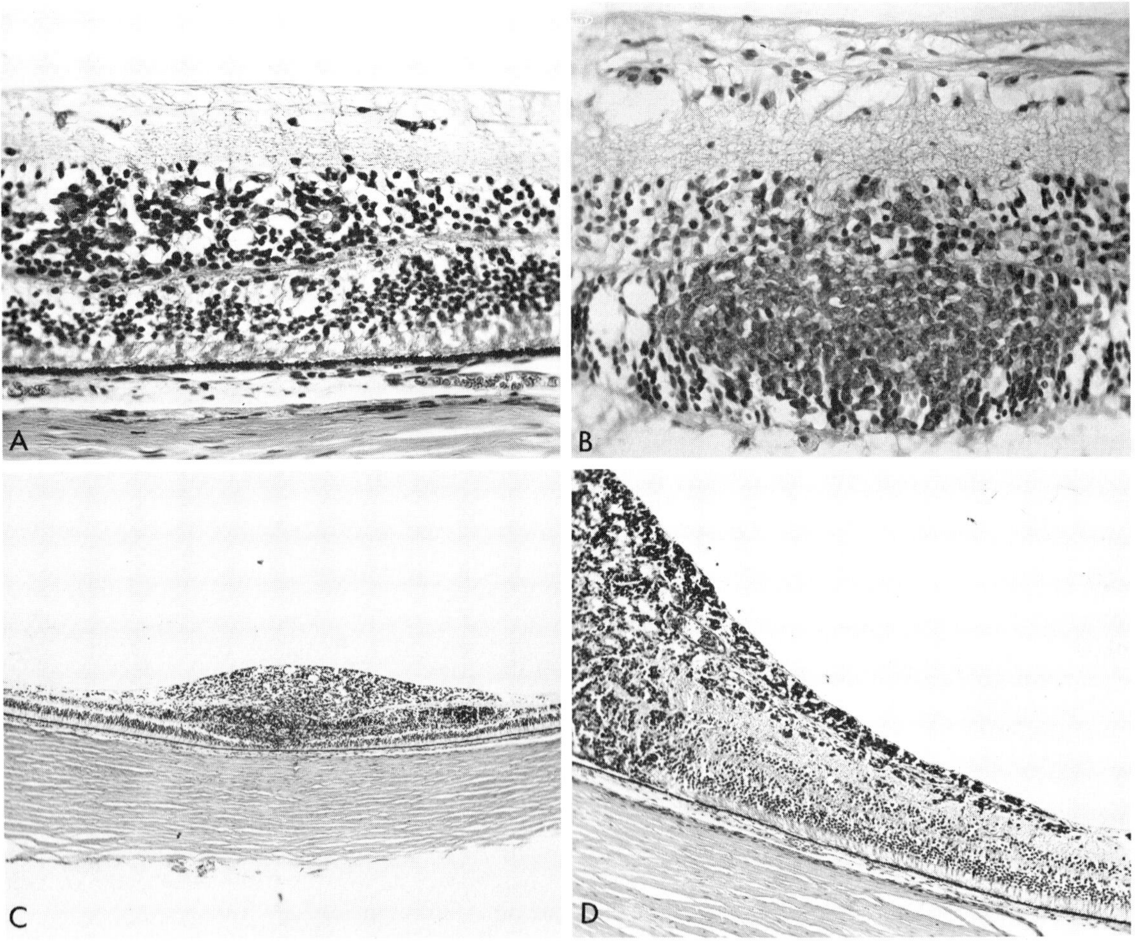

Figure 8–579. Minute foci of retinoblastomatous alteration, involving the inner nuclear layer in *A,* the outer nuclear layer in *B,* and all layers in *C* and *D.* The neoplastic cells possess nuclei that are larger and more basophilic than those of the adjacent normal retina. *A,* × 305. AFIP Neg. 57-13186. B, × 305. AFIP Neg. 61-4415. C, × 50. AFIP Neg. 57-13184. D, × 115. AFIP Neg. 57-13187.

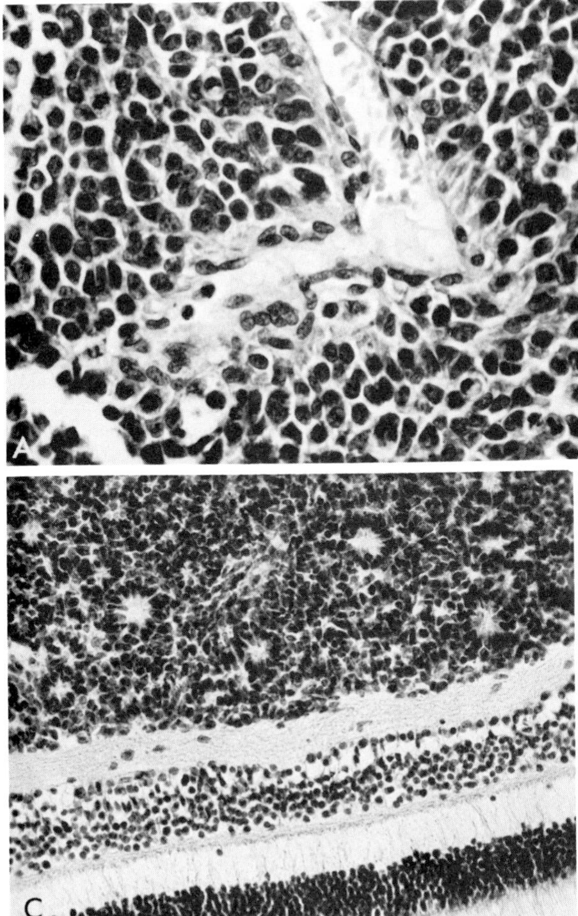

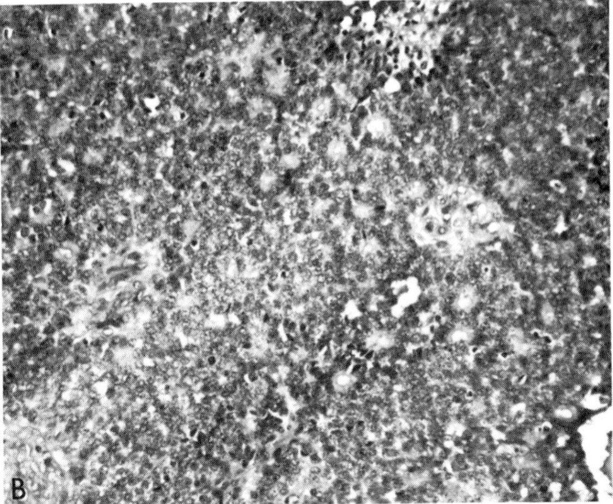

Figure 8–580. These highly anaplastic **retinoblastoma cells** have very large, irregular hyperchromatic nuclei that are densely packed, reflecting the fact that the neoplastic cells have scanty cytoplasm except where they form rosettes. Mitotic figures are typically numerous. *A,* ×400. AFIP Neg. 190088-02101. *B,* ×160. AFIP Neg. 82-7564. *C,* ×280. AFIP Neg. 59-611.

pair of normal genes at the retinoblastoma locus tends to protect against the development of retinoblastoma and other tumors whereas its absence or alteration in one allele predisposes to the formation of malignant neoplasms, especially retinoblastoma. When a vulnerable cell becomes homozygous for the tumor-predisposing recessive allele, the cell undergoes malignant transformation.

These concepts may be portrayed symbolically as follows: let P_t represent the normal, dominant gene at the retinoblastoma locus, which prevents or protects against the formation of tumors, while p_t represents the inactive recessive allele and − represents a missing allele, as in the deletion forms of retinoblastoma. Using these symbols, the following represent the various genotypic possibilities:

Somatic cells of normal individuals and patients with nonheritable retinoblastoma	$P_t/\ P_t$
Somatic cells of patients with heritable retinoblastoma	$P_t/\ p_t$
Somatic cells of patients with chromosomal deletion retinoblastoma	$P_t/-$
Retinoblastoma tumor cells (depending on type of retinoblastoma)	$p_t/\ p_t$ $p_t/-$ $-/-$

PATHOLOGY

Histologic Features

Retinoblastomas are essentially undifferentiated malignant neuroblastic tumors that may arise in any of the nucleated retinal layers (Fig. 8–579). The predominant cell has a large basophilic nucleus of variable size and shape and scanty cytoplasm (Fig. 8–580). Mitotic figures are typically numerous. The tumor cells have a striking tendency to outgrow their blood supply. Consequently, a characteristic pattern is usually observed, especially in larger tumors (Fig. 8–581). Sleeves of viable cells are present along dilated blood vessels, but as the tumor cells become displaced more than 90 to 110 microns away from the nutrient vessel, they undergo ischemic coagulative necrosis (Burnier, McLean, Zimmerman,

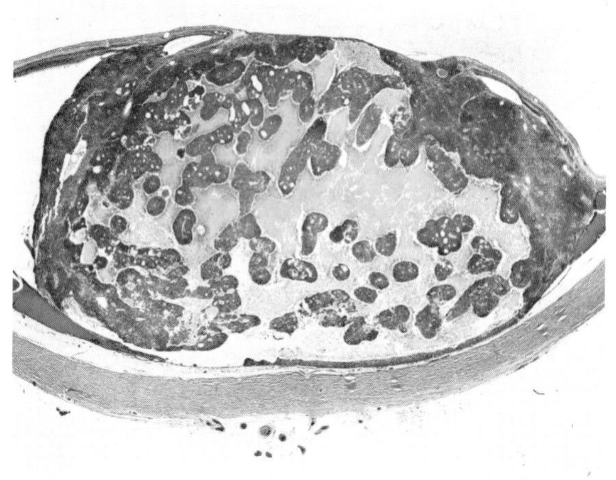

Figure 8–581. The typical histologic pattern of retinoblastoma is characterized by hyperchromatic viable neoplastic cells forming sleeves about capillaries, with pale-staining necrotic tumor tissue in between the islands of non-necrotic tumor. ×8. AFIP Neg. 68-7842.

1984; Schipper, 1980) (Fig. 8–582). This is a remarkably constant finding from one tumor to the next, though the degree of necrosis does vary considerably. Calcification occurs almost constantly, mainly within the areas of necrosis (Figs. 8–582 and 8–583). Albert, Craft, and Sang (1978), in describing their electron microscopic findings in retinoblastoma, noted that calcification seemed to begin in the mitochondria of degenerating tumor cells. While much has been written about the tumor angiogenesis factor in retinoblastoma (Albert, Sang, Craft, 1978; Folkman, 1974; Schipper, 1980), it appears that, almost without exception, the tumor's intrinsic blood vessels cannot keep pace with the proliferation of the neoplastic cells. This results in extensive areas of coagulative necrosis.

When viable tumor cells are shed into the vitreous or into subretinal fluid, they may grow into spheroidal aggregates (Fig. 8–584) with diameters that rarely exceed 1 mm (Folkman, 1974; Schipper, 1980). The more peripherally situated cells derive their nutrition from the vitreous or subretinal fluid, but as such free-floating spheroidal aggregates grow, the most centrally situated cells exhibit the same cytologic alterations as do the tumor cells that become necrotic as they are displaced away from nutrient vessels in the primary tumor. If viable cells in the vitreous become attached to the retina, they may invade the retina (Fig. 8–585) or stimulate the proliferation of capillaries from the retina into the tumor. Similarly, tumor cells in the subretinal exudate may seed onto the outer surface of the retina (Fig. 8–586)

Text continued on page 1304

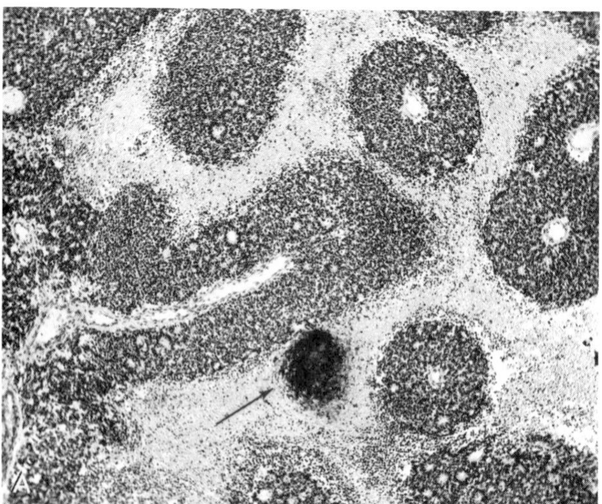

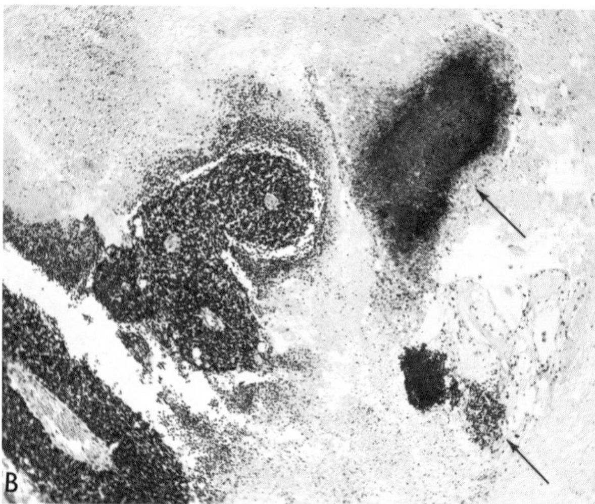

Figure 8–582. *A* and *B*, **The retinoblastoma pattern** is even more obvious as the relationship of viable tumor cells to patent blood vessels is more readily observed: sleeves of viable tumor averaging 100 microns in thickness surround prominent vessels. Deeply basophilic deposits of calcium salts are indicated by arrows in areas of necrosis. *A*, ×80. AFIP Neg. 58-14174. *B*, ×50. AFIP Neg. 39579-02101.

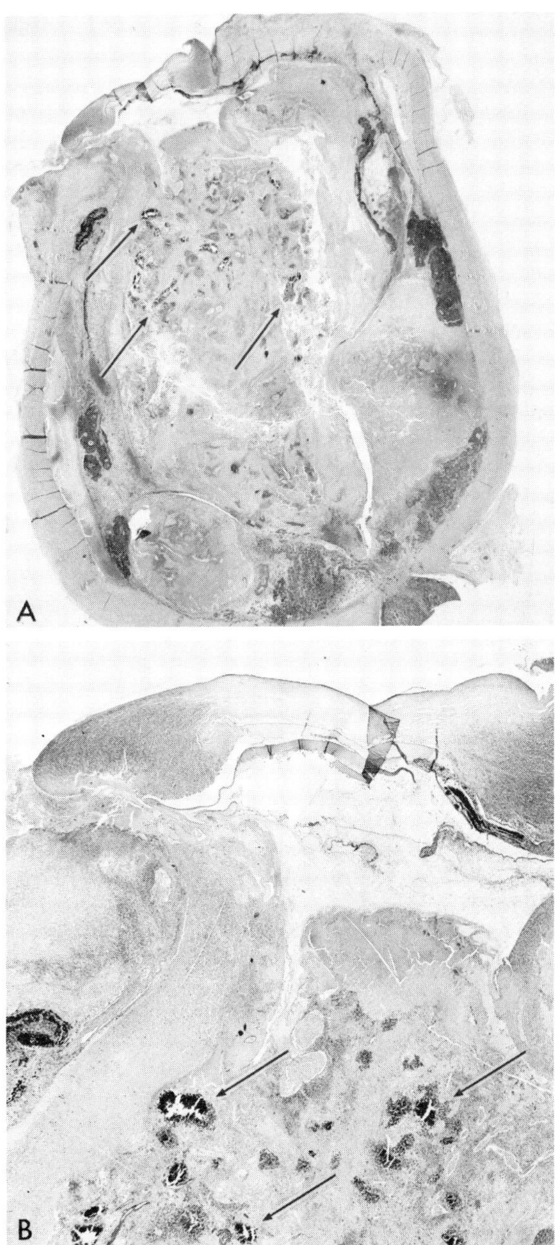

Figure 8–583. The eye is filled with an almost totally necrotic **retinoblastoma,** viable tumor being present only in the uvea and optic nerve. Many foci of calcification (arrows) are present in the necrotic central mass. *A,* ×3. AFIP Neg. 65-12528. *B,* ×11. AFIP Neg. 65-12529.

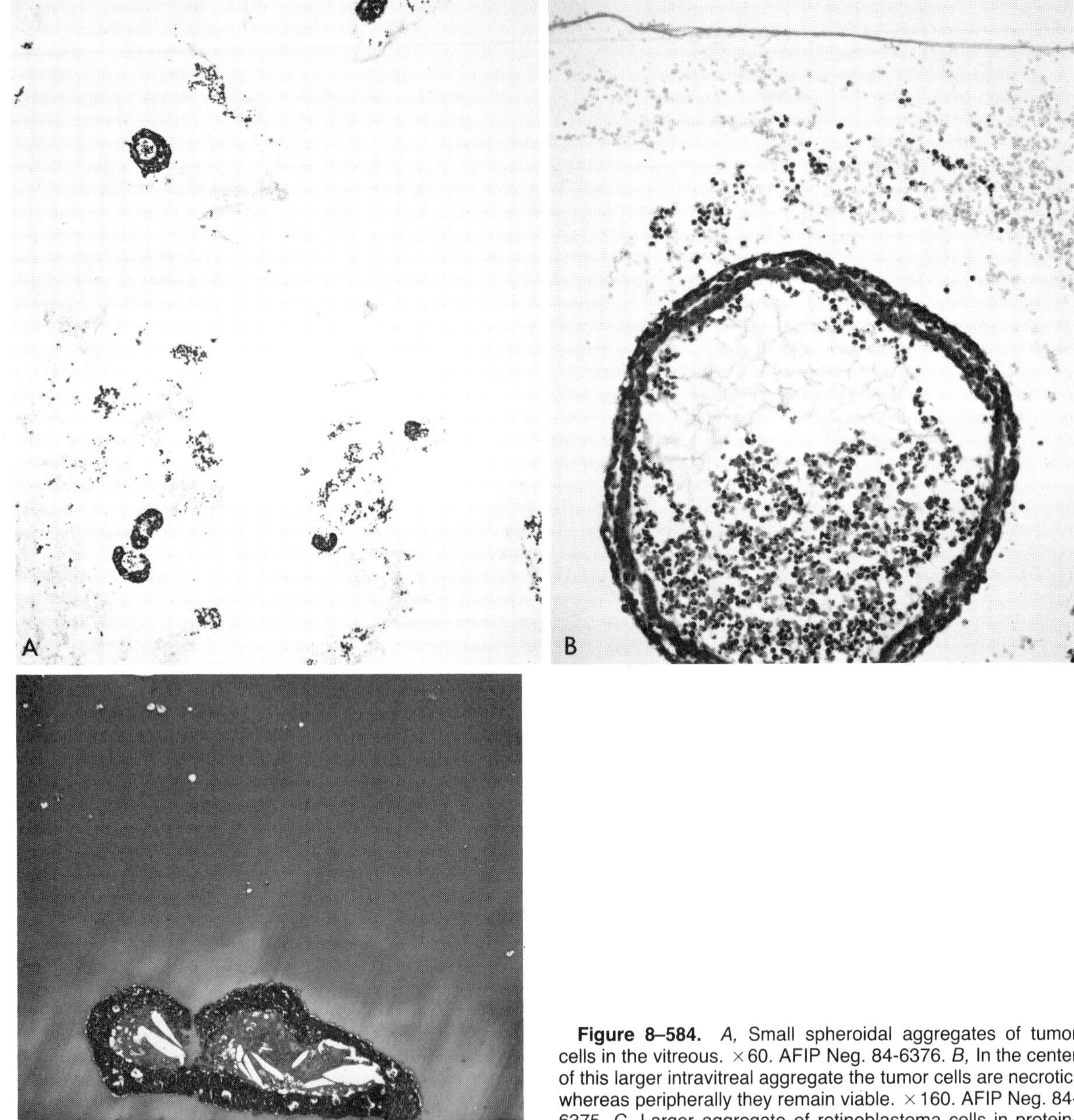

Figure 8–584. *A,* Small spheroidal aggregates of tumor cells in the vitreous. ×60. AFIP Neg. 84-6376. *B,* In the center of this larger intravitreal aggregate the tumor cells are necrotic, whereas peripherally they remain viable. ×160. AFIP Neg. 84-6375. *C,* Larger aggregate of retinoblastoma cells in protein-rich subretinal exudate. The most peripherally situated cells within the aggregate remain viable while those located centrally have become necrotic; cholesterol clefts may be seen in the necrotic center. ×60. AFIP Neg. 82-7566.

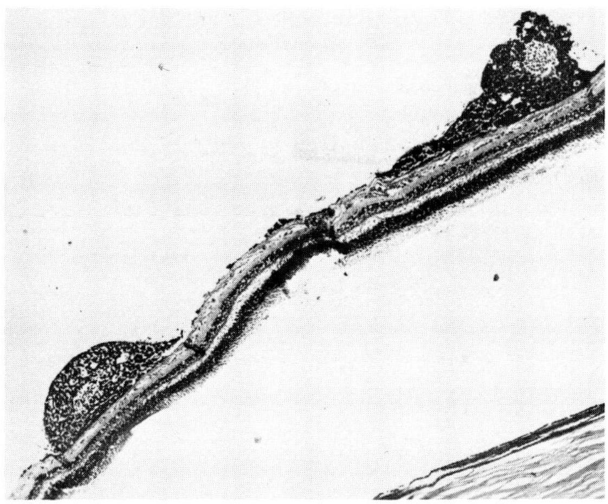

Figure 8–585. Invasion of nerve fiber layer from implants of tumor cells that had been dispersed into the vitreous. ×50. AFIP Neg. 59-5231.

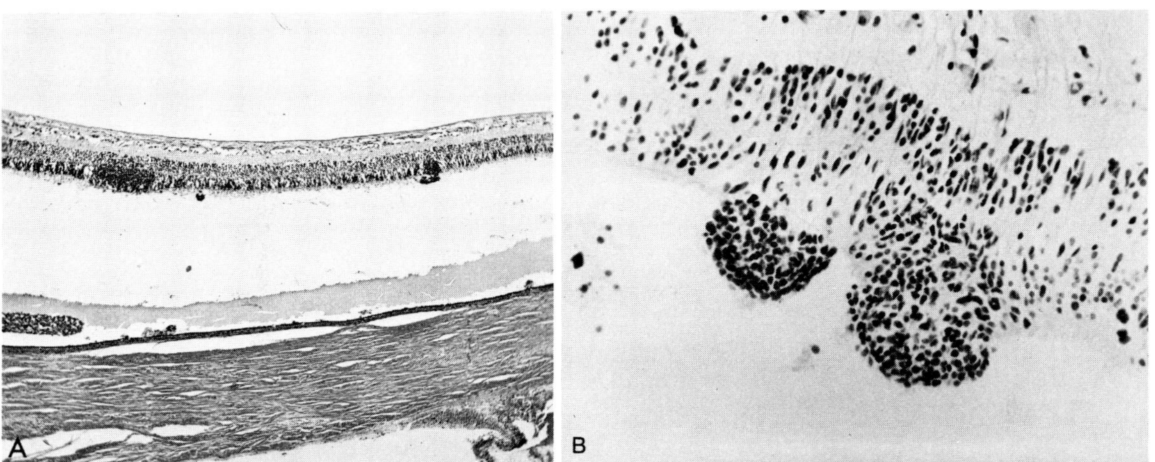

Figure 8–586. Invasion of outer retinal layers by tumor cells dispersed in the subretinal exudate. *A,* × 50. AFIP Neg. 61-4414. *B,* ×610. AFIP Neg. 45945.

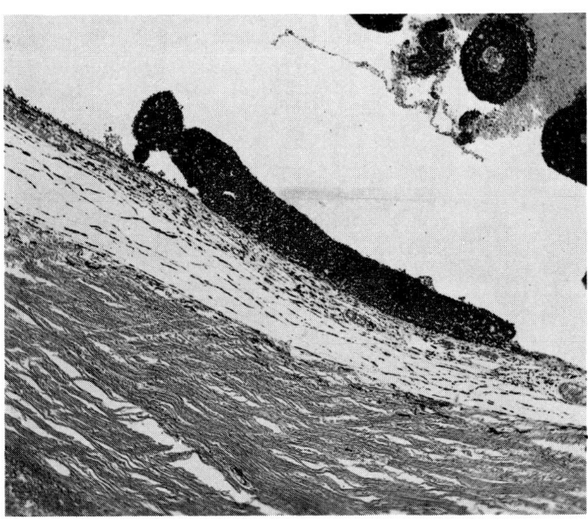

Figure 8–587. Implantation onto and replacement of the retinal pigment epithelium by tumor cells from the subretinal exudate. ×50. AFIP Neg. 57-351.

or onto the inner surface of the retinal pigment epithelium (Fig. 8–587), remaining viable by deriving nutrition from the retina or the choriocapillaris.

In most instances, the necrotic portions of retinoblastomas do not seem to provoke much of an inflammatory response. With marked necrosis and the liberation of much DNA from the tumor's nuclei, DNA may become absorbed preferentially in the walls of blood vessels or by the internal limiting membrane of the retina, giving a deep blue (hematoxylinophilic) staining reaction to their tissues (Albert, Sang, Craft, 1978; Datta, 1974; Mullaney, 1969) (Fig. 8–588). One may also observe similar deep blue staining of the lens capsule, vessels in the iris, or the tissues adjacent to Schlemm's canal, suggesting that much of the disintegrated DNA escapes into the aqueous and gets absorbed from the aqueous by the affected tissues.

The formation of rosettes (Fig. 8–589) is highly characteristic of retinoblastomas, a feature that has been widely recognized since the classic descriptions of Flexner and Wintersteiner, whose names are now attached to these rosettes. No other neural neoplasm so frequently contains rosettes in such abundance, nor are the rosettes of other neural tumors so highly differentiated. The most significant exception is observed in rare examples of pineoblastoma, such as the one that was so beautifully illustrated by Stefanko and Manschot (1979) (Fig. 8–590).

The typical Flexner-Wintersteiner rosette is lined by cuboidal cells, the apical ends of which are held together by terminal bars, circumscribing a lumen. In the most highly differentiated rosettes, some cells have cytoplasmic projections into the lumen of the rosette, representing primitive inner segments of photoreceptor cells, as has been demonstrated by electron microscopy (Tso, Fine, Zimmerman, 1969; Tso, Zimmerman, Fine, 1970) (Fig. 8–591). Stains for acid mucopolysaccharides reveal a coating of hyaluronidase-resistant acid mucopolysaccharide along the apical surface of tumor cells, forming well-differentiated rosettes (Zimmerman, 1958) (Fig. 8–592). The basal ends of the cells that form the rosettes contain the nuclei. Tso and coworkers (1969, 1970), who studied Flexner-Wintersteiner rosettes by electron microscopy, were impressed by several features that the cells forming rosettes share with retinal photoreceptors: terminal bars of the luminal limiting membrane analogous to those that form the outer limiting membrane of the retina (Fig. 8–591), cytoplasmic microtubules, cilia with the 9 + 0 pattern (Fig. 8–593), lamellated mem-

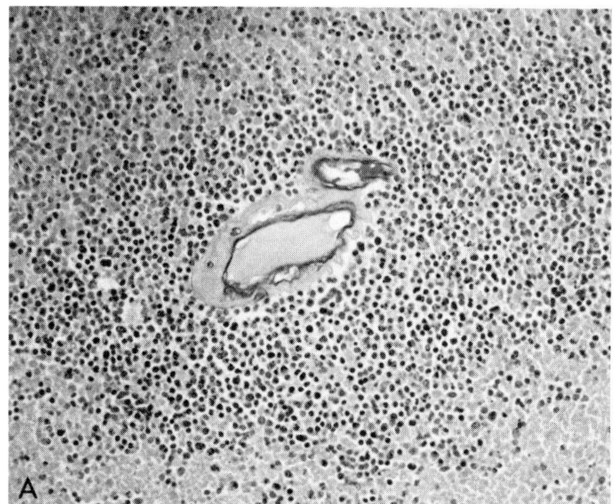

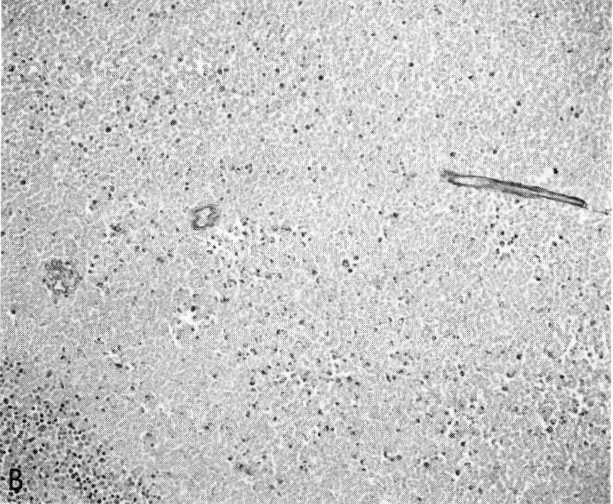

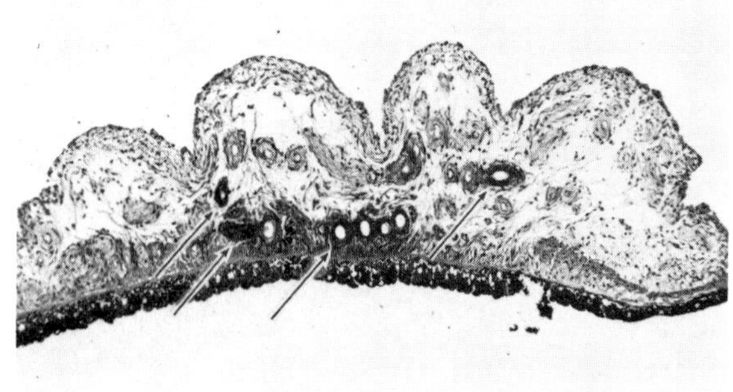

Figure 8–588. Deposits of DNA derived from nuclei of necrotic retinoblastoma cells give an intensely basophilic staining reaction to walls of blood vessels. *A,* ×250. AFIP Neg. 84-6499. *B,* ×160. AFIP Neg. 84-6498. *C,* Similar basophilic staining of vessels in iris (arrows). ×80. AFIP Neg. 65-12118.

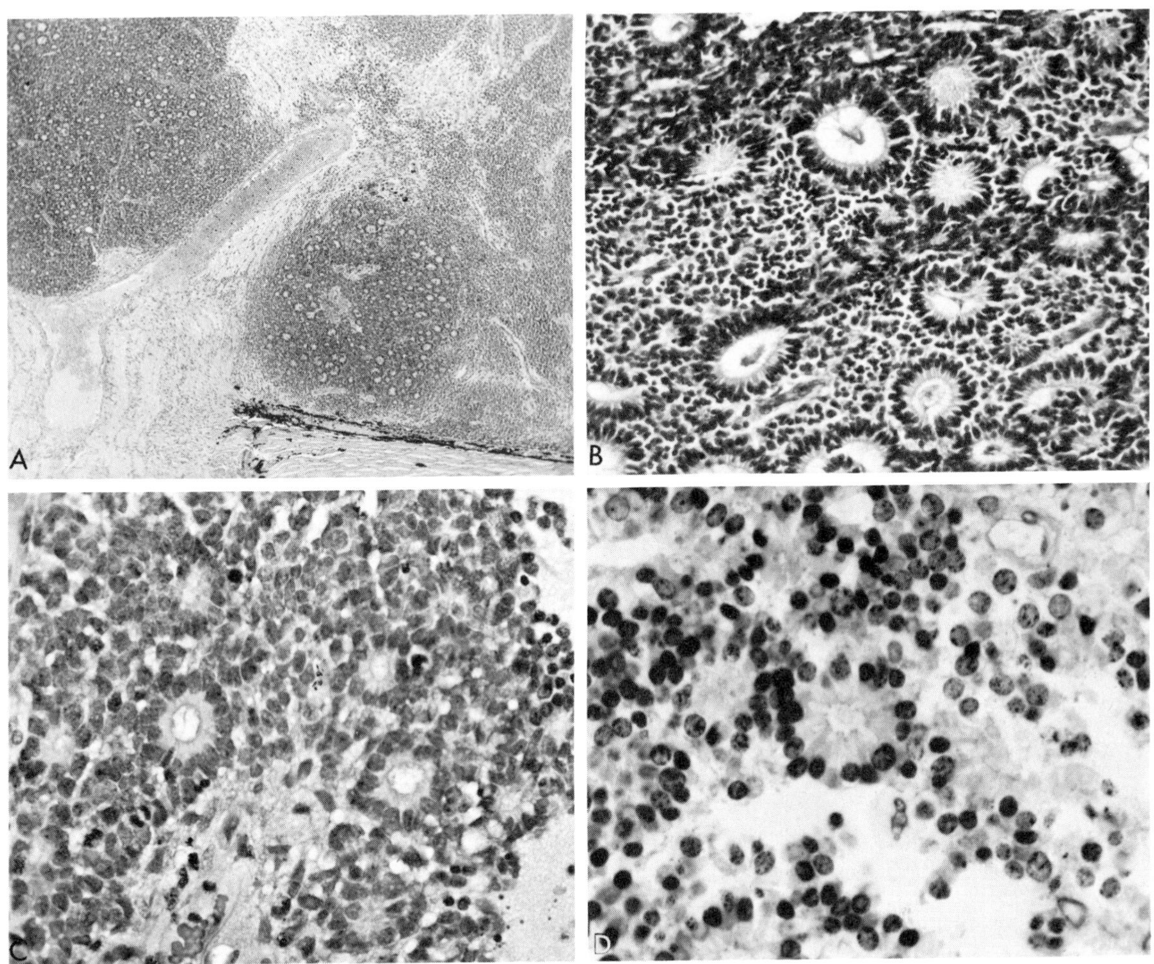

Figure 8–589. *A* and *B*, Numerous well-formed **Flexner-Wintersteiner rosettes,** a distinctive feature of many retinoblastomas, stand out against a background of undifferentiated neuroblastic cells. *A*, ×50. AFIP Neg. 56-11408. *B*, ×250. AFIP Neg. 84-6219. *C*, and *D*, The **Flexner-Wintersteiner rosette** is formed by a single layer of cuboidal or short columnar cells, the apical ends of which are united by terminal bars, delineating the lumen of the rosette. The round nuclei are contained at the basal end of the cell. *C*, ×440. AFIP Neg. 69-3354. *D*, ×615. AFIP Neg. 69-3351.

branous structures, and acid mucopolysaccharide resistant to hyaluronidase in the lumina of rosettes.

Glial differentiation also has been described (Popoff, Ellsworth, 1971; Smith, 1974; Taylor et al, 1979; Schipper, 1980; Lane, Klintworth, 1983; Messmer, Font, Kirkpatrick, 1984), but in our experience it is very exceptional (Figs. 8–594 and 8–595) and difficult to differentiate from reactive gliosis (Tso, 1980). Immunohistochemical studies for glial fibrillary acidic protein have been made in an effort to support the view that retinoblastomas and retinocytomas may show astroglial differentiation (Fig. 8–595). As Kyritsis, Tsokas, Triche, et al have recently stated (1984), the neoplastic nature of glial cells in retinoblastoma has so far been a moot point. Lane and Klintworth (1983), who used the immunoperoxidase reaction to demonstrate glial fibrillary acidic protein, found foci of positive staining in some retinoblastomas, but they could not convince themselves that they saw definite glial differentiation in tumor cells. Messmer and coworkers, however, were convinced that a small number of tumor cells do exhibit glial differentiation (Fig. 8–595).

Kyritsis and coworkers have shown that with specific variations in the composition of culture media used to grow retinoblastoma cells, they could induce the typically undifferentiated cells to undergo neuronal differentiation, with the formation of neuritic-type processes and rosettes, or to develop as glial cells. When they studied these three cell populations for neuron-specific enolase (NSE) and glial fibrillary acidic protein (GFAP) by immunofluorescence, they found that both markers were present in the undifferentiated cells; whereas the cells that exhibit neuronal differentiation lose GFAP, those that grow as glial cells lose NSE. These investigators also studied neuroblastomas and other neural tumors, but so far, they have found no other tumor simultaneously exhibiting markers for both neuronal and glial cells. This new work provides the most convincing support for the concept that retinoblas-

Text continued on page 1314

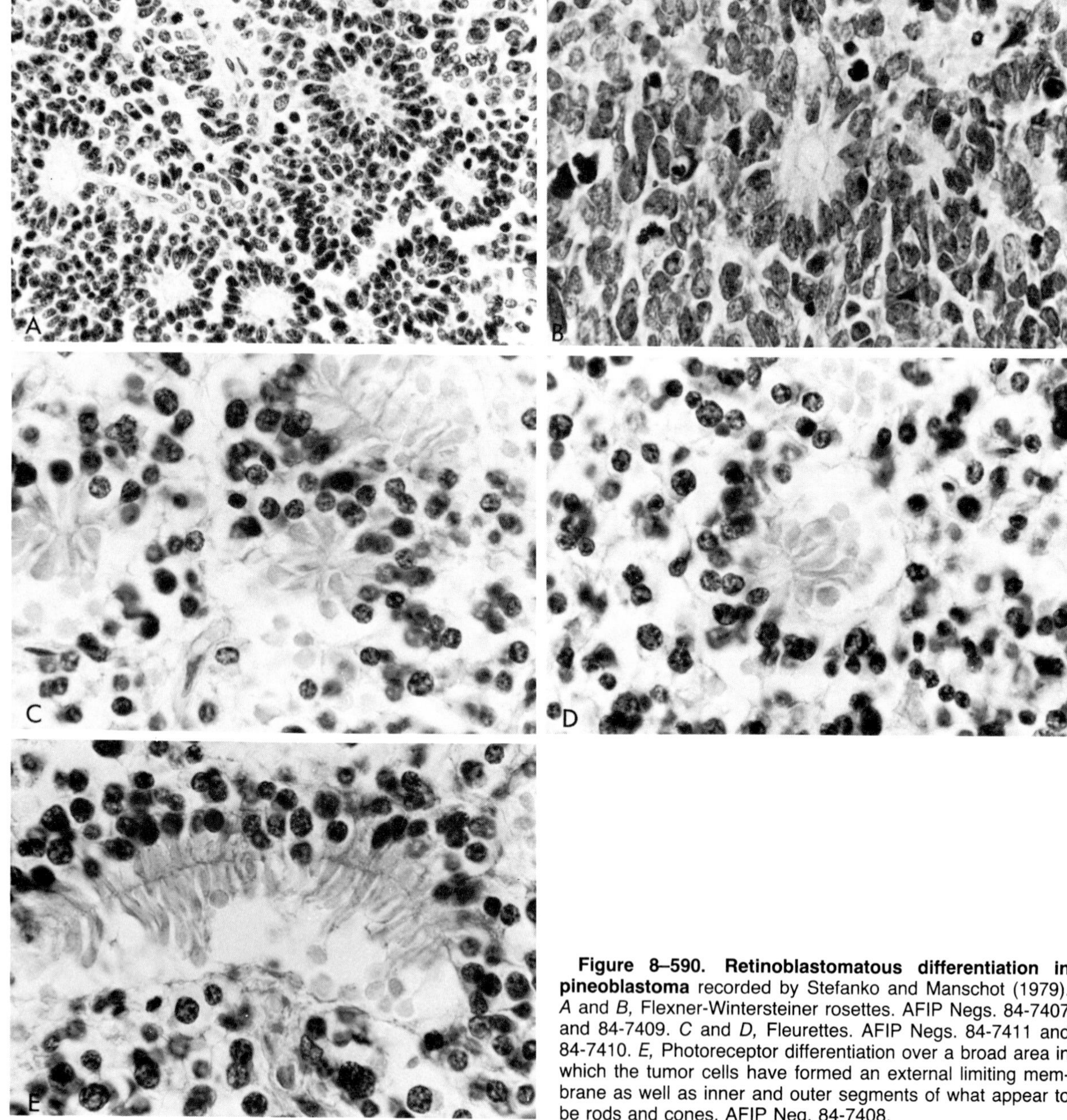

Figure 8–590. Retinoblastomatous differentiation in pineoblastoma recorded by Stefanko and Manschot (1979). *A* and *B,* Flexner-Wintersteiner rosettes. AFIP Negs. 84-7407 and 84-7409. *C* and *D,* Fleurettes. AFIP Negs. 84-7411 and 84-7410. *E,* Photoreceptor differentiation over a broad area in which the tumor cells have formed an external limiting membrane as well as inner and outer segments of what appear to be rods and cones. AFIP Neg. 84-7408.

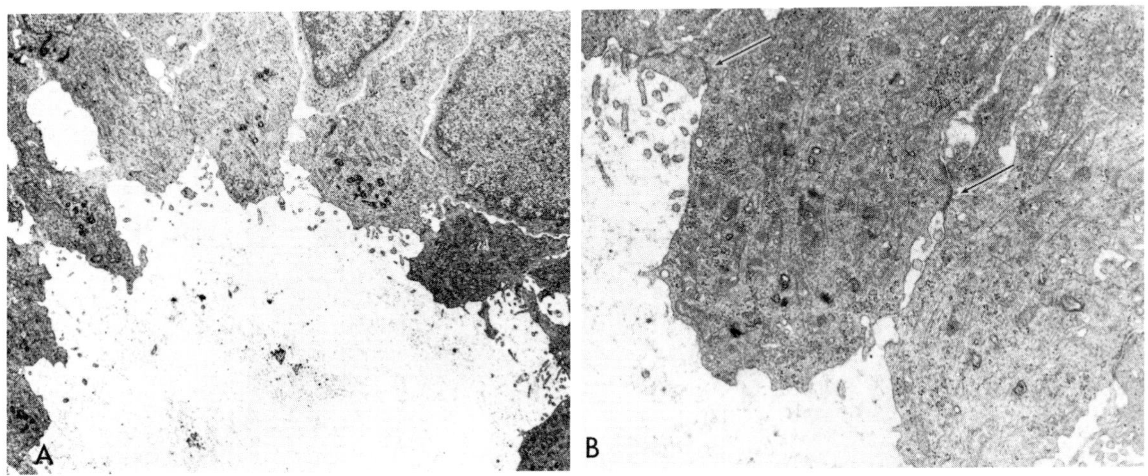

Figure 8–591. *A* and *B*, **Tumor cells of Flexner-Wintersteiner rosette** joined by terminal bars (arrows), which are zonula adherens–like cell attachments. The apical ends of tumor cells with their villous projections into the lumen of the rosette contain many mitochondria and correspond to the inner segments of photoreceptor cells. *A*, ×7000. AFIP Neg. 69-3792-2. *B*, ×17,000. AFIP Neg. 69-3792-1. (From Tso MOM, Fine BS, Zimmerman LE: The Flexner-Wintersteiner rosettes in retinoblastoma. Arch Pathol *88*:665–671, 1969.)

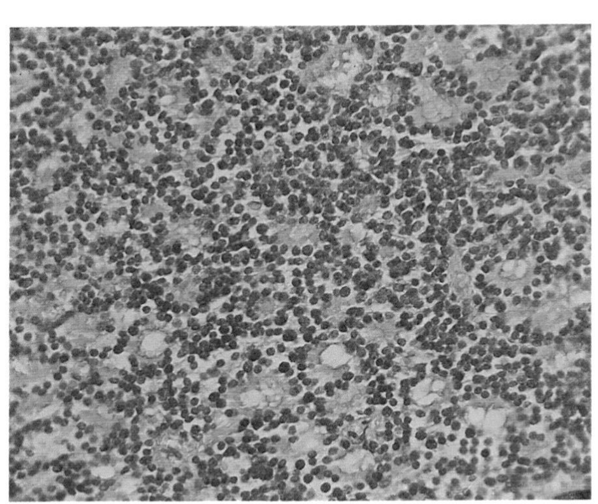

Figure 8–592. A layer of mucopolysaccharide, resistant to hyaluronidase, coats the inner surface to the rosettes. Alcian blue, ×540. AFIP Neg. 57-14082.

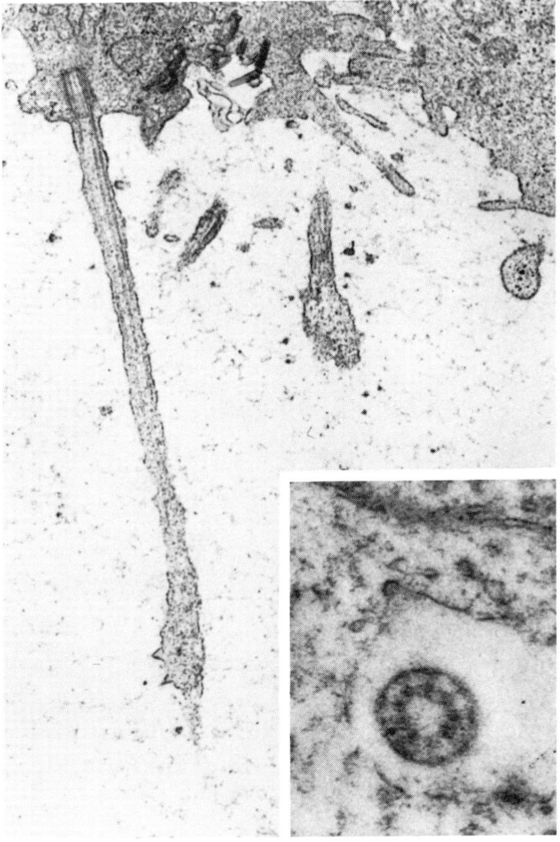

Figure 8–593. Cilium at apex of tumor cell projects into lumen of rosette. ×17,000. Inset: Cross-section of shaft of cilium beyond apical plasmalemma, showing 9+0 pattern. ×39,000. AFIP Neg. 69-3794-4. (From Tso MOM, Fine BS, Zimmerman LE: The Flexner-Wintersteiner rosettes in retinoblastoma. Arch Pathol *88*:665–671, 1969).

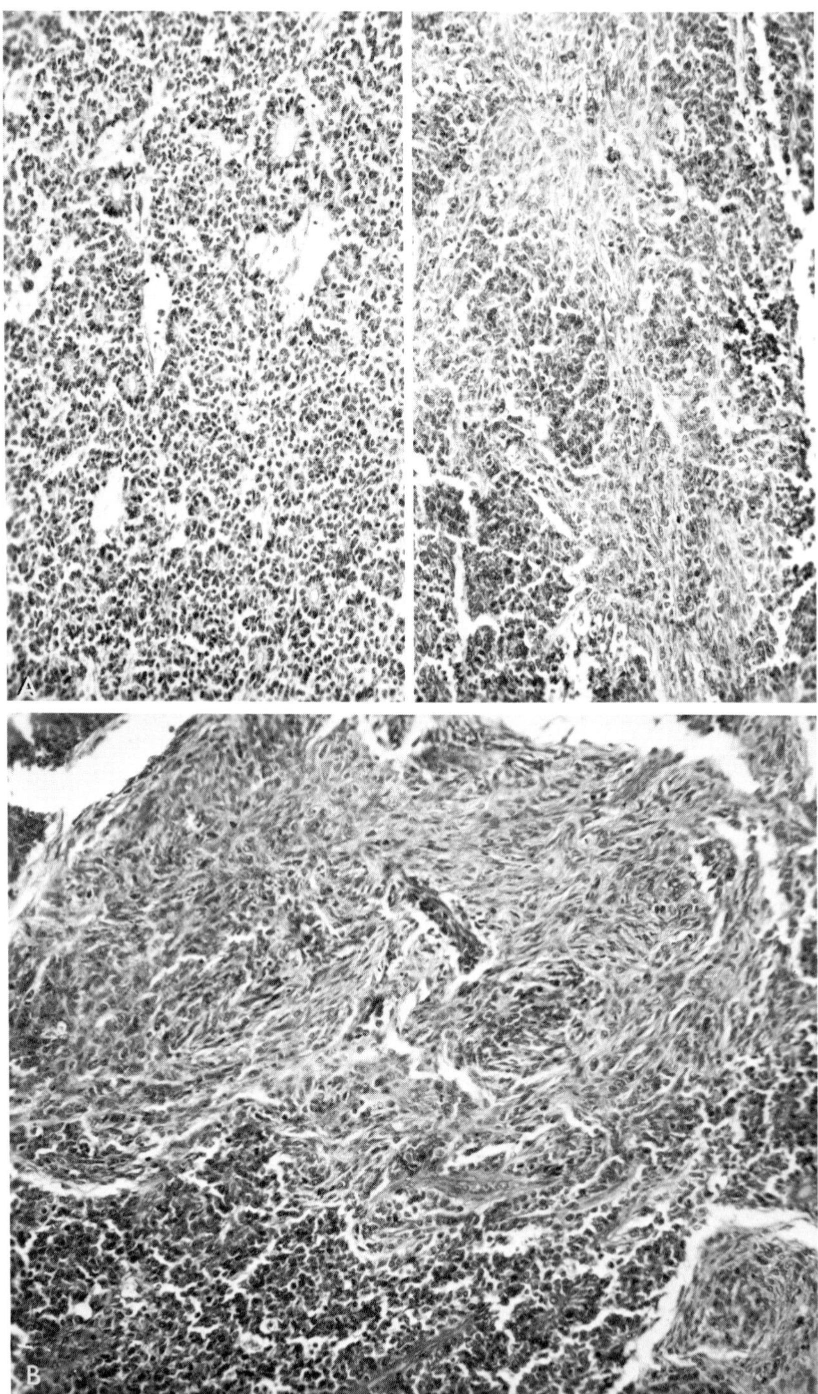

Figure 8–594. *A,* Two different areas from the same retinoblastoma: on the left the tumor is composed mainly of undifferentiated neuroblastic cells and some rosettes, whereas on the right the tumor cells exhibit a spindle cell transformation interpreted as **glial differentiation**. ×250. AFIP Neg. 77-6340. *B,* Higher magnification of cells exhibiting the spindle-shaped glial transformation. ×250. AFIP Neg. 77-6341.

Illustration continued on opposite page

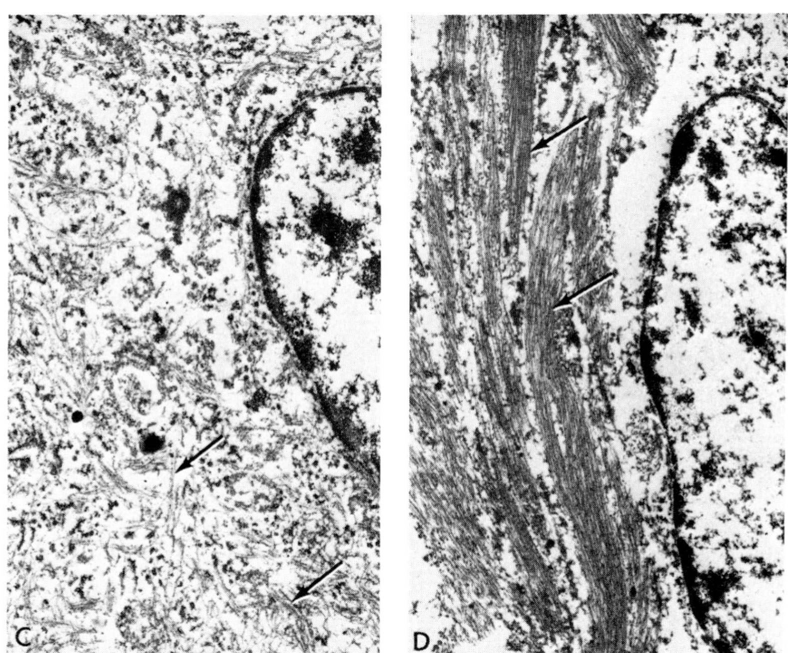

Figure 8–594 *(Continued) C*, Electron micrograph of a neoplastic cell from the same tumor shown in *A* and *B* reveals scattered intracytoplasmic glial filaments (arrows). *D*, Electron micrograph of another neoplastic cell from the same tumor shows bundles of aggregated intracytoplasmic glial filaments (arrows). (From Tso MOM: Clues to the cells of origin in retinoblastoma. Int Ophthalmol Clin *20*:191–210, 1980.)

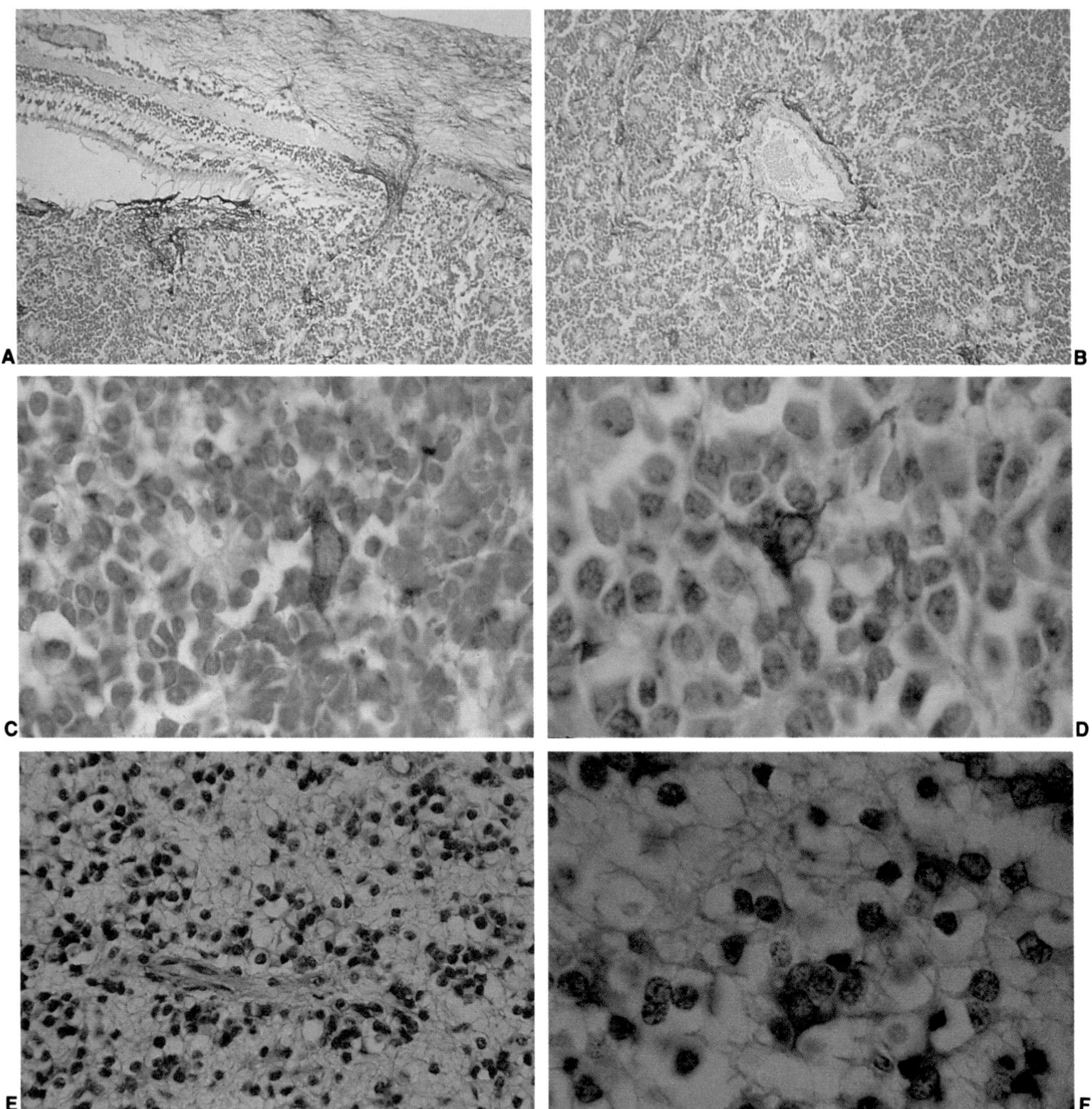

Figure 8–595. Glial differentiation (cells stained brown) in retinoblastoma (*A, B, C,* and *D*) and in retinocytoma *(F)*, demonstrated by immunoperoxidase staining for glial fibrillary acidic protein. *A,* Reactive gliosis in retina adjacent to tumor. ×40. *B,* Perivascular reactive gliosis. ×40. *C,* Positive staining in one neoplastic cell. ×250. *D,* Positive staining in several neoplastic cells. ×400. *E,* Retinocytoma stained by PAS reaction. ×100. *F,* Positive staining for glial fibrillary acidic protein in same tumor shown in *E.* ×250. (From Messmer EP, Font RL, Kirkpatrick JB, Höpping W: Immunohistochemical demonstration of neuronal and astrocytic differentiation in retinoblastoma. Ophthalmology, in press; Invest Ophthalmol Vis Sci (Arvo Abstr) *25*:83, 1984.)

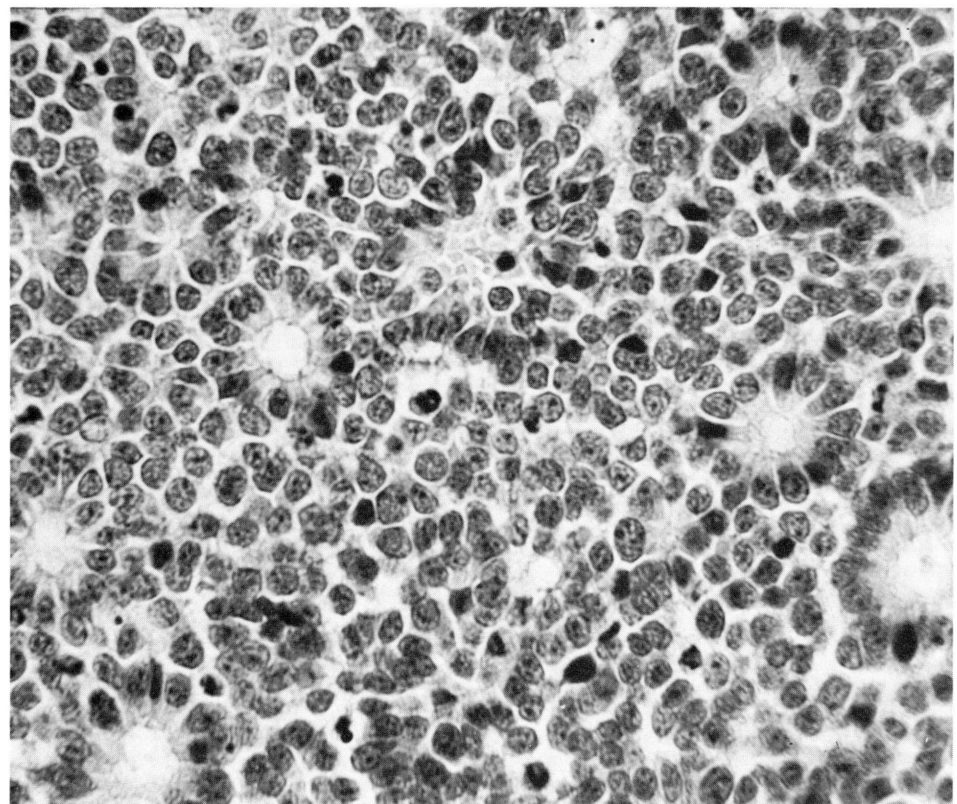

Figure 8–596. Although the **Flexner-Wintersteiner rosettes** are well differentiated, they are in a milieu of undifferentiated malignant neuroblastic cells exhibiting nuclear pleomorphism and marked mitotic activity. ×700. AFIP Neg. 293627-2.

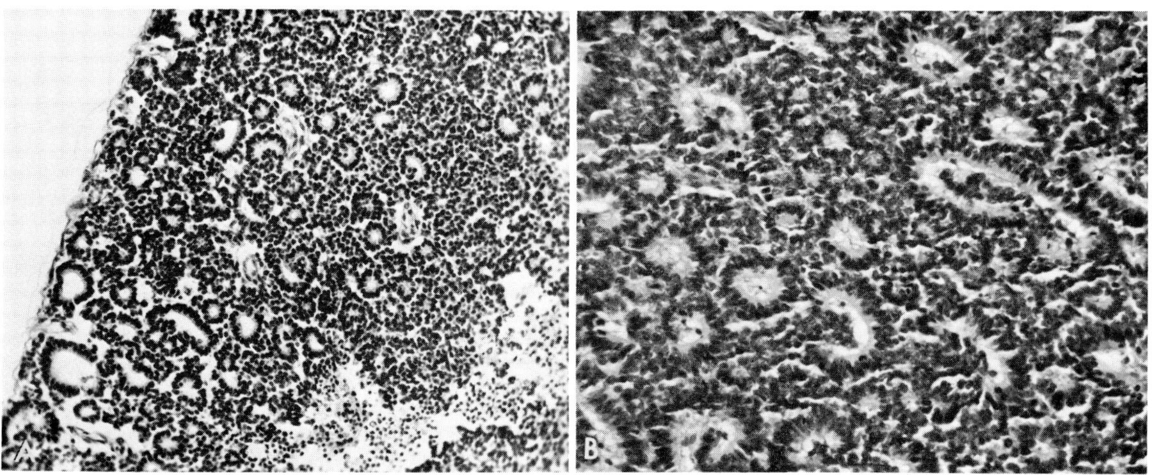

Figure 8–597. Incompletely formed rosettes and ribbon-like arrangements of more highly differentiated tumor cells. A, ×200. AFIP Neg. 56-11407. *B,* ×250. AFIP Neg. 84-2616.

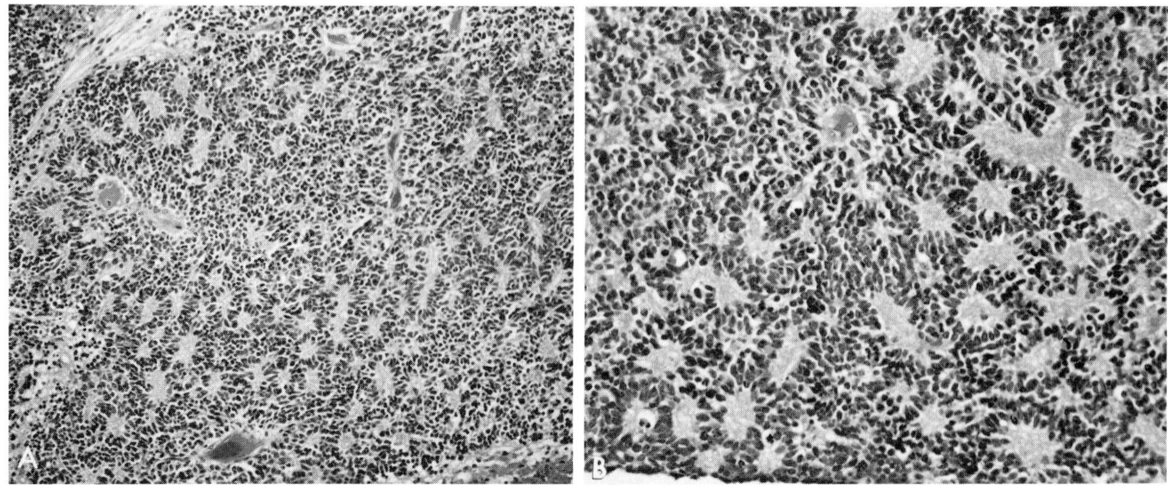

Figure 8–598. **Homer-Wright rosettes** differ from Flexner-Wintersteiner rosettes in being formed by less highly differentiated cells that have a less epithelial configuration, and by the absence of a central lumen. The non-nucleated center of the Homer-Wright rosette is formed by a tangle of cytoplasmic processes of the cells that form the rosettes. *A,* ×160. AFIP Neg. 84-6504. *B,* ×250. AFIP Neg. 84-6501.

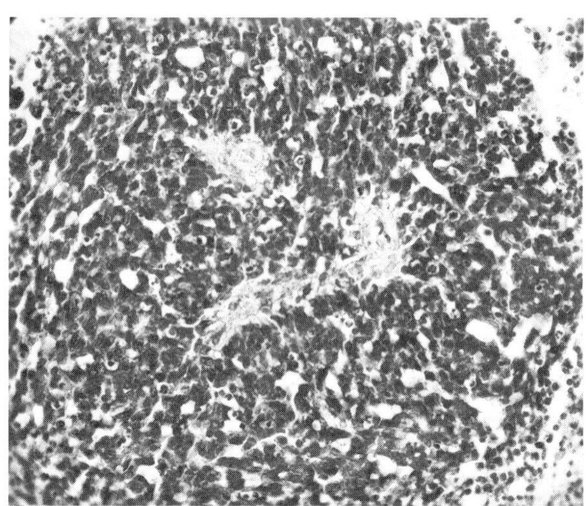

Figure 8–599. Degenerative changes, including minute foci of necrosis involving only a few cells, may produce empty spaces that are sometimes confused with rosettes (**"pseudorosettes"**), such as those shown here. ×305. AFIP Neg. 58-13693.

Figure 8–600. Portions of retinoblastomas composed of much more mature, benign-appearing tumor cells exhibiting photoreceptor differentiation, with formation of bouquet-like clusters, termed **"fleurettes."** *A,* Photoreceptor differentiation is indicated by the bulbous cytoplasmic expansions (arrows) in benign-appearing tumor cells. ×350. AFIP Neg. 68-7185. *B,* Uniformly benign-appearing tumor cells, a few of which exhibit photoreceptor differentiation. ×660. AFIP Neg. 68-7161. *C,* A large proportion of these benign-appearing tumor cells exhibits an exceptional degree of photoreceptor differentiation with the formation of fleurettes. ×575. AFIP Neg. 68-9466. *D* and *E,* Groups of tumor cells held together by terminal bars (arrows) corresponding to the outer limiting membrane of the retina. Photoreceptor cell processes project past the terminal bars into a lumen. Both, ×600. AFIP Negs. 68-9467 and 68-7853. All fields (*A* through *E*) are from the small, pale-staining foci of the otherwise typical retinoblastoma shown in Figure 8–601, *D.* (From Tso MOM, Zimmerman LE, Fine BS: The nature of retinoblastoma. I. Photoreceptor differentiation. A clinical and histologic study. Am J Ophthalmol *69*:339–350, 1970.)

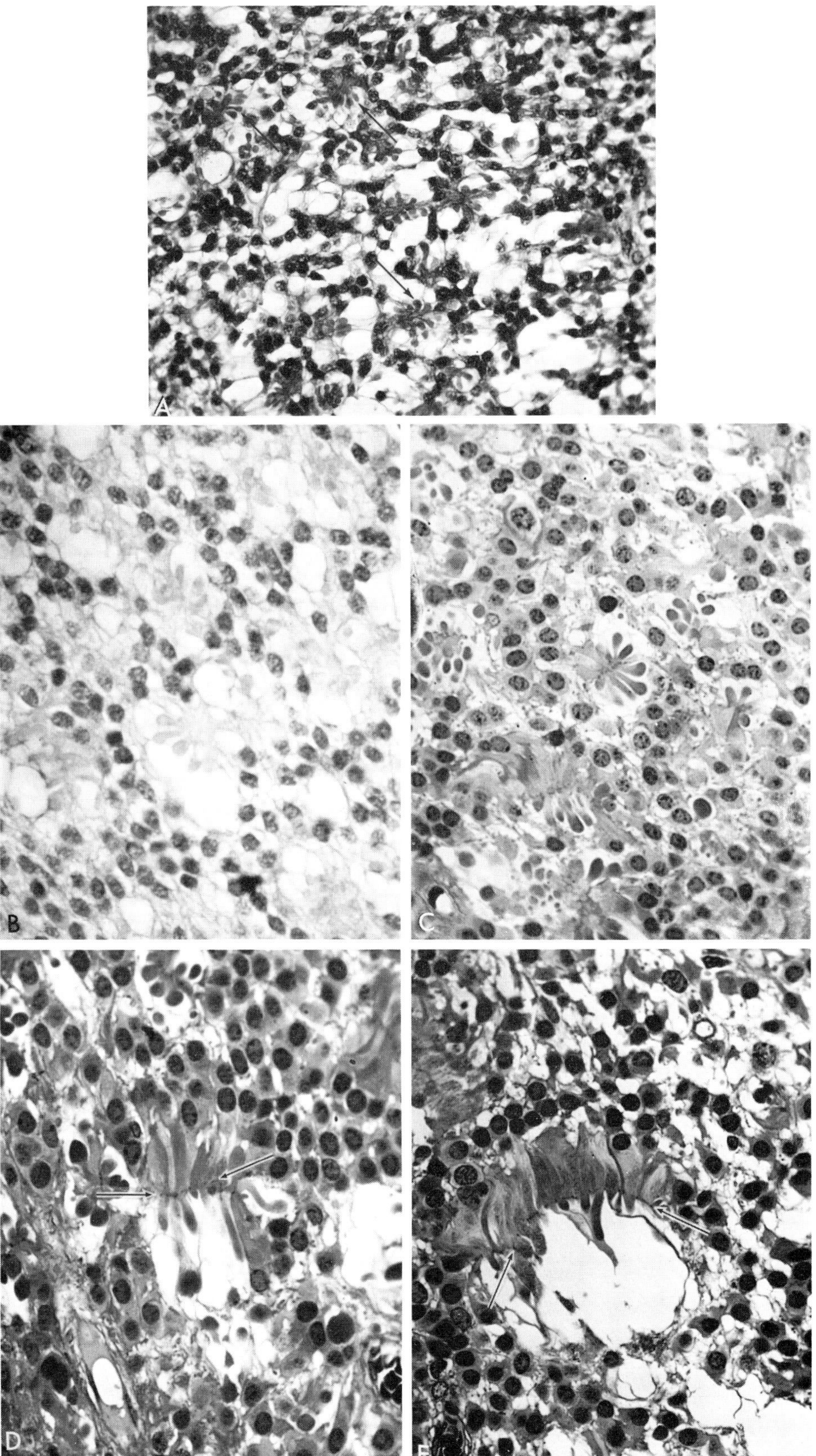

Figure 8–600 *See legend on opposite page*

toma is a specific retinal tumor derived from retinoblasts that have the potential to differentiate along both neuronal and glial pathways. It is also of interest that in these in vitro studies, glial differentiation was induced in a much smaller proportion of cells compared with neuronal differentiation.

Very characteristically, Flexner-Wintersteiner rosettes are contained within a milieu of undifferentiated malignant cells exhibiting mitotic activity (Figs. 8–589 and 8–596), and the cells that form rosettes also may contain mitotic figures. Some rosettes are incompletely formed (Fig. 8–597). A much less common and less characteristic rosette is the Homer-Wright type, which was first described in sympathicoblastomas and which is also highly characteristic of cerebellar medulloblastomas (Rubinstein, 1972). In these rosettes the cells are not arranged about a lumen but instead, send out cytoplasmic processes, a tangle of which occupies the center of the rosette (Fig. 8–598).

Generally, the more numerous and more highly differentiated the rosettes, the better the prognosis. The smaller retinoblastomas are more likely to have a greater concentration of well-formed rosettes than are the larger, more advanced tumors; hence the prognostic significance of rosettes may reflect the fact that the larger, more advanced tumors, especially those with extraocular extension, tend to have a smaller, less conspicuous complement of rosettes.

"Pseudorosette" is a term that has crept into the retinoblastoma literature only to confuse students and mislead readers. The problem is that different writers have used the term to designate different phenomena, each of which can be more appropriately and more specifically identified by other descriptive terms. Some writers have used the term to designate poorly differentiated rosettes (Fig. 8–597) or rosettes of the Homer-Wright type (Fig. 8–598). Others have in mind tiny foci of necrosis surrounded by viable malignant cells that might be misinterpreted as rosettes (Fig. 8–599). Still others have referred to the collar of viable tumor cells surrounding capillaries (Fig. 8–582) as pseudorosettes. These are described and illustrated in Rubinstein's Fascicle on Tumors of the Central Nervous System (1972). I see no need for the term and advocate its deletion from the vocabulary of ophthalmic pathologists.

In 1970 Tso and coworkers described and illustrated (Figs. 8–600 through 8–602) an even higher degree of maturation, with evidence of photoreceptor differentiation by individual tumor cells and small, bouquet-like clusters of benign-appearing tumor cells ("fleurettes") in 18 of 300 retinoblastomas treated only by enucleation. In most of these 18 tumors, the areas exhibiting photoreceptor differentiation could easily be spotted at low magnification as discrete, comparatively pale-staining islands of viable tumor tissue standing out in contrast with the much more intensely basophilic portions of the tumor in which the histologic features were typical of retinoblastoma. Where the tumor cells exhibited photoreceptor differentiation, they appeared benign. The cells had more abundant cytoplasm and smaller, less basophilic nuclei that were much less densely packed. Mitotic figures were rarely observed, and necrosis was not present in these areas of greatest differentiation, but some calcification in nonnecrotic areas was observed. Figure 8–603 reproduces drawings from Tso et al (1970) depicting the highest degrees of differentiation they observed in some retinoblastomas.

In a subsequent study, Tso, Zimmerman, Fine, and Ellsworth (1970) re-evaluated 54 eyes enucleated after having been irradiated. Only 42 contained viable tumor, and 17 of these (40 per cent) exhibited photoreceptor differentiation. In seven cases, the residual tumor consisted entirely of cells showing photoreceptor differentiation. Consequently these investigators suggested that tumors containing such benign components might be incompletely radioresponsive because—as with many other tumors—the more highly malignant and poorly differentiated the tumor, the more radiosensitive it is likely to be, whereas the more benign and highly differentiated, the less radioresponsive the tumor generally is. Follow-up information was obtained in 13 of the 17 cases; there was only one tumor death. Figure 8–604 shows a tumor judged to have been only partially

Text continued on page 1320

Figure 8–601. *A*, Macroscopic appearance of a typical multicentric retinoblastoma. AFIP Neg. 59-4278. *B*, Histologic section through one of the tumors shown in *A* reveals mainly the typical pattern of an ordinary retinoblastoma, but arrows indicate tiny foci in which the constituent cells appear to be benign and exhibit photoreceptor differentiation. ×8. AFIP Neg. 68-7842. *C*, One of the foci marked by arrows in *B*, showing in the upper part of the field the benign component with cells exhibiting photoreceptor differentiation, contrasted with the population of undifferentiated malignant cells in the lower half. ×300. AFIP Neg. 68-7160. *D*, Another example of what is mainly a rather typical retinoblastoma, but the pale-staining areas marked by arrows are the ones in which the fields shown in Figure 8–600, *A* through *E* were found. ×5. AFIP Neg. 68-7851. *E*, An unusually large, pale-staining area (arrows) in which cystoid spaces are present within a highly differentiated, benign part of an otherwise typical retinoblastoma. ×8. AFIP Neg. 68-7192. (From Tso MOM, Zimmerman LE, Fine BS: The nature of retinoblastoma. I. Photoreceptor differentiation. A clinical and histologic study. Am J Ophthalmol *69*:339–350, 1970.)

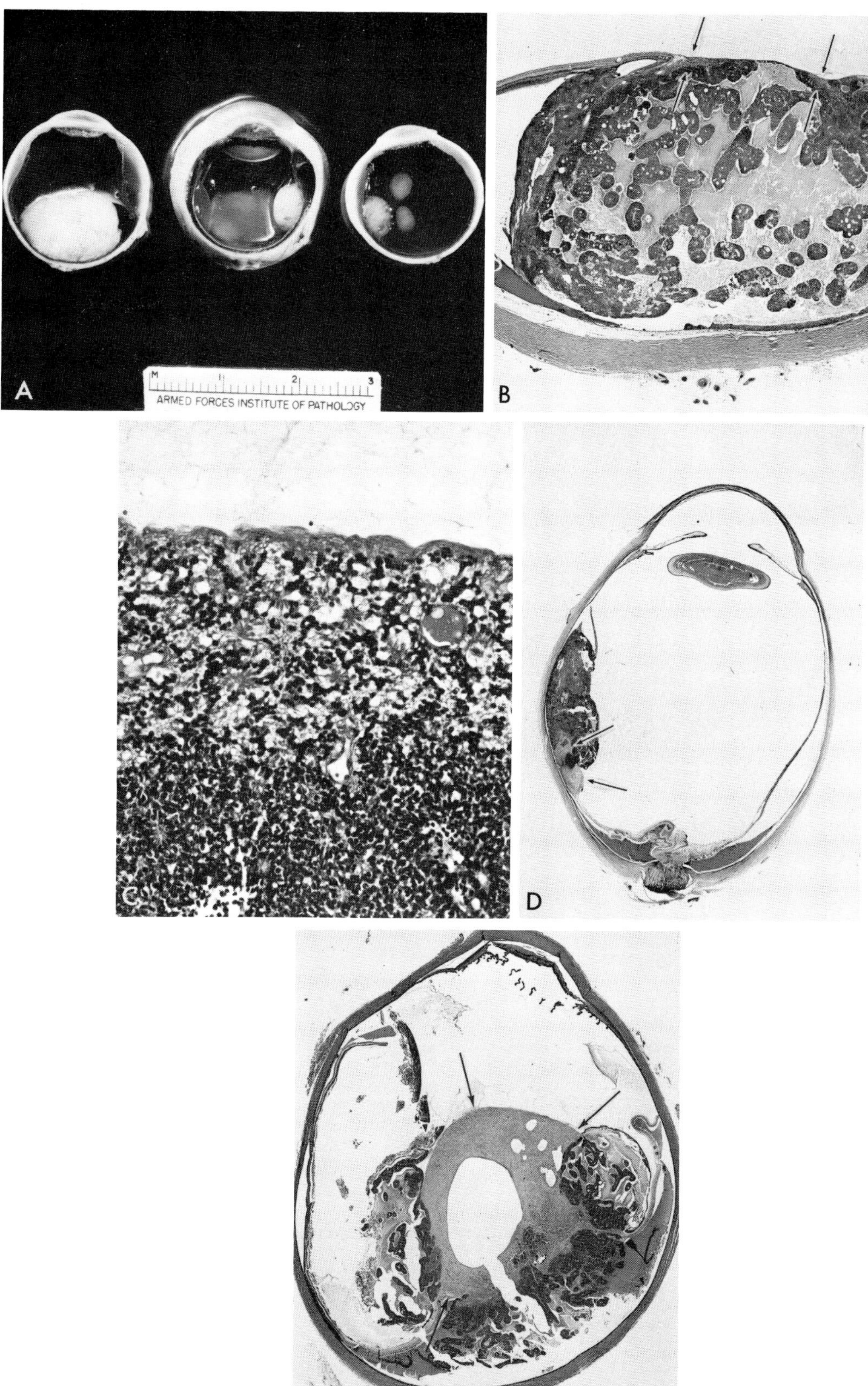

Figure 8–601 *See legend on opposite page*

See legend on opposite page

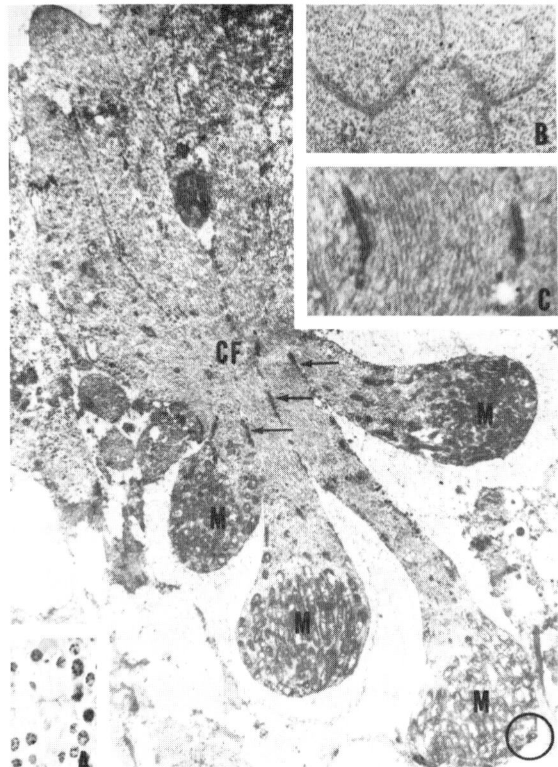

Figure 8–602. Electron micrographs of **fleurette** in retinoblastoma. The highly differentiated tumor cells have produced long conducting fibers *(CF)*. Adjacent cells are attached to one another by zonular adherents (arrows), shown in cross-section in inset *B* and in longitudinal section in inset *C*. The bulbous ends of the cells in the fleurette are packed with mitochondria *(M)*. Inset *A* reveals the light microscopic counterpart of such a fleurette. ×5400. *A*, ×440. *B*, ×6800. *C*, ×16,000. AFIP Neg. 69-4552-8. (From Tso MOM, Fine BS, Zimmerman LE: The nature of retinoblastoma. II. Photoreceptor differentiation. An electron microscopic study. Am J Ophthalmol *69*:350–359, 1970.)

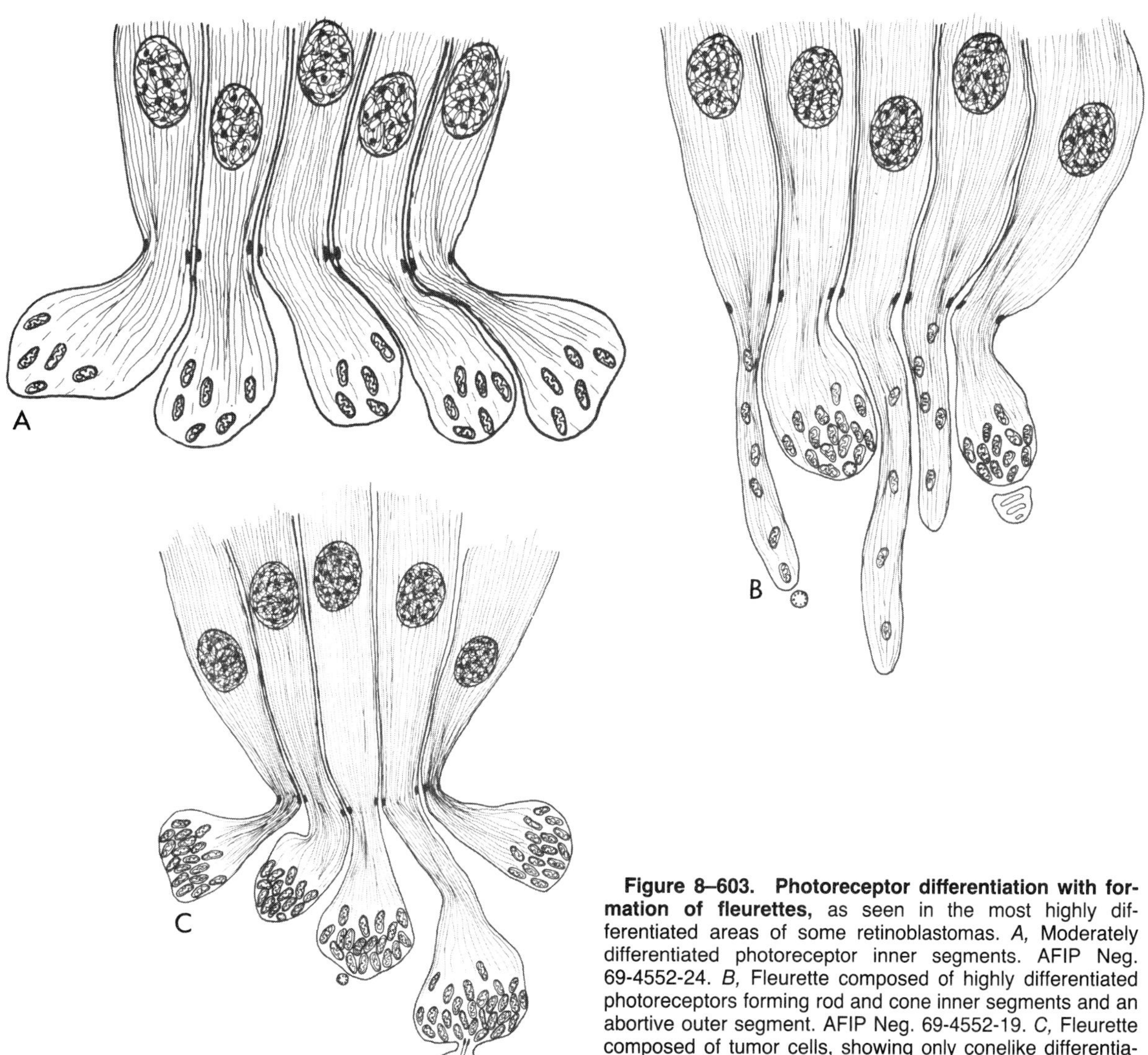

Figure 8–603. Photoreceptor differentiation with formation of fleurettes, as seen in the most highly differentiated areas of some retinoblastomas. *A,* Moderately differentiated photoreceptor inner segments. AFIP Neg. 69-4552-24. *B,* Fleurette composed of highly differentiated photoreceptors forming rod and cone inner segments and an abortive outer segment. AFIP Neg. 69-4552-19. *C,* Fleurette composed of tumor cells, showing only conelike differentiation. AFIP Neg. 69-4552-20. (From Tso MOM, Fine BS, Zimmerman LE: The nature of retinoblastoma. II. Photoreceptor differentiation. An electron microscopic study. Am J Ophthalmol *69*:350–359, 1970.)

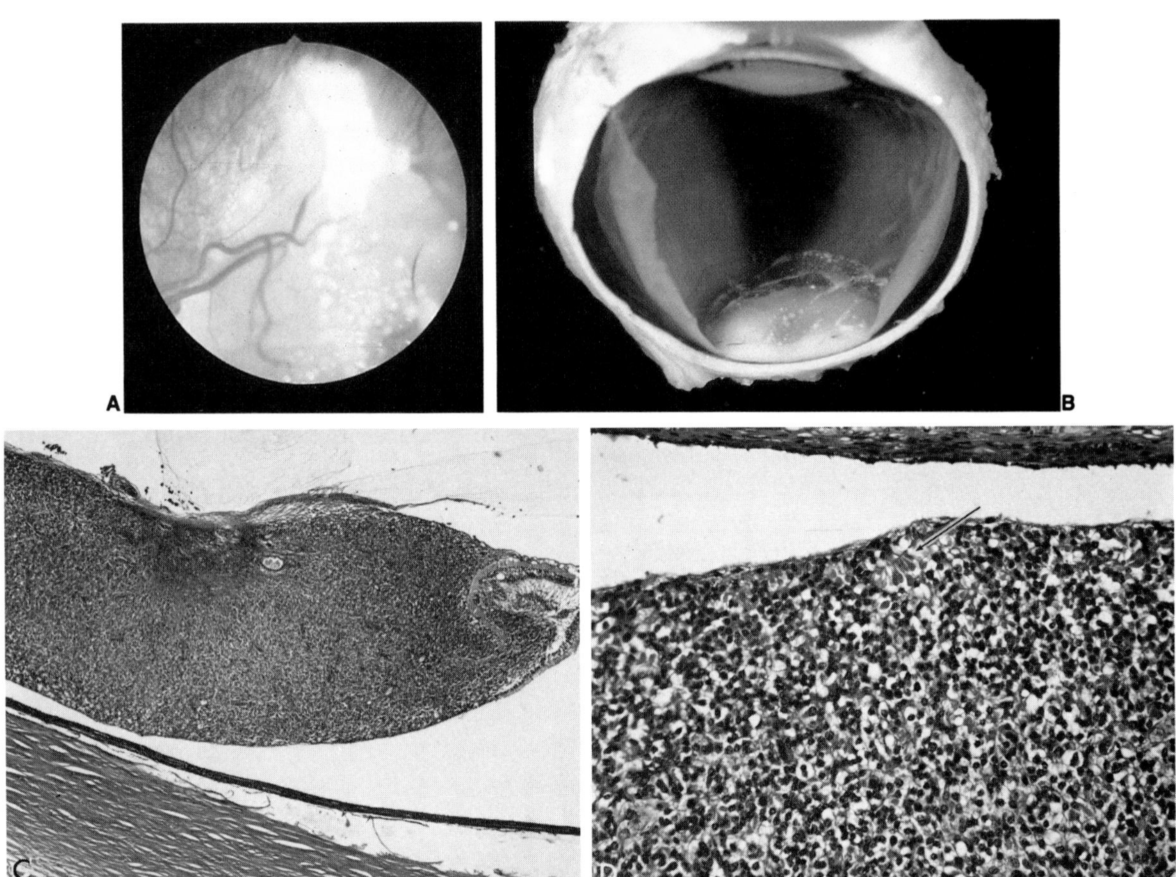

Figure 8–604. *A,* This tumor had shown an incomplete response to radiation therapy, and the eye was therefore enucleated. *B,* Macroscopic appearance of the tumor. *C,* The tumor is composed almost entirely of viable cells. ×40. AFIP Neg. 79-11107. *D,* The constituent cells appear to be benign and exhibit photoreceptor differentiation with the formation of fleurettes (arrow). ×250. AFIP Neg. 79-11105.

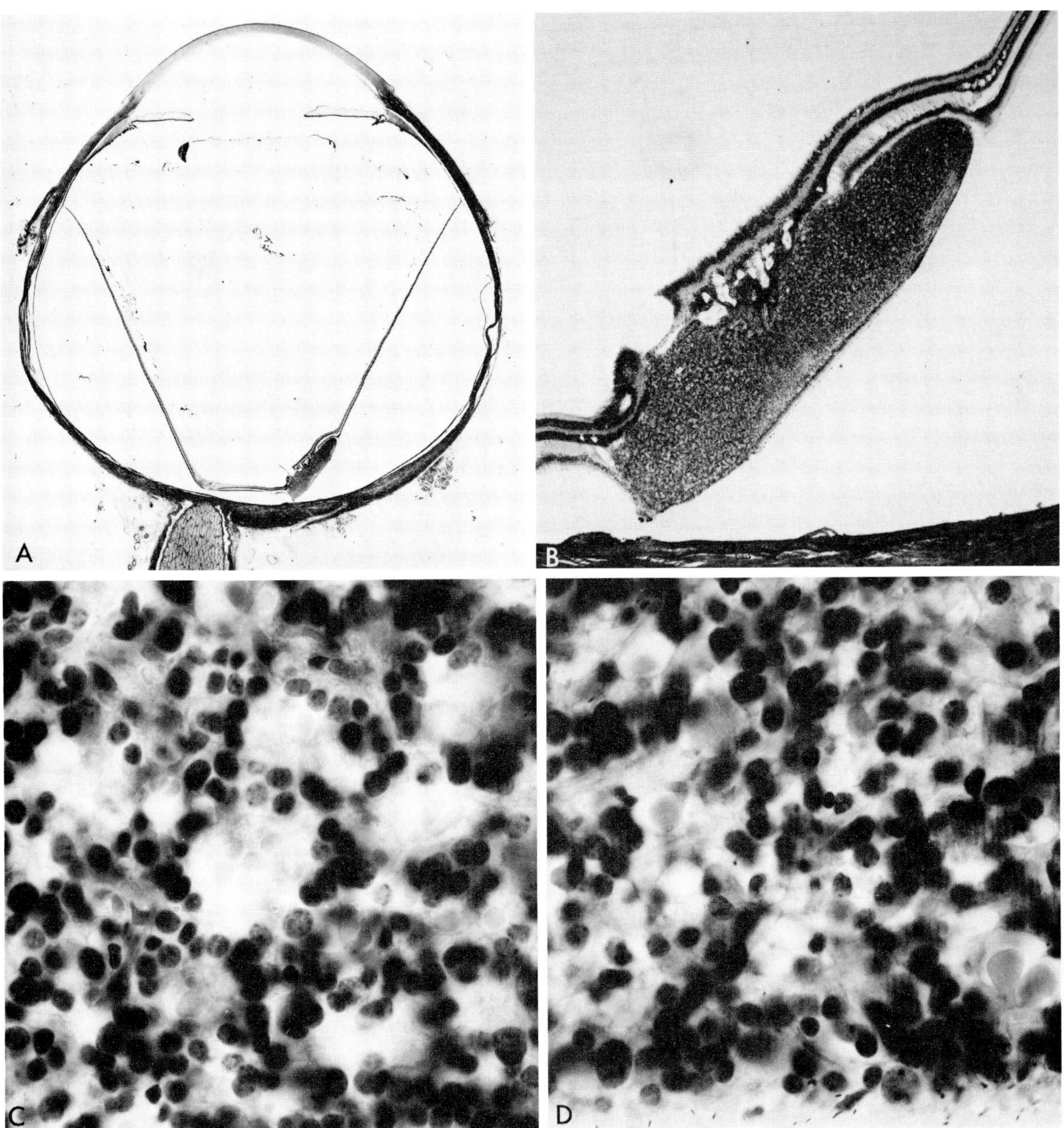

Figure 8–605. Retinocytoma. The small placoid tumor at the posterior pole is composed entirely of benign-appearing cells exhibiting photoreceptor differentiation. *A,* ×2.5. AFIP Neg. 82-6410. *B,* ×15. AFIP Neg. 82-6393. *C,* ×630. AFIP Neg. 84-6578. *D,* ×630. AFIP Neg. 84-6580. (From Margo C, Hidayat A, Kopelman J, Zimmerman LE: Retinocytoma; A benign variant of retinoblastoma. Arch Ophthalmol *101*:1519–1531, 1983.

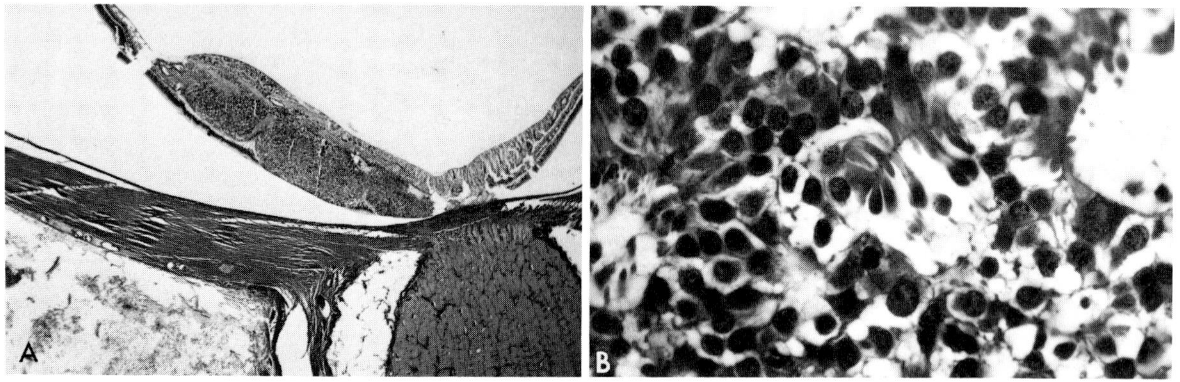

Figure 8–606. Retinocytoma. Another placoid tumor at the posterior pole. *A,* ×15. AFIP Neg. 82-6926. *B,* Fleurette in same tumor. ×630. AFIP Neg. 82-12126. (From Margo C, Hidayat A, Kopelman J, Zimmerman LE: Retinocytoma; A benign variant of retinoblastoma. Arch Ophthalmol *101*:1519–1531, 1983.)

responsive to radiation therapy and which, therefore, was subsequently treated by enucleation. Histologic study revealed the tumor to be composed entirely of benign-appearing cells that exhibited photoreceptor differentiation.

Histologically, similar benign-appearing tumors have been described in eyes that had not been irradiated prior to enucleation (Figs. 8–605 through 8–608). Margo, Hidayat, Kopelman, and Zimmerman (1983) have suggested that when the entire tumor appears to be benign and exhibits photoreceptor differentiation, the term *retinocytoma* would be appropriate for this benign variant of retinoblastoma. This represents a modification of Offret and coworkers' use of Mawas' term (see page 1292), restricting its use to those tumors believed to be cytologically benign. Thus, if one conceives of retinoblastomas as having a broad spectrum of malignant potential, ranging from very highly malignant, totally undifferentiated neuroblastic tumors to completely benign, highly differentiated tumors, retinocytomas would represent the benign end of the spectrum. Glial differentiation also may be observed in these benign variants of retinoblastoma (Margo, Hidayat, Kopelman, Zimmerman, 1983; Smith, 1974), but it is difficult to be certain whether this represents reactive gliosis in the adjacent retina or glial differentiation of tumor cells. In any case, glial tissue is seldom found and is rarely conspicuous. Table 8–9 compares the cytologic characteristics of retinoblastomas and retinocytomas. At least one retinocytoma has been recorded as an oligodendroglioma of the retina (Boniuk, Bishop, 1969).

Growth Patterns

While there is no significant evidence that the growth pattern provides any indication of the origin of a retinoblastoma from either the inner or outer retinal layers, the growth pattern does ex-

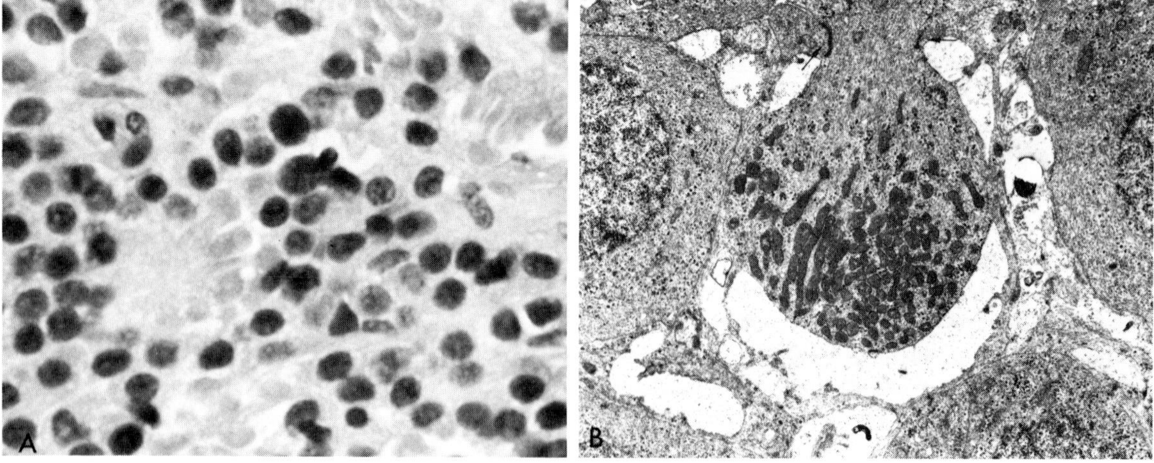

Figure 8–607. Retinocytoma. The tumor is composed of uniformly benign-appearing cells exhibiting photoreceptor differentiation and formation of fleurettes. *A,* ×630. AFIP Neg. 82-9998. *B,* Electron microscopy reveals the clublike cytoplasmic expansions to be packed with mitochondria as in the inner segments of photoreceptors. ×6000. AFIP Neg. 82-12137. (From Margo C, Hidayat A, Kopelman J, Zimmerman LE: Retinocytoma; A benign variant of retinoblastoma. Arch Ophthalmol *101*:1519–1531, 1983.)

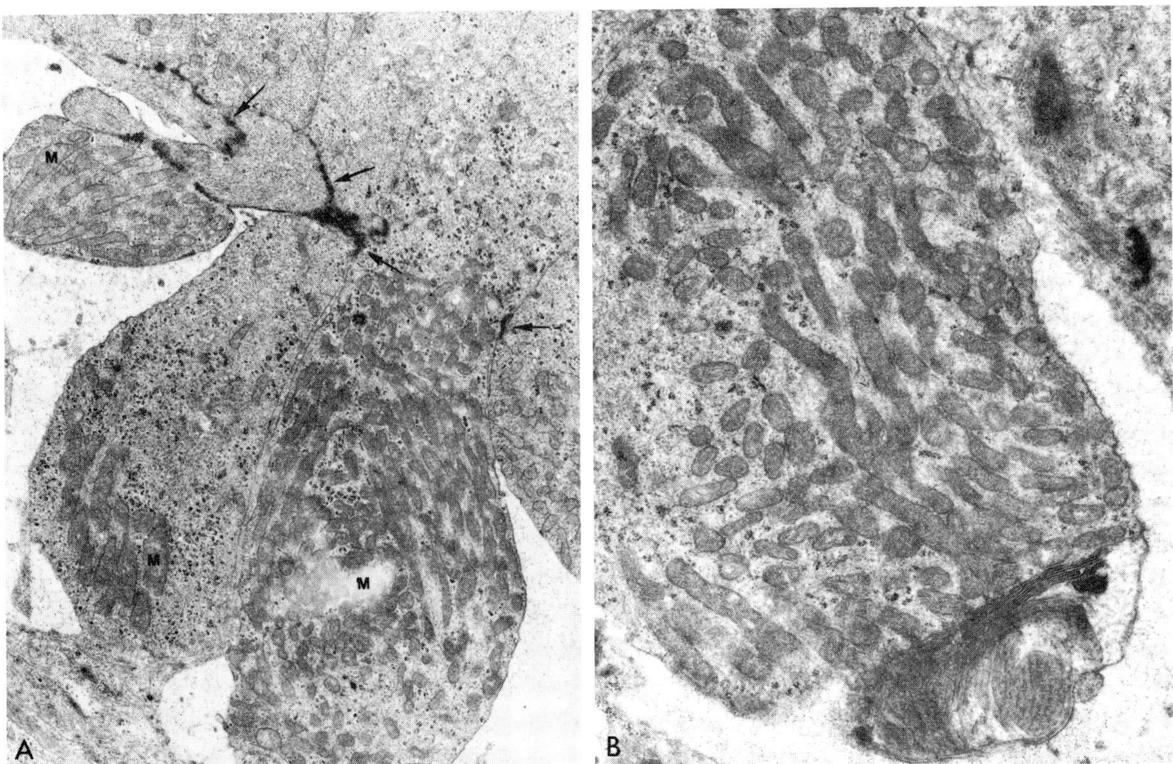

Figure 8–608. Retinocytoma. Electron micrographic evidence of photoreceptor differentiation presented by Margo et al (1983) from the same tumor shown in Figure 8–607. *A,* In a fleurette arrangement, several tumor cells are attached by zonula adherens (arrows) beyond which cytoplasmic expansions filled with mitochondria *(M)* bear a striking resemblance to inner segments of photoreceptor cells. ×6700. AFIP Neg. 82-12140. *B,* Conelike differentiation with formation of a stack of lamellae (bottom right corner), suggestive of formation of an outer segment. ×14,000. AFIP Neg. 82-12134. (From Margo C, Hidayat A, Kopelman J, Zimmerman LE: Retinocytoma; A benign variant of retinoblastoma. Arch Ophthalmol *101*:1519–1531, 1983.)

plain certain clinical variations as well as differences in intraocular and extraocular spread.

Endophytic retinoblastomas grow mainly from the inner surface of the retina into the vitreous (Figs. 8–609 and 8–610). Thus, on ophthalmoscopic examination, one views the tumor directly (Fig. 8–611). Retinal vessels are typically lost from view as they enter the tumor. As endophytic tumors grow large and become friable, tumor cells tend to be shed from the tumor into the vitreous where they grow into separate tiny spheroidal masses that may be confused clinically with the "fluff balls" or "cotton balls" of inflammatory conditions, such as mycotic or nematodal endophthalmitis (Fig. 8–612). Tumor cells in the vitreous also may become secondarily deposited

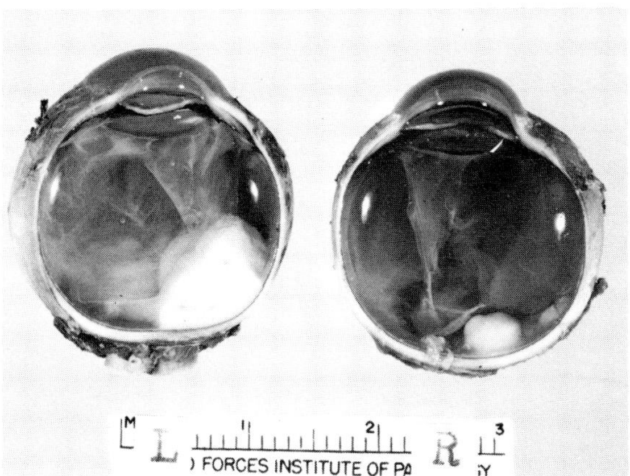

Figure 8–609. Bilateral multicentric endophytic retinoblastomas. In both eyes the tumors have grown preferentially in toward the vitreous; the retina remains in place. AFIP Neg. 56-20185-2.

Table 8–9. HISTOLOGIC COMPARISON OF RETINOBLASTOMAS AND RETINOCYTOMAS

Retinoblastoma	Retinocytoma
Larger and more hyperchromatic nuclei	Smaller and less hyperchromatic nuclei
Scanty cytoplasm and intercellular matrix	Abundant cytoplasm and intercellular matrix
Numerous mitotic figures	Mitotic figures absent or very rare
Necrosis highly characteristic	Necrosis typically absent
Calcification in areas of necrosis	Calcification in non-necrotic tumor
Differentiation into Flexner-Wintersteiner rosettes	Differentiation into fleurettes
Cytologically malignant	Cytologically benign

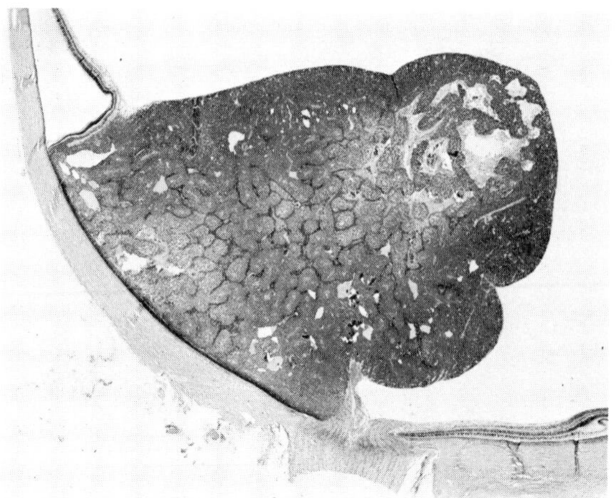

Figure 8–610. Comparatively small **endophytic retinoblastoma** showing small areas of necrosis in the innermost apical part of the tumor. ×12. AFIP Neg. 56-11404.

onto the inner surface of the retina, where they may give rise to clinical difficulty in differentiation from independent new tumors of multicentric retinoblastoma, such as those shown in Figure 8–579,*A* and *C*, which are from the same case shown in Figure 8–609. If one can discern that the tumor lies mainly on the inner surface of the retina rather than within it (as in Fig. 8–585), and if one can also see tumor cell clusters within the vitreous, retinal seeding has occurred. Tumor cells in the vitreous also may spread into the posterior chamber and become disseminated by aqueous flow. Secondary deposits on the lens, zonular fibers, ciliary epithelium, iris, and trabecular meshwork may be observed, and tumor cells may follow the aqueous outflow pathways out of

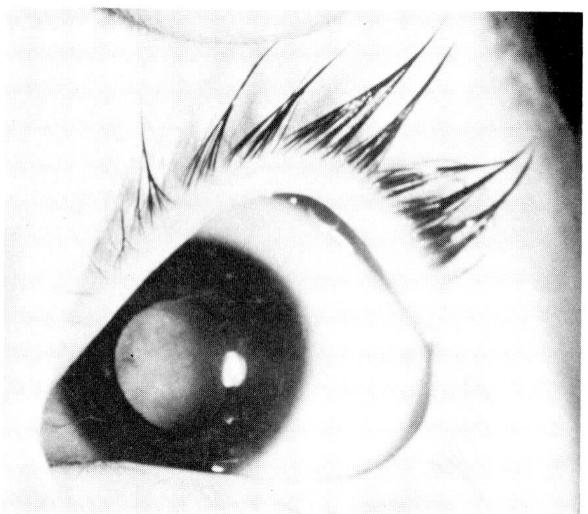

Figure 8–611. Clinical appearance of **endophytic retinoblastoma**. On ophthalmoscopic examination one looks in directly upon tumor tissue growing from the inner retina, obscuring the normal retinal vessels. AFIP Neg. 69-1770.

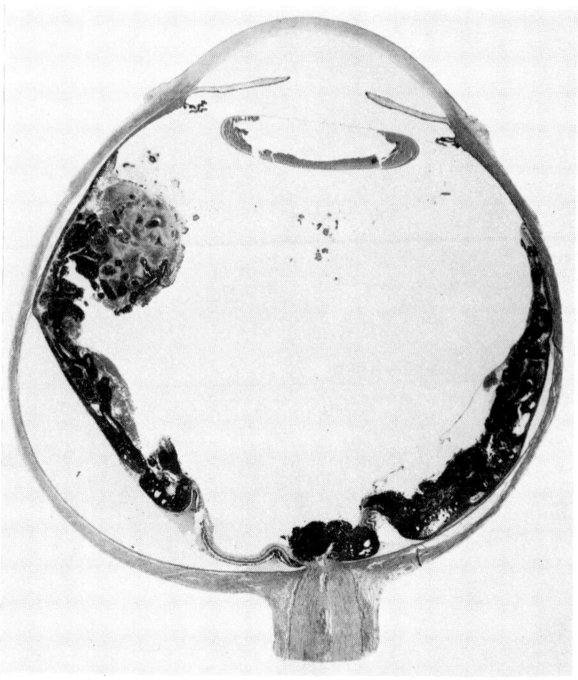

Figure 8–612. Diffusely **infiltrative retinoblastoma** that involves almost the entire retina. In multiple areas the tumor has invaded through the internal limiting membrane, and many small secondary deposits are present in the vitreous. ×6. AFIP Neg. 50319.

the eye. In such cases the anterior segment changes may be misinterpreted clinically as those of granulomatous iridocyclitis (Fig. 8–613).

Exophytic retinoblastomas grow primarily from the outer retinal surface toward the choroid, producing at first a solid elevation of the retina (Fig. 8–614). In such cases, on ophthalmoscopic examination one can see the retinal vessels coursing over the tumor (Fig. 8–615). As the tumor grows larger, it may give rise to a total retinal detachment (Figs. 8–616 and 8–617), and tumor cells may escape into the subretinal exudate. Second-

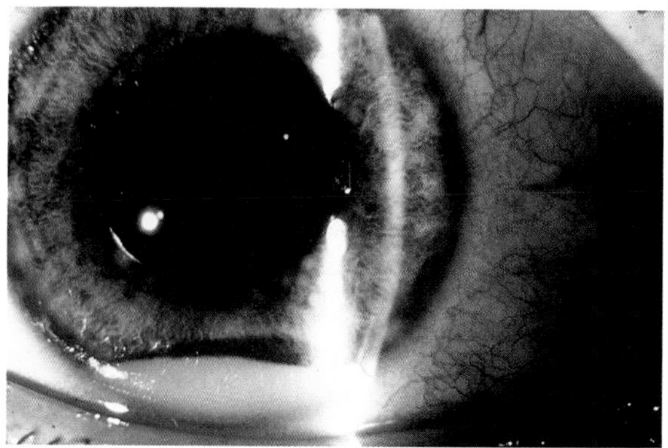

Figure 8–613. Clinical appearance of **retinoblastoma cells** in the anterior chamber angle and implanted on the iris of an 8 year old child who presented a 2 month history of an inflamed eye. AFIP Neg. 72-3750.

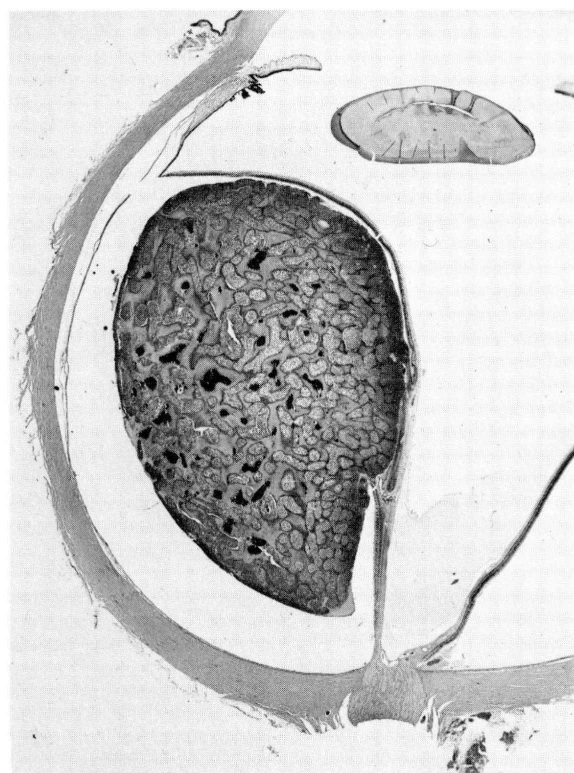

Figure 8–614. Exophytic retinoblastoma. The tumor has grown preferentially outward into the subretinal space, producing a solid elevation of the retina. ×6. AFIP Neg. 65-3319.

ary implants may then develop on the outer retinal surface or onto the inner surface of the retinal pigment epithelium (Figs. 8–586, 8–587, 8–616, 8–617). Such implants may then replace the pigment

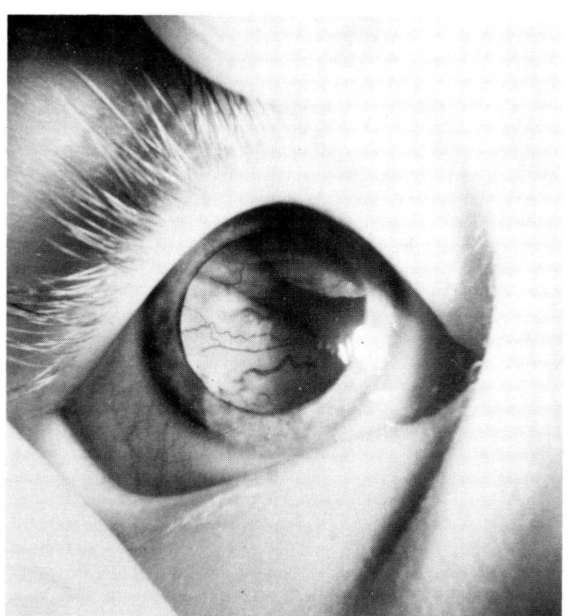

Figure 8–615. Clinical appearance of **exophytic retinoblastoma,** with the retina and its retinal vessels pushed forward against the lens, which typically remains transparent. AFIP Neg. 69-1768-1.

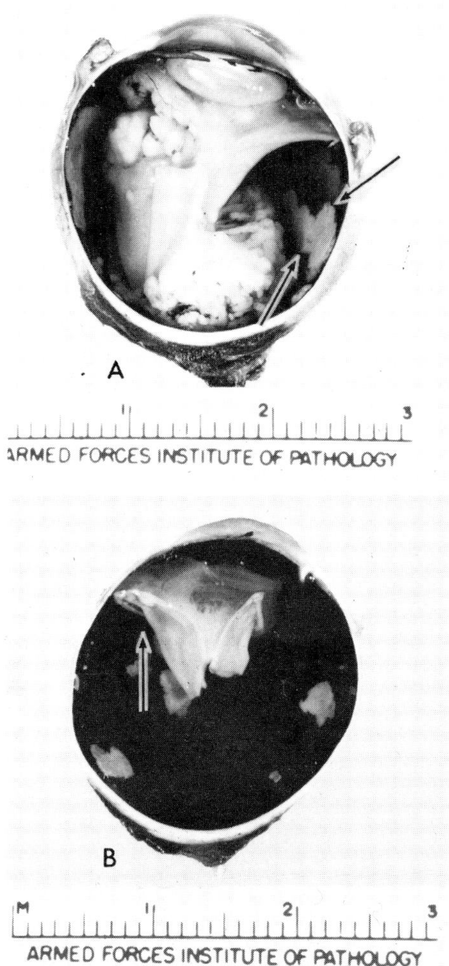

Figure 8–616. *A* and *B*, **Total retinal detachment associated with extensive exophytic retinoblastoma.** Whereas the vitreous is free of tumor, large white plaques of implanted tumor are growing on the inner surface of the retinal pigment epithelium (arrows). *A*, AFIP Neg. 64-397-1. *B*, AFIP Neg. 64-397-2.

epithelium and eventually infiltrate through Bruch's membrane into the choroid (Fig. 8–618). From the choroid, tumor cells may escape along ciliary vessels and nerves into the orbit, or they may invade choroidal blood vessels and become disseminated hematogenously.

Mixed endophytic-exophytic tumors (Fig. 8–619) are probably more common than either purely endophytic or exophytic retinoblastomas, especially among the larger tumors. The combined features of both groups just described characterize these tumors.

Diffuse infiltrating retinoblastomas are the least common and often give rise to the greatest difficulty in clinical diagnosis (Morgan, 1971; Nicholson, Norton, 1980; Schofield, 1960). These tumors grow diffusely within the retina without greatly thickening it (Fig. 8–620) and may, therefore, escape clinical recognition. They also may be overlooked on macroscopic examination.

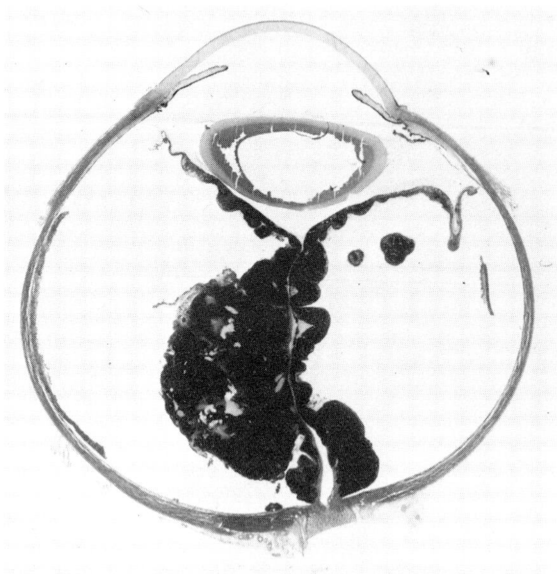

Figure 8–617. Extensive and diffusely infiltrative **retinoblastoma** that has grown mainly in an exophytic fashion, producing a total retinal detachment. The internal limiting membrane is intact and no tumor has spread into the vitreous, but there is a large placoid deposit on the inner surface of the retinal pigmant epithelium (arrows). ×5. AFIP Neg. 183030.

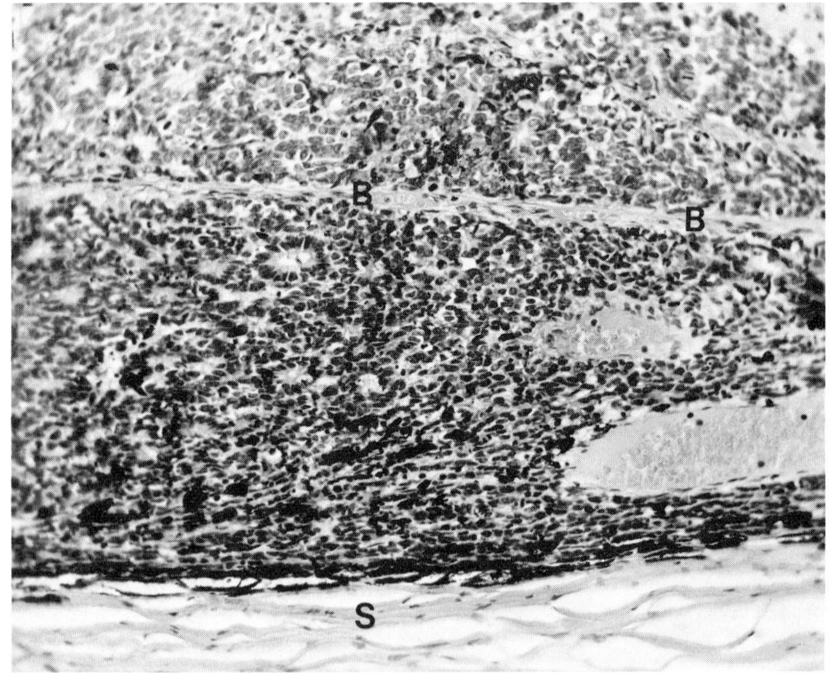

Figure 8–618. Retinoblastoma in choroid. Tumor in subretinal space has replaced the retinal pigment epithelium; only Bruch's membrane *(B)* and sclera *(S)* remain as histologic landmarks. ×190. AFIP Neg. 56-11410.

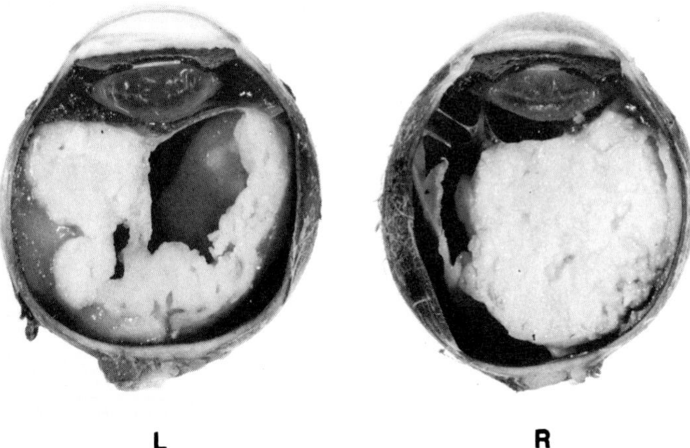

Figure 8–619. Bilateral retinoblastomas exhibiting mixed patterns of endophytic and exophytic growth. AFIP Neg. 54-6959.

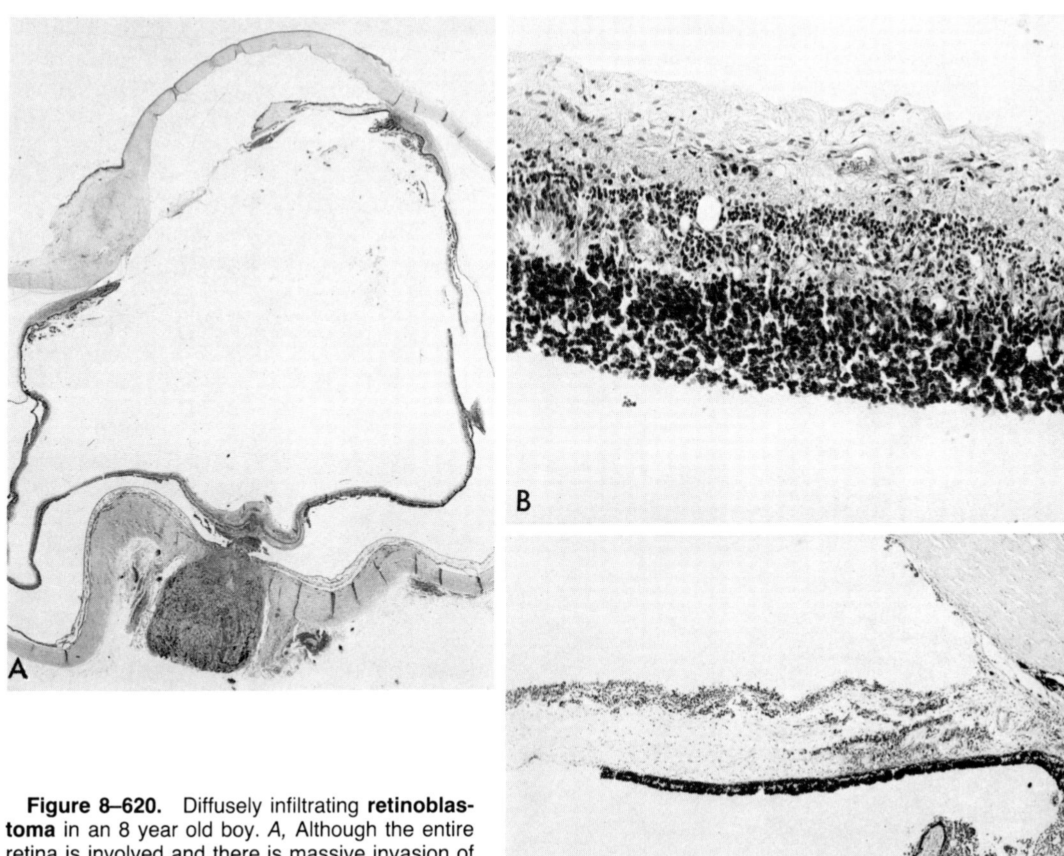

Figure 8–620. Diffusely infiltrating **retinoblastoma** in an 8 year old boy. *A,* Although the entire retina is involved and there is massive invasion of optic nerve, a definite mass was not observed clinically, and the child had been treated for "uveitis" with secondary glaucoma. ×7. AFIP Neg. 56-19953. *B,* Diffuse infiltration of retina. ×145. AFIP Neg. 56-19961. *C,* Infiltration of iris and ciliary body. ×50. AFIP Neg. 56-19960. (From Weizenblatt S: Differential diagnostic difficulties in atypical retinoblastoma; Report of a case. Arch Ophthalmol *58*:699–709, 1957.)

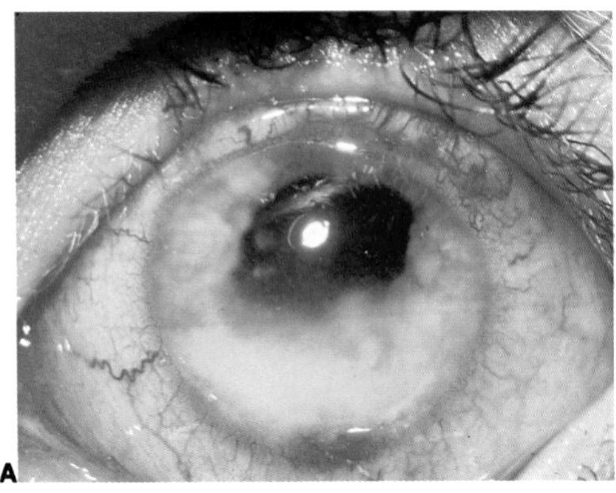
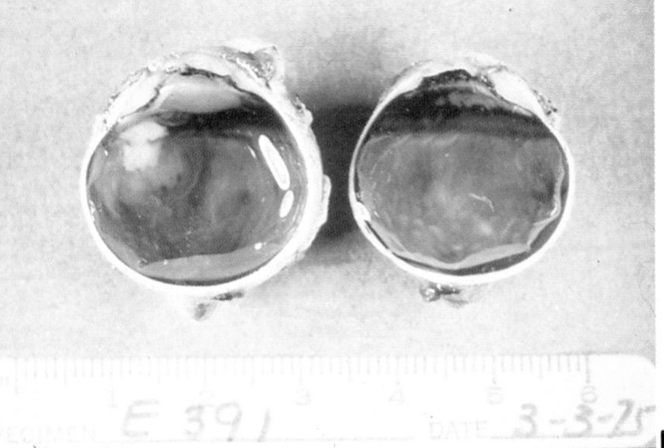

Figure 8–621. *A,* Massive involvement of anterior segment that gave rise to prolonged difficulty in clinical and histopathologic diagnosis despite repeated aspirations of exudate from anterior chamber and biopsies of iris, secondary to invasion from *B. B,* Small peripheral area of **infiltrative retinoblastoma**. (From Reeser F: Iris spread from a peripheral retinoblastoma; case presented at the Verhoeff Society, Washington, DC, April, 1975.)

Nevertheless, tumor cells often are discharged into the vitreous, masquerading as inflammatory cells of a retinitis, vitritis, or *Toxocara* endophthalmitis. With anterior chamber involvement, hyperacute iritis with hypopyon, juvenile xanthogranuloma, or tuberculosis may be suspected (Fig. 8–621) (Reeser, 1975; Soll, Turtz, 1960; Weizenblatt, 1957). There is some suggestion that such diffuse retinoblastomas may carry a more favorable prognosis despite long delays in establishing a diagnosis and a greater median age of patients with this type of tumor (Morgan, 1971; Nicholson, 1980; Schofield, 1960), but Weizenblatt's patient, an 8 year old boy, died with extensive spread to the brain 1 year after he was first examined for an inflamed eye (Fig. 8–620). Other lethal diffuse retinoblastomas are on file in the Registry of Ophthalmic Pathology.

Complete spontaneous necrosis leading to regression and a "cure" is a well-known phenomenon that is said to occur more frequently in retinoblastoma than in any other malignant neoplasm (Abramson, 1983; Gallie, Ellsworth, Abramson, Phillips, 1982). Typically there is a severe inflammatory reaction followed by phthisis bulbi (Fig. 8–622) (Boniuk, Zimmerman, 1962). Although many theories have been advanced, the specific pathogenetic mechanism responsible for total necrosis of the tumor is unknown. Verhoeff (1966) believed calcification caused necrosis and suggested that hypervitaminosis D might have therapeutic value, whereas today most patholo-

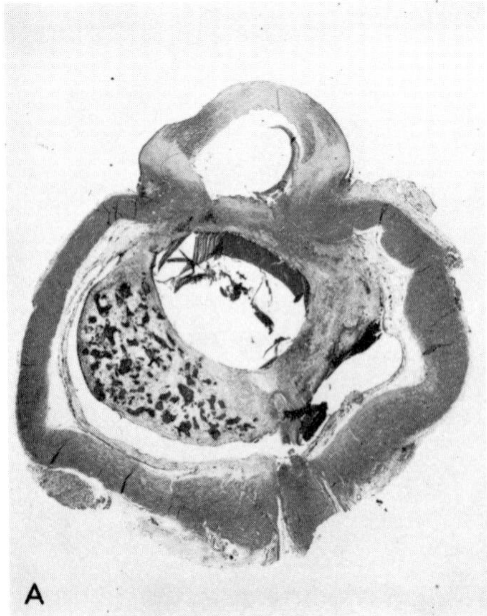
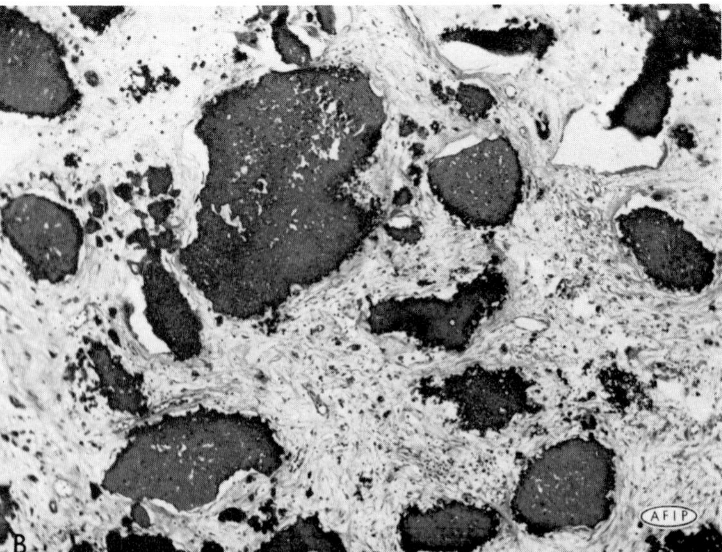

Figure 8–622. **Phthisis bulbi** resulting from total spontaneous necrosis of retinoblastoma. *A* and *B,* Extensive calcification in the totally necrotic tumor. *A,* ×4. AFIP Neg. 235121-1. *B,* ×75. AFIP Neg. 235121-2.

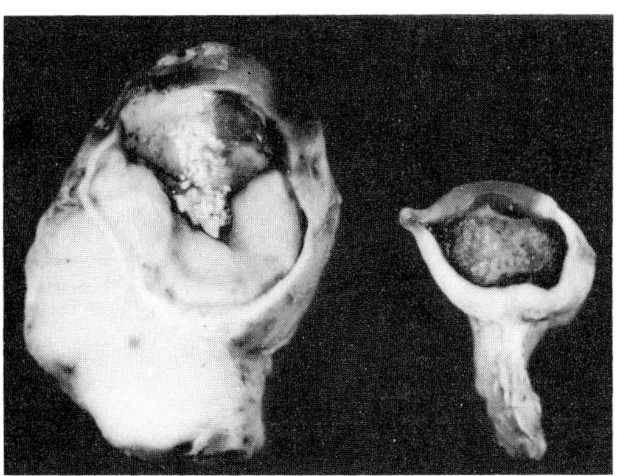

Figure 8–623. Bilateral retinoblastoma. On one side the tumor has spontaneously undergone complete necrosis and the eye became phthisical, while on the opposite side the tumor massively invaded the choroid, sclera, and orbit. AFIP Neg. 53-5707.

gists believe calcification occurs in areas that have already become necrotic. Some have suggested an immunopathologic mechanism, perhaps accompanied by severe inflammation that destroys most of the eye as well as the tumor. We have, on several occasions, observed bilateral retinoblastoma in which there was total necrosis and phthisis bulbi on one side whereas on the other, a viable tumor massively filled the eye and invaded the orbit (Fig. 8–623) (Boniuk, Zimmerman, 1962). Such cases seem to exclude the possibility of a systemic mechanism (e.g., production of antibodies against the tumor, a circulating toxin, hypercalcemia, and so on). Occlusion of the central retinal artery (Fig. 8–624) has been observed in eyes with necrotic retinoblastomas, but whether this occurs before or after the tumor becomes necrotic cannot always be established. Andersen and Jensen (1974) ascribed massive necrosis of a retinoblastoma to occlusion of the central retinal vessels by the tumor, and Gallie et al (1983) believe that all spontaneous regressions resulting in phthisis are the result of central vessel occlusion, a mechanism also favored by Reese (1976).

In phthisical eyes with totally regressed retinoblastomas, histologic examination reveals dense calcification in a tumor that exhibits such complete coagulative necrosis that definitive diagnosis may be difficult. Under high magnification, one can usually make out the ghostly outlines of fossilized tumor cells (Fig. 8–625). Further confusion may be created by exuberant reactive proliferation of pigmented retinal and ciliary epithelial cells (Fig. 8–626), and by ossification.

Until recently, some smaller, often calcified tumors, now called retinomas (Aaby, Price, Zakov, 1983; Gallie, Ellsworth, Abramson, Phillips, 1982) or retinocytomas (Margo, Hidayat, Kopelman, Zimmerman, 1983) (see page 1320, and Figs. 8–605 and 8–606), typically found in eyes retaining useful vision, were lumped together with the group just described in blind, phthisical eyes, under the heading "regressed retinoblastoma." This confusion came about as a consequence of the similar ophthalmoscopic appearance of these smaller lesions to retinoblastomas that had previously been treated by radiation (Reese, 1967, 1976). Gallie and coworkers (1982) have presented clinical criteria for separating these small, benign variants of retinoblastoma from genuine regression of retinoblastoma (Table 8–10). Both spontaneous regression leading to phthisis bulbi and benign retinomas (retinocytomas) in eyes retaining useful vision may be observed unilaterally in nongenetic or bilaterally in genetically determined cases of retinoblastoma. The genetic implication of these variants is nicely demonstrated by the case reported by Gangwar, Jain, Gupta, et al

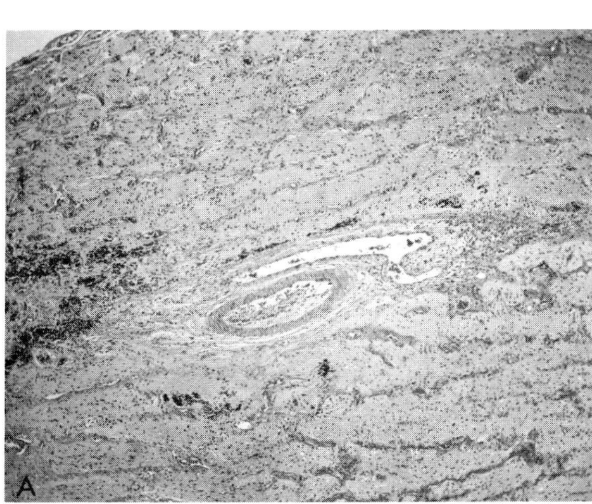

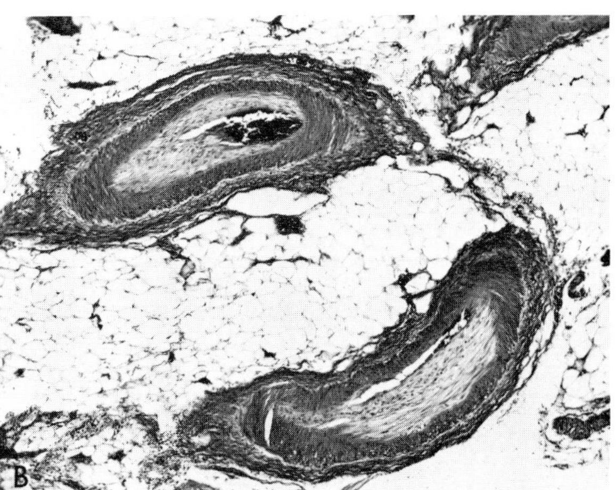

Figure 8–624. Severe fibroblastic thickening of intima with extreme narrowing of the lumen of the central retinal artery. *A,* In an optic nerve invaded by tumor. ×100. AFIP Neg. 74-13607. *B,* In a phthisical eye following radiation therapy. ×70. AFIP Neg. 69-7168.

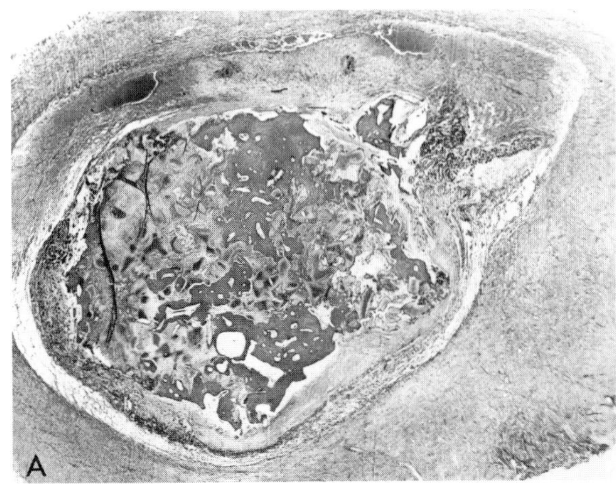

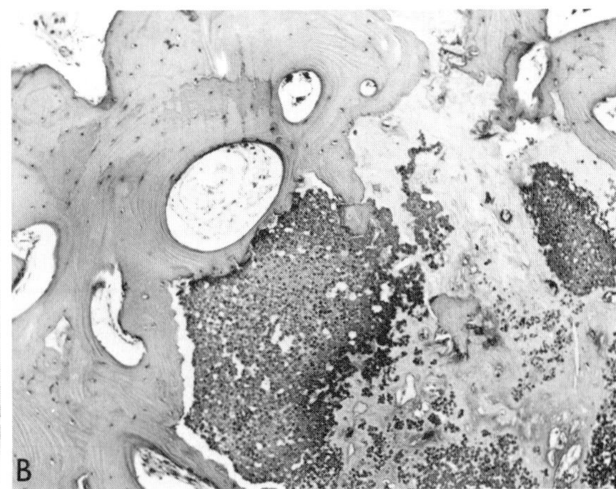

Figure 8–625. Mineralized necrotic tumor cells in a spontaneously regressed retinoblastoma, also showing dystrophic ossification. *A,* ×11. AFIP Neg. 61-3514. *B,* ×115. AFIP Neg. 61-3518.

(1982). The subject of their report, a 29 year old man, gave a history of having had a leukocoria before developing acute inflammation that progressed to phthisis bulbi in his right eye during infancy. He had retained good vision in his left eye, but when his newborn daughter was found to have a typical retinoblastoma that produced a total retinal detachment in one eye, ophthalmoscopic examination of his "good" left eye revealed three separate small retinal tumors typical of retinomas.

Intraocular Spread and Extraocular Extension

Most retinoblastomas exhibit the relentlessly progressive, invasive growth that is generally associated with malignant neuroblastic tumors of childhood. Although they may grow progressively, mainly in toward the vitreous or outward toward the choroid, many grow in all directions. If left untreated, they usually fill the eye and completely destroy the internal architecture of the globe (Fig. 8–627). Endophytic tumors and the diffusely infiltrating retinoblastomas (Figs. 8–620 and 8–621) tend to spread anteriorly, invading the iris, anterior chamber angle, and ciliary body. Exophytic tumors grow preferentially into the choroid (Fig. 8–628). Once the tumor has invaded the choroid, it may then spread into the orbit via the scleral canals or by massively replacing the sclera (Fig. 8–629). Owing to the vascularity of the choroid, the chances of hematogenous dissemination are greatly increased once the tumor has invaded the choroid. The tumor shown in Fig. 8–628 is exemplary: there is no involvement of the optic disk or nerve, but this tumor became widely disseminated to skin and bones about 6 months after enucleation. Anterior uveal invasion also may lead to hematogenous dissemination or to regional lymphatic spread via the aqueous outflow pathways and the conjunctival lymphatic vessels.

All retinoblastomas, regardless of their pattern of growth, show a striking tendency to invade the optic disk and to spread into the optic nerve (Figs. 8–630, 8–631, and 8–632). Once into the

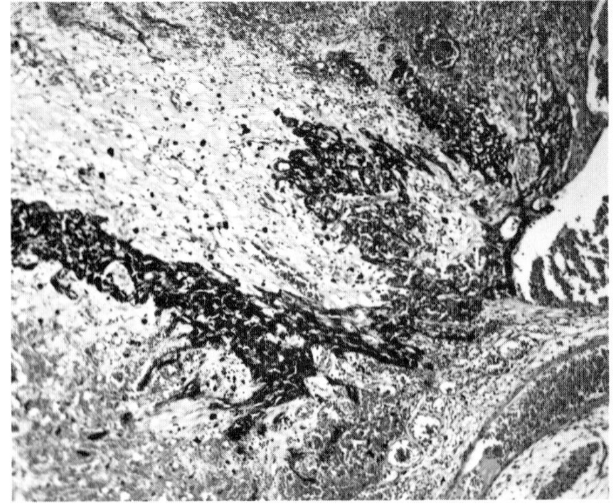

Figure 8–626. Exuberant reactive proliferation of pigmented ciliary epithelium. Clinically, a black, retrolental mass had been observed to develop in this eye. ×60. AFIP Neg. 74-11047.

Table 8–10. CLINICAL CHARACTERISTICS OF RETINOMAS (RETINOCYTOMAS)

1. Comparatively small, homogenous, translucent, gray, slightly elevated placoid mass with functional retinal blood vessels looping into the mass
2. Opaque, white calcified flecks having appearance of cottage cheese
3. Proliferation and migration of retinal pigment epithelium in areas underlying or adjacent to the tumors
4. Functional eye with clear media and no retinal detachment

(After Gallie BL, Phillips RA, Ellsworth RM, Abramson DH: Significance of retinoma and phthisis bulbi for retinoblastoma. Ophthalmology *89*:1393–1399, 1982.)

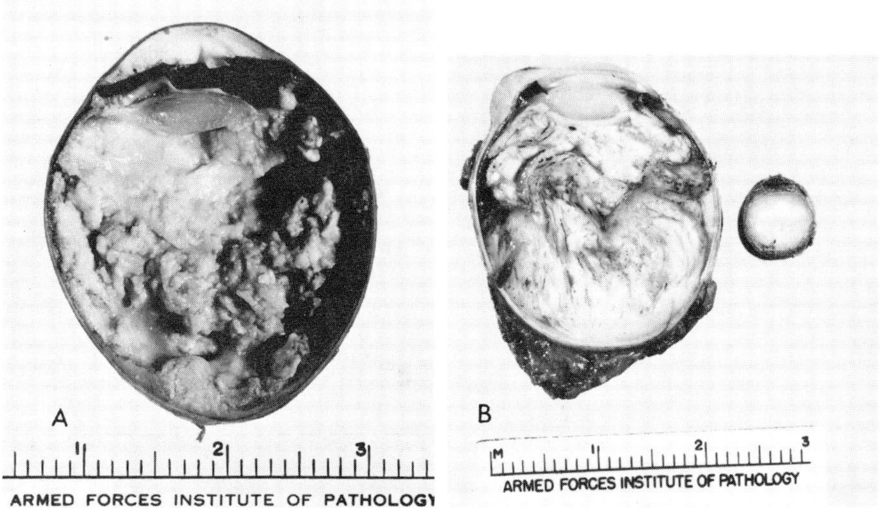

Figure 8–627. Advanced **intraocular growth of retinoblastomas,** with destruction of internal architecture of eyes and glaucomatous enlargement of globes. Both tumors are markedly necrotic and have produced a panophthalmitis. In *A,* the optic nerve (shown in cross-section) is massively replaced by the tumor. *A,* AFIP Neg. 62-1528-2. *B,* AFIP Neg. 54-11537.

nerve, the tumor may spread directly along the nerve fiber bundles back toward the chiasm, or it may infiltrate through the pia into the subarachnoid space. Tumor cells may be carried via the circulating cerebrospinal fluid to the brain. Infiltrating along the central retinal vessels, tumor cells in the nerve pass into meninges or into the orbit.

Metastasis and Recurrence

Retinoblastomas exhibit metastatic potential in four ways:

(1) Direct infiltrative spread may occur along the optic nerve from the eye to the brain. Once the orbital soft tissues have been invaded, the tumor also may spread directly into the orbital bones or via the various foramina into the cranium.

(2) Dispersion of tumor cells may occur after cells in the optic nerve have invaded the leptomeninges and gained access to the circulating subarachnoid fluid. The cerebrospinal fluid may carry tumor cells from the eye to the brain and spinal cord, and even to the optic nerve on the opposite side (Fig. 8–633), as described by de-Buen (1960) and Espiritu (1970).

(3) Hematogenous dissemination leads to widespread metastasis to the lungs, bones, brain, and other organs. Massive uveal invasion greatly increases the risk for hematogenous spread.

(4) Lymphatic spread occurs mainly in those advanced cases in which there has been massive invasion of the anterior segment with anterior ex-

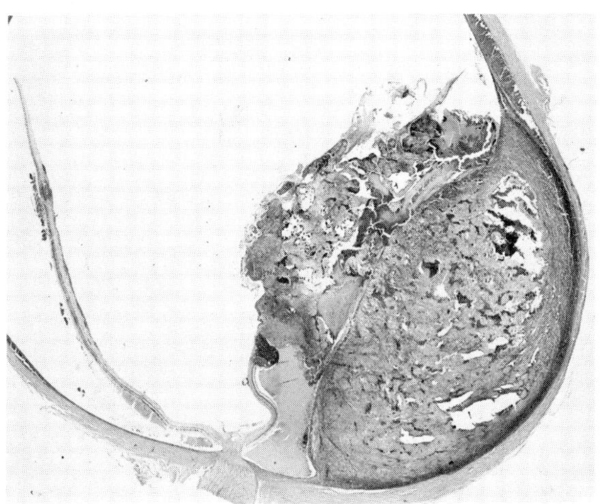

Figure 8–628. This **retinoblastoma,** which has spread into and massively thickened the choroid, metastasized hematogenously to skin and bones. Note that the optic disk and nerve are not involved. ×6. AFIP Neg. 67-795.

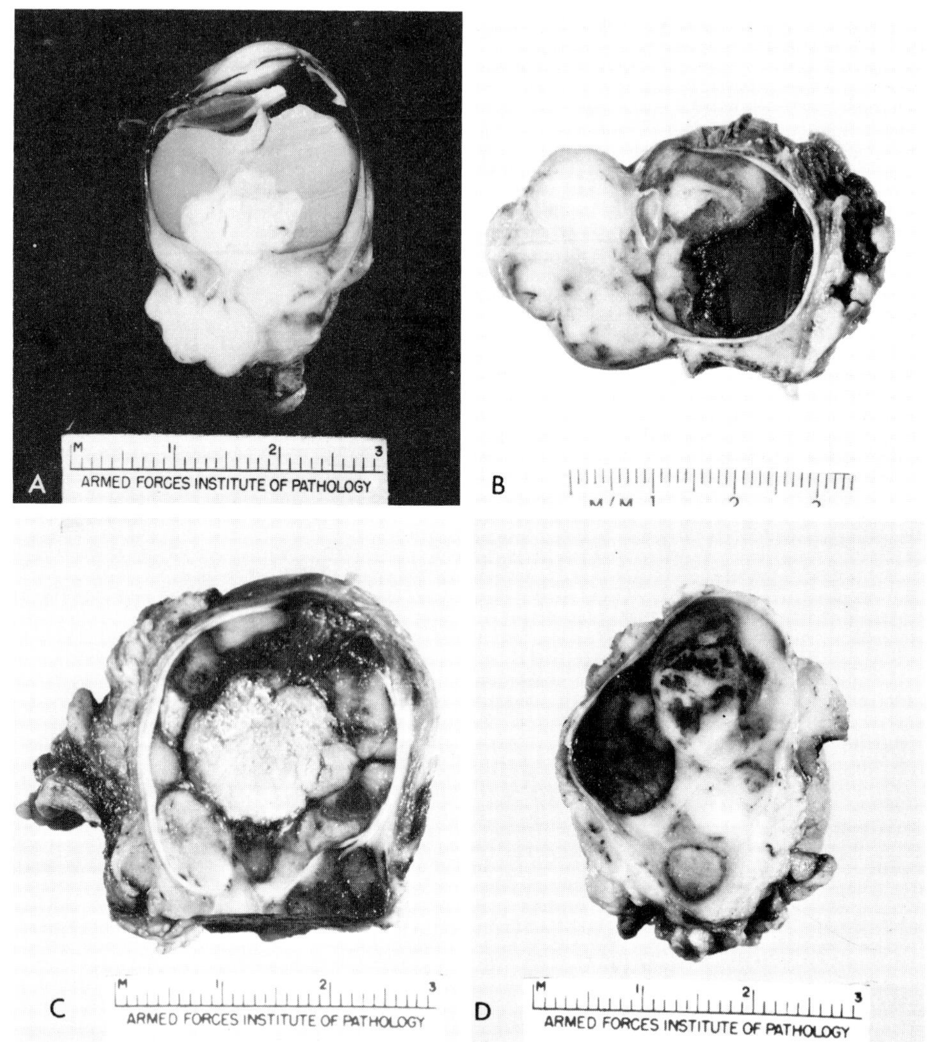

Figure 8–629. Retinoblastomas that have massively invaded the choroid, sclera, and orbit. *A,* AFIP Neg. 60-3807. *B,* AFIP Neg. 70-1068. *C,* AFIP Neg. 62-5820-2. *D,* AFIP Neg. 62-5860-1.

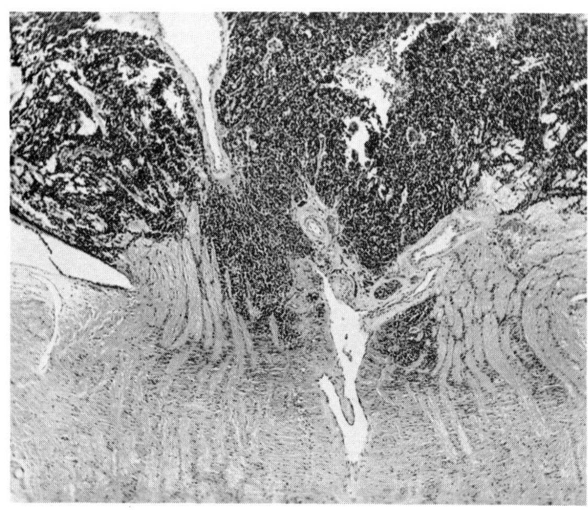

Figure 8–630. Invasion of optic nerve head by neoplastic cells to level of the lamina scleralis, but the retrolaminar optic nerve is spared. ×56. AFIP Neg. 56-11411.

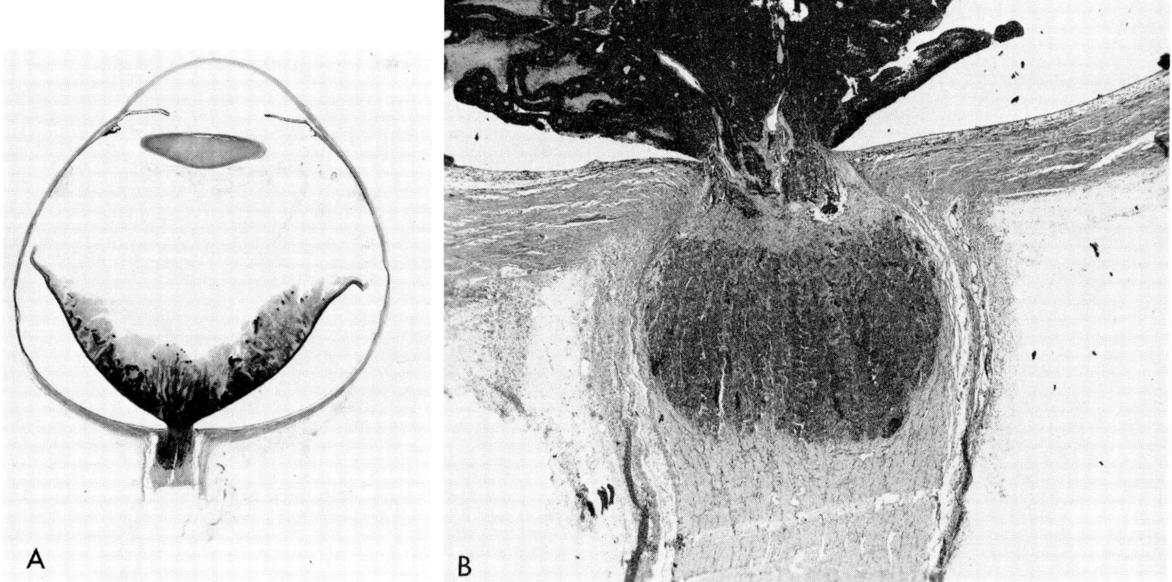

Figure 8–631. Invasion of retrolaminar optic nerve, but there is a significant margin of uninvolved optic nerve between the posterior edge of the infiltrating tumor and the plane of surgical transection. Transverse histologic sections at the plane of surgical transection revealed no tumor in either case. *A,* ×3. AFIP Neg. 211405. *B,* ×14. AFIP Neg. 57-344.

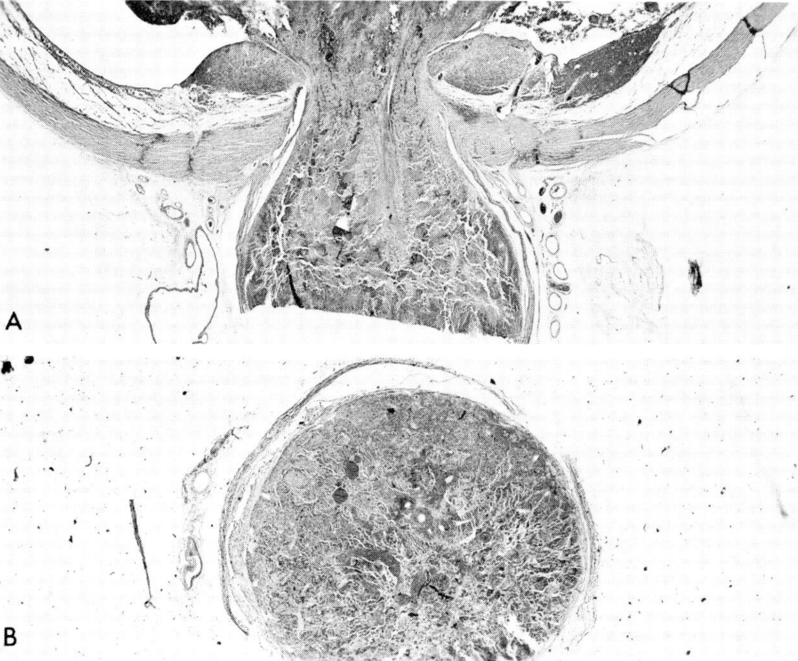

Figure 8–632. *A and B,* **Massive invasion of optic nerve** to the level of the surgical transection, indicating that residual tumor remains in the optic nerve stump left in the orbit. Both, ×7. AFIP Neg. 68-9154.

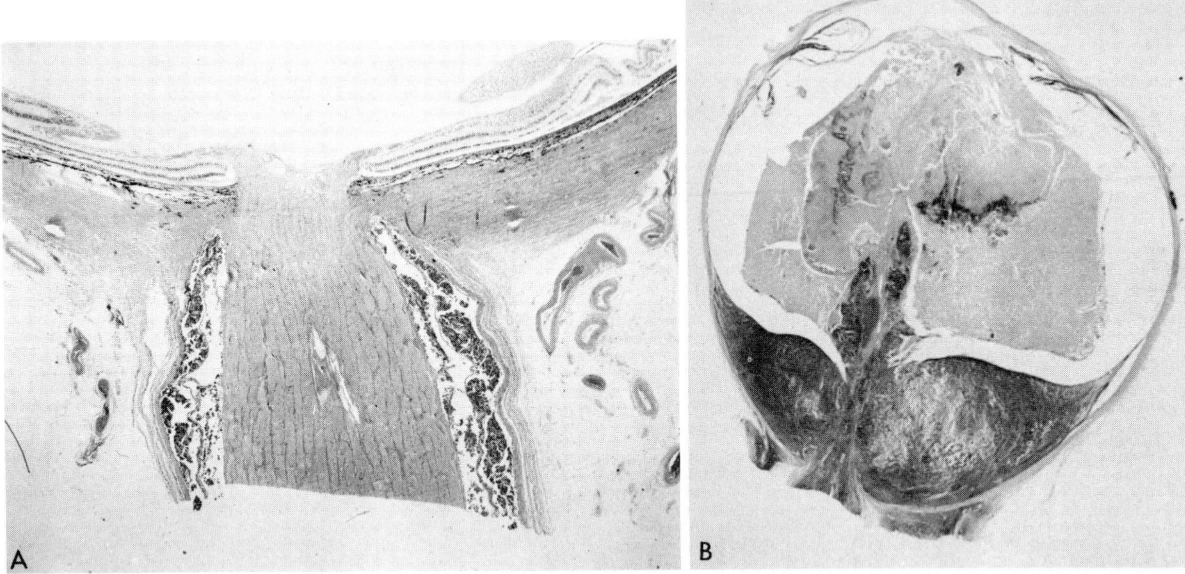

Figure 8–633. *A,* **Spread of retinoblastoma cells** in subarachnoid space to uninvolved eye from a primary located in the fellow eye (see *B*). This eye was obtained post mortem. ×14. AFIP Neg. 60-1454. *B,* Surgically enucleated eye showing massive invasion of choroid, optic nerve, and orbit. ×3. AFIP Neg. 60-1455. (From deBuen S: Retinoblastoma with spread by direct continuity to the contralateral optic nerve. Am J Ophthalmol *49*:815–819, 1960.)

traocular extension. It is generally believed that there are no intraocular lymphatic channels, but the bulbar conjunctiva, eyelids, and anterior orbital tissues are richly supplied with lymph vessels. Massive preauricular and cervical lymph node involvement (Fig. 8–634) may be observed in neglected cases with massive anterior extraocular extension or with orbital recurrence following enucleation.

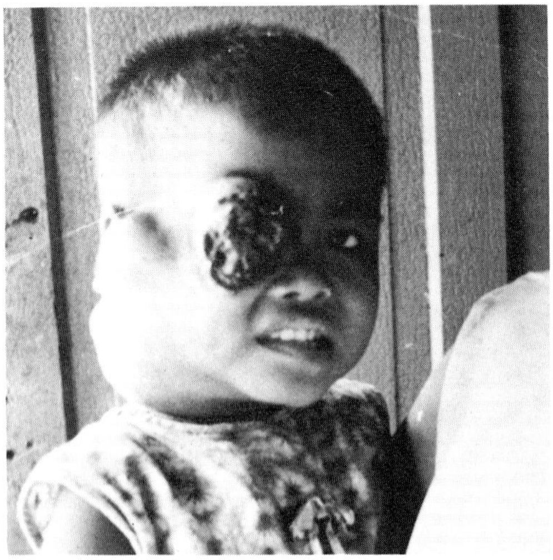

Figure 8–634. Massive preauricular, submandibular, and cervical **lymphadenopathy** from advanced retinoblastoma that destroyed the eye and filled the orbit in a Laotian girl. AFIP Neg. 66-216. (From Zimmerman LE: Retinoblastoma, including a report of illustrative cases. Med Ann Dist Colum *38*:366–374, 1969.)

When metastasis occurs, it is generally within the first year or two following treatment (Taktikos, 1966). Late metastasis, which occurs so frequently following enucleation for uveal melanomas, is so rare after treatment for retinoblastoma that, when it is suspected, the question of an in-

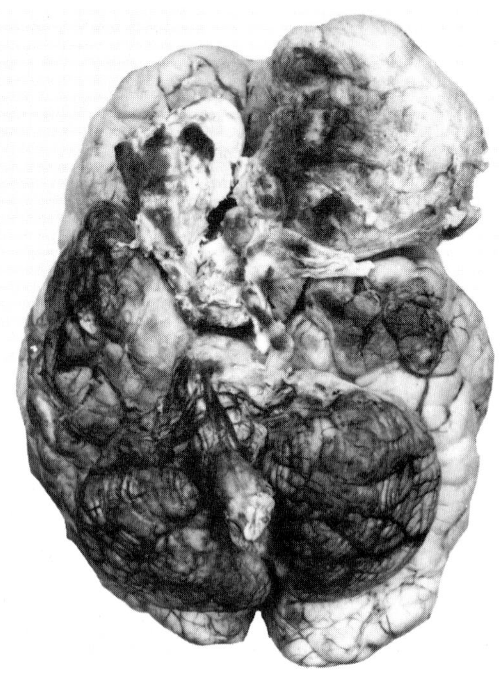

Figure 8–635. Metastatic spread of retinoblastoma to leptomeninges of brain. AFIP Neg. 62019.

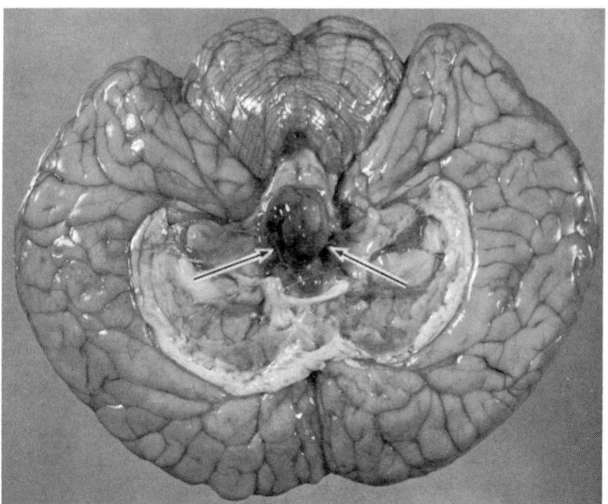

Figure 8–636. Post-mortem demonstration of a discrete **pineal tumor** (arrows) that had produced dilation of the lateral ventricles in a child who had been treated successfully for bilateral retinoblastoma 2 years earlier. AFIP Neg. 62-12516. (From Jakobiec FA, Tso MOM, Zimmerman LE, Danis P: Retinoblastoma and intracranial malignancy. Cancer *39*:2048–2058, 1977.)

dependent new primary tumor must be considered. Metastasis from retinoblastoma is also characteristically widespread. The brain may be selectively affected, especially when spread has occurred via the optic nerve or by dispersion of tumor cells in the cerebrospinal fluid. The latter typically gives rise to a thick accumulation of tumor cells in the meninges along the basilar surface of the brain and in the ventricles—a "tumor meningitis" (Fig. 8–635).

Typically in metastatic lesions, retinoblastoma appears much more highly malignant and less well differentiated than in the intraocular primary tumor. Rosettes, which are often so numerous and highly organized in the primary tumors, are typically very difficult to find and are poorly formed in metastatic lesions; fleurettes are not observed.

The solitary midline ectopic retinoblastomas observed in the pineal (Figs. 8–636 through 8–639) and in parasellar sites (Figs. 8–640 and 8–641) of patients with trilateral retinoblastoma (Bader, Meadows, Zimmerman, et al, 1982) have been confused with metastatic retinoblastoma, but in contrast with the latter, these tumors are solitary and not accompanied by other tumors as one would expect with metastatic disease (Bader et al, 1982; Brownstein, deChadarevian, Little, 1984; Easterbrook, Wehunt, Zimmerman, 1984, Jakobiec, Tso, Zimmerman, Danis, 1977). They often appear several years after the successful treatment of the intraocular tumors and may ex-

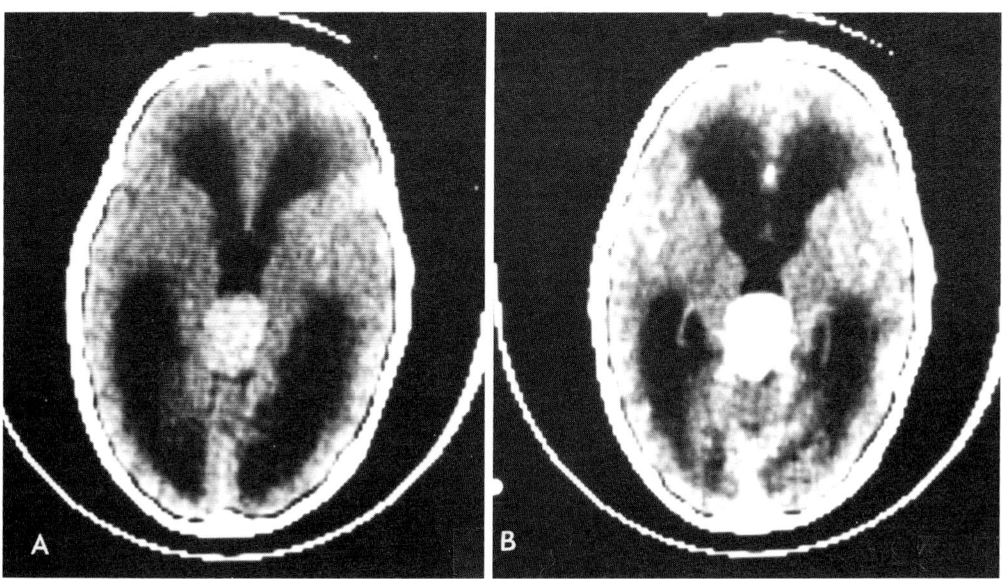

Figure 8–637. Pineal tumor demonstrated by computed tomography in a child who had had bilateral enucleations for retinoblastoma. The tumor has obstructed the flow of cerebrospinal fluid and produced a symmetric dilatation of the ventricles. *A,* Without contrast enhancement. *B,* With contrast enhancement. AFIP Neg. 81-2278. (From Zimmerman LE, Burns RP, Wankum G, et al: Trilateral retinoblastoma: Ectopic intracranial retinoblastoma associated with bilateral retinoblastoma. J Pediatr Ophthalmol Strab *19*:320–325, 1982.)

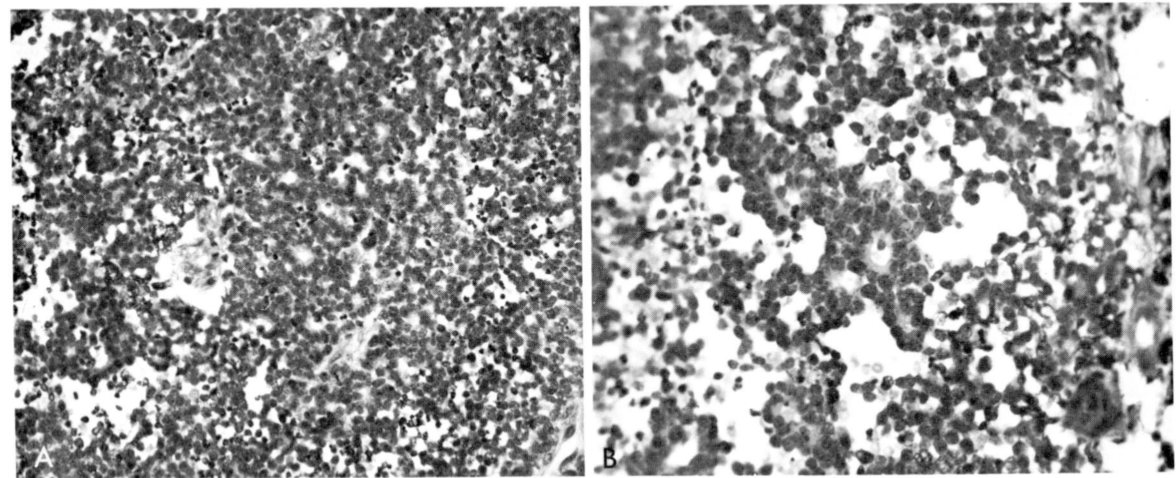

Figure 8–638. **Rosettes** are conspicuous in these fields **of the pineal tumor** shown in Figure 8–637. *A,* ×250. AFIP Neg. 81-18543. *B,* ×400. AFIP Neg. 81-18541.

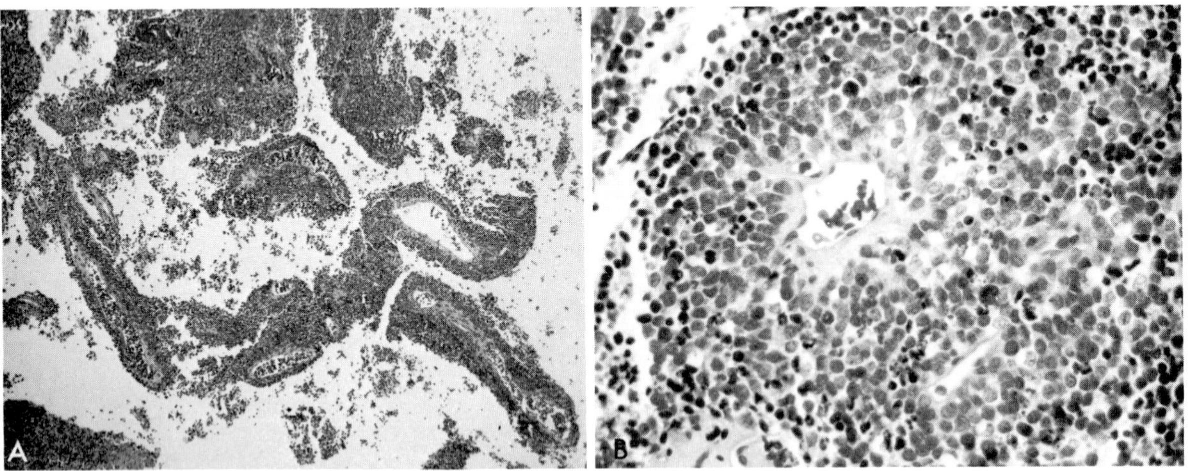

Figure 8–639. Poorly differentiated neuroblastic **pineal tumor** of a child who had been treated successfully with radiation for very small, multicentric, bilateral retinoblastomas. She had been considered cured when she developed her neurologic manifestations. The perivascular proliferation of undifferentiated neuroblastic cells resembles the characteristic pattern shown in Figures 8–581 and 8–582. *A,* ×60. AFIP Neg. 84-7823. *B,* ×400. AFIP Neg. 84-7826.

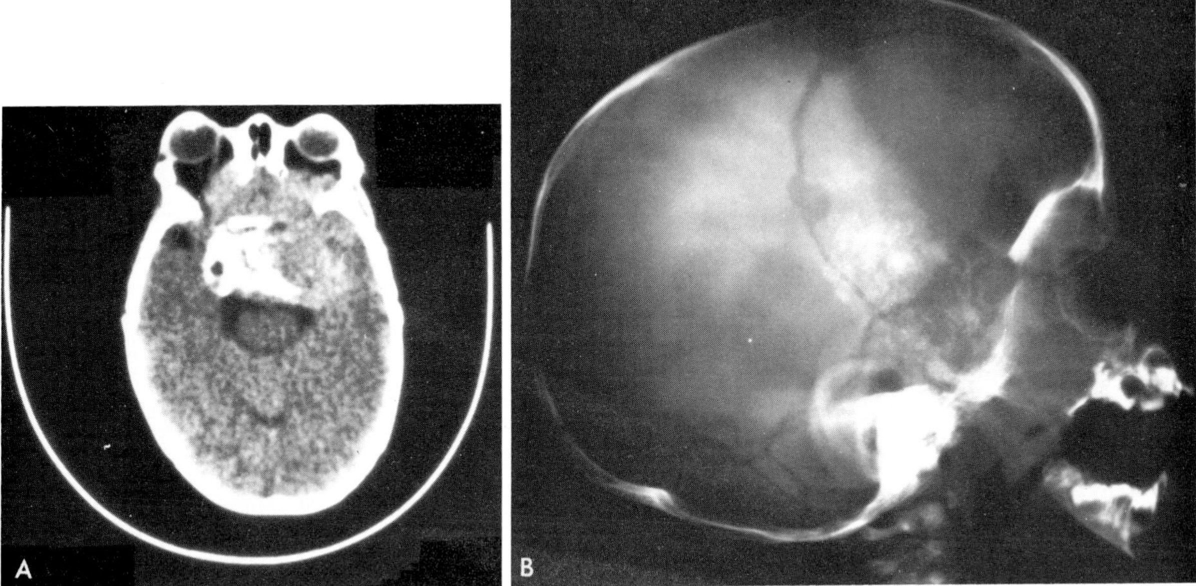

Figure 8–640. Huge **parasellar tumor** that destroyed the posterior wall of both orbits in an infant who had multiple small retinoblastomas in both eyes. *A,* CT scan. AFIP Neg. 82-861. *B,* Plain x-ray film: lateral view of mass. AFIP Neg. 82-861.

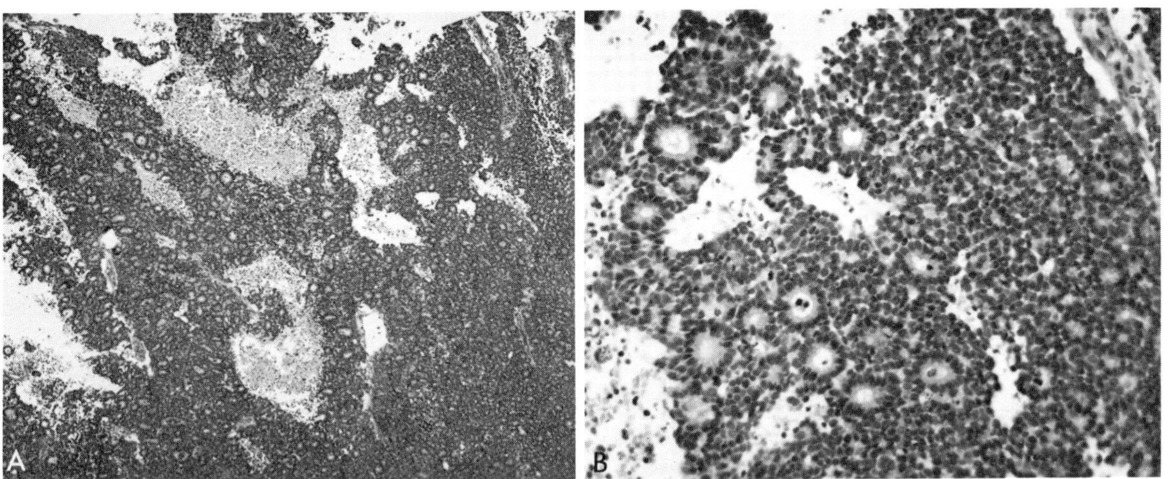

Figure 8–641. A. **Multiple rosettes observed in suprasellar tumor of** child with familial bilateral retinoblastoma. *A,* ×60. AFIP Neg. 81-18989. *B,* ×250. AFIP Neg. 81-18992.

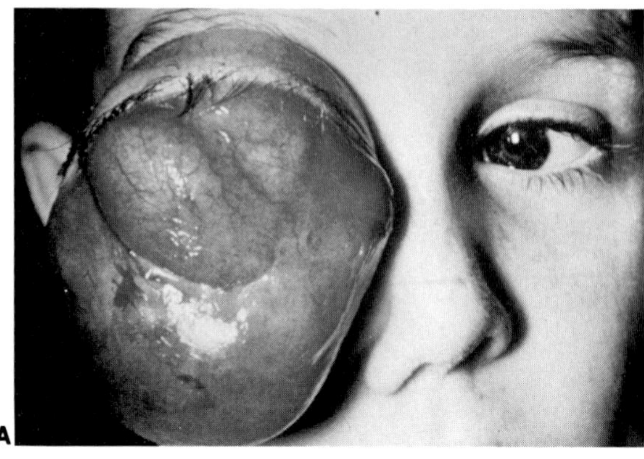

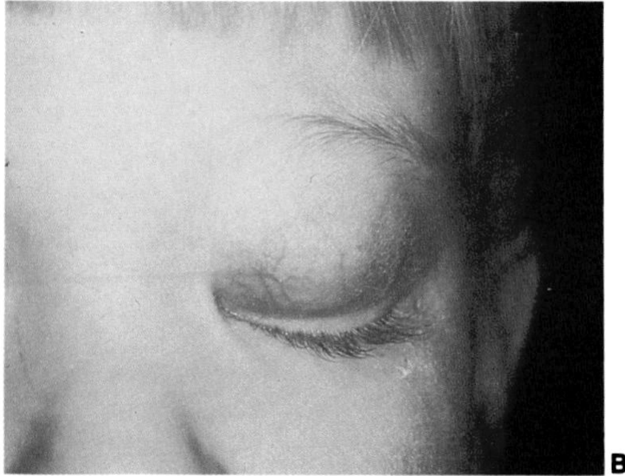

Figure 8–642. *A,* Massive orbital recurrence of retinoblastoma. AFIP Neg. 69-1767-3. *B,* Localized tumor in eyelid of anophthalmic orbit, probably representing a local metastasis rather than the usual type of recurrence that follows incomplete removal of tumor cells in the orbit or optic nerve.

hibit far greater differentiation with numerous rosettes, fleurettes, and individual cells exhibiting photoreceptor differentiation than one would expect to observe in a metastatic tumor.

Recurrence of retinoblastoma in the orbit following enucleation (Fig. 8–642,*A*) is almost always the result of tumor cells that were left untreated in the orbit. In some instances this may be the result of subclinical orbital involvement that also may have escaped histopathologic recognition, but much more frequently it is a consequence of incomplete removal of the orbital component or invasion of the optic nerve beyond the plane of surgical transection. Rarely, orbital recurrence may be the result of lymphatic or hematogenous spread to the bony wall or soft tissue of the orbit to the lids (Fig. 8–642,*B*).

Figure 8–643. Small **retinoblastoma** in macular area of an infant with esotropia. ×4. AFIP Neg. 260992-2. (From Zimmerman LE: Retinoblastoma, including a report of illustrative cases. Med Ann Dist Colum *38*:366–374, 1969.)

Ocular Complications

Ocular complications produced by retinoblastomas are many, and they affect virtually all ocular tissues and functions of the eye.

Visual loss from replacement of retina by neoplastic tissue, retinal detachment, or opacification of the media is observed to some degree in almost every case. Small tumors in the macular area (Fig. 8–643) as well as larger tumors may give rise to strabismus (Fig. 8–644).

Rubeosis iridis (Fig. 8–645) is very commonly present (Minoda, 1971; Spaulding, 1978; Walton, Grant, 1968), possibly attributable to an angiogenesis factor derived from the tumor itself or from anoxic, non-neoplastic retina. It may give rise to spontaneous hyphemas, and when it affects much of the anterior chamber angle, it may lead to a severe neovascular angle-closure glaucoma.

Secondary glaucoma is often present in advanced cases. In addition to rubeosis of the chamber angle, other common mechanisms are forward dislocation of the lens-iris diaphragm causing a pupillary block, accumulation of tumor cells in the anterior chamber obstructing the outflow channels, and inflammatory processes producing synechias.

Inflammation of the eye is usually attributable to necrosis of the tumor (Fig. 8–646), although many tumors with extensive necrosis are not significantly inflamed. The clinical signs of inflammation include those of a low grade endophthalmitis, iritis with hypopyon, keratitis, or a full-blown panophthalmitis with orbital cellulitis. When tumor cells spread into the anterior chamber, they may accumulate in the chamber angle, inferiorly, and be mistaken for a true hypopyon, a

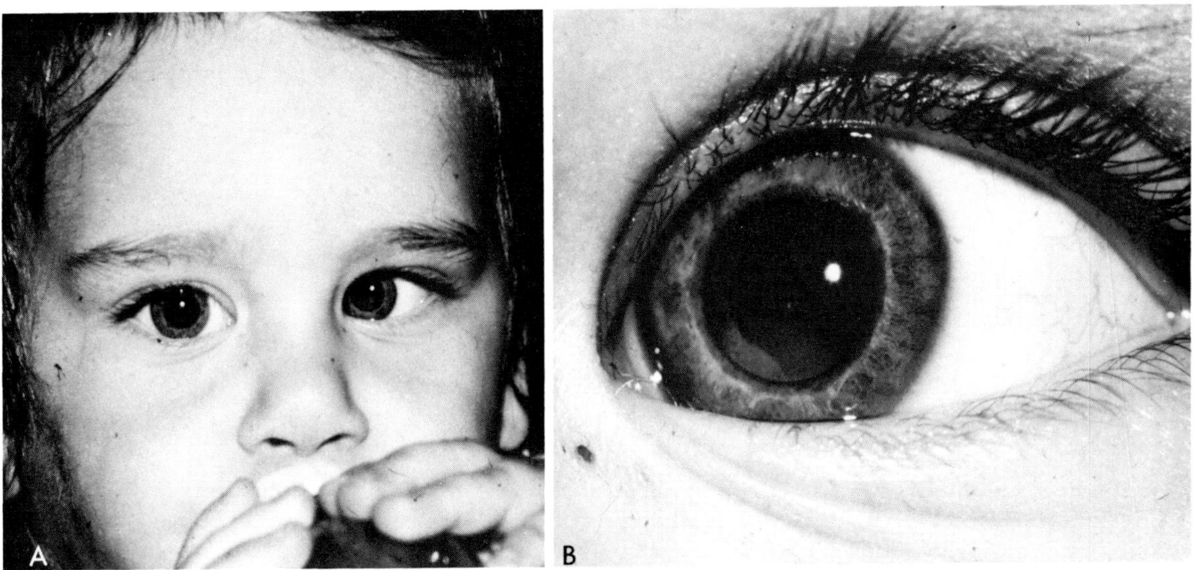

Figure 8–644. Combination of **esotropia and leukocoria** as presenting manifestations of a large retinoblastoma. AFIP Negs. 84-6092-1&2.

situation called pseudohypopyon (Fig. 8–647). In many such cases, however, cytologic study of the aqueous will reveal a mixture of inflammatory exudate and tumor cells (Fig. 8–648). In such cases, one often sees discrete nodular infiltrates in the iris, which may be misinterpreted as granulomatous lesions suggestive of tuberculosis, sarcoidosis, or juvenile xanthogranuloma (Fig. 8–613).

Corneal changes of great severity are seen mainly in very advanced stages in which large tumors have given rise to a combination of secondary glaucoma, hyphema, severe inflammation, and/or extraocular extension (Fig. 8–649). In such cases, the spectrum of corneal changes includes enlargement with loss of transparency, bullous keratopathy with formation of a pannus, bloodstaining, vascularization and scarring of the stroma, necrosis with ulceration, perforation, and extraocular extension of tumor through large areas of necrosis (Fig. 8–649,*B*).

Cataract formation is characteristically a late complication of advanced tumors that have produced one or more of the previously discussed complications.

Phthisis bulbi is another complication that is generally considered a late manifestation of advanced tumors that have produced severe endophthalmitis or panophthalmitis (Figs. 8–622

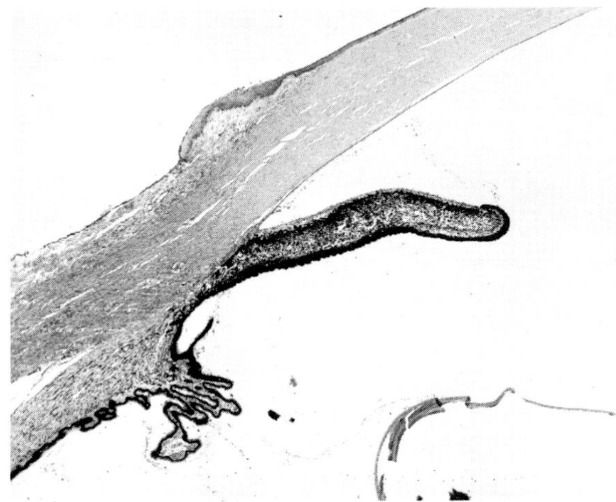

Figure 8–645. Rubeosis iridis with secondary angle-closure glaucoma in an eye enucleated for retinoblastoma. The anterior surface of the iris is covered by a prominent neovascular membrane, and there is ectropion of the pupillary margin. ×28. AFIP Neg. 57-343.

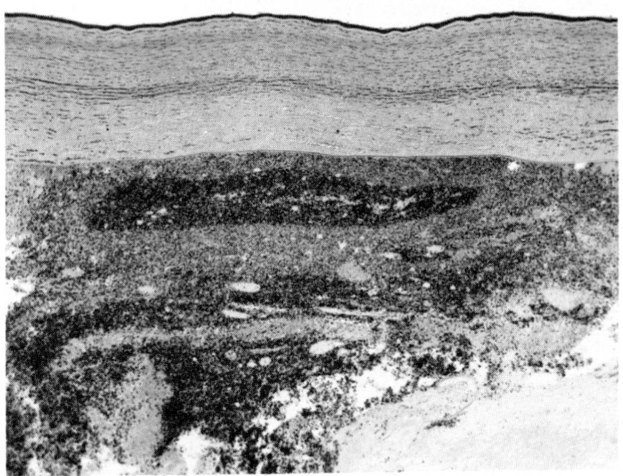

Figure 8–646. Necrotic tumor and inflammatory exudate fill the anterior chamber. There is a diffuse leukocytic infiltration of the corneal stroma. × 50. AFIP Neg. 60-7160.

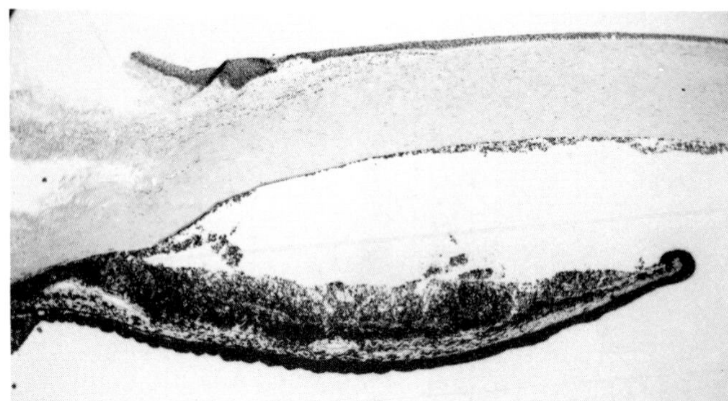

Figure 8–647. Retinoblastoma cells in the anterior chamber may be mistaken for inflammatory cells ("pseudohypopyon"). × 75. AFIP Neg. 60-7158.

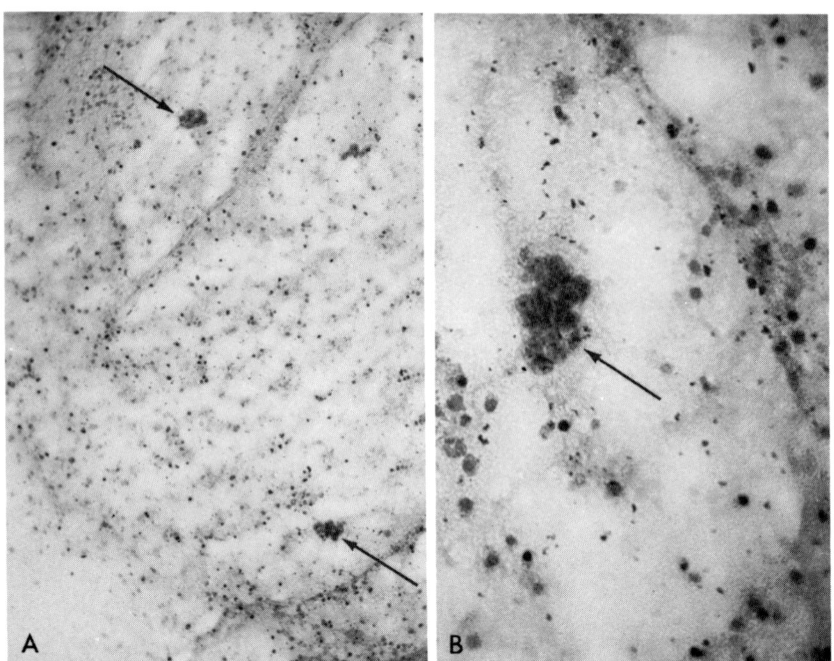

Figure 8–648. Cytologic study of material aspirated from the anterior chamber reveals inflammatory exudate containing clumps of neoplastic cells (arrows). *A,* × 85. *B,* × 280. AFIP Neg. 60-1269.

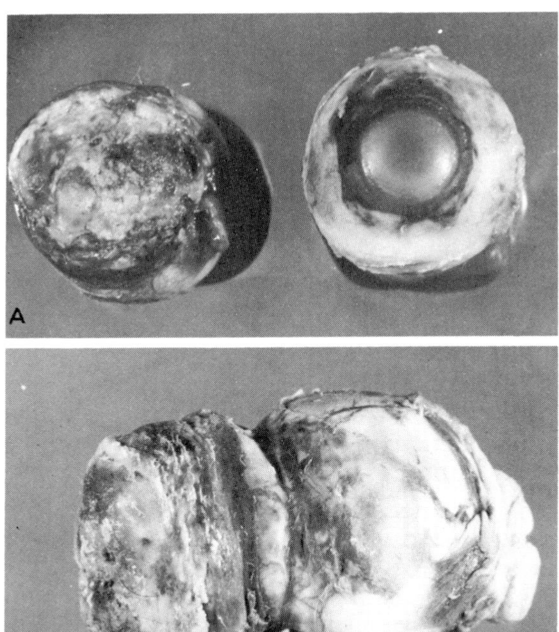

Figure 8–649. Advanced bilateral retinoblastoma. *A,* In the eye shown on the left, there was massive extraocular extension of tumor through the necrotic cornea; in the fellow eye, there was secondary glaucoma with blood-staining of the cornea. AFIP Neg. 63-2302. *B,* Profile view of the eye shown on left in A to demonstrate the massiveness of the transcorneal extension of the tumor. AFIP Neg. 63-2302-3.

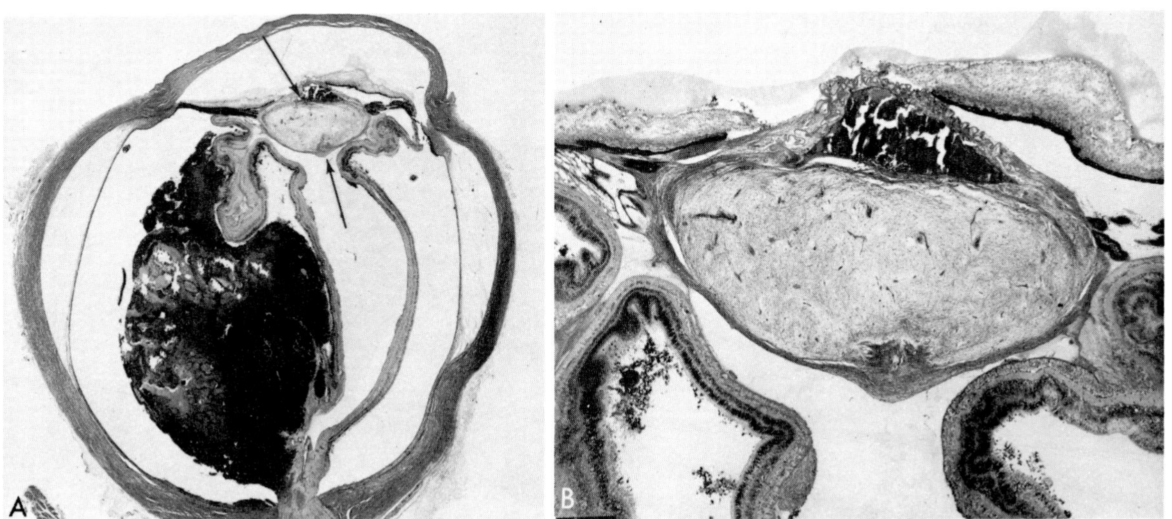

Figure 8–650. Retinoblastoma in an eye with persistence and hyperplasia of primary vitreous (PHPV). Arrows indicate a mass of vascularized mesenchymal tissue just behind a remnant of cataractous lens. *A,* × 4. AFIP Neg. 70-3918. *B,* × 16. AFIP Neg. 3921. (From Irvine AR, Albert DM, Sang DN: Retinal neoplasia and dysplasia. II. Retinoblastoma occurring with persistence and hyperplasia of the primary vitreous. Invest Ophthalmol Visual Sci *16*:403–407, 1977).

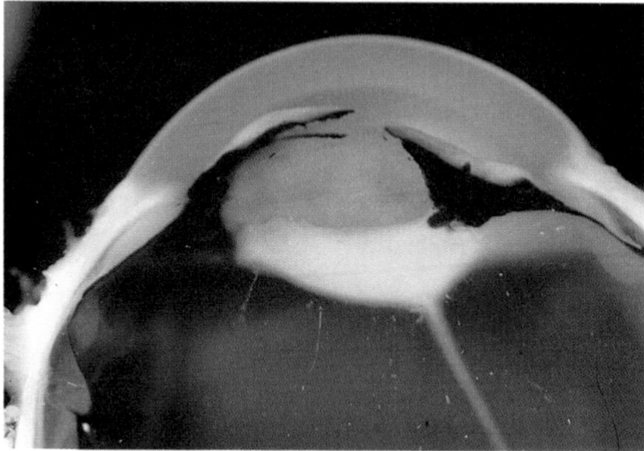

Figure 8–651. This retrolental mass, attributable to persistence and hyperplasia of primary vitreous with associated patent hyaloid vessels, was observed in an infant with a family history of retinoblastoma.

and 8–623), but one may see such phthisic eyes in remarkably young infants. Unexplained phthisis bulbi dating back to early infancy has been recognized in parents of children with retinoblastoma. In family studies of retinoblastoma patients, phthisis bulbi must always be regarded as a possible manifestation of total necrosis ("spontaneous regression") of retinoblastoma (Gallie, Phillips, Ellsworth, Abramson, 1982; Gangwar, Jain, Gupta, et al, 1982).

Associated Chromosomal Disorders and Other Abnormalities

Although chromosomal abnormalities are observed in only about 5 per cent of retinoblastoma patients, deletions of the long arm of chromosome 13 involving the 14 band have an almost constant association with retinoblastoma (Fig. 8–578,*A*), whereas other deletions of chromosome 13 that spare the 14 band are not associated with retinoblastoma. This important observation and its genetic implications are discussed in the earlier section on epidemiology and genetics.

Chromosomal aneuploidy and other chromosomal disorders, including trisomy 21 (Down's syndrome), have been associated with retinoblastoma but much less frequently than with deletions of the long arm of chromosome 13 (Schipper, 1980). Because of the frequency of trisomy 21, the number of retinoblastoma patients who have also had Down's syndrome is considered too few to represent more than a chance association (Dryja, personal communication).

Mental retardation was the only congenital defect associated with retinoblastoma more frequently than expected in a review of 1077 cases at the National Cancer Institute (Jensen, Miller, 1971), but other studies have established that most patients with retinoblastomas have normal or above average mentality. Therefore, the association of mental retardation with or without other developmental malformations and retinoblastoma suggests a chromosomal disorder for which appropriate studies are indicated.

Retinoblastoma may be observed in association with other heritable conditions, as in the case described by Friendly and Parks (1970). Their patient inherited congenital cataracts from one parent and bilateral retinoblastoma from the other parent who had had bilateral enucleations in infancy. The parents, who had met in a school for the blind, had not received appropriate genetic counseling.

Persistence and hyperplasia of the primary vitreous (PHPV) has been observed in a slightly microphthalmic eye containing a retinoblastoma (Fig. 8–650) (Irvine, Albert, Sang, 1977). In an-

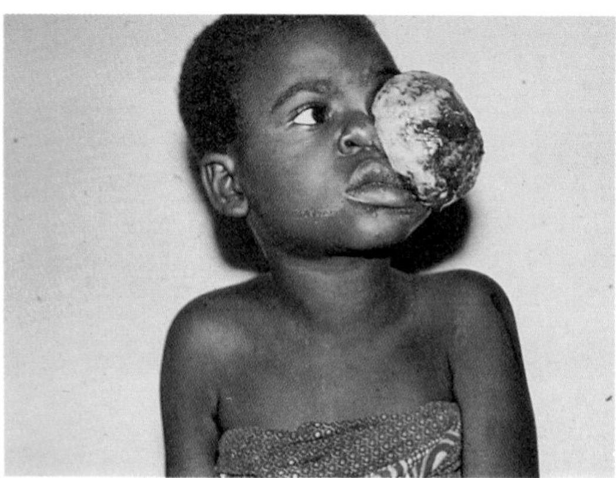

Figure 8–652. Advanced retinoblastoma with massive extraocular involvement in an African child. AFIP Neg. 68-7834-14. (From Zimmerman LE: Retinoblastoma, including a report of illustrative cases. Med Ann Dist Colum *38*:366–374, 1969.)

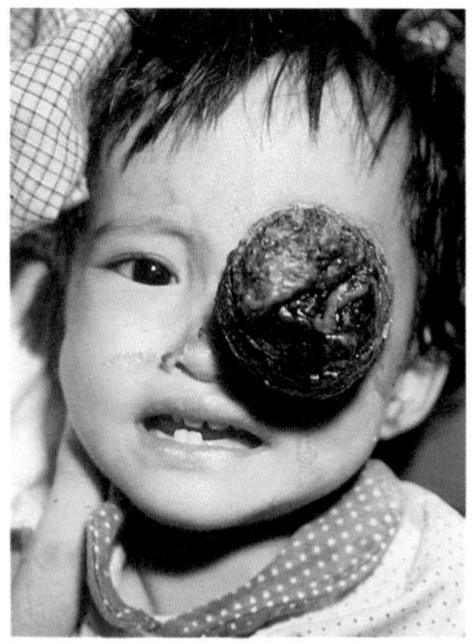

Figure 8–653. Advanced retinoblastoma with massive extraocular involvement in a Vietnamese child.

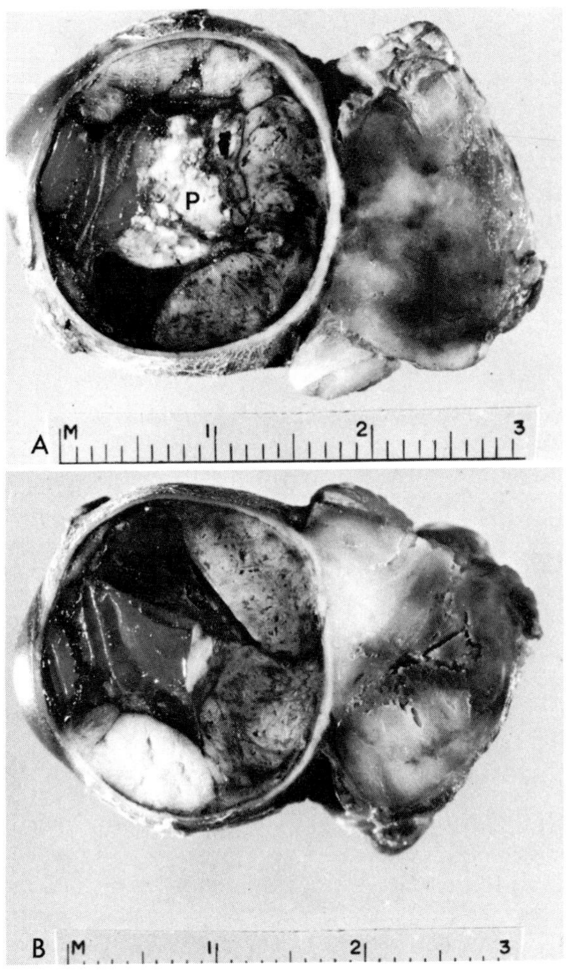

Figure 8–654. This **retinoblastoma** has diffusely invaded and greatly thickened the choroid and ciliary body, infiltrated through the sclera, and produced a huge orbital mass; the primary site of origin *(P)* in the retina in necrotic and calcified. Specimen received from Equatorial Africa. AFIP Neg. 56-2297.

other recently recorded case, an infant with bilateral leukocoria was found to have an exophytic retinoblastoma in one eye that had a total retinal detachment and PHPV in the other eye (Morgan, McLean, 1981). In still another case in which there was a family history of retinoblastoma, enucleation revealed PHPV in a microphthalmic eye with a large patent hyaloid artery (Fig. 8–651).

CLINICAL ASPECTS

The clinical manifestations of retinoblastoma vary with the stage of the disease at the time of clinical evaluation, and this in turn varies in different parts of the world. In underdeveloped regions, the typical case is so far advanced that some degree of extraocular extension is the rule and treatment is largely palliative (Figs. 8–634 and 8–652 through 8–655). In such cases, fungating masses presenting through corneal perforations, proptosis caused by posterior orbital invasion, buphthalmos from advanced secondary glaucoma, optic nerve invasion to the plane of surgical transection, and neurologic manifestations related to brain or leptomeningeal involvement are common. Before the turn of the century such manifestations were also commonly observed in Europe and North America (Figs. 8–656, 8–657, and 8–658), but with improvement in the general medical education of the public, the greater awareness on the part of physicians of the early signs of retinoblastoma, and the increased availability of eye care, there has been a great change in the typical presenting signs and symptoms. Neglected cases such as those illustrated in Figures 8–659 and 8–660 are now seldom seen in

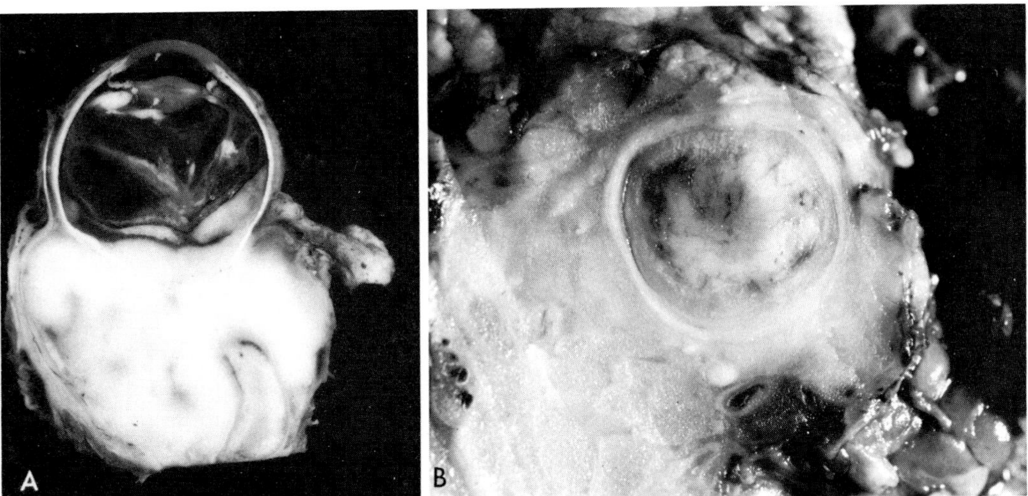

Figure 8–655. *A.* This **advanced retinoblastoma** with extensive choroidal, scleral, and optic nerve invasion had produced an orbital tumor that is much larger than the intraocular component. AFIP Neg. 71-6131-1. *B,* Transverse section near posterior edge of specimen shown in *A* reveals complete replacement of optic nerve by the tumor as well as extensive perineural orbital invasion. Specimen received from Equatorial Africa. AFIP Neg. 71-6131-5.

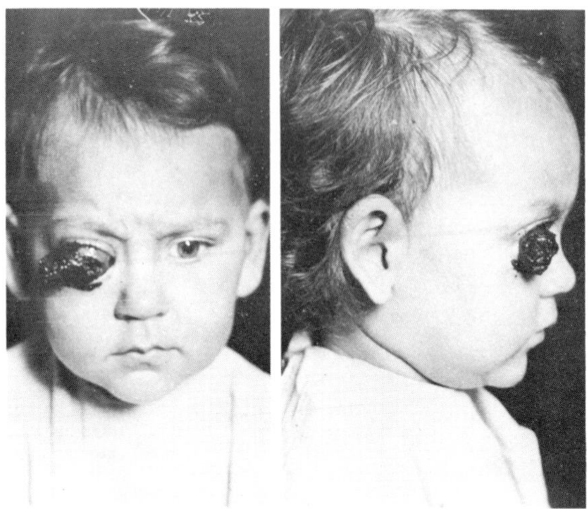

Figure 8–656. Advanced retinoblastoma from the old Wilmer Institute collection. Wilmer Neg. A-3353.

the United States. For example, in Shields' review of 60 consecutive new cases seen at Wills Eye Hospital between 1974 and 1978, there were no cases presenting with extraocular extension, buphthalmos, or manifestation of metastatic disease. In fact, in four cases there were no external signs, the tumor having been discovered on a routine examination (Shields, 1983).

Today, in most of North America and Europe, the great majority of cases are discovered as a result of someone, usually a parent, having become concerned about the abnormal appearance of one or both pupils or strabismus (Fig. 8–644). In Shields' review of 60 consecutive recent cases, 90 per cent had leukocoria, a convenient term used to indicate that the pupil is not black and that the fundus has an abnormal light reflex. Most often the pupil appears white, pink, or grayish-yellow. Strabismus was present in 35 per cent, with exotropia being more frequent than esotropia, an observation that is at variance with the experience of Reese (1976), who found esotropia to be more frequent. Other presenting signs observed in a very few cases included a dilated and fixed pupil, hyphema, and heterochromia iridis.

Leukocoria is most frequently the consequence of an intravitreal, often retrolental, mass that reflects the incidental light back through the pupil. A discrete intraretinal tumor situated at the posterior pole also may reflect light back, producing a white pupil. When light is reflected back from the intraocular tumor in a dark or semidarkened

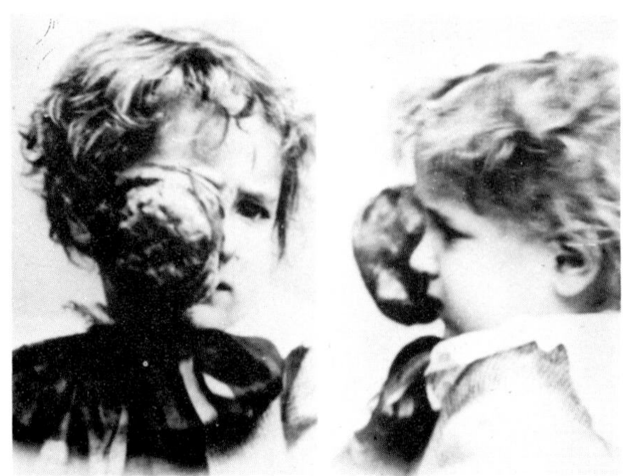

Figure 8–657. Advanced retinoblastoma from the de Schweinitz collection. AFIP Neg. 84-7564. (Courtesy of Dr. Daniel Albert.)

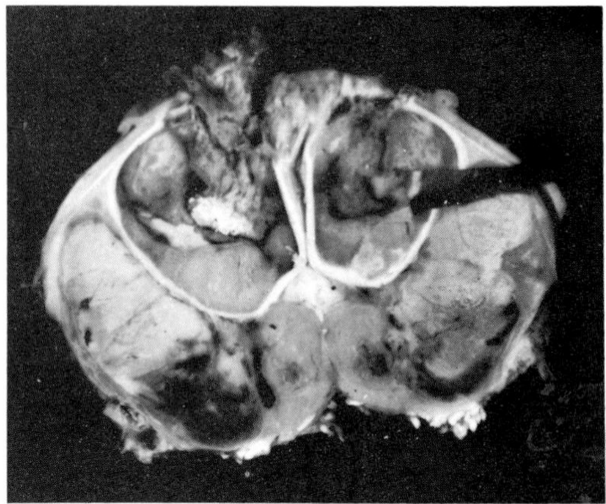

Figure 8–658. Old Army Medical Museum mounted specimen of historic interest. (a) It was the first surgical specimen as well as the first ophthalmologic case (AFIP Acc. No. 6) contributed to what is now a series of 2 million accessions at the AFIP; (b) until about 1960 the specimen had been on display in the Museum with an incorrect pathologic diagnosis; and (c) it illustrates the typically advanced state of retinoblastoma that was associated with nearly 100 per cent lethality in the early days of this century. The eye had been enucleated in April, 1917, in Washington, DC. AFIP Neg. 60-5429. (From Zimmerman LE: The Registry of Ophthalmic Pathology: Past, present, and future. Trans Am Acad Ophthalmol Otolaryngol *65*:51–113, 1961.)

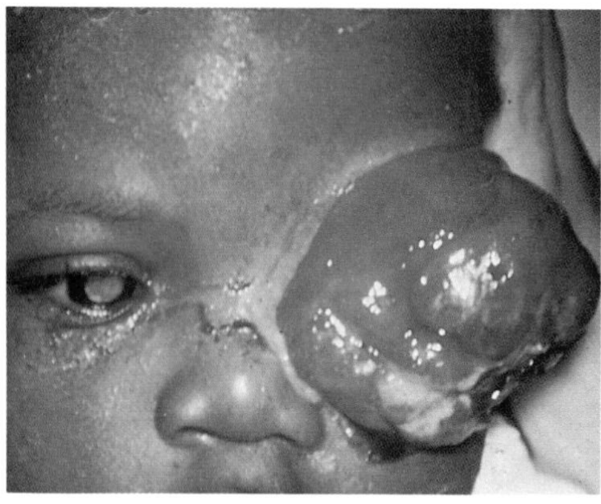

Figure 8–659. A neglected case of **bilateral retinoblastoma** observed in the United States. A year earlier a physician informed the parents that the pupillary abnormality they had observed in the right eye would disappear! (From Zimmerman LE: Retinoblastoma, including a report of illustrative cases. Med Ann Dist Colum *38*:366–374, 1969).

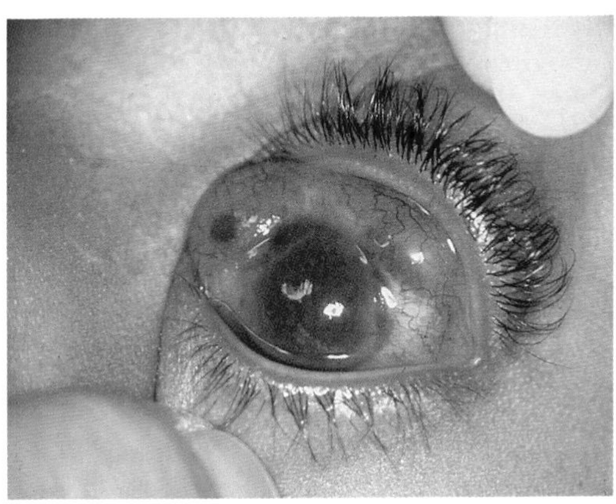

Figure 8–660. Subconjuctival extension of an **advanced retinoblastoma** in a child who had been treated for conjunctivitis until the eye became proptotic.

Table 8–11. MEDIAN AGES AND MORTALITY RATES OF 618 RETINOBLASTOMA PATIENTS RELATED TO DELAYS IN ENUCLEATION

	Prompt Diagnosis	Delayed Diagnosis
Total cases	526	92
Median age at diagnosis	23.2 months	23.9 months
Median age at enucleation	23.3 months	29.9 months
Mortality rate	25.5 %	55.4 %

(From Stafford WR, Yanoff M, Parnell B: Retinoblastoma initially misdiagnosed as primary ocular inflammation. Arch Ophthalmol *82*:771–773, 1969.)

room, the appearance may resemble that of the normal cat's eye reflex produced by the tapetum lucidum in certain animals. Obviously, all leukocorias are not indicative of a retinoblastoma as a broad spectrum of developmental, inflammatory, degenerative, and other pathologic conditions may be detected as a result of leukocoria. *Toxocara canis* infections, persistence and hyperplasia of the primary vitreous (PHPV), and Coats' disease account for over 60 per cent of such pseudoretinoblastomas (Shields, 1983).

In a review of 257 eyes enucleated because of the clinical suspicion of retinoblastoma during the period 1947 through 1960, Kogan and Boniuk (1962) found that about one fourth had non-neoplastic lesions such as Coats' disease, other retinal detachments, glaucoma, and so on. In a more recent study covering the period 1974 through 1980, Margo and Zimmerman (1983) found essentially the same frequency of pseudoretinoblastomas. Both these studies were based on cases in the Registry of Ophthalmic Pathology, which can be considered representative of the average state-of-the-art of ophthalmologic diagnosis in the United States. As might be expected, in those institutions where the staffs have had greater experience and specialization in ocular oncology, the frequency of simulating lesions observed in enucleated eyes is significantly less (Howard, 1969; Robertson and Campbell, 1977). To further document the value of a referral center for differential diagnosis, one can cite the experience reported from the Pediatric Tumor Clinic at the Eye Institute of Columbia-Presbyterian Hospital in New York City and from the Ocular Oncology Unit at Wills Eye Hospital. At the former, 53 per cent of 500 retinoblastoma suspects were judged to have other conditions (Howard, Ellsworth, 1965), and at the latter institution 56 per cent of 136 suspects were diagnosed as having simulating lesions (Shields, 1983).

The clinical and pathologic characteristics of ocular toxocariasis, PHPV, Coats' disease, and other pseudoretinoblastomas are detailed in other sections of these volumes.

Although the largest diagnostic problem concerns pseudoretinoblastomas, a more important though less frequent problem is the failure to suspect retinoblastoma when it is present. Stafford, Yanoff, and Parnell (1969), in their analysis of 618 histologically proved cases in which adequate clinical data were available, found that almost 15 per cent had been misdiagnosed initially. In 6.6 per cent, the initial diagnosis had led to delays in enucleation while treatment was for panophthalmitis, endophthalmitis, tuberculosis, or other forms of uveitis. In another 8.3 per cent, a variety of noninflammatory, non-neoplastic conditions had been diagnosed. These delays in diagnosis had typically led to delays in enucleation and were associated with a much greater mortality than in the cases in which a correct initial diagnosis had been followed promptly by enucleation (see Table 8–11).

When in addition to misleading inflammatory signs, the patient is a child older than 5 years who gives a history of recent injury to the symptomatic eye, the chances for failure to consider retinoblastoma in the differential diagnosis becomes very great.

ASSOCIATED MALIGNANCIES

The genetic abnormality that predisposes affected individuals to the development of multifocal retinoblastoma is one that is also associated with a number of other neoplasms, not only in retinoblastoma survivors but also in other members of their families. Almost all new nonocular malignancies in retinoblastoma patients carry a poor prognosis, as there have been very few survivors of these second tumors.

1. Radiation therapy has been used successfully in treatment of retinoblastoma since 1918 when Verhoeff had the second eye of one of his

patients treated with subcataractogenic doses of x-rays. Recently, Albert, McGhee, Seddon, and Weichselbaum (1984) reported the 60 year survival of this patient who developed multiple skin cancers of the lids on the irradiated side. Postirradiation cancers constitute the largest, best-known group of secondary tumors, accounting for 70 to 80 per cent of second tumors (Schipper, 1980). While they have been recognized for well over 35 years (Cahan, Woodward, Higinbotham, et al, 1948; Reese, Merriam, Martin, 1949; Zimmerman, Ingalls, 1957), it has only been rather recently that a genetic factor has been suspected in their pathogenesis. For many years the occurrence of these new tumors in previously irradiated tissues was thought to be solely attributable to excessive radiation to young, rapidly growing cells, and a genetic predisposition was not seriously considered.

Following Schoenberg's dictum "...to use x-ray or radium in massive doses without delay, on the better eye, as soon as a small mass is discovered in the retina..." (Forrest, 1962), many clinicians prescribed two or more courses of 7000 to 10,000 r orthovoltage x-ray administered through two or more portals. By 1961, Forrest had been able to identify 25 cases (16 previously unreported and 9 from the literature) in which tumors had developed in the irradiated tissues. Typically, in these cases, the new tumors were highly lethal neoplasms that appeared 4 to 27 years after treatment. Sarcomas of bone were most frequent but other sarcomas and carcinomas of the skin were also represented in Forrest's series. Following recognition of the magnitude of this and other complications of radiation therapy, over a period of many years a progressive reduction in the dosage levels and the development of supervoltage therapy ensued. Up to 1945, it was customary to deliver a tumor dose of 11,000 to 14,000 r by means of an ipsilateral direct field and a contralateral oblique field. In 1945, the orthovoltage tumor dose was reduced to 6000 to 6500 r, using a single direct lateral field. In the late 1950s kilovoltage was replaced by supervoltage therapy. Radiation therapists expressed great confidence that the combined effects of the change from orthovoltage to megavoltage therapy and the significantly lowered total dose would reduce the incidence of radiogenic osteosarcomas from over 30 per cent to less than 2 per cent (Sagerman, Cassady, Tretter, Ellsworth, 1969; Schipper, 1980).

In many centers the use of triethylene melamine (TEM) was employed along with the reduced levels of radiation. Unfortunately, new tumors continued to develop with regularity and, strangely, after shorter latent periods than had been observed in the earlier cases (Abramson, Ellsworth, Zimmerman, 1976; Abramson, Ellsworth, Kitchin, Tung, 1984). Schipper (1980) has discussed the possibility that TEM may act as a carcinogenic drug. He pointed out that the age at first exposure to chemical carcinogens has been shown to be an important risk factor and that bilateral retinoblastoma patients, who are typically treated during the first year of life, might be especially susceptible to the "carcinogenicity of anticancer drugs."

Until the 1970s, virtually every new malignancy that arose in a survivor of treatment for retinoblastoma met the criteria for a diagnosis of radiation-induced neoplasia, including the two most important: very high doses of radiation and a long latent interval (mean of 11 years) between completion of therapy and the appearance of the new tumor (Abramson et al, 1984).

In 1948, Cahan, Woodward, Higinbotham, and coworkers concluded from their extensive review of the literature and large personal experience that development of sarcomas in irradiated bone is an uncommon sequel. It is interesting that one of their 11 cases followed treatment for retinoblastoma. Several recent papers have also stressed that, in general, postirradiation sarcomas of bone are very rare (Coia, Fazekas, Kramer, 1980; Tountas, Fornasier, Harwood, Leong, 1979; Weatherby, Dahlin, Irvins, 1981). In striking contrast, however, are the facts that over 10 per cent of patients who have survived treatment for bilateral retinoblastoma have developed a second nonocular tumor (Abramson, Ellsworth, Zimmerman, 1976), and 20 per cent of all postirradiation sarcomas have been in patients treated for retinoblastoma, a relatively uncommon cancer (Abramson, personal communication). Another curious discrepancy is the fact that in the series of 80 cases recorded by Abramson et al in 1976, 13 patients developed new tumors in the field of radiation after comparatively low doses (average of 3631 rads). Of prime significance is the fact that 78 of the 80 patients in that series were known to have had bilateral (i.e., genetically determined) retinoblastoma. In a more recent analysis Abramson, Ellsworth, Kitchin, and Tung (1984) reported that 89 of 94 patients with second tumors had been treated for bilateral retinoblastoma. Furthermore, one of the five tumors that developed in patients who had received no radiation arose in what would have been considered the field of irradiation had they been so treated. A life table analysis of patients whose second tumors had developed out of the field of irradiation and of those who had received no radiation therapy indicated that the incidence of new tumors increases with length of survival: 10 per cent at 10 years, 30 per cent at 20 years, and 68 per cent at 32 years. Abramson and coworkers concluded, therefore, that even without radiation or chemotherapy 70 per cent of survivors of heritable retinoblastoma would develop second tumors eventually.

Obviously, therefore, we are faced with a very complex problem in which multiple factors appear to play a role in the pathogenesis of post-irradiation tumors in survivors of retinoblastoma. The most significant of these are (1) genetic hypersusceptibility to the development of sarcomas and other malignancies in general, (2) an especially heightened degree of hypersusceptibility of the orbital and periorbital tissues to this genetic predisposition, and (3) genetic hypersensitivity to such oncogenic agents as ionizing radiation and perhaps chemotherapeutic agents.

One curious and as yet unexplained observation is that with the reduction in radiation dosage and the switch from orthovoltage to supervoltage therapy, there has been a significant increase of new tumors that have appeared after a short latent period. Schipper (1980) has predicted that megavoltage therapy should not induce osteosarcomas but that radiogenic tumors of other types are to be expected.

Support for the thesis that patients with heritable retinoblastoma have a particular susceptibility to develop other malignant tumors upon exposure to radiation is provided by reports that cultured fibroblasts from patients with heritable retinoblastoma are more susceptible to the effects of radiation when compared with either normal controls or fibroblasts from patients with nonheritable retinoblastoma (Gallie, 1980; Nove, Weichselbaum, Nichols, et al, 1980; Schipper, 1980). As Nove and coworkers pointed out, the increased incidence of radiogenic malignancies and the shortened latency in patients with heritable retinoblastoma, coupled with the absence of any perturbation in their immune system, make retinoblastoma an excellent model for the study of the relationship between what is perceived to be a defective DNA repair process and tumorigenesis.

In addition to osteogenic sarcomas, tumors arising in the field of irradiation include chondrosarcomas, a variety of soft tissue sarcomas, carcinomas of the upper respiratory passages and nasopharynx, and malignant melanomas and carcinomas of the skin, including sebaceous carcinomas of the lids. We have even seen three examples of one of the rarest of all orbital tumors —leiomyosarcoma—following radiation therapy in patients who had been treated for bilateral retinoblastoma (Folberg, Cleasby, Flanagan, et al, 1983).

2. Second cancers arisen outside the field of irradiation have been recognized with increasing frequency since the reports of Jensen and Miller (1971) and Abramson, Ellsworth, and Zimmerman (1976). The latter study, based on 84 nonocular new cancers in 80 survivors of retinoblastoma, included 18 cases in which the new tumor arose outside the field of radiation. Of these, three patients had received no radiation at all. The most common of these new cancers were osteosarcomas of the lower extremities. Subsequently, François (1977) and Meadows, D'Angio, Mike, et al (1977) reported similar observations. According to Schipper (1980), at least half of the nonradiogenic new primaries have been osteogenic sarcomas, and Abramson et al (1976) have estimated that the frequency of osteogenic sarcoma of the femur in retinoblastoma patients is increased to 500 times the expected rate. Schimke, Lowman, and Dowan (1974) reported a family in which two siblings with bilateral retinoblastoma subsequently developed osteogenic sarcomas of the femur. Abramson, Ellsworth, and Kitchin (1980) also have recorded the occurrence of an osteogenic sarcoma of the humerus that arose 6 years after cobalt plaque treatment of the right eye of a child whose left eye had been enucleated. Other sarcomas and carcinomas arisen outside the field of radiation have also appeared. Abramson and his colleagues believe that with longer follow-up data on survivors of heritable retinoblastoma, the frequency of second cancers unrelated to radiation will increase to 50 per cent.

Included among the 80 cases in the study of Abramson, Ellsworth, and Zimmerman (1976), were 5 in which a clear clinicopathologic distinction between an exceptionally late metastasis from retinoblastoma and an independent, new, undifferentiated neuroblastic neoplasm could not be made. The average latent period for the appearance of the new tumor in these cases was 9.2 years, suggesting strongly that these were new primaries rather than metastases from retinoblastomas, which very rarely prove lethal after a latent period of more than 2 years. It is conceivable that panels of monoclonal antibodies might be used to assist the pathologist in this difficult diagnostic problem as has been suggested for the differential diagnosis between neuroblastoma and lymphoblastic disorders (Kemshead, Fritschy, Goldman, et al, 1983). Using hybridoma-produced monoclonal antibodies, Char, Wood, Huhta, et al (1984) showed that retinoblastoma cell lines established from different tumors share retinoblastoma-specific antigens, but much remains to be determined before practical use can be made of this potentially valuable method. For example, we need to know how sensitive the technique is in differentiating among retinoblastoma, neuroblastoma, and pineoblastoma, and whether the same tumor-associated antigens are present in metastases as in the primary tumors.

3. Ectopic retinoblastoma in the pineal or in a parasellar location ("trilateral retinoblastoma"). For many years, pathologists have been confronted periodically with the diagnostic problem

posed by a solitary midline intracranial tumor histologically consistent with retinoblastoma in a child who had a past history of retinoblastoma. In those cases in which the retinoblastomas had been small and successfully treated and in which there was a latent period of several years before the development of symptoms of the brain tumor, it seemed very unlikely that the latter could represent a metastasis, especially in the absence of such poor prognostic signs as extraocular extension, orbital recurrence, or optic nerve invasion, and with no other evidence of metastatic disease. When such solitary midline intracranial tumors were encountered in the pineal (Figs. 8–636 and 8–637), as most of them have been, the tendency was to consider them as pineoblastomas, unrelated to retinoblastomas. When such intracranial tumors were discovered either concurrently with or soon after treatment of the retinoblastoma, they would be judged as metastatic.

Jakobiec, Tso, Zimmerman, and Danis (1977) recorded two exemplary cases, one in which a pineal tumor appeared more than 2 years after successful treatment of bilateral retinoblastoma (Fig. 8–636), and one in which clinical investigations made because of a parasellar tumor in an infant led to the discovery of an unsuspected tiny retinoblastoma. These and another previously recorded case from the series of Jensen and Miller (1971) were included among those that were the basis of the reports of Bader, Miller, Meadows, et al (1980) and Bader, Meadows, Zimmerman, et al (1982), in which they proposed the term "*trilateral retinoblastoma*" for such associations of a solitary midline intracranial tumor with heritable retinoblastoma. Although this new diagnostic term is admittedly inappropriate for the rare case in which retinoblastoma is unilateral, almost without exception the retinoblastoma has been either bilateral or familial. If these cases had represented late metastases rather than new, independent primaries, one would have expected many more cases to have been sporadic unilateral retinoblastomas since the latter are twice as frequent as heritable retinoblastomas. Furthermore, metastases to the brain rarely present as solitary midline tumors.

These ectopic retinoblastomas in the brain often exhibit a remarkable degree of differentiation with the formation of rosettes or fleurettes (Figs. 8–638, 8–639, and 8–641). As it is extremely unusual to observe more than a very rare, poorly differentiated rosette in metastatic retinoblastoma, the degree of differentiation observed in about half of these brain tumors favors their being independent primary tumors (i.e., ectopic retinoblastomas).

The question of these brain tumors representing the chance occurrence of pineoblastoma and retinoblastoma was also addressed by Bader and colleagues. Calculations based on the known very low frequencies of retinoblastoma and pineoblastoma in the United States excluded beyond any doubt the possibility that this was a chance occurrence. That eight were discovered in the United States in a 13 year period was far too many to be accounted for by random association. Two other considerations added support to this conclusion: (1) if this had been a chance association, one would have expected most of the retinoblastomas to have been unilateral and sporadic; and (2) too many of the brain tumors exhibited retinoblastomatous differentiation.

Retinoblastomatous differentiation has been observed in pineal tumors of patients who have not had known retinoblastoma or a family history of retinoblastoma. Stefanko and Manschot (1979) recently recorded and beautifully illustrated a case in which classic Flexner-Wintersteiner rosettes and fleurettes, indistinguishable from those described and illustrated by Tso, Fine, and Zimmerman, (1970), were conspicuous (Fig. 8–590). Such pineal tumors are very rare, however, and only a very few descriptions of Flexner-Wintersteiner rosettes in pinealomas have appeared (Zimmerman, Burns, Wankum, et al, 1982).

The pineal has long been regarded as a "third eye" or "median eye" because in primitive reptiles and certain amphibia its histologic appearance resembles an eye (Warwick, 1976), and it has photoreceptor activity (Wurtman, Moskowitz, 1977). In most higher species, the pineal has lost most of its structural and functional similarities to a photoreceptor organ, but in guinea pigs, the pineal shares the retina-specific S antigen (Kalsow, Wacker, 1977). Furthermore, the pineal responds to immunization with retinal S antigen in rats and guinea pigs (Kalsow, Wacker, 1979; Mochizuki, Charley, et al, 1983). Zimmerman and Tso (1975) were able to demonstrate morphologic evidence of transient photoreceptor differentiation in the neonatal rat pineal. It is suspected that, in the infant pineal and more rarely elsewhere in the parasellar region, cells with latent potential for development as "retinoblasts" are capable of being affected by the same mutagens responsible for multicentric retinoblastoma in the retina. The comparatively small numbers of such retinoblastic cells in the pineal and their even smaller numbers in the parasellar tissues would account for the relative rarity of ectopic retinoblastomas, even in genotypically affected individuals.

Since the publications of Bader and coworkers, additional reports of cases of trilateral retinoblastomas have appeared (Brownstein, de Chadarevian, Little, 1984; Donoso, Shields, Felberg, 1981; Dudgeon, Lee, 1984; Judisch, Patil, 1981; Zimmerman, Burns, Wankim, et al, 1982). Zimmerman (1984) has recently summarized information based on all available published and unpublished data that he has collected. Brownstein et al (1984) and Dudgeon and Lee (1984) have recorded examples of cases that in the past had been considered metastatic retinoblastoma to the brain. With the introduction of CT scanning it is now possible to identify ectopic retinoblastomas in the pineal (Fig. 8–637) or in a parasellar (Fig. 8–640) location. With increasing awareness of this new syndrome by radiologists, neurosurgeons, and pathologists as well as by ophthalmologists, one must anticipate a rising incidence of trilateral retinoblastoma based on improved diagnosis.

4. Malignant tumors in other family members of retinoblastoma patients provide additional support for the thesis that the genetic abnormality leading to the development of multicentric retinoblastomas may be expressed by the development of other tumors, the most conspicuous of which is, again, osteosarcoma. Several striking examples were provided by Gordon (1974) in his paper on family studies in retinoblastoma. In one family, a man who had had unilateral retinoblastoma had one child with bilateral retinoblastoma, another with unilateral retinoblastoma, and a third with osteogenic sarcoma. He subsequently developed bronchogenic carcinoma and his brother had a small cell cancer of the liver of uncertain type. Another remarkable pedigree was one in which an apparently normal man fathered two children with retinoblastoma by different mothers and then developed osteogenic sarcoma of the femur at age 38. The bone tumor was discovered at the Mayo Clinic when he was there mainly for an ophthalmoscopic examination seeking evidence of a regressed retinoblastoma. None was found, but because the man was complaining of discomfort and swelling of his knee, a radiograph revealed the osteogenic sarcoma of the distal femur.

Chan and Pratt (1977) described their findings in the extraordinary family of a survivor of bilateral retinoblastoma who developed multiple osteosarcomas of the extremities. Of 36 family members through six generations, 10 relatives on the maternal side had had malignant tumors, mainly genitourinary cancers, but the patient's mother had had unilateral retinoblastoma and her great-great-grandfather had died of a bone cancer of the jaw.

Smith (1974) mentioned an interesting family in his fine paper dealing primarily with spontaneous regression of retinoblastomas. A man in his early fifties was examined ophthalmoscopically because he had had one son who died of bilateral retinoblastoma and another who had survived retinoblastoma only to die of a tibial sarcoma. The ophthalmoscopic examination revealed 5 "spontaneously arrested" retinoblastomas involving both eyes. Shortly thereafter the patient died with carcinomas of the bladder and bronchus in his 54th year.

PROGNOSIS

Many risk factors affect prognosis. In an analysis of over 500 cases of retinoblastoma treated by enucleation, Kopelman and McLean (1983) reported that 7 of 31 possible risk factors were independently associated with mortality: invasion of optic nerve, invasion of sclera, bilaterality, invasion of choroid, large size, basophilic staining of vessels, and incorrect clinical diagnosis. When the data were evaluated by multivariate analysis and compared with univariate analysis, bilaterality was the only variable that proved to be more significantly associated with a fatal outcome, suggesting that bilaterality is related to death for reasons unrelated to the primary tumor. The investigators suspected that new intracranial primary tumors might have been responsible in some of the cases.

From the clinical point of view, the most important predictor, by far, is the degree of progression of the tumor at the time of its discovery. For the purpose of this presentation, risk factors will be grouped in four categories indicative of most favorable, intermediate, and poorest prognosis *for life*. This discussion, based on histologic findings, should not be confused with the Reese-Ellsworth (1963) prognostic classification, which was designed to provide clinical guidelines for planning appropriate therapy.*

In cases of bilateral retinoblastoma, prognosis is judged mainly on the basis of the eye exhibiting features indicative of the least favorable prognosis. Bilaterality in itself is a bad risk factor because of its genetic implications and the associated high frequency of new nonocular cancers (Kopelman, McLean, 1983).

1. Most favorable prognosis:
   a. Cytologically benign retinocytomas, regardless of size, are considered to have no potential for metastasis.
   b. Small tumors confined to the retina, with no evidence of seeding into the vitreous or into the subretinal space and no involvement of the optic disk, carry a very favorable prognosis.
   c. Larger tumors that are also still confined to the retina but which may have seeded cells into the vitreous or subretinal space

*In this discussion, favorable and unfavorable are used entirely with respect to life expectancy, whereas in the Reese-Ellsworth classification these adjectives relate to expectancy for control with conservative measures, mainly radiation therapy.

also carry a favorable prognosis if they have not invaded the optic nerve or uveal tract.

d. Highly differentiated tumors exhibiting many well-formed Flexner-Wintersteiner rosettes in almost all viable areas, with or without fleurettes, carry a favorable prognosis, especially when they are also associated with features 1b and 1c.

2. An intermediate group with relatively favorable prognosis includes the following:

   a. Tumors that have invaded the optic disk but have not infiltrated behind the lamina cribosa,
   b. Tumors that have minimally invaded the uveal tract,
   c. Large tumors that are composed mainly of undifferentiated cells exhibiting marked mitotic activity, but showing no invasion of optic disc or uvea, and
   d. Flat, diffusely infiltrating tumors.

3. An intermediate group with relatively unfavorable prognosis includes the following:

   a. Tumors that have invaded the optic nerve beyond the lamina cribrosa but not to the plane of surgical transection,
   b. Tumors that have invaded the uvea more massively,
   c. Tumors that have seeded onto the iris, cornea, or anterior chamber angle,
   d. Large tumors that fill the eye,
   e. Tumors that have produced secondary glaucoma as a consequence of:
      (1) neovascularization of anterior chamber angle,
      (2) pupillary block,
      (3) inflammatory complications,
      (4) intraocular hemorrhage, and
   f. Tumors that are totally undifferentiated, exhibiting marked cytologic atypia and mitotic activity.

4. Worst prognosis. The following are characteristics associated with 80 to 100 per cent lethality:

   a. Distant metastasis,
   b. Malignant cells demonstrable in cerebrospinal fluid,
   c. Regional (preauricular and/or cervical) lymph node involvement,
   d. Extension into optic nerve to plane of surgical transection and/or into leptomeninges,
   e. Trans-scleral extension into the orbit, and
   f. Associated intracranial ectopic retinoblastoma ("trilateral retinoblastoma"), even though the intraocular tumors might have features indicative of a favorable prognosis.

References

Aaby AA, Price RL, Zakov ZN: Spontaneously regressing retinoblastomas, retinoma, or retinoblastoma group 0. Am J Ophthalmol *96*:315–320, 1983.

Abiose A, Adido J: Childhood malignancies of the eye and orbit in Northern Nigeria. Cancer, in press.

Abramson DH: Retinoma, retinocytoma, and the retinoblastoma gene. Arch Ophthalmol *101*:1517–1518, 1983.

Abramson DH, Ellsworth RM, Kitchin FD: Osteogenic sarcoma of the humerus after cobalt plaque treatment for retinoblastoma. Am J Ophthalmol *90*:374–376, 1980.

Abramson DH, Ellsworth RM, Kitchin FD, Tung G: Second non-ocular tumors in retinoblastoma survivors: Are they radiation induced? Ophthalmology, in press.

Abramson DH, Ellsworth RM, Zimmerman LE: Nonocular cancer in retinoblastoma survivors. Trans Am Acad Ophthalmol Otolaryngol *81*:454–456, 1976.

Abramson DH, Ronner HJ, Ellsworth RM: Nonocular cancer in nonirradiated retinoblastoma. Am J Ophthalmol *87*:624–627, 1979.

Albert DM, Craft J, Sang DN: Ultrastructure of retinoblastoma: Transmission and scanning electron microscopy, *in* Jakobiec FA (ed): Ocular and Adnexal Tumors. Birmingham, AL, Aesculapius Publishing Company, 1978, pp 157–171.

Albert DM, McGhee CNJ, Seddon JM, Weichselbaum RR: Development of additional primary tumors after 62 years in the first patient with retinoblastoma cured by radiation therapy. Am J Ophthalmol *97*:189–196, 1984.

Albert DM, Reid TW: RNA-directed DNA polymerase activity in retinoblastoma: Report of its presence and possible significance. Trans Am Acad Ophthalmol Otolaryngol *77*:630–640, 1973.

Albert DM, Robinson N: Wardrop Lecture, 1974. James Wardrop: A brief review of his life and contributions. Trans Ophthalmol Soc UK *94*:892–908, 1974.

Albert DM, Sang DN, Craft JL: Clinical and histopathologic observations regarding cell death and tumor necrosis in retinoblastoma. Jap J Ophthalmol *22*:358–374, 1978.

Andersen SR, Jensen OA: Retinoblastoma with necrosis of central retinal artery and vein and partial spontaneous regression. Acta Ophthalmol *52*:183–193, 1974.

Arlett CF, Harcourt SA: Survey of radiosensitivity in a variety of human cell strains. Cancer Res *40*:926–932, 1980.

Bader JL, Meadows AT, Zimmerman LE, et al: Bilateral retinoblastoma with ectopic intracranial retinoblastoma: Trilateral retinoblastoma. Cancer Genet Cytogenet *5*:203–213, 1982.

Bader JL, Miller RW, Meadows AT, et al: Trilateral retinoblastoma. Lancet *2*:582–583, 1980.

Balaban G, Gilbert F, Nichols W, et al: Abnormalities of chromosome 13 in retinoblastoma from individuals with normal constitutional karyotypes. Cancer Genet Cytogenet *6*:213–221, 1982.

Benedict WF, Murphree AL, Banerjee A, et al: Patient with chromosome deletion: Evidence that the retinoblastoma gene is a recessive cancer gene. Science *219*:973–975, 1983.

Bishop JO, Madsen EC: Retinoblastoma: Review of current status. Surv Ophthalmol *19*:342–366, 1975.

Boniuk M, Bishop DW: Oligodendroglioma of the retina. Surv Ophthalmol *13*:284–289, 1969.

Boniuk M, Zimmerman LE: Spontaneous regression of retinoblastoma. Int Ophthalmol Clin *2*:525–542, 1962.

Brownstein S, deChadarevian J-P, Little JM: Trilateral retinoblastoma: Report of two cases. Arch Ophthalmol *102*:257–262, 1984.

Burnier M Jr, McLean IW, Zimmerman LE: Viability of retinoblastoma cells: Spatial relationship to blood vessels. Invest Ophthalmol Vis Sci, in press.

Cahan WG, Woodward HQ, Higinbotham NL, et al: Sarcoma arising in irradiated bone; Report of 11 cases. Cancer *1*:3–29, 1948.

Carbajal UM: Metastasis in retinoblastoma. Am J Ophthalmol *48*:47–69, 1959.

Cavenee WK, Dryja TP, Phillips RA, et al: Expression of recessive alleles by chromosomal mechanisms in retinoblastoma. Nature *305*:779–784, 1983.

Chan H, Pratt CB: A new cancer syndrome? A spectrum of malignant and benign tumors including retinoblastoma, carcinoma of the bladder and other genitourinary tumors, thyroid adenoma, and a probable case of multifocal osteosarcoma. J Natl Cancer Inst *58*:205–207, 1977.

Char DH, Wood IS, Huhta K, et al: Retinoblastoma; Tissue culture lines and monoclonal antibody studies. Invest Ophthalmol Vis Sci *25*:30–40, 1984.

Coia LR, Fazekas JT, Kramer S: Postirradiation of the head and neck. Cancer *46*:1982–1985, 1980.

Comings DE: A general theory of carcinogenesis. Proc Natl Acad Sci USA *70*:3324–3328, 1973.

Connolly MJ, Payne RH, Johnson G, et al: Familial EsD-linked retinoblastoma with reduced penetrance and variable expressivity. Hum Genet *65*:122–124, 1984.

Datta BN: DNA coating of blood vessels in retinoblastoma. Am J Clin Pathol *62*:94–96, 1974.

DeBuen S: Retinoblastoma with spread by direct continuity to the contralateral optic nerve: Report of a case. Am J Ophthalmol *49*:815–819, 1960.

Donoso LA, Felberg NT, Shields JA, et al: Immunodiagnosis of late, recurrent retinoblastoma. Retina *1*:107–112, 1981.

Donoso LA, Shields JA, Felberg NT, et al: Intracranial malignancy in patients with bilateral retinoblastoma. Retina *1*:67–74, 1981.

Dryja TP, Bruns GAP, Gallie B, et al: Low incidence of deletion of the esterase D locus in retinoblastoma patients. Hum Genet *64*:151–155, 1983.

Dryja TP, Bruns GAP, Orkin SH, et al: Isolation of DNA fragments from chromosome 13. Retina *3*:121–125, 1983.

Dryja TP, Cavenee W, White R, et al: Homozygosity of chromosome 13 in retinoblastoma. N Engl J Med *310*:550–553, 1984.

Dryja TP, Rapaport JM, Weichselbaum R, Bruns GAP: Chromosome 13 restriction fragment length polymorphisms. Hum Genet *65*:320–324, 1984.

Dudgeon J, Lee WR: The trilateral retinoblastoma syndrome. Trans Ophthalmol Soc UK, in press.

Duke-Elder S, Dobree JH: Diseases of the Retina. Vol X. St Louis, CV Mosby Company, 1967, pp. 672–729.

Dunphy EB: The story of retinoblastoma. Trans Am Acad Ophthalmol Otolaryngol *68*:249–264, 1964.

Easterbrook J, Wehunt W, Zimmerman LE: Trilateral retinoblastoma: Radiologic, clinical, and pathologic features. In preparation.

Folberg R, Cleasby G, Flanagan JA, et al: Orbital leiomyosarcoma after radiation therapy for bilateral retinoblastoma. Arch Ophthalmol *101*:1562–1565, 1983.

Folkman J: Tumor angiogenesis factor. Cancer Res *34*:2109–2113, 1974.

Forrest AW: Tumors following radiation about the eye. Trans Am Acad Ophthalmol Otolaryngol *65*:694–717, 1961; Int Ophthalmol Clin *2*:543–553, 1962.

François J: Retinoblastoma and osteogenic sarcoma. Ophthalmologica *175*:185–191, 1977.

Freedman J, Goldberg L: Incidence of retinoblastoma in the Bantu of South Africa. Br J Ophthalmol *60*:655–656, 1976.

Friendly DS, Parks MM: Concurrence of hereditary congenital cataract and hereditary retinoblastoma. Arch Ophthalmol *84*:525–527, 1970.

Gallie BL: Gene carrier detection in retinoblastoma. Ophthalmology *87*:591–594, 1980.

Gallie BL, Ellsworth RM, Abramson DH, Phillips RA: Retinoma: Spontaneous regression of retinoblastoma or benign manifestation of the mutation? Br J Cancer *45*:513–521, 1982.

Gallie, BL, Phillips RA: Multiple manifestations of the retinoblastoma gene. Birth Defects *18*:689–701, 1982.

Gallie BL, Phillips RA: Retinoblastoma: A model of oncogenesis. Ophthalmology *91*:666–672, 1984.

Gallie BL, Phillips RA, Ellsworth RM, Abramson DH: Significance of retinoma and phthisis bulbi for retinoblastoma. Ophthalmology *89*:1393–1399, 1982.

Gangwar DN, Jain IS, Gupta A, et al: Bilateral spontaneous regression of retinoblastoma with dominant transmission. Ann Ophthalmol *14*:479–480, 1982.

Godbout R, Dryja TP, Squire J, et al: Somatic inactivation of genes on chromosome 13 is a common event in retinoblastoma. Nature *304*:451–453, 1983.

Gomez-Leal A: Causas de remocion de globos oculares en relacion con retinoblastoma. Arch Asoc Evit Ceguera Mexico *87*:7–13, 1978.

Gordon H: Family studies in retinoblastoma. Birth Defects *10*:185–190, 1974.

Hashem N, Khalifa S: Retinoblastoma: A model of hereditary fragile chromosomal regions. Hum Hered *25*:35–49, 1975.

Hatfield PM, Schultz MD: Post-irradiation sarcoma including five cases after x-ray therapy of breast carcinoma. Radiology *96*:593–602, 1970.

Howard GM: Erroneous clinical diagnosis of retinoblastoma and uveal melanoma. Trans Am Acad Ophthalmol Otolaryngol *73*:199–203, 1969.

Howard GM, Ellsworth RM: Differential diagnosis of retinoblastoma. A statistical survey of 500 children. I. Relative frequency of the lesions which simulate retinoblastoma. Am J Ophthalmol *60*:610–617, 1965.

Howard RO, Breg WR, Albert DM, Lesser RL: Retinoblastoma and chromosome abnormality; Partial deletion of the long arm of chromosome 13. Arch Ophthalmol *92*:490–493, 1974.

Irvine AR, Albert DM, Sang DN: Retinal neoplasia and dysplasia. II. Retinoblastoma occurring with persistence and hyperplasia of the primary vitreous. Invest Ophthalmol Visual Sci *16*:403–407, 1977.

Jakobiec FA, Tso MOM, Zimmerman LE, Danis P: Retinoblastoma and intracranial malignancy. Cancer *39*:2048–2058, 1977.

Jensen RD, Miller RW: Retinoblastoma: Epidemiologic characteristics. N Engl J Med *285*:307–311, 1971.

Judisch GF, Patil SR: Concurrent heritable retinoblastoma, pinealoma, and trisomy X. Arch Ophthalmol *99*:1767–1769, 1981.

Kalsow CM, Wacker WB: Pineal reactivity of anti-retina sera. Invest Ophthalmol Vis Sci *16*:181–184, 1977.

Kalsow CM, Wacker WB: The pineal gland in experimental allergic uveitis, *in* Silverstein AM, O'Conner GR (eds): Immunology and Immunopathology of the Eye. New York, Masson Publishing, 1979, pp 113–120.

Kemshead JT, Fritschy J, Goldman A, et al: Use of panels of monoclonal antibodies in the differential diagnosis of neuroblastoma and lymphoblastic disorders. Lancet *1*:12–17, 1983.

Klein D: Genetic prognosis in retinoblastoma. J Genet Hum *11*:71–75, 1962.

Knudson AG Jr: Mutation and cancer: A statistical study of retinoblastoma. Proc Natl Acad Sci USA *68*:820–823, 1971.

Knudson AG Jr: Retinoblastoma: A prototypic hereditary neoplasm. Semin Oncol *5*:57–60, 1978.

Knudson AG Jr, Hethcote HW, Brown BW: Mutation and childhood cancer. A probabilistic model for the incidence of retinoblastoma. Proc Natl Acad Sci USA *71*:5116–5120, 1975.

Kodilinye HC: Retinoblastoma in Nigeria: Problems of treatment. Am J Ophthalmol *63*:469–481, 1967.

Kogan L, Boniuk M: Causes for enucleation in children with special reference to pseudoglioma and unsuspected retinoblastoma. Int Ophthalmol Clin *2*:507–524, 1962.

Kopelman JE, McLean IW: Multivariate analysis of clinical and histological risk factors for metastatis in retinoblastoma. Invest Ophthalmol Vis Sci *24*:50, 1983.

Kyritsis AP, Tsokos M, Triche TJ, et al: Retinoblastoma—origin from a primitive neurectodermal cell? Nature *307*:471–473, 1984.

Lane JC, Klintworth GK: A study of astrocytes in retinoblastomas using the immunoperoxidase technique and antibodies to glial fibrillary acidic protein. Am J Ophthalmol *95*:197–207, 1983.

Margo C, Hidayat A, Kopelman J, Zimmerman LE: Retinocytoma; A benign variant of retinoblastoma. Arch Ophthalmol *101*:1519–1531, 1983.

Margo CE, Zimmerman LE: Retinoblastoma: The accuracy of clinical diagnosis in children treated by enucleation. J Pediatr Ophthalmol Strabis *20*:227–229, 1983.

Matsunaga ER: Retinoblastoma: Host resistance and 13q− chromosomal deletion. Hum Genet *56*:53–58, 1980.

Meadows AT, D'Angio CJ, Mike V, et al: Patterns of second malignant neoplasms in children. Cancer *40*:1903–1911, 1977.

Messmer EP, Font RL, Kirkpatrick JB: Immunohistochemical demonstration of neuronal and astrocytic differentiation in retinoblastoma. Invest Ophthalmol Vis Sci (Arvo Abstr) *25*:83, 1984.

Messmer EP, Font RL, Kirkpatrick JB, Höpping W: Immunohistochemical demonstration of neuronal and astrocytic differentiation in retinoblastoma. Ophthalmology; in press.

Michaud J, Jacob JL, Demers J, Dumas J: Trilateral retinoblastoma: Bilateral retinoblastoma with pinealoblastoma. Can J Ophthalmol *191*:36–39, 1984.

Minoda KC: Retinoblastoma and iris neovascularization; A light and electron microscopic study. Jap J Ophthalmol *15*:215–222, 1971.

Mochizuki M, Charley J, Kuwabara T, et al: Involvement of the pineal gland in rats with experimental autoimmune uveitis. Invest Ophthalmol Vis Sci *24*:1333–1338, 1983.

Molnar ML, Stefansson K. Marton LS, et al: Immunohistochemistry of retinoblastoma in humans. Am J Ophthalmol *97*:301–307, 1984.

Morgan G: Diffuse infiltrating retinoblastoma. Br J Ophthalmol *55*:600–606, 1971.

Morgan KS, McLean IW: Retinoblastoma and persistent hyperplastic primary vitreous occurring in the same patient. Ophthalmology *88*:1087–1091, 1981.

Mukai S, Rapaport JM, Shields JA, et al: Linkage of genes for human esterase D and hereditary retinoblastoma. Am J Ophthalmol 000:000–000, 1984.

Mullaney J: Retinoblastomas with DNA precipitation. Arch Ophthalmol *82*:454–456, 1969.

Murphree AL, Benedict WF: Retinoblastoma: Clues to human oncogenesis. Science *223*:1028–1033, 1984.

Murphree AL, Gomer CJ, Doiron DR, Benedict WF: Recent developments in the genetics and treatment of retinoblastoma. Birth Defects *18*:681–687, 1982.

Nicholson DH: Retinoblastoma: Current concepts, *in* Nicholson DH (ed): Ocular Pathology Update. New York, Masson Publishing, 1980, pp 235–243.

Nicholson DH, Norton EW: Diffuse infiltrating retinoblastoma. Trans Am Ophthalmol Soc *78*:265–289, 1980.

Nielson M, Goldschmidt E: Retinoblastoma among offspring of adult survivors in Denmark. Acta Ophthalmol (Kbh) *46*:736–741, 1968.

Nove J, Weichselbaum RR, Nichols WW, et al: In vitro studies of fibroblasts from patients with retinoblastoma. Int Ophthalmol Clin *20*:211–222, 1980.

Offret G, Dhermy P, Brini A, Bec P: Anatomie Pathologique de L'Oeil et de Ses Annexes. Paris, Masson Publishing, 1974, pp 345–347.

Parkhill EM, Benedict WB: Gliomas of the retina; A histopathologic study. Am J Ophthalmol *24*:1354–1373, 1941.

Popoff NA, Ellsworth RM: The fine structure of retinoblastoma. *In vivo* and *in vitro* observations. Lab Invest *25*:389–402, 1971.

Paterson ML, Torben Bech-Hansen N: Survey of human hereditary and familial disorders for x-ray response in vitro: Occurrence of both cellular radiosensitivity and radioresistance in cancer prone families, *in* Nygaard OF, Simic MG (eds): Radioprotectors and Anticarcinogens. New York, Academic Press, 1983, pp 615–638.

Pratt CB, George SL: Second malignant neoplasms among children and adolescents treated for cancer. Proc Am Assoc Cancer Res *22*:151, 1981; and personal communication, 1983.

Reese AB: Tumors of the Eye. 2nd ed. Hagerstown, MD, Harper and Row Publishers, 1967.

Reese AB: Retinoblastomas and other neuroectodermal tumors of the eye, *in* Tumors of the Eye. 3rd ed. Hagerstown, MD, Harper and Row Publishers, 1976, pp 89–132.

Reese AB, Ellsworth RM: The evaluation and current concept of retinoblastoma therapy. Trans Am Acad Ophthalmol Otolaryngol *67*:164–172, 1963.

Reese AB, Merriam GR Jr, Martin HE: Treatment of bilateral retinoblastoma by irradiation and surgery: Report on 15-year results. Am J Ophthalmol *32*:175–190, 1949.

Reeser F: Iris spread from a peripheral retinoblastoma. Presented at the Verhoeff Society Meeting, Washington, DC, April, 1975.

Reid TW, Albert DM: RNA-dependent DNA polymerase activity in human tumors. Biochem Biophys Res Commun *46*:383–390, 1972.

Reid TW, Russell P: Recent observations regarding retinoblastoma. III. An enzyme study of retinoblastoma. Trans Ophthalmol Soc UK *94*:929–937, 1974.

Robertson DM, Campbell RJ: Analysis of misdiagnosed retinoblastoma in a series of 726 enucleated eyes. Mod Probl Ophthalmol *18*:156–159, 1977.

Rubinstein LJ: Tumors of the central nervous system, *in* Atlas of Tumor Pathology. 2nd Series, Fascicle 6. Washington, DC, Armed Forces Institute of Pathology, 1972, pp 125–139.

Rubinstein LJ: Tumors of the central nervous system, *in* Atlas of Tumor Pathology. Suppl to 2nd Series, Fascicle 6. Washington, DC, Armed Forces Institute of Pathology, 1982, pp 15–20.

Sagerman RH, Cassady JR, Tretter P, Ellsworth RM: Radiation-induced neoplasia following external beam therapy for children with retinoblastoma. Am J Roentgenol *105*:529–535, 1969.

Salem LE, Travezan R: Retinoblastoma: Am J Surg *114*:577–581, 1967.

Sang DN, Albert DM: Recent advances in the study of retinoblastoma, *in* Peyman GA, Apple DJ, Sanders DR (eds): Intraocular Tumors. New York, Appleton-Century-Crofts, 1977, pp 285–329.

Sang DN, Albert DM: Retinoblastoma: Clinical and histopathologic features. Hum Pathol *13*:133–147, 1982.

Schappert-Kimmijser J, Hemmes GD, Nijland R: The heredity of retinoblastoma. Ophthalmologica *152*:197–213, 1966.

Schimke RN, Lowman JT, Dowan GAB: Retinoblastoma and osteogenic sarcoma in siblings. Cancer *34*:2077–2079, 1974.

Schipper J: Retinoblastoma: A medical and experimental study. Thesis, University of Utrecht, 29 April, 1980, p 144.

Schofield PG: Diffuse infiltrating retinoblastoma. Br J Ophthalmol *44*:35–41, 1960.

Shields JA: Diagnosis and Management of Intraocular Tumors. St. Louis, CV Mosby Company, 1983, pp 437–533.

Smith JLS: Histology and spontaneous regression of retinoblastoma. Trans Ophthalmol Soc UK *94*:953–967, 1974.

Soll DB, Turtz AI: Retinoblastoma diagnosed as granulomatous uveitis. Arch Ophthalmol *63*:687–691, 1960.

Sparkes RS, Murphree AL, Lingua RW, et al: Gene for hereditary retinoblastoma assigned to human chromosome 13 by linkage to esterase D. Science *219*:971–973, 1983.

Sparkes RS, Sparkes MC, Wilson MG, et al: Regional assignment of genes for human esterase D and retinoblastoma in chromosome band 123 of 14. Science *208*:1042–1044, 1980.

Spaulding AG: Rubeosis iridis in retinoblastoma and pseudoglioma. Trans Am Ophthalmol Soc *76*:584–609, 1978.

Stafford WR, Yanoff M, Parnell B: Retinoblastoma initially misdiagnosed as primary ocular inflammation. Arch Ophthalmol *82*:771–773, 1969.

Stefanko SZ, Manschot WA: Pinealoblastoma with retinoblastomatous differentiation. Brain *102*:321–332, 1979.

Takahashi T, Tamura S, Inoue M, et al: Retinoblastoma in a 26-year-old adult. Ophthalmology *90*:179–183, 1983.

Taktikos A: Investigation of retinoblastoma with special reference to histology and prognosis. Br J Ophthalmol *50*:225–234, 1966.

Tarkkanen A, Tuovinen E: Retinoblastoma in Finland 1912–1964. Acta Ophthalmol *49*:293–300, 1971.

Taylor HR, Carroll N, Jack I, Crock GW: A scanning electron microscopic examination of retinoblastoma in tissue culture. Br J Ophthalmol *63*:551–559, 1979.

Terret M, Vawter GF, Mitus A: Second primary neoplasm in children. Am J Roentgenol *103*:800–822, 1968.

Tountas AA, Fornasier VL, Harwood AR, Leong PMK: Postirradiation sarcoma of bone: A perspective. Cancer *43*:182–187, 1979.

Tso MOM: Clues to the cells of origin in retinoblastoma. Int Ophthalmol Clin *20*:191–210, 1980.

Tso MOM, Fine BS, Zimmerman LE: The Flexner-Wintersteiner rosettes in retinoblastoma. Arch Pathol *88*:665–671, 1969.

Tso MOM, Fine BS, Zimmerman LE: The nature of retinoblastoma. II. Photoreceptor differentiation. An electron microscopic study. Am J Ophthalmol *69*:350–359, 1970.

Tso MOM, Fine BS, Zimmerman LE, Vogel MH: Photoreceptor elements in retinoblastoma. A preliminary report. Arch Ophthalmol *82*:57–59, 1969.

Tso MOM, Zimmerman LE, Fine BS: The nature of retinoblastoma. I. Photoreceptor differentiation. A clinical and histologic study. Am J Ophthalmol *69*:339–350, 1970.

Tso MOM, Zimmerman LE, Fine BS, Ellsworth RM: A cause of radioresistance in retinoblastoma: Photoreceptor differentiation. Trans Am Acad Ophthalmol Otolaryngol *74*:959–969, 1970.

Tsukahara I: A histopathological study on the prognosis and radiosensitivity of retinoblastoma. Arch Ophthalmol *63*:1005–1008, 1960.

Verhoeff FH: Retinoblastoma: Report of a case in a male age forty-eight. Arch Ophthalmol *2*:643–650, 1929.

Verhoeff FH: Retinoblastoma undergoing spontaneous regression: Calcifying agent suggested in the treatment of retinoblastoma. Am J Ophthalmol *62*:573–574, 1966.

Verhoeff FH, Jackson E: Minutes of Proceedings, 62nd Annual Meeting. Trans Am Ophthalmol Soc *24*:38, 1926.

Vogel F: Genetics of retinoblastoma. Hum Genet *52*:1–54, 1979.

Walton DS, Grant WM: Retinoblastoma and iris neovascularization. Am J Ophthalmol *65*:598–599, 1968.

Warburg M: Retinoblastoma, *in* Goldbert M: Genetic and Metabolic Disease. Boston, Little, Brown, 1974, pp 447–461.

Warwick R: Parietal and pineal eyes, *in* Wolff E (ed): Anatomy of the Eye and Orbit. Philadelphia, WB Saunders Company, 1976, pp 506–509.

Weatherby RP, Dahlin DC, Irvins JC: Postirradiation sarcoma of bone: Review of 78 Mayo Clinic cases. Mayo Clin Proc *56*:294–306, 1981.

Weichselbaum RR, Zakov ZN, Albert DM, et al: New findings in the chromosome 13 long-arm deletion syndrome and retinoblastoma. Trans Am Acad Ophthalmol Otolaryngol *86*:1191–1198, 1979.

Weizenblatt S: Differential diagnostic difficulties in atypical retinoblastoma; Report of a case. Arch Ophthalmol *58*:699–709, 1957.

Wurtman RJ, Moskowitz MA: The pineal organ. N Engl J Med *296*:1329–1333 and 1383–1386, 1977.

Yunis JJ, Ramsay N: Retinoblastoma and subband deletion of chromosome 13. Am J Dis Child *132*:161–163, 1978.

Zimmerman BL, Tso MOM: Morphologic evidence of photoreceptor differentiation of pinealocytes in the neonatal rat. J Cell Biol *66*:60–75, 1975.

Zimmerman LE: Application of histochemical methods for the demonstration of acid mucopolysaccharide to ophthalmic pathology. Trans Am Acad Ophthalmol Otolaryngol *62*:697–710, 1958.

Zimmerman LE: The Registry of Ophthalmic Pathology: Past, present, and future. Trans Am Acad Ophthalmol Otolaryngol *65*: 51–113, 1961.

Zimmerman LE: Retinoblastoma, including a report of illustrative cases. Med Ann Dist Colum *38*:366–374, 1969.

Zimmerman LE: Changing concepts concerning the pathogenesis of infectious diseases. Am J Ophthalmol *69*:947–964, 1970.

Zimmerman LE: Trilateral retinoblastoma, *in* Blodi FC (ed): Contemporary Issues in Ophthalmology. Vol II, Retinoblastoma. New York, Churchill Livingstone, in preparation.

Zimmerman LE, Burns RP, Wankum G, et al: Trilateral retinoblastoma: Ectopic intracranial retinoblastoma associated with bilateral retinoblastoma. J Pediatr Ophthalmol Strab *19*:310–315, 1982.

Zimmerman LE, Ingalls R: Clinical pathologic conference: A case of osteogenic sarcoma of the orbit following radiation therapy of retinoblastoma. Am J Ophthalmol *43*:417–426, 1957.

INDEX

Note: Page numbers in *italics* indicate figures; page numbers followed by t refer to tables.